W0254689

HANDBUCH DER MEDIZINISCHEN RADIOLOGIE

ENCYCLOPEDIA OF MEDICAL RADIOLOGY

HERAUSGEGEBEN VON · EDITED BY

L. DIETHELM   F. HEUCK

O. OLSSON   F. STRNAD   H. VIETEN

A. ZUPPINGER

BAND/VOLUME XV
TEIL/PART 1B

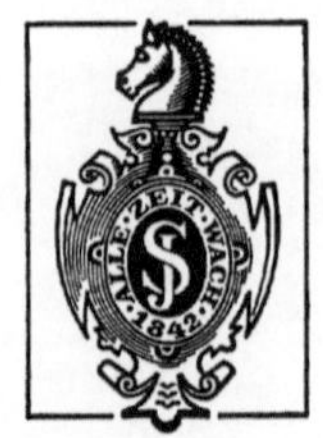

SPRINGER-VERLAG BERLIN · HEIDELBERG · NEW YORK

NUKLEARMEDIZIN

TEIL 1B
EMISSIONS-COMPUTERTOMOGRAPHIE
MIT KURZLEBIGEN ZYKLOTRON-PRODUZIERTEN RADIOPHARMAKA

NUCLEAR MEDICINE

PART 1B
EMISSION COMPUTER TOMOGRAPHY
WITH SHORT-LIVED CYCLOTRON-PRODUCED RADIOPHARMACEUTICALS

VON · BY

J. FITSCHEN · F. HELUS · K. JORDAN · D. JUNKER · G.-J. MEYER
O. SCHOBER · G. STÖCKLIN

REDIGIERT VON · EDITED BY

H. HUNDESHAGEN
HANNOVER

MIT 214 ABBILDUNGEN (277 EINZELDARSTELLUNGEN)
WITH 214 FIGURES (277 SEPARATE ILLUSTRATIONS)

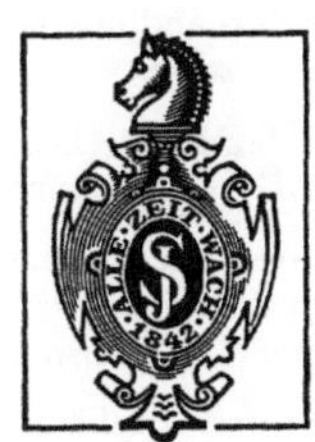

SPRINGER-VERLAG BERLIN · HEIDELBERG · NEW YORK

Professor Dr. H. HUNDESHAGEN
Medizinische Hochschule Hannover, Abteilung Nuklearmedizin
und spezielle Biophysik, Zentrum Radiologie
Konstanty-Gutschow-Straße 8, D-3000 Hannover 61

ISBN-13:978-3-642-83147-8   e-ISBN-13:978-3-642-83146-1
DOI: 10.1007/978-3-642-83146-1

CIP-Kurztitelaufnahme der Deutschen Bibliothek
Handbuch der medizinischen Radiologie = Encyclopedia of medical radiology
hrsg. von L. Diethelm... – Berlin; Heidelberg; New York
Teilw. mit d. Erscheinungsorten Berlin; Heidelberg; New York; Tokyo
NE: Diethelm, Lothar [Hrsg.]; PT Bd. 15. Nuklearmedizin. Teil 1. B. Emissions-Computertomographie. – 1988
Nuklearmedizin = Nuclear medicine/red. von H. Hundeshagen. – Berlin; Heidelberg; New York: Springer
(Handbuch der medizinischen Radiologie; Bd. 15) Teilw. mit d. Erscheinungsorten Berlin, Heidelberg, New York, Tokyo
NE: Hundeshagen, Heinz [Hrsg.]; PT Teil 1. B. Emissions-Computertomographie. – 1988
Emissions-Computertomographie: mit kurzlebigen zyklotron-produzierten Radiopharmaka = Emission computer tomography
von J. Fitschen... Red. von H. Hundeshagen. – Berlin; Heidelberg; New York: Springer, 1988
(Nuklearmedizin; Teil 1, B) (Handbuch der medizinischen Radiologie; Bd. 15)
ISBN-13:978-3-642-83147-8
NE: Fitschen, J. [Mitverf.] ; Hundeshagen, Heinz [Red.]; PT

Dieses Werk ist urheberrechtlich geschützt. Die dadurch begründeten Rechte, insbesondere die der Übersetzung, des Nachdrucks, des Vortrags, der Entnahme von Abbildungen und Tabellen, der Funksendung, der Mikroverfilmung oder der Vervielfältigung auf anderen Wegen und der Speicherung in Datenverarbeitungsanlagen bleiben, auch bei nur auszugsweiser Verwertung, vorbehalten. Eine Vervielfältigung dieses Werkes oder von Teilen dieses Werkes ist auch im Einzelfall nur in den Grenzen der gesetzlichen Bestimmungen des Urheberrechtsgesetzes der Bundesrepublik Deutschland vom 9. September 1965 in der Fassung vom 24. Juni 1985 zulässig. Sie ist grundsätzlich vergütungspflichtig. Zuwiderhandlungen unterliegen den Strafbestimmungen des Urheberrechtsgesetzes.

© Springer-Verlag Berlin·Heidelberg 1988
Softcover reprint of the hardcover 1st edition 1988

Die Wiedergabe von Gebrauchsnamen, Handelsnamen, Warenbezeichnungen usw. in diesem Werk berechtigt auch ohne besondere Kennzeichnung nicht zu der Annahme, daß solche Namen im Sinne der Warenzeichen- und Markenschutz-Gesetzgebung als frei zu betrachten wären und daher von jedermann benutzt werden dürften

Produkthaftung: Für Angaben über Dosierungsanweisungen und Applikationsformen kann vom Verlag keine Gewähr übernommen werden. Derartige Angaben müssen vom jeweiligen Anwender im Einzelfall anhand anderer Literaturstellen auf ihre Richtigkeit überprüft werden.

Gesamtherstellung: Universitätsdruckerei H. Stürtz AG, Würzburg
2122/3130-543210

Mitarbeiter von Band XV/1 B
Contributors to Volume XV/1 B

Dipl. Phys. J. FITSCHEN, Medizinische Hochschule Hannover, Abteilung Nuklearmedizin und spezielle Biophysik, Zentrum Radiologie, Konstanty-Gutschow-Straße 8, D-3000 Hannover 61

Dr. F. HELUS, Deutsches Krebsforschungszentrum, Institut für Nuklearmedizin, Im Neuenheimer Feld 280, D-6900 Heidelberg 1

Professor Dipl.-Ing. K. JORDAN, Medizinische Hochschule Hannover, Abteilung Nuklearmeßtechnik und Strahlenschutz, Zentrum Radiologie, Konstanty-Gutschow-Straße 8, D-3000 Hannover 61

Dr. rer. nat. D. JUNKER, Medizinische Hochschule Hannover, Abteilung Nuklearmedizin und spezielle Biophysik, Zentrum Radiologie, Konstanty-Gutschow-Straße 8, D-3000 Hannover 61

Privatdozent Dr. G.-J. MEYER, Medizinische Hochschule Hannover, Abteilung Nuklearmedizin und spezielle Biophysik, Zentrum Radiologie, Konstanty-Gutschow-Straße 8, D-3000 Hannover 61

Professor Dr.Dr. O. SCHOBER, Medizinische Hochschule Hannover, Abteilung Nuklearmedizin und spezielle Biophysik, Zentrum Radiologie, Konstanty-Gutschow-Straße 8, D-3000 Hannover 61

Professor Dr. G. STÖCKLIN, Kernforschungsanlage Jülich GmbH, Institut für Chemie, Institut 1: Nuklearchemie, D-5170 Jülich 1

Vorwort

Die nuklearmedizinische Funktionsdiagnostik wird durch den Einsatz von zyklotron-produzierten Radionukliden in der Zukunft wesentlich beeinflußt und erweitert.

Gerade zu dem Zeitpunkt, zu dem dieser Band erscheint, sind sowohl aus technischer, als auch aus medizinischer Sicht bedeutende Entwicklungen im Gange. Die Produktion der positronen-strahlenden Radionuklide, die Synthesen von Radiopharmaka, sowie ihre Quali-tätskontrolle sind dabei ein Faktor. Andererseits muß durch eine aufwendige Geräteentwick-lung zur Messung und Darstellung des Radiopharmaka-Stoffwechsels die Möglichkeit ge-schaffen werden, daß nuklearmedizinische Zentren ihre bisherigen großen Erfahrungen in die Funktionsanalyse einbringen können. Das wesentliche für die Diagnostik ist, die Funktion einzelner Organabschnitte bildhaft darzustellen, dies dreidimensional und quantitativ.

Die Entwicklungs- und Erprobungsphase für die Anwendung der Emissionstomographie ist noch nicht beendet. Dieser Band beinhaltet dies und gibt einen Einblick in die gesamte Problematik.

Hannover   H. Hundeshagen

Preface

Functional diagnosis employing nuclear medicine will in the future be influenced and extended through the use of radionuclides produced in a cyclotron. Just as this book is being published, developments are taking place which are significant from both technical and clinical points of view. Examples are the production of radionuclides emitting positrons, the synthesis of radiopharmaceuticals, and the supervision of the quality of the latter. On the other hand, it is necessary for equipment to be developed in order to measure and depict the metabolism of radiopharmaceuticals, in order to let the centers for nuclear medicine contribute their great experience to the analysis of function. Essential for diagnosis is the ability to present the function of individual sections of organs as an image which is three dimensional and quantitative.

The phase of the development and testing of emission tomography is not yet complete. This is reflected in this volume, which provides insight into the current issues.

Hannover   H. HUNDESHAGEN

Inhaltsverzeichnis – Contents

3. Klinische Anwendung der Positronen-Emissionstomographie.
Von O. SCHOBER und G.-J. MEYER 315

1.1 Target Technique

By

F. HELUS

With 14 Figures and 5 Tables

A. Introduction

In the past three decades enormous advances have been made in the production of radioactive tracers, especially with regard to their applications in medical and biological studies (WAGNER 1968; WOLF and FOWLER 1979; LARSON and CARASQUILLO 1984; SILVESTER 1976; RUTH and KROHN 1981). Instrumentally it is a very long way for a radioactive tracer from its place of origin to delivery for use as a radiopharmaceutical. Between the physics, as source of the bombarding particles, and the physicians, as users of the tracers, the position of radiochemistry is of great importance.

The major roles of radiochemistry as applied in bioscientific research are (a) to discover, develop, and produce radioactive materials as radioisotopes or labeled compounds for direct use in biochemical research and medical clinical diagnostics, and (b) to obtain information from inside the human body without surgical intervention. In order to carry out these tasks some basic conditions have to be fulfilled. For the production of radioactive tracers it is essential to have:
1. A source of particles for a nuclear reactions
2. Sophisticated targetry based on modern technology
3. Optimal target material
4. The services of an excellent chemistry department specialized in the study of separation procedures and synthetic methods facilitating the labeling of the produced radioactive tracers on the desired position in the biomolecule.

The target is one of the most important parts in the radionuclide production process. Sometimes the preparation of targets needs more time than the irradiation itself. Very briefly the target may be defined as follows: Target is the apparatus consisting of the target material and the target holder where the projectiles interact with target nuclei resulting in the production of desired radioactive nuclides.

The word *target* is metaphorically derived from military vocabulary. Target, projectile, bombardment, and other such terms were adopted by scientists during the Second World War, in the improvisational period when nuclear science was in pursuit of the development of nuclear weapons. The problems in the army and the science are similar; you can aim at the target and either hit it or miss it. There are many kinds of targets and it is a task for scientists to choose one which will fit the bill and hit the goal spot-on; this requires choosing the appropriate element which can produce the desired radionuclides economically, while taking into account the occupational health and safety of personnel. Production, by irradiation or activation, is only one part of the problem. Once the short-lived radionuclides

Table 1. Important reactor produced radionuclides

Radio-nuclide	Stable target isotope	Isotope enrichment [%]		Typical target material	Nuclear reaction	Cross-section [barn]	Final chemical form
^{18}F	^{6}Li	enr.	96.00	Li_2CO_3	$^6Li(n,^4He)^3H$ $^{16}O(^3H,n)^{18}F$	950.00	NaF
^{24}Na	^{23}Na	nat.	100.00	Na_2CO_3	(n,γ)	0.53	NaCl
^{32}P	^{32}S	nat.	95.02	S	(n,p)	0.06	H_3PO_4
^{35}S	^{35}Cl	nat.	75.77	KCl	(n,p)	0.98	H_2SO_4
^{45}Ca	^{44}Ca	enr.	>98.00	$^{44}CaCO_3$	(n,γ)	0.80	$CaCl_2$
^{64}Cu	^{63}Cu	enr.	>99.00	^{64}CuO	(n,γ)	9.50	$Ca(NO_3)_2$
^{75}Se	^{74}Se	enr.	77.70	^{74}Se	(n,γ)	52.00	H_2SO_4 ; H_2SeO_3
^{125}I	^{124}Xe	enr.	>10.00	^{124}Xe	(n,γ)	110.00	NaI
^{131}I	^{130}Te	nat.	34.50	TeO_2	(n,γ)	0.20	NaI
^{198}Au	^{197}Au	nat.	100.00	Au	(n,γ)	99.00	$AuCl_3$
^{99m}Tc	^{98}Mo	nat. enr.	24.01 97.23	MoO_3 Mo	(n,γ)	0.51	^{99}Mo
	^{235}U	enr.	99.00	U	(n,f)	580.00	$^{99}Mo/Al_2O_3$ generator

have been produced, the race is on to get them to where they finally will be used; this starts with removing the target material from the beam line of the cyclotron. Every step that takes place from this point on must be planned and executed with great precision. All should be planned and prepared before the projectiles – nucleons – hit the target and if possible the operation should be rehearsed with nonactive material.

Renewed interest in the production, synthesis, and use of radiotracers and labeled compounds has come about as a result of the greater availability of cyclotrons to biomedical investigators – who recognized the utility of labeling metabolites with short-lived positron emitters of their natural elements (^{11}C, ^{13}N, ^{15}O, and, because there is no positron-emitting isotope of hydrogen, ^{18}F, which behaves similarly is used instead; FERRIERI and WOLF 1983). In addition to the "biological" (also called physiological) radioisotopes, there is a significant variety of very important cyclotron-produced radioisotopes, for example, ^{34m}Cl (HELUS et al. 1985), ^{121}I (HELUS et al. 1979), ^{123}I, ^{67}Ga, ^{75}Br, ^{76}Br, ^{77}Br (STÖCKLIN 1977), ^{111}In (THAKUR 1977), and ^{201}Tl (LEBOWITZ et al. 1975). From the nuclear point of view ^{123}I is, for example, preferable to the most commonly available ^{131}I which has been used up to now in many important diagnostic and scientific procedures. Occasionally cyclotron-produced radionuclides are preferred to ^{99m}Tc (characterized by its repeated short-interval applications, difficult chemistry of technetium, and the fact that it is not a biological element).

The reactor target technique will not be considered in this section in any detail. Not only is it being regarded as a topic of minor importance, but also there is fundamentally no difference between the reactor or cyclotron procedures for producing radionuclides by irradiating materials. Particle accelerators were extraordinarily important as tools for producing radionuclides in the very early years of the applications of radionuclides (1935–1945). In the past 20 years, however, use of radioactive tracers has declined more and more in favor of short-lived and positron-emitting radionuclides produced on the new type of cyclotrons. These cyclotrons, sometimes also called medical cyclotrons, have been developed especially for the production of radionuclides for beneficial application as tracers in medical and biological studies and diagnostics. Therefore, further attention in this report will be restricted to conditions primarily affecting cyclotron targetry.

Table 2. Typical cyclotron produced radionuclides

Nuclide	T	Reaction	Target	Product
		I. Positron emitting radionuclides		
^{11}C	20m	$^{14}N(p,\alpha)^{11}C$	N_2	$^{11}CO_2(^{11}CO)$
		$^{11}B(p,n)^{11}C$	B_2O_3	$^{11}CO_2$
^{13}N	10m	$^{16}O(p,\alpha)^{13}N$	H_2O	$^{13}N;^{13}NOx;^{13}NH_3$
		$^{13}C(p,n)^{13}N$	$^{13}C^a$	$C^{13}N(He)$
^{15}N	2m	$^{14}N(d,n)^{15}O$	N_2	$^{15}O_2$
		$^{15}N(p,n)^{15}O$	$N_2{}^b$	$^{15}O_2$
^{18}F	110m	$^{20}Ne(d,\alpha),^{18}F$	$Ne/F_2{}^c$	$^{18}F_2$
		$^{18}O(p,n)^{18}F$	$H_1{}^{18}O;B_2{}^{18}O_3{}^b$	$H^{18}F$
^{30}P	2.3m	$^{32}S(d,\alpha)^{30}P$	S	$^{30}PH_3$
^{34m}Cl	32m	$^{34}S(p,n)^{34m}Cl$	NiS;MoS	$^{34m}Cl^-$
^{61}Cu	3.3h	$^{60}Ni(d,n)^{61}Cu$	Ni foil	$^{61}Cu^{2+}$
^{68}Ga	68m	$^{69}Ga(p,2n)^{68}Ge$	Ga/Cu alloy	$^{68}Ge-^{68}Ga^d$
^{75}Br	1.6h	$^{76}Se(p,2n)^{75}Br$	$^{76}Se^b$	$^{75}Br^-$
		$^{78}Kr(p,4n)^{75}Rb\rightarrow^{75}Kr\rightarrow^{75}Br$	$^{78}Kr^b$	$^{75}Br^-$
^{76}Br	16.0h	$^{77}Se(p,2n)^{76}Br$	$^{77}Se^b$	$^{76}Br^-$
^{82}Sr	26d	$^{85}Rb(p,4n)^{82}Sr$		
		$^{80}Kr(\alpha,2n)^{82}Sr$	$^{80}Kr^b$	$^{82}Sr-^{82}Rb^d$
		II. Gamma emitting radionuclides		
^{67}Ga	78.3h	$^{68}Zn(p,2n)^{67}Ga$	Zn	
		$^{68}Ga(p,3n)^{67}Ge\rightarrow^{67}Ga$	Ga alloy	$^{67}Ga^{3+}$
		$^{68}Cu(\alpha,2n)^{67}Ga$	Cu foil	
^{77}Br	56h	$^{78}Se(p,2n)^{77}Br$	$^{78}Se^b$	$^{77}Br^-$
^{81}Rb	4.7h	$^{82}Kr(p,2n)^{81}Rb$	$^{82}Kr^b$	$^{81}Rb-^{81}Kr^d$
^{111}In	2.83d	$^{112}Cd(p,2n)^{111}In$	$^{112}Cd^b$	^{111}In
^{123}I	13.2h	$^{124}Te(p,2n)^{123}I$	$^{124}TeO_2{}^b$	$^{123}I^-$
		$^{124}Xe(p,2n)^{123}Cs\rightarrow^{123}Xe\rightarrow^{123}I$	$^{124}Xe^b$	$^{123}I^-$
^{127}Xe	36.4d	$^{127}I(p,n)^{127}Xe$	I	^{127}Xe
^{195m}Hg	9.5h	$^{197}Au(p,3n)^{195m}Hg$	Au foil	^{195m}Hg
^{201}Tl	73.5h	$^{203}Tl(p,3n)^{201}Pb\rightarrow^{201}Tl$	Tl	^{201}Tl

[a] charcoal enriched
[b] enriched material
[c] non-active tracer
[d] generator

Table 1 shows the most important reactor-produced radionuclides and when they were used. A special position in applications in clinical diagnostics is held by ^{99m}Tc, for its almost ideal physical characteristics (SMITH 1964).

For comparison, Table 2 lists the cyclotron-produced radioisotopes which are of present and likely to be of future clinical and research importance. Radionuclides are divided into those employed principally for their β^+ emissions and those for their gamma emissions.

The second great advantage of cyclotron-produced radionuclides is that nuclear reaction induced with charged particles produces neutron-deficient isotopes, resulting in products different from target nuclides. This implies that "carrier-free" products of high specific activity are the normal products of a cyclotron. Radiopharmaceuticals prepared from "carrier-free" radionuclides may be applied to biological systems without significantly changing the physiology of their stable counterparts already present in the system.

In general, radionuclides are produced by disturbing a preferred neutron-proton ratio in the nuclei of elements. This is done by adding or removing (or both) neutrons or charged particles such as protons, deuterons, alphas, or others. The nuclear processes are based on (n,gamma) reactions, using the nuclear reactor as a source of the particles. The (n,gamma) is the type of nuclear reaction which is used most frequently in reactor radionuclide production. This activation generally gives the so-called neutron-rich radionuclides, which usually decay with the emission of negatively charged β particles, often, but not necessarily, accompanied by gamma radiation. The supplier of accelerated particles (protons, deuterons, alphas, and others) is the cyclotron (AMPHLET et al. 1970).

The production of radionuclides results from the interaction of bombarding particles with the nuclei of a target, whereby the bombarding particle comes close enough to the target nucleus to react with it, forming various intermediates which:
1. Unite with the target nucleus, forming a compound nucleus,
2. Knock particles out of the target nucleus (high-energy reaction only), or
3. Cause nucleons to be stripped from the bombarding particle (^{2}H, ^{3}He, ^{4}He), transferring the nucleons to the target nucleus.

B. Target Definition

Target systems are the vital interfaces between the sources of particles, the cyclotron or reactor, and the chemistry. Target is a restricted area (space) containing target material. Target material is situated in a closed space separated from the vacuum of the beam line and from the cyclotron by a thin foil. The required radioactive isotope originates through the nuclear reaction initiated by the projectiles (accelerated particle beam). The accelerated particles are allowed to bombard the selected target material in order to induce the desired nuclear reaction. The target material holder is constructed ideally from nonactivated material with a high melting point and high heat conductivity (pure aluminum is preferred).

According to the facility used as the source of projectiles (neutrons, protons, deuterons, and others) the targets, used for routine production of radionuclides, are classified into two basic groups:
1. Reactor targets, and
2. Accelerator-cyclotron targets.

Although in biomedical research and nuclear medicine there are advantages in the use of cyclotron radionuclides, at present the most widely used radionuclide in diagnostic practice is still ^{99m}Tc. For this reason the next part will discuss the production of reactor radionuclides, with special attention given to the production of ^{99m}Tc (BOYD 1983).

C. Reactor Target Technique

The use of reactor-produced radionuclides is limited practically to the production of ^{99}Mo (produced mainly from fission products) and a handful of other radionuclides (^{131}I, ^{64}Cu, and others). This, together with the fact that reactor target technology is simpler than cyclotron technology, explains why description of the reactor target technique will be restricted to a minimum.

Nuclear reactors and ion particle accelerators are the best primary sources of radionuclides. Most of the manmade radionuclides, by far, originate from the application of one of these two irradiation techniques. Practically all commercially available radionuclides used in medicine, industry, and as tracers in various scientific fields have been prepared in one of these two ways.

In the nuclear reactor, uranium (natural ^{238}U or enriched ^{235}U) and plutonium (^{239}Pu) undergo fission and produce heat, fission neutrons, and radionuclides in the form of fission products. Therefore, the nuclear reactor is the most useful source of thermal and fast neutrons. Since the neutron has no electrical charge, it is possible for neutrons with a very low kinetic energy to interact with stable target nuclei and cause nuclear reactions. Of the various reaction mechanisms caused by thermal, epithermal, or fast neutrons, the most frequently occurring is the (n,gamma) type of nuclear reaction. Since the products of (n,gamma) type reactions are isotopically identical with the target material element, chemical separation from target material generally can not be carried out and the obtainable specific activity is limited, unless a special separation procedure (for example Szillard-Chalmers reaction; SZILLARD and CHALMERS 1934) is used. The cross-sections for most of the (n,p) and (n,alpha) processes are usually small and therefore the yields of these reactions are low. The products of these two processes are chemically different from the target element. It is possible to separate products from the target material and thereby produce radioactive species of a higher specific activity than could be produced with other methods.

The second source of radionuclides from the target reactor are the fission products. The fission process splits an excited heavy nucleon into two nuclei of approximately equal size; many of these are radioactive. Fission produces a wide variety of different radionuclides, each with a maximum yield of about 6%. Since the required radionuclides represent only a small fraction of the total activity, the recovery of the specific radionuclides requires a complicated chemical procedure. In acquiring the desired radioactive product, a great amount of radioactive waste is produced – which is one of the great disadvantages of this production method. Examples of radionuclides obtained and routinely produced from the fission products are ^{131}I, ^{133}Xe, and especially ^{99}Mo (ARROL et al. 1956), which is used for the preparation of $^{99}Mo - ^{99m}Tc$ generators. In the past four decades a wide range of applications in nuclear medicine have been found for ^{99m}Tc, because of its optimal physical characteristics.

The reactor target system consists of:
1. Target material
2. Irradiation capsules and containers
3. A hydraulic or pneumatic target transfer system
4. Target processing facility and chemistry.

First the appropriate target material must be selected and then the target must be prepared for irradiation. Some aspects of this are common for both irradiation techniques, reactor and cyclotron. However, because of the differences the reactor target technique will be considered separately.

One of the most important considerations in choosing the reactor target material is safety, from the standpoint of preventing damage to the reactor, i.e., by overheating, the development of gases, and rupture of the target container. The use of ultrapure materials is essential because radioactive impurities which have a long life may be coproduced by long irradiations. The following factors are important for the *selection* of appropriate target material:
1. For routine production the target material should be commercially available. Metallic elements, stable oxides, carbonates, and other mechanically and thermally stable compounds are generally the best target materials. It is important to choose a target material

of known and reproducible chemical composition in order to minimize control for each irradiation.

2. Radiation decomposition, chemical stability, and thermal conductivity of the target material should be considered before irradiation. The experimental irradiation should supply information about the physical and chemical stability. Starting with a small amount, the temperature of the material should be estimated at the intended irradiation position in the reactor.

3. It is important to obtain all nuclear reaction data for the appropriate target isotope and for all other isotopes in the target material. All possible nuclear reactions in the target material should be surveyed. Activation analysis of the target material before the actual production procedure is helpful in many cases. Possible impurities have to be removed before irradiation to minimize the purification procedure after the irradiation.

4. After irradiation the target material used for the production of radionuclides which have a short life must be chemically processed very quickly. Therefore it is sometimes preferable to use soluble compounds instead of metallic material, or material which can be made inactive during the irradiation.

The general requirements for the *preparation* of target material are more or less known and are described in comprehensive monographs, where further information can be found.

After selecting the most appropriate target material and its method of preparation for irradiation, it is usual to determine the irradiation conditions. For producing radionuclides it is very important to get all available data on the target materials, irradiation conditions, applications of the product, and nuclear cross-sections. Neutron reaction data have been extensively measured and evaluated with regard to needs in various fields, fission reactors, breeder systems, etc. Under the heading "nuclear reaction data" we placed all data arising from the interactions of nuclei with matter: elastic and nonelastic cross-sections, capture cross-section, total cross-section, excitation functions, fission yields, and microscopic data. Four regional data centers work actively on the compilation, evaluation, and dissemination of nuclear data, mainly neutron data. There are data files on topics such as fission products, dosimetry, and activation. The nuclear data relevant to the production of radionuclides via neutron-induced reaction, especially in nuclear reactors are known and accurate to a fairly high degree.

I. Irradiation Containers and Activation Loops

To prevent unnecessary contamination or possible loss, and where volatile products are expected, the reactor target material is closed off or sealed in small plastic or high purity quartz or aluminum tubes or ampules. Plastic ampules and plastic sample containers are particularly advantageous for short irradiations, since they do not acquire appreciable amounts of induced activity. In longer irradiations or irradiations with high neutron flux, many plastics become brittle and tend to disintegrate. For such types of irradiations, mostly performed in the central irradiation position, the target material is sealed in quartz ampules mounted in a special reactor purity aluminum holder. To avoid activation of the argon in the air, the target material should be prepared, if possible, under vacuum or in a helium atmosphere.

Target material holders – the hardware of the reactor irradiation system – vary not only for different types of reactors, but also for different types of irradiation positions in the same reactor. In standard operating techniques the samples are irradiated in two types of containers:

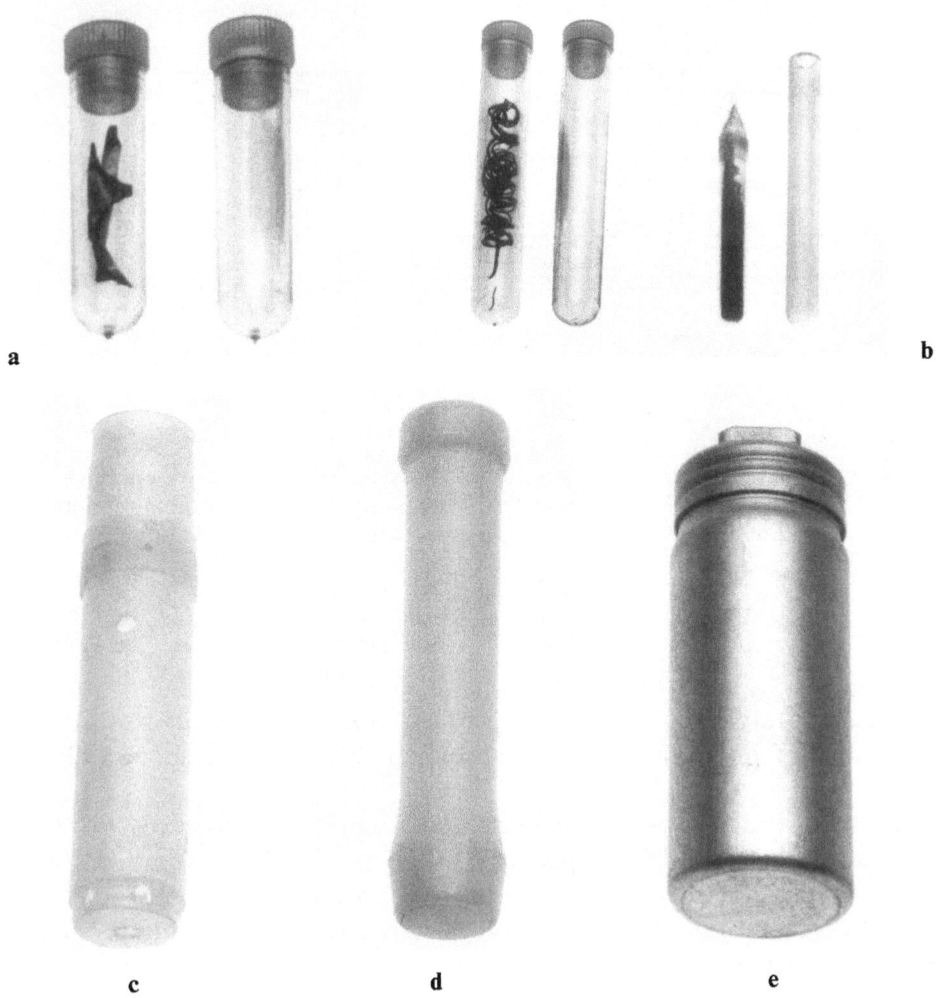

Fig. 1 a–e. Typical reactor irradiation containers and transport containers

1. Sample containers. These cover the target material and protect it from the surroundings during the irradiation; they are mostly plastic or quartz ampules.
2. Transport rabbits. These are holders of sample containers made mostly from high purity aluminum, enabling insertion of samples from the hot laboratory into the reactor as well as their removal from the reactor core after irradiation.

Figure 1 shows a typical sample container and transport container for insertion and irradiation as used in the Triga Heidelberg II type of research reactor.

Reactors used for the production of radionuclides have basically two different positions for irradiation. The first are the fixed positions in the reactor core, including the central irradiation position with the highest neutron flux, as well as a couple of other positions in the core. The second are the mobile positions typical with the research reactors. These positions are in a special irradiation system – the rotary specimen rack, also called "lazy Susan" – located around the core; they rotate and provide a supplemental facility for irradiation of about 40 samples in an uniform neutron flux. Rotation of the specimen rack eliminates flux variation from position to position in the reactor, and permits equal irradiations of different samples with flux variations lower than 1%. The ring also has a lower neutron flux and provides better cooling of the samples, therefore the overheating and radiation

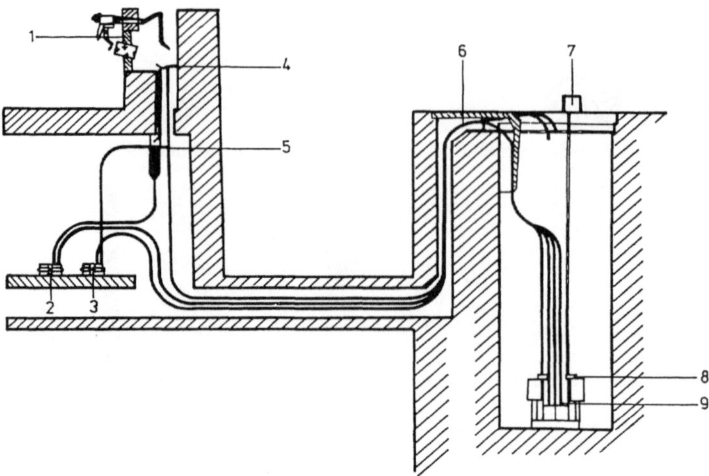

Fig. 2. General arrangement of hydraulic target transport system on the Heidelberg TRIGA II reactor. *1* loading cell with *4* loading station, *2* suction and *3* pressure pumps, *5* transport tubing system, *6* monitoring system, *7* position distributor, *8* rotary specimen rack, *9* in-core irradiation positions

damage of irradiated samples is not a serious problem. Figure 2 presents a schematic drawing of the Triga II reactor pool with a rotary specimen rack and transport hydraulic tubing system.

In addition to the straightforward reactions, for example, the direct reactions (n,gamma), (n,p), and (n,alpha), it is possible for the reactor to produce radioisotopes by secondary reactions. After irradiation the desired radioactive product of the secondary reaction is separated from the reaction mixture. These types of reactor radionuclide production procedures, based on successive reactions, require the development of special irradiation devices. The ^{18}F reactor production method is typically used for routine production over successive reactions. The first reaction ^{6}Li(n,^{4}He)^{3}H has a cross-section of 950 barn for thermal neutrons and produces 2.73 MeV tritons and 2.05 MeV alpha particles. The tritons are sufficiently energetic to initiate (t,p) and (t,n) reactions, which can be used for the production of ^{18}F, taking as target material compounds containing enriched ^{6}Li and oxygen. Lithium carbonate is recommended because of its thermal stability, chemical purity, and good yields (Helus and Maier-Borst 1973). The disadvantage of this ^{18}F production method, in comparison with the ^{18}F cyclotron production method, is the coproduction of high amounts of tritium, which complicates the chemical separation of ^{18}F and its use in human medicine (Clark and Silvester 1955). Because the yield of ^{18}F produced by this method is limited, using a thick layer of target mixture and a special target capsule has been developed and constructed. Figure 3 shows a quartz capsule which enables a threefold increased yield of ^{18}F.

Another type of irradiation in reactors involves the activation loop. It is a special apparatus for irradiation of circulating gases, solutions, or molten salt samples. The irradiated materials pass through the core of the reactor and after or during the irradiation it is possible to get them directly into a hot cell or a system outside the reactor. This type of irradiation may be used for the preparation of short-lived radionuclides in the liquid or gaseous phase. The production of ^{85m}Kr, which can be used in ventilation studies in medical diagnostics, is a practical example of the use of the activation loop in the production of radionuclides.

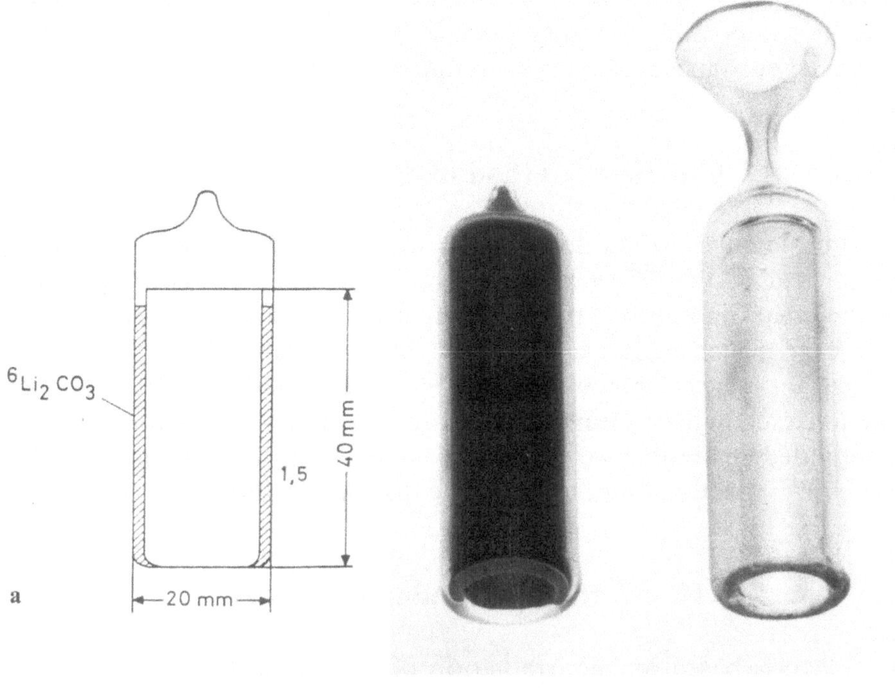

Fig. 3a, b. Special quartz capsule for the irradiation of Lithium carbonate for the production of ^{18}F

II. Target Transfer Systems

The irradiated target material should, if possible, be delivered directly from the reactor to the processing laboratory or in the shielded manipulation hood without manual transfer. Short irradiations under well-defined conditions, as well as fast delivery of irradiated highly active samples, are most conveniently achieved with the use of the so-called rabbit systems, which can be either pneumatic or hydraulic. The end station of this system is usually in the hot laboratory, where the chemical separation is done.

D. A Special Position of ^{99m}Tc

Technetium, being an artificial element, has many advantages over other radioactive elements. These include its physical characteristics, half-life (6.02 h), simple decay scheme (140 keV photon), very low radiation doses with regard both for the object being studied the personnel, and simple preparation. The fact that Tc is not known to biological organisms can be seen either as an advantage or a disadvantage. However, ^{99m}Tc cannot solve all the problems in biological studies and nuclear medicine, because of its very complicated chemistry and because it does not take part in any specific metabolic reaction. The distribution of ^{99m}Tc is similar to that of its longer-lived parent ^{99}Mo, which is loaded as a solution of ammonium molybdate onto an aluminum chromatographic column (RICHARDS 1966). This so-called generator can be eluted with isotonic saline solution to remove ^{99m}Tc as required, in the chemical form of pertechnetate ion. The product may then be used in the eluted form or for labeling of many different compounds. The disadvantage of technetium is that its chemistry is not simple and ^{99m}Tc labeling of typical biomolecules and complicated organic molecules is impossible. Mother nuclide ^{99}Mo used for the preparation of these generators is routinely produced in reactors in one of two ways:

I. The First Method of Producing ^{99}Mo

The first method involves irradiation of ^{238}U or ^{235}U and separation from fission products. The fission yield of the ^{99}Mo is only about 6%, while the second disadvantage of this method is the great amount of other coproduced radionuclides – some of them volatile – which complicates the chemical separation. ^{99}Mo produced from the fission products has the advantage that it is very high with regard to specific activity of the product, enabling sorption on the ion exchange column. Uranium for irradiation is used in the form of UO_2 pellets; it is irradiated in double-welded, stainless-steel capsules, with the pellets packed in powdered reactor grade aluminum to assist the dissipation of heat.

II. Method of Producing ^{99}Mo

The second ^{99}Mo is based on the irradiation of MoO_3 via the ^{98}Mo (n,gamma) ^{99}Mo reaction. If enriched ^{98}Mo is used this method is not as effective as the previously described method. Large amounts of target material have to be irradiated (from 10 to 100 grams of molybdenum oxide enriched on ^{98}Mo). Using molybdenum hexacarbonyl in a matrix of oxalic acid as the target material is another example of this method of producing ^{99}Mo (Colonomos and Parker 1969). In this case, one makes use of a recoil technique, whereby the recoil products are trapped in the oxalic acid. Upon completion of the irradiation, the target material is dropped into water, whereupon the oxalic acid dissolves, together with any recoil fragments it might contain. The large amount of irradiated material produced in the preparation of ^{99}Mo $-$ ^{99m}Tc generators makes ion exchange chromatography impossible due to the low capacity of the aluminum columns, and other methods, mostly solvent extraction with MEK (Methyl-Ethyl-Keton), have to be used (Belkas and Perricos 1969).

E. Cyclotron Targets

For physiological studies of various biochemical functions in living systems, the use of cyclotron-produced radionuclides is advantageous. This is because of the high specific activity of the positron emitters produced in minute concentrations from the nonisotopic target material. Typically these radionuclides are all positron emitters and have very short half-lives. These facts require new production procedures, methods, organization, and logistics. The use of positron-emitting radionuclides has been increasing rapidly in the past two decades. The tremendous progress in the development of imaging techniques in particular has led the way to the development of positron-emission transaxial tomography.

Generally, cyclotron radionuclides are produced by nuclear reactions initiated by charged particles. A simple nuclear reaction can be described as:

$$A(x,y)B + Q$$

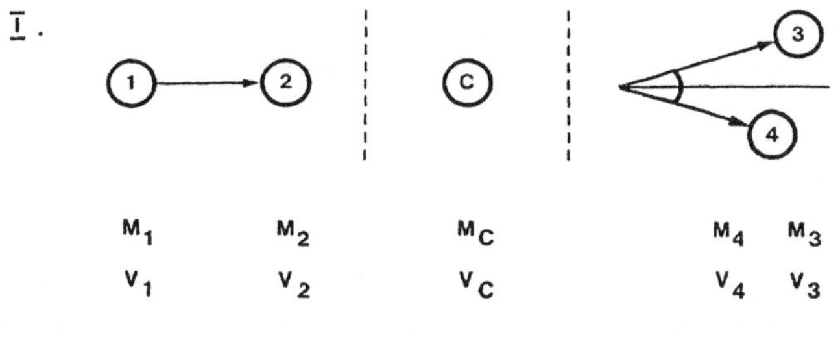

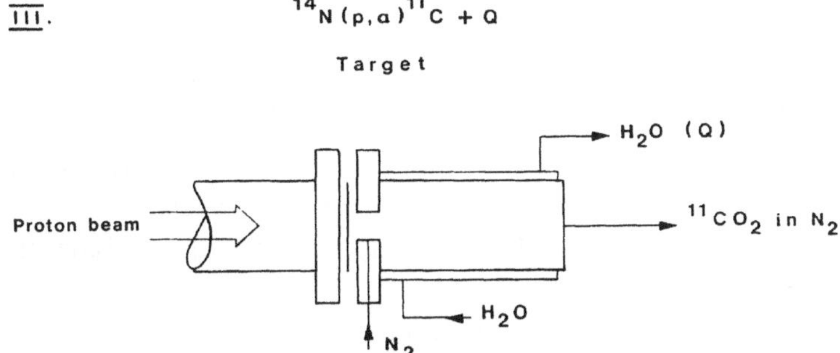

Fig. 4. Schema of the $^{14}N(p,\alpha)^{11}C$ reaction with the simple gas target system

where

A = target material nucleus

B = produced radioactive nuclei

x = bombarding particle (proton, deuteron, etc.)

y = resulting particle

Q = resulting reaction energy.

To produce radionuclide B, the stable nuclide A must be present as target for irradiation (the terms bombardment or activation are also used). Target may contain pure nuclide A or material which predominantly contains nuclide A, or, finally, artificially enriched nuclide A.

Figure 4 shows an example of the typical nuclear reaction for cyclotron production of the very important radionuclide carbon-11. At the bottom of this schematic presentation of different styles of writing nuclear reactions a sketch of a simple gas target system is shown.

The overall goal in using the various techniques of producing radionuclides is to obtain maximum yields of the desired nuclides in a chemical form well suited for fast processing and labeling, with a minimum of accompanying contaminants.

The yield of radionuclide activity can be roughly estimated before preparation and irradiation by using known physical data on the target-projectile system. The dependence on parameters relevant to the activation procedure, however, has to be verified by a series of experiments.

The production of radionuclides depends on a number of factors. Primary consideration must be given to the quantity that can be prepared. Theoretical yield relates only to the maximum yield obtainable, as determined by the limitations of the nuclear process itself. Theoretical yields, without regard to chemical form, depend on:

1. The probable energy of the thick target
2. The beam current used
3. The duration of bombardment.

These conditions can vary with local needs. Target design and target substrate can be varied, to optimize yield of radionuclides. However, what is not taken into account in most published works is the actual yield of radionuclides obtainable from the target. The radionuclides must be extracted from the target matrix in a chemical form which is of immediate use or synthetically useful as a precursor for further chemical synthesis. The actual yield will vary from 10% to 95% of the theoretical, depending on the target itself, irradiation conditions, and purity or chemical form of the target material used.

Obtaining a high yield with the highest specific activity chemically possible in an identified radioactive species remains the primary objective for the radiochemist in the field of targetry and target chemistry.

With regard to charged particle-induced reactions, the fundamental considerations are (KELLER et al. 1979; NORTHCLIFF and SHILLING 1970; WILLIAMSON et al. 1973):

- The choice of an adequate type of nuclear reaction, as mainly determined by
- The reaction cross-sections for the particles and energies available
- The Q-value or threshold energy, and the Coulombic repulsion barrier, i.e., the starting point of the reaction
- The stopping power defining energy loss and range of the particles in the target and the covering foil(s)
- The optimum energy dissipated in the target with respect to undesired concurrent reactions, and, in special cases,
- Scattering effects resulting in beam broadening which could determine the physical dimensions of the thick target.

The resulting compromise is a target thickness as great as possible for maximum yield of the desired nuclides accompanied by minimum yield of possible contaminants. The "thick target yield" thus obtained is the sum of more or less "thin target yields." All of these features are extensively dealt with in nuclear physics or nuclear chemistry textbooks (LIESER 1980; CHOPIN and RYDBERG 1980).

Radioactive nuclides may be prepared by a wide variety of particle accelerators. However, only cyclotrons accommodating at least moderate particle flux are able to produce radioactive sources with sufficiently high specific radioactivities to be of practical interest. The production principles are the same for all types of accelerators. The main steps are target preparation, irradiation and its secondary effects (recoil and hot-atom effects), target processing, and isolation and specification (labeling, purifying, etc.) of the radionuclides.

In cyclotrons, the product of charged particles such as protons, deuterons, alpha, and ^{3}He particles bombarding the target nuclei, and after emission of one or more particles to remove the excess excitation energy, may be radioactive nuclides. The capture of positively charged particles and the subsequent emission of neutrons results in isotopes which are neutron deficient in comparison with the stable isotopes of the element. Another important point in cyclotron bombardments is that normally the product is non-isotopic with the target. As a result, after chemical separations a product of high specific activity is obtained, since it has not been diluted by the target material. This is in contrast to the situation with nuclear reactors, where product and target are usually isotopic. Even if the same radioactive nuclides can be produced in a nuclear reactor, cyclotron production may be preferred where high specific activity is necessary for particular biomedical experiments.

I. The Cyclotron Production Facility

Routinely reliable production of cyclotron radionuclides depends on optimum parameters and reliable functioning of the cyclotron itself, as well as on the functioning of all the other components in this technologically sophisticated process (MARTIN 1979). To facilitate discussion about the cyclotron radionuclide production, the following brief outline detailing the different parts of the cyclotron production facility is given:

- Cyclotron, cyclotron vault, operation room
- Beam transport system
- Targetry and target rooms
- Target and radioactivity transport systems
- Hot-cell chemistry, automation, and labeling
- Quality control and distribution of the product
- Workshop and other nonactive areas or rooms.

Some important points to be taken into consideration in the building design are:
1. The transfer pathways for the radioactive products, especially those for the short-lived radionuclides and irradiated parts, should be as short as possible and in separate areas in the building.
2. The exterior shielding concrete walls should be so high that the radiation can not reach higher buildings in the neighborhood. The main sources of the highest radioactive radiation are the cyclotron itself and the target in the target rooms during bombardment.
3. It is important to have an electricity and water supply that is independent of other services (for emergencies).
4. Careful planning of the entire facility is to be recommended. The vault and target rooms should not be designed merely to meet minimum requirements as perceived at the outset, but some allowance should be made for future additions or expansions.

II. The Cyclotron

The average daily demand for radionuclides will be the determining factor in the choice of cyclotron (SILVESTER and WATERS 1979). It is advisable to purchase completely automated, computer-controlled equipment with a proven record of reliable performance (no experiments, no prototypes). A well-tested product should be selected from a cyclotron-manufacturing firm which is financially stable enough to guarantee maintenance and spare parts for the near future. A medical cyclotron for the production of short-lived positron-emitting radionuclides (mainly for PET studies) and other typical cyclotron gamma-emitters (see Table 2) should have the following basic parameters:

- The maximum energy of the proton beam should be 40 MeV
- The guaranteed beam current for long proton runs should be about 50 µA

As can be seen from Table 2, practically all important production routes are initiated by protons, based on three nuclear reactions:
1. (p,n)
2. (p,2n)
3. (p,3n).

Cross-sections of these reactions are maximal for protons with an energy range of up to 40 MeV. For heavy nuclei it is also possible with 40 MeV protons to initiate the (p,4n) reaction. Higher energy machines are too expensive. To purchase a machine with 60 or 70 MeV only for the possibility of producing pure ^{123}I via $^{127}I(p,5n)^{123}Xe \rightarrow ^{123}I$ reaction is neither economical nor reasonable (CUNINGHAME et al. 1976). ^{123}I may be produced more economically by other processes utilizing lower proton beams. In the future radioisotope laser separators may bring in a revolution in the production of pure radioactive species. On the other hand, the low-energy cyclotrons (20 to 30 MeV) impose limitations on the application of very important (p,2n) reactions; the (p,3n) reactions are practically impossible with this energy level. Use of low energy beams also demands the use of very thin foils to reduce energy losses in the foil system; this, in turn, limits the beam current.

Purely economic considerations to use low cost cyclotrons prompted the design of very small "baby cyclotrons" with restricted capabilities adapted to the production of low Z positron emitters exclusively for PET. The operating limitations of these cyclotrons imposed by the 10 MeV ceiling on proton energy make this option impractical; thus, today most manufacturers of "minicyclotrons" accelerate protons to 17 MeV.

There are some good arguments for manufacturing and using a medium proton energy machine with the "optimum" energy of proton particles at 35–40 MeV. This argumentation is based on 20 years of experience with radionuclide production and the following facts:

1. Most radionuclides are produced via the (p,2n) nuclear reactions (see Table 2). Threshold energies for these processes are about 16–18 MeV, and the optimum energy range for the (p,2n) reactions in comparison with the (p,n) and (p,3n) reactions gives the highest yields of desired radionuclides.

2. The half-lives of the preferred positron emitters preclude medical investigations of processes with biological (observation) time constraints greater than a few hours. It is to be expected that at least in the field of labeled antibodies, PET will need longer-lived radionuclides (like ^{75}Br, ^{76}Br, ^{121}I, or others). A look at the cross-sections shows that protons in the 25–35 MeV range are needed for effective production of these nuclides.

3. Using a higher initial particle energy makes it possible to use thicker foil windows on the target chamber. This in turn gives more target security, while partially eliminating some hot spots by dispersion throughout the foil, and making the beam more homogeneous. It is generally recommended to have some reserve in particle beam energy rather than to work with the maximum energy and a very narrow energy range.

4. Succesful PET groups will attract scientists and institutes from nearby with nuclear medical instrumentation. This extended cooperation will require either more batches per day or higher activities per batch of short-lived radionuclides. These requirements can be better satisfied with a machine of medium energy than with a "baby cyclotron."

5. To optimize the yields of positron emitters from gas targets (the most elegant production method), it is possible to simply raise gas pressure or use tandem targets. For the safe handling of high-pressure targets, a thicker entrance foil must be used.

From these arguments it follows that, in choosing a cyclotron which is to produce radionuclides for PET studies in addition to gamma-cyclotron radionuclides, and still have some reserve for future development work, one cyclotron with proton energies in the range of 35–40 MeV is to be recommended. It must be taken into account, however, that the expense for the cyclotron itself is nearly proportional to the energy range and the costs for the whole enterprise, including the laboratory facilities, etc., will go up correspondingly.

Figure 5 shows the major components of the beam transport system, the location of the diagnostic devices, and the target positions at the end of the beam lines.

After being magnetically deflected (horizontal bending X^0), the beam crosses the diagnostic components situated immediately in front of target(s). The beam profile, i.e., the current density across the beam, is an important characteristic, influencing heat dissipation throughout the entrance foils and target material. "Hot spots" can cause serious problems, such as leaks or the evaporation of (sometimes very expensive) target material through a damaged entrance foil. Homogeneous spatial current distribution is essential in the use of high current irradiations and for the longer life of target foils. A beam profile monitor in front of the target allows control and correction of beam quality, without significantly interfering with

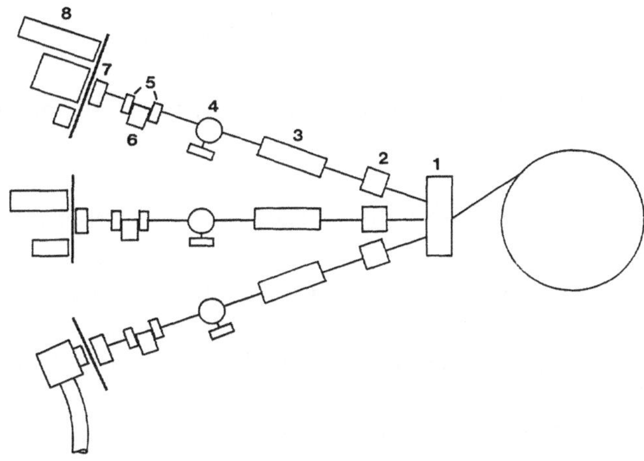

Fig. 5. Components of the cyclotron beam transport system with three target beam lines. *1* horizontal switching magnet, *2* fast closing valve, *3* quadrupole magnetic lenses, *4* diffusion pumps, *5* faraday cup/ diaphragm, *6* beam viewer, *7* twin foils cooling system, *8* target system

irradiation conditions. The water-cooled diaphragm operated by remote control has one or more circular bores (depending on the diameter of the target foil, usually with a diameter of about 10–25 mm). A second diaphragm can be used to obtain a better beam, in combination with a Faraday cup. The arrangement of the components of the beam transport system presents no particular problem with respect to machine vacuum. To separate the vacuum in the beam transport system from the target chamber, a twin-foil system is used which is situated at a short distance from the front of the target. The space between both foils is flushed by helium gas, precooled to about −25° C. Using this set-up, the target can be irradiated with a beam current of up to 25–35 µA, depending on the diaphragm used and the material of the irradiated target.

III. Choosing a Cyclotron

The following is a list of factors which should be taken into consideration in choosing a cyclotron:
1. Applications
   a) Average daily demand for radionuclides
   b) Neutron therapy only
   c) Multipurpose machine: production of radionuclides, activation analysis, material testing, neutron therapy (most of these cyclotrons exist in the planning stages only)
   d) Production of positron-emitting radionuclides only (low-energy machine)
2. Price-to-output ratio (to get the best cost-benefit relationship)
3. Reliability of the product (cyclotron)
   - Proven record of reliable performance
   - Information from other users
   - General experience with different manufacturers
   - Commercial stability of manufacturing firm
4. Additional costs, such as beam line periphery, beam transport system, as well as power and cooling supplies – are these included in the purchase price?
5. Quality and reliability of components
6. Guarantee period
7. Training of operators
8. Installation and testing within a short period of time.

F. Cyclotron Targetry

In practice the targets themselves consist of the following main parts:
a) Target material
b) Holder of the target material
c) Foil or double-foil system, enclosing the target material separated by a vacuum from the machine
d) Cooling system with water cooling circuit for the target, and helium cooling loop for the entrance foils
e) Clamps or automatic coupling system for the fixing of the target at the end of the beam line
f) Measuring and control instruments and sensors.

I. Targets and Target Periphery

The target is the place where the energetic accelerated particles touch the target material and any other kind of material which gives rise to various physical and chemical processes, such as:
a) Nuclear reactions, with target nuclides as well as with isotopical and nonisotopical contaminants of the target material in solid, liquid, and gaseous phase; coproduced ultrashort-lived radionuclides give rise to high energy photons
b) Reaction heat (Q) and the heat of other physical phenomena
c) Target itself is a source of fast neutrons
d) Activation of the target holder, the foils, and cooling media.

From these reasons (whether the radioactivity is of direct or indirect origin) the target to be bombarded should be enclosed in a shielded room. The installation of only a one-target system at the end of the beam line is not efficient. Therefore it is advantageous for methodologically similar target systems to be housed in independent vaults, constituting a multiple irradiation station. Also, in the event of accidental contamination in one beam room, irradiation can be carried out in the other beam room.

The reasons for attaching more targets at the end of the beam line can be summarized by the following points:
1. Optimum beam quality can be adjusted once for repeated irradiation of various targets
2. Efficiency in preparation of the next irradiation in another beam room and in the components for adjustment of the beam optics used for more targets
3. Reliability of the irradiation
4. Ease of operation, as all targets for irradiation may be prepared and maintained before hand
5. Remotely controlled fast change in the production is possible, an advantage for the production of short-lived radionuclides.

All similar target assemblies should be housed in independent vaults, or target rooms. For a cyclotron producing radionuclides for nuclear medicine, it is possible to divide the produced radionuclides into three groups which are similar in function or production procedure:
1. Short-lived, positron-emitting radionuclides (^{11}C, ^{13}N, ^{15}O, and ^{18}F)
2. Targets with complicated periphery and targets using enriched target material (^{123}I, ^{75}Br, ^{76}Br, ^{81}Rb, etc.)
3. Long-lived, gamma-emitting radionuclides (^{67}Ga, ^{111}In, ^{201}Tl, and others).

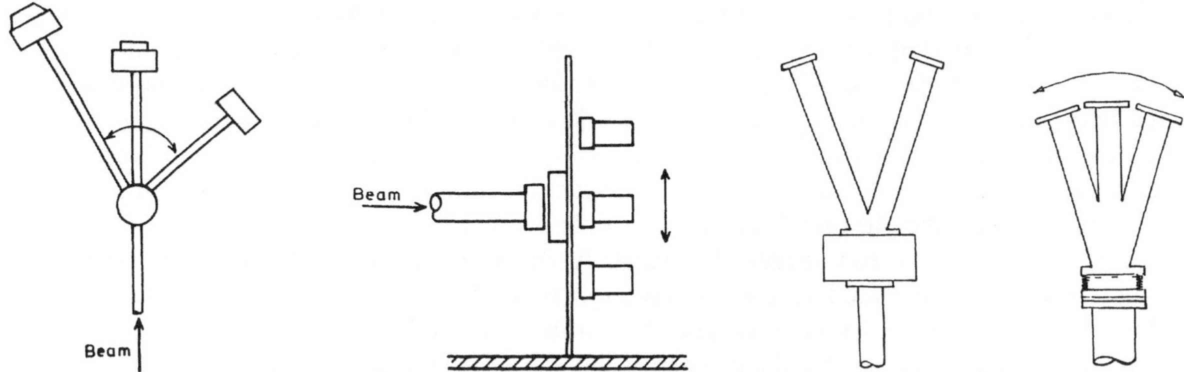

Fig. 6. Multiple irradiation set-up, situated on the end of the beam line

It is recommended, to have, if possible, a minimum of three target rooms. The experiment can then be set up, and a target changed or maintained during bombardment of another target. In this way cyclotron operation will be more efficient with respect to beam-on-target time. The smaller number of beam lines and separate target rooms can be compensated by using versatile equipment at the end of the beam lines.

The problem of multiple irradiation stations at the end of the beam line may be solved in different ways as shown in Fig. 6.

Various kinds of equipment enable the installation two or more targets at the end of the beam line, while remotely controlling the irradiation of each of these targets (Burton 1970). Generally there are three ways to solve this problem:

1. Installation of a changeable mechanism situated at the end of the beam line and operated by remote control from the operator's room. This target support system may be situated horizontally or vertically. Three targets on the support frame are optimal.
2. Installation of a target transport system for the transfer of the target from the loading station in the processing room to the irradiation position in the target room. This consists of two major components, a transport mechanism and an irradiation station. The support frame slide guides the target to the selected irradiation position. The target entrance flange is pneumatically depressed on the end flange of the beam line. This system should be advantageous for the routine production of long-lived radionuclides, where the separation of the product must not be done immediately after the bombardment.
3. Installation of a stationary target system which simultaneously produces different radionuclides using a special operation mode. Sophisticated, sequential, and multipurpose target systems are represented by this group.

II. Design and Construction of the Targets

The target material may be irradiated in any of the three phases, gas, liquid, or solid, and, correspondingly there are gaseous targets, liquid targets, and targets for metal foil and solid materials.

Generally there are two sources of cyclotron targets:

1. Some target assemblies are available for the production of important radionuclides (^{11}C, ^{13}N, ^{15}O, ^{18}F, and others) and may be purchased from the cyclotron producer together with the machine itself (Instrument AB Scanditronix 1985). As of now there are no special commercial suppliers of this nonstandardized equipment.

2. Targets may be designed and constructed in the workshops of the cyclotron. In constructing targets, workshop personnel learn the special problems associated with this new technology. This experience can be helpful in the future improvement, repair, and maintenance of irradiated targets. In any event this work must be done in the workshop near the cyclotron. The handling of targets after a long production period (more than 1000 μAh) can be very tricky and dangerous. It is better to change the target system for another one and then let the old one decay for a couple of days before maintenance.

The design of cyclotron targets is primarily determined by the target material to be irradiated and the estimated rate of production of the required radionuclides. The shape and size of the particle beam may also be important. The price of the target material, which can be very high, particularly if enriched material is used, will also affect the final target design.

Success in achieving efficient radionuclide production frequently depends largely upon the design of suitable target systems. Some important factors must be considered in designing cyclotron targets for the production of radionuclides. These include:

1. The nature of the target material
2. The provision of cooling adequate to prevent damage of the target and entrance foil from overheating
3. The method of recovering the product, during or after irradiation
4. The thickness of the target material required to maximize the yield of the required product, while minimizing possible impurities
5. The nature of the target holder construction material and foils for entry windows
6. The selection of irradiation conditions (energy of the particles and beam current).

In the production of radionuclides, the targets are normally exposed for long periods of time to high-intensity particle beams and gamma-ray fluxes. It is therefore desirable to select for targets and target holders materials which have the following characteristics:
– High melting point
– High thermal conductivity
– Will not decompose by heating
– Inorganic
– No aqueous solution in solid target materials
– Will not yield gaseous byproducts
– Material of target will not react chemically with material of the target holder
– Stable with regard to irradiation environment
– Chemical and physical form that will permit simple chemical and physical manipulations to remove the target material from the target holder, and which will subsequently allow postirradiation processing to be performed simply and rapidly with remote handling manipulators or automation.

Cyclotron targets can sometimes be of very simple construction, especially if the target material is a metal foil with a high melting point and if the resulting radioactive product is not volatilized in vacuum. For economic reasons, automation of production processes and handling by remote control, which are aspects of the construction of targets that require highly sophisticated technology, should be aimed at by most cyclotron radionuclide production laboratories.

However, most target materials and practical irradiation conditions differ from these optimal situations and thus for most routine production processes targets are very complicated systems. An example of such a sophisticated system is the production of ^{123}I via the $^{124}Xe(p,2n)^{123}Cs \rightarrow ^{123}Xe \rightarrow ^{123}I$ reaction (Grabmayr and Novotny 1978; Graham et al. 1984). This method, using highly enriched Xe as target gas, (the price of the enriched ^{124}Xe is at this time very high) will be described later on.

In summary, the design of the cyclotron target is primarily determined by the target material to be irradiated and the desired rate of production of the required radionuclides. In addition, the shape and size of the particle beam may be important factors. The price of the target material also affects the final design. Tight cooperation between the cyclotron physicist, radiochemist, operators, and precision mechanic is advisable in the construction of a new target system. The main problem for the radiochemist in the field of target chemistry is to determine how to reproduce high yields of the highest specific activity of the chemically identified species. A very important factor in the production of radionuclides for applications in nuclear medicine is the reproducibility of the production processes in the target and in subsequent chemical processing. The ideal case will be when radionuclides may be extracted from the target matrix in a chemical form which is of direct utility (^{15}O in $^{15}O_2$ form) or is synthetically useful as a precursor (^{11}C in $^{11}CO_2$ form) in labeling other chemical compounds. Surprising as it is, we cannot claim complete understanding of any single phenomenon in the target system used in the field (example, $^{14}N(p,alpha)^{11}C$ in $^{11}CO_2$ form), although we can prepare it. Clearly, basic hot-atom chemistry research into the nature of nuclear processes and chemistry in the target will always contribute significantly to new developments in targetry and target chemistry.

III. Classification of Cyclotron Targets

Cyclotron targets may be subdivided into different groups, according to their use. There are:

- Targets for the production of radionuclides. This is probably the largest group and includes the typical production targets used in routine production of radionuclides for applications in various research fields.
- Targets which are themselves objects of investigation. These targets may include substances which are bombarded in the cyclotron for the purpose of studying their physical properties. The use of targets from this group is limited exclusively to scientific investigation in nuclear physics studies.
- Targets for the production of other nucleons. These targets are produced for generating radiation used for further investigation or other purposes. This group includes the targets for generating neutrons used in neutron therapy.

According to the site of irradiation, targets may be subdivided into external and internal targets. External targets are irradiated outside the cyclotron vacuum chamber in which the target material is separated by the foil from the machine or beam-line vacuum. Internal targets are irradiated inside the machine. The use of internal targets is limited to nonvolatile radioactive products and target materials with high melting points.

According to the state of aggregation of the irradiated materials, targets are classified as solid, liquid, and gaseous.

Figure 7 shows a schematic view of common target assembly and all the important components constituting the target system.

The entire simple target assembly shown in Fig. 7 is attached to the end of the beam line. The diaphragm (made from aluminum, tantalum, or other pure and nonactivated material) prevents the beam from striking the beam line, electron suppressor ring, and O-ring support structure. By focusing the beam on a small aperture, a section of reasonably uniform power density is selected to hit the target material. The beam profile behind the diaphragm should have a diameter smaller than the surface of the target material to be irradiated. The beam should be homogeneous over the entire surface of the target material. The electron suppressor is used to prevent back-streaming of electrons from the target to enable exact

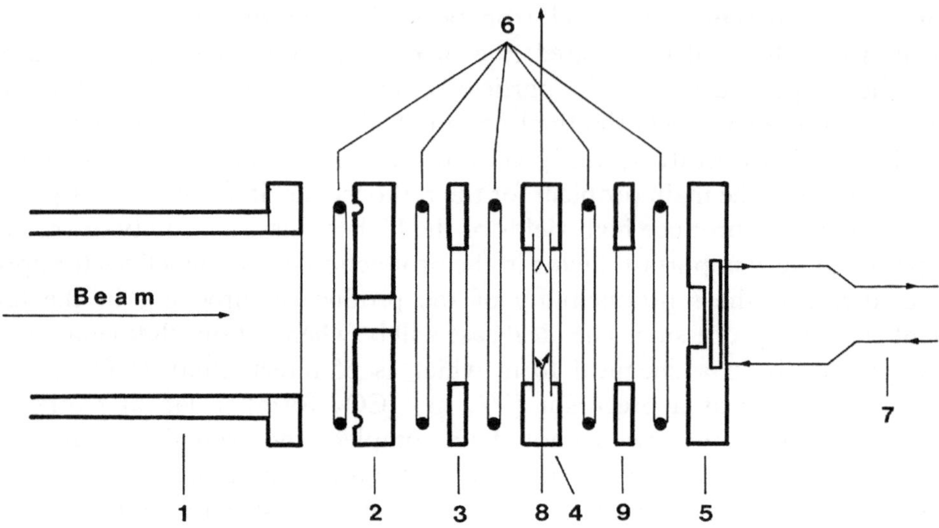

Fig. 7. Schematic view of the external target system. *1* beam line, *2* diaphragm, *3* insulator, *4* double foil system, *5* target head, *6* O-rings system, *7* water cooling, *8* He gas foil cooling, *9* electron suppressing ring

measurement of the beam current. The foil system can be cooled by spraying the foils with precooled helium gas. The target backing plate is regularly cooled with water. The insulator makes the beam current measurements possible, using the principle of the Faraday cup.

Target heating in charged particle irradiation is calculated from the power dissipation in the target:

$$\text{power (watts)} = \text{energy (MeV)} \times \text{current (µA)}$$

For example, consider a thick target bombarded with 50 µA of protons from a 35-MeV cyclotron in which the beam is completely stopped within the target, then: $P = (35 \text{ MeV}) \times (50 \text{ µA}) = 1750$ watts; since

$$1 \text{ watt} = 0.24 \text{ cal/sec}$$

$$P = (0.24)\,(1750) = 420 \text{ cal/sec}$$

The target cooling system must be sufficient to remove 420 cal/sec to prevent target overheating during the bombardment (HELUS and WOLBER 1983).

For practical considerations targets are classified mostly into three main groups: solid, liquid, and gaseous.

For the preparation of *solid targets*, target material with relatively good physical and mechanical properties, especially with a high melting point and good heat conductivity, should be used. For example, for the production of ^{68}Ge via ^{69}Ga(p,2n)^{68}Ge reaction, a special Ga—Cu alloy is used instead of Ga (or Ga compounds; LOCH et al. 1980). This alloy has a melting point at about 800° C. As the range of the bombarding particles in solid target materials does not exceed a few hundred microns, a relatively thin layer of target material is sufficient to provide "thick target" status. Metal foils, blocks, thin films on different backgrounds, pills, or pressed tablets on an appropriate support are generally used as targets.

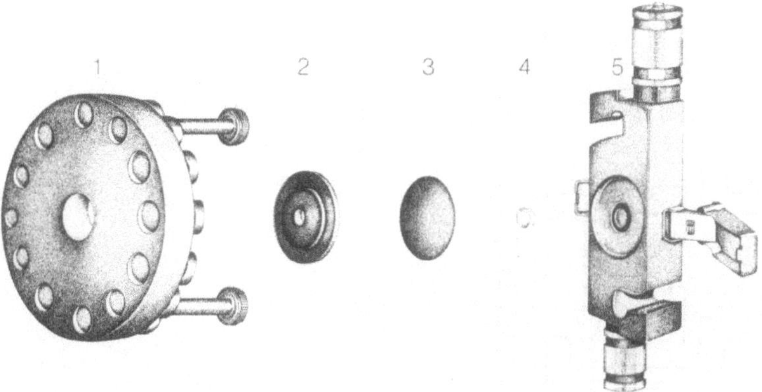

Fig. 8. Expanded view of the target for irradiation of solid target materials. *1* flange, *2* foil holder, *3* Havar foil, *4* Ca disc, *5* target

As a support for the target material, aluminum, tantalum, or titanium are used. The target material is attached to the backing plate by different methods. The important factor is suitable cooling and good heat conductivity between target material and backing plate. Figure 8 shows an expanded view of a target system used for irradiation of pressed pills, melted material in the target cavity ($^{124}TeO_2$ for production of ^{123}I), or tablets. The target can be quickly mounted onto the flange with clamps.

Typical radionuclides produced by irradiation of solid targets include ^{123}I (via irradiation of enriched tellurium targets), ^{77}Br, ^{67}Ga, ^{201}Tl, and others.

There are two reasons for using *liquid targets*. The first is that the water or other solvent may be used directly for cooling the entry beam window. For example, the water is used as target material for the production of ^{13}N via the $^{16}O(p,alpha)^{13}N$ reaction (TILBURY et al. 1971) and water enriched with ^{18}O (up to 99%) is used for the production of the very important radionuclide ^{18}F via the $^{18}O(p,n)^{18}F$ reaction (NICKLES et al. 1984). In both cases, the irradiated target water is pumped through the target cavity and used as cooling medium for the entrance foil. The second reason is connected with the subsequent chemical processing. After the end of the bombardment, the irradiated solution can be pumped through the tubing system directly into the hot cell where further chemical steps will occur. The irradiated solution may be also transferred to the chemical laboratory in a vial using a rabbit pneumatic system. Figure 9 presents a schematic view of a target system for the production of ^{13}N which could be representative of other liquid target systems.

Irradiating the water solution with high beam currents may give rise to problems connected with the occurrence of radiolytically induced reactions and radiolysis, which produce hydrogen and oxygen. These then have to be recombined with the aid of catalysts (on a Pd basis) in order to prevent dangerous pressure increases in the target.

Gas targets are especially advantageous in the production of short-lived radionuclides. Practically all positron emitters produced for PET studies (BEANEY 1984), including ^{11}C, ^{13}N, ^{14}O and ^{15}O, ^{18}F, and ^{19}Ne, are swept out of the target with target gas. These targets typically combine a gaseous target material with a gaseous product nuclide. To this group also belongs an important target for the production of the ^{81}Rb used in the preparation of the $^{81}Rb-^{81m}Kr$ generator, which represents the type of generator where the target material is gaseous and the product solid (JONES and CLARK 1969). Some of these targets are very simple in their construction, especially when the target gas is not expensive. For the expensive enriched target gases (for example, ^{124}Xe for the production of high purity ^{123}I), special safety precautions must be undertaken.

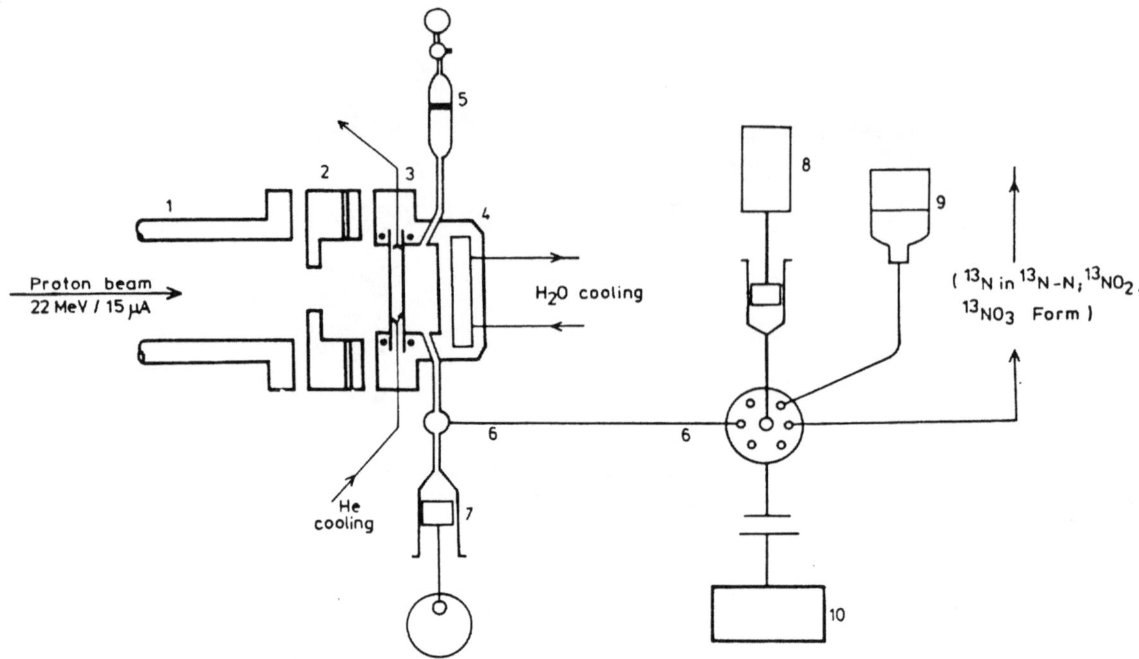

Fig. 9. External liquid target system for the production of ^{13}N via the $^{16}O(p,\alpha)^{13}N$ reaction using water as target material. *1* beam line, *2* collimator, insulator, *3* double foil system, *4* target body with target cavity, *5* volume compensation vessel, *6* remotely operated valves, *7* reciprocating pump, *8* injection pump, *9* target sterile water, *10* remotely handling control system

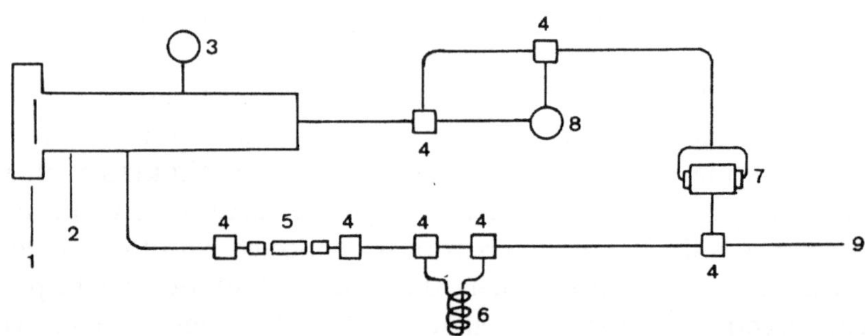

Fig. 10. Gas recirculating target system. *1* foil, *2* stainless steel, target chamber, *3* pressure gauge, *4* three way valves, *5* ^{18}F adsorbtion trap, *6* ^{18}O recovery trap, *7* pump, *8* flow meter, *9* vacuum

The scheme in Fig. 10 shows an ^{81}Rb recirculating gas target system.

Gas targets fall into two classes: those in which a gas is the target material and those in which target material is solid but the activity produced is in gaseous form and can be removed from the target by sweeping gas (for example, B_2O_3 as solid target material produces ^{11}C and ^{13}N by proton bombardment, while both may be swept away be He gas). Figure 11 shows a schematic view of this type of target.

The advantages of gas targets are:

1. Target design is simpler than for solid targets
2. There is no dismantling of the target and target material after irradiation and the transport of produced radioactive nuclides is done simply via a tubing system.
3. The range of particle energy in the target material is increased and facilitates the optimization of target length to avoid contaminating reactions and to increase the yield of desired radionuclides.

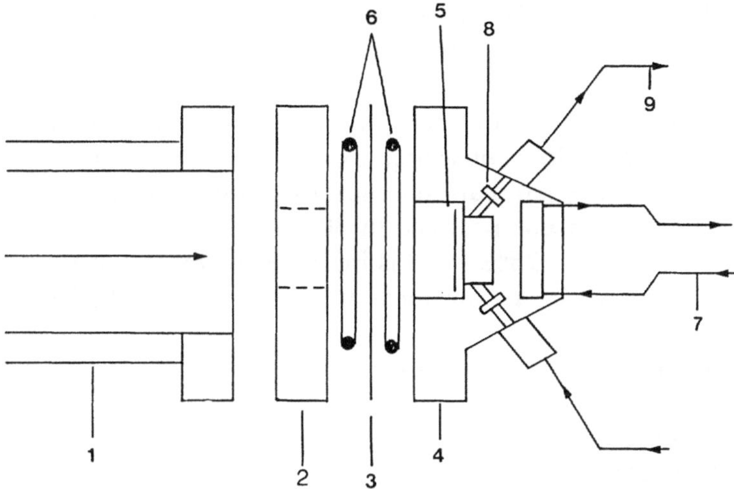

Fig. 11. Target system for the extraction of volatile products from the solid matrix. *1* beam line, *2* diaphragm, *3* foil, *4* target body, *5* target material, *6* O-Rings, *7* water cooling, *8* porous metal disc, *9* carrier gas

It is recommended that the handling of radioactive gases (0.5 to 2.0 Ci of ^{11}C is a normal batch of the produced activity) should be done in closed hot cells. In the event of an accident involving a release of gaseous activity, the cell atmosphere is to be vented to an evacuated shielded container and the activity allowed to decay.

G. Examples of Routine Production Methods

As typical examples of the routine production of high demand radionuclides and the targetry used, the production of ^{11}C, ^{81}Rb, and ^{123}I, will be commented up on.

Table 3 lists some of the more common reactions along with the requirements for incident particle energy and the production reaction.

Carbon-11 (20 min half-life) as a metabolic tracer has acquired great importance in the labeling of biologically active molecules for use in the PET technique.

The most useful nuclear reactions for ^{11}C production, from a technical standpoint, are the proton bombardment of pure nitrogen gas and the irradiation of natural or enriched B_2O_3. The irradiation of nitrogen gas with protons (energy lower than 13 MeV) is a less

Table 3. ^{11}C production reactions

	Natural abundance (%)	Treshold energy (MeV)	Maximum cross-section (mb)	Particle energy at maximum cross-section (MeV)
^{10}B (d,n) ^{11}C	20.00	6.47	180	11.87
^{11}B (p,n) ^{11}C	80.00	3.02	100	9.52
^{14}N (p,α) ^{11}C	99.63	3.13	250	7.43
^{12}C (p,pn) ^{11}C	98.90	20.30	100	42.30
^{9}Be (α,2n) ^{11}C	100.00	18.80	17	–
^{12}C (γ,n) ^{11}C	98.90	–	–	–

complicated method at present. The presence of oxygen contaminant in N_2 target gas (1–10 ppm) is of sufficient concentration to scavenge the recoil ^{11}C atoms in $^{11}CO_2$ form (Wolf and Redwandly 1977).

The target is a simple, about 25 cm long, stainless-steel chamber combined with a tubing and electronic sensor system (flow, pressure, valves, etc.) connected directly to a hot cell in the chemical laboratory. The irradiation conditions of 40 bar N_2, 13 MeV proton initial energy, and a 25-μA beam current produce in 30 minutes irradiation time approximately 600 to 800 mCi of ^{11}C as $^{11}CO_2$ (96%–97% is in $^{11}CO_2$ form, the rest is ^{11}CO).

Total yield of ^{11}C produced via the most used $^{14}N(p,alpha)^{11}C$ reaction depends on the following parameters:
1. Reaction cross-section, excitation function
2. Beam current
3. Initial energy of bombarding particles
4. Homogenity of the beam
5. Thickness of the target material, pressure of the target gas
6. Flow of the target (or sweeping) gas, if the flow method of irradiation is used; the stop-flow technique gives higher specific activity
7. Impurities of the target gas (moisture and chemical composition of the target or sweeping gas)
8. Isotopic abundance of the target material
9. Temperature of the target material, cooling problems.

The produced ^{11}C is in a "carrier-free" form. However, in practice true carrier-free conditions are difficult to achieve, because of contamination with stable carbon isotopes during production. Carbon is so abundant in nature that practically any contact with organic material will result in a lower specific activity of the ^{11}C-labeled compounds. The achievable activities for $^{11}CO_2$ have been reported to range from 1000–5000 Ci/mmol and 200–500 Ci/mmol for subsequent steps. $^{11}CO_2$ as parent precursor can be easily transformed on-line (catalytically) into other important precursors (for example, ^{11}CO, $H^{11}CN$, $^{11}CH_3OH$, $^{11}CH_4$, and $^{11}CH_3I$).

The production of ^{81}Rb via the $^{82}Kr(p,2n)^{81}Rb$ reaction is an example of the special case where the target material is a gas and the product is solid. As the target gas (pure krypton) is expensive, and only small quantities are available, special construction with an excellent cooling facility for the foil entry window and target chamber must be assured. As a safety precaution, if enriched gases are used, the target chamber is fitted with a trap (with molecular sieve and cooled by liquid air) into which, by decreasing the pressure (through a foil leak or other accident), the gas can be withdrawn.

At the end of the bombardment the activity deposited on the walls inside the target chamber or on the internal liner can be washed out and collected. After drying and evacuating the chamber, the gas can be released into the target by heating the molecular sieve. The irradiation may be then repeated, (generally a useful system for production of ^{81}Rb and ^{123}I if the enriched target material is used). For multiple use of one loading of nonenriched krypton gas, we have developed a target system as described in Fig. 12 (Helus et al. 1980).

This design has been used for a number of years for the production of ^{81}Rb and preparation of $^{81}Rb-^{81m}Kr$ generators. It is remotely controlled and the target consists of a stainless-steel liner inside a cylindrical stainless-steel vessel. The liner is connected to a rotor which is coupled magnetically to an external multipole magnet.

By mechanical rotation of the external multipole magnet, the internal liner is rotated, allowing the inner surface of the liner to be washed by a solvent (sterile water). After washing the activity from the walls, the ^{81}Rb is transferred into a vessel outside the target and the generators are loaded. All these operations have been fully automated under micro-

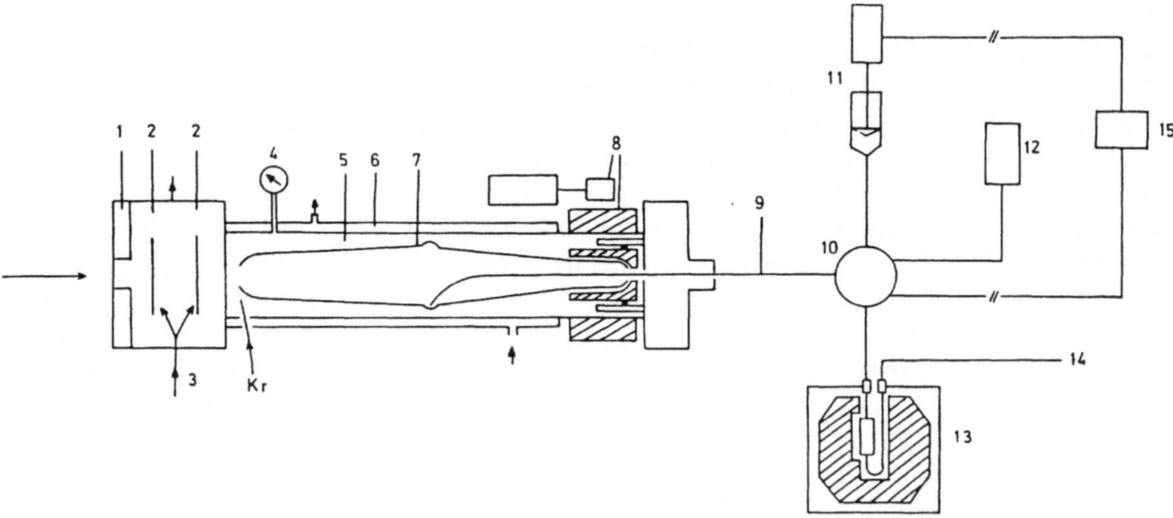

Fig. 12. Scheme of ^{81}Rb production system. *1* collimator, *2* foils, *3* foil cooling, *4* pressure gauge, *5* target body, *6* water cooling, *7* quartz liner, *8* magnetic rotation system, *9* solvent line, *10* remote operated valve, *11* injection pump, *12* reservoire with sterile water, *13* ^{81}Rb$-^{81m}$Kr generator, *14* waste, *15* electronic control

processor control. In a three-hour irradiation with a proton beam of 20.5 MeV initial energy and 15 μA beam current, 180 mCi of ^{81}Rb may be produced (actual yield). Using enriched target material, the yield may increase about 5 to 6 times (or irradiation time may be shorter).

The third example is the routine production of the very important radionuclide ^{123}I. A large number of production methods for ^{123}I have been reported. The overriding problems in the production of ^{123}I by many of these processes have been the coproduction of ^{124}I and low yields. Table 4 lists the nuclear reactions studied on a low-energy cyclotron ($E_p = $ max 21.5 MeV), together with the calculated production rates.

A widely used method for the production of ^{123}I on the medium-energy cyclotron is the ^{124}Te(p,2n)^{123}I nuclear reaction (KONDO et al. 1977). The target material ^{124}Te in the

Table 4. Methods of ^{123}I-production

Reaction	Energy of Incident Beam (MeV)	Target	Isotopic Enrichment	^{123}I Thick Target Yield (mCi/μAh)	^{124}I (%)	^{125}I (%)	Other Impurities
^{121}Sb(α,2n)^{123}I	31.0	Sb-nat.	98.4%	0.930	0.8	0.015	0.03% ^{126}I
^{122}Te(d,n) ^{123}I	7.0	Te[a]	95.4%	0.100	0.09	0.013	0.04% ^{126}I (and others)
^{122}Te(^{3}He,2n)^{123}Xe (β^+,EC) → ^{123}I	27.0	Te[a]	90.9%	0.530	–	1.0	–
^{123}Te(p,n)^{123}I	19.5	Te[a]	79.0%	0.440	0.88	0.08	0.24% ^{126}I
^{124}Te(p,2n) ^{123}I	27.8	Te[a]	96.2%	0.540	0.05	(1)	0.50% ^{121}I
^{124}Xe(p,2n)^{123}Cs (β^+)→^{123}Xe→^{123}I	30.0	^{124}Xe[a]	70–90%	8.0	–	–	–

(1) not indicated
[a] enriched

TeO$_2$ form enriched to 94%–99% was used (supplied by Oak Ridge National Laboratory). Using an initial proton energy of 22 MeV, the production of ^{123}I exhibits strong discrepancies in the ratio ^{124}I/^{123}I. Contaminant ^{124}I is coproduced via the ^{124}Te(p,n)^{124}I reaction even if the highest enrichment possible, 99.0% ^{124}Te, is used. ^{123}I was separated from the molten ^{124}TeO$_2$ matrix by dry distillation. Unfortunately, this separation method is always accompanied by a significant loss of enriched material, which quantitatively depends on separation time, temperature, sweeping gas flow, and TeO$_2$ surface area. In suppressing volatilization of tellur dioxide during the separation and ensuring the best uniformity in target thickness, the optimal target thickness plays a very important role. A high-frequency oven has also been used for the heating of the target; the loss of target material was considerably reduced by heating for only 30 seconds. The product was contaminated with 0.8% to 1.2% ^{124}I at EOB (End of bombardment) and must be prepared and used within 24 hours.

Evidently the best of all production procedures for pure ^{123}I is the ^{124}Xe(p,2n)^{123}Cs→ ^{123}Xe→^{123}I reaction. It has only one small fault – the price of the enriched ^{124}Xe target material. Using this method, ^{123}I is produced in the three cyclotron laboratories (KfK Karlsruhe, Eindhoven, and Vancouver).

I. Automation of the Production Processes

The main advantage of the automation and remotely controlled target systems is that production can be controlled from outside the target room, resulting in reduced radiation exposure to personnel. Sometimes remote control is satisfactory; in other cases, when repeated identical operations are involved, full automation is preferable. The comfort of the operator, reduced preparation time (which for short-lived isotopes results in higher activity), more reliable production processes, and careful control of all parameters may result in increased chemical yields and reproducibility. Usually "intelligent" automation under microprocessor control is preferable. On the other hand, the development of automated systems is only worthwhile for products in routine production (twice a week or more).

II. Multipurpose and Sequential Targets

Some clinical studies require the rapid sequential delivery of two or three radiopharmaceuticals labeled with short-lived radionuclides. This needs short bombardment with high yields and quick change over from target to target. Typical physical solutions involve the fast switching system or scanning system over more targets or movable target platforms (see Fig. 13).

Another solution may be found in the choice of target material to produce more radionuclides at once and their subsequent sophisticated separation from one another. Reports of some multipurpose or sequentially operated target systems have been just published.

As an example of the function of a multipurpose target system, the simultaneous production of ^{11}C, ^{13}N, and ^{18}F from the proton irradiation of boron trioxide on a special vertical beam-line construction (HELUS and MAHUNKA 1986) will be described.

Figure 13 shows a vertically situated beam transport line and new target system for the production of useful radionuclides by separation from melted target materials.

The volatile reaction products may be recovered from the target material with nonreactive carrier gas. The thermochromatographic chemical separation method is the most appropriate for the production and separation of short-lived radionuclides. It has the following advantages:

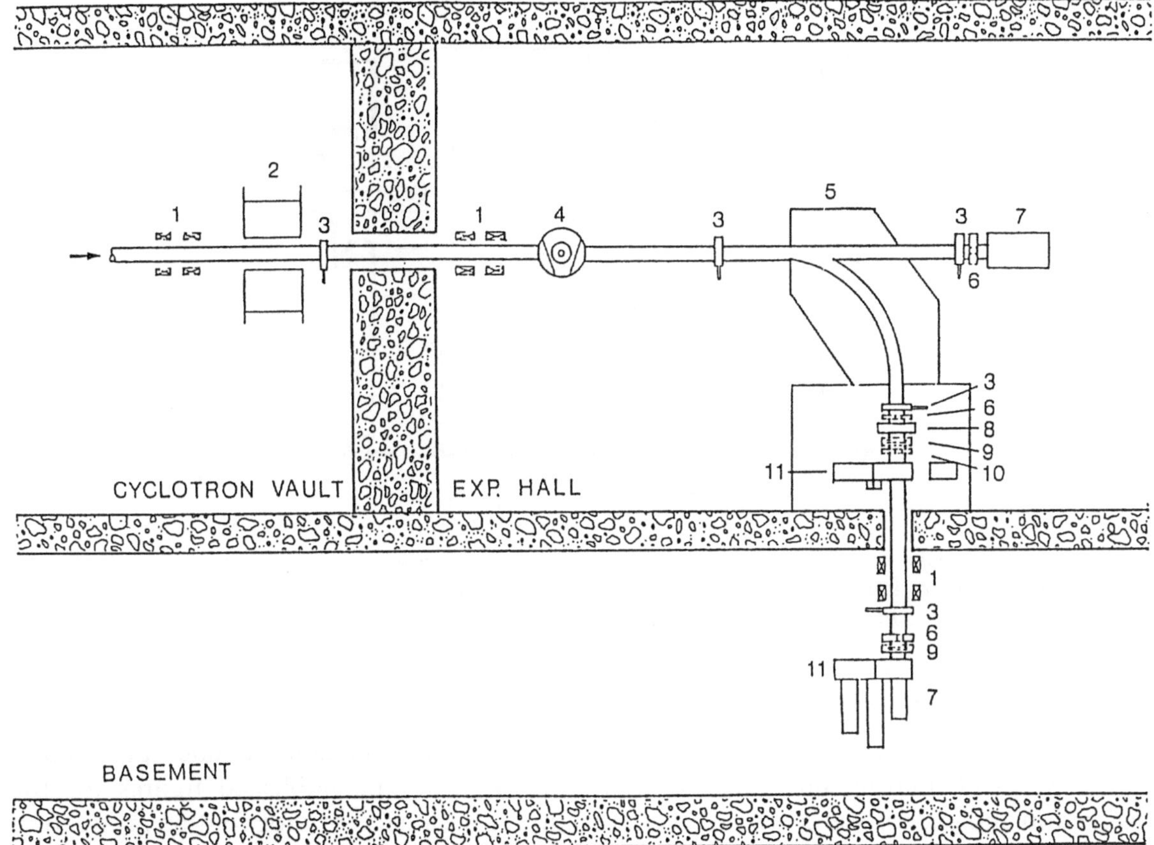

Fig. 13. An elevation view of the beam transport system. *1* quadrupoldublet, *2* switching-magnet, *3* valve, *4* turbomolecular pump, *5* deflecting magnet, *6* diaphragm fixed, *7* target, *8* beam profile monitor, *9* double foil system, *10* variable diaphragm, *11* target changing device

Table 5. Remote sequential production of ^{11}C, ^{13}N and ^{18}F using B_2O_3 as target material

Target isotope	Natural abundance %	Nuclear reaction	Product chemical form	Sweeping gas	Maximum cross-section (mb)
^{11}B	80,00	^{11}B(p,n)^{11}C	^{11}CO$_2$	He	360
^{16}O	99,75	^{16}O(p,α)^{13}N	^{13}N$-$N, ^{13}NO$_x$	He	19
^{18}O	0,20[a]	^{18}O(p,n)^{18}F	H^{18}F(?)	Xe(?)	~700

[a] enrichment on ^{18}O is possible

- The energy carried by the particle beam is used for melting the target material, which is not possible with targets installed at horizontal beam lines;
- The target can be used many times without any recovery procedure and dismounting after the irradiation;
- The separation is fast and can be carried out online with irradiation;
- The yield of the nuclear production processes, (described in Table 5) – the radionuclides produced – can be easily separated from each other and chemically processed;
- The target system can be remotely controlled and automation is possible.

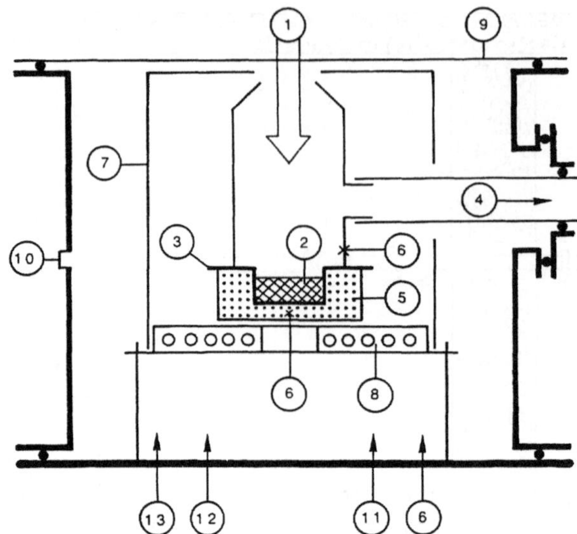

Fig. 14. Schematic design of target chamber. *1* beam, *2* target material, *3* target frame, *4* sweep gas and product nuclei, *5* temperature controlled oven, *6* thermopars, *7* heat reflector, *8* water cooled target mounting plate, *9* foil, *10* vacuum gauge, *11* heating current, *12* sweep gas, *13* cooling water

Proton irradiation of boron trioxide is advantageous for the simultaneous production of three positron-emitting nuclides, as shown in Table 5. The published figures for the cross-section and experimental yield of these reactions are satisfactory for routine production of these radionuclides.

The construction and design of the target system were dictated by the properties of the target material and the radioactive species produced, which have to have sufficient stability to be transported via the tubing system with nonreactive carrier gas. A schematic arrangement of this target system is shown in Fig. 14.

The target material is placed in a small cavity constructed from Mo (or Ta) metal and surrounded by a heater which keeps the temperature at the appropriate level. This is partially achieved through the energy carried by the particle beam and additional electrical heating or water cooling. Precautions have been taken to minimize background diffusion of the volatile product to regions of low temperatures. The cylindrical part situated on the top of the target material holder works as a heat reflector and separates the chamber from the beam entry with thin Havar foil. The helium carrier gas is preheated to a higher temperature to avoid cooling of the target material surface. The target allows temperatures of up to 1000° C. The produced radioactivity of ^{11}C and ^{13}N is transported to the traps outside the target room. With the use of enriched boron trioxide, the production and discontinuous separation of ^{18}F from the target material is possible.

In the meantime the study and development of multipurpose target systems continues (Ruth et al. 1984; Wieland et al. 1984; Blessing et al. 1984). Understanding the phenomena in the targets needs more experimental work in the fields of target construction and target chemistry and requires an enormous amount of intellectual and material resources. It is necessary for scientists (from hot-atom chemists to cyclotron physicists) to get together and develop lively contacts and cooperation in order to conduct research properly and at the best cost-benefit relationship.

References

Amphlett C, Vonberg DD et al (1970) The use of cyclotron in chemistry, metalurgy and biology. Butterworths, London

Arrol WJ, Chadwick J, Eakins J (1956) The preparation from irradiated uranium of iodine-131 and certain other fission products. Progress in Nucl Energy, Ser III, Process Chemistry 1. Pergamon, London

Beaney RP (1984) Positron emission tomography in the study of humane tumors. Seminars in nuclear medicine, vol XIV, no 4 (October), pp 324–341

Belkas HP, Perricos DC (1969) ^{99m}Tc production based on the extraction with methyl ethyl ketone. Radiochimica Acta 11:56

Blessing G et al (1984) A multipurpose target system for high-current irradiations. Fifth Int Symp on Radiopharmaceutical Chemistry, July 9–13, Tokyo, p 270

Boyd RE (1983) The special position of ^{99m}Tc in nuclear medicine. In: Helus F (ed) Radionuclide production, vol II. CRC Press, Florida, pp 126–150

Burton G (1970) Cyclotron beam sharing for multiple irradiations. In: McIlroy RW (ed) Butterworths, London, p 250

Choppin GR, Rydberg J (1980) Nuclear chemistry. Pergamon, Oxford, pp 173–188

Clark JC, Silvester DJ (1966) A cyclotron method for the production of ^{18}F. Int J Appl Radiat Isot 17:151

Colonomos M, Parker W (1969) Preparation of carrier-free ^{99}Mo by neabs of (n,gamma) recoil. Radiochimica Acta 12:163

Cuninghame JG et al. (1976) Large scale production of ^{123}I from a flowing liquid target using the (p,5n) reaction. Int J Appl Radiat Isot 27:597–603

Ferrieri RA, Wolf AP (1983) The chemistry of positron emitting nucleogenic atoms with regard to preparation of labelled compounds of practical utility. Radiochimica Acta 34:69–83

Grabmayr P, Nowotny R (1978) Statistical-model based evaluation of reactions producing ^{123}Xe and ^{127}Xe. Int J Appl Radiat Isot 29:261–267

Graham D et al (1984) Enriched Xenon-124 for the production of high-purity Iodine-123 using a CP-42 cyclotron. J Nucl Med 25:32

Helus F, Mahunka I (1986) Cyclotron production of positron emitters in vertical target system. J Radio Analyt Chem (in press)

Helus F, Maier-Borst W (1973) Erhöhte Ausbeute und schnellere, halbautomatische Präparation für in Forschungsreaktoren dargestelltes ^{18}F. Nuklearmedizin 38:336–339

Helus F, Wolber G (1983) Nuclear data; simple calculus with practical examples and optimum irradiation conditions. In: Helus F (ed) Radionuclide production, vol I. CRC Press, Florida

Helus F, Sahm U et al (1979) Production of ^{121}I on the Heidelberg compact cyclotron and aspects of ^{121}I dosimetry. Radiochem Radioanal Letters 39:9–18

Helus F, Maier-Borst W et al. (1980) Remotely controlled target system for the routine production of ^{81}Rb. Radiochem Radioanal Letters 44:187

Helus F, Gasper H et al. (1985) Cyclotron production of ^{34m}Cl for biomedical use. J Radioanal Nucl Chem Letters 94:149–160

Jones T, Clark JC (1969) A cyclotron produced ^{81}Rb$-^{81m}$Kr generator and its uses in gamma camera studies. Br J Radiol 42:237

Keller KA et al (1973) Q-Values and excitation functions for nuclear reactions. In: Schopper H (ed) Landolt-Börnstein New Series, group I, vol 5. Springer, Berlin Heidelberg New York

Kondo K et al (1977) Improved target and radiochemistry for production of ^{123}I and ^{124}I. Int J Appl Radiat Isot 28:765–771

Larson SM, Carasquillo JA (1984) Nuclear oncology. In: Freeman LM, Blaufox MO (eds) Seminars in nuclear medicine, vol XIV, no 4 (October). Grune and Stratton, Orlando/Florida, pp 268–276

Lebowitz E et al (1975) Thallium-201 for medical use. J Nucl Med 16:151–155

Lieser KH (1980) Einführung in die Kernchemie. Chemie, Weinheim, S 239–261

Loch C, Maziere B, Comar D (1980) A new generator for ionic ^{68}Ga. J Nucl Med 21:171–173

Martin JA (1979) Cyclotrons. IEEE Trans Nucl Sci 26:2443–2651

Nickles RJ, Daube ME, Ruth TJ (1984) An ^{18}O$_2$ target for the production of ^{18}F$_2$. Int J Appl Radiat Isot 35:117–122

Northcliff LC, Shilling RF (1970) Range and stopping-power tables for heavy ions. In: Nuclear data tables, vol 7. no 3–4 (January 1970). Academic, New York London

Richards P (1966) Radioactive pharmaceuticals (Proc Symp Oak Ridge), USAEC Div Techn Inform. Extension, Oak Ridge, p 323

Root J, Krohn K (eds) (1981) Short-lived radiopharmaceuticals in chemistry and biology. ACS Adv in chemistry series monograph. Am Chem Soc Washington/DC

Ruth TH, Adam MJ et al (1984) Radionuclide production on the Triumf CP$-$42: A gas target for sequential production of ^{18}F$-$F$_2$, and ^{15}O$-$O$_2$. Fifth Int Symp on Radiopharmaceutical Chemistry, July 9–13, Tokyo, p 282

Silvester DJ (1976) Preparation of radiopharmaceuticals and labelled compounds using short-lived radionuclides. In: Newton GWA, Fox BW, Harbottle GR, Heslap JA (eds) Radiochemistry, vol 3. The Chemical Society, Burlington House, London, p 73

Silvester DJ, Waters S (1979) Second international symposium on radiopharmaceuticals, March 19–22 1979, Seattle

Smith EM (1964) Properties, uses, radiochemical purity, and calibration of ^{99m}Tc. J Nucl Med 5:871

Stöcklin G (1977) Bromine-77 and Iodine-123 radiopharmaceuticals. Int J Appl Radiat Isot 28:131–148

Szillard L, Chalmers TA (1934) Chemical separation of the radioactive element from its bombarded isotope in the Fermi effect. Nature 134:462

Thakur ML (1983) Radioactive compounds of Gallium and Indium. In: Rayudu GVS (ed) Radiotracers for medical applications, vol 1. CRC Press, Florida, pp 187–218

Tilbury RS, Dahl JR et al (1971) The production of ^{13}N labelled ammonia for medical use. Radiochem Radioanal Letters 8:317

Wagner HN (ed) (1968) Principles of nuclear medicine. Saunders, Philadelphia

Wieland BW et al (1984) Multipurpose target unit for small cyclotrons. Fifth Int Symp on Radiopharmaceutical Chemistry, July 9–13, Tokyo, p 268

Williamson CF et al (1973) Tables of range and stopping powers of chemical elements for charged particles of energy 0.5 to 500 MeV. CEA-R 3042 Report Commissariat d'energy Atomique, Centre d'etudes Nucleaires. Saclay, Essone

Wolf AP, Fowler JS (1979) Organic radiopharmaceuticals, recent advances, in radiopharmaceuticals II. Society of Nuclear Medicine, New York, p 73

Wolf AP, Redwanly CS (1977) Carbon-11 and radiopharmaceuticals. Int J Appl Radiat Isot 28:29–48

^{11}C, ^{13}N, ^{15}O and ^{18}F target and processing systems. Prospect from Instrument AB Scanditronix. Huysborg, Uppsala/Sweden

1.2 Spezielle Syntheseverfahren mit kurzlebigen Radionukliden und Qualitätskontrolle

Von

G. Stöcklin

Mit 11 Abbildungen, 9 Schemata und 16 Tabellen

A. Einleitung

Kurzlebige Zyklotron-produzierte Radionuklide gewinnen in der modernen nuklearmedizinischen Funktionsdiagnostik zunehmend an Bedeutung. Das ideale Radionuklid für in-vivo Anwendungen sollte möglichst folgende Voraussetzungen erfüllen:
- kein α- oder β^--Strahler sein,
- γ-Quanten mit Energien im Bereich von 100–300 keV oder Positronen emittieren,
- eine Halbwertzeit von einigen Minuten bis zu einigen Stunden besitzen,
- möglichst stabile kovalente Bindungen mit Kohlenstoffatomen bilden.

Die Vorteile kurzlebiger Radionuklide sind evident:
- geringe Dosis für den Patienten,
- Wiederholung der Anwendung in relativ kurzen Intervallen (Therapiekontrolle etc.) prinzipiell möglich,
- keine Störung der biochemischen Gleichgewichte, sofern das Produkt praktisch trägerfrei oder trägerarm ist (nca = no-carrier-added); auch Einsatz toxischer oder zentralwirksamer Radiopharmaka möglich,
- keine bzw. geringe Probleme der Abfallbeseitigung.

Die Kurzlebigkeit bringt aber auch signifikante Probleme bei der Herstellung, Markierung und Anwendung mit sich:
- hohe Anfangsaktivitäten (einige GBq) erforderlich,
- automatisierte oder fernbediente Chemie in Bleizellen insbesondere im Falle von Positronenstrahlern (511 keV Vernichtungsstrahlung),
- down-scaling der Synthese bis in den Subnanogrammbereich,
- Durchführung von Synthese und Qualitätskontrolle innerhalb von maximal etwa drei Halbwertszeiten,
- nur relativ schnelle Funktionen erfaßbar,
- in vielen Fällen sog. „in-house"-Zyklotron erforderlich.

Die moderne nuklearmedizinische Funktionsdiagnostik führt in zunehmendem Maße zu biochemischen Ansätzen der Radiopharmakaentwicklung. Die Erfassung regionaler Funktionen mit Hilfe moderner Methoden der Emissionstomographie unter Verwendung körpereigener Substrate oder deren Analoga sowie Pharmaka stehen im Vordergrund dieser Entwicklung. Das biochemische Konzept umfaßt im wesentlichen die folgenden Stoffgruppen:
- Stoffwechselsubstrate oder deren Analoga,
- Enzym-Inhibitoren,
- Rezeptor-bindende Liganden,
- Antikörper-Antigen-Systeme.

So werden z.B. markierte Stoffwechselsubstrate wie Glukose, Fettsäuren oder Aminosäuren sowie deren Analoga zum Studium von Herz- bzw. Hirnfunktionen sowie in der Tumordiagnostik eingesetzt, Rezeptor-bindende Radiopharmaka insbesondere zentralwirksame Verbindungen, Neurotransmitter und ihre Antagonisten zur Erfassung von Rezeptordichten, um nur einige der bedeutendsten zu nennen.

Stoffwechselprodukte und andere körpereigene Verbindungen bestehen im allgemeinen aus C-, H-, N-, O-, P- und S-Atomen verschiedener Kombination. Die Anzahl der Radionuklide dieser Elemente mit geeigneten nuklearen Eigenschaften ist begrenzt. Nur die organischen Positronenstrahler wie $^{11}C(T_{1/2} = 20$ min), $^{13}N(T_{1/2} = 10$ min), $^{15}O(T_{1/2} = 2,1$ min) und $^{30}P(T_{1/2} = 2,3$ min) können hier die wünschenswerte Voraussetzung erfüllen, daß nach deren Einbau anstelle ihres stabilen Isotops in eine körpereigene Verbindung die Biochemie bzw. die Zellphysiologie völlig unverändert bleibt. Man hat deshalb nach Analoga gesucht, d.h. Verbindungen, in denen H-, C- oder andere Atome bzw. Gruppen durch Fremdatome ersetzt sind. Bei einer solchen Fremdmarkierung kann vor allem das Struktur-Analogie-Prinzip hilfreich sein. Während die Einführung eines Halogenatoms in ein Molekül bei guter Syntheseplanung sterisch keine wesentliche Veränderung hervorrufen muß (räumlich entspricht ein Br- oder I-Atom einer CH_3-Gruppe und ein F-Atom einem H-Atom), so können die Veränderungen der Ladungsverteilung des markierten Moleküls gravierend sein: die $C - X$ Bindungen sind polarisiert, die Verbindungen werden durch die Halogensubstitution u.a. lipophiler, so daß trotz der erhaltenen sterischen Eigenschaften des Moleküls sein physiologisches Verhalten oft stark verändert ist. Im allgemeinen eignen sich Halogene jedoch gut, um Analoga herzustellen, zumal ihre kovalenten Bindungen zum Kohlenstoff relativ stabil sind. Deshalb spielen einige Radiohalogene wie die Positronenstrahler $^{18}F(T_{1/2} = $ 110 min), $^{75}Br(T_{1/2} = 96$ min) und der Photonenstrahler $^{123}I(T_{1/2} = 13$ h) eine bedeutende Rolle. Aber auch andere Radionuklide können prinzipiell zur Synthese isosterer Verbindungen eingesetzt werden, so etwa Se und Te als Ersatz für $-HC=CH-$ und Sn in Form von $-Sn(CH_3)_3$ als Ersatz eines quarternären C-Atoms. Bei metallischen Radionukliden wie z.B. ^{67}Ga oder ^{99m}Tc gelten andere Regeln. Bei diesen anorganischen Fremdmarkierungen müssen geeignete Komplexliganden gefunden und Chelate eingesetzt werden. Ein biochemisches Konzept, z.B. im Falle des bedeutenden Generator-Nuklids ^{99m}Tc, konnte bisher nicht verwirklicht werden.

Zur regionalen Erfassung von Funktionen sind – wie bereits erwähnt – Radionuklide geeignet, die entweder vorwiegend Positronen emittieren oder aber eine stark dominante γ-Linie mit einer Energie im Bereich von 100 bis 300 keV besitzen. Im ersteren Falle kann die PET oder PECT (positron emission computed tomography) im zweiten die SPECT-Technik (single photon emission computed tomography) eingesetzt werden. Markierungsnuklide für die regionale Funktionstomographie mit PET sind ^{11}C, ^{13}N, ^{15}O und ^{18}F; für SPECT ist dies insbesondere ^{123}I und prinzipiell ^{99m}Tc. Tabelle 1 zeigt eine Zusammenstellung derjenigen kurzlebigen „organischen" Radionuklide, die sich für ein biochemisches Konzept eignen (vgl. Qaim 1982; Qaim u. Stöcklin 1983).

Die für die Synthese und Qualitätskontrolle mit solchen kurzlebigen Radionukliden zur Verfügung stehende Zeitskala ist in Schema I für die wichtigsten kurzlebigen Markierungsnuklide vereinfacht dargestellt. Man sieht, daß im Falle von ^{15}O nur wenige Minuten, beim ^{11}C schon 1 bis 2 Stunden und beim ^{18}F bereits mehrere Stunden zur Verfügung stehen. Dies gilt allerdings nur bei sehr hohen Anfangsaktivitäten von der Größenordnung einiger GBq. Beim ^{15}O sind praktisch nur einfache Moleküle wie CO, CO_2 und H_2O zugänglich. Beim ^{30}P gibt es bisher noch keine Anwendungen. Auch der Einsatz des 3,6 min Positronenstrahlers und Generatornuklids ^{122}I dürfte begrenzt bleiben. Der Positronenstrahler ^{75}Br ist kein ideales Nuklid für PET. Die 286 keV γ-Linie des 1,3 nsec angeregten Zustandes des ^{75}Se führt zu zufälligen Koinzidenzen und damit zu einem schlechten Bildkontrast,

Tabelle 1. Kurzlebige Radionuklide zur Molekülmarkierung für die regionale Funktionsdiagnostik mit PET und SPECT

Radionuklid	$T_{1/2}$	Zerfallsart (%)	E_β max keV (rel. %)	Haupt-γ-Linien keV (% Häufigkeit)
^{11}C	20,3 min	β^+ (99,8) EC (0,2)	960 (100)	511 (199,6)
^{13}N	9,96 min	β^+ (100)	1190 (100)	511 (200)
^{15}O	2,03 min	β^+ (99,9) EC (0,1)	1723 (100)	511 (200)
^{18}F	109,7 min	β^+ (96,9) EC (3,1)	635 (100)	511 (193,8)
^{30}P	2,5 min	β^+ (100)	3245 (100)	511 (200)
^{75}Br	1,6 h	β^+ (75,5) EC (24,5)	1740 (82)	286 (91,6) 511 (151)
^{77}Br	57 h	β^+ (0,7) EC (99,3)	340 (100)	239 (22,8) 297 (4,1) 521 (22,1)
^{73}Se	7,1 h	β^+ (65) EC (35)	1320 (91,3)	511 (130)
^{122}I via ^{122}Xe→^{122}I-Generator	3,6 min	β^+ (77) EC (23)	3120	564 (18)
^{123}I	13,02 h	EC (100)		159 (83) 529 (1,05)

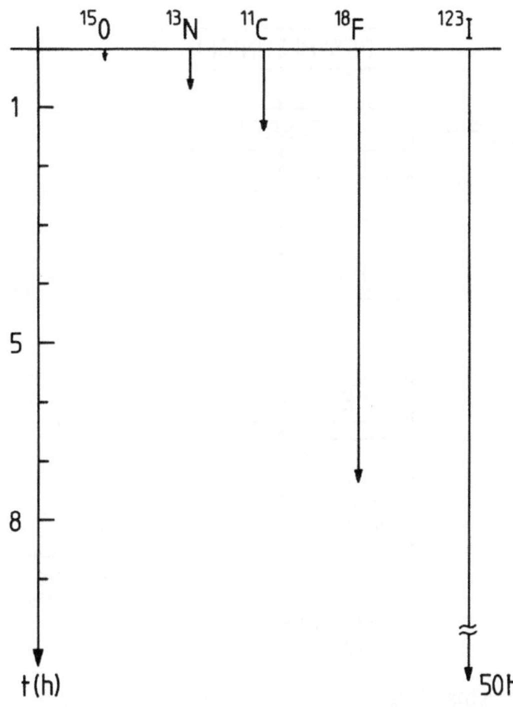

Schema I. Zeitskala für Synthese und Qualitätskontrolle mit einigen kurzlebigen organischen Radionukliden

sofern das PET-Gerät nicht mit einer Flugzeit-Meßeinrichtung ausgestattet ist. Darüber hinaus ergibt die unvermeidbare Verunreinigung (2–6% am Bestrahlungsende) mit dem längerlebigen Positronenstrahler ^{76}Br ($T_{1/2} = 16$ h) eine erhöhte Strahlendosis für den Patienten. Auch das Tochternuklid ^{75}Se ($T_{1/2} = 120$ d) trägt zur Erhöhung der Strahlendosis bei. Obwohl die Chemie des trägerfreien Broms wesentlich einfacher ist als die des Fluors, ist die Einsatzmöglichkeit dieses Radionuklids begrenzt. Dies liegt auch schon daran, daß für seine Erzeugung relativ hohe Teilchenenergien (Mittelenergie-Zyklotron) erforderlich sind. Auch ^{77}Br eignet sich weniger gut für abbildende Verfahren und vor allem für tomographische Verfahren wie SPECT, da seine relativ hohe γ-Energie einen Hochenergiekolimator erforderlich macht. Es besitzt jedoch als „Auger-Strahler" potentielle Bedeutung als therapeutisches Radionuklid. Es handelt sich hier allerdings nicht um ein kurzlebiges Radionuklid im Sinne der Thematik.

In diesem Kapitel sollen spezielle Syntheseverfahren mit kurzlebigen Radionukliden beschrieben werden. Als obere Grenze der Halbwertszeit wird willkürlich diejenige von ^{123}I gewählt. Anorganische Nuklide wie etwa ^{99m}Tc, Perfusions-Tracer wie Alkali und Alkali-ähnliche Ionen sowie Edelgase sollen nicht einbezogen werden.

B. Synthese von Vorläufern und einfachen Ausgangsprodukten

Im Falle der sehr kurzlebigen Positronenstrahler ist – mit Ausnahme von ^{18}F und ^{75}Br – ein „in-house" Zyklotron erforderlich. Bei der notwendigerweise schnellen Markierung ist man stets bestrebt, ein geeignetes Ausgangsprodukt für die Synthese bereits während der Bestrahlung entweder als Rückstoßprodukt im Target selbst oder aber mittels on-line Synthese zu erzeugen. Ein generelles Fließschema für den gesamten Ablauf von der Radionukliderzeugung bis zum medizinischen Einsatz zeigt Schema II. Markierte Vorläufer können

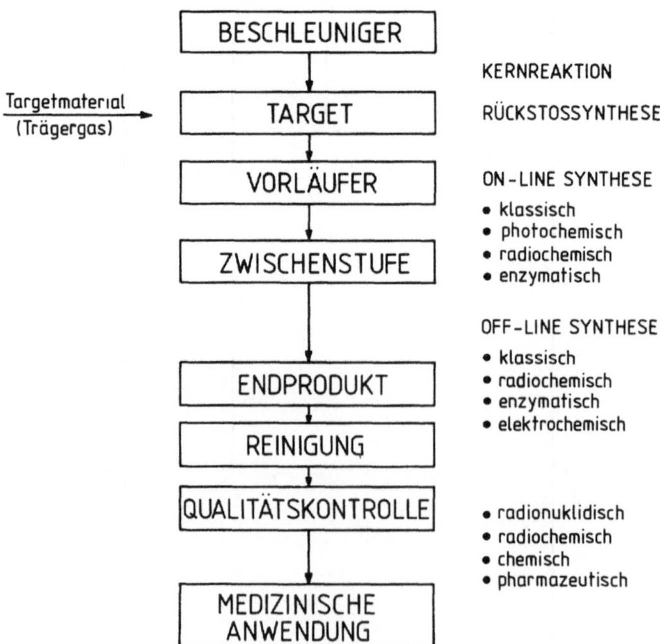

Schema II. Fließschema für den Ablauf der Herstellung eines kurzlebigen Tracers für den medizinischen Einsatz

bereits in-situ durch Bestrahlung einer geeigneten Verbindung oder eines Substanzgemisches im Target gebildet werden. Grundlage der Erzeugung von Verläufern im Target selbst sind die chemischen Folgereaktionen von Kernumwandlungen. Diese Chemie heißer Atome, d.h. die Reaktion von Atomen hoher kinetischer Energie, führt in Nanosekunden nach dem Kernprozeß zu chemischen Reaktionen (zur Übersicht s. STÖCKLIN 1969, 1972 sowie TOMINAGA u. TACHIKAWA 1981; FERRIERI u. WOLF 1983). Die hierbei entstehenden Vorläufer können in einigen Fällen on-line zu Ausgangsverbindungen für weitere Synthesen umgewandelt werden. Hierbei müssen wiederum möglichst schnelle Verfahren eingesetzt werden. Das markierte Ausgangsprodukt wird entweder direkt oder nach Abtrennung und Reinigung für weitere Synthesen verwendet. Diese off-line Synthesen finden zweckmäßigerweise in unmittelbar an den Targetraum angrenzenden Bleizellen möglichst voll- oder teilweise automatisiert statt. Eine Fernbedienung oder Automatisierung ist im Falle der kurzlebigen Positronenstrahler bei ständig sich wiederholender Routineproduktion unerläßlich, da wegen der Kurzlebigkeit die Anfangsaktivität sehr hoch sein muß, und die 511 keV Vernichtungsstrahlung eine ausreichende Abschirmung erfordert. Dies, die notwendigerweise schnellen chemischen Arbeitsschritte und die erforderliche Zuverlässigkeit beim Routineeinsatz machen eine Fernbedienung oder besser eine Automatisierung notwendig. Bei Positronenstrahlern muß deshalb meist ein relativ hoher Aufwand an Verfahrenstechnik und elektronischer Steuerung betrieben werden. Allerdings werden für häufig gebrauchte PET-Radiopharmaka und Vorläufer von den Zyklotron-liefernden Firmen vollautomatische Syntheseapparaturen angeboten.

Sie sind jedoch relativ teuer und meist nicht anpaßbar, wenn bessere Synthesen bekannt werden. Man sollte deshalb die Auswahl auf wenige dringend erforderliche Produkte beschränken.

I. Kohlenstoff-11

Durch geeignete Wahl von Kernreaktion und Targetmaterial kann man im Falle des kurzlebigen Kohlenstoff-11 flüchtige Vorstufen wie ^{11}CO, $^{11}CO_2$, $H^{11}CN$ etc. in-situ, d.h. im Target selbst während der Bestrahlung erzeugen (zur Übersicht s. WOLF et al. 1973; WOLF u. REDVANLY 1977; FERRIERI u. WOLF 1983). Der meist verwendete Prozeß zur Erzeugung von Kohlenstoff-11 ist die $^{14}N(p,\alpha)^{11}C$-Reaktion. Die Rückstoßkohlenstoffatome, die mit Rückstoßenergien von einigen MeV entstehen, können nach Verlust ihrer hohen Anfangsenergien schließlich im eV-Bereich als sog. heiße Atome chemische Reaktionen eingehen. So laufen in einem Stickstoff-Gastarget in Gegenwart von Spuren Sauerstoff (1–10 ppm), die stets im Stickstoff vorhanden sind, u.a. folgende sehr schnelle Reaktionen ab ($[\ ]^{\neq}$ hohe kinetische Energie, $[\ ]^*$ angeregter Zustand):

$$[^{11}C]^{\neq} + O_2 \longrightarrow {}^{11}CO + O \tag{1}$$

$$^{11}CO \xrightarrow{O_2} {}^{11}CO_2 \tag{2}$$

$$[^{11}C]^{\neq} + N_2 \longrightarrow [^{11}C\!-\!N\!-\!N]^* \longrightarrow {}^{11}CN + N \tag{3}$$

$$^{11}CN + O_2 \longrightarrow [^{11}CON] + O \tag{4}$$

$$[^{11}CON] + O_2 \longrightarrow {}^{11}CO_2 + NO \tag{5}$$

Primär erhält man ein Gemisch aus ^{11}CO und $^{11}CO_2$. Hierbei spielen die Strahlströme und damit die absorbierte Strahlendosis eine wesentliche Rolle, da auf strahlenchemischem Wege eine Umwandlung von ^{11}CO in $^{11}CO_2$ stattfindet (ACHE u. WOLF 1968; ANDERSON et al. 1966). Da man meist mit Hochstromtargets arbeitet, um möglichst hohe Aktivitäten zu erreichen, liegen zumindest beim statischen Betrieb mehr als 90% des ^{11}C in Form von

$^{11}CO_2$ vor. Der Zusatz größerer Mengen O_2 ändert das CO/CO_2-Verhältnis nur wenig, führt jedoch zur Bildung von NO_x und zu störender ^{13}N-Aktivität, die über die $^{16}O(p,\alpha)^{13}N$-Reaktion entsteht. Daneben wird ^{13}N auch über die $^{14}N(p,pn)^{13}N$-Reaktion gebildet, wenn die Protonenenergie oberhalb etwa 12 MeV liegt. Bei einem offenen Kreislauf mit Durchfluß-Target ist die Strahlendosis und damit die relative $^{11}CO_2$-Ausbeute klein. Man arbeitet deshalb auch aus Gründen der spezifischen Aktivität (s.u.) meist mit einem statischen Target. Zur Ausbeuteerhöhung des $^{11}CO_2$ kann im Anschluß an das Gastarget on-line eine Konvertierung des ^{11}CO zu $^{11}CO_2$ in einem Oxidationsofen vorgenommen werden.

$$^{11}CO \xrightarrow[\text{800 °C}]{\text{CuO}} \ ^{11}CO_2 \tag{6}$$

Wird ^{11}CO gewünscht, so reduziert man mit Zink, indem man das Gasgemisch im Anschluß an das Target durch einen Reduktionsofen leitet, in dem sich z.B. Zn-Pulver gemischt mit einem inerten nicht-schmelzenden Trägermaterial befindet:

$$^{11}CO_2 \xrightarrow[\text{300 °C}]{\text{Zn auf Träger}} \ ^{11}CO \tag{7}$$

Um eine zu starke Verdünnung mit dem allgegenwärtigen Kohlenstoff-12 (bzw. CO_2 oder CO) zu verhindern, vermeidet man jedoch solche Durchflußsysteme möglichst. Um die Verdünnung mit dem stabilen Kohlenstoff klein zu halten, verwendet man als Targetmaterial i. allg. Aluminium und für das Fenster Titanfolie. Das Stickstoffgas sollte von höchster Reinheit bezüglich der Verunreinigung an Kohlenstoffverbindungen sein. Als Vorsichtsmaßnahme gegen CO_2 Einschleppung kann das Gas noch über ein Absorbens (Lithiumhydroxid, Molekularsieb (4Å oder 5Å) oder Poropak (P oder Q) geleitet werden. Das Leitungssystem sollte möglichst aus Stahl oder Kupfer sein und nur kleine Volumina umfassen. Auf diese Weise können spezifische Aktivitäten von > 1 TBq/µMol erhalten werden. Die Produktionsausbeuten liegen bei 4–5 GBq/µAh für 16 MeV Protonen. Für weitere experimentelle Details, s. Clark u. Buckingham (1975) sowie neue Standardisierungsvorschläge eines Workshops der EUROPÄISCHEN GEMEINSCHAFT (1987). Synthetisch ist $^{11}CO_2$ die wichtigste Ausgangsverbindung für weitere sekundäre Vorläufer:

$$
\begin{array}{lll}
 & ^{11}CH_4 \longrightarrow & H^{11}C\equiv CH \\
 & & H^{11}C\equiv N \\
^{11}CO_2 \longrightarrow & ^{11}CO \longrightarrow & ^{11}COCl_2 \\
 & ^{11}CH_3OH \longrightarrow & ^{11}CH_2O \\
 & & ^{11}CH_3I
\end{array}
\tag{8}
$$

Der markierte Vorläufer $H^{11}CN$ entsteht in einem N_2-H_2 Target direkt durch eine Kombination von Rückstoß- und Strahlenchemie. In einer Mischung aus N_2-H_2 reagieren die nach Gleichung (2) entstandenen ^{11}CN-Radikale durch H-Abstraktion:

$$^{11}CN + H_2 \longrightarrow H^{11}CN + H \tag{9}$$

Die direkte Bestrahlung von N_2-H_2 Gemischen (Ache u. Wolf 1968) führt jedoch zu relativ kleinen Ausbeuten, da $H^{11}CN$ radiolytisch während der Bestrahlung zu $^{11}CH_4$ konvertiert wird:

$$H^{11}CN + 3 H_2 \rightsquigarrow \ ^{11}CH_4 + NH_3 \tag{10}$$

Im Zusammenhang mit der ebenfalls über die Radiolyse des $N_2 - H_2$ Gemisches entstehenden Ammoniaks läßt sich dieser Umstand dennoch zur on-line Synthese von $H^{11}CN$ durch chemische Konversion des $^{11}CH_4$ außerhalb des Targets ausnutzen (CHRISTMAN et al. 1975):

$$^{11}CH_4 + NH_3 \xrightarrow[1000\,°C]{Pt\text{-}Wolle} H^{11}CN + 3\,H_2 \qquad (11)$$

Das mit $>95\%$iger radiochemischer Ausbeute entstehende $^{11}CH_4$ wird hierbei on-line nahezu quantitativ in $H^{11}CN$ umgewandelt. Eine andere Möglichkeit bietet die off-line Umwandlung von $^{11}CO_2$ auf klassischem Wege in $K^{11}CN$ (FINN et al. 1971):

$$^{11}CO_2 + K + NH_3 \longrightarrow K^{11}CN + H_2O \qquad (12)$$

Auch ^{11}C-markiertes Methyliodid, die wichtigste Ausgangsverbindung zur Methylierung von OH-, NH- und SH-Gruppen, kann in-situ über Rückstoßreaktionen hergestellt werden (WAGNER et al. 1981), indem man ein $HI - N_2$-Gasgemisch (1:4) bestrahlt. Hierbei gehen die Rückstoßkohlenstoffatome bereits im Target Einschiebungs- und H-Abstraktionsreaktion mit dem HI ein, wobei im wesentlichen $^{11}CH_3I$ und $^{11}CH_4$ entstehen. Dieses Verfahren ist allerdings durch die begleitende Strahlenchemie, d.h. die Zerstörung des $^{11}CH_3I$ durch Protonenradiolyse nicht für die Produktion hoher Aktivitätsmengen geeignet. Besser geeignet ist deshalb die Herstellung von $^{11}CH_3I$ auf klassischem Wege (s.u. Gl. 13). Die begleitende Radiolyse ist meist eine nicht zu überwindende Schwierigkeit, wenn man versucht, komplexere Ausgangsverbindungen in hinreichender Aktivität über direkte Rückstoßreaktionen im Target zu erzeugen. In den meisten Fällen werden deshalb diese Produkte off-line im batch-Verfahren erzeugt. Die wichtigen ^{11}C-markierten Methylierungsreagenzien Formaldehyd und Methyliodid können in einer schnellen zweistufigen Synthese erhalten werden (s. z.B. MARAZANO et al. 1977 und dort zitierte Literatur):

$$^{11}CO_2 \xrightarrow{LiAlH_4} {}^{11}CH_3OH \begin{cases} \xrightarrow{Ag_2O} H^{11}CHO \\ \xrightarrow{HI} {}^{11}CH_3I \end{cases} \qquad (13)$$

Zur Erreichung hoher spezifischer Aktivitäten sind wiederum Maßnahmen erforderlich, die ein Einschleppen von Kohlenstoff-12 minimieren können. Hierzu wird das kryogen oder mittels Molekularsieb abgetrennte $^{11}CO_2$ mit N_2 oder He langsam (10–20 ml/min) über ein Trockenmittel ($MgClO_4 \cdot H_2O$ oder P_2O_5) in ein kleines konisches Gefäß geleitet (s. Abb. 1), das Lithiumaluminiumhydrid ($LiAlH_4$) in Tetrahydrofuran oder Diethylether enthält. Detaillierte Informationen können wiederum einer EG Standardisierungsanleitung (EUROPÄISCHE GEMEINSCHAFT 1987) entnommen werden. Im Hinblick auf die Bedeutung von $[^{11}C]$-Methyliodid als Markierungsreagenz soll die Synthese hier ausführlich behandelt werden.

In Abb. 1 ist das Schema einer Apparatur wiedergegeben, die als Basis für eine Fernbedienung oder automatisierte Synthese verwendet wird (SCHÜLLER u. BLESSING 1987). Etwa 37 GBq $^{11}CO_2$ werden in der Sammelschleife bei $-196°\,C$ ausgefroren und vom N_2-Gas abgetrennt. Im Reaktor I werden ca. 1 mg $LiAlH_4$ in 100 µl Tetrahydrofuran vorgelegt. Das $^{11}CO_2$ wird mit dem Fön aufgetaut und im He-Strom bei $-35°\,C$ durch die Reaktionslösung geleitet. Das Lösungsmittel wird bei $130°\,C$ abdestilliert. Mit 0.5 ml 30%iger HI erfolgt der Umsatz zu $^{11}CH_3I$. Zur Abtrennung von H_2O und HI wird das $^{11}CH_3I$ über einen Rückflußkühler mit nachgeschalteten Trockenrohren T3–T4 ($NaOH/P_2O_5$) geleitet und für nachfolgende Synthesen im Reaktor II gesammelt. Die Synthesezeit beträgt ca.

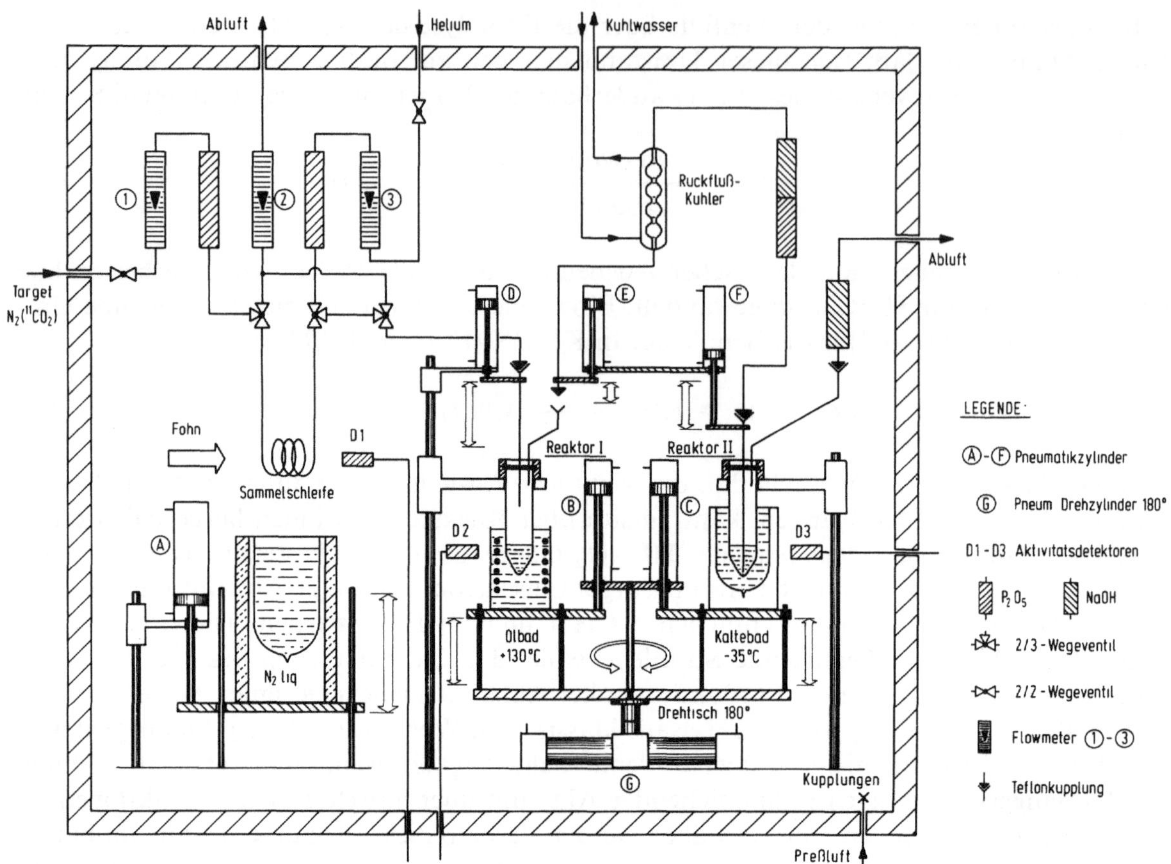

Abb. 1. Ferngesteuerte Syntheseapparatur zur Produktion von $^{11}CH_3I$. (Nach Schüller u. Blessing 1987)

10 min bei einer radiochemischen Ausbeute von ca. 90%. Spezifische Aktivitäten von $>3{,}7\cdot10^5$ GBq/mMol sind erreichbar (Schüller u. Blessing 1986). Alle Bewegungsabläufe der Apparatur sind fernbedient und automatisierbar. Sie werden durch pneumatische Stellglieder ausgeführt (A–F). Der Reaktionsverlauf wird mittels Aktivitätsdetektoren D1–D3 kontrolliert.

Neben [^{11}C]-Methyliodid sind in ähnlicher Weise auch [1-^{11}C]-Ethyl-, Propyl-, Butyl-, Isobutyliodid (Langström et al. 1986) als [^{11}C]-Alkylierungsmittel synthetisiert worden.

^{11}C-markiertes Acetylen entsteht als Rückstoßprodukt bei Verwendung der $^{12}C(p,pn)^{11}C$-Reaktion bei der Bestrahlung von Kohlenwasserstoffen (zur Übersicht s. Stöcklin 1969), jedoch sind die erzeugbaren Aktivitäten infolge der begleitenden Protonenradiolyse wiederum begrenzt. Höhere Aktivitäten erhält man jedoch über klassische off-line Synthesen durch Hydrolyse von [^{11}C]$-BaC_2$ aus [^{11}C]$-BaCO_3$ (Cramer u. Kistiakowsky 1941) oder über die Hydrolyse von [^{11}C]$-CaC_2$, das auch durch Rückstoßsynthese erzeugt werden kann (Myers 1972). Eine interessante Variante ist die Pyrolyse von $^{11}CH_4$, das zunächst über Rückstoßsynthese (vgl. Gl. 9 u. 10) hergestellt wird (Crouzel et al. 1979):

$$N_2 + H_2 \xrightarrow{\ ^{14}N(p,\,\alpha)^{11}C\ } {}^{11}CH_4 \tag{14}$$

$$^{11}CH_4 \xrightarrow{\ \Delta\ } {}^{11}CH\equiv CH \tag{15}$$

Ein weiteres wichtiges Ausgangsprodukt für Synthesen von ^{11}C-markierten Dialkylkarbonaten, -karbamaten, Harnstoff und dessen Derivaten ist Phosgen, das ausgehend von ^{11}CO

hergestellt werden kann. Die Anlagerung von Cl_2 über Cl-Atome kann entweder katalytisch durch $PtCl_4$ (ROEDA et al. 1978) oder aber mit Hilfe von UV-Licht erfolgen (ROEDA u. WESTERA 1981):

$$^{11}CO \xrightarrow[380\,°C]{PtCl_4} {}^{11}COCl_2 \tag{16}$$

$$^{11}CO \xrightarrow[h\nu]{Cl_2} {}^{11}COCl_2 \tag{17}$$

Eine on-line Synthese von [^{11}C]-Phosgen ohne Trägerzusatz ist ebenfalls beschrieben worden (DIKSIC et al. 1982).

Auch komplexere Vorläufer sind durch Rückstoß- und Strahlenchemie in-situ erzeugt worden. So erhält man über die $^{14}N(p,\alpha)^{11}C$-Reaktion in flüssigem NH_3 gute radiochemische Ausbeuten an [^{11}C]-Guanidin insbesondere beim Zusatz von N_2O als Radikalfänger (IWATA et al. 1981). Das [^{11}C]-Guanidin läßt sich durch Zyklokondensation mit Trimethiniumsalzen leicht in [^{11}C]-Pyrimidinderivate, insbesondere 2-Amino-2-[^{11}C]-pyrimidin umsetzen. In festem NH_3 (77K), $LiNH_2$ und Ammoniumhalogeniden entstehen neben [^{11}C]-Methylamin und [^{11}C]-Guanidin auch ein relativ hoher Anteil an [^{11}C]-Formamidin und [^{11}C]-Cyanamid (RÖSSLER et al. 1981; RÖSSLER et al. 1982), die zu Imidiazolen, Barbituraten und Purinderivaten umgesetzt werden können. [^{11}C]-Methanol entsteht durch Reaktionen von ^{11}C-Rückstoßatomen in festen H_2O-NH_3 Gemischen (RÖSSLER et al. 1986). Problematisch bleibt stets die erreichbare Gesamtaktivität sowie zusätzliche Abtrennverfahren. Eine Zusammenfassung der wichtigsten ^{11}C-Synthesevorläufer gibt Tabelle 2.

Tabelle 2. Wichtigste ^{11}C-markierte Synthesevorläufer

Targetfüllung	Kernreaktion	Vorläufer im Target	Konversion außerhalb des Targets	Literatur
B_2O_3	$^{10}B(d,n)^{11}C$ $^{11}B(p,n)^{11}C$	$^{11}CO_2(^{11}CO)^a$		
N_2 (1–10ppm O_2)	$^{14}N(p,\alpha)^{11}C$	$^{11}CO_2(^{11}CO)^a$	$^{11}CO_2 \rightarrow {}^{11}CH_3I \rightarrow {}^{11}CH_3Li$	MAZIERE et al. (1977)
			$^{11}CO_2 \rightarrow {}^{11}CH_2O$	BERGER et al. (1980a)
			$^{11}CO_2 \rightarrow {}^{11}CO \rightarrow {}^{11}COCl_2$	ROEDA et al. (1978) ROEDA u. WESTERA (1981) DIKSIC et al. (1982)
			$^{11}CO_2 \rightarrow K^{11}CN$	FINN et al. (1971)
N_2(5% H_2)	$^{14}N(p,\alpha)^{11}C$	$^{11}CH_4(H^{11}CN)^a$	$^{11}CH_4 \rightarrow H^{11}CN$	CHRISTMAN et al. (1975)
			$^{11}CH_4 \rightarrow H^{11}C \equiv CH$	MYERS (1972) CROUZEL et al. (1979)

^{a} Kleine Ausbeuten bei hohen Dosen.

II. Stickstoff-13

Synthesen komplizierter Verbindungen sind mit dem 10 Minuten-Stickstoff-13 äußerst schwierig und bisher im wesentlichen auf enzymatische Synthesen von Aminosäuren beschränkt geblieben. Dagegen können einfache ^{13}N-haltige Gase wie z.B. ^{13}NN und $^{13}NH_3$ relativ einfach und schnell produziert werden (CLARK u. BUCKINGHAM 1975; STRAATMAN

1977). ^{13}N-markierter molekularer Stickstoff für die regionale Lungenfunktionsprüfung mit Hilfe der PET-Technik läßt sich am einfachsten über die ^{12}C(d,n)^{13}N-Reaktion in CO_2-Gas erzeugen (Crouzel u. Comar 1975; Jones et al. 1977). Die Rückstoßreaktionen von ^{13}N in Gasen wie CO_2, N_2, O_2 etc. sind ausführlich untersucht worden (Stewart et al. 1974). Im CO_2 entstehen in Gegenwart von N_2- und O_2-Verunreinigungen die Produkte sowohl über radiolytische als auch über hochenergetische Rückstoßreaktionen, wobei die primäre Reaktion mit N_2 zu angeregtem [^{13}NN]* führt, das entweder zu ^{13}NNO oxidiert oder zu molekularem ^{13}NN stabilisiert wird:

$$[^{13}N]^{\ddagger} + N_2 \longrightarrow [^{13}NN]^* \quad \begin{array}{c} \xrightarrow{\text{O}_2 \text{ oder CO}_2} \quad ^{13}NNO + O(CO) \\ \\ \xrightarrow{+\,M} \quad ^{13}NN + M^* \end{array} \tag{18}$$

Bei hohen Strahlströmen wird im CO_2-Gastarget mit fast 100%iger radiochemischer Ausbeute molekularer Stickstoff, [^{13}N]$-N_2$, erhalten. Das [^{13}N]$-$NO wird dabei offensichtlich radiolytisch zu [^{13}N]$-N_2$ zurückverwandelt. Auch feste Targets aus Graphit oder Aktivkohle werden verwendet (zur Übersicht s. Clark u. Buckingham 1975). Durch die starke Aufheizung des Festkörpertargets (bei 60 µA und 14 MeV ca. 840 W) werden Temperaturen von $> 1400°$ C erreicht, wobei die Graphit-Matrix durch die Reaktion $C + CO_2 \rightarrow 2CO$ aufgebrochen, und der entstandene Stickstoff-13 abgegeben wird. Wesentlich höhere spezifische Aktivitäten (ca. 740 MBq ml^{-1}) [^{13}N]$-N_2$ können bei Verwendung von mit ^{13}C angereichertem Kohlepulver als Target und Nutzung der ^{13}C(p,n)^{13}N-Reaktion (Krohn u. Mathis 1981; Ferrieri et al. 1983) erhalten werden. Diese Reaktion ist besonders für kleine medizinische Zyklotrone mit niedrigen Protonenenergien (10–11 MeV) geeignet.

Unterschiedliche Wege werden zur Abtrennung des CO_2 beschritten. Nach Oxidation der CO-Verunreinigung zu CO_2 mit CuO wird das CO_2 entweder durch Absorption in NaOH oder durch Ausfrieren mit flüssigem Stickstoff abgetrennt und das [^{13}N]$-N_2$ direkt in physiologischer Kochsalzlösung gelöst. Gesamtaktivitäten von etwa 1 TBq und spezifische Aktivitäten bis zu 37 MBq ml^{-1} Kochsalzlösung können erreicht werden. Eine Zusammenstellung der Methoden zur Produktion von [^{13}N]$-N_2$ zeigt Tabelle 3.

Größere Bedeutung kommt dem ^{13}N-markierten Ammoniak zu. ^{13}NH$_3$ wird vor allem zur Messung des regionalen Blutflusses im Herzen eingesetzt. Außerdem dient es als Ausgangsmaterial für weitere Synthesen. Als Targetmaterial kann bei der ^{12}C(d,n)^{13}N-Reaktion gasförmiges Methan verwendet werden. Hierbei entsteht ^{13}NH$_3$ als Rückstoßprodukt mit hoher radiochemischer Ausbeute (95%) zusammen mit $H_3C^{13}NH_2$, $HC^{13}N$ (Tilbury et al. 1971; Straatman u. Welch 1973b). Bei höheren Dosen werden die primären Produkte offensichtlich radiolytisch zu ^{13}NH$_3$ reduziert. Am besten geeignet ist die ^{13}NH$_3$-Produktion über die ^{16}O(p,α)^{13}N-Reaktion unter Verwendung eines H_2O-Targets. Hierbei entstehen als Endprodukte der Bestrahlung vorwiegend $^{13}NO_2^-$ und $^{13}NO_3^-$. Bei kleinen Dosen reagieren die Rückstoßstickstoffatome unter sukzessiver H-Abstraktion und Hydratisierung mit dem Wasser unter Bildung von NH_3 bzw. NH_4^+:

$$^{13}N \xrightarrow{\text{H}_2\text{O}} \longrightarrow \, ^{13}NH_3 \tag{19}$$

$$^{13}NH_3 + HOH \rightleftharpoons \, ^{13}NH_4^+ + OH^- \tag{20}$$

Bei höheren Dosen und/oder in Gegenwart von Sauerstoff erfolgt eine radiolytische Oxidation zu $^{13}NO_3^-$ und $^{13}NO_2^-$ (zur Übersicht s. Krohn u. Mathis 1981; Tilbury 1981):

$$NH_3 \xrightarrow{\text{H}_2\text{O}} H^{13}NO_2, \, H^{13}NO_3, \text{ etc.} \tag{21}$$

Tabelle 3. Methoden zur Produktion von ^{13}NN

Target-füllung	Kernreaktion	Vorläufer im Target	Nachbehandlung bzw. Konversion	Literatur
Graphit, A-Kohle (1450° C)[b]	$^{12}C(d,n)^{13}N$	$C^{13}N$ $[^{13}N]-N_2$	CO_2-Strom über CuO-Ofen bei 700° C (on-line)	BUCKINGHAM u. CLARK (1972) CLARK u. BUCKINGHAM (1975)
	$^{13}C(p,n)^{13}N$[a]	$[^{13}N]-N_2$	He od. CO_2 Spülung on-line	KROHN u. MATHIS (1981) FERRIERI u. WOLF (1983)
O_2 (450° C 10–15 atm)	$^{16}O(p,\alpha)^{13}N$	$[^{13}N]-N_2$, $^{13}NO_X$	Kryogene Abtrennung von $^{13}NO_X$ (on-line)	PARKS et al. (1975)
CO_2-Gas (N_2-Spuren)	$^{12}C(d,n)^{13}N$	$[^{13}N]-N_2$	CuO-Ofen, Abtrennung des CO_2 durch NaOH (on-line flow system) oder kryogene Abtrennung	JONES et al. (1977) CROUZEL u. COMAR (1975)
H_2O (0,1 M NH_3)	$^{16}O(p,\alpha)^{13}N$	$[^{13}N]-N_2$		SUZUKI u. IWATA (1977) PARKS u. KROHN (1978)

[a] ^{13}C angereichertes Kohlepulver als Targetfüllung.
[b] Aufbrechen der Graphit-Matrix zu CO durch Aufheizen durch den Strahlstrom führt zur Freisetzung von $[^{13}N]-N_2$.

Diese Produkte müssen also off-line auf klassischem Wege wieder zu $^{13}NH_3$ reduziert werden. Die Bestrahlung einer wäßrigen Ammoniaklösung führt übrigens fast ausschließlich zu molekularem Stickstoff $[^{13}N]-N_2$ (SUZUKI u. IWATA 1977). Die chemische Konversion der im H_2O Target gebildeten radiolytischen Oxidationsprodukte geschieht nach der Bestrahlung z.B. mit DeVarda Legierung:

$$^{13}NO_2^-, \quad ^{13}NO_3^- \xrightarrow[\text{deVarda}]{\text{Red.}} {}^{13}NH_3 \tag{22}$$

Eine Zusammenstellung der wichtigsten Produktionsmethoden für $^{13}NH_3$ zeigt Tabelle 4. Die Routineproduktion von $^{13}NH_3$ wird heute meist mit einem H_2O-Target und anschließen-

Tabelle 4. Methoden zur Produktion von $^{13}NH_3$

Target-füllung	Kernreaktion	Vorläufer im Target	Nachbehandlung bzw. Konversion	Literatur
CH_4 (Durchfluß)	$^{12}C(d,n)^{13}N$	$^{13}NH_3$, $CH_3{}^{13}NH_2$ $HC^{13}N$ etc.	on-line Abtrennung von $^{13}NH_3$	TILBURY et al. (1971) STRAATMAN u. WELCH (1973a) HARPER et al. (1973)
H_2O	$^{16}O(p,\alpha)^{13}N$	$^{13}NO_2^-$, $^{13}NO_3^-$	Red. mit $TiCl_3$ zu $^{13}NH_3$	LATHROP et al. (1973)
H_2O	$^{16}O(p,\alpha)^{13}N$	$^{13}NO_2^-$, $^{13}NO_3^-$	Red. nach KJELDAHL zu $^{13}NH_3$	KRIZEK et al. (1973)
H_2O	$^{16}O(p,\alpha)^{13}N$	$^{13}NO_2^-$, $^{13}NO_3^-$	Red. mit DeVARDA Leg. zu $^{13}NH_3$	VAALBURG et al. (1975) PARKS u. KROHN (1978)

der Reduktion mittels $TiCl_3$ (Lathrop et al. 1973) oder DeVarda Legierung (Vaalburg et al. 1975) durchgeführt. Die in-target Rückstoß-Strahlensynthese durch Deuteronenbestrahlung von Methan kann zwar ohne wesentliche Nachbehandlung on-line erfolgen, das organische Targetmaterial hat jedoch den Nachteil der stärkeren Radiolyseempfindlichkeit, die bei hohen Strahlströmen und/oder mehrmaliger Bestrahlung zur Polymerenbildung führt und eine reibungslose on-line-Abtrennung erschwert.

III. Sauerstoff-15

Die kurze Halbwertszeit des Sauerstoff-15 von nur 2 Minuten beschränkt die Anwendung auf einige einfache Verbindungen wie $[^{15}O]-O_2$, $[^{15}O]-CO$, $[^{15}O]-CO_2$ und $H_2^{15}O$, die in der regionalen Funktionsdiagnostik mit PET Bedeutung erlangt haben. Molekularer Sauerstoff $[^{15}O]-O_2$ wird insbesondere zur Messung des regionalen zerebralen Sauerstoffumsatzes, und ^{15}O-markiertes Wasser bzw. $[^{15}O]-CO_2$ zur Bestimmung der regionalen zerebralen Perfusion verwendet. Mit ^{15}O-markiertem Sauerstoff oder Kohlenmonoxid können durch einfaches Lösen in Blut auch ^{15}O-markiertes Oxyhämoglobin bzw. Carboxyhämoglobin erzeugt werden. Die kontinuierliche Inhalation von $[^{15}O]-CO_2$ stellt durch den schnellen ^{15}O-Austausch mit H_2O eine stetige Infusion von $H_2^{15}O$ dar (Jones et al. 1976). $[^{15}O]-CO_2$ durchdringt leicht die Alveolarmembran und tauscht unter dem katalytischen Einfluß der Carboanhydrase (CbA) über die intermediäre Bildung von Kohlensäure Sauerstoff-15 mit dem Wasser aus:

$$C^{15}OO + H_2O \rightleftharpoons H_2CO_2^{15}O \tag{23}$$

$$H_2CO_2^{15}O \overset{CbA}{\rightleftharpoons} CO_2 + H_2^{15}O \tag{24}$$

Auf diese Weise gelingt es, durch einfache Inhalation von $[^{15}O]-CO_2$ (Gleichgewichtsmethode) über das venöse Blut der Lunge $H_2^{15}O$ in den Kreislauf einzuführen. $H_2^{15}O$, das als frei diffundierendes Molekül die Blut-Hirnschranke durchdringt und zur regionalen Blutflußmessung verwendet wird, kann auch direkt hergestellt (s.u.) und injiziert werden (Bolus-Injektionsmethode).

Die einzig praktisch bedeutende Kernreaktion zur Produktion von Sauerstoff-15 ist der $^{14}N(d,n)^{15}O$-Prozeß. Für kleine Maschinen, die nur über niederenergetische Protonen (10 MeV) verfügen, ist darüber hinaus die $^{15}N(p,n)^{15}O$-Reaktion mit angereicherten ^{15}N-Targets von Interesse. Hier ist allerdings eine Wiedergewinnung des Targetmaterials erforderlich. Im allgemeinen werden N_2-O_2, N_2-H_2 oder N_2-CO_2 Gemische bestrahlt. Hierbei empfiehlt es sich, bei der meist verwendeten (d,n)-Reaktion die Deuteronenenergie unterhalb etwa 6 MeV zu halten, da oberhalb dieser Energie zunehmende Aktivitätsmengen an ^{13}N und ^{11}C über die $^{14}N(d,dn)^{13}N$ und $^{14}N(d,\alpha n)^{11}C$-Reaktion gebildet werden. Der entstehende ^{15}O-Rückstoßsauerstoff reagiert sehr schnell mit molekularem Sauerstoff unter Bildung von markiertem Sauerstoff und Ozon:

$$[^{15}O]^{\ddagger} + O_2 \longrightarrow [^{15}OO_2]^* \overset{M}{\longrightarrow} \begin{cases} ^{15}OO + O \\ ^{15}OO_2 + M^* \end{cases} \tag{25}$$

Daneben entsteht durch Reaktionen mit dem molekularen Stickstoff auch NO_x:

$$[^{15}O]^{\ddagger} + N_2 \longrightarrow [N_2^{15}O]^* \underset{-N}{\longrightarrow} N^{15}O \overset{O_2}{\longrightarrow} N^{15}OO + O \tag{26}$$

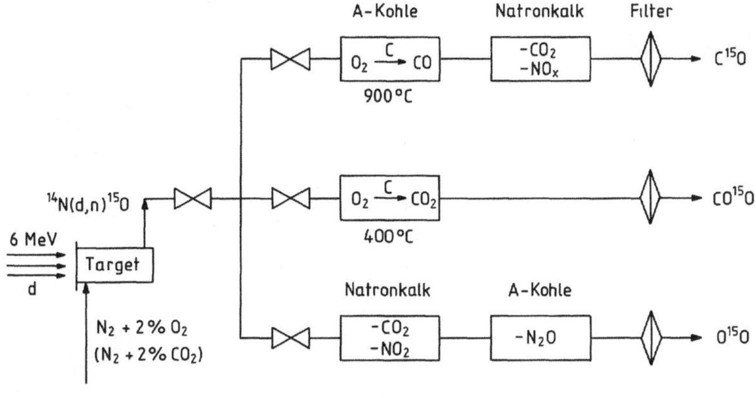

Abb. 2. Fließschema der on-line-Konversion und -Reinigung ^{15}O-markierter Gase

Auch durch strahlenchemische Oxidation von N_2 kommt es zur Bildung von $[^{15}O]-N_2O$, $[^{15}O]-NO$ und $[^{15}O]-O_3$. Darüber hinaus entstehen ebenfalls durch strahlenchemische Prozesse inaktive NO_x-Verunreinigungen und Ozon. Diese unerwünschten radioaktiven und inaktiven Nebenprodukte können durch geeignete Fallen chemisch abgetrennt werden. Abbildung 2 zeigt ein Fließdiagramm für eine automatische Herstellung der verschiedenen ^{15}O-markierten Gase.

Die Bildung von $[^{15}O]-CO$ bzw. $[^{15}O]-CO_2$ aus $[^{15}O]-O_2$ gelingt durch einen Aktivkohle-Ofen, wobei je nach Temperatur überwiegend $[^{15}O]-CO$ (900° C) oder $[^{15}O]-CO_2$ (400° C) entstehen (Boudouard Gleichgewicht):

$$^{15}OO \xrightarrow[\text{400, 900 °C}]{\text{A-Kohle}} C^{15}O, \ C^{15}OO \qquad (27)$$

Vollständige Oxidation von $C^{15}O$ zu $[^{15}O]-CO_2$ kann auch on-line mittels eines CuO-Ofens bei 500° C erreicht werden. Durch die Gegenwart von inaktivem O_2 sind die ^{15}O-markierten Produkte mehr oder weniger stark geträgert. Die Abhängigkeit der Gesamtausbeute an $[^{15}O]-O_2$, $[^{15}O]-NO$ und $[^{15}O]-O_3$ vom O_2 Trägerzusatz in einem N_2-Target zeigt die Abb. 3 (MEYER 1984). Anstelle von O_2 kann dem N_2-Target auch CO_2 zugesetzt werden. Der nukleogene Sauerstoff stabilisiert sich dann als $[^{15}O]-O_2$ und $[^{15}O]-CO_2$. Das O_2/CO_2-Verhältnis ist stark von der Strahlstromdichte, d.h. von der Dosis abhängig (Abb. 4) (MEYER 1984).

$H_2^{15}O$ kann aus $[^{15}O]-O_2$ on-line erzeugt werden, indem man es gemeinsam mit Wasserstoff über erhitzten Pd-Katalysator leitet (WEST u. DOLLERY 1961; CLARK u. BUCKINGHAM 1975). Abbildung 5 zeigt eine Apparatur zur Herstellung und konstanten Infusion von $[^{15}O]-H_2O$ (MEYER et al. 1986). Der vom Target kommende Gasstrom (0,2% Sauerstoff in Stickstoff [ca 200 ml/min]) wird mit Wasserstoff versetzt (ca. 10 ml/min) und über einen Pd Katalysator bei 150° C geleitet. Das Gas-Wasserdampf Gemisch wird dann in ein Vorlagegefäß mit ca 7 ml gekühlter physiol. NaCl Lösung geleitet. Das Restgas wird einer kontrollierten Abluft zugeführt. Eine doppelte Schlauchpumpe entnimmt der Vorlage 4,5 ml/min und führt die gleiche Menge frischer physiol. NaCl Lösung wieder zu. Schwankungen in der Strahlstromführung am Zyklotron, d.h. Änderungen im Aktivitätsniveau des Infusates, werden über die Vorlagemenge mit einer motorgesteuerten Spritze reguliert.

Ausgehend von $[^{15}O]-CO_2$ kann ^{15}O-markiertes Wasser auch durch schnellen Carbo-anhydrase-katalysierten Austausch mit H_2O hergestellt werden (WELCH et al. 1969). Die

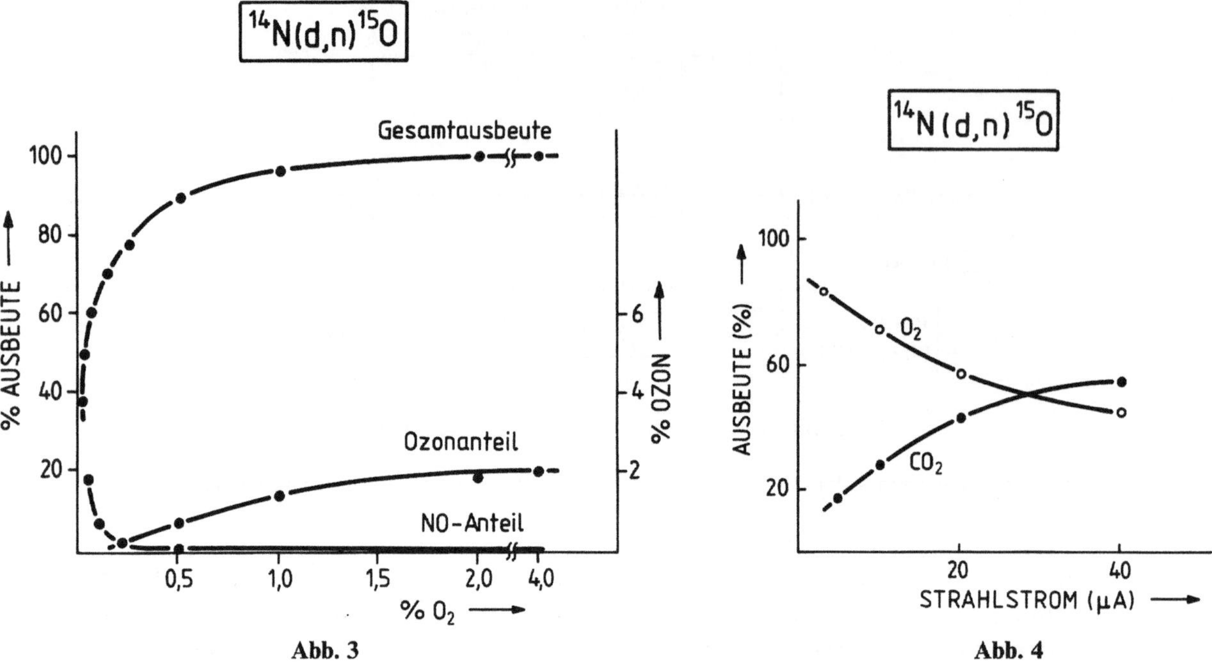

Abb. 3. Abhängigkeit der radiochemischen Ausbeuten an ^{15}O-markierten Produkten im System N_2/O_2 vom O_2-Anteil (Nach MEYER 1984)

Abb. 4. Abhängigkeit der radiochemischen Ausbeuten an $[^{15}O]-O_2$ und $[^{15}O]-CO_2$ vom Strahlstrom (Target 2% CO_2 in N_2) (Nach MEYER 1984)

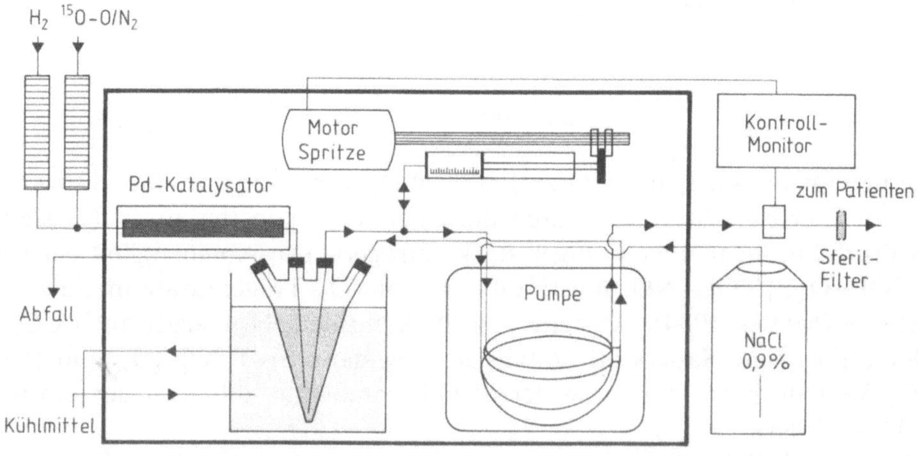

Abb. 5. On-line Produktion von $[^{15}O]-H_2O$. (Nach MEYER et al. 1986)

direkte Rückstoßsynthese von $H_2^{15}O$ mit hoher spezifischer Aktivität im Durchflußtarget wird durch Bestrahlung eines N_2-H_2-Gemisches erreicht (RUIZ u. WOLF 1978). Eine Übersicht der Herstellungsmethoden einfacher ^{15}O-markierter Produkte zeigt Tabelle 5.

IV. Fluor-18

^{18}F ist wegen seiner etwas längeren Halbwertzeit von 110 min und seiner relativ kleinen Positronenenergie ($E_{\beta_{max}} = 635$ keV) ein außerordentlich nützliches Radionuklid für die PET-Technik.

Tabelle 5. Methoden zur on-line Produktion von $[^{15}O]-O_2$, $[^{15}O]-CO$, $[^{15}O]-CO_2$ und $H_2{}^{15}O$ im Anschluß an die Kernreaktion $^{14}N(d,n)^{15}O$

Targetfüllung	Primäre Produkte im Target	Nachbehandlung bzw. Konversion	Endprodukt	Literatur
$N_2+4\%\ O_2$	$[^{15}O]-O_2$	Abtrennung von $[^{15}O]-NO_x$ durch Adsorptionsfallen	$[^{15}O]-CO_2$ $[^{15}O]-O_2$ $[^{15}O]-CO_2$	CLARK u. BUCKINGHAM (1975) MEYER (1984) DEL FIORI et al. (1979)
N_2+O_2-Spuren	$[^{15}O]-O_2$	A-Kohle 800° C	$C^{15}O$	WELCH et al. (1969)
$N_2+2\%\ O_2$	$[^{15}O]-O_2$	A-Kohle 800° C	$C^{15}O$	CLARK u. BUCKINGHAM (1975)
$N_2+2,5\%\ O_2$		A-Kohle 900° C	$C^{15}O$	DEL FIORI et al. (1979)
$N_2+2,5\%\ CO_2$	$[^{15}O]-CO_2$	Reinigung	$[^{15}O]-CO_2$	CLARK u. BUCKINGHAM (1975)
$N_2+4\%\ O_2$	$[^{15}O]-O_2$	A-Kohle 500° C	$[^{15}O]-CO$	BUCKINGHAM u. FORSE (1963)
$N_2+2\%\ O_2$	$[^{15}O]-O_2$	A-Kohle 600° C 1000° C	$[^{15}O]-CO_2$ $C^{15}O$	SUBRAMANYAM et al. (1977)
$N_2+5\%\ H_2$		Pd-Katalysator	$H_2{}^{15}O$	CLARK u. BUCKINGHAM (1975)
N_2+ Spuren O_2	$[^{15}O]-O_2$	A-Kohle 500° C CbA-katal. Austausch von $[^{15}O]-CO_2$ mit H_2O	$H_2{}^{15}O$	WELCH et al. (1969)
$N_2+0,2\%\ O_2$		$+H_2$ Pd-Katalysator	$H_2{}^{15}O$	WEST u. DOLLERY (1961), MEYER et al. (1986)
$N_2+5\%\ H_2$	$H_2{}^{15}O$		$H_2{}^{15}O$	RUIZ u. WOLF (1978)

In den meisten Fällen handelt es sich bei der Einführung von ^{18}F in ein Biomolekül um eine Fremdmarkierung, die prinzipiell zu einer Veränderung der physiologischen Eigenschaften führen kann. Die physiologische Akzeptanz muß deshalb in jedem Einzelfalle überprüft und das Schicksal des Markierungsisotops im Tierexperiment verfolgt werden.

Markierungssynthesen mit ^{18}F sind mit einer Reihe von Schwierigkeiten verbunden. Dies gilt insbesondere für ^{18}F ohne Trägerzusatz. In diesem Falle müssen oft spezielle Gefäßmaterialien verwendet werden, um Wandverluste zu vermeiden. Dies gilt vor allem auch für das $[^{18}F]$-Fluoridion. Hier haben sich besonders Gefäße aus Glaskohlenstoff, Platin oder Polyethylen bewährt. Außerdem empfiehlt sich die Zugabe eines nichtisotopen Trägers wie z.B. Carbonat in Form von K_2CO_3. Bei homogenen Lösungen mit Anionen-aktivierenden Katalysatoren wie Tetrabutylammoniumhydroxid oder Aminopolyether 2.2.2 (s.u.) spielt das Material des Behältnisses meist nur noch eine untergeordnete Rolle.

Als primäre Vorläufer stehen je nach Kernreaktion $[^{18}F]$-F_2, $[^{18}F]-HF$ und $[^{18}F]-F_{aq}^-$ zur Verfügung (s.u. Tabelle 6). Kernreaktionen am Neon können zu wasserfreien Spezies führen, wenn man dem Neon kleine Mengen eines reaktiven Gases (z.B. F_2 oder H_2) zusetzt, mit denen die Rückstoßfluoratome im Target reagieren können:

$$^{18}F + F_2 \longrightarrow {}^{18}FF + F \tag{28}$$

$$^{18}F + H_2 \longrightarrow H^{18}F + H \tag{29}$$

$[^{18}F]-F_2$ kann in einem Neon Gastarget bei kleinen F_2 Partialdrucken (0,1–1%) erzeugt (LAMBRECHT et al. 1978; BIDA et al. 1980; CASELLA et al. 1980; SHAUGNESSY et al. 1981; BLESSING et al. 1986) und entweder direkt oder nach Umwandlung in sekundäre Spezies (s.u.) zur Synthese verwendet werden (s. Abschnitt D.I.). Die von $[^{18}F]-F_2$ ausgehenden Produkte sind jedoch in ihrer spezifischen Aktivität auf einige 10 GBq mMol^{-1} begrenzt. Die Ausbeute beträgt bei einer Energiedegradation im Target von 11,3 auf 0 MeV und einem Strahlstrom von 25 µA bei einer einstündigen Bestrahlung 9,2 GBq entsprechend 370 MBq/µAh (Blessing et al. 1986), d.h. ca. 40% der Theorie.

Wasserfreies $H^{18}F$ kann ohne Trägerzusatz in einem $Ne-H_2$ Target erzeugt werden (Lambrecht et al. 1978; Clark et al. 1973; Straatman u. Welch 1977; Blessing et al. 1986). Auch durch Bestrahlung von reinem Neon kann $H^{18}F$ durch anschließendes Ausheizen des adsorbierten ^{18}F mit H_2 erhalten werden (Dahl et al. 1981). Der einfachste Weg zur Erzeugung von $H^{18}F$ ohne Trägerzusatz ist die Bestrahlung eines $Ne-H_2$ Gemisches, wobei das $H^{18}F$ nach der Bestrahlung ausgeheizt (Crouzel u. Comar 1978; Ehrenkaufer et al. 1983; Blessing et al. 1986) oder während der Bestrahlung durch Zirkulieren des Targetgases über CsOH auf Glas- oder Silberwolle als $Cs^{18}F$ fixiert wird (Tewson et al. 1978). Das Ausheizen eines statischen Targets nach der Bestrahlung geschieht am besten bei 800° C für etwa 5 Minuten, wobei das Target insgesamt für etwa 15 Minuten mit H_2 gespült wird. Auf diese Weise können etwa 80% des ^{18}F aus dem Target entfernt werden. Die Gesamtausbeute beträgt bei einer Energiedegradation von 11,3–0 MeV für einen Strahlstrom von 25 µA nach einstündiger Bestrahlung etwa 9,2 GBq entsprechend 370 MBq/µAh, d.h. etwa 48% der Theorie.

Beim $[^{18}F]-HF$ Gastarget sollten lange Transportstrecken wegen der Sorptionsgefahr vermieden werden. Es empfiehlt sich, sowohl beim offenen als auch beim zirkulierenden geschlossenen Kreislauf, direkt hinter dem Target zu absorbieren, auszufrieren oder im Lösungsmittel zu lösen. Als Targetmaterial wird häufig Ni (poliert oder im Falle der Produktion von $[^{18}F]-F_2$ mit F_2 passiviert), bzw. vernickelte Cu-Be-Legierungen empfohlen, um eine gute Extraktion zu gewährleisten. Es hat sich jedoch gezeigt, daß in vielen Fällen auch vernickelter Edelstahl verwendet werden kann. Zum Passivieren oder zum Abfüllen des Targets werden Vakuumapparaturen mit Conel oder Inconel-Rohren verwendet (Lambrecht et al. 1978; Casella et al. 1980). Die beschriebenen Verfahren leiden oft unter schlechter Reproduzierbarkeit der Ausbeuten. Besonders wichtig ist die Abwesenheit von Luft und insbesondere von organischen Verunreinigungen im Ne-Target.

Die Herstellung von n.c.a. $[^{18}F]$-Fluorid für nukleophile Substitutionen kann etwa über das o.g. $Ne-H_2$ oder über ein Wassertarget erfolgen. Im $Ne-H_2$ Target wird nach der Bestrahlung das an der Wandung haftende $H^{18}F$ bzw. $^{18}F^-$ durch H_2O ausgespült (Helus et al. 1979; Blessing et al. 1986). Auf diese Weise können bei geeignetem Targetmaterial (nicht Quarz!) etwa 60–70% der Fluoraktivität aus dem Target entfernt werden. Die Gesamtausbeute nach einer einstündigen Bestrahlung bei 25 µA beträgt etwa 7,4 GBq entsprechend 296 MBq/µAh (Blessing et al. 1986). Zur Erzeugung möglichst hoher spezifischer Aktivitäten sind Kontaminationen mit inaktivem Fluor zu vermeiden. Neon enthält häufig Spurenverunreinigungen verschiedener Freone. Diese entfernt man zweckmäßigerweise beim Füllen des Targets, indem man das Neon vorher durch eine Molekularsiebfalle ($-78°$ C) leitet. Im allgemeinen wird $[^{18}F]$-Fluorid am kleinen Zyklotron durch Protonenbestrahlung von ^{18}O-angereichertem Wasser hergestellt:

$$H_2^{18}O \xrightarrow{\ ^{18}O\,(p,\,n)^{18}F\ } {}^{18}F_{aq}^- \tag{30}$$

Die $^{18}O(p,n)^{18}F$-Reaktion hat schon bei 10 MeV einen sehr großen Wirkungsquerschnitt, und mit Eintrittsenergien von 15 MeV können Ausbeuten von 3,3 GBq/µAh erhalten werden (Ruth u. Wolf 1979). Gesamtaktivitäten von 37 GBq pro ml Wasser können mit einer spezifischen Aktivität von $3,7 \cdot 10^5$ GBq mMol^{-1} produziert werden (Kilbourn et al. 1984). Wenn ein Zyklotron zur Verfügung steht, das ^{3}He-Teilchen beschleunigt, so kann auch die $^{16}O(^3He,p)^{18}F$-Reaktion an natürlichem Wasser genutzt werden (TILBURY et al. 1970). Allerdings sind hier die Wirkungsquerschnitte und damit die Ausbeuten erheblich kleiner (zur Übersicht s. QAIM u. STÖCKLIN 1983).

Im Falle eines Wassertargets sind nukleophile Synthesen mit trägerfreiem Fluorid unter Verwendung von Anionen-aktivierenden Phasentransferkatalysatoren wie Oniumsalze, Kronenether bzw. Aminopolyether besonders geeignet (GNADE et al. 1981; IRIE et al. 1982; LANDVATER et al. 1983; KIESEWETTER et al. 1984; BLOCK et al. 1986 a, b; COENEN et al. 1986a, b), da sie die Reaktivität des Fluorids in nukleophilen Reaktionen entscheidend erhöhen. Heute wird fast ausschließlich entweder Tetraalkylammoniumhydroxid oder Aminopolyether 2.2.2 verwendet. Hierzu setzt man schon dem $^{18}F^-$-haltigen Wasser z.B. eine wäßrige Lösung von K_2CO_3 und den Aminopolyether 2.2.2 zu, dampft bis zur Trockne ein und nimmt dann mit dem gewünschten Lösungsmittel auf. Das CO_3-Ion wirkt hier gleichzeitig als nichtisotoper Träger und als Base und verhindert das Entweichen der ^{18}F-Aktivität in Form von $H^{18}F$.

Eine Reihe von $[^{18}F]$-Fluorierungsreagenzien können, ausgehend von den primären Vorläufern, über einfache Austauschreaktionen synthetisiert werden, so z.B. $[^{18}F]$-Trifluormethylhypofluorit (NEIRINCKX et al. 1978) durch den katalysierten F-Austausch zwischen $Cs^{18}F$ und CF_3OF:

$$Cs^{18}F + CF_3OF \longrightarrow [^{18}F]\text{-}CF_3OF \qquad (31)$$

$[^{18}F]$-Methylhypofluorit wurde zur Synthese von 5-Fluoruracil verwendet. Mit dieser elektrophilen Substitutionsreaktion konnte gleichzeitig gezeigt werden, daß nur 33% der ^{18}F-Aktivität des Fluorierungsreagenz in der OF-Funktion vorliegen. Dieses Fluorierungsreagenz hat jedoch bisher keine wesentliche Bedeutung erlangt. Durch Isotopenaustausch konnte on-line, ausgehend von $H^{18}F$, auch Diäthylaminoschwefeltrifluorid (DAST) markiert werden, das zur Substitution der Hydroxygruppe in Alkoholen durch Fluor geeignet ist (STRAATMAN u. WELCH 1977). Auch das zur elektrophilen Einführung von Fluor-18 geeignete $[^{18}F]-XeF_2$ kann über einen F-Isotopenaustausch ausgehend vom $H^{18}F$ mit relativ guter radiochemischer Ausbeute (31%) hergestellt werden (SCHROBILGEN et al. 1981):

$$XeF_2 + H^{18}F \rightleftharpoons Xe^{18}FF + HF \qquad (32)$$

Das $[^{18}F]-XeF_2$ ist zur Synthese von $[6\text{-}^{18}F]$-Fluordopa und $[2\text{-}^{18}F]$-FDG verwendet worden (s. Abschnitt D). Aber auch hier besteht das inhärente Problem der geringen spezifischen Aktivität. Deswegen und wegen der Schwierigkeit ihrer Herstellung bei fehlendem synthetischem Vorteil, haben die elektrophilen Spezies aus Isotopenaustauschreaktionen praktisch keine Bedeutung erlangt.

Ein sehr nützliches elektrophiles Fluorierungsreagenz ist Acetylhypofluorit, das milder ist als F_2 und syn-Addition sowie Regiospezifität zeigt (ROZEN et al. 1981). Es ist auch zur direkten Fluorierung von Aromaten eingesetzt worden (LERMAN et al. 1981). Dieses Reagenz kann mit guter Ausbeute hergestellt werden, wenn man $[^{18}F]$-F_2 aus einem $Ne-F_2$ Gastarget nach der Bestrahlung in eine Lösung von Ammoniumacetat in Eisessig leitet (SHIUE et al. 1982; FOWLER et al. 1982b):

$$[^{18}F]\text{-}F_2 + CH_3CO_2NH_4 \xrightarrow{\ CH_3CO_2H\ } CH_3CO_2^{18}F + NH_4^{(18)}F \qquad (33)$$

$[^{18}F]$-Acetylhypofluorit wird in-situ zur Synthese von $[^{18}F]$-2-FDG verwendet (s.u. Abschnitt D.I.). Gasförmiges Acetylhypofluorit kann auch durch Reaktion von $[^{18}F]-F_2$ mit einem festen Salz der Essigsäure für Reaktionen in verschiedenen polaren Lösungsmitteln

Tabelle 6. Erzeugung der wichtigsten primären ^{18}F-Vorläufer

Targetfüllung	Kernreaktion	Produkt	Literatur
Ne+0,1% F$_2$ 18–24 bar	^{20}Ne(d,α)^{18}F	[^{18}F]−F$_2$	LAMBRECHT et al. (1978) CASELLA et al. (1980), BLESSING et al. (1986)
Ne+15% H$_2$ 8 bar	^{20}Ne(d,α)^{18}F	[^{18}F]−HF Ausheizen des Targets	LAMBRECHT et al. (1978), CROUZEL u. COMAR (1978), DAHL et al. (1981) EHRENKAUFER et al. (1983), BLESSING et al. (1986)
Ne+15% H$_2$	^{20}Ne(d,α)^{18}F	[^{18}F]−F$_{aq}^{-}$ nach Ausspülen des Targets mit H$_2$O	HELUS et al. (1979), BLESSING et al. (1986)
H$_2$^{18}O	^{18}O(p,n)^{18}F	[^{18}F]−F$_{aq}^{-}$	RUTH u. WOLF (1979), NICKLES et al. (1983)
H$_2$O	^{16}O(^{3}He,p)^{18}F		TILBURY et al. (1970)

erzeugt werden (EHRENKAUFER et al. 1984). Da elektrophile Fluorierungsspezies wie [^{18}F]-Acetylhypofluorit ausgehend vom trägerhaltigen [^{18}F]−F$_2$ hergestellt werden oder im Falle von [^{18}F]−XeF$_2$ über Fluoraustausch, sind sie a priori trägerhaltig. Bisher führt der einzige Weg zur Einführung von ^{18}F ohne Trägerzusatz über die nukleophile Substitution ausgehend von [^{18}F]-Fluorid. Eine Zusammenstellung der wichtigsten primären ^{18}F-Markierungsvorläufer zeigt Tabelle 6.

V. Brom-75,77, Jod-123 Zerfallsinduzierte Markierung

Bei den schweren Halogenen wie ^{75}Br ($T_{1/2}=1,6$ h), ^{77}Br ($T_{1/2}=56$ h) oder ^{123}I ($T_{1/2}=13$ h) ist soviel Zeit für eine Markierung vorhanden, daß in vielen Fällen auf klassische Reaktionen zurückgegriffen werden kann. Allerdings gilt dies nur mit Einschränkungen, und es bleiben die Probleme der Trägerfreiheit (vgl. Abschnitt C.I.). Als Ausgangsform bietet sich für die Markierung ohne Trägerzusatz das Halogenidion an, das durch in-situ Oxidation in elektrophile Spezies umgewandelt werden kann. Dennoch hat man versucht, Methoden der Direktmarkierung zu entwickeln. Besonders geeignet ist für ein solches Vorgehen die Ausnutzung des radioaktiven Zerfalls geeigneter Vorläufer (auch excitation labelling genannt). Im Falle von Brom und Iod bietet sich hierzu z.B. der Zerfall von ^{77}Kr bzw. ^{123}Xe an. Der β-Zerfall führt nämlich zu angeregten Tochteratomen oder Ionen, die u.a. in der Lage sind, Substitutionsreaktionen einzugehen (zur Übersicht s. STÖCKLIN 1977; TOMINAGA u. TACHIKAWA 1981). So zerfällt ^{77}Kr durch β^+-Emission und Elektroneneinfang (EC) zu reaktiven ^{77}Br-Spezies:

$$^{77}\text{Kr} \xrightarrow{1,2 \text{ h}} \begin{array}{c} \xrightarrow{16\% \text{ EC}} \text{Auger Effect} \\ \xrightarrow{84\% \ \beta^+} \text{Anregung} \end{array} \begin{array}{c} ^{77}\text{Br}^{n+} \to \to \to \ ^{77}\text{Br}^+(^{77}\text{Br}^\circ) \\ \\ ^{77}\text{Br}^-(^{77}\text{Br}^+, \ ^{77}\text{Br}^\circ) \end{array} \tag{34}$$

und ^{123}Xe ebenfalls durch EC- und β^+-Zerfall zu reaktiven ^{123}I-Spezies:

$$^{123}\text{Xe} \xrightarrow{\;2,1\,\text{h}\;} \begin{cases} \xrightarrow[\text{Auger Effect}]{78\%\ \text{EC}} \;^{123}\text{I}^{n+} \to\to\to\; ^{123}\text{I}^+(^{123}\text{I}^\circ) \\[2ex] \xrightarrow[\text{Anregung}]{22\%\ \beta^+} \;^{123}\text{I}^-(^{123}\text{I}^+,\,^{123}\text{I}^\circ) \end{cases} \qquad (35)$$

Diese äußerst reaktiven Zerfallsspezies reagieren allerdings sehr unspezifisch, und die radiochemischen Ausbeuten des gewünschten markierten Produktes sind meist klein (einige Prozent), so daß sich i. allg. die direkte Markierung einer komplexen Verbindung nicht lohnt. Das Verfahren selbst ist allerdings extrem einfach: das feste, flüssige oder gasförmige Substrat wird direkt dem radioaktiven Edelgas in einer Ampulle bis zur optimalen Zerfallszeit ausgesetzt. Größere Schwierigkeiten kann die chromatographische Trennung des oft unspezifisch markierten Substanzgemisches darstellen. Einfacher und für die Praxis lohnender ist die zerfallsinduzierte Präparierung von Halogenierungsreagenzien. Dies bietet sich vor allem im Fall von ^{123}I an, da hier die wichtigsten Produktionsprozesse zunächst den Xenon-123 Vorläufer liefern, der dann in Iod-123 zerfällt (s. Gl. 35). Dieser ^{123}Xe$-^{123}$I-Generator kann hier genutzt werden, um klassische elektrophile Iodierungsreagenzien herzustellen (LAMBRECHT et al. 1972; EL-GARHY u. STÖCKLIN 1974; MACHULLA et al. 1977)

$$^{123}\text{Xe} \xrightarrow{\;\beta^+,\ \text{EC}\;} {}^{123}\text{I}^* \xrightarrow{\;\text{Cl}_2\;} {}^{123}\text{ICl} \qquad (36)$$

$$^{123}\text{Xe} \xrightarrow{\;\beta^+,\ \text{EC}\;} {}^{123}\text{I}^* \xrightarrow{\;\text{KIO}_3\;} {}^{123}\text{II} \qquad (37)$$

In beiden Fällen kann die ohnehin notwendige Zerfallszeit für das ^{123}Xe (optimal 6,5 h) genutzt werden, um ein einfaches Reagenz für die elektrophile Iodierung zu präparieren, indem man das ^{123}Xe in Cl$_2$ oder an KIO$_3$ zerfallen läßt. Tabelle 7 zeigt für den Fall der Modellsysteme Phenol, Anilin und Tyrosin sehr deutlich die gegenüber der direkten Exponierungsmethode höhere Ausbeute und Selektivität. Das ^{123}Xe/KIO$_3$ Verfahren ist lediglich eine Variante der klassischen Iodid/Iodat-Methode.

Tabelle 7. Vergleich der direkten zerfallsinduzierten Radioiodierung durch Exponieren mit ^{123}Xe mit der Reagenzmarkierung Xenon-123/ KIO$_3$. (Nach EL-GARHY u. STÖCKLIN 1974; MACHULLA et al. 1977)

Substrat	Methode	% Radiochemische Ausbeute		
		ortho	meta	para
Phenol	^{123}Xe-direkt[a]	3,7	0,7	3,3
	^{123}Xe$-$KIO$_3$[b]	66	–	12
Anilin	^{123}Xe-direkt[a]	23	–	5,5
	^{123}Xe$-$KIO$_3$[b]	1,3	0,7	55
Tyrosin	^{123}Xe-direkt[a]	2	(Monoiod-L-tyrosin)	
	^{123}Xe$-$KIO$_3$[b]	81	(Monoiod-L-tyrosin)	

[a] 100 mg Substrat exponiert mit 10 MBq ^{123}Xe (10 h) in einer 200 µl Glasampulle; anschließend Reinigung durch HPLC.

[b] 1 mg ^{123}Xe exponiertes (6,5 h) KIO$_3$, gelöst in 1 ml 0,1 N HCl 1 mg Substrat enthaltend. Reaktionszeit: 1 min (22° C); anschließend Reinigung durch HPLC.

C. Einige grundlegende Synthesen zur Markierung mit kurzlebigen organischen Radionukliden

I. Das Problem der Trägerfreiheit

Unter den Positronenstrahlern bietet ^{11}C den Vorteil, daß die Moleküle nach der Markierung keinerlei Änderung in den biochemischen Eigenschaften aufweisen. Andererseits sind durch die Halbwertszeit und die in der Praxis erreichbare spezifische Aktivität der Anwendung Grenzen gesetzt. Die spezifische Aktivität spielt vor allem bei toxischen, zentral wirksamen und bei Rezeptor-bindenden Produkten eine wesentliche Rolle, da diese Radiopharmaka häufig nur in Nanogramm-Mengen eingesetzt werden können. Theoretisch besitzen zwar die kurzlebigen Zyklotron-erzeugten Radionuklide extrem hohe spezifische Aktivitäten (s. Tabelle 8), jedoch wird auf vielfältigen Wegen durch Verunreinigungen isotoper Träger aufge-

Tabelle 8. Spezifische Aktivitäten einiger kurzlebiger „trägerfreier" markierter Vorläufer für Markierungssynthesen

Vorläufer	Kernreaktion	Target	Spezifische Aktivität	
			Theoretisch trägerfrei GBq mmol^{-1}	Praktisch (n.c.a.) GBq mmol^{-1}
$[^{11}C]-CO_2$	$^{14}N(p,\alpha)^{11}C$	$N_2(O_2)$	$3,4\cdot10^8$	10^4–10^5
$[^{11}C]-CH_3I$	$^{14}N(p,\alpha)^{11}C$			10^3–10^4
$[^{11}C]-HCN$	$^{14}N(p,\alpha)^{11}C$	$N_2(H_2)$		10^4
$[^{18}F]-F_{aq}^-$	$^{18}O(p,n)^{18}F$	H_2O	$6,4\cdot10^7$	10^5–10^6
$[^{18}F]-F_2$	$^{20}Ne(d,\alpha)^{18}F$	$Ne(0,1\% F_2)$		10^1–10^2
$[^{75}Br]-Br^-$	$^{75}As(^3He,3n)^{75}Br$	Cu_3As	$7,2\cdot10^7$	10^5–10^6
	$^{76}Se(p,2n)^{75}Br$	$^{76}SeO_2$		10^4
$[^{123}I]-I^-$	$^{127}I(p,5n)^{123}Xe\rightarrow^{123}I$	KI, CH_2I_2	$8,9\cdot10^6$	10^4–10^5

(n.c.a. = no-carrier-added am Ende der Synthese)

nommen, so daß tatsächlich meist eine Verdünnung um einen Faktor 10 bis 10000 stattfindet. Dies gilt insbesondere für ^{11}C. Hier müssen gründliche Vorsichtsmaßnahmen getroffen werden (s. Abschnitt B.I.). Aber auch bei den Halogenen ist es trotz ihrer geringen Häufigkeit nicht leicht, in die Nähe des theoretischen Wertes der spezifischen Aktivität zu gelangen. Eine Verdünnung um einen Faktor 10 ist bereits optimal. Der isotope Träger wird durch Gefäße, Targetmaterialien, Synthesechemikalien etc. eingeschleppt, so daß die spezifische Aktivität sich auch im Laufe der Synthese verändern kann. Zur Angabe der spezifischen Aktivität gehört auch die Angabe des Zeitpunktes ihrer Messung (EOB = end of bombardment oder EOS = end of synthesis). Eine völlig trägerfreie Markierung ist grundsätzlich nur bei künstlichen Elementen wie etwa Astat möglich. Man spricht deshalb im allgemeinen von Markierungen ohne Trägerzusatz (n.c.a. = no-carrier-added). Über die Bestimmung der spezifischen Aktivität wird in Abschnitt E.III. berichtet.

Während hohe spezifische Aktivität in vielen Fällen eine wichtige Voraussetzung für die Anwendung des Radiopharmakons darstellt, z.B. beim Einsatz von Rezeptor-bindenden

Radioliganden, bringen die damit verbundenen kleinen Konzentrationen für die Synthese erhebliche Probleme. Hierzu gehören u.a.:
- Verluste durch Adsorption an Gefäßwänden oder Niederschlägen,
- Nebenreaktionen mit Lösungsmitteln oder Verunreinigungen,
- Reaktionen entfernt vom Gleichgewicht und von stöchiometrischen Bedingungen,
- begrenzte Möglichkeiten der Qualitätskontrolle.

Der Einfluß von zugesetztem Träger auf die Ausbeute einer Reaktion läßt sich nicht immer vorhersagen. Das sog. down-scaling vom Gramm- zum Nanogrammbereich ist deshalb ebenso schwierig wie das up-scaling zum Tonnenbereich, vor allem, wenn die Synthese wegen der hohen Anfangsaktivitäten fernbedient oder automatisiert in Bleizellen durchgeführt werden muß, wie das bei kurzlebigen Positronenstrahlern im Falle einer Routineproduktion aus Strahlenschutzgründen erforderlich ist.

II. Basissynthesen mit ^{11}C-Vorläufern

1. Ausgehend vom $^{11}CO_2$, $^{11}CH_3I$

Die einfachste Möglichkeit, eine $C-C$ Bindung zu schaffen, bietet die Carboxylierung metallorganischer Vorstufen wie z.B. Grignard Verbindungen. Hierdurch gelangt man u.a. zu Carbonsäuren, Aminosäuren, Ketonen und Aldehyden mit einer ^{11}C-markierten Carbonylgruppe. Der einfachste Weg führt zu Carbonsäuren:

$$R-MgX \quad \xrightarrow{\ ^{11}CO_2\ } \quad R-^{11}CO_2MgX \quad \xrightarrow{\ H^+\ } \quad R-^{11}CO_2H \qquad (38)$$
$$(RLi) \qquad\qquad\qquad (R-^{11}CO_2Li)$$

Die Reaktion ist schnell und einfach und deshalb für Kohlenstoff-11 im allgemeinen gut geeignet. Man kann $^{11}CO_2$ im Trägergas direkt durch die Grignard-Lösung leiten oder besser zunächst in den Reaktionskolben kondensieren und dann die Grignard-Lösung in dem gewünschten minimalen Volumen zusetzen. Die Ausbeuten sind oft nahezu quantitativ. Besondere Vorsichtsmaßnahmen (s.o.) sind erforderlich, um eine Kontamination mit inaktivem CO_2 zu vermeiden und damit die spezifische Aktivität möglichst hoch zu halten.

Ausgehend von α-Lithioisonitrilen erhält man durch Carboxylierung Aminosäuren:

$$R-CH_2-\bar{N}{=}\bar{C} \quad \xrightarrow{\ n\text{-BuLi}\ } \quad R\underset{\underset{\displaystyle Li}{|}}{C}H-\bar{N}{=}\bar{C} \qquad (39)$$

$$\xrightarrow{\ ^{11}CO_2\ } \quad R\underset{\underset{\displaystyle ^{11}COOLi}{|}}{C}H-\bar{N}{=}\bar{C} \quad \xrightarrow{\ H^+\ } \quad R-\underset{\underset{\displaystyle NH_2}{|}}{C}H-^{11}COOH \qquad (40)$$

Die Carboxylierung der Li-Isonitrile erfolgt bei niedrigen Temperaturen mit extrem kleinen Mengen der feuchtigkeitsempfindlichen Verbindung. Eine sehr vorsichtige Handhabung unter Schutzgas ist deshalb erforderlich (VAALBURG et al. 1976).

Zahlreiche aliphatische und aromatische Carbonsäuren und Aminosäuren sind auf diese Weise mit guter Ausbeute mit ^{11}C in der Carboxylgruppe markiert worden (s. Abschnitt D). Bei den Aminosäuren erhält man allerdings Racemate, die erst aufgetrennt werden müssen.

Mit Hilfe von Methyllithium gelangt man ausgehend vom $^{11}CO_2$ auch zu [1-^{11}C]-Essigsäure bzw. zu [2-^{11}C]-Aceton (BERGER et al. 1980):

$$^{11}CO_2 + LiCH_3 \longrightarrow CH_3{}^{11}CO_2Li \tag{41}$$

$$\xrightarrow{LiCH_3} (CH_3)_2{}^{11}C(OLi)_2 \xrightarrow{H_2O} (CH_3)_2{}^{11}C{=}O \tag{42}$$

Die Acetonausbeute hängt empfindlich von der CH_3Li-Konzentration ab. Bei einem zu hohen Überschuß erhält man vorwiegend den tert. Alkohol. ^{11}C-markierte tertiäre Alkohole erhält man allgemein durch Alkylierung des entsprechenden Ketons z.B. mit $^{11}CH_3MgI$ oder $^{11}CH_3Li$:

$$\underset{R}{\overset{R'}{>}}C{=}O + {}^{11}CH_3MgI \longrightarrow \underset{R}{\overset{R'}{>}}C\underset{{}^{11}CH_3}{\overset{OH}{<}} \tag{43}$$
$$({}^{11}CH_3Li)$$

Die Addition von $^{11}CH_3Li$ an Ketone hat u.a. bei der Markierung von Steroiden Anwendung gefunden (s. Abschnitt D). [^{11}C]-Methyllithium läßt sich ausgehend vom $^{11}CH_3I$ z.B. mit n-Butyllithium herstellen (REIFFERS et al. 1980):

$$n\text{-BuLi} + {}^{11}CH_3I \underset{}{\overset{-80°}{\rightleftharpoons}} {}^{11}CH_3Li + n\text{-BuI} \tag{44}$$

Wegen des hohen Überschusses an n-BuLi erhält man nahezu quantitative Ausbeuten. Das Gleichgewicht stellt sich innerhalb von 10 min ein. Bei allen Reaktionen mit metallorganischen Verbindungen ist wegen der unerwünschten Isotopenverdünnung mit ^{12}C ein möglichst völliger Ausschluß von inaktivem CO_2 anzustreben. Die metallorganischen Verbindungen müssen stets frisch hergestellt werden. Arbeiten unter Schutzgas von höchstem Reinheitsgrad und die Verwendung von entgasten Lösungsmitteln bieten die Möglichkeit, spezifische Aktivitäten von mindestens einigen zehn TBq mMol^{-1} zu erhalten (s.o. Tabelle 8).

Sehr wichtige Vorläufer, die über $^{11}CO_2$ hergestellt werden, sind [^{11}C]-Methyliodid und [^{11}C]-Formaldehyd (s.o. Gl. 13). Sie erlauben eine einfache Methylierung der NH-, SH- und OH-Funktion:

$$R{-}NH_2 + {}^{11}CH_3I \longrightarrow RNH^{11}CH_3 \tag{45}$$
$$({-}SH) \qquad\qquad ({-}S^{11}CH_3)$$
$$({-}OH) \qquad\qquad ({-}O^{11}CH_3)$$

Auch andere [^{11}C]-Alkylierungen ausgehend von Alkyliodiden sind beschrieben worden (LANGSTRÖM et al. 1986). Die N-Methylierung sekundärer und primärer Amine mit $^{11}CH_3I$ erfordert zuweilen erhebliche Reaktionszeiten oder relativ hohe Temperaturen, die zu Nebenreaktionen führen können. In diesen Fällen ist der Umweg über die reduktive Formylierung vorzuziehen:

$$R{-}N\underset{R'}{\overset{H}{<}} \xrightarrow{{}^{11}CH_2O} \underset{R'}{\overset{R}{>}}\overset{+}{N}{=}^{11}CH_2 \xrightarrow{Red.} \underset{R}{\overset{R'}{>}}N{-}^{11}CH_3 \tag{46}$$

Als Reduktionsmittel können Ameisensäure, Natriumborhydrid ($NaBH_4$) oder Natriumcyanoborhydrid ($NaCNBH_3$) verwendet werden. Empfindliche und komplexe Moleküle wie Albumin, Fibrinogen (STRAATMAN u. WELCH 1975), Chlorpromazin, Imipramin und Nikotin (BERGER et al. 1979) lassen sich mit dieser Methode leicht methylieren. Eine Zweitmethylierung im Falle von primären Aminen findet wegen des großen Überschusses des Amins praktisch nicht statt. Häufiger angewendet als die reduktive Formylierung wird die einfache direkte Methylierung mit [^{11}C]-Methyliodid.

Mit Hilfe von [^{11}C]-Aceton (vgl. Gl. 41) kann auch die Isopropylgruppe eingeführt werden:

$$R-N\overset{R}{\underset{H}{\diagup}} \xrightarrow{CH_3{}^{11}COCH_3} \overset{R'}{\underset{R}{\diagdown}}N\overset{+}{=}{}^{11}C\overset{CH_3}{\underset{CH_3}{\diagup}} \xrightarrow{Red.} \overset{R'}{\underset{R}{\diagdown}}N-{}^{11}CH\overset{CH_3}{\underset{CH_3}{\diagup}} \qquad (47)$$

Die Isopropylierung ist jedoch im Vergleich zur Methylierung deutlich erschwert, und die Ausbeuten sind wesentlich kleiner.

Ausgehend von metallorganischen Verbindungen gelangt man mit [^{11}C]-Methyliodid auch zu um ein C-Atom verlängerten [^{11}C]-markierten Kohlenwasserstoffen:

$$RMgX + {}^{11}CH_3I \longrightarrow R{}^{11}CH_3 \qquad (48)$$
$$(RLi)$$

2. Ausgehend vom H^{11}CN

[^{11}C]-Cyanwasserstoff ist ein weiterer wichtiger Vorläufer (vgl. Gl. 11), von dem zahlreiche Synthesen ausgehen. Durch nukleophile Substitution an Alkylhalogeniden werden Nitrile zugänglich,

$$RX + {}^{11}CN^- \longrightarrow R{}^{11}CN + X^- \qquad (49)$$

die ihrerseits wieder den Weg zu Verbindungen mit Amin- oder Carbonylfunktionen zugänglich machen:

$$R{}^{11}CN \longrightarrow \begin{cases} R-{}^{11}CH_2NH_2 \\ R-{}^{11}CHO \\ R-\overset{}{\underset{\underset{O}{\|}}{{}^{11}C}}-R' \\ R-{}^{11}COOH \end{cases} \qquad (50)$$

Mit Cyanhydrinen gelangt man zu 2-Hydroxycarbonsäuren bzw. -aminen:

$$R-\underset{\underset{OH}{|}}{C}-{}^{11}CN \longrightarrow \begin{cases} R-\underset{\underset{OH}{|}}{CH}-{}^{11}COOH \\ R-\underset{\underset{OH}{|}}{CH}-{}^{11}CH_2-NH_2 \end{cases} \qquad (51)$$

Ein Weg, der bei der Synthese von [1-^{11}C]-Dopamin (FOWLER et al. 1973a) und [1-^{11}C]-Norepinephrin (FOWLER et al. 1974) angewendet wurde. Auch Aminosäuren, die in der Carboxylgruppe mit ^{11}C markiert sind, können ausgehend vom [^{11}C]-Cyanid und dem entsprechenden Aldehyd oder Keton erhalten werden:

$$R_1-\overset{\overset{O}{\|}}{C}-R_2 \xrightarrow[NH_4Cl]{K^{11}CN, (NH_4)_2CO_3} R_1\overset{R_2}{\underset{\underset{\underset{O}{\|}}{HN\diagup\diagdown NH}}{|}}{}^{11}C\mathord{=}O \xrightarrow[-CO_2\; -NH_3]{OH^-} \overset{R_1}{\underset{R_2}{\diagdown}}C\underset{NH_2}{-}{}^{11}CO_2H \qquad (52)$$

Man erhält zunächst ein Hydantoin, das anschließend zur Aminosäure hydrolysiert wird. Zahlreiche Aminosäuren sind auf diesem Wege mit ^{11}C markiert worden. Wie bei der vom CO_2 ausgehenden Isonitrilsynthese erhält man auch hier Racemate (s.u. Abschnitt D.II.).

3. Ausgehend von ^{11}CO, $^{11}COCl_2$

Im Vergleich zu $^{11}CO_2$ und $H^{11}CN$ wird ^{11}CO als Vorläufer für Markierungssynthesen bisher kaum eingesetzt. Ausgehend von dem leicht zugänglichen ^{11}C-Phosgen (s.o. Gl. 16,17) sind hierüber durch Kondensation mit Alkoholen, Ammoniak und Aminen interessante Synthesevorläufer wie Carbonsäureester, Säurechloride, -amide, Isocyanate etc. zugänglich:

$$
\begin{array}{ll}
& \xrightarrow{\;2\,EtOH\;} \quad Et-O-^{11}C(=O)-OEt \\[4pt]
& \xrightarrow{\;EtOH\;} \quad Et-O-^{11}C(=O)-Cl \xrightarrow{\;NH_3\;} H_2N-^{11}C(=O)-OEt \\[4pt]
O=^{11}C(Cl)_2 & \xrightarrow{\;2\,NH_3\;} \quad H_2N-^{11}C(=O)-NH_2 \\[4pt]
& \xrightarrow{\;RNH_2\;} \quad R-N=^{11}C=O \\[4pt]
& \xrightarrow{\;2\,\varnothing NH_2\;} \quad \varnothing NH-^{11}C(=O)-NH\varnothing
\end{array}
\tag{53}
$$

Diese Produkte können z.B. zur ^{11}C-Markierungssynthese von Heterozyklen genutzt werden. Ausgehend von ^{11}CO können auch ^{11}C-Amide über die Carbonylierung von Li-dialkylaminen erhalten werden (Kilbourn u. Welch 1982):

$$
\begin{array}{c}
\text{(Piperidin)}NH \xrightarrow{\;n-BuLi\;} \text{(Piperidin)}N-Li \\[8pt]
\xrightarrow{\;^{11}CO\;} \text{(Piperidin)}N-^{11}C(=O)-Li
\begin{cases}
\xrightarrow{\;H_2O\;} & \text{(Piperidin)}N-^{11}CHO \\[4pt]
\xrightarrow{\;RI\;} & \text{(Piperidin)}N-^{11}C(=O)-R
\end{cases}
\end{array}
\tag{54}
$$

Die Zwischenstufe kann mit H_2O in das Formamid bzw. mit einem Alkyliodid in das Carbonsäureamid umgewandelt werden. Auch die Carbonylierung durch Einschiebung von ^{11}CO in eine Kohlenstoff-Bor Bindung ist potentiell nützlich. So ist z.B. $[1-^{11}C]$-Octanal durch Reaktion von ^{11}CO mit n-Heptyl-9-borabicyclo[3.3.1]nonan (B-heptyl-9-BBN) und $(CH_3O)_3LiAlH$ hergestellt worden. Das Addukt wurde oxidativ hydrolysiert (Tang et al. 1979):

$$
\text{B-heptyl-9-BBN} + (CH_3O)_3HLiAl + {}^{11}CO \xrightarrow[\;H_2O_2\,(30\%)\;]{\;\text{Hydrolyse (pH 7)}\;} C_7H_{15}{}^{11}CHO \tag{55}
$$

III. Einige Basissynthesen mit ^{18}F-Vorläufern

Die elektrophile Einführung von ^{18}F geht insbesondere von Vorläufern wie F_2, CH_3CO_2F und seltener von XeF_2 aus. In zunehmendem Maße werden jedoch – wo immer möglich – nukleophile Synthesen ausgehend von [^{18}F]-Fluorid angewendet, da sich nur hier die Möglichkeit bietet, zu praktisch trägerfreien (n.c.a.) Produkten zu gelangen. Darüber hinaus stehen, anders als im Falle von [^{18}F]$-F_2$, wo maximal nur 50% des ^{18}F genutzt werden können, bei der nukleophilen Fluorierung 100% des ^{18}F zur Verfügung. Dennoch ist man in zahlreichen Fällen auf die elektrophile Fluorierung angewiesen.

1. Elektrophile Fluorierung

Eine Reihe von Techniken ist entwickelt worden, auch F_2 unter geeigneten Bedingungen zur Reaktion zu bringen (ALKER et al. 1980). [^{18}F]$-F_2$, [^{18}F]$-XeF_2$ und [^{18}F]$-CH_3CO_2F$ werden als Reagenzien für die elektrophile Fluorierung verwendet, wenn Trägerfreiheit oder extrem hohe spezifische Aktivitäten nicht erforderlich sind. Mit Interhalogenverbindungen wie BrF und IF sind nur Additionsreaktionen möglich (CHI et al. 1985), die hier zu trägerfreien Produkten führen. Die hohe Reaktivität und die geringe Ausbeute bei der Präparation der n.c.a. ^{18}F-Interhalogene, lassen diese Methode als wenig geeignet erscheinen. Auch andere elektrophile Spezies wie CF_3OF, ClO_3F oder NOF haben bisher bei Markierungssynthesen kaum Anwendungen gefunden. Die Verwendung von F_2 geschieht wegen seiner hohen Reaktivität nach Verdünnung mit einem inerten Gas. Auch die Lösungsmittel, in denen die Reaktionen durchgeführt werden, sollten gegenüber elementarem Fluor weitgehend inert sein. So

Tabelle 9. Selektivität und Reaktivität von [^{18}F]$-F_2$ und [^{18}F]$-CH_3CO_2F$ in monosubstituierten Benzolen bei 0° C in Trifluoressigsäure (COENEN et al. 1986c)

$$[^{18}F] - F_2$$

	CF_3	F	OCH_3
ortho / meta (oben)	11 / 11	15 / 15	32 / 32
ortho / meta (unten)	30 / 30	6 / 6	0,5 / 0,5
para	18	58	35
% RCA H–Subst.	32 ± 3	34 ± 3	48 ± 2

$$[^{18}F] - CH_3CO_2F$$

	CF_3	F	OCH_3
ortho / meta (oben)	10 / 10	12 / 12	30 / 30
ortho / meta (unten)	32 / 32	3 / 3	0,5 / 0,5
para	16	70	39
% RCA H–Subst.	55 ± 2	74 ± 5	85 ± 3

eignen sich HF, Freon, Tetrachlorkohlenstoff und insbesondere Trifluoressigsäure. Die Temperaturen werden so niedrig wie möglich gehalten, meist im Bereich zwischen -78 und $0°$ C. Acetylhypofluorit, $[^{18}F]-CH_3CO_2F$ wird als milderes Fluorierungsreagenz dem $[^{18}F]-F_2$ vorgezogen. Der Unterschied in der Reaktivität und Selektivität zwischen den beiden Spezies ist jedoch gering (Coenen et al. 1986c; Franken 1987), wie Tabelle 9 für einfache monosubstituierte Benzole zeigt. Die Fluorierung ist wenig selektiv, und man erhält in aktivierten Aromaten vorwiegend ortho- und para-Substitution, in desaktivierten Systemen sind die Ausbeuten erwartungsgemäß kleiner. Hier erhält man auch eine beachtliche Substitution in der meta-Position. Die Ausbeuten sind beim Acetylhypofluorit im allgemeinen sehr ähnlich denen, die mit elementarem Fluor erhalten werden, wenn man die Bildung des AcOF aus F_2 (Verlust 50%) berücksichtigt.

Eine schnelle, regiospezifische elektrophile aromatische Fluorierung mit $[^{18}F]-F_2$ oder $[^{18}F]-CH_3CO_2F$ gelingt in speziellen Fällen auch über Demetallierungsreaktionen (Adam et al. 1981, 1986; Visser et al. 1984; Coenen u. Moerlein 1987):

$$\text{(56)}$$

In der Reihe M = Si, Ge, Sn erhält man für M = Sn die höchsten radiochemischen Ausbeuten (Coenen u. Moerlein 1987). Tabelle 10 zeigt darüber hinaus, daß auch im Falle der Destannylierung der Unterschied zwischen $[^{18}F]-F_2$ und $[^{18}F]-CH_3CO_2F$ bezüglich der radiochemischen Ausbeuten bei nicht zu tiefen Temperaturen vernachlässigbar klein ist. Protische Lösungsmittel sind weniger geeignet, und die Ausbeute wird deutlich kleiner. Die Desaktivierung durch den Erstsubstituenten (X) macht sich bei der Demetallierung deutlich weniger bemerkbar als bei der direkten Fluorierung.

Tabelle 10. Einfluß von Erstsubstituent und Metall auf die chemische Ausbeute der Fluordemetallierung in einfachen Aromaten. (Nach Coenen u. Moerlein 1987)

X/M	Sn	Ge	Si
OCH$_3$	70,4$\pm$6,6 (66,0$\pm$4,3)	35,4$\pm$1,4	19,8$\pm$3,0
CH$_3$	78,4$\pm$6,4	40,6$\pm$5,8 (16,4$\pm$1,8)	22,4$\pm$4,0 (9,1$\pm$1,1)
F	73,8$\pm$6,8	55,8$\pm$3,6	30,4$\pm$3,2
H	64,4$\pm$7,0 (68,2$\pm$5,7)	40,4$\pm$4,0 (8,5$\pm$0,5)	23,0$\pm$4,0 (3,5$\pm$0,3)
CF$_3$	35,0$\pm$2,8 (36,3$\pm$1,6)	10,4$\pm$1,6	2,4$\pm$0,5

Reaktionsbedingungen: 6–8 mM Lösung des Substrates in $CFCl_3$; 3–5 µMol $[^{18}F]-F_2$ bzw. $^{18}F-CH_3CO_2F$ (Werte in Klammern); Temperatur: $-78°$ C für F_2, $0°$ C für CH_3CO_2F. Die maximale theoretische radiochemische Ausbeute beim $[^{18}F]-F_2$ kann nur 50% betragen. Zum besseren Vergleich von $[^{18}F]-F_2$ und $[^{18}F]-AcOF$ wird deshalb die chemische Ausbeute angegeben.

Auch die Fluorierung über Organoquecksilberverbindungen bietet eine Möglichkeit zur Einführung von Fluor-18 (zur Übersicht s. ADAM 1986), die u.a. zur Präparation von [6-^{18}F]-Fluordopa genützt wurde (LUXEN et al. 1986, s. Abschnitt D.II.). Im allgemeinen ist die Demercurierungsreaktion nicht regioselektiv (VISSER et al. 1984).

Wie bei der direkten Fluorierung so sind auch bei der Fluordemetallierung die Produkte stark geträgert. Ein weiterer Nachteil bei komplexen Molekülen ist der Umstand, daß meist alle gegenüber dem Fluorierungsreagenz reaktiven funktionellen Gruppen geschützt werden müssen. Einführung und Hydrolyse der Schutzgruppen erfordern zusätzlich Zeit und erniedrigen die verfügbare ^{18}F-Produktaktivität stark. Hier ist stets der Aufwand der Isomerentrennung bei der direkten elektrophilen Fluorierung mit dem der Fluorodemetallierung gegeneinander abzuwägen. Speziell in stark aktivierten aromatischen Systemen ist der Vorteil der Demetallierung gegenüber der Direktfluorierung gering. So sind eine Reihe von komplexen Molekülen in hinreichender Ausbeute durch elektrophile Fluorierung erhalten worden (s.u. Abschnitt D). Die Anwendungen sind allerdings auf das Studium metabolischer Vorgänge mit relativ großen Stoffumsätzen von etwa 10^{-5}–10^{-3} Mol begrenzt. Vorgänge in kleineren Konzentrationsbereichen können mit hinreichender Empfindlichkeit in-vivo nur mit n.c.a. Radiopharmaka beobachtet werden.

2. Nukleophile Fluorierung

Die direkte nukleophile Fluorierung bereitet wegen der geringen Nukleophilie des Fluoridions in Gegenwart von aciden Protonen aufgrund seiner hohen Ladungsdichte große Schwierigkeiten. Zur direkten nukleophilen Fluorierung sind daher nur Substrate ohne H-acide funktionelle Gruppen und Lösungsmittel mit dipolar aprotischem Charakter geeignet. Darüber hinaus findet in aprotischen Lösungsmitteln oder in der Schmelze aufgrund der hohen Basizität des Fluoridions leicht eine konkurrierende Eliminierungsreaktion statt:

$$R\text{—}CH_2CH_2\text{—}X \ + \ ^{18}F^- \ \xrightarrow{\begin{array}{c} -\,X^- \\[2pt] \\[2pt] -\,H^{18}F \end{array}} \ \begin{array}{l} R\text{—}CH_2CH_2\text{—}^{18}F \\[8pt] R\text{—}CH{=}CH_2 \end{array} \tag{57}$$

Liegt das Fluoridion trägerfrei vor, so werden die Probleme der Solvatation und der Nebenreaktionen drastisch verstärkt. In Gegenwart des basischen, nichtisotopen Trägers CO_3^{2-} kann das durch Eliminierung entstehende $H^{18}F$ allerdings rezykliert und als $^{18}F^-$ erneut zur Reaktion gebracht werden. Das Carbonatanion hat darüber hinaus den Vorteil, daß es nicht als Nukleophil mit trägerfreiem Fluorid konkurriert. Leider kann es jedoch bei sehr Basen-empfindlichen Molekülen nicht verwendet werden. Hier muß ein weniger basisches Puffersystem eingesetzt werden.

Verschiedene Alkalifluoride wie $K^{18}F$, $Rb^{18}F$ und $Cs^{18}F$, Ammoniumfluoride $R_4N^{18}F$ sowie Übergangsmetallfluoride wie $Ag^{18}F$, $Ag^{18}F_2$, $Hg^{18}F_2$ sind zur direkten nukleophilen Fluorierung eingesetzt worden. Befriedigende Ausbeuten wurden außer mit $R_4N^{18}F$ als Phasentransferkatalysator mit diesen Verbindungen jedoch meist nicht erhalten.

Zur Anionenaktivierung und zur Fixierung des ^{18}F-Fluorids eignen sich vor allen Phasentransferkatalysatoren wie Tetrabutylammoniumhydroxid und andere Oniumsalze insbesondere der Aminopolyether (APE) 2.2.2. (z.B. Kryptofix 2.2.2. von Merck) in Verbindung mit K_2CO_3 als basische Matrix. So wurde der APE 2.2.2.-K_2CO_3-Komplex erfolgreich zur effizienten nukleophilen n.c.a.-Fluorierung eingesetzt (BLOCK et al. 1986a, 1987; COENEN et al. 1986a; HAMACHER et al. 1986). Bei Verwendung der üblichen dipolar aprotischen Lösungsmittel wie THF, Dioxan, Acetonitril, DMSO, Aceton und halogenierten Kohlenwasserstoffe können ^{18}F-Aktivitätsverluste durch einen unlöslichen und damit kaum noch reaktiven Bodenkörper hervorgerufen werden. Dies sollte möglichst vermieden werden, da bei vollständiger Lösung meist auch die Wandsorptionsprobleme entfallen. Die Löslichkeiten des K_2CO_3-APE 2.2.2.-Komplexes, die mit zunehmender Polarität der verschiedenen Lösungsmittel steigen, sind deshalb weitgehend auch für die Fluorierungsausbeuten verantwortlich (BLOCK et al. 1987).

Der Aminopolyether hat gegenüber bekannten Phasentransfer-Katalysatoren wie 18-Krone-6 oder Oniumsalzen den Vorteil, daß er die Löslichkeit der anorganischen Fluoride in dipolar aprotischen Lösungsmitteln aufgrund seiner dreidimensionalen Komplexierung des Kaliumions stärker erhöht. Durch die besseren Komplexierungseigenschaften des APE 2.2.2. wird der Anteil an wenig solvatisierten und damit hoch reaktiven Fluoridionen erhöht und somit die Reaktion beschleunigt. Bei der aliphatischen nukleophilen n.c.a. Fluorierung wird die optimale Ausbeute meist schon nach 10 min erreicht. Nachteile des Aminopolyethers sind sein relativ hoher Preis und eine geringe Toxizität. Letztere erfordert eine saubere Abtrennung vom hergestellten Radiopharmakon.

In Spezialfällen bietet die nukleophile Substitution auch eine Möglichkeit, ^{18}F in aromatische Ringe mit stark elektronenziehenden Gruppen (Hal., NO_2, CN) einzuführen (CACACE et al. 1981; ATTINA et al. 1983; BERRIDGE et al. 1982a; KNUST et al. 1982; SHIUE et al. 1984a; OBERDORFER et al. 1984; COENEN et al. 1985):

$$Y-C_6H_4-X \xrightarrow[-Y^-]{+\,^{18}F^-} {}^{18}F-C_6H_4-X \tag{58}$$

$$Y = Hal, NO_2, NR_3^+ ClO_4^-$$

$$X = NO_2, CN, -\overset{O}{\overset{\|}{C}}-R$$

Die Reaktion kann in aprotischen, polaren Lösungsmitteln wie DMSO bei Temperaturen von 80 bis 160° C oder in einer Acetamidschmelze durchgeführt werden. Vorteilhafter ist wiederum der aktivierte Austausch mittels Aminopolyether 2.2.2. in Gegenwart von K_2CO_3 (COENEN et al. 1985). Mit $[K/2.2.2.]^{+\,18}F^-$ gelingt z.B. der nukleophile Austausch elektronenziehender Gruppen schon bei 80° C mit guten radiochemischen Ausbeuten (s. Tabelle 11), so daß auch temperaturempfindliche Moleküle auf die Weise mit hoher spezifischer Aktivität (n.c.a.) markiert werden können.

Tabelle 11. Nukleophile aromatische n.c.a. $[^{18}F]$-Fluorierung in DMSO bei 80° C, mit APE 2.2.2./K_2CO_3. (Nach COENEN et al. 1985)

$$X-C_6H_4-Y + {}^{18}F^- \to X-C_6H_4-{}^{18}F + Y^-$$

X	Y	% Radiochemische Ausbeute
NO_2	NO_2	78 ± 5
CN	NO_2	72 ± 5
$COCH_3$	NO_2	38 ± 3
NO_2	Br	30 ± 2
CN	F	70 ± 4
CN	Br	33 ± 1
CN	Cl	24 ± 1
CN	NR_3^+	68 ± 4

Ein allgemeiner Weg, ^{18}F ausgehend vom Fluorid in aromatische Verbindungen einzuführen, geht über Dediazonierungsreaktionen wie etwa die Balz-Schiemann Reaktion.

$$R-\bigcirc-N_2^+ + [B^{18}FF_3]^- \xrightarrow{\Delta} R-\bigcirc-^{18}F \tag{59}$$

Allerdings ist sie durch die Verwendung von BF_4^- schlecht geeignet, da die spezifischen Aktivitäten a priori niedrig und die erreichbaren radiochemischen Ausbeuten gering sind (theoretisch 25%). Man hat deshalb andere Dediazonierungsreaktionen wie die Triazenmethode herangezogen, die prinzipiell zur regioselektiven, praktisch trägerfreien Einführung von ^{18}F ausgehend von [^{18}F]-Fluorid geeignet ist. Triazene bilden sich bei der Reaktion der Diazoniumverbindung mit sekundären Aminen in Gegenwart einer Base (B, Gl. 60) und können als stabile Quelle der Diazoniumkationen betrachtet werden, die im sauren Medium zu den üblichen Halodediazonierungsprodukten führen (Gl. 61)

$$ArN_2^+ + HNR_2 \xrightarrow[- HB]{B} Ar-N=N-NR_2 \tag{60}$$

$$R-\bigcirc-N=N-N\bigcirc + {}^{18}F^- \xrightarrow{H^+} R-\bigcirc-{}^{18}F + N_2 + HN\bigcirc \tag{61}$$

Bei allen bisherigen Anwendungen waren auch hier die radiochemischen Ausbeuten ohne Trägerzusatz extrem niedrig (maximal einige Prozent). Dennoch bietet die höhere Stabilität des Triazens und die chemische Ausgangsform des Fluors hier grundsätzliche Vorteile gegenüber der Schiemann-Reaktion. Die extrem geringen Ausbeuten bei der n.c.a. ^{18}F-Fluorierung sind auf die zahlreichen Nebenreaktionen zurückzuführen, die die intermediären sehr reaktiven Spezies, die bei der Zersetzung der Diazoniumverbindung entstehen, mit anderen Nukleophilen (Lösungsmittel, Substrat, Verunreinigungen) eingehen können, da das n.c.a. Fluorid nur in nano- bis mikromolaren Konzentrationen vorliegt.

3. Fluoralkylierung und Fluoracylierung

Die Einführung von ^{18}F über kleinere prosthetische Gruppen gelingt über die Fluoralkylierung und in speziellen Fällen über die Fluoracylierung. Die Fluoralkylierung stellt eine längerlebige Alternative zur ^{11}C-Alkylierung insbesondere zur ^{11}C-Methylierung dar. Als Alkylierungsmittel eignen sich radiofluorierte bifunktionelle Alkane, die über die anionenaktivierte nukleophile Substitution erhalten werden (BLOCK et al. 1987 a):

$$X-(CH_2)_n-X + n.c.a.\ ^{18}F^- \xrightarrow[\text{MeCN, 80 °C}]{[K/2.2.2.]^+} {}^{18}F-(CH_2)_n-X \tag{62}$$

$$X = Br, OMes, OTos$$

Besonders gute radiochemische Ausbeuten von >80% erhält man innerhalb von 10 min mit Bistosyloxyethan und -propan. Das n.c.a. [^{18}F]-Fluortosyloxyalkan wird in einem nachfolgenden Schritt zur Fluoralkylierung mit einer H-aciden Verbindung kondensiert (BLOCK et al. 1987 b):

$$^{18}F-(CH_2)_n-X + R-Y-H \xrightarrow[CO_3^{2-},\ \text{MeCN}]{[K/2.2.2.]^+} {}^{18}F-(CH_2)_n-Y-R \tag{63}$$

$$Y = O, S, N, P, C$$

Als Base für die Kondensationsreaktion wird das gleiche $APE - K_2CO_3$ System eingesetzt, das zur Fixierung und Anionenaktivierung des aktiven Fluorids (Gl. 62) dient. Der pK_a-Wert des Lösungsmittels muß größer sein als der des zu fluoralkylierenden Substrats, um eine Konkurrenz mit dem Substrat in der Deprotonierungsreaktion durch das Basensystem zu vermeiden. Da sowohl bei der Fluorierung (Gl. 62) als auch bei der nachfolgenden Fluoralkylierung (Gl. 63) das gleiche Basensystem verwendet wird, können die beiden Reaktionen in vielen Fällen als Eintopfreaktion durchgeführt werden und sind deshalb für eine Automatisierung besonders gut geeignet. Die n.c.a. Fluoralkylierung hat gegenüber der direkten nukleophilen Fluorierung den Vorteil, daß auch H-acide Verbindungen markiert werden können. Die Methode ist durch die unterschiedlichen Aciditäten der funktionellen Gruppen sehr selektiv. Da Biomoleküle oder Pharmaka häufiger H-acide als nukleofuge Gruppen besitzen, ist eine relativ breite Anwendungsmöglichkeit gegeben. Bei sehr Basen-empfindlichen Verbindungen muß das K_2CO_3 durch weniger basische Puffer ersetzt werden.

Im Hinblick auf die notwendigerweise schnelle Kondensationsreaktion, die eine Deprotonierung erforderlich macht, können Moleküle, die sich nur im wäßrigen Milieu lösen, nicht fluoralkyliert werden, da die Acidität des Wassers hoch ist und somit eine Konkurrenz zum Substrat bei der Deprotonierung darstellt. In diesen Fällen, die z.B. für Antikörper und andere Polypeptide von Interesse sind, bietet die Fluoracylierung eine Markierungsmöglichkeit. Als geeignetes Acylierungsreagenz eignet sich – besser als der wenig stabile und toxische Fluoressigsäureester – vor allem der Propiosäureester (BLOCK et al. 1987 c), der mit 95%iger radiochemischer Ausbeute n.c.a. erhalten werden kann:

$$H_3C\!-\!\underset{\underset{\displaystyle Br}{|}}{CH}\!-\!CO_2CH_3 \; + \; n.c.a. \; {}^{18}F^- \quad \xrightarrow[H^+]{2.2.2.} \quad H_3C\!-\!\underset{\underset{\displaystyle {}^{18}F}{|}}{CH}\!-\!CO_2CH_3 \qquad (64)$$

Mit Aminen wie z.B. n-Butylamin als Modellsubstanz können in wäßriger Lösung mit 0,1% NH_4Cl als Säure bei Rückflußtemperatur innerhalb von 10 min radiochemische Ausbeuten von 80% erhalten werden.

4. Einige Basissynthesen mit kurzlebigem n.c.a. Radiobromid und -iodid

Wie bei der Einführung von ${}^{18}F$, so ist auch bei der Markierung mit Radiobrom und -iod zweckmäßig, vom Radiohalogenid und nicht vom elementaren Radiohalogen auszugehen, um möglichst hohe spezifische Aktivitäten zu erhalten. Die einfachste Reaktion ist wiederum die nukleophile Substitution an Aliphaten (s. z.B. Abschnitt D.III.), auf die hier nicht näher eingegangen werden soll.

Anders als bei der Fluorierung kann man beim Bromid und Iodid folgende Methoden einsetzen (zur Übersicht s. SEEVERS u. COUNSELL 1982; COENEN et al. 1983):
- direkte elektrophile Substitution
  (über Oxidationsmittel, auch enzymatische),
- elektrophile Demetallierung,
- nukleophile Substitution
  (Halogenaustausch, Dediazonierung etc.).

Bei der direkten elektrophilen Substitution besteht das Problem im wesentlichen darin, ein geeignetes Oxidationsmittel zu finden, um das Elektrophil X in-situ zu erzeugen:

$$*X^- \xrightarrow{\text{Oxidation}} *X^{\delta+} \xrightarrow{R-\text{\Large$\bigcirc$}} R-\underset{\displaystyle X^*}{\text{\Large$\bigcirc$}} \qquad (65)$$

Tabelle 12. Milde organische Oxidationsmittel zur elektrophilen Radiobromierung und -iodierung ausgehend von Radiohalogenid ohne Trägerzusatz. (Nach COENEN et al. 1983)

Oxidationsmittel	Lösungsmittel	Bemerkung
Chloramin-T (CAT) Dichloramin-T (DCT)	H_2O, AcOH TFA, TFAA AcOH, CH_2Cl_2, CH_3OH CCl_4, TFA, DMF, TFAA	kurze Reaktionszeiten (Minuten) und kleine Reagenskonzentration (10^{-3} M)
N-Chlorsuccinimid (NCS)	EtOH, TFA, TFAA	lange Reaktionszeiten
N-Chlortetrafluorsuccinimid (NCTFS)	TFA, TFAA	lange Reaktionszeiten; wasserempfindlich
Trifluormethansulfonylhypochlorit (CF_3SO_3Cl)	Nitrobenzol	höhere Temperaturen ($70–150°$ C);
Trifluoracetylhypochlorit (CF_3CO_2Cl)	TFA	wasserempfindlich

TFA = Trifluoressigsäure, TFAA = Trifluoressigsäureanhydrid, DMF = Dimethylformamid

Diese Reaktion verläuft im allgemeinen nicht regiospezifisch, sondern man erhält je nach Art des Erstsubstituenten und des Elektrophils eine entsprechende Isomerenverteilung. Dennoch sind diese elektrophilen Substitutionsreaktionen über die Oxidation des Halogenids zumindest an aktivierten Aromaten einfach und schnell durchzuführen, und das gewünschte Isomere kann mit Hilfe der HPLC meist schnell abgetrennt werden.

Zahlreiche anorganische Oxidationsmittel wie $KMnO_4$, MnO_2, $CH_3CO_3H(H_2O_2/ CH_3COOH)$, HNO_3, $CeCl_4$, $TlCl_3$, KIO_3 werden zu diesem Zweck eingesetzt. Aufgrund ihrer hohen Oxidationskraft führen sie jedoch häufig zu Oxidationsnebenprodukten; milde organische Reagenzien sind deshalb oft vorteilhafter, obwohl auch sie vor allem im Falle der trägerfreien n.c.a. Halogenierung zu Nebenprodukten führen. In Tabelle 12 sind die wichtigsten organischen Oxidationsmittel sowie einige geeignete Lösungsmittel aufgeführt, die eine relativ milde elektrophile Halogenierung ausgehend vom Halogenid gestatten.

Zahlreiche Iodierungsmethoden sind speziell für die Proteinmarkierung mit den längerlebigen Iodisotopen ^{125}I ($T_{1/2} = 60$ d) und ^{131}I ($T_{1/2} = 8$ d) entwickelt worden. Eine der bekanntesten ist die Chloramin-T-Methode (HUNTER u. GREENWOOD 1962; GREENWOOD u. HUNTER 1963). Die Anwendung von Chloramin-T (CAT) oder Dichloramin-T (DCT) ist einfach und schnell und sowohl für die praktisch trägerfreie Iodierung als auch Bromierung geeignet (PETZOLD u. COENEN 1981; HE YOUFENG et al. 1982; COENEN et al. 1983). Gute radiochemische Ausbeuten erhält man ohne Trägerzusatz, allerdings nur in aktivierten aromatischen Systemen. Problematisch ist insbesondere beim Arbeiten ohne Trägerzusatz, daß die zur Oxidation verwendeten Chlorverbindungen (s. Tabelle 12) leicht auch zu chlorierten Nebenprodukten führen. Deshalb erweist sich in einigen Fällen Peroxyessigsäure (CH_3CO_3H) als geeigneteres Oxidationsmittel (KATZENELLENBOGEN et al. 1981; FRIEDMAN et al. 1982; MOERLEIN et al. 1986 a).

Elektrophile Demetallierungsreaktionen bieten gegenüber der direkten Halogenierung einige Vorteile. Da die Kohlenstoff-Metall Bindung empfindlicher ist gegenüber einem elektrophilen Angriff, erhält man in vielen Fällen bei kurzer Reaktionszeit und milden Reaktionsbedingungen hohe Ausbeuten. Wegen der leichten Reaktion an der Kohlenstoff-Metall Bindung im Vergleich zu anderen Positionen ist diese Radiohalogenierung praktisch regiospezifisch. Anders als die Fluorodemetallierung kann die Bromo- und Iododemetallierung durch die hier mögliche in-situ Oxidation des eingesetzten Bromids und Iodids ohne Trägerzusatz erfolgen. Geeignete Metalle sind B, Si, Ge, Sn, Tl und Hg. Elektrophile Halogen-Spezies reagieren schnell mit Organoboranen zu Alkyl- oder Arylhalogeniden. Unter Verwendung von Chloramin-T (CAT) als Oxidationsmittel sind Alkylhalogenide (Kabalka et al. 1982a, b) und Arylhalogenide (Kabalka et al. 1982c) ausgehend von [^{82}Br]-Bromid oder [^{123}I]-Iodid ohne Trägerzusatz mit guter radiochemischer Ausbeute markiert worden:

$$R\text{-}C_6H_4\text{-}B(OR')_2 \quad \xrightarrow[\text{H}_2\text{O}]{\text{*Br}^-/\text{CAT}} \quad R\text{-}C_6H_4\text{-*Br} \;+\; HOB(OR')_2 \qquad (66)$$

Auch Organosiliziumverbindungen wie Trimethylsilylarene sind zur Radiobromierung und -iodierung unter Verwendung von N-Chlorsuccinimid (NCS) als Oxidationsmittel eingesetzt worden (Wilbur et al. 1982):

$$CH_3\text{-}C_6H_4\text{-}Si(CH_3)_3 \quad \xrightarrow{\text{*I}^-/\text{NCS}} \quad CH_3\text{-}C_6H_4\text{-*I} \;+\; ClSi(CH_3)_3 \qquad (67)$$

Die relativ hohe C−Si Bindungsenergie begrenzt allerdings diesen Reaktionstyp auf weniger aktivierte Aromaten, da im Falle der stark aktivierten Substrate weitgehender Verlust der Regiospezifität auftritt. Besser geeignet sind zinnorganische Verbindungen, da die Zinn-Kohlenstoff Bindung gegenüber einem elektrophilen Angriff reaktiver ist als die Kohlenstoff-Silizium Bindung. Trialkylarylzinn-Verbindungen sind ohne Trägerzusatz mit hoher radiochemischer Ausbeute in Arylbromide überführt worden (Adam et al. 1982):

$$MeO\text{-}C_6H_4\text{-}Sn(CH_3)_3 \quad \xrightarrow{\text{*Br}^-/\text{CAT}} \quad MeO\text{-}C_6H_4\text{-*Br} \;+\; Cl\,Sn(CH_3)_3 \qquad (68)$$

Für die Halodemetallierung ausgehend von den entsprechenden Trimethylzinn-, -germanium- oder -siliziumverbindungen konnte im Falle der n.c.a. Bromierung und Iodierung wie bei der Fluorierung gezeigt werden (Moerlein u. Coenen 1985), daß die Destannylierung am effektivsten verläuft und die Reaktivität der Halogenierung linear vom aktivierenden Einfluß des Erstsubstituenten abhängt. Die in-situ Oxidation des n.c.a. Halogenides kann durch ein organisches Oxidationsmittel (s. Tabelle 12) erfolgen. Zur Vermeidung der hierbei entstehenden chlorierten Nebenprodukte kann auch hier Peroxyessigsäure verwendet werden (Moerlein et al. 1986a). In diesem Falle entstehen zwar u.a. auch protonierte Nebenprodukte, die sich aber leichter von den halogenierten Produkten abtrennen lassen als die chlorierten. Die Verwendung von Peroxyessigsäure, die in-situ aus Essigsäure und H_2O_2 entsteht, erlaubt eine regiospezifische Halodestannylierung innerhalb von wenigen Minuten. Die Ioddestannylierung erfolgt in Modellsystemen mit 95%iger Ausbeute und zwar sowohl mit Dichloramin-T als auch mit H_2O_2 praktisch sofort, ein Umstand, der auch zur Markierung mit dem sehr kurzlebigen Generatornuklid ^{122}I ($T_{1/2}=3{,}6$ min) ausgenutzt wurde (Moerlein et al. 1987).

Eine selektivere Halogenierung als die direkte elektrophile Substitution bietet auch die Halodemercurierung (zur Übersicht s. Adam 1986). Allerdings erhält man immer noch ein Substitutionsmuster, das der elektrophilen Merkurierung entspricht. Die isomeren Hg-organischen Verbindungen sind jedoch in vielen Fällen so stabil, daß sie z.B. chromatographisch aufgetrennt werden können. Darüber hinaus gestattet die Verwendung besonders stabiler

Aryl-Mercaptyl-Quecksilberverbindungen (ArHgSR) ihre Fixierung an Säulenmaterial. Nach der Reaktion mit dem elektrophilen Halogen kann so das Produkt (ArX) eluiert werden, während das Mercaptylsalz auf der Säule bleibt (FLANAGAN et al. 1986a). Verschiedene Steroide sind über Quecksilbervorläufer mit Erfolg radiohalogeniert worden (FLANAGAN et al. 1986b, s. Abschnitt D.IV).

In vielen Fällen gelingt die selektive Einführung eines Radiohalogens in einen aromatischen Ring über die nukleophile Substitution. Anders als beim ^{18}F sind im Falle des Radiobroms und -iods Dediazonierungsreaktionen, insbesondere die Triazenmethode (s. Abschnitt C.III.2.) auch praktisch trägerfrei (n.c.a.) mit guter Ausbeute anwendbar (zur Übersicht s. COENEN et al. 1983). Eine andere Möglichkeit, die nukleophile Substitution in dafür nicht aktivierten aromatischen Verbindungen zu katalysieren, bietet die Anwendung von Cu(I) Salzen. Verschiedene Radiopharmaka wie Hippursäure (WANEK 1981), Phenylfettsäuren (FRITZBERG u. ESHIMA 1982; MERTENS 1986; DOUGAN et al. 1986), N-Isopropyl-p-iodamphetamine (MERTENS 1985) sowie Steroide (TARLE et al. 1978, 1979; FLANAGAN 1981) sind durch Cu(I)-katalysierten Iod-Isotopenaustausch auf einfache Weise markiert worden. Diese einfachen Austauschmethoden eignen sich insbesondere für Markierungsbestecke (kits) (MERTENS et al. 1985, 1986). Hierbei ist allerdings die spezifische Aktivität inhärent niedrig, jedoch für Fluß- oder Metabolismus Tracer meist ausreichend.

Eine weitere Möglichkeit, den aromatischen Halogenaustausch zu beschleunigen, besteht in der Verwendung eines geschmolzenen Systems. Polare Lösungsmittel mit niedrigem Schmelzpunkt wie Acetamid oder Benzoesäure sind in einigen Fällen verwendet worden, um Radiopharmaka zu radioiodieren (ELIAS u. LOTTERHOS 1976; THAKUR et al. 1975; WESTERA u. GIJLSWIJK 1979; EISENHUT 1982).

Eine milde und schnelle Methode des Iodisotopenaustauschs bietet auch die Festkörperreaktion in einer Ammoniumsulfat-Matrix (MANGNER et al. 1982; OTTO et al. 1986).

D. Spezielle Synthesen ausgewählter organischer Radiopharmaka

I. Kohlenhydrate

Kohlenhydrate sind wichtige Substrate für den Energiestoffwechsel von Herz und Hirn. Das Hirn benötigt ausschließlich D-Glukose, um daraus seine Energie zu gewinnen. Für D-Glukose besteht ein Transportsystem über die Blut-Hirn-Schranke, auf dem auch einige ähnliche Zucker durch erleichterte Diffusion transportiert werden (PARDRIDGE u. OLDENDORF 1975). Allerdings bestehen für Zuckeranaloge enge strukturelle Anforderungen: es werden nur Analoge transportiert, die eine all-trans, all-äquatoriale Anordnung der elektronegativen Substituenten enthalten, wie dies für D-Glukose typisch ist. Auch kann nicht an jeder Position die Hydroxygruppe gegen Halogen ersetzt werden. Daher ist die Zahl der in Frage kommenden und bisher untersuchten Substanzen relativ begrenzt (Tabelle 13).

Als erstes ist die ^{11}C-markierte D-Glukose selbst eingesetzt worden, die über die Photosynthese mit $^{11}CO_2$ synthetisiert werden kann (LIFTON u. WELCH 1971). Bei der medizinischen Anwendung der [^{11}C]-D-Glukose zur nichtinvasiven Untersuchung des regionalen Glukosestoffwechsels im Hirn zeigte sich, daß es äußerst schwierig ist, aus den gemessenen Verteilungsdaten Rückschlüsse auf den Stoffwechsel zu ziehen. Durch Wiederverwendung des Kataboliten $^{11}CO_2$ und anderen Kataboliten der Glukose für andere Stoffwechselwege liegen viele verschiedene markierte Verbindungen nebeneinander vor (RAICHLE et al. 1978), zwi-

Tabelle 13. ^{11}C- bzw. ^{18}F-markierte Glukose und Analoge zur nichtinvasiven Bestimmung des regionalen Glukosestoffwechsels bzw. -transports mittels PET

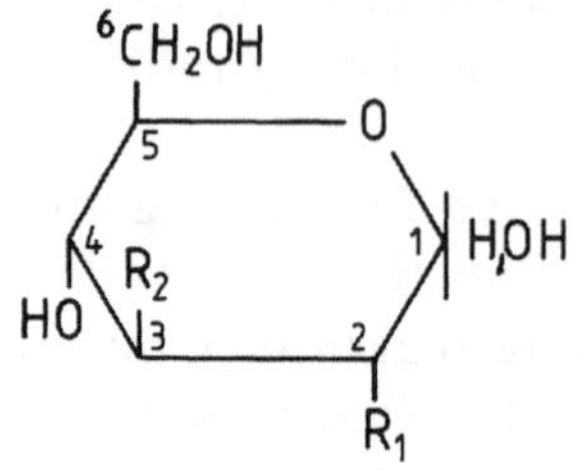

^{6}CH$_2$OH — 5 — O — 1 — H,OH — ^{4} R$_2$ — HO — 3 — 2 — R$_1$

Glukose und Analoge	R$_1$	R$_2$	Synthese
[U-^{11}C]-D-Glukose (G)	OH	OH	Lifton und Welch (1971) Goulding und Palmer (1973) Ehrin et al. (1980)
[1-^{11}C]-D-Glukose	OH	OH	Shiue und Wolf (1981)
[1-^{11}C]-Desoxy-D-glukose (DG)	H	OH	Shiue et al. (1979) Mestelan et al. (1979) MacGregor et al. (1981)
3-O-[^{11}C]-Methyl-D-glukose (MG)	OH	O^{11}CH$_3$	Kloster et al. (1982)
[2-^{18}F]-2-Fluor-2-desoxy-D-glukose (2-FDG)	^{18}F	OH	s. Tabelle 14
[3-^{18}F]-3-Fluor-3-desoxy-D-glukose (3-FDG)	OH	^{18}F	Tewson et al. (1978)

schen denen das PET-Gerät natürlich nicht unterscheiden kann. Dennoch sind Modelle zur Quantifizierung entwickelt worden (Blomquist et al. 1985).

Anders als die Glukose wird die 2-Desoxy-D-glukose (DG) nur im ersten Schritt des Glukosestoffwechsels umgesetzt. DG wird wie die Glukose über den gleichen Transportmechanismus in die Zelle transportiert und dort ebenfalls phosphoryliert, sie kann dann aber die Zelle nicht mehr verlassen (blockierter Stoffwechsel), da sie nicht weiter verstoffwechselt wird, und die Rückreaktion vernachlässigbar langsam ist. Auf diese Weise wird die DG entsprechend dem Glukoseumsatz in der Zelle akkumuliert. Mit ^{14}C-markierter DG konnte so der Glukosestoffwechsel des Gehirns im Tierexperiment quantitativ autoradiographisch erfaßt werden (Sokoloff et al. 1977). Es wurde schließlich gezeigt, daß der Ersatz des H-Atoms in der 2 Position der DG durch ein Fluoratom (Gallagher et al. 1977) die biochemischen Eigenschaften der DG praktisch nicht verändert. Die ^{18}F-markierte Verbindung [2-^{18}F]-Fluor-2-desoxy-D-glukose (2-FDG) konnte so auch zur regionalen Erfassung des Glukosestoffwechsels mittels PET eingesetzt werden (Reivich et al. 1979; Phelps et al. 1979).

Auch das Glukose-Analoge 3-O-Methylglukose (MG) wird über den gleichen Träger wie D-Glukose durch die Blut-Hirn-Schranke transportiert. Anders als Glukose oder DG wird MG jedoch überhaupt nicht verstoffwechselt, sondern sie verläßt das Hirn wieder unverändert. Damit bietet sich die Möglichkeit zur Messung des Glukosetransports in Herz und Hirn (Vyska et al. 1982; Feinendegen et al. 1986). Auch [3-^{18}F]-Fluor-3-desoxy-D-glukose (3-FDG) ist ein Substrat für den Hexose-Träger und wird durch die Blut-Hirn-Schranke transportiert. Die Phosphorylierungsrate ist jedoch zu langsam für die Messung des Glukoseumsatzes und zu schnell für einen guten Transport-Tracer (Holden et al. 1983).

Gleichmäßig markierte [U-^{11}C]-D-Glukose kann wie das ^{14}C-markierte Produkt durch Photosynthese hergestellt werden (Lifton u. Welch 1971; Goulding u. Palmer 1973; Ehrin et al. 1980):

$$^{11}CO_2 + \text{Blattgrün oder Grünalgen} \quad \xrightarrow[\text{2. Alkohol-Extraktion}]{\text{1. Photosynthese}} \quad \begin{array}{l} [^{11}C]\text{-D-Glukose} \\ [^{11}C]\text{-D-Fruktose} \\ [^{11}C]\text{-Saccharose} \\ \quad \text{Phosphate} \end{array}$$

$$\xrightarrow[\substack{\text{4. Neutralisation} \\ \text{5. Entfernung der} \\ \text{Pigmente durch} \\ \text{Chloroform-Extr.} \\ \text{6. Entfernung der} \\ \text{Salze durch} \\ \text{Ionenaustauscher}}]{\text{3. Hydrolyse, H}^+} \quad \begin{array}{l} [^{11}C]\text{-D-Glukose} \\ [^{11}C]\text{-D-Fruktose} \end{array} \quad \xrightarrow{\text{7. HPLC}} [^{11}C]\text{-D-Glukose} \qquad (69)$$

Hierzu wird $^{11}CO_2$ unter UV-Beleuchtung z.B. über Spinatblätter zirkuliert (ca. 20 min). Schneller (max. 3 min) verläuft die Inkorporation bei Verwendung von Grünalgen (Scenedesmus obtusiusculus Chod), denen $H^{11}CO_3^-$ angeboten wird (EHRIN et al. 1980). Die D-Glukose kann mit Hilfe der Hochleistungsflüssigkeitschromatographie (HPLC = high performance liquid chromatography) ebenfalls innerhalb von wenigen Minuten abgetrennt werden (GOULDING 1979; STRAATMAN u. WELCH 1973a; ISHIWATA et al. 1982). Eine automatisierte Photosynthese von $[U-^{11}C]$-D-Glukose für die Routineproduktion ist beschrieben worden (ISHIWATA et al. 1982). $[1-^{11}C]$-D-Glukose ist über die Cyanhydrin-Methode ausgehend von $[^{11}C]-NaCN$ und D-Arabinose hergestellt worden (SHIUE u. WOLF 1981). Das Cyanhydrin wird durch kontrollierte Reduktion mittels Raney-Nickel zu $[1-^{11}C]$-D-Glukose und $[1-^{11}C]$-D-Mannose konvertiert (Kiliani Reaktion), die mit Hilfe der HPLC getrennt werden.

Von besonderem Interesse im Hinblick auf die mögliche Quantifizierung und die Wiederholbarkeit der Untersuchung am selben Tag ist die ^{11}C-markierte 2-Desoxy-D-glukose und ihre Analoga. $[1-^{11}C]$-2-Desoxy-D-glukose kann über die nukleophile Substitution durch das $[^{11}C]$-Cyanidion am geschützten Substrat, einem 2,3:4,5-Di-O-isopropyliden-D-arabinitol mit geeigneter Abgangsgruppe (Tosylat, Trifluormethansulfonat) erhalten werden (SHIUE et al. 1979; MESTELAN et al. 1979; MACGREGOR et al. 1981; VAN HAVER et al. 1985):

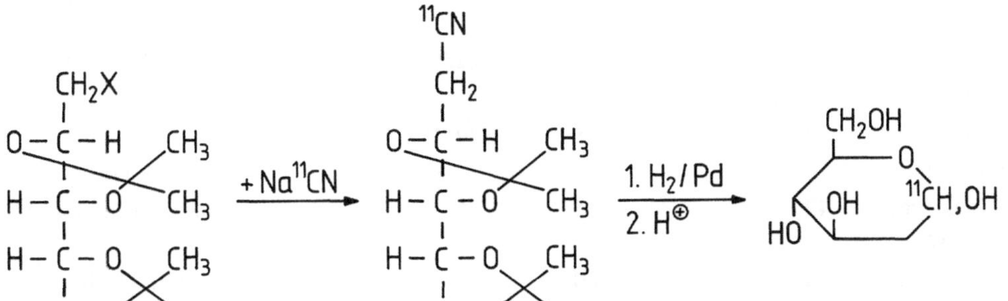

$$\text{(70)}$$

$$X = OSO_2C_7H_7 \, , \, I \, , \, OSO_2CF_3$$

Das reine Produkt kann innerhalb von etwa einer Stunde mit radiochemischen Ausbeuten von 20–30% erhalten werden.

Die nicht-metabolisierbare 3-O-$[^{11}C]$-Methyl-D-glukose kann durch Methylierung des Kalium-Salzes der Diaceton-D-glukose und anschließende hydrolytische Entfernung der

Schutzgruppen synthetisiert werden (Kloster et al. 1980):

$$
\text{(71)}
$$

Synthese und Abtrennung der MG von der D-Glukose mittels HPLC können innerhalb von 40 Minuten abgeschlossen werden. Die Synthese von 3-O-[^{11}C]-Methyl-D-glukose kann im Routinebetrieb in einer Zelle fernbedient durchgeführt werden (Laufer u. Kloster 1982).

Das bisher im Zusammenhang mit PET Studien (Hirn, Herz, Tumor) am meisten eingesetzte Glukosederivat ist die [2-^{18}F]-FDG, das Fluoranaloge der 2-Desoxy-D-glukose. Während die oben beschriebene [1-^{11}C]-2-Desoxy-D-glukose den Vorteil hat, daß die Untersuchungen am selben Tag wiederholt werden können (Kontrolle am Patienten), bietet [2-^{18}F]-FDG die Möglichkeit, die längere Halbwertszeit des ^{18}F ($T_{1/2} = 110$ min) zu nutzen. Dies ist nicht nur für den Transport zu entfernteren Anwendungsorten, sondern auch im Hinblick auf die maximale Anreicherung vorteilhaft, da letztere erst 45–60 min nach Injektion erreicht ist. Wegen der relativ breiten Anwendung der [2-^{18}F]-FDG sind zahlreiche elektrophile und nukleophile Synthesen durchgeführt worden. Eine Zusammenstellung mit den wichtigsten Parametern gibt die Tabelle 14. Die erste Markierungssynthese wurde über die elektrophile

Tabelle 14. Die wichtigsten Synthesemethoden für [2-^{18}F]-FDG

Methode	Radiochemische Ausbeute (%)	Zeit (min)	2-FDG/2-FDM (Bida 1984, Shiue 1985a)	Literatur
F_2 + TAG[a] in Freon	10	90	90/10	Ido et al. (1978) Fowler et al. (1981)
F_2 + Glucal in H_2O	30	30	65/35	Bida et al. (1984)
CH_3COOF + TAG in CH_3COOH	20	70	84/16	Shiue et al. (1982)
XeF_2 + TAG in Ether BF_3OEt_2	20	45	79/21	Shiue et al. (1983) Sood et al. (1983)
CH_3COOF (gasförmig) + Glucal in H_2O	40	15	45/55	Ehrenkaufer et al. (1984)
CH_3COOF (gasförmig) + TAG in Freon	20	60	95/5	Bida et al. (1984)
F^- + 2-Triflat	10	120	n.b.	Levy et al. (1982)
F^- + zykl. Sulfatester	40 20	40 150	n.b. >99	Tewson (1983) Vora et al. (1985)
F^- + 1,6 Anhydro-hexopyranose	(60)	–	n.b.	Haradahira et al. (1985)
F^- + 1-NO$_2$-Epoxid	10	105	n.b.	Beeley et al. (1984)
F^- + 2-Triflat	80	50	>99	Hamacher et al. (1986a)

[a] Triacetylglucal

Addition von $[^{18}F]$-F_2 an das geschützte Glucal 3,4,6-Tri-O-acetyl-D-glucal (TAG) erreicht (GALLAGHER et al. 1977, 1978; IDO et al. 1978):

$$(72)$$

Die cis-Addition von $[^{18}F]$-F_2 führt zu den zwei Epimeren. Diese Derivate der D-Glukose und D-Mannose können z.B. durch Filtration über Silicagel getrennt werden. Nach Hydrolyse erhält man $[2\text{-}^{18}F]$-FDG nach chromatographischer Reinigung in radiochemischen Ausbeuten von etwa 10 bis 12%. Eine deutliche Verbesserung, d.h. etwas höhere radiochemische Ausbeuten (20%) an ^{18}F-markierter 2-FDG brachte die Verwendung von $[^{18}F]$-AcOF (s.o. Gl. 33). Das $[^{18}F]$-Acetylhypofluorit wird wie erwähnt entweder in-situ aus $[^{18}F]-F_2$ und Ammoniumacetat in Essigsäurelösung erzeugt (SHIUE et al. 1982) oder aber in einer heterogenen Gas-fest-Reaktion beim Durchleiten von $Ne-[^{18}F]-F_2$ durch eine Säule mit KOAc/HOAc (EHRENKAUFER et al. 1984) oder $NaOAc \cdot 3H_2O$ (BIDA et al. 1984). Während im allgemeinen elementares Fluor mit organischen Verbindungen in möglichst inerten organischen Lösungsmitteln zur Reaktion gebracht wird, zeigen neuere Untersuchungen, daß die relativ geringen Konzentrationen an $[^{18}F]-F_2$ im inerten Targetgas Neon auch in wäßrigen Lösungen des ungeschützten D-Glucals zur Reaktion gebracht werden können (z. Übersicht s. BIDA et al. 1984). Die Synthesezeit kann hierdurch wesentlich verkürzt werden. Der stereochemische Verlauf der elektrophilen Anlagerung hängt sehr stark von der Polarität des Lösungsmittels, der Art des Fluorierungsagens und der Struktur des Substrates ab. In allen Fällen entsteht neben 2-FDG ein mehr oder weniger großer Anteil der Mannose (2-FDM, s. Tabelle 14). Dies ist vor allem bei der Fluorierung des ungeschützten Glucals mit Acetylhypofluorit zu beachten. Hier entstehen neben den entsprechenden acetylierten Produkten beide Epimere 2-FDG und 2-FDM (EHRENKAUFER et al. 1984):

$$(73)$$

Auch die Synthese von $[^{18}F]-FDG$ über $[^{18}F]-XeF_2$ (SHIUE et al. 1983; SOOD et al. 1983) führt nur zu mäßigen Ausbeuten. Die Herstellung von $[^{18}F]-XeF_2$ in hohen radiochemischen Ausbeuten und hinreichender spezifischer Aktivität ist darüber hinaus relativ aufwendig. Im Hinblick auf die Einfachheit der Synthese und die Reinheit des Produktes ist unter den elektrophilen Methoden der 2-FDG Synthese vor allem die von BIDA et al. (1984)

zu empfehlen, die von gasförmigem $[^{18}F]$-Acetylhypofluorit und TAG ausgeht. Die Synthese kann als Eintopfverfahren durchgeführt werden (Schema III), in dem man on-line Acetylhypofluorit durch die Lösung von TAG in Freon leitet. Entfernung des Freons und anschließende Hydrolyse kann im selben Gefäß durchgeführt werden.

0.1% $[^{18}F]-F_2$ in Ne im Hochdrucktarget, expandiert zur on-line Reaktion mit festem $CH_3COOK \cdot 1.5\ CH_3COOH$ zu $[^{18}F]$-Acetylhypofluorit

Vorläufer | Strömungsgeschwindigkeit:
Präparation | 100 ml Ne/min

Durchleiten durch Lösung von TAG in Freon

Additionsreaktion | Zimmertemperatur

Zugabe von 1 N HCl, Entfernung des Freons durch Erhitzen

Hydrolyse | 15 min, 130° C, Rückfluß

Durch Säulen-Serie von AG11A8, Al_2O_3, C-18 Sep-Pak leiten

Deionisation | Elution mit Wasser

Einstellen einer isotonischen Lösung, Sterilfitration

$[2-^{18}F]$-FDG + $[2-^{18}F]$-FDM

Schema III. Fließschema der $[2-^{18}F]$-FDG-Synthese via Addition von $[^{18}F]$-Acetylhypofluorit. (Nach EHRENKAUFER et al. 1984)

n.c.a. $^{18}F^-$ in wäßriger Lösung; Zugabe von APE 2.2.2./K_2CO_3

Trocknung des $^{18}F^-$ | 5–10 min, 100° C, He-Strom oder Vakuum

Zugabe von 1,3,4,6,tetra-O-acetyl-2-O-triflyl-β-D-Mannose in CH_3CN

Substitution | 5–10 min, 100° C, Rückfluß

Zugabe von H_2O, C-18 Sep-Pak Filtration

Abtrennung von APE 2.2.2. und $^{18}F^-$ | Elution mit 0.01 N HCl, Elution des geschützten Zuckers mit Acetonitril

Eindampfen zur Trockne, Zugabe von 1 N HCl

Hydrolyse | 15 min, 130° C, Rückfluß

C-18 Sep-Pak Filtration, AG11A8 Verzögerungssäule + Al_2O_3

Deionisation | Elution mit H_2O

Einstellen einer isotonischen Lösung, Sterilfiltration

$[2-^{18}F]$-FDG

Schema IV. Fließschema der $[2-^{18}F]$-FDG-Synthese via APE 2.2.2. gestützter nukleophiler Substitution mit $^{18}F^-$. (Nach HAMACHER et al. 1986a, c)

Beachtung verdienen Markierungssynthesen für $[2-^{18}F]$-FDG, die anstelle von $[^{18}F]-F_2$ vom leichter zugänglichen und handhabbaren $[^{18}F]$-Fluorid ausgehen (LEVY et al. 1982; TEWSON 1983). Diese Methode hat den Vorteil, daß theoretisch 100% des Radiofluorids umgesetzt werden können, während beim $[^{18}F]-F_2$ die radiochemische Ausbeute nur maximal 50% betragen kann. Sie ist für Niederenergie-Protonenbeschleuniger besonders gut geeignet, da diese nur $[^{18}F]$-Fluorid in hinreichender Ausbeute leicht erzeugen können (s. Abschnitt B.IV). Außerdem können hier sehr hohe spezifische Aktivitäten erhalten werden. Beide Methoden verlaufen stereoselektiv und gehen deshalb von D-Mannose Derivaten aus, bei denen alle

OH-Gruppen gegen eine nukleophile Substitution geschützt werden außer der in der C-2 Position. Die erste Methode (LEVY et al. 1982) verwendet das Triflat am C-2 als Abgangsgruppe. Sie hat allerdings den Nachteil, daß der Methylether am C-3 sehr stabil gegen die hydrolytische Abspaltung ist und daher relativ drastische Reaktionsbedingungen erforderlich sind, die zu sehr kleinen radiochemischen Ausbeuten von nur etwa 10% führen. Bei der zweiten Methode (TEWSON 1983) wird ein zyklischer Sulfatester am C-2, C-3 verwendet, der durch nukleophile Substitution das 2-Fluor-3-sulfat bildet. Nach Hydrolyse der Schutzgruppen und chromatographischer Reinigung erhält man 2-FDG in 40%iger Ausbeute. Von den nukleophilen Methoden ist zweifellos die von HAMACHER et al. (1986a) die effizienteste und einfachste. Der Vorläufer, die tetraacetylierte-2-triflylmannose ist leicht zugänglich, und die radiochemische Ausbeute ist hoch. Die Anionenaktivierung kann wieder mit dem Aminopolyether 2.2.2. erfolgen:

$$[\text{K}/2.2.2.]^{+\,18}\text{F}^- \qquad (74)$$

Wichtig ist bei dieser Synthese, daß die Konzentration an kaltem Fluorid klein gehalten wird (Fluorid/Edukt $\leq 10^{-3}$), da andernfalls durch die Basizität des Carbonat/Fluoridsystems konkurrierende Eliminationsreaktionen überhand nehmen. Bei zu hoher Fluoridkonzentration ist die Abnahme der Eduktkonzentration durch Parallelreaktionen so rasch, daß mit steigendem Fluorid/Edukt-Verhältnis die Ausbeute des Substitutionsproduktes 2-FDG schließlich drastisch abnimmt (HAMACHER et al. 1986c). Im Hinblick auf die Bedeutung der Synthese ist in Schema IV der detaillierte Reaktionsverlauf wiedergegeben.

Mehrere automatisierte bzw. fernbediente $[2-^{18}\text{F}]$-FDG-Synthesen sind beschrieben worden (BARRIO et al. 1981a; FOWLER et al. 1981; ADAM et al. 1984; IWATA et al. 1984; ALEXOFF et al. 1986; DIKSIC u. JOLLY 1986). Sie sind für die jeweils angewandte Syntheseart spezifisch. In Abb. 6 ist das Schema eines fernbedienbaren Verfahrens wiedergegeben, das bei der nukleophilen APE 2.2.2. gestützten Einführung von $[^{18}\text{F}]$-Fluorid (Schema IV) verwendet wird (HAMACHER et al. 1986a, c). Das Kernstück der FDG-Syntheseapparatur ist ein geschlossenes Reaktionsgefäß, bestehend aus einem chemisch inerten Glaskohlenstoffzylinder (Sigradur) von 15 ml Inhalt und einem säureresistenten Reaktorkopf aus Inconel. Der Reaktor ist von einem elektrisch heizbaren Kupfermantel umgeben und mit einer Druck- und Temperaturmeßsonde ausgerüstet. Die Kühlung des Reaktionsgefäßes erfolgt durch gekühlte Preßluft. In den peripheren Einheiten, die über PE- bzw. Teflonleitungen mit dem Reaktor verbunden sind, gehören:

a) Vakuumanschluß, kombiniert mit einem Kondensor zur Rückgewinnung des ^{18}O-angereicherten Wassers.

b) PE-Vorratsbehälter mit den für die Reaktion erforderlichen Lösungen bzw. Lösungsmitteln.

c) SEP-PAK C18 Kartusche zur Separierung der acetylierten FDG und des Aminopolyethers.

d) Säulenchromatographische Deionisierung und Mischung der FDG-Lösung mit NaCl-Lösung sowie Sterilfiltration der isotonischen FDG-Lösung.

Die Apparatur ist fernbedienbar und so konzipiert, daß die Synthese rechnergesteuert durchgeführt werden kann.

Für die Qualitätskontrolle, die im Falle dieses wichtigen Radiopharmakons ausführlicher beschrieben werden soll, stehen eine Reihe von chromatographischen Verfahren zur Verfü-

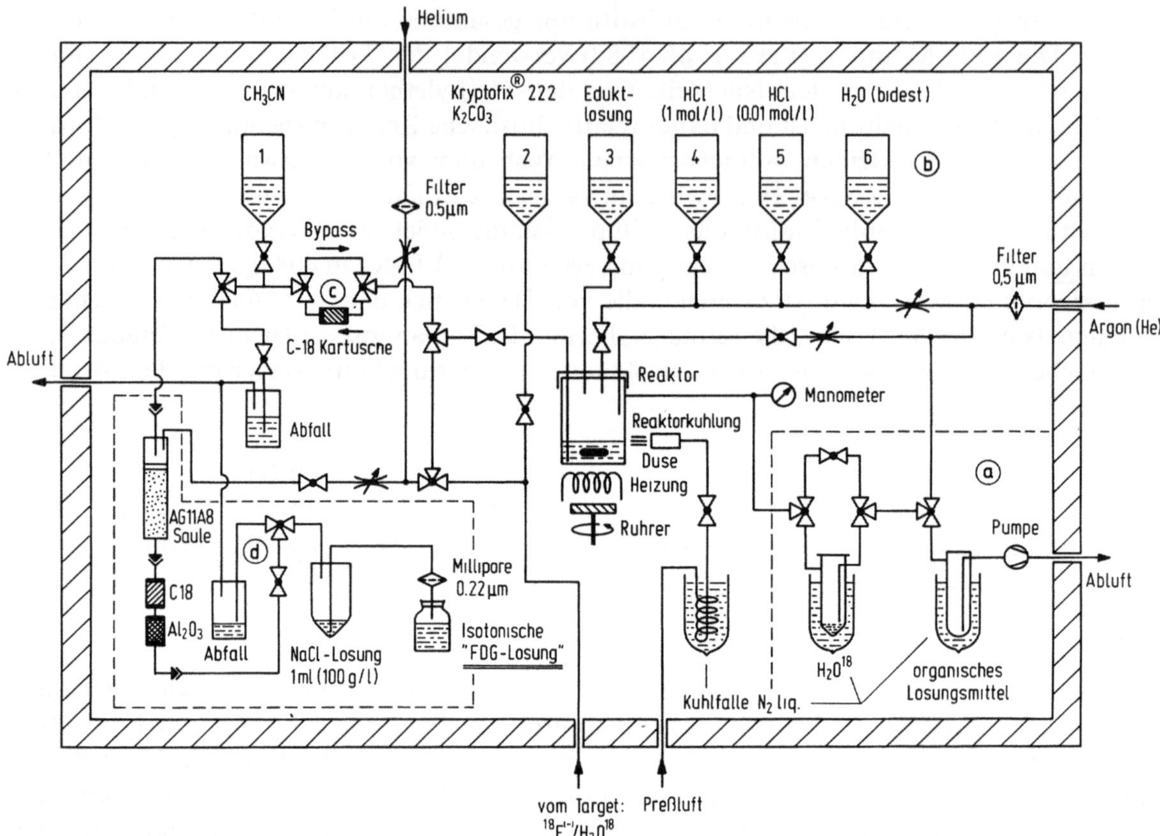

Abb. 6. Ferngesteuerte Syntheseapparatur zur Produktion von [2-^{18}F]-FDG. (Nach Hamacher u. Blessing 1987)

Tabelle 15. Chromatographische Routineverfahren zur Qualitätskontrolle von [2-^{18}F]-FDG

Methode	Bedingungen	Trennung von	Literatur
GLC	4% SE 30 + 6% OV210 auf Chromosorb WHP 2 m, 3 mm $\varnothing$, 150° C, 15 ml He/min	FDG/FDM nach Silylierung	Shiue et al. (1985a)
TLC	NaH$_2$PO$_4$-imprägnierte Silica-Gel-Platten, CH$_3$CN, H$_2$O 95/5, wiederholte Entwicklung	FDG/FDM	Van Rijn et al. (1985)
TLC	Silica-Gel-Platten, CH$_3$CN/H$_2$O 85/15, oder 95/15	FDG/FDM von F$^-$ und teilweise hydrolysierten Produkten	Fowler et al. (1981)
TLC	Silica-Gel-Platten (CHCl$_3$/CH$_3$OH) H$_2$O, 30/9/1	FDG/FDM von F$^-$ und teilweise hydrolysierten Produkten	Fowler et al. (1981)

gung (s. Tabelle 15). Die Prüfung auf radiochemische Reinheit sollte zumindest mit Hilfe einer der in Tabelle 15 aufgeführten Methoden durchgeführt werden. Auch HPLC-Systeme zur Abtrennung von Fluorid und nur teilweise hydrolysierten Produkten sind eingesetzt worden (Vora et al. 1985; Levy 1982). Die Isomerenreinheit, d.h. das Verhältnis 2-FDG/2-FDM wird bei den trägerhaltigen elektrophilen Methoden im allgemeinen mit Hilfe der

^{19}F-NMR Spektroskopie geprüft (BIDA et al. 1984; PHILIPPS u. WRAY 1971). Bei trägerfreien Mengen kann eine radiogaschromatographische Trennung der silylierten Produkte vorgenommen werden (SHIUE et al. 1985). Eine relativ einfache Methode zur direkten Trennung der trägerfreien Epimeren ohne Derivatisierung bietet ein TLC-Verfahren (VAN RIJN et al. 1985).

Auch andere Kohlenhydrate sind mit ^{18}F markiert worden. So wurde 2-Deoxy-2-fluor-D-galactose synthetisiert (TADA et al. 1984) und als Träger zur Erfassung des Leberstoffwechsels mittels PET vorgeschlagen (FUKADA et al. 1986). Weiterhin wurde 2-Deoxy-2-fluoro-L-fucose, ein potentieller Tracer zur Erfassung des Glycoproteinstoffwechsels synthetisiert (IMAHORI et al. 1986).

Iod- oder Bromanaloge der Glukose, die sich physiologisch ähnlich wie FDG oder MG verhalten würden, wären wegen der längeren Halbwertszeit in Verbindung mit der SPECT-Technik eine interessante Alternative für Kliniken, die nicht über ein Zyklotron verfügen. Die Bemühungen waren jedoch bisher wenig erfolgreich, da die Iodanalogen wie 2-Deoxy-2-iod-D-glukose (FOWLER et al. 1979) und 3-Deoxy-3-iod-D-glukose (KLOSTER et al. 1983a) in-vitro oder in-vivo sehr schnell Iod abspalten. Stabil dagegen sind die Methylglukoside Methyl-2-deoxy-2-iod-β-D-glucopyranosid und Methyl-2-deoxy-2-brom-β-D-glucopyranosid sowie das acetylierte Methyl 3,4,6-tri-O-acetyl-2-deoxy-2-iod-β-D-glucopyranosid und das entsprechende Bromanaloge (KLOSTER et al. 1983a). Die beiden letzteren ^{75}Br- bzw. ^{123}I-markierten Verbindungen zeigen eine brauchbare Anreicherung im Hirn (KLOSTER et al. 1983b). Die Präparation der Verbindungen gelingt über eine interessante elektrophile Anlagerungsreaktion, bei der ausgehend von Dichloramin-T und trägerfreiem Halogenid (X = *Br$^-$, *I$^-$) in Methanol das Halogen und eine Methoxygruppe an die Doppelbindung im Tri-O-acetyl-D-glucal angelagert werden:

$$\text{Tri-O-acetyl-D-glucal} \xrightarrow[\text{X}^{\ominus}/\text{CH}_3\text{OH}]{\text{Dichloramin T}} \text{(Zwischenprodukt)} \xrightarrow{\text{NaOMe}} \text{Produkt} \qquad (75)$$

$$X = {}^{75,77}\text{Br}, \ {}^{123}\text{I}$$

Das Produkt ist möglicherweise für die Messung des regionalen Glykosetransports im Hirn von Interesse, da es sich gut im Zielorgan anreichert und wahrscheinlich nicht verstoffwechselt wird (KLOSTER et al. 1983b). Ein anderer Weg zur Stabilisierung des Iods im Zuckermolekül ist die Einführung einer Iodvinylgruppe. So konnten 2-Deoxy-2-iodvinyl Altrose Derivate hergestellt werden, von denen vor allem [^{123}I]-Methyl-2-deoxy-2-(E)-iod-vinyl-2,4,6-O-triacetyl-β-D-altropyranosid eine gute Anreicherung im Hirn zeigt (GOODMAN et al. 1986).

II. Aminosäuren

Im Rahmen des biochemischen Konzeptes der Radiopharmakaentwicklung spielen Aminosäuren und ihre Analoga eine große Rolle. Sie können zur regionalen Erfassung der Proteinsynthese mittels PET eingesetzt werden (zur Übersicht s. BUSTANY u. COMAR 1985; SOKOLOFF 1986), so z.B. im Pankreas (SYROTA et al. 1979, 1981, 1982; HÜBNER et al. 1980), im Hirn (BUSTANY et al. 1981, 1983; PHELPS et al. 1984) und im Herzen (BARRIO et al. 1982; HENZE et al. 1982; SCHELBERT u. SCHWAIGER 1986) sowie zur Erfassung des Stoffwechsels von Tumoren (SMITH et al. 1980; HÜBNER et al. 1982; BERGSTRÖM et al. 1983; MEYER et al.

1985; Schober et al. 1986). Bisher sind Markierungen deshalb vor allem mit ^{11}C, ^{13}N, und für Analoge mit ^{18}F und ^{75}Br sowie für SPECT mit ^{123}I durchgeführt worden.

Bei den ^{13}N-markierten Aminosäuren ist zu beachten, daß einer ihrer Hauptabbauwege die Transaminierung ist. Man beobachtet deshalb bei der in-vivo Anwendung durch externe Messung in vielen Fällen das Schicksal der markierten Metabolite. Das Problem des mit der Proteinsynthese konkurrierenden Abbaus und der Wiederverwertung der Katabolite stellt sich auch bei ^{11}C-markierten Aminosäuren. Im Falle der in der Carboxylgruppe mit ^{11}C-markierten Aminosäuren wird das Markierungsisotop durch Decarboxylierung relativ schnell als ^{11}CO$_2$ abgespalten und schließlich ausgeatmet, so daß prinzipiell eine differentielle Messung der relativ langsamen Proteinsynthese möglich sein sollte (zur Übersicht s. Barrio 1986).

Zwei Synthesewege werden zur ^{11}C-Markierung von Aminosäuren in der Carboxylgruppe angewendet, die Carboxylierung von α-Lithioisonitrilen ausgehend von ^{11}CO$_2$ sowie die modifizierte Bucherer-Strecker Synthese ausgehend von K^{11}CN (s. Abschnitt C.II.1. Gl. 40 und 52). Das Isonitril-Verfahren wurde zur ^{11}C-Markierung von Phenylalanin und Phenylglycin (Vaalburg et al. 1976) sowie von DOPA (Reiffers et al. 1977) verwendet. Mit Hilfe der Bucherer-Strecker Synthese wurde u.a. [^{11}C]-Valin, -Leucin, -Tryptophan und -Phenylalanin markiert (Washburn et al. 1978; Hübner et al. 1979; Zalutsky et al. 1981; Casey et al. 1981). Beide Methoden führen zu Racematen. Diese müssen entweder chromatographisch (Gil-Av et al. 1980; Wu et al. 1981; Washburn et al. 1982) oder enzymatisch (Casey et al. 1981; Barrio et al. 1981b, 1982) aufgetrennt werden. Hierbei verliert man allerdings die Hälfte der ^{11}C-Aktivität. Asymmetrische chemische Synthesen, d.h. stereoselektive Reaktionen, die bevorzugt zum gewünschten Enantiomeren führen, sind wegen der relativ langen Synthesezeit im allgemeinen nicht für kurzlebige Radionuklide geeignet. Die Verwendung enzymatischer Synthesen (s.u.) sind deshalb vorzuziehen. Die Gegenwart von möglicherweise pyrogenen Enzymen macht jedoch solche Synthesen oft für medizinische Anwendungen unmöglich. Die Verwendung immobilisierter Enzyme umgeht diese Probleme. Enzyme, an eine geeignete feste Matrix gebunden, sind wasserunlösliche, hochspezifische Reagenzien, die den Vorteil haben, daß sie leicht vom Reaktionsgemisch abgetrennt werden können und so eine schnelle Produktisolierung gestatten. Darüber hinaus können sie wiederverwendet werden (zur Übersicht s. Goldstein u. Katchalski-Katzir 1976; Barrio 1986). Eine stereospezifische Synthese optisch aktiver Aminosäuren gelingt durch enzymatische Reaktionen oder durch Reaktion eines optisch aktiven Substrates mit einer radioaktiven Vorstufe. So kann z.B. durch ^{11}C-Methylierung von L-Homocystein L-Methionin erhalten werden. Hierbei wird entweder S-Benzyl-Homocystein (Langström u. Lundquist 1976) oder Homocystein-Thiolacton (Comar et al. 1976; Berger et al. 1979) mit [^{11}C]-Methyliodid umgesetzt:

$$\text{L} \quad \overline{\text{S}-\text{CH}_2-\text{CH}_2-\underset{\underset{\text{NH}_2}{|}}{\text{CH}}-\text{C}}=\text{O} \quad \xrightarrow{\overset{^{11}\text{CH}_3\text{I}}{\text{OH}^-}} \quad \text{L-} \ ^{11}\text{CH}_3\text{S}-\text{CH}_2-\text{CH}_2-\underset{\underset{\text{NH}_2}{|}}{\text{CH}}\text{CO}_2\text{H} \quad (76)$$

In ähnlicher Weise sind Metenkephalin (Nägren et al. 1986) und andere Peptide (Langström et al. 1981a) durch ^{11}C-Methylierung von SH-Gruppen erhalten worden.

Ausgehend von ^{11}CO$_2$ sind vor allem enzymatische Methoden zur schnellen spezifischen Synthese von optisch aktiven ^{11}C-markierten Aminosäuren eingesetzt worden. So ist L-[4-^{11}C]-Asparaginsäure in Anlehnung an die ^{14}C-Markierung enzymatisch präpariert worden (Hara et al. 1971). In neuerer Zeit ist L-[4-^{11}C]-Asparaginsäure als potentieller Tracer für die Untersuchung des regionalen Myokardstoffwechsels über immobilisierte Phosphoenolpyrovat-(PEP)-Carboxylase markiert worden (Barrio et al. 1982). Der Reaktion zwischen dem Phosphoenolpyruvat und ^{11}CO$_2$ unter Bildung von [4-^{11}C]-Oxalacetat folgt die Transaminierung durch immobilisierte Glutamat-Oxalat Transaminase (GOT), wobei das Oxalacetat in die Asparaginsäure umgewandelt wird:

$$\underset{\substack{|\\ \text{OPO}_3\text{H}_2}}{\text{H}_2\text{C}=\text{C}}-\text{CO}_2\text{H} \;+\; {}^{11}\text{CO}_2 \;\xrightarrow[]{\substack{\text{PEP}\\ \text{Carboxylase}}}\; \text{HO}_2{}^{11}\text{C}-\text{CH}_2\overset{\overset{\text{O}}{\|}}{\text{C}}-\text{CO}_2\text{H}$$

$$\xrightarrow[\text{L-Glutamat}]{\text{GOT}}\; \text{HO}_2{}^{11}\text{C}-\text{CH}_2\underset{\substack{|\\ \text{NH}_2}}{\text{CH}}-\text{CO}_2\text{H} \tag{77}$$

Ähnlich konnte [3-^{11}C]-Phenylalanin über die enzymatische Transaminierung von [3-^{11}C]-Phenylpyruvat erhalten werden, das zuvor ausgehend vom ^{11}CO$_2$ über [^{11}C]-Benzaldehyd hergestellt wurde (HALLDIN u. LANGSTRÖM 1986):

$$\text{(Gl. 78)} \tag{78}$$

$$\text{(Gl. 79)} \tag{79}$$

Hierbei wird die α-Ketosäure über eine Kondensationsreaktion von [^{11}C]-Benzaldehyd und 2-Phenyl-5-oxazolon unter Verwendung von Diazabicyclooctan (DABCO) als Base erhalten. Das Kondensationsprodukt wird über basische Hydrolyse in das [3-^{11}C]-Phenylpyruvat umgewandelt. Dieser erste Teil der Synthese (Gl. 78) verläuft in 40 min mit einer radiochemischen Ausbeute von 40%. Die Transaminierung (Gl. 79) erfolgt wiederum durch Glutamat-Oxalat Transaminase (GOT) (EC 2.6.1.1), die immobilisiert auf CNBr-aktivierter Sepharose vorliegt.

Racemate von in der 2- oder 3-Position der Seitenkette mit ^{11}C markierten aromatischen Aminosäuren wie D,L-Phenylalanin, D,L-Dopa (HALLDIN u. LANGSTRÖM 1984a) sowie D,L-[2-^{11}C]-Phenylglycin (HALLDIN u. LANGSTRÖM 1985) waren zuvor schon durch mehrstufige Synthesen über [^{11}C]-Benzaldehyd hergestellt worden. Eine asymmetrische Synthese von L-[3-^{11}C]-Phenylalanin mit chiralen Hydrierungskatalysatoren über die Hydrierung von [α-^{11}C]-4-Arylen-2-aryl-5-oxazolon ist ebenfalls beschrieben worden (HALLDIN u. LANGSTRÖM 1984b). Innerhalb von 60 min konnte die Aminosäure mit einer radiochemischen Ausbeute von 10–15% in einer optischen Reinheit von 60–80% erhalten werden.

Enzymatische Methoden sind vor allem zur schnellen Markierung mit ^{13}N eingesetzt worden. Hierbei wird, ausgehend von ^{13}NH$_3$, das Enzymsystem, das auch für den Stoffwechsel von Ammoniak in lebenden Organismen verantwortlich ist, zur stereospezifischen Markierungssynthese genutzt. Drei Reaktionstypen können grundsätzlich verwendet werden. Die direkte Aminierung einer α-Ketosäure durch Glutaminsäuredehydrogenase (GAD),

$$\text{R}-\underset{\substack{\|\\ \text{O}}}{\text{C}}-\text{CO}_2\text{H} \;+\; {}^{13}\text{NH}_3 \;\xrightarrow{\text{GAD}}\; \text{R}-\underset{\substack{|\\ {}^{13}\text{NH}_2}}{\text{CH}}-\text{CO}_2\text{H} \tag{80}$$

die Transaminierung mit markierter Glutaminsäure unter Verwendung von Glutamat-Oxal-acetat-Transaminase (GOT),

$$HO_2C(CH_2)_2\text{--}\underset{{}^{13}NH_2}{CH}\text{--}CO_2H \;+\; R\text{--}\overset{O}{\underset{}{C}}\text{--}CO_2H \;\xrightarrow{\;GOT\;}\; R\text{--}\underset{{}^{13}NH_2}{CH}\text{--}CO_2H \qquad (81)$$

$$+\; HO_2C\text{--}(CH_2)_2\text{--}\overset{O}{\underset{}{C}}\text{--}CO_2H$$

und die Einführung einer markierten Amidgruppe in eine Dicarbonsäure über Glutamin (GS) – oder Asparagin Synthetase (AS).

$$HO_2C(CH_2)_n\text{--}\underset{NH_2}{CH}\text{--}CO_2H \;+\; {}^{13}NH_3 \;\xrightarrow{\;AS\;}\; H_2{}^{13}N\text{--}\underset{O}{\overset{}{C}}(CH_2)_n\text{--}\underset{NH_2}{CH}CO_2H \qquad (82)$$

Glutamin, Asparagin und Glutaminsäure wurden auf diesem Wege entweder in Lösung (Elmaleh et al. 1979; Cohen et al. 1972) oder immobilisiert auf aktivierter Sepharose (Barrio et al. 1981 b; Cohen et al. 1981; Gelbard et al. 1981) markiert. Auch L-Alanin, L-Valin, L-Methionin und L-α-Aminobuttersäure sind auf enzymatischem Wege mit ^{13}N markiert worden (Gelbard 1981). Ausgehend von $[^{13}N]$-Glutaminsäure wurden durch Transaminierung (Gl. 81) verschiedene aromatische Aminosäuren markiert (Gelbard u. Cooper 1979).

Einige aromatische Aminosäuren sind für PET Untersuchungen mit ^{18}F am aromatischen Ring markiert worden. Vor allem L-p-Fluorphenylalanin und L-6-Fluordopa sind für Untersuchungen des Hirnstoffwechsels von Bedeutung. L-Dopa ist ein Vorläufer von Dopamin. Anders als Dopamin gelangt es leicht durch die Blut-Hirn-Schranke und wird schnell zu Dopamin decarboxyliert. L-$[1\text{-}^{11}C]$-Dopa verliert jedoch dabei sein Markierungsisotop, so daß es nicht mehr geeignet ist, etwa den Dopaminpool zu markieren und dopaminerge Zentren sichtbar zu machen (Reiffers et al. 1977). L-6-Fluordopa mit ^{18}F markiert hat sich dagegen als ein geeignetes Analoges zur Erfassung des zerebralen Dopamingehaltes erwiesen (Garnett et al. 1983). L-6-Fluordopa ist ausgehend von L-3-Methoxy-4-hydroxy-phenylalanin direkt mit $[^{18}F]\text{--}XeF_2$ in Methylenchlorid markiert worden. Nach Entfernung der Schutzgruppe erhält man L-6-Fluordopa (Firnau et al. 1981):

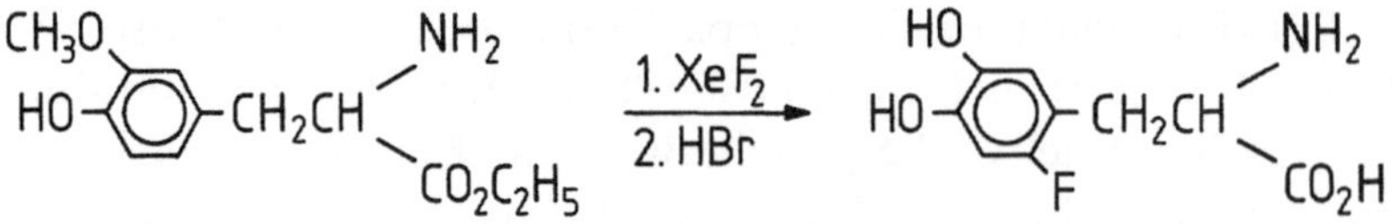

$$(83)$$

Eine weitere methodische Vereinfachung ist die direkte Einwirkung von $[^{18}F]\text{--}F_2$ auf L-Dopa in flüssigem HF (Chirakal et al. 1986). Bei diesen direkten Fluorierungen entstehen naturgemäß Isomerengemische, die im Falle des Fluors häufig schwer zu trennen sind.

Die wahrscheinlich effizienteste Synthese von $[6\text{-}^{18}F]$-Fluordopa ist die regioselektive Fluordemerkurierung ausgehend von dem geschützten Organoquecksilber-Vorläufer, der mit $[^{18}F]$-Acetylhypofluorit elektrophil demerkuriert und anschließend entschützt wird (Luxen et al. 1986):

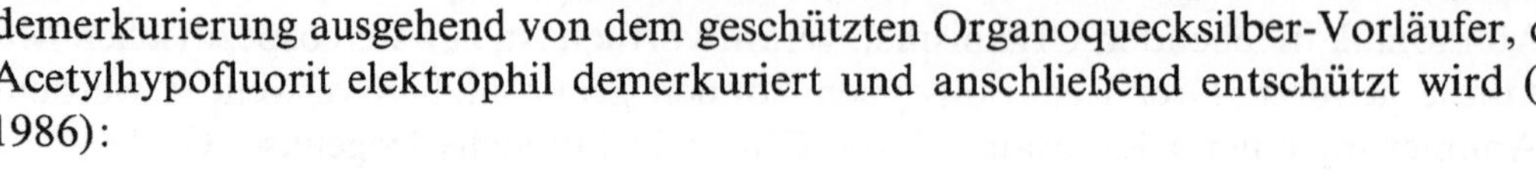

$$(84)$$

p-Fluorphenylalanin erscheint als Aminosäureanaloges geeignet, um die Proteinsynthese mit Hilfe der PET Technik zu erfassen (COENEN et al. 1986d; BODSCH et al. 1987). Anders als bei ^{11}C-markierten Aminosäuren, bei denen der Metabolismus die Erfassung der Proteinsynthese erschwert, ist eine Reutilisation nach eventueller Abspaltung des Fluoratoms nicht möglich.

Über die Balz-Schiemann-Reaktion (vgl. Abschnitt C.III) erhält man nur kleine radiochemische Ausbeuten von etwa 10% und niedrige spezifische Aktivitäten. Nach Entfernung der Schutzgruppen liegt die gewünschte Aminosäure als racemisches Gemisch vor. Über die Balz-Schiemann Reaktion sind p-[^{18}F]-Fluorphenylalanin (GOULDING u. PALMER 1972), o-, m-, und p-Fluorphenylalanin (HOYTE et al. 1971) sowie 5- und 6-Fluortryptophan (ATKINS et al. 1972) hergestellt worden. Eine direkte elektrophile Fluorierung von Phenylanin mit [^{18}F]$-$F$_2$ in CF$_3$COOH ist ebenfalls möglich (COENEN et al. 1986c). Allerdings entsteht dabei ein Isomerengemisch (ortho:meta:para$=60:15:25$), aus dem die para-Fraktion nur mit großem Aufwand chromatographisch abgetrennt werden kann. Einen eleganteren Weg stellt die Fluordestannylierung dar (s. Schema V), wobei das gewünschte Isomere regioselektiv

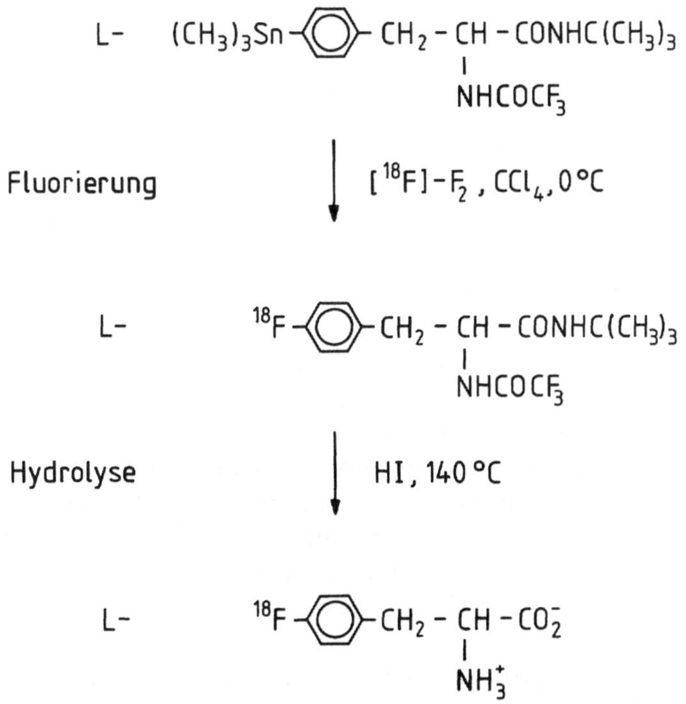

$$\text{L-} \quad (CH_3)_3Sn-\!\!\bigcirc\!\!-CH_2-CH-CONHC(CH_3)_3$$
$$| \qquad\qquad\qquad$$
$$NHCOCF_3$$

Fluorierung $\qquad\downarrow\quad$ [^{18}F]$-$F$_2$, CCl$_4$, 0 °C

$$\text{L-} \qquad ^{18}F-\!\!\bigcirc\!\!-CH_2-CH-CONHC(CH_3)_3$$
$$| \qquad\qquad\qquad$$
$$NHCOCF_3$$

Hydrolyse $\qquad\downarrow\quad$ HI , 140 °C

$$\text{L-} \qquad ^{18}F-\!\!\bigcirc\!\!-CH_2-CH-CO_2^-$$
$$| \qquad$$
$$NH_3^+$$

Schema V. Synthese von L-p-[^{18}F]-Fluorphenylalanin. (Nach COENEN et al. 1986c)

mit 25%iger radiochemischer Ausbeute erhalten wird (COENEN et al. 1986c). Trifluoracetylamid und tert-Butylamid erwiesen sich als geeignete Schutzgruppen für die Vorläuferverbindung L-p-Trimethylzinn-phenylalanin, die in einer Pd-katalysierten Reaktion mit Hexamethyldizinn hergestellt wurde (METWALLY et al. 1987). Eine alternative Methode geht analog der Synthese von [3-^{11}C]-Phenylalanin von der Markierung von Benzaldehyd mit ^{18}F-Fluorid aus (LEMAIRE et al. 1986). Durch die dreistufige Aktivsynthese und die notwendige Racemattrennung wird hier nur eine sehr kleine radiochemische Ausbeute erhalten.

Aminosäure-Analoga sind auch mit ^{75,77}Br und ^{123}I markiert worden (s. z.B. PETZOLD u. COENEN 1981). Erwähnenswert sind hier vor allem die 3-Halo-L-α-methyltyrosine, die sich sowohl zur Pankreas-Szintigraphie (TISLJAR et al. 1979; RITZL et al. 1981; KLOSTER et al. 1982), als auch zur Erfassung von Augenmelanomen (BOCKSLAFF et al. 1980; BOCKSLAFF et al. 1982) eignen. Die ^{123}I- oder ^{75}Br-markierte Verbindung läßt sich sehr einfach und schnell über elektrophile Halogenierung (X = ^{75}Br, ^{123}I) mit Chloramin-T erhalten:

$$HO-\langle\bigcirc\rangle-CH_2-\underset{NH_2}{\overset{CH_3}{\underset{|}{\overset{|}{C}}}}-CO_2H \quad\xrightarrow[-H^+]{X^-/\text{Chloramin T}}\quad HO-\underset{X}{\langle\bigcirc\rangle}-CH_2-\underset{NH_2}{\overset{CH_3}{\underset{|}{\overset{|}{C}}}}-CO_2H \qquad (85)$$

Zu den analogen Aminosäuren, die in der Nuklearmedizin eine Rolle spielen, gehören auch die Selenanalogen. Im Hinblick auf den Positronenstrahler ^{73}Se ($T_{1/2} = 7{,}2$ h) (s.o. Tabelle 1) ist das früher zur Pankreas-Szintigraphie verwendete Selenomethionin erneut von Interesse. Die Markierung mit dem verwendeten langlebigen ^{75}Se ($T_{1/2} = 125$ d) wurde i. allg. über eine biochemische Synthese vorgenommen (BLAU u. BENDER 1962), die allerdings mehr als 30 Stunden dauert. Kürzlich wurde eine schnelle Synthese von L-Selenomethionin beschrieben (PLENEVAUX et al. 1987), die das L-Isomere in einer optischen Reinheit von $>99\%$ innerhalb von 3 Stunden mit einer radiochemischen Ausbeute von 80% liefert:

$$*Se \quad\xrightarrow{\text{CH}_3\text{Li}}\quad CH_3*SeLi \qquad (86)$$

$$\xrightarrow[\text{THF/EtOH}]{\text{ARB—HBr}}\quad CH_3-*Se-CH_2-CH_2-\underset{NH_2HBr}{\overset{|}{CH}}-COOH \qquad (87)$$

Ausgehend von L-α-Amino-γ-brombuttersäure (ARB) in HBr Form kann diese Synthese als Eintopfsynthese durchgeführt werden. Falls die biochemischen Voraussetzungen erfüllt sind, würde sich [^{73}Se]-L-Selenomethionin als längerlebige Alternative zu [^{11}C]-Methionin anbieten.

Zahlreiche Enzyme und Blutproteine sind radioiodiert und als mögliche Tracer untersucht worden. Auf die Methoden zur Iodierung von Proteinen und zur Markierung mit ^{99m}Tc soll hier nicht näher eingegangen werden, da sie nicht direkt zum Thema dieses Kapitels gehören. Die Voraussetzungen bei der Markierung mit kurzlebigen Radionukliden für in-vivo Anwendungen sind jedoch im wesentlichen die gleichen:

- Stabilität der Markierung in-vivo für die Zeit der Untersuchung (Problem des Blutuntergrundes),
- keine Veränderung der biologischen Aktivität (keine selektive Inaktivierung durch Fremdmarkierung oder makroskopische Veränderung durch den Markierungsprozeß, biochemische Akzeptanz),
- nur Proteine mit sehr spezifischer Mitwirkung an dem zu untersuchenden Prozeß geeignet (selektive Anreicherung).

Milde Halogenierungsmethoden sind erforderlich, um die biologische Aktivität zu erhalten. Dies gilt insbesondere für die Bromierung, die schwer ohne Verlust der biologischen Aktivität durchführbar ist. Hier sind enzymatische Methoden gegenüber den üblichen Oxidationsmitteln wie Chloramin-T vorteilhaft. So sind Bromoperoxidase oder Myeloperoxidase erfolgreich zur Radiohalogenierung von Proteinen eingesetzt worden (MCELVANY et al. 1980; MCELVANY u. WELCH 1980).

Für die Einführung von ^{18}F in Peptide eignet sich die Fluoracylierung. Hier sind zwei Verfahren beschrieben worden. Das erste geht von [^{18}F]-Fluoracetat aus, das durch ein wasserlösliches Carbodiimid als aktivierte Säure an freie Aminogruppen gebunden wird (MÜLLER-PLATZ et al. 1982). Das zweite einfachere Verfahren ist eine direkte Fluoracylierung unter Verwendung eines α-substituierten Carbonsäureesters wie [2-^{18}F]-Fluorpropionsäuremethylester (BLOCK et al. 1987c):

$$H_3C-\underset{\underset{^{18}F}{|}}{\overset{\overset{H}{|}}{C}}-CO_2CH_3 \; + \; H_2N-R \; \underset{}{\overset{H_2O,\ H^+}{\rightleftharpoons}} \; H_3C-\underset{\underset{^{18}F}{|}}{\overset{\overset{H}{|}}{C}}-\underset{\underset{NH-R}{\diagdown}}{\overset{\overset{O}{\diagup\!\!\diagup}}{C}} \tag{88}$$

Das Fluoracylierungsmittel, [2-^{18}F]-Fluorpropionsäuremethylester, kann praktisch trägerfrei durch APE-2.2.2. gestützten nukleophilen Austausch von Brom gegen n.c.a. [^{18}F]-Fluorid aus analogen 2-Brompropionsäuremethylester erhalten werden (s. Abschnitt C.III.3, Gl. 64).

III. Fettsäuren

Der Herzmuskel deckt seinen hohen Energiebedarf unter aeroben Bedingungen vorwiegend (ca. 60% in Ruhe) durch langkettige freie Fettsäuren und in geringerem Maße durch Glukose und Laktat. Es bietet sich deshalb an, geeignet markierte Fettsäuren zur Erfassung des regionalen Stoffwechsels des Herzens einzusetzen. Man hat schon relativ früh verschiedene markierte Fettsäuren evaluiert (EVANS et al. 1965; POE et al. 1976; WEISS et al. 1976; MACHULLA et al. 1978). Dies gilt sowohl für ^{11}C-markierte Fettsäuren (zur Übersicht s. SCHELBERT 1982; SCHELBERT u. SCHWAIGER 1986), als auch für Fettsäureanaloge insbesondere für Halogenfettsäuren (zur Übersicht s. STÖCKLIN 1982; STÖCKLIN et al. 1980; FREUNDLIEB et al. 1980; STÖCKLIN u. KLOSTER 1982; DUDCZAK et al. 1983; VISSER et al. 1985a).

^{11}C-markierte Fettsäuren, wie die [1-^{11}C]-Palmitinsäure, die durch einfache Grignard-Synthese ausgehend von ^{11}CO$_2$ hergestellt wird (KLEIN et al. 1979; MACHULLA et al. 1978; POE et al. 1975; WELCH et al. 1981), sind bisher die einzigen mit einem Positronenstrahler markierten Fettsäuren, die klinisch erprobt wurden (zur Übersicht s. SCHELBERT u. SCHWAIGER 1986). Im Tierexperiment evaluiert wurden auch ω-^{18}F-Fettsäuren (KNUST et al. 1979) und ^{75}Br-markierte aromatische Fettsäuren (STÖCKLIN et al. 1980; COENEN et al. 1981, 1986a). Für die planare Szintigraphie sowie für SPECT sind insbesondere ^{123}I-markierte Analoge entwickelt und evaluiert worden. Hier stehen z.Zt. vor allem die [17-^{123}I]-Iodheptadecansäure (IHA), die 15-(p-[^{123}I]-Iodphenyl)pentadecansäure (p-IPPA) und die 15-(p-[^{123}I]-Iodphenyl)-3,3-dimethylpentadecansäure (DMIPP) im Vordergrund.

Bei den fremdmarkierten Fettsäuren ist besonders zu berücksichtigen, daß durch externe Messung der Eliminationskinetik im wesentlichen das Schicksal der markierten Metabolite erfaßt wird, das ein komplexes Stoffwechselgeschehen widerspiegelt (s. z.B. KLOSTER u. STÖCKLIN 1982; COENEN et al. 1981; VISSER et al. 1985b; SCHÖN et al. 1986). Seine Kenntnis ist für quantitative Aussagen über den Stoffwechsel unentbehrlich.

Die natürlichen ^{11}C-markierten langkettigen Fettsäuren bieten prinzipiell den Vorteil, daß ihr Stoffwechsel gut bekannt ist. Eine Markierung in der Carboxylgruppe führt über die β-Oxidation letztlich zu ^{11}CO$_2$, das die Zelle verläßt und ausgeatmet wird. Die β-Oxidation selbst ist sehr schnell, ihre metabolischen Zwischenstufen können kaum erfaßt werden. Ein je nach Versorgungslage des Herzmuskels mehr oder weniger großer Teil der markierten Fettsäure wird zunächst in Form von Lipiden gespeichert und gelangt erst später zur β-Oxidation. Man beobachtet deshalb nach einer schnellen Aufnahme zunächst eine schnelle Elimination durch die direkte β-Oxidation gefolgt von einer langsamen späten Elimination der β-Oxidation des aus den Speicherlipiden zurückkehrenden Anteils (zur Übersicht s. SCHELBERT u. SCHWAIGER 1986).

Die ^{11}C-Markierung langkettiger Fettsäuren in der Carboxylgruppe erfolgt am einfachsten über geeignete Grignard Reaktionen ausgehend vom ^{11}CO$_2$ (Gl. 38, Abschnitt C.II.1). Auf diesem Wege sind Palmitinsäure (Poe et al. 1975; Weiss et al. 1976; Machulla et al. 1978), Ölsäure (Poe et al. 1975) sowie auch kürzerkettige Carbonsäuren wie Octansäure (Weiss et al. 1976) und Essigsäure (Pike et al. 1982) hergestellt worden.

Fettsäuren mit einer Methylgruppe in der β-Position sind im Hinblick auf eine Metabolisierung durch die β-Oxidation inhibiert und werden deshalb länger retendiert. Aus diesem Grunde ist auch die [1-^{11}C]-β-Methylheptadecansäure synthetisiert und evaluiert worden (Livni et al. 1982). Auch diese Fettsäure ist ausgehend von ^{11}CO$_2$ und dem entsprechenden Alkylhalogenid über eine Grignard Reaktion hergestellt worden.

Als Fettsäureanaloge für PET kommen u.a. ^{18}F-markierte Fluorfettsäuren in Frage. Während ungeradzahlige ω-Fluorfettsäuren das Fluoratom im letzten Schritt der β-Oxidation verlieren, und das freie Fluoridion die Zelle verläßt (Knust et al. 1979; Kloster u. Stöcklin 1982), werden die geradzahligen ω-Fluorfettsäuren zur toxischen 2-Fluoressigsäure abgebaut. Die ω-Fluorfettsäuren wie z.B. die [17-^{18}F]-Fluorheptadecansäure werden ebensogut wie die analogen [^{11}C]-markierten Fettsäuren im Herzmuskel angereichert (Knust et al. 1979). Sie können durch Aminopolyether (APE 2.2.2. Kryptofix) praktisch trägerfrei (n.c.a.) in hoher Ausbeute synthetisiert werden (Coenen et al. 1986). Ausgehend vom entsprechenden Methylester wird zunächst die nukleophile ^{18}F-für-Br Substitution und anschließend die Esterhydrolyse durchgeführt:

$$\text{BrCH}_2\text{---}(\text{CH}_2)_{15}\text{---COOCH}_3 \quad \xrightarrow[\substack{\text{CH}_3\text{CN} \\ -\ \text{Br}^-}]{[\text{K}/2.2.2.]^{+18}\text{F}^-} \quad {}^{18}\text{FCH}_2(\text{CH}_2)_{15}\text{---COOCH}_3 \qquad (89)$$

$$^{18}\text{FCH}_2\text{---}(\text{CH}_2)_{15}\text{---COOCH}_3 \quad \xrightarrow{\text{KOH}} \quad {}^{18}\text{FCH}_2(\text{CH}_2)_{15}\text{---COOH} + \text{CH}_3\text{OH} \quad (90)$$

Innerhalb von etwa 90 Minuten erhält man das Produkt mit einer radiochemischen Ausbeute $>80\%$ und einer spezifischen Aktivität $>5\cdot10^2$ TBq mMol^{-1}. ^{18}F-markierte Fettsäuren stellen prinzipiell eine längerlebige Alternative zu den ^{11}C-Fettsäuren dar. Durch die praktisch trägerfreie Herstellung können prinzipiell auch toxische geradzahlige Fluorfettsäuren eingesetzt werden.

Zahlreiche Radiobrom- und Radioiod-markierte Fettsäuren sind synthetisiert und evaluiert worden (zur Übersicht s. Westera 1981; Machulla et al. 1986). Die heute bereits kommerziell erhältliche ω-[^{123}I]-Iodheptadecansäure (IHA) kann auf mehreren Wegen hergestellt werden (Schema VI). Der nukleophile Austausch kann homogen in polaren aprotischen Lösungsmitteln (s. z.B. Robinson 1977; Robinson u. Lee 1975; Machulla et al. 1978) oder in nicht-polaren Lösungsmitteln mit Hilfe von Phasentransferkatalysatoren (Argentini et al. 1981; Laufer et al. 1981) oder auch in der Schmelze durchgeführt werden (Stöcklin 1977; Laufer et al. 1981). Schmelz- und Phasentransfermethode laufen besonders schnell ab (5–10 min) und liefern radiochemische Ausbeuten von 80–90%.

Trägerhaltige Produkte können durch Isotopenaustausch erhalten werden. Wenn man die Mengen der inaktiven Iodfettsäure auf einige 10 µg begrenzt, so lassen sich auch hier spezifische Aktivitäten von einigen GBq pro 10 µg erhalten. Der I-für-Br Austausch liefert prinzipiell trägerfreie Produkte, da die ω-Iodfettsäure von der ω-Bromfettsäure mittels HPLC getrennt werden kann. In der Praxis enthält die radioiodierte Fettsäure jedoch oft nicht nur Spuren der inaktiven Iodfettsäure durch Spurenverunreinigungen an Iod, sondern auch den nichtisotopen Träger der analogen Bromfettsäure. Hierdurch sind die spezifischen Aktivitäten im allgemeinen nicht größer als etwa 2,6 GBq mg^{-1} Fettsäure (Argentini et al. 1981). Dies ist weniger für die in-vivo Anwendung als für die Lösung der Fettsäure ein Problem

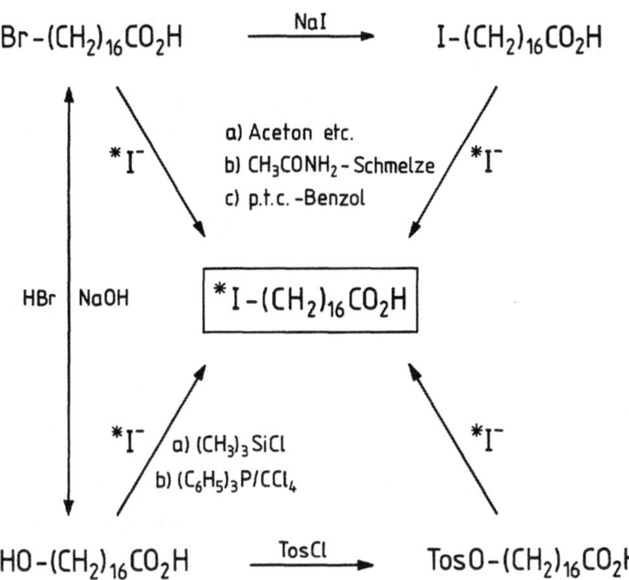

Schema VI. Verschiedene Möglichkeiten zur Präparation von ω-[^{123}I]-Fettsäuren

(s.u.). Bei Verwendung geeigneter HPLC-Methoden (LAUFER et al. 1981) kann die Abtrennung auch nahezu quantitativ erfolgen. Darüber hinaus kann die Halogenfettsäure auch über das Tosylat hergestellt werden, wobei man von der entsprechenden ω-Hydroxyfettsäure ausgeht. In diesem Falle kann das Tosylat der ω-Hydroxyfettsäure mittels HPLC völlig von der Iodfettsäure abgetrennt werden (ARGENTINI et al. 1981).

Auch über Organoborane lassen sich langkettige Halogenfettsäuren herstellen (KABALKA et al. 1981).

$$H_2C\!=\!CH\!-\!(CH_2)_n\!-\!COOH \xrightarrow{R_2BH} R_2B\!-\!CH_2\!-\!(CH_2)_{n+1}\!-\!COOBR_2$$
$$\xrightarrow[\text{MeOH}]{^*ICl} {}^*ICH_2\!-\!(CH_2)_{n+1}\!-\!COOH \tag{91}$$

Die Wahl der Synthese wird u.a. auch durch die verfügbaren Ausgangsmaterialien bestimmt. Einige ω-Iodfettsäuren verschiedener Kettenlänge (n = 18, 21, 26) sind durch Kopplung olefinischer Grignard Reagenzien mit ω-Bromfettsäuren in Gegenwart von Li_2CuCl_4 als Katalysator, anschließender HBr-Addition über den Br-für-I Austausch hergestellt worden (OTTO et al. 1981). So wurde u.a. die β-methylierte Iodfettsäure 13-Jod-3-methyltridecansäure über eine Malonesterkondensation ausgehend von 2-Brom-11-dodecen hergestellt. ω-Halogenfettsäuren können auch ausgehend von kommerziell erhältlichen makrozyklischen Laktonen über die entsprechenden Hydroxyfettsäuren erhalten werden (DOUGAN et al. 1985).

Langkettige Radiobrom-markierte ω-Bromfettsäuren, die sich allerdings nur etwa halb so gut im Herzmuskel anreichern wie die analogen Iodfettsäuren (MACHULLA et al. 1978), können z.B. durch *Br-für-I Austausch ausgehend von der inaktiven Iodfettsäure hergestellt werden. Auch haloaromatische Fettsäuren wie die 15-(p-[^{123}I]-Iodphenyl)pentadecansäure (p-IPPA, MACHULLA et al. 1980) und die ω-(p-[^{75}Br]-Bromphenyl)pentadecansäure (STÖCKLIN et al. 1980; COENEN et al. 1981) sind präpariert und evaluiert worden. Die p-IPPA hat gegenüber der IHA den Vorteil, daß nicht freies Radioiodid als Katabolit auftritt, sondern organische Katabolite insbesondere p-[^{123}I]-Iodbenzoesäure. Eine Blockierung der Schilddrüse ist deshalb nicht erforderlich. Eine Quantifizierung von Stoffwechselvorgängen dürfte jedoch schwierig sein, da die Kamera nicht zwischen den verschiedenen nebeneinander vorliegenden chemischen Formen des Tracers unterscheiden kann.

Die Markierung kann über die elektrophile Substitution, ausgehend vom Halogenid (X^-) und einem geeigneten Oxidationsmittel (vgl. Abschnitt C.IV) erfolgen:

$$C_6H_5—(CH_2)_{14}—COOH \quad \xrightarrow{\ X^-/Oxid.\ } \quad X—C_6H_4—(CH_2)_{14}—COOH \qquad (92)$$

Hierbei entsteht ein Isomerengemisch aus dem ortho- und para-Produkt, das mit Hilfe der HPLC getrennt werden kann. Bei der Bromierung mit $^{75}Br^-$ und Trifluormethansulfonylhypochlorit als Oxidationsmittel erhält man vorwiegend (93%) das para-Isomere (Coenen et al. 1981). Eine ähnliche Selektivität wird auch bei Verwendung von Dichloramin-T in Trifluoressigsäure gefunden. Bei den direkten elektrophilen Iodierungen ist eine Isomerentrennung mittels HPLC erforderlich. Die Halogenierung kann auch regiospezifisch, z.B. über die entsprechende metallorganische Verbindung durch Demetallierung erfolgen (vgl. Abschnitt D.IV). So wurde IPPA durch Ioddestannylierung (Kulkarni u. Parkey 1982) sowie über Organoborverbindungen (Kabalka et al. 1981) hergestellt. Eine Iodierung über Organothalliumvorläufer ist nicht regiospezifisch und eine Isomerentrennung wiederum erforderlich. Auch die regiospezifische Triazenmethode erfordert eine Abtrennung des überschüssigen Triazens; darüber hinaus sind die radiochemischen Ausbeuten relativ niedrig (Goodman et al. 1983). Von Interesse ist auch der Isotopenaustausch am aromatischen Ring in einer Benzoesäureschmelze (Eisenhut 1982). Dieser Austausch verläuft bei 170° C mit einer hohen radiochemischen Ausbeute von 95%. Allerdings muß die Benzoesäure abgetrennt werden. Ein katalysierter Isotopenaustausch in der festen Phase mit einer Ammoniumsulfat-Matrix bei 145–170° C stellt die bisher einfachste Markierung der IPPA dar, die innerhalb von 1 h zu radiochemischen Ausbeuten von 95% führt (Otto et al. 1986). Eine spezifische Aktivität von 200 MBq/mg kann bei diesem Verfahren leicht erhalten werden. Der Vorteil dieses Verfahrens liegt u.a. in der leichten Reinigungsprozedur, die lediglich eine Abtrennung des überschüssigen Radioiodids mittels einer Ionenaustauschersäule erfordert. Eine sehr einfache und effiziente Markierung des IPPA kann auch über den Cu(I)-katalysierten Isotopenaustausch erhalten werden (Dougan et al. 1986; Mertens et al. 1986).

Wie bereits im Zusammenhang mit den ^{11}C-markierten Fettsäuren erwähnt, führt eine Methylierung der Fettsäure in der 3-Position zu einer Inhibierung der β-Oxidation und damit zu einer stärkeren Retention und im Extremfall zu einem „Trapping" der Fettsäure im Herzmuskel. Es sind aus diesem Grunde auch die entsprechenden [^{123}I]-Iodphenylfettsäuren 15-(p-[^{123}I]-Iodphenyl)-3-methylpentadecansäure (BMIPP) und 15-(p-[^{123}I]-Iodphenyl)-3,3-dimethylpentadecansäure (DMIPP) synthetisiert und evaluiert worden (Knapp et al. 1986). Während im Falle von [^{123}I]-BMIPP zwar eine stark verlangsamte Elimination aber noch kein Trapping beobachtet wird, bleibt die [^{123}I]-DMIPP weitgehend im Herzmuskel liegen. Sie zeigt darüber hinaus das beste Herz/Blut Aktivitätsverhältnis. Beide Fettsäuren können im letzten Syntheseschritt durch Iodierung der entsprechenden Methyl- bzw. Dimethylfettsäure erhalten werden, wobei die Iodierung entweder elektrophil über das Thallium-(III)trifluoracetat (Knapp et al. 1986) oder durch Isotopenaustausch in Gegenwart von CuCl als Katalysator (Machulla et al. 1986) erfolgt.

Ein Problem bei der medizinischen Anwendung aller beschriebenen Fettsäuren stellt die Herstellung einer geeigneten Injektionslösung dar. Die einfachste Möglichkeit bietet sich, wenn die Anwendung am Herstellungsort erfolgt, da eine Lösung im Serum des Patienten erfolgen kann. Auch die Verwendung von Humanserum-Albumin, das zur verdünnten ethanolischen Lösung der Fettsäure gegeben wird, ist möglich. Allerdings treten hierbei durch mikroaggregiertes Albumin gelegentlich Anreicherungen der Fettsäure in der Lunge auf.

Die IHA ist kommerziell im allgemeinen in einer isotonischen Kochsalzlösung erhältlich, die 50–80 mg Ethanol und 10–16 mg Tween 80 pro ml Lösung enthält. In jedem Falle sollte die Fettsäure in möglichst hoher spezifischer Aktivität vorliegen, um den Lösevorgang zu erleichtern und zu beschleunigen.

IV. Steroide

Auch Steroide stellen eine wichtige Klasse endogener Substanzen dar. Sie spielen deshalb ebenfalls in der modernen Radiopharmakaentwicklung eine Rolle. Rezeptorbindende Steroidhormone sind vor allem in der Tumorforschung von Bedeutung, so z.B. Östrogen-Rezeptor-bindende Steroide im Falle von Brustkrebs und Androgen-Rezeptor-bindende Steroide beim Prostata-Krebs. Veränderungen an den Rezeptoren gehen mit der Entstehung der Krankheit einher, und die nichtinvasive Erfassung von Rezeptorarealen (s. Abschnitt D.V) kann neue Möglichkeiten in der Tumorforschung eröffnen. Außerdem spielen geeignete Steroide auch zur Darstellung der Nebenniere oder der Prostata als Radiopharmaka eine Rolle. Im Falle der Rezeptorliganden liegt die Begrenzung in der notwendigerweise hohen spezifischen Aktivität (s. Abschnitt D.V), bei anderen Anwendungen, etwa der Nebennierendarstellung, in der relativ langen Zeit (einige Tage), die erforderlich ist, bis der Blutuntergrund hinreichend niedrig ist, damit gute Bilder gemacht werden können. Hier sind oft Radionuklide wie ^{123}I noch zu kurzlebig. Markierungen mit längerlebigen Radionukliden wie ^{131}I, ^{75}Se und ^{123m}Te sollen hier nicht behandelt werden.

Eine Reihe von Markierungssynthesen ist im Hinblick auf die Entwicklung von Östrogen-Rezeptor-Liganden mit ^{11}C und ^{18}F durchgeführt worden. Einen Syntheseweg bietet die Ethinylierung mit [^{11}C]-Acetylen. So ist [^{11}C]-Moxöstrol durch Ethinylierung von β-Methoxyöstron mit [^{11}C]-Acetylen markiert worden (VAALBURG et al. 1977, 1981). Höhere spezifische Aktivitäten können durch [^{11}C]-Methylierung von 17-Ketosteroiden mit Methyllithium erhalten werden (REIFFERS et al. 1980). Ohne Trägerzusatz konnte 17-α-Methyltestosteron in analoger Weise jedoch unter Verwendung von Butyllithium und ^{11}CH$_3$Li mit ausreichender spezifischer Aktivität von 37 bis 74 TBq mMol^{-1} markiert werden (BERGER et al. 1981):

$$\tag{93}$$

Die ersten Markierungssynthesen von Steroiden mit ^{18}F sind über die Balz-Schiemann Reaktion (vgl. Abschnitt C.III.) durchgeführt worden (PALMER et al. 1977; PALMER u. WIDDOWSON 1979). Auf diese Weise konnten [^{18}F]-Fluoröstron und [^{18}F]-Fluoröstradiol mit sehr kleinen spezifischen Aktivitäten von nur 1,7 bis 5 MBq mMol^{-1} erhalten werden. Auf ähnlichem Wege konnten verschiedene andere Steroide mit spezifischen Aktivitäten von 2 bis 10 GBq mMol^{-1} mit ^{18}F markiert werden (SPITZNAGLE u. MARINO 1977). Über die nukleophile Substitution mit Hilfe von Kronenether (18-Krone-6) konnten auch [^{18}F]-21-

Fluorprogesteron (Irie et al. 1982) und [^{18}F]-Pregnenolon (Eng et al. 1983) mit höherer spezifischer Aktivität hergestellt werden. Mit guten radiochemischen Ausbeuten (30–60%) und brauchbaren spezifischen Aktivitäten (4–6 TBq mMol^{-1}) konnten innerhalb 70–110 min verschiedene [^{18}F]-Fluoröstrogene als Östrogen-Rezeptor-Liganden synthetisiert und evaluiert werden (Landvater et al. 1983; Kiesewetter et al. 1984). Die Präparation gelang durch einfachen nukleophilen Austausch der Triflat-Gruppe (OTf) gegen [^{18}F]-Fluorid in Gegenwart von Tetrabutylammoniumhydroxid als Anionenaktivator:

$$1) \text{ n–Bu}_4\text{NF} \qquad 2) \text{ LiAlH}_4 \tag{94}$$

Die Markierungssynthese des (2R*, 3S*)-1-[^{18}F]-Fluor-2,3-bis(4-hydroxyphenyl)-pentan ([^{18}F]-Fluornorhexöstrol) beinhaltet zwei aktive Reaktionsschritte: der nukleophile Austausch der Triflatgruppe am aliphatischen Kohlenstoff und die anschließende reduzierende Abspaltung der aromatischen Triflatgruppen. Sie kann jedoch als Eintopfreaktion durchgeführt werden.

16-α-Halogenöstradiole sind zur szintigraphischen Darstellung von Mamakarzinomen markiert worden. Sie ermöglichen die in-vivo Unterscheidung Östradiol-abhängiger Tumore von nicht-enzymstimulierten. Die Radioiodierung gelingt durch nicht-isotopen I-für-Br Austausch an 16α-Iodöstradiol-17β mit einer spezifischen Aktivität von 5,2 TBq mMol^{-1} (Hochberg 1979). Höhere spezifische Aktivitäten von 33 bis 55 TBq mMol^{-1} konnten bei der Radiobromierung von Östradiol-17β und dem 11-β-Methoxy-Derivat erhalten werden (Katzenellenbogen et al. 1981; Senderoff et al. 1982). Dabei wurde die Enol-diacetat-Ausgangsverbindung mit Na^{77}Br und H$_2$O$_2$ in-situ elektrophil bromiert. Anschließende Reduktion mit LiAlH$_4$ lieferte das gewünschte Produkt in weniger als zwei Stunden in 50%iger Ausbeute:

$$\xrightarrow[\text{H}_2\text{O}_2/\text{HOAc}]{^*\text{Br}^-} \qquad \xrightarrow[\text{THF}]{\text{LiAlH}_4} \tag{95}$$

$$R = H, OCH_3; \quad R^1 = OH, H; \quad R^2 = H, OH$$

Diese Synthese ist auch für den kurzlebigen Positronenstrahler Brom-75 geeignet. Eine vergleichende Studie zeigt, daß 16α-[^{77}Br]-Bromöstradiol-17β und 16α-[^{125}I]-Iodöstradiol-17β etwa gleich gut geeignet sind (McElvany et al. 1982).

V. Rezeptor-Liganden

Die nichtinvasive Untersuchung von Rezeptorarealen in-vivo ist eines der wichtigsten Anliegen der heutigen Radiopharmaka-Entwicklung für die PET Technik. Neben der bildlichen Darstellung der regionalen Verteilung bietet sich mit Hilfe geeigneter Modelle vor allem die Möglichkeit der quantitativen in-vivo Messung der Bindungskinetik von Liganden und von Rezeptordichten am lebenden Primaten (z. Übersicht s. Eckelman 1982; Wagner 1986; Maziotta u. Phelps 1986). Agonisten und Antagonisten, die mit hoher Affinität und Spezifität als Liganden für spezielle Rezeptoren geeignet sind, stehen im Vordergrund der Markierungschemie. Hier sind bisher neben Steroiden (Onkologie) vor allem Liganden adrenerger und cholinerger (Kardiologie), dopaminerger und serotonerger Systeme (Neurologie) sowie der Benzodiazepin-, GABA- und Opiat-Rezeptoren (Pharmakologie, Neurologie) untersucht worden.

Neben den Steroiden, die vor allem in der Tumorforschung eine Rolle spielen (vgl. Abschnitt D.IV), betreffen die anderen Gruppen vor allem Störungen in Herz- und Hirn-Rezeptorarealen. Die nichtinvasive Messung α- und β-adrenerger Rezeptordichten des Herzens und die in-vivo Erfassung und pharmakologische Beeinflussung des Herzens auf Kreislaufänderungen, also von Prozessen, die durch Rezeptoren gesteuert werden, bieten neue Ansätze für die Neurokardiologie (z. Übersicht s. SCHELBERT u. SCHWAIGER 1986). Die frühe Erkennung von Veränderungen in der Dichte von Dopamin-Rezeptorarealen (z.B. bei Schizophrenie, Chorea Huntington) und Serotonin-Rezeptorarealen (Schizophrenie) ist für die Neurologie von großer Bedeutung (s. Übersicht MAZIOTTA u. PHELPS 1986; WAGNER 1986). In der Arzneimittelforschung schließlich kann die Verteilung und Kinetik von zentralwirksamen Pharmaka nichtinvasiv in Primaten mittels der PET-Technik erfaßt werden.

Für die Auswahl der markierten Liganden gelten sehr strikte Randbedingungen. Zunächst sollte er eine hohe Affinität zum Rezeptor haben und chemisch so stabil sein, daß er durch den Körper zum Rezeptor transportiert werden kann und sich auch während der Messung nicht verändert. Für die Markierungssynthese ist vor allem wichtig, daß der Ligand in extrem hoher spezifischer Aktivität hergestellt werden muß. Dabei sind neben nicht-isotopen Verbindungen auch chemisch ähnliche z.B. die Ausgangssubstanz, die oft selbst hohe Rezeptoraffinitäten haben, zu berücksichtigen. Dies ist leicht einzusehen, wenn man bedenkt, daß z.B. die Rezeptordichte in der Hirnrinde nur in der Größenordnung von 10 pmol g^{-1} Hirnprotein entsprechend einer Konzentration von etwa 10^{-9} M liegt. Aufgrund der physiologischen Randbedingungen läßt sich abschätzen (ECKELMAN et al. 1979), daß bei einer applizierten Dosis von 370 MBq und hohen Rezeptoraffinitäten (K_D etwa 1 bis 10 nM) der markierte Ligand eine spezifische Aktivität von 10^4 bis 10^5 GBq mMol^{-1} besitzen muß. Selbst bei kurzen Halbwertzeiten von 20–110 min stellt dies im Hinblick auf die inhärenten isotopen Verunreinigungen und die Schwierigkeiten einer Synthese ohne Trägerzusatz (vgl. Abschnitt C.I) eine beträchtliche Anforderung dar. In vielen Fällen haben sich allerdings auch spezifische Aktivitäten von einigen 10^3 GBq mMol^{-1} (>hundert mCi mMol^{-1}) als ausreichend erwiesen.

Markierte Neurotransmitter selbst (z.B. Dopamin, Serotonin oder GABA) sind wegen ihrer bereits hohen regionalen Konzentration in einzelnen Organen des Körpers und der damit verbundenen Verdünnung meist nicht geeignet, postsynaptische Rezeptorareale mittels der PET Technik zu evaluieren, sondern nur um ihren präsynaptischen Vorrat bzw. ihren Stoffwechsel sichtbar zu machen (s. Dopamin-Abschnitt D.II.). Besser geeignet sind Antagonisten, die mit hoher Affinität an einen spezifischen Rezeptor gebunden werden. Viele zentralwirksame Pharmaka, die in der Neurologie eingesetzt werden, sind Antagonisten eines oder mehrerer Neurotransmitter-Rezeptoren. Diese haben oft eine vom Agonisten völlig verschiedene Struktur. Sie durchdringen die Blut-Hirn-Schranke durch passiven Transport aufgrund ihrer hohen Lipophilie. Eine Reihe von pharmakologischen Kriterien müssen erfüllt sein, damit ein Ligand als Rezeptor-spezifisches Radiopharmakon eingesetzt werden kann (z. Übersicht s. ECKELMAN 1982). Für die Bewertung stehen invasive in-vivo und in-vitro Verfahren zur Verfügung.

Wegen der Bedeutung des dopaminergen Stoffwechsels bei verschiedenen neurologischen Erkrankungen spielen prae- und postsynaptische Tracer eine besondere Rolle. Auf das präsynaptische [6-^{18}F]-Fluordopamin bzw. seinen Vorläufer [6-^{18}F]-Fluordopa und seine Markierung wurde bereits in Abschnitt D.II. hingewiesen. Für die Bestimmung von Dopamin Rezeptordichten sind – wie bereits erwähnt – exogene Agonisten und Antagonisten geeignet. Dopamin-Rezeptorliganden sind für bildgebende Verfahren besonders günstig, da z.B. die dopaminergen Zellen im Hirn in einem sehr eng begrenzten Bereich, dem Striatum, in besonders hoher Dichte vorkommen. Hier sind vor allem Butyrophenon-Neuroleptika eingesetzt worden, Dopamin Antagonisten mit hoher Affinität zum D-2 Rezeptor. Bei den Butyrophenon-Neuroleptika stellt der p-Fluor-ω-aminobutyrophenonrest die pharmakophore Gruppe dar (Schema VII). In diesem Molekülteil darf eigentlich eine Fremdmarkierung, die zur Veränderung des Molekülteils führen würde, nicht vorgenommen werden. Dennoch konnte kürzlich gezeigt werden, daß eine Iodierung in der 2′-Position die Rezeptor-bindenden Eigenschaften eher verbessert (Saji et al. 1986). Darüber hinaus bietet sich für die PET die Möglichkeit, entweder das inaktive Fluoratom durch ein ^{18}F oder z.B. den Kohlenstoff der

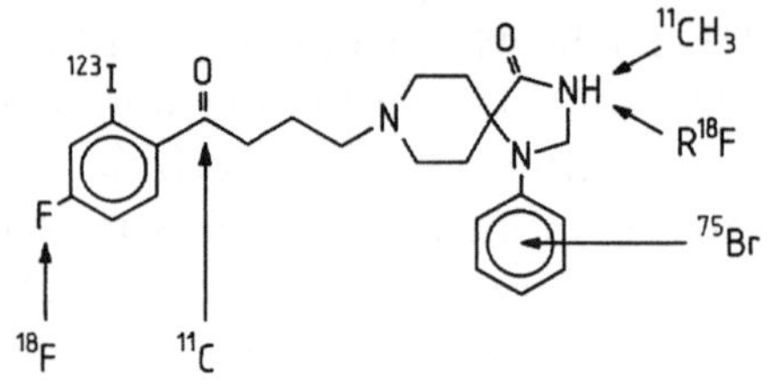

Schema VII. Markierungsmöglichkeiten von Spiroperidol für PET und SPECT

Carbonylgruppe durch ^{11}C zu ersetzen. Im sogenannten nichtessentiellen Teil des tertiären Amins dagegen kann auch eine Fremdmarkierung, z.B. mit ^{75}Br, vorgenommen werden. Diese Markierungsmöglichkeiten sind am Beispiel des Spiroperidols in Schema VII angedeutet. Die 3-N-Methylierung oder die Bromierung des aktivierten Phenylrings sind synthetisch besonders einfach. So wurde mit klassischen Methoden der elektrophilen Bromierung das p-Bromspiroperidol mit verschiedenen Bromisotopen markiert (Kulmala et al. 1981; Friedman et al. 1982; Maziere et al. 1984). Für eine Radiobromierung ohne Trägerzusatz ist vor allem die in-situ Oxidation von n.c.a. Bromid mit Dichloramin-T geeignet, wie im Falle des [^{75}Br]-Brombenperidol gezeigt werden konnte (Moerlein u. Stöcklin 1984). Eine Markierung mit ^{11}C in der Carboxylposition ist schwierig. Unter Verwendung von [^{11}C]-HCN als Vorläufer wurden nur kleine Ausbeuten erhalten (Fowler et al. 1982a). Einfacher ist die 3-N-Methylierung mit [^{11}C]-CH$_3$I, die mit guter Ausbeute zum Analogen [3-N-^{11}C]-Methylspiroperidol führt (Wagner et al. 1983; Burns et al. 1984; Dannals et al. 1986a). Im Hinblick auf die relativ langsame in-vivo Kinetik ist ^{11}C nur bedingt geeignet, da die Sättigungsanreicherung im spezifischen Rezeptorareal meist erst nach mehreren Stunden erreicht wird. ^{18}F und ^{75}Br sind deshalb und auch im Hinblick auf die meist leichter erreichbare hohe spezifische Aktivität oft bessere Tracer. Die Bromierung im nichtessentiellen, aktivierten Benzolring von Butyrophenon-Neuroleptika führt allerdings aufgrund der erhöhten Lipophilie oft zu einem erheblichen Verlust der Spezifität (Moerlein et al. 1986b).

Die ^{18}F-Markierung in der pharmakophoren p-Fluorbutyrophenon-Gruppe gelingt ohne Trägerzusatz durch nukleophile aromatische ^{18}F-für-NO$_2$ Substitution am p-Nitrobenzonitril (Arnett et al. 1985; Shiue et al. 1985b). Ausgehend vom Vorläufer p-[^{18}F]-Fluorbenzonitril erreicht man in einer mehrstufigen Synthese die ^{18}F-markierten Neuroleptika Pipamperon, Benperidol, Haloperidol, Spiroperidol und N-Methylspiroperidol (Shiue et al. 1985b) mit einer radiochemischen Ausbeute von 10–20% (EOB) und einer spezifischen Aktivität von 10^5 GBq mMol^{-1} innerhalb von etwa 90 min (Schema VIII). Diese Synthese ist der Einführung von ^{18}F über die Triazenmethode (Corley et al. 1981; Welch et al. 1983), die nur zu Ausbeuten von einigen wenigen Prozent führt, überlegen. Mit Milfe der Aminopo-

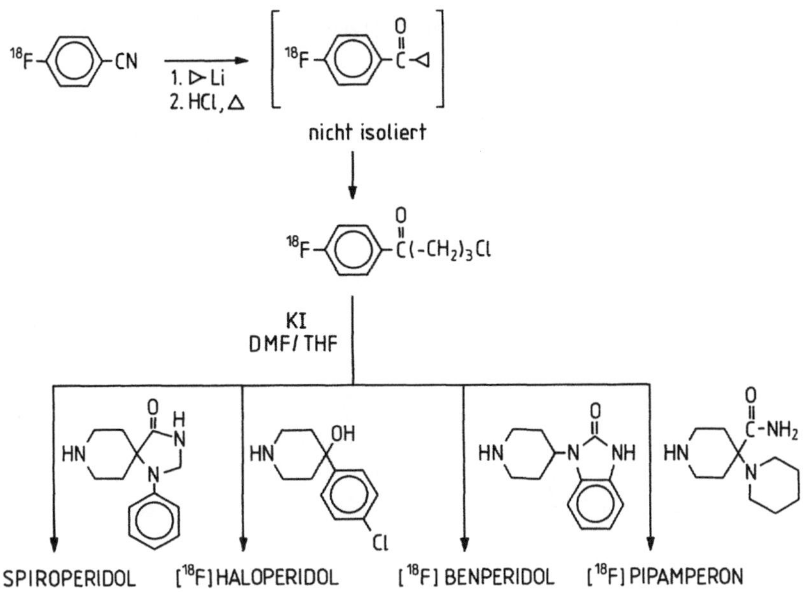

Schema VIII. Synthese von ^{18}F-Butyrophenon-Neuroleptika. (Nach SHIUE et al. 1985b)

lyether-gestützten nukleophilen aromatischen Substitution läßt sich sogar der direkte Austausch nukleofuger Gruppen gegen [^{18}F]-Fluorid am Neuroleptikum selbst bewerkstelligen (HAMACHER et al. 1986b). Auf diese Weise konnten Spiroperidol und Methylspiroperidol mit radiochemischen Ausbeuten von mehr als 30% markiert werden:

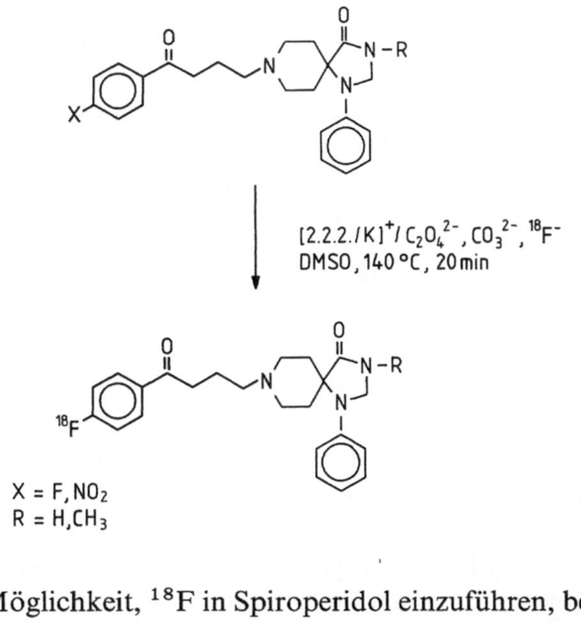

$$X = F, NO_2$$
$$R = H, CH_3$$

(96)

Eine andere elegante Möglichkeit, ^{18}F in Spiroperidol einzuführen, besteht in der Fluoralkylierung (BLOCK et al. 1986; CHI et al. 1986; KIESEWETTER et al. 1986; SHIUE et al. 1987). Die [^{18}F]-Fluoralkylierung ist generell eine längerlebige Alternative zur [^{11}C]-Methylierung (s. Abschnitt C.III.3.). Prinzipiell können hier zwei Wege beschritten werden. Eine zweistufige Synthese, bei der zunächst ein [^{18}F]-markiertes bifunktionelles Alkan hergestellt wird (s.o. Gl. 62), das dann mit der H-aciden Verbindung kondensiert wird, wobei im Falle des Spiroperidols z.B. das 3-N-([2-^{18}F]-Fluorethyl)-spiroperidol (^{18}F-FESP) entsteht (Block et al. 1986b):

$$^{18}F-(CH_2)_2-OTos \quad + \qquad\qquad\qquad\qquad\qquad\qquad\qquad\qquad\qquad\qquad\qquad$$

$$\xrightarrow[\substack{MeCN\\82\,°C}]{\substack{[K/2.2.2.]^+\\CO_3^{2-}\\10\,min}} \qquad\qquad\qquad\qquad\qquad\qquad\qquad\qquad\qquad\qquad\qquad (97)$$

Bezogen auf das eingesetzte [^{18}F]-Fluorid verläuft die 2-Stufenreaktion mit 20%iger radiochemischer Ausbeute mit spezifischen Aktivitäten von $\geq 10^5$ GBq mMol^{-1}. Sie kann auch als Eintopfsynthese durchgeführt werden. In diesem Falle betragen die Ausbeuten 40% (Block 1987b), die spezifischen Aktivitäten sind jedoch kleiner ($\geq 10^4$ GBq mMol^{-1}). Die Fluorierung kann auch mit [2-^{18}F]-Fluoralkylbromiden in Gegenwart von n-Bu$_4$NOH vorgenommen werden (Chi et al. 1986; Shiue et al. 1987). Während bei der nukleophilen Fluorierung des Alkylierungsmittels das Aminopolyether 2.2.2./K$_2$CO$_3$-System höhere Ausbeuten liefert (Block et al. 1987a), führt die Verwendung von n-Bu$_4$NOH als Base bei der Fluoralkylierung zu besseren Ausbeuten. Alternativ läßt sich das [^{18}F]-FESP auch in einer einstufigen Aktivsynthese herstellen (Kiesewetter et al. 1986; Satyamurthy et al. 1986), indem man zunächst in einer mehrstufigen kalten Synthese das 3-N-(2-Hydroxyethyl)-spiroperidol und daraus z.B. das entsprechende Mesylat herstellt. Die Mesylatgruppe wird sodann nukleophil gegen [^{18}F]-Fluorid ausgetauscht. Die relativ aufwendige kalte Synthese führt zu einem nicht sehr stabilen Vorläufer, der jeweils unmittelbar vor der Aktivsynthese präpariert oder gereinigt werden muß. 3-N-(2-[^{18}F]-Fluorethyl)-spiroperidol hat ähnlich gute D$_2$-Rezeptor-bindende Eigenschaften wie 3-N-[^{11}C]-Methylspiperon (Kiesewetter et al. 1986; Coenen et al. 1987).

Auch ^{11}C-markierte substituierte Benzamide wie z.B. Raclopride sind potente Dopamin D$_2$-Rezeptor-Antagonisten (Farde et al. 1986; Ehrin et al. 1985). Raclopride (s-($-$)-3,5-Dichlor-N-[(1-ethyl-2-pyrrolidinyl)]methyl-2-hydroxy-6-methylbenzamid) ist mit [^{11}C]-Ethyliodid am Stickstoffatom des Pyrrolidinringes (Ehrin et al. 1985) und mit ^{11}CH$_3$I an der OH-Gruppe der Desmethylverbindung (Farde et al. 1985) alkyliert worden. Die radiochemischen Ausbeuten betragen ca. 40% und die spezifische Aktivität ca. $2 \cdot 10^4$ GBq mMol^{-1} bei einer Präparationszeit von 50–60 min.

Als selektiver Dopamin D-1 Rezeptor Antagonist ist das Benzazepine SCH 23390, (R)$-$($+$)$-$8-Chlor-2,3,4,5-tetrahydro-3-methyl-5-phenyl-1H-3benzazepin-7-ol-hemilat, evaluiert (Billard et al. 1984) und mit ^{11}C markiert worden (Halldin et al. 1986a). Die Markierung erfolgte über eine einfache [^{11}C]-Methylierung der Desmethyl-Verbindung mit ^{11}CH$_3$I in 80%iger radiochemischer Ausbeute und einer spezifischen Aktivität von 11 GBq mMol^{-1} bei einer Synthesezeit von 40 min.

Zahlreiche andere Rezeptorliganden sind mit ^{123}I für SPECT-und insbesondere mit den Positronenstrahlern ^{11}C, ^{18}F und ^{75}Br für PET-Anwendungen markiert worden. Die wichtigsten sind in Tabelle 16 mit Angaben über Ausbeuten und spezifische Aktivität zusammenge-

Tabelle 16. Rezeptor-Liganden für PET und SPECT

Ligand	Synthese-vorläufer	Radio-chemische Ausbeute [%]	Spez. Aktivität [TBq mMol^{-1}] EOS	Literatur
Dopaminerge				
[^{11}C]-Spiroperidol	H^{11}CN		24	FOWLER et al. (1982a)
[^{11}C]-N-Methylspiroperidol	^{11}CH$_3$I		10	WAGNER et al. (1983), BURNS et al. (1984)
		21	100	DANNALS et al. (1986a)
[^{18}F]-Haloperidol	^{18}F$^-$		n.c.a.	TEWSON et al. (1980), WELCH et al. (1983), KILBOURN et al. (1984)
[^{18}F]-Benperidol	^{18}F$^-$		n.c.a.	CORLEY et al. (1981)
		10–20	> 100	ARNETT et al. (1985)
		10–20	> 100	SHIUE et al. (1985b)
[^{18}F]-Spiroperidol	^{18}F$^-$	10–20	> 100	ARNETT et al. (1985), SHIUE et al. (1985b)
[^{18}F]-3-N-Methylspiro-peridol	^{18}F$^-$	10–20	100	ARNETT et al. (1985)
		10–20	100	SHIUE et al. (1985b)
		30	> 100	HAMACHER et al. (1986b)
3-N-[^{18}F]-Fluorethylspiro-peridol	^{18}F$^-$	20–50	10–100	BLOCK et al. (1986b), SATYAMURTHY et al. (1986), CHI et al. (1986), SHIUE et al. (1987), COENEN et al. (1987)
		30–40	40–100	
3-N-[^{18}F]-Fluorpropylspiro-peridol				COENEN et al. (1987)
		30–40	40–100	CHI et al. (1986)
		15–20	40	SATYAMURTHY et al. (1986)
		10–20		SHIUE et al. (1987)
[^{77,75}Br]-p-Bromspiroperidol	*BrBr			KULMALA et al. (1981), DeJESUS et al. (1983), MAZIERE et al. (1984a)
	^{75}Br$^-$	20–30	> 70	MOERLEIN et al. (1986b)
[^{75}Br]-Brombenperidol	^{75}Br$^-$	30	300	MOERLEIN u. STÖCKLIN (1984)
[^{75}Br]-Bromperidol	^{75}Br$^-$	35	370	MOERLEIN u. STÖCKLIN (1985)
[2'-*]-Iodspiroperidol	*I$^-$		1	SAJI et al. (1986)
[4-*I]-Iodspiroperidol	*I$^-$		80	LANDVATTER (1985)
[^{11}C]-Pimozid	^{11}COCl$_2$	20	10	CROUZEL et al. (1980)
[^{11}C]-Chlorpromazin	H^{11}CHO		22	BERGER et al. (1979)
[^{11}C]-Thioproperazin	H^{11}CHO		22	MAZIERE et al. (1977)
[^{11}C]-Raclopride	[^{11}C]−C$_2$H$_5$I	30–40		EHRIN et al. (1985)
	^{11}CH$_3$I	40–50	5	FARDE et al. (1985)
SCH 23390	^{11}CH$_3$I	80	30	HALLDIN et al. (1986a)
Serotonerge				
[^{11}C]-O-Methylbufotenin	H^{11}CHO		20	BERGER et al. (1978)
[^{11}C]-Ketanserin	^{11}COCl$_2$	25–50	90	BERRIDGE et al. (1983)
[^{11}C]-N-Methylketanserin	^{11}CH$_3$I	10	50	DANNALS et al. (1986b)
[^{18}F]-Ritanserin	^{18}F$^-$			BOULLAIS et al. (1986)

Tabelle 16. (Fortsetzung)

Ligand	Synthese-vorläufer	Radio-chemische Ausbeute [%]	Spez. Aktivität $[TBq\ mMol^{-1}]$ EOS	Literatur
Cholinerge				
$[^{123}I]$-3-Quinuclidinyl -4-iodbenzylat (4-IQNB)	$^{123}I^{-}$	20	40	ECKELMAN et al. (1984), GIBSON et al. (1984)
$[^{11}C]$-Methioidid-quinuclidinyl benzylat (^{11}C-MQMB)	$^{11}CH_3I$			MAZIERE et al. (1981), SYROTA et al. (1984)
$[^{11}C]$-Dexetimid	$C_6H_5{}^{11}CH_2I$	8	30	DANNALS et al. (1986c)
$[^{11}C]$-Levetimid	$C_6H_5{}^{11}CH_2I$	8	30	DANNALS et al. (1986c)
Adrenerge				
$[^{123}I]$-m-Iodbenzylguanidin (^{123}I-mIBG)	$^{123}I^{-}$			MANGNER et al. (1982), McEWAN et al. (1986), SISSON u. WIELAND (1986)
$[^{11}C]$-Noradrenalin	$H^{11}CN$		n.c.a.	FOWLER et al. (1974)
$[^{11}C]$-Propanolol	$(CH_3)_2{}^{11}CO$		70	BERGER et al. (1982)
$[^{11}C]$-Prazosin	$^{11}CO_2$	30	7	EHRIN et al. (1986)
$[^{11}C]$-Practolol	$^{11}CO_2$		n.c.a.	BERGER et al. (1983)
Benzodiazepine				
$[^{11}C]$-Diazepam	$^{11}CH_3I$		40	MAZIERE et al. (1980)
$[^{11}C]$-Flunitrazepam	$^{11}CH_3I$		30	MAZIERE et al. (1980)
$[^{11}C]$-Fludiazepam	$^{11}CH_3I$		n.c.a.	ARIYOSHI et al. (1982)
$[^{11}C]-$Ro 15-1788	$^{11}CH_3I$		60	MAZIERE et al. (1984b)
		51	>100	SUZUKI et al. (1985)
$[^{75}Br]$-7-Brombenzodiazepin	$^{75}Br^{-}$	20	700	SCHOLL et al. (1983)
$[^{123}I]$-7-Iodbenzodiazepin	$^{123}I^{-}$		n.c.a.	FOSTER et al. (1981)
Opiate				
$[^{11}C]$-Carfentanyl	$^{11}CH_3I$	30	40	DANNALS et al. (1985)
$[^{11}C]$-Morphin	$^{11}CH_3I$	70–80		SVÄRD et al. (1982)
		9	0,6	KLOSTER et al. (1979)
$[^{11}C]$-Heroin	$^{11}CH_3I$	4	0,6	KLOSTER et al. (1979)
$[^{18}F]$-3-Acetylcyclofoxy	^{18}F	35	7	CHANNING et al. (1985)
$[^{11}C]$-Diprenorphin	$^{11}CO_2$	35	n.c.a.	LUTHRA et al. (1985)

faßt. Die Liste erhebt keinen Anspruch auf Vollständigkeit, und nicht alle der dort aufgeführten Liganden erfüllen die Kriterien für eine Bestimmung von Rezeptordichten am lebenden Hirn. Fast alle Verbindungen sind Produkte der pharmazeutischen Industrie, und ihre Rezeptorbindenden Eigenschaften wurden zuvor in-vitro oder invasiv in-vivo mit $[^3H]$-markierten Liganden untersucht.

Die radiochemischen Ausbeuten in Tabelle 16 beziehen sich auf die Summe aller Synthesestufen, d.h. auf den Primärvorläufer (z.B. $^{11}CO_2$) und nicht auf den letzten Synthesevorläufer (z.B. $^{11}CH_3I$). Die Mehrzahl der ^{11}C-markierten Liganden ist durch einfache ^{11}C-Methylierung der entsprechenden Desmethylverbindung synthetisiert worden, da die meisten komplexeren Liganden OH oder NH Gruppen besitzen. In einigen Fällen wird auch der ursprüngliche Ligand durch zusätzliche ^{11}C-Alkylierung oder ^{18}F-Fluoralkylierung in einer OH oder NH Funktion in einen neuen homologen Liganden mit oft besseren Eigenschaften umgewandelt, da durch Einführung einer Alkylgruppe die Lipophilie erhöht wird. Die Synthesezeiten für die ^{11}C-Alkylierungen – ausgehend von $^{11}CO_2$ – liegen meist nur im Bereich von 20–60 min. Erhebliche Anstrengungen sind allerdings erforderlich, um die notwendigen spezifischen Aktivitäten von mindestens 10 TBq mMol^{-1} zu erhalten (s. Abschnitt B.I. und E.III.). Im Falle der Halogenierungen kommt deshalb nur das Radiohalogenid als Vorläufer in Frage.

VI. Verschiedenes

Zahlreiche Radiopharmaka, die mit kurzlebigen Nukliden für Anwendungen in der SPECT oder PET markiert worden sind, lassen sich nicht in die bisher behandelten Stoffgruppen einordnen. Einige wichtige sollen hier erwähnt werden.

1. Tracer für die Blutflußmessung

Neben den frei diffusiblen Edelgasen werden in der klinischen Routine vor allem N-Isopropyl-[^{123}I]-p-iodamphetamin (IMP) und neuerdings ^{99m}Tc-Hexamethyl-propylen-amin-oxim (HM-PAO) für die Messung des zerebralen Blutflusses mittels SPECT eingesetzt. Diese Produkte sind kommerziell erhältlich, und ihre Herstellung soll hier nicht beschrieben werden. Zahlreiche Verbindungen sind für die Messung des regionalen zerebralen Blutflusses für die PET entwickelt worden. Neben $H_2^{15}O$ (s. Abschnitt B.III) und ^{77}Kr als frei diffusible Tracer sind andere nahezu frei diffusible Moleküle wie [^{11}C]-Methan, [^{11}C]-Acetylen, [^{11}C]-Butanol, [^{18}F]-Fluorethanol und [^{18}F]-Fluormethan sowie „chemische Mikrospären" wie [^{11}C]-Iodantipyrin, [4-^{18}F]-Fluorantipyrin verwendet worden. Von diesen sind vor allem [^{18}F]-Fluormethan, [4-^{18}F]-Fluorantipyrin und [^{11}C]-Butanol evaluiert worden.

Zahlreiche ^{11}C-markierte Alkohole sind im Hinblick auf ihre Anwendbarkeit zur Flußmessung untersucht worden (RAICHLE et al. 1976; DISCHINO et al. 1983). Die ^{11}C-markierten Alkohole lassen sich leicht über Grignard Reaktion herstellen. Im Falle des [1-^{11}C]-Butanol (HELUS et al. 1982) konnte gezeigt werden, daß die Carboxylierung von 1-Propylmagnesiumbromid schneller verläuft als die Synthese über Organoborane (KOTHARI et al. 1985). Hierbei konnten innerhalb von 25 min radiochemische Ausbeuten von 55–74% erhalten werden.

Als Inhalationstracer ist vor allem [^{18}F]$-CH_3F$ geeignet (HOLDEN et al. 1981; KOEPPE et al. 1985). [^{18}F]-Fluormethan kann z.B. über die nukleophile Silber-katalysierte ^{18}F-für-I Substitution am CH_3I (GATLEY et al. 1981) erhalten werden oder in einer Modifikation dieser Methode ausgehend von [^{18}F]$-F_2$, das in eine Suspension von Ag_2O und Tetraethyl-ammoniumhydroxid in Acetonitril geleitet wird (WAGNER 1984). Letztere Reaktion, die innerhalb von 20 min mit einer 80%igen radiochemischen Ausbeute verläuft, führt zu einem trägerhaltigen Produkt. Da das eingeatmete [^{18}F]$-CH_3F$ nicht metabolisiert wird und den Körper in kurzer Zeit wieder durch Respiration verläßt, wird ein trägerfreies Produkt hier nicht benötigt. Als injizierbarer Tracer wurde in Anlehnung an das [^{123}I]Iodantipyrin, das früher in der Szintigraphie verwendet wurde, für die PET auch das [4-^{18}F]-Fluorantipyrin entwickelt. Es kann durch direkte elektrophile Substitution von Antipyrin mit [^{18}F]$-F_2$ (SHIUE u. WOLF 1981) oder [^{18}F]-Acetylhypofluorit (DICSIC u. DIRADDO 1985; WAGNER 1986) sowie regiospezifisch durch Spaltung der Si$-$C Bindung in 4-(Trimethylsilyl)antipyrin mit [^{18}F]$-F_2$ (DIRADDO u. DICSIC 1985) hergestellt werden. Bei der direkten Fluorierung entstehen neben dem Hauptprodukt [4-^{18}F]-Fluorantipyrin auch das markierte 4,4-Difluorantipyrin, das sich jedoch leicht durch HPLC abtrennen läßt. Das [4-^{18}F]-Antipyrin wird innerhalb von 40–50 min in radiochemischen Ausbeuten von 20–30% erhalten.

2. Stoffwechselzwischenprodukte

Auch Zwischenprodukte des Kohlenhydratstoffwechsels wie [^{11}C]-Pyruvat, das Endprodukt der anaeroben Glykolyse, [^{11}C]-Lactat oder auch [^{11}C]-Acetat sind neben 2-FDG und Fettsäuren als Tracer zur Beurteilung des Herzmuskel-Stoffwechsels verwendet worden.

[1-^{11}C]-Pyruvat ist durch enzymatische Synthese ausgehend von ^{11}CO$_2$ durch Austausch der Carboxylgruppe des Pyruvats mittels Pyruvat-Ferredoxin Oxidoreductase hergestellt worden (Cohen et al. 1980; Hara et al. 1985). Es kann durch Milchsäure-Dehydrogenase in L-[3-^{11}C]-Laktat umgewandelt werden (Cohen et al. 1980). L-[3-^{11}C]-Laktat kann enzymatisch auch über D,L-[3-^{11}C]-Alanin mittels ^{11}C-Methylierung von tert.-Butyl-2-isocyanoacetat erhalten werden (Kloster u. Laufer 1980). Die radiochemische Ausbeute beträgt 26% bei einer Synthesezeit von 45 Minuten.

[1-^{11}C]-Acetat kann über die Grignard Synthese innerhalb von 10 min mit hoher radiochemischer Ausbeute synthetisiert werden (Pike et al. 1982). Eine fernbediente Synthese dieses Tracers ist ebenfalls beschrieben worden (Pike et al. 1984).

Zum Studium des Lungenstoffwechsels wurden ^{11}C-markierte Amine insbesondere [1-^{11}C]-Octylamin (Fowler et al. 1976) und [^{11}C]-Serotonin (Fowler et al. 1977) ausgehend von H^{11}CN synthetisiert.

Putrescin (1,4-Diaminobutan) ist der Vorläufer der natürlichen Polyamine Spermin und Spermidiñ. Er ist u.a. als Indikator für maligne Hirntumore evaluiert worden (Volkow et al. 1983). [1-^{11}C]-Putrescin ist mit 20%iger radiochemischer Ausbeute ausgehend von [^{11}C]-Cyanid innerhalb von 50 min synthetisiert worden (McPherson et al. 1985). Eine verbesserte Eintopfsynthese, die innerhalb von 35 min eine radiochemische Ausbeute von 35–40% [1-^{11}C]-Putrescin lieferte, ist kürzlich beschrieben worden (Fowler et al. 1986).

3. DNS-, RNS-Vorläufer

Markierte DNS-Vorläufer und ihre Halogenanaloga spielen in der Tumorforschung eine bedeutende Rolle. Das in der Krebstherapie verwendete 5-Fluoruracil wurde durch direkte elektrophile Addition von [^{18}F]$-$F$_2$ an Uracil mit ^{18}F markiert (Fowler et al. 1973b; Vine et al. 1979). Intermediär entsteht in Essigsäure als Lösungsmittel [5-^{18}F]-6-Acetoxy-5,6-dihydrouracil (Schema IX). Die radiochemische Ausbeute beträgt 28% und die spezifische Aktivität 18,5 GBq mg^{-1} (Vine et al. 1979). Markierte Uracil- oder Uridin-Analoge zur Messung der RNA Syntheserate und des Tumorwachstums (Therapiekontrolle) sind ebenfalls mit ^{18}F markiert worden. Hierzu wurden die peracetylierten Nukleoside mit [^{18}F]$-$F$_2$ (Shiue et al. 1984b; Ishiwata et al. 1984) oder mit [^{18}F]$-$CH$_3$CO$_2$F (Shiue et al. 1984) mit radiochemischen Ausbeuten von 15–20% fluoriert. Kürzlich wurde über die Fluorierung der ungeschützten Nukleoside mit [^{18}F]$-$CH$_3$CO$_2$F in Ausbeuten von 20–30% berichtet (Visser et al. 1986).

Auch ^{11}C-markierte Nukleoside sind synthetisiert worden. So konnte durch enzymatische Methylierung von Desoxyuridilat mit ^{11}C-Formaldehyd [^{11}C]-Thymidylat hergestellt werden (Crawford et al. 1978), das durch enzymatische Dephosphorylierung in [^{11}C]-Thymidin umgewandelt wurde. [Methyl-^{11}C]-Thymidin konnte auch durch Bildung einer C$-$C Bindung ausgehend vom geschützten 5-Bromdesoxyuridin und dessen Umwandlung in das Lithiumsalz durch anschließende Methylierung erhalten werden (Langström et al. 1981b). Hierbei wurde das Trimethylsilylderivat des Lithiumsalzes des Desoxyuridins verwendet. Besser geeignet erscheint das Tetrahydropyranylderivat des 5-Bromdesoxyuridins (Sundoro-

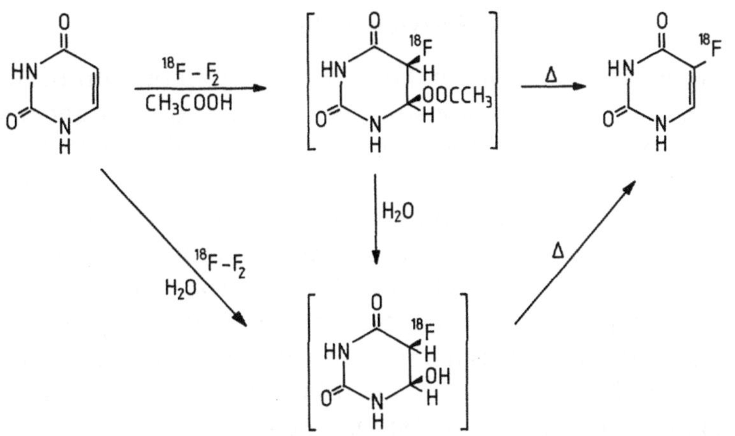

Schema IX. Synthese von [5-^{18}F]-Fluoruracil. (Nach Vine et al. 1979)

Wu et al. 1984). Diese Schutzgruppen sind stabil gegenüber der Halogen-Metall-Austausch-reaktion. Die Verbindung hat gegenüber den Trimethylsilyl- und methoxyisopropylderivaten den Vorteil, daß sie leicht präpariert und in kristalliner Form ohne Zersetzung für mehrere Monate gelagert werden kann.

4. Tracer für die Bestimmung des pH-Wertes

Änderungen des regionalen pH-Wertes stellen interessante physiologische Parameter dar. Das normale Hirngewebe, in dem das Säure-Basen-Gleichgewicht genau aufrechterhalten wird, hat einen intrazellulären pH-Wert von 7,0–7,1. Er ist niedriger als der des Plasmas mit 7,4. Der pH-Gradient zwischen Blut und Hirn oder auch zwischen Plasma und Lunge (pH etwa 6,7) kann eine Akkumulation des Tracers in der ionisierten, nicht diffusiblen Form hervorrufen. Dies kann wiederum genutzt werden, um lokale intrazelluläre pH Unter-schiede zu bestimmen. Eine Reihe von Aminen ist deshalb vorgeschlagen und evaluiert wor-den (Sargent et al. 1978; Braun et al. 1978; Tramposch et al. 1981; Winchel et al. 1980). Für die PET ist vor allem [^{11}C]-markiertes DMO (5,5-Dimethyloxazolidin-2,4-dion) erwäh-nenswert. DMO (pK$_a$ = 6,13) ist eine nicht metabolisierbare ungiftige Verbindung, die inner-halb einer mit der Halbwertszeit des ^{11}C kompatiblen Halbwertszeit Gleichgewichtsverteilung erreicht (Syrota et al. 1985; Rottenberg et al. 1985; Yamamoto et al. 1985). Als schwache Säure reichert sich DMO in alkalischem Gewebe in höheren Konzentrationen an, saures enthält im Gleichgewichtszustand geringere Konzentrationen. [2-^{11}C]-DMO kann ausgehend von [^{11}C]-Phosgen in hohen radiochemischen Ausbeuten innerhalb kurzer Zeit hergestellt werden (Berridge et al. 1982b; Ginos et al. 1982; Diksic 1984):

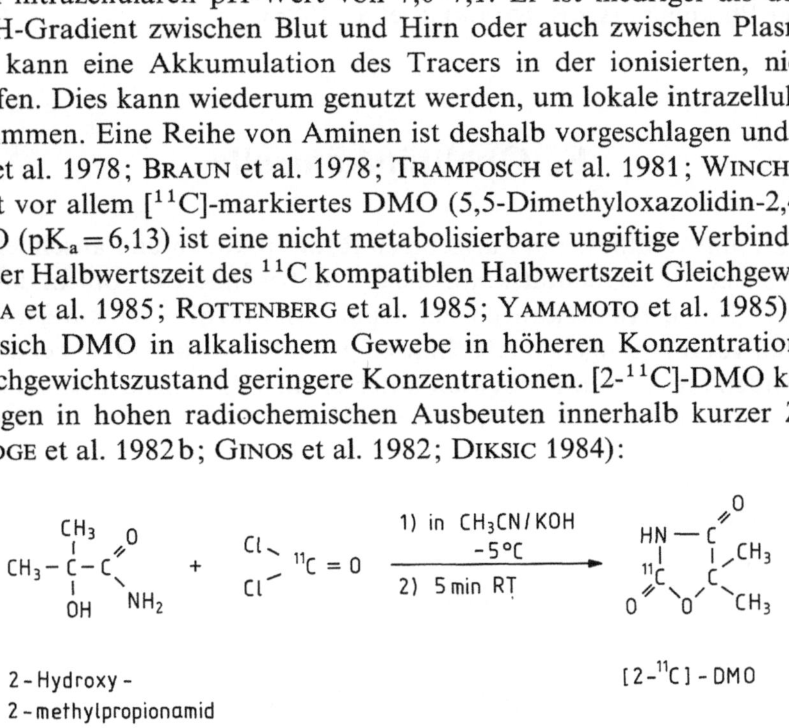

$$\text{(98)}$$

2-Hydroxy-
2-methylpropionamid   [2-^{11}C]-DMO

Da die Einstellung des Gewebe-Plasma-Gleichgewichts von DMO etwa 50–60 min erfor-dert, müssen relativ hohe Aktivitäten von einigen 0,7–1 GBq eingesetzt werden. Die ein-fachste und effizienteste Synthese (Diksic 1984) führt innerhalb von 30 min zu radioche-mischen Ausbeuten von 40–60% und einer spezifischen Aktivität von 3 TBq mMol^{-1}.

5. Enzyminhibitoren

Die in-vivo Erfassung von Enzymaktivitäten oder Enzymkonzentrationen stellt eine weitere interessante Anwendung der Emissionstomographie dar, die vor allem auch für pharmakologische bzw. toxikologische Untersuchungen am lebenden Primaten von Bedeutung ist (z.B. Therapiekontrolle). Die irreversible Inhibition (Suizid-Inhibition) wird auch als Anreicherungsmechanismus bei der Anwendung von Radiopharmaka in der Diagnostik genutzt. Beispielhaft sollen hier nur einige Inhibitoren der Monoamin-Oxidase (MAO) erwähnt werden, die für Anwendungen mit der PET mit ^{11}C markiert worden sind. Es sind dies in erster Linie die Propinylamine wie Pargylin, N-Benzyl-N-methyl-2-propinylamin, ein MAO-B-Inhibitor, der ausgehend von N-Desmethyl-pargylin mit radiochemischen Ausbeuten von 22–45% und einer spezifischen Aktivität von 37–148 GBq mMol^{-1} innerhalb von 50–60 min markiert werden konnte (Ishiwata et al. 1985). Auch Chlorgylin und L-Deprenyl sind als MAO-A bzw. MAO-B Inhibitoren mit Kohlenstoff-11 markiert worden, um die MAO-Aktivität in vivo mittels PET zu erfassen (MacGregor et al. 1985). Die Markierung konnte durch ^{11}C-Methylierung der Desmethylverbindung innerhalb von 40 min mit einer radiochemischen Ausbeute von 93 bzw. 85% und einer spezifischen Aktivität von 7,4 TBq mMol^{-1} erreicht werden (Halldin et al. 1986b).

Auch das dopaminerge Neurotoxin 1-Methyl-4-phenyl-1,2,3,6-tetrahydropyridin (MPTP), das durch MAO zum entsprechenden Pyridiniumion (MPP^{+}) oxidiert wird, das die nigrostratialen Zellen im Gehirn zerstört und die Symptome von Parkinsonismus hervorruft (Davis et al. 1979; Langston et al. 1983) wurde nach ^{11}C-Methylierung der Desmethylverbindung im Hinblick auf seine zerebrale in-vivo Pharmakokinetik mittels PET untersucht (Moerlein et al. 1986). Die bevorzugte Anreicherung in den Basalganglien konnte durch einen MAO Inhibitor stark unterdrückt werden. Diese und andere Anwendungen sind auch Beispiele für den Einsatz von PET zur quantitativen in-vivo Messung der Pharmakokinetik zentralwirksamer Pharmaka (s.z.B. Stöcklin et al. 1986).

E. Qualitätskontrolle

Bei der Markierungssynthese mit kurzlebigen Radionukliden und anschließender Anwendung am Patienten stellt die Qualitätskontrolle oft ein besonderes Problem dar, das spezieller Lösungen bedarf. Einige Anmerkungen zur Qualitätskontrolle bei kurzlebigen Produkten sind bereits in den vorangegangenen Abschnitten gemacht worden. Wie bei den mit längerlebigen Radionukliden markierten Produkten unterscheidet man prinzipiell auch bei den kurzlebigen folgende Einzelaspekte der Qualitätskontrolle:
– radionuklidische Reinheit,
– radiochemische Reinheit,
– chemische Reinheit,
– spezifische Aktivität,
– pharmazeutische Reinheit (Sterilität und Pyrogenfreiheit).

I. Radionuklid-Reinheit

Die Radionuklid-Reinheit betrifft die isotopen und nichtisotopen radioaktiven Verunreinigungen, und zwar unabhängig von der chemischen Form, in der diese Radioaktivität auftritt. Diese radionuklidischen Verunreinigungen entstehen im allgemeinen bei der Radio-

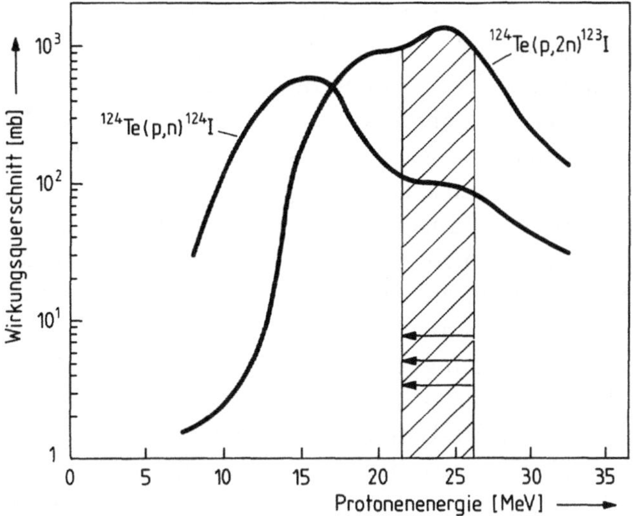

Abb. 7. Anregungsfunktionen der ^{124}Te(p,n)^{124}I- und ^{124}Te(p,2n)^{123}I-Reaktionen. (Nach Kondo et al. 1977)

nuklidproduktion durch konkurrierende Kernreaktionen. Dies kann am Targetisotop selbst geschehen, wie etwa im Falle der ^{11}C-Produktion:

$$\text{Produktionsreaktion} \quad ^{14}\text{N}(p,\alpha)^{11}\text{C}$$
$$\text{Störreaktion} \quad ^{14}\text{N}(p,pn)^{13}\text{N},$$

wenn mit Energien oberhalb der Schwelle der Störreaktion (11,4 MeV) bestrahlt wird. Ähnliches gilt für die ^{123}I Produktion:

$$\text{Produktionsreaktion} \quad ^{124}\text{Te}(p,2n)^{123}\text{I}$$
$$\text{Störreaktion} \quad ^{124}\text{Te}(p,n)^{124}\text{I}.$$

Hier überlappen sich die Anregungsfunktionen (vgl. Abb. 7), so daß selbst bei Auswahl eines optimalen Energiebereichs (s. schraffierter Teil in Abb. 7) ^{124}I-Verunreinigungen nicht vermieden werden können (Kondo et al. 1977). Daneben laufen im vorliegenden Falle auch Störreaktionen an isotopen Verunreinigungen ab. So enthält z.B. das hochangereicherte ^{124}Te u.a. kleine Mengen ^{125}Te, so daß eine Reaktion an diesem Isotop ebenfalls zum unerwünschten ^{124}I führt:

$$\text{Störreaktion am Nachbarisotop} \quad ^{125}\text{Te}(p,2n)^{124}\text{I}.$$

Schließlich können radionuklidische Verunreinigungen auch durch andere chemische Elemente im Target entstehen, so etwa bei der ^{11}C-Produktion in N_2-Targets in Gegenwart von Sauerstoff:

$$\text{Produktionsreaktion} \quad ^{14}\text{N}(p,\alpha)^{11}\text{C}$$
$$\text{Störreaktion} \quad ^{16}\text{O}(p,\alpha)^{13}\text{N}.$$

Die radionuklidische Verunreinigung wird in % der Gesamtaktivität angegeben. Eine Verunreinigung von 1% ^{124}I ($T_{1/2}=4{,}15$ d) im ^{123}I bedeutet, daß zu einer gegebenen Zeit 1% aller Zerfälle vom ^{124}I stammen. Die radionuklidische Verunreinigung ist vom Zeitpunkt der Messung abhängig, da Verunreinigung und Hauptaktivität unterschiedliche Halbwertszeiten besitzen. Im allgemeinen wird sie auf Bestrahlungsende (EOB = end of bombardment) bezogen.

Die Minimierung der radionuklidischen Verunreinigungen erfolgt bereits bei der Produktionsoptimierung mit Hilfe der γ-Spektrometrie und Absolutzählung (zur Einführung s. z.B. Lieser 1981). Bei Gemischen aus reinen Positronenstrahlern ist man zur Identifizierung auf die Halbwertszeit angewiesen, da nur die 511 keV Vernichtungsstrahlung zur Verfügung steht. Die radionuklidische Qualitätskontrolle erfolgt bei den kurzlebigen Positronenstrahlern on-line und eine Abtrennung von nichtisotopen radionuklidischen Verunreinigungen ist meist einfach. Oft kann darauf auch verzichtet werden, wenn das andere Nuklid sich unter den Bedingungen der anschließenden Synthese chemisch inert oder völlig anders verhält, so daß es bei vorgegebener chromatographischer Reinigung (s.u.) nicht stört. Dies gilt z.B. für ^{13}N bei ^{11}C-Markierungssynthesen. Insgesamt ist bei einer routinemäßigen bereits eingefahrenen Radionuklidproduktion die nicht-isotope Radionuklidreinheit kein Problem und gut bekannt, da man es immer mit dem gleichen Produktionsprozeß zu tun hat. Es ist dennoch notwendig, die Radionuklidreinheit regelmäßig zu überwachen, da durch Veränderungen der Bestrahlungsvorrichtung Bedingungen entstehen, die zu Verschiebung der Teilchenenergie und zur Änderung des Energieverlusts im Target führen können. Dies kann wiederum zu veränderten Konzentrationen der Radionuklidverunreinigungen führen, insbesondere in festen Targets, bei denen darüber hinaus die Gefahr des Schmelzens und damit der Veränderung der Targetdicke besteht. Bei den kurzlebigen leichten Positronenstrahlern wie ^{11}C, ^{13}N, ^{15}O, ^{18}F spielen Radionuklidverunreinigungen eine untergeordnete Rolle, bei ^{75}Br und ^{123}I dagegen eine sehr bedeutende (zur Übersicht s. BLESSING et al. 1982; QAIM u. STÖCKLIN 1983).

II. Radiochemische und chemische Reinheit

Bei der Reinigung des gewünschten Produktes muß man zwischen chemischer und radiochemischer Verunreinigung unterscheiden. Chemische Verunreinigungen, wie die inaktive Ausgangssubstanz oder inaktive Neben- oder Zersetzungsprodukte, müssen in den meisten Fällen ebenso wie die radiochemischen Verunreinigungen entfernt werden.

Die radiochemische Reinheit bezieht sich auf die gewünschte chemische Form des Markierungsisotops. Unterschiedlich vom klassischen chemischen Reinheitsbegriff umfaßt die radiochemische Reinheit nicht nur geringste, makroskopisch oft kaum nachweisbare Verunreinigungen an radioaktiven Nebenprodukten, sondern auch Verunreinigungen, die Markierungsatome in einer unerwünschten Position aufweisen. Letzteres ist z.B. dann möglich, wenn das Markierungsreagens mehrere radioaktive Atome enthalten kann, wie im Falle von Acetylen oder wenn bei der Markierungsreaktion über eine Austauschreaktion mehrere austauschbare Gruppen betroffen sind. Das gilt insbesondere für die sehr unspezifische Rückstoßmarkierung. Die in unterschiedlichen Positionen im gleichen Molekül markierten Produkte können natürlich nicht voneinander getrennt werden. Im allgemeinen tritt das Problem der Markierungsposition nicht auf, da meist die Syntheseführung positionsspezifische Produkte liefert. Im Falle einer Fremdmarkierung, die etwa bei der aromatischen Halogenierung zur Bildung von ortho-, meta- und para-Isomeren führen kann, handelt es sich um unterschiedliche Moleküle, deren Trennung im allgemeinen eine analytisch lösbare Aufgabe darstellt.

Häufiger entstehen nichtisomere Verunreinigungen, die bei Synthesen ohne Trägerzusatz oft nur mit Hilfe radioanalytischer Methoden erfaßt werden können, da die oft nicht vorhersagbaren Nebenprodukte in Subnanogramm-Mengen vorliegen. Schwierigkeiten treten insbesondere immer dann auf, wenn die Verunreinigung dem Markierungsprodukt chemisch sehr ähnlich ist, so daß ihre Identifizierung bei einer chromatographischen Qualitätskontrolle mißlingt. Es empfiehlt sich deshalb zumindest beim Einfahren der Synthese, mehrere Trennverfahren, d.h. im Falle der Chromatographie, mehrere Säulen mit unterschiedlichen Trenneigenschaften einzusetzen. Schnelle chromatographische Trennmethoden in Verbindung mit einer Strahlendetektion (Radiochromatographie) sind für die Qualitätskontrolle von Verbindungen, die mit kurzlebigen Radionukliden markiert sind, unentbehrlich. Zur Einführung in die verschiedenen Techniken sei auf einschlägige Lehrbücher verwiesen (s. z.B. ROBERTS 1978; SIMON 1974).

1. Qualitätskontrolle gasförmiger Produkte

Die radiochemische Reinheit von kurzlebigen gasförmigen Produkten wie $[^{11}C]$-CO, $[^{11}C]$-CO$_2$, $[^{13}N]$-N$_2$, $[^{13}N]$-NH$_3$, $[^{15}O]$-O$_2$, $[^{15}O]$-CO, $[^{15}O]$-CO$_2$ etc. erfolgt fast ausschließlich mit Hilfe der Radiogaschromatographie. Hierbei wird ein Radioaktivitätsdetektor unmittelbar hinter dem Säulenausgang, oder bei gleichzeitiger Detektion von inaktiven Produkten z.B. hinter einem Wärmeleitfähigkeitsdetektor (WLF oder WLD) angebracht. Abbildung 8 zeigt eine schematische Darstellung eines Radiogaschromatographen. Als Detektor wird im Falle der hier vorliegenden γ-Strahler bzw. Positronenstrahler mit der 511 keV Vernichtungsstrahlung meist ein NaI-Szintillationsdetektor verwendet, wobei die Gasleitung entweder durch ein Bohrloch oder an zwei Detektoren vorbeigeführt wird, um eine günstige Geometrie zu erreichen. Für den meist qualitativen und halbquantitativen Nachweis sehr hoher Aktivitäten bei der Routineproduktion eignen sich auch einfache G.M.-Zähler, Ionisationskammern etc., an denen das Gas vorbeigeleitet wird.

Die in der gaschromatographischen Säule aufgetrennten Fraktionen (Produkte) durchströmen zunächst die WLF-Zelle und je nach Abstand und Strömungsgeschwindigkeit einige Sekunden später den Strahlendetektor, so daß eine nahezu synchrone Messung von

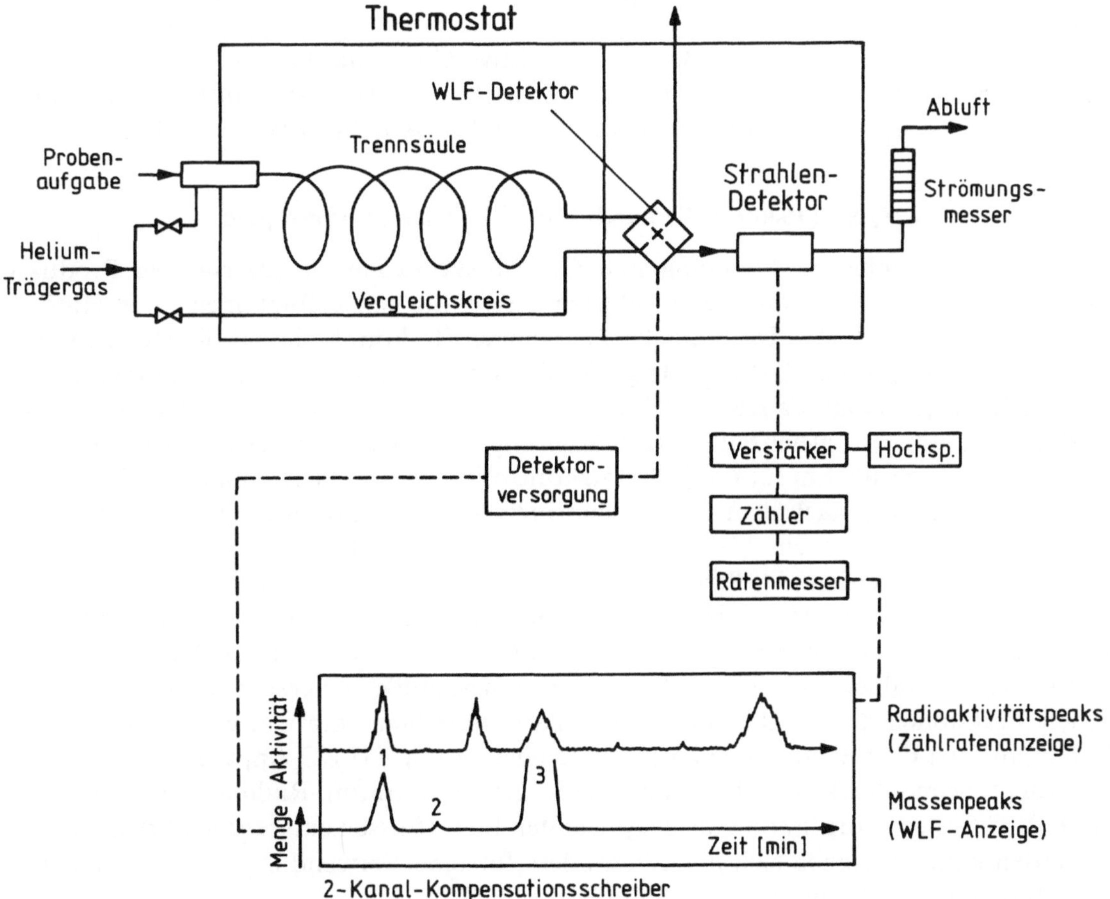

Abb. 8. Schema einer einfachen Anordnung zur radiogaschromatographischen Analyse mit Wärmeleitfähigkeits- und Strahlendetektor

Wärmeleitfähigkeit (Masse) und Radioaktivität erfolgt. Trägerfreie radioaktive Produkte erscheinen also nur als Radioaktivitätspeak, während bei geträgerten Produkten Massen- und Radioaktivitätspeak simultan erscheinen. Ein „masseloses" radioaktives Produkt ist durch seine Retentionszeit, d.h. durch die Lage seines Radioaktivitätspeaks im Gaschromatogramm charakterisiert und kann durch nachträgliche oder gleichzeitige Chromatographie des vermuteten Produktes mit einer durch den WLF-Detektor erfaßbaren Menge identifiziert werden. Dabei ist auf eine mögliche Mengenabhängigkeit der Retentionszeit zu achten.

Auch eine quantitative Erfassung der Radioaktivität der Produkte ist nach Eichung des Detektors möglich. Ist V das der Strahlendetektion ausgesetzte Volumen in cm^3 und f die Strömungsgeschwindigkeit in $cm^3\ min^{-1}$, so beträgt die Anzahl der beim Durchgang der Fraktion insgesamt registrierten Impulse I:

$$I = A\frac{V}{f}a \tag{99}$$

wobei A die absolute Aktivität, d.h. die Zerfallsrate in Zerfällen pro Minute und a der charakteristische Ausbeutefaktor des Detektors ist.

Eine routinemäßige regelmäßige radiogaschromatographische Analyse ist bei der Produktion der o.g. kurzlebigen Gase für medizinische Anwendungen unbedingt notwendig, da sich durch Änderung der Bestrahlungsbedingungen und/oder der Zusammensetzung des Gastargets sowie durch Veränderung von Parametern bei der chemischen Konversion (z.B. in den Reduktions- oder Oxidationsöfen) die Aktivitätsverteilung auf verschiedene Produkte ändern kann. Die radiogaschromatographische Qualitätskontrolle erfolgt hier on-line im Bypass.

Auch die chemische Reinheit in Bezug auf inaktive Gase muß beachtet werden. So kann im Falle der ^{15}O-Produktion durch strahlenchemische Prozesse NO_x auftreten, das durch entsprechende Absorptionsfallen entfernt werden muß (s. Abschnitt B. III, Abb. 2).

2. Qualitätskontrolle durch Flüssigkeitschromatographie

Die chromatographische Trennung und Qualitätskontrolle von markierten Produkten mit kleinen Dampfdrucken oder von gelösten festen Stoffen erfolgt meist mit Hilfe der Flüssigkeitschromatographie. Im Falle der kurzlebigen Radionuklide hat die Hochleistungsflüssigkeitschromatographie (HPLC = High Performance Liquid Chromatography) eine besondere Bedeutung erlangt, da sie hohe Auflösung bei der Trennung mit großer Schnelligkeit verbindet. Trennung und gleichzeitige Identifizierung erlauben Aufarbeitung, Reinigung und Analyse in einem Schritt. Ein für die Qualitätskontrolle kurzlebiger Radiopharmaka geeignetes HPLC-System kann nach dem Baukastenprinzip nach Bedarf zusammengesetzt werden, wobei als Massendetektor ein UV- und/oder ein RI (Refractive Index = Brechungsindex) Detektor verwendet werden. Als Strahlendetektor sind im Prinzip wie bei der Radiogaschromatographie alle für den Nachweis von γ-Strahlen geeigneten Detektoren verwendbar. Bei kleinen Aktivitäten oder präparativer Anwendung kann direkt oder im Anschluß an den kontinuierlichen Strahlennachweis auch ein Fraktionssammler eingesetzt werden, wobei die einzelnen Fraktionen der Strahlenmessung diskontinuierlich unterworfen werden können. In Abbildung 9 ist die schematische Anordnung einer Radio-HPLC-Apparatur mit verschiedenen Detektionsmöglichkeiten (Brechungsindex, UV-Absorption, Radioaktivität) wiedergegeben. HPLC-Systeme, die im Baukastensystem den Bedürfnissen entsprechend zusammengestellt werden können, eignen sich auch besonders für eine Verwendung im Zusammenhang mit Fernbedienung und Automatisierung in Bleizellen.

Für Radiopharmaka ist die Frage der Lösungsmittel im Hinblick auf die weitere Anwendung von Bedeutung. Bei der konventionellen Verteilungschromatographie fällt das Produkt

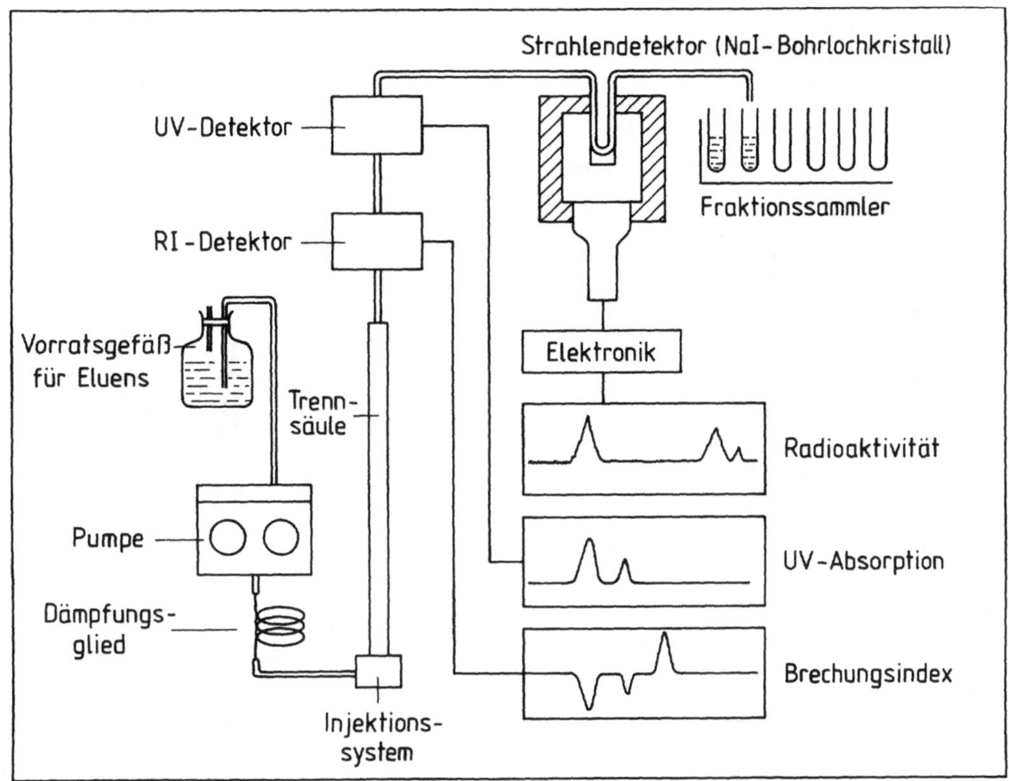

Abb. 9. Schema einer Anordnung zur Radio-Hochdruckflüssigkeitschromatographie mit UV-, IR- und Strahlendetektor (Bohrlochkristall) sowie Fraktionssammler

meist in organischen Lösungsmitteln an, d.h. das Eluens muß erst völlig verdampft und das Produkt in einer wäßrigen isotonen Lösung wiedergelöst werden. Bei diesen Manipulationen kommt es oft zu Verlusten durch Zersetzung, Verdampfung, Adsorption, Löserückstände und radioaktiven Zerfall.

Bei der Abtrennung von Verunreinigungen ist es für die Trennung am günstigsten, wenn die gewünschte Verbindung vor der Verunreinigung eluiert wird. Im umgekehrten Falle besteht die Gefahr, daß durch den noch erhöhten Untergrund des Vorpeaks (tailing) ein entsprechender Anteil der Verunreinigung in die Produktfraktion gelangt. In diesem Falle kann man durch Umkehrung der Phasenpolaritäten die Reihenfolge der Fraktionen oft vertauschen.

Auch bei der Routineproduktion ist eine ständige Qualitätskontrolle bzw. Reinigung meist nicht zu entbehren, da durch leicht veränderte Produktionsbedingungen der Anteil an radiochemischen Verunreinigungen stark verändert werden kann. Bei der Herstellung von [^{11}C]-Methionin z.B. tritt [^{11}C]-Aceton in wechselnden Mengen auf (BERGER et al. 1980b), und eine Abtrennung ist unerläßlich. Abbildung 10 zeigt eine HPLC-Trennung der entstehenden Produkte (MEYER 1982). Das Chromatogramm links gibt die präparative Trennung des Reaktionsgemisches wieder. Man sieht als inaktive Produkte Homocystein und Aceton sowie [^{11}C]-Methanol und [^{11}C]-Methionin als radioaktive Produkte. Je nach Syntheseführung kann die [^{11}C]-Methanol-Verunreinigung zwischen 2 und 30% schwanken. Die Effizienz der Trennung und gleichzeitig die Identität des Produktes Methionin zeigt das Chromatogramm rechts, das nach Reinjektion der Methionin-Fraktion erhalten wurde. Hierbei wurden Aceton, Methionin und Homocystein als Träger zugesetzt. Man sieht, daß der [^{11}C]-Methanolpeak verschwunden ist, und daß der Trägerpeak des Methionin mit dem Radioaktivitätspeak des gewünschten Produktes synchron erscheint.

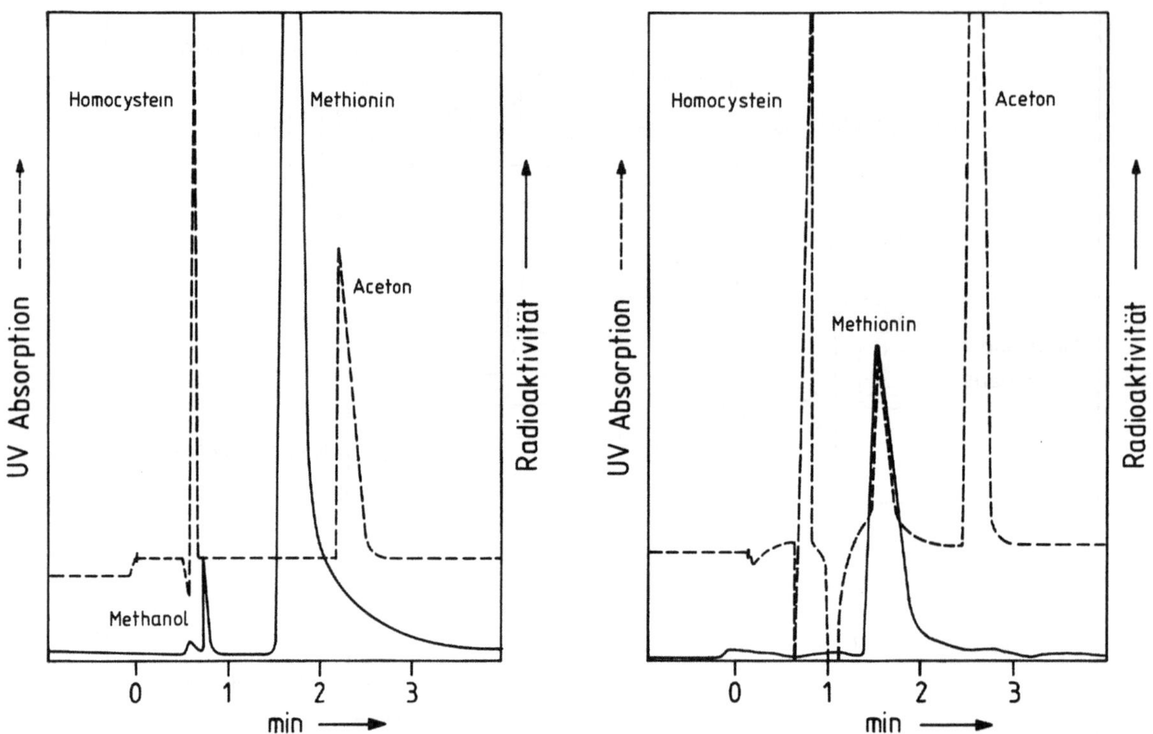

Abb. 10. *Links:* Radio-HPL-Chromatogramm der präparativen Trennung von [^{11}C]-Methionin von radioaktivem [^{11}C]-Methanol und inaktivem (gestrichelt) Homocystein und Aceton. *Rechts:* Radio-HPL-Chromatogramm nach Reinjektion der Methionin-Fraktion. Aceton und Homocystein wurden als Träger zugesetzt (Nach Meyer 1982)

Die Abtrennung von inaktiven chemischen Verunreinigungen ist immer dann dringend erforderlich, wenn es sich um toxische oder zentralwirksame Substanzen handeln kann. Insbesondere ist dies im Falle von rezeptorbindenden Radiopharmaka notwendig, da die meist chemisch ähnlichen inaktiven Produkte mit den radioaktiven Liganden um die Rezeptorstellen konkurrieren können. Abbildung 11 zeigt am Beispiel der Radiobromierung eines Benzodiazepins ohne Trägerzusatz über Triazenzersetzung (Scholl et al. 1983), daß neben dem bromierten Produkt (*3*) auch das protonierte (*1*), das chlorierte (*2*) und das dimerisierte Produkt (*4*) in makroskopischen Mengen entstehen. Sie können mit Hilfe des UV-Detektors sehr empfindlich nachgewiesen werden. Im Radioaktivitätschromatogramm erscheint nur das gewünschte Produkt BFB (*3*), das unter den verwendeten chromatographischen Bedingungen gut abgetrennt werden kann.

Zur Optimierung der HPLC-Bedingungen ebenso wie zur Qualitätskontrolle im Anschluß an eine präparative Trennung eignet sich auch die Dünnschichtchromatographie (TLC = Thin Layer Chromatography). Sie ist weniger aufwendig und genügt in vielen Fällen den Anforderungen. In Verbindung mit einem Strahlendetektor (scanner) kann die Dünnschichtplatte abgetastet werden, und man erhält auch hier ein Radiochromatogramm. Auf die Bedeutung der TLC bei der Optimierung im Entwicklungsstadium eines Produktes ist an anderer Stelle dieses Handbuches hingewiesen worden (Cohen u. Besnard 1980).

Bei einer Reihe von wichtigen Radiopharmaka-Präparationen kann die HPLC-Reinigung entfallen. Dies gilt z.B. für die Routineproduktion von [2-^{18}F]-FDG (s. Abschnitt D.I., Schema III, Tabelle 15). Hier sind einfache säulenchromatographische Trennungsstufen ausreichend: die erste zur Trennung der cis-trans-Isomeren, die zweite zur Reinigung des hydrolysierten Endproduktes. Kurze Silicagel-Säulen eignen sich in beiden Fällen, im zweiten Falle kann auch eine Al$_2$O$_3$-Säule verwendet werden. Eine anschließende Qualitätskontrolle des gereinigten Produktes durch TLC ist jedoch erforderlich.

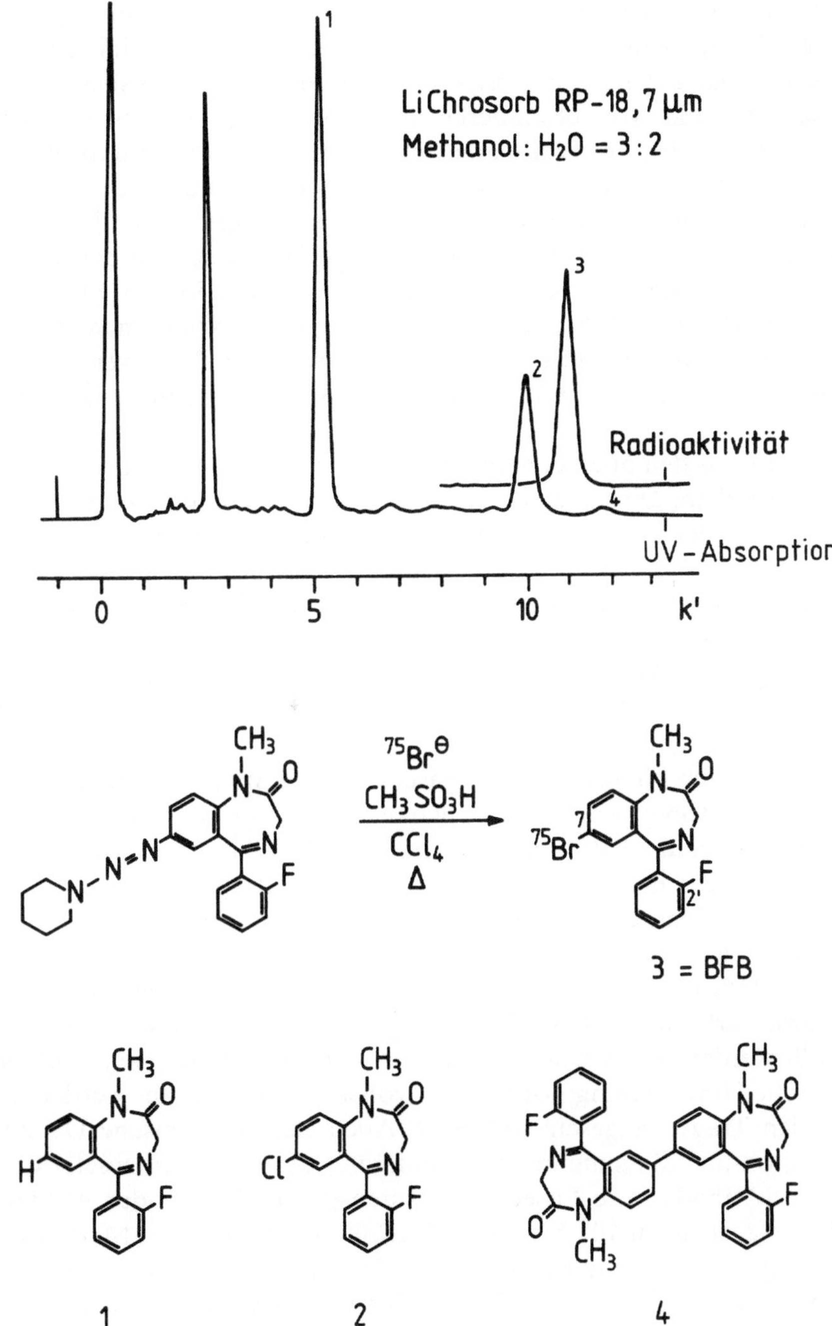

Abb. 11. Radiochromatogramm (HPLC) eines Reaktionsgemisches nach Triazenzersetzung. Neben dem radioaktiven Produkt *3* treten die inaktiven Nebenprodukte *1*, *2* und *4* auf (Nach SCHOLL et al. 1983)

III. Spezifische Aktivität

Auf die Bedeutung der spezifischen Aktivität ist bereits mehrfach hingewiesen worden (s. z.B. Abschnitt C.I., Tabelle 8 und Abschnitt D.V.). Die spezifische Aktivität bezieht sich i. allg. auf die Verdünnung der markierten Moleküle mit isotopen inaktiven Molekülen, und die Angabe erfolgt in TBq/mMol (Ci/mMol). Oft liegt aber auch eine Verdünnung mit nicht-isotopen analogen Molekülen vor, z.B. bei Fremdmarkierungen eine nicht völlig abgetrennte Ausgangsverbindung. Auch diese Information ist bei medizinischen Anwendungen sehr wichtig. Schließlich wird nach dem Vorliegen einer Injektionslösung auch die Angabe der Aktivität pro Volumeneinheit erforderlich. Die spezifische Aktivität ist also für die Anwendung von Radiopharmaka, die mit organischen Radionukliden insbesondere mit Positronenstrahlern markiert sind, von besonderer Bedeutung. Dies gilt vor allem für die neuen Anwendungsgebiete, d.h. bei der Erfassung physiologischer Organfunktionen. Ein trägerarmes Produkt (s. Tabelle 8) ist bei den kurzlebigen Radionukliden vor allem deshalb wünschenswert, weil es biologische Gleichgewichte nicht stört und sogar den Einsatz toxischer und zentralwirksamer Verbindungen ermöglicht. Auf die Bedeutung bei der Erfassung von Rezeptorarealen ist ebenfalls bereits hingewiesen worden. Wie in Abschnitt C.I. ausgeführt, ist eine absolute Trägerfreiheit bei den betrachteten Radionukliden nicht erhältlich, und Verdünnungen von 10–10.000 sind meist nicht zu vermeiden. Man verwendet deshalb hier nicht mehr den Ausdruck „trägerfrei" (carrier-free), sondern „ohne Trägerzusatz" (no-carrier-added = n.c.a.).

Für die Praxis ist aus den oben erwähnten Gründen die Kenntnis der spezifischen Aktivität unbedingt erforderlich. Dies bedingt aber neben der Absolutmessung der Radioaktivität auch eine Bestimmung der kleinsten Mengen an isotopen oder nicht-isotopen inaktiven Trägern. Während die Absolutmessung der Radioaktivität mit Hilfe geeichter Detektoren unproblematisch ist und routinemäßig mit Hilfe kommerziell erhältlicher Curiemeter erfolgt, stellt die Bestimmung der inaktiven Verbindungen in vielen Fällen erhebliche analytische Anforderungen, und relativ hohe Aktivitätsmengen müssen eingesetzt werden, um die spezifische Aktivität nahezu trägerfreier Produkte zu bestimmen. Im Prinzip eignen sich viele klassische Analysemethoden hoher Empfindlichkeit.

Gasförmige Vorläufer können bei der gaschromatographischen Analyse mit Hilfe von FID- oder ECD-Detektoren sehr empfindlich nachgewiesen werden. Im Falle von [^{18}F]-Fluorethanol (Tewson et al. 1980) konnte die spezifische Aktivität mittels eines FID-Detektors bestimmt werden, der in diesem speziellen Falle eine Empfindlichkeit von $2 \cdot 10^{-13}$ Mol Kohlenstoff sec^{-1} mV^{-1} hatte. Hierdurch konnten mit einer nur 13 MBq enthaltenden Probe entsprechend einem Signal von 1 mVsec eine nur 10fache Trägerverdünnung nachgewiesen werden. Auch die HPLC eignet sich zum empfindlichen Nachweis mittels UV-Detektor, wenn die Substanz stark im UV-Bereich absorbiert. Auf diese Weise können nMol-Mengen noch leicht erfaßt werden. Bei Verbindungen, die nicht im UV-Bereich absorbieren, ist eine vorherige chemische Umwandlung notwendig, wobei darauf geachtet werden muß, daß hierbei nicht zusätzlich Träger eingeschleppt wird. Auch elektrochemische Detektoren können zur empfindlichen on-line Messung in Verbindung mit der HPLC eingesetzt werden. Weitere hochempfindliche Methoden wie Laser-IR, Massenspektroskopie oder Aktivierungsanalyse sind prinzipiell geeignet, noch 10^8 bis 10^{10} Moleküle nachzuweisen. Meist wird dieser Aufwand nicht benötigt, und es genügt, eine obere Grenze etwa mit Hilfe der GC oder HPLC zu bestimmen, wenn diese die zulässige Grenze der Verdünnung nicht überschreitet.

IV. Pharmazeutische Qualitätskontrolle

Die pharmazeutische Qualitätskontrolle betrifft Sterilität und Pyrogenität. Der offizielle Test entsprechend der Pharmakopöe dauert im Falle der Sterilitätskontrolle etwa eine Woche, der Pyrogentest mindestens einen Tag. Der Limulus Test (Cooper et al. 1971; Yin et al. 1972; McAuley et al. 1974; Servian 1977) kann zwar innerhalb von etwa einer Stunde Auskunft über Pyrogenfreiheit geben und ist auch empfohlen worden (Cohen u. Besnard 1980; Nickoloff 1978), er ist jedoch in Europa nicht offiziell anerkannt. Dies macht im Prinzip die pharmazeutische Qualitätskontrolle bei den kurzlebigen Radiopharmaka unmöglich, und man muß nach neuen Wegen suchen. Die meisten Labors gehen wie folgt vor:

Ein und dieselbe Apparatur wird für eine spezielle Syntheseart immer wieder verwendet. In dieser Apparatur werden zunächst eine Reihe von Aktivsynthesen durchgeführt, wobei immer die gleichen Chemikalien, Trennsäulen und Reaktionsschritte verwendet werden, wie in der geplanten Markierungssynthese, einschließlich Sterilfiltration in eine sterilisierte Ampulle. Mit diesem kalten Produkt werden dann nach dem Abklingen der Radioaktivität die offiziellen Tests durchgeführt. Gleichzeitig wird auch der Limulus Test angewendet. Bei der Markierungssynthese in derselben Apparatur und mit den gleichen Chemikalien darf angenommen werden, daß durch Zugabe der praktisch gewichtslosen radioaktiven Mengen, die außerdem noch eine Art Strahlensterilisation bei der Herstellung erfahren haben, auch das radioaktive Produkt unverändert pyrogenfrei ist, solange der Limulus Test negativ ist. Im übrigen sind die injizierten Volumina stets klein, und die Pharmakopöe (Europäisches Arzneibuch 1978) fordert die Prüfung auf Pyrogenfreiheit nur, wenn das wäßrige Probenvolumen 15 ml übersteigt. Dies bedeutet allerdings nicht, daß der Pyrogentest bei der Radiopharmakaproduktion unterbleiben kann, zumal während der Synthesen auch Einengungen durchgeführt werden. Es muß deshalb das oben beschriebene Procedere häufiger durchgeführt werden.

F. Schlußfolgerungen und Ausblick

Aus der Vielfalt der Markierungssynthesen für die Herstellung von Vorläufern und komplizierten organischen Verbindungen sind einige der wichtigsten in den vorangegangenen Abschnitten aufgezeigt worden. Die Auswahl erhebt keinen Anspruch auf Vollständigkeit. Dies gilt einmal für die Vielfalt der Verfahren und Techniken zur Erzeugung von einfachen Synthesevorläufern. Hier verläuft die Entwicklung sehr schnell, so daß viele der behandelten Techniken in einigen Jahren durch noch bessere ersetzt sein werden. Die Devise lautet: einfacher, schneller, zuverlässiger und mit möglichst hoher spezifischer Aktivität. Ähnliches gilt auch für die Entwicklung von Radiopharmaka. Auch hier werden in den nächsten Jahren weitere Fortschritte und viele neue Produkte zu erwarten sein. Einige bedeutende Radiopharmaka, wie markierte Antikörper für die Tumorforschung, wurden nicht behandelt, da es sich hierbei meist um Markierungen mit längerlebigen oder anorganischen Radionukliden handelt, die nicht Gegenstand dieses Kapitels sind.

Synthesen mit kurzlebigen Radionukliden für die Emissionstomographie erfordern einen hohen Aufwand an Investitions- und Personalkosten. Nur wenige der beschriebenen Produkte sind oder werden jemals für eine routinemäßige Frühdiagnose im größeren Ausmaß zur Verfügung stehen. Der heutige Zustand kann im wesentlichen als Grundlagenforschung beschrieben werden. Hier stehen vor allem die Neurologie und die Kardiologie im Vordergrund des Interesses. Die Erforschung normaler und gestörter, dynamischer physiologischer Funktionsabläufe stellen jedoch eine wesentliche Vorraussetzung für Diagnose und Therapie dar. Der erhebliche Aufwand wird allerdings derartige Untersuchungen auf relativ wenige Zentren beschränken müssen. Hier sind bereits heute drei Kategorien unterscheidbar:
1. Kliniken, die nur über ein PET Gerät, nicht aber über einen Beschleuniger verfügen. Die Anwendung ist hier im wesentlichen auf ^{18}F und das Generator-Nuklid ^{81}Rb beschränkt. Die Versorgung mit ^{18}F-markierten Produkten kann über einen im Umkreis von bis zu etwa 200 km vorhandenen Beschleuniger erfolgen.
2. Kliniken mit einem kleinen Ein- oder Zwei-Teilchenbeschleuniger niedriger Energie (≤ 17 MeV p), die sich weitgehend auf die Routineproduktion mit einfachen Produkten beschränken. Hierbei werden in zunehmendem Maße automatisierte Syntheseapparaturen zur Anwendung gelangen.

3. Zentren mit einem Mehrteilchenbeschleuniger relativ hoher Energie (≥ 30 MeV p), die eine Vielfalt von Radionukliden und Produkten herstellen können und im wesentlichen Entwicklungsarbeit aber auch Radionuklidproduktion für Dritte betreiben. Die Entwicklungsarbeiten sollten sich hier nicht nur auf die kurzlebigen Positronenstrahler beschränken, sondern auch auf Tracer für SPECT wie etwa ^{123}I ausdehnen, denn bei positiver Entwicklung der SPECT-Technik und unter der Voraussetzung, daß neue [123]I- und ^{99m}Tc-Radiopharmaka für die Funktionsdiagnostik zur Verfügung stehen, werden unabhängig vom Ort der Produktion in zunehmendem Maße auch kleinere Kliniken diese Technik annehmen. Hier könnte ein relativ breiter Einsatz erfolgen, wenn geeignete Produkte entwickelt und diese entweder direkt oder in Form von sog. Bestecken kommerziell verfügbar werden.

Danksagung: Den Herren Dres. H.H. Coenen, G. Kloster, K. Hamacher, S.M. Qaim und K. Rössler danke ich für die Durchsicht des Manuskriptes sowie für zahlreiche Anregungen.

Literatur

Ache HJ, Wolf AP (1968) The effect of radiation on the reactions of recoil carbon-11 in the nitrogen-oxygen system. J Phys Chem 72:1988–1993

Adam MJ (1986) The demetallation reaction in radiohalogen labelling: Synthesis of bromine and fluorine labelled compounds. Int J Appl Radiat Isot 37:811–815

Adam MJ, Pate BD, Ruth TJ, Berry JM, Hall LD (1981) Cleavage of aryl-tin bonds with elemental fluorine: rapid synthesis of [18F]fluorobenzene. J Chem Soc Chem Comm 733

Adam MJ, Ruth TJ, Pate BD, Hall LD (1982) Site-specific bromination of aromatic compounds: a rapid method for radiobromine labelling. J Chem Soc Chem Comm 625–626

Adam MJ, Ruth TJ, Jiva S, Pate BD (1984) The use of C-18 SEP PAK cartridges to simplify routine production of 2-deoxy-2-fluoro-D-glucose. Int J Appl Radiat Isot 35:985–986

Alexoff DL, Russell JAG, Shiue C-Y, Wolf AP, Fowler JS, MacGregor RR (1986) Modular automation in PET tracer manufacturing: Application of an autosynthesizer to the production of 2-deoxy-2-[18F]-fluoro-D-glucose. Int J Appl Radiat Isot 37:1045–1061

Alker D, Barton DHR, Hesse RH, Listerja J, Markwell RE, Pecht MM, Rozen S, Takeshit T, Toli HT (1980) Selective fluorination at tertiary centres in steroids and adamantanoids using fluorooxytrifluoromethane and using molecular fluorine. Nouveau J Chim 4:239–254

Anderson AR, Best JVF, Willet MJ (1966) Proton radiolysis of carbon monoxide. Trans Farad Soc 62:595–609

Argentini M, Zahner M, Schubiger PA (1981) Comparison of several methods for synthesis of ω-^{123}I-heptadecanoic acid. J Radioanalyt Chem 65:131–137

Ariyoshi Y, Maeda M, Kojima M, Suehiro M, Ito M (1982) Carbon-11 labeling of fludiazepam. Radioisotopes 31:431–433

Arnett CD, Shiue C-Y, Wolf AP, Fowler JS, Logan J, Watanabe M (1985) Comparison of three [18F]-labeled buryrophenone neuroleptic drugs in the baboon using positron emission tomography. J Neurochem 44:835–844

Atkins HL, Christman DR, Fowler JS, Hanser W, Hoyte RM, Klopper JF, Lin SS, Wolf AP (1972) Organic radiopharmaceuticals labeled with isotopes of short half-lifes. V. [18F]-labeled 5- and 6-fluorotryptophan. J Nucl Med 13:713–719

Attina M, Cacace F, Wolf AP (1983) Displacement of a nitrogroup by [18F]-fluoride ion. A route to aryl fluorides of high specific activity. J Chem Soc Chem Comm 108–109

Barrio JR (1986) Biochemical principles in radiopharmaceutical design and utilization. In: [Phelps ME, Maziotta JC, Schelbert HR (eds)] Positron emission tomography and autoradiography. Raven, New York

Barrio JR, MacDonald NS, Robinson GD, Najafi A, Cook JS, Kuhl DE (1981a) Remote, semiautomated production of F-18 labeled 2-deoxy-2-fluoro-D-glucose. J Nucl Med 22:372–375

Barrio JR, Egbert JE, Baumgärtner FJ, Henze E, Schelbert HR, Phelps ME, Kuhl DE (1981b) Enzymatic synthesis of N-13, C-11 labeled amino acids and related tricarboxylic acid cycle intermediates. J Nucl Med 22:P77

Barrio JR, Egbert JE, Henze E, Schelbert HR, Baumgärtner FJ (1982) L-[4-11C]-Aspartic acid: enzymatic synthesis, myocardial uptake and metabolism. J Med Chem 25:93–96

Beeley PA, Szarek WA, Hay GW, Perlmutter MM (1984) A synthesis of 2-deoxy-2-[18F]fluoro-D-glucose using accelerator-produced [18F]F-fluoride ion generated in a water target. Can J Chem 62:2709–2711

Berger G, Maziere M, Marazano C, Comar D (1978) Carbon-11 labeling of the psychoactive drug O-methyl-bufotenine and its distribution in the animal organism. Eur J Nucl Med 3:101–104

Berger G, Maziere M, Knipper R, Prenant C, Comar D (1979) Synthesis of ^{11}C-labeled radiopharmaceuticals: imipramine, chloropromazine, nicotine and methionine. Int J Appl Radiat Isot 30:393–399

Berger G, Maziere M, Sastre J, Comar D (1980a) Carrier-free ^{11}C-formaldehyde: an approach. J Label Comp Radiopharm 17:59–71

Berger G, Maziere M, Prenant C, Comar D (1980b) Synthesis of carbon-11 labelled acetone. Int J Appl Radiat Isot 31:577–578

Berger G, Maziere M, Prenant C, Sastre J, Comar D (1981) Synthesis of high specific activity ^{11}C-17α-methyl-testosterone. Int J Appl Radiat Isot 32:811–815

Berger G, Maziere M, Prenant C, Sastre J, Syrota A, Comar D (1982) Synthesis of ^{11}C-propranolol. J Radioanalyt Chem 74:301–306

Berger G, Prenant C, Sastre J, Syrota A, Comar D (1983) Synthesis of a β-blocker for heart visualization: [^{11}C]Proctolol. Int J Appl Radiat Isot 34:1556–1557

Bergström M, Collins VP, Ehrin E, Ericson K, Eriksson L, Greitz T, Halldin C, Holst H, Langström B, Lilja A, Lundquist H, Nagren K (1983) Discrepancies in brain tumor extent as shown by computed tomography and positron emission tomography using ^{68}Ga-EDTA, ^{11}C-glucose, and ^{11}C-methionine. J Comp Assist Tomography 7:1062–1066

Berridge M, Crouzel C, Comar D (1982a) No-carrier-added ^{18}F-fluoride in organic solvents: production and labeling results. J Label Comp Radiopharm 19:1639–1640

Berridge M, Comar D, Roeda D, Syrota A (1982b) Synthesis and in vivo characteristics of [2-^{11}C]5,5-dimethyloxyzolidine-2,4-dione (DMO). Int J Appl Radiat Isot 33:647–651

Berridge M, Comar D, Crouzel C, Baron JC (1983) ^{11}C-labeled ketanserin: a selective serotonin S_2-antagonist. J Label Comp Radiopharm 20:73–78

Bida GT, Ehrenkaufer RL, Wolf AP, Fowler JS, MacGregor RR, Ruth TJ (1980) The effect of target gas purity on the chemical form of ^{18}F during ^{18}F-F$_2$ production using neon/fluorine target. J Nucl Med 21:758–762

Bida GT, Satyamurthy N, Barrio JR (1984) The synthesis of 2-[^{18}F]fluoro-2-deoxy-D-glucose using glycals. A reexamination. J Nucl Med 25:1327–1334

Billard W, Ruperto V, Crosby G, Iorio LC, Barnett A (1984) Characterization of the binding of ^{3}H-SCH 23390, a selective D-1 receptor antagonist ligand, in rat brain. Life Sci 35:1885–1893

Blau M, Bender MA (1962) ^{75}Se-Selenomethionine for visualization of the pancreas by isotope scanning. Radiology 78:974

Blessing G, Weinreich R, Qaim SM, Stöcklin G (1982) Production of ^{75}Br and ^{77}Br via the ^{75}As(^{3}He, 3n)^{75}Br and ^{75}As(α, 2n)^{77}Br reactions using Cu$_3$As-alloy as high-current target material. Int J Appl Radiat Isot 33:333–339

Blessing G, Coenen HH, Franken K, Qaim SM (1986) Production of [^{18}F]F$_2$, H^{18}F, and ^{18}F$^-_{aq}$ using the ^{20}Ne(d, α) process. Int J Appl Radiat Isot 37:1135–1139

Block D, Klatte B, Knöchel A, Beckmann R, Holm U (1986a) Nca [^{18}F]-Labeling of aliphatic compounds in high yields via aminopolyether-supported nucleophilic substitution. J Label Comp Radiopharm 23:467–477

Block D, Coenen HH, Laufer P, Stöcklin G (1986b) Nca [^{18}F]-Fluoroalkylation via nucleophilic fluorination of disubstituted alkanes and application to the preparation of N-[^{18}F]-fluoroethylspiperone. J Label Comp Radiopharm 23: 1042–1044

Block D, Coenen HH, Stöcklin G (1987a) The nca nucleophilic ^{18}F-fluorination of 1,N-disubstituted alkanes as fluoroalkylation agents. J Label Comp Radiopharm (in press)

Block D, Coenen HH, Stöcklin G (1987b) Nca ^{18}F-fluoroalkylation of H-acidic compounds. J Label Comp Radiopharm (in press)

Block D, Coenen HH, Stöcklin G (1987c) Nca ^{18}F-fluoroacylation via fluorocarboxylic acid esters. J Label Comp Radiopharm (in press)

Blomquist G, Bergström K, Bergström M, Ehrin E, Eriksson L, Garmelius B, Lindberg B, Lilja A, Litton J-E, Lundmark L, Lundquist H, Malmborg P, Moström U, Nilsson L, Stone-Elander S, Widén L (1985) Models for ^{11}C-Glucose. In: Greitz T et al. (eds) The metabolism of the human brain studied with positron emission tomography. Raven, New York, pp 185–194

Bockslaff H, Kloster G, Stöcklin G, Safi N, Bornemann H (1980) Studies on L-3-^{123}iodo-α-methyltyrosene: a new potential melanoma seeking compound. Nuklearmedizin [Suppl] 17:179–182

Bockslaff H, Kloster G, Dausch D, Schad K, Hundeshagen H (1982) Noncontact detection of ocular melanoma with L-3-^{123}I-iodo-α-methyltyrosine: first clinical results. Graefes Arch Clin Exp Ophthalmol 219:149–154

Bodsch W, Coenen HH, Stöcklin G, Takahashi K, Hossmann K-A (1987) Biochemical and autoradiographic study of cerebral protein synthesis with ^{18}F- and ^{14}C-fluorophenylalanine. J Neurochem (in press)

Boullais C, Frie T, Crouzel C (1986) No-carrier-added fluorine-18 labelling of neuroleptics with different ^{18}F-sources. J Label Comp Radiopharm 23:1424–1425

Braun G, Shulgin AT, Sargent T (1978) Synthesis of ^{123}I-labelled 4-iodo-2,5-dimethoxyphenylisopropylamine. J Label Comp Radiopharm 14:767–773

Buckingham PD, Clark JC (1972) Nitrogen-13 solutions for research studies in pulmonary physiology. Int J Appl Radiat Isot 23:5–8

Buckingham PD, Forse GR (1963) The preparation and processing of radioactive gases for clinical uses. Int J Appl Radiat Isot 14:439–445

Burns HD, Dannals RF, Langström B, Ravert HT, Zemyan SE, Duelfer T, Wong DF, Frost JJ, Kuhar MJ, Wagner HN (1984) (3-N-[11C]methyl) spiperone, a ligand to dopamine receptors: Radiochemical synthesis and biodistribution studies in mice. J Nucl Med 25:1222–1227

Bustany P, Comar D (1985) Protein synthesis evaluation in brain and other organs in humans by PET. In: Reivich M, Alavi A (eds) Positron emission tomography. Riss, New York, pp 183–201

Bustany P, Sargent T, Saudubray J, Henry JF, Comar D (1981) Regional human brain uptake and protein incorporation of 11C-L-methionine studied in-vivo with PET. J Cereb Blood Flow Metab [Suppl 1] 1:S17–S18

Bustany P, Henry JF, Sargent T, Zarifian E, Cabanis E, Collard P, Comar D (1983) Local brain protein metabolism in dementia and schizophrenia: In vivo studies with [11C]-L-methionine and positron emission tomography. In: Heiss W-D, Phelps ME (eds) Positron emission tomography of the brain. Springer, Berlin Heidelberg New York

Cacace F, Speranza M, Wolf AP, Fowler JS (1981) Labeling of fluorinated aromatics by isotopic exchange with [18F]-fluoride. J Label Comp Radiopharm 18:1721–1730

Casella V, Ido T, Wolf AP, Fowler JS, McGregor RR, Ruth TJ (1980) Anhydrous F-18 labeled elemental fluorine for radiopharmaceutical preparation. J Nucl Med 21:750–757

Casey DL, Digenis GA, Wesner DA, Washburn LC, Chaney JE, Hayes RL, Callahan AP (1981) Preparation and preliminary tissue studies of optically active 11C-D- and L-phenylalanine. Int J Appl Radiat Isot 32:325–330

Channing MA, Eckelman WC, Bennet JM, Burke TR, Rice KC (1985) Radiosynthesis of [18F]3-acetylcyclofoxy: a high affinity opiate antagonist. Int J Appl Radiat Isot 36:429–433

Chi DY, Katzenellenbogen JA, Kilbourn MR, Welch MJ (1985) [18F]Halofluorination: a rapid and effective method for the incorporation of radiofluorine into organic molecules. J Nucl Med 26:P37

Chi DY, Kilbourn MR, Katzenellenbogen JA, Brodack JW, Welch MJ (1986) Synthesis of no-carrier-added N-([18F]fluoroalkyl) spiperone derivatives. Int J Appl Radiat Isot 37:1173–1180

Chirakal R, Firnau G, Garnett ES (1986) High yield synthesis of 6-[18F]fluor-L-dopa. J Nucl Med 27:417–421

Christman DR, Finn RD, Karlstrom KI, Wolf AP (1975) The production of ultra-high activity 11C-labeled hydrogen cyanide, carbon dioxide, carbon monoxide and methane via the 14N(p, α)11C reaction. Int J Appl Radiat Isot 26:435–442

Clark JC, Buckingham PD (1975) Short-lived radioactive gases for clinical use. Butterworths, London Boston

Clark JC, Goulding RW, Roman M, Palmer AJ (1973) The preparation of fluorine-18 labelled compounds using a recirculatory neon target. Radiochem Radioanal Lett 14:101–108

Coenen HH, Moerlein SM (1987) Regiospecific aromatic fluorodemetallation of group IVb metalloarenes using elemental fluorine or acetyl hypofluorite. J Fluor Chem 36:63–65

Coenen HH, Harmand MF, Kloster G, Stöcklin G (1981) 15-(p-[75Br]-bromophenyl)pentadecanoic acid: pharmacokinetics and potential as heart agent. J Nucl Med 22:891–896

Coenen HH, Moerlein SM, Stöcklin G (1983) No-carrier-added radiolabelling methods with heavy halogens. Radiochimica Acta 34:47–68

Coenen HH, Colosimo M, Schüller M, Stöcklin G (1985) Mild and effective aliphatic and aromatic nca 18F-fluorination using crown ether. J Nucl Med 26:P37

Coenen HH, Klatte B, Knöchel A, Schüller M, Stöcklin G (1986a) Preparation of nca [17-18F]-fluoroheptadecanoic acid in high yield via aminopolyether supported, nucleophilic substitution. J Label Comp Radiopharm 23:455–466

Coenen HH, Colosimo M, Schüller M, Stöcklin G (1986b) Preparation of nca [18F]-CH2BrF via aminopolyether supported nucleophilic substitution. J Label Comp Radiopharm 23:587–595

Coenen HH, Franken K, Metwally S, Stöcklin G (1986c) Electrophilic radiofluorination of aromatic compounds with [18F]-F2 and [18F]-CH3CO2F and regioselective preparation of L-p-[18F]-fluorphenylalanine. J Label Comp Radiopharm 23:1179–1180

Coenen HH, Bodsch W, Takahashi K, Hossmann A, Stöcklin G (1986d) Synthesis, autoradiography and biochemistry of L-[18F]-fluorophenylalanines for probing protein synthesis. Nuklearmedizin [Suppl] 21:600–602

Coenen HH, Laufer P, Stöcklin G, Wienhard K, Pawlik G, Böcher-Schwarz HG, Heiss W-D (1987) 3-N-(2-[18F]-Fluoroethyl)-spiperone: a novel ligand for cerebral dopamine receptor studies with PET. Life Sci 40:81–88

Cohen MB, Spolter L, Chang CC, MacDonald NS (1972) Enzymatic synthesis of 13N-L-glutamine. J Nucl Med 13:422

Cohen MB, Spolter L, Chang CC, Cook JS, MacDonald NS (1980) Enzymatic synthesis of 11Cpyruvic acid and ^{11}C-L-lactic acid. Int J Appl Radiat Isot 31:45–49

Cohen MB, Spolter L, Chang CC, MacDonald NS, Cook J (1981) Synthesis and distribution of ^{11}C-L-glutamic acid (α and γ carboxyl labeled): comparison to N-13-L-glutamic acid. J Nucl Med 22:P77

Cohen YI, Besnard MR (1980) Radionuclides, pharmacokinetics. In: Hundeshagen H (Redig von) Radiopharmaka, Gerätetechnik, Strahlenschutz. Springer, Berlin Heidelberg New York (Handbuch der medizinischen Radiologie, Bd XV/1A, S 3–76)

Comar D, Cartron JC, Maziere M, Marazano C (1976) Labeling and metabolism of methionine methyl [11]C. Eur J Nucl Med 1:11–14

Cooper JF, Levin J, Wagner HN (1971) Quantitative comparison of in-vitro and in vivo methods for the detection of endotoxin. J Lab Clin Med 78:138–148

Corley EG, Burns HD, Frost JJ, Duelfer T, Kuhar MJ, Wagner HN (1981) Synthesis of radiotracers for in vivo mapping and quantification of dopamine receptors. J Nucl Med 22:P12

Cramer RD, Kistiakowsky GB (1941) The synthesis of radioactive lactic acid. J Biol Chem 137:549–555

Crawford EJ, Christman D, Atkins H, Friedkin M, Wolf AP (1978) Scintigraphy with positron-emitting compounds. I. Carbon-11 labeled thymidine and thymidilate. Int J Nucl Med Biol 5:61–69

Crouzel C, Comar D (1975) Production of nitrogen-13 solution for injection by means of a medical compact cyclotron. Radiochem Radioanal Letters 20:273–278

Crouzel C, Comar D (1978) Production of carrier-free ^{18}F-hydrofluoric acid. Int J Appl Radiat Isot 29:407–408

Crouzel C, Sejourne C, Comar D (1979) Production of ^{11}C-acetylene by methane pyrolysis. Int J Appl Radiat Isot 30:566–568

Crouzel C, Mestelan G, Kraus E, Lecomte JM, Comar D (1980) Synthesis of a ^{11}C-labelled neuroleptic drug: pimozide. Int J Appl Radiat Isot 31:545–548

Dahl JR, Lee R, Schmall B, Bigler RE (1981) A novel target for the preparation of anhydrous H[18]F with no added carrier. J Label Comp Radiopharm 18:34–35

Dannals RF, Raver HT, Frost JJ, Wilson AA, Burns HD, Wagner HN (1985) Radiosynthesis of an opiate receptor binding radio tracer: [11]C]carfentanil. Int J Appl Radiat Isot 36:303–306

Dannals RF, Ravert HT, Wilson AA, Wagner HN (1986a) An improved synthesis of (3-N-^{11}C]-methylspiperone. Int J Appl Radiat Isot 37:433–434

Dannals RF, Frost JJ, Ravert HT, Wilson AA, Wagner HN (1986b) Radiosynthesis and biodistribution of a serotonin receptor radiotracer for positron emission tomography: ^{11}C-N-methyl-ketanserin. J Nucl Med 27:983

Dannals RF, Langström B, Frost JJ, Ravert HT, Wilson AA, Wagner HN (1986c) Synthesis of radiotracers for studying muscarinic cholinergic receptors in the living human brain using positron emission tomography: [^{11}C]-dexetimide and [^{11}C]-levetimide. J Label Comp Radiopharm 23:1407–1409

Davis GC, Williams AC, Markey SP, Ebert MH, Caine ED, Reichert CM, Kopin IJ (1979) Chronic parkinsonism secondary to intravenous injection of meperidine analogues. Psychiat Res 1:249–254

DeJesus OT, Friedman AM, Prasad A, Revenaugh JR (1983) Preparation and purification of [77]Br-labelled p-bromspiroperidol suitable for in-vivo dopamine receptor studies. J Label Comp Radiopharm 20:745–755

Del Fiori G, Depresseux J-C, Bartsch P, Quaglia L, Peters J-M (1979) Production of oxygen-15, nitrogen-13 and carbon-11 and of their low molecular weight derivatives for biomedical application. Int J Appl Radiat Isot 30:543–549

Diksic M (1984) A new, simple, high-yield synthesis of "no carrier added" ^{11}C-labeled DMO. Int J Appl Radiat Isot 35:1035–1038

Diksic M, Diraddo P (1985) A convenient, high-yield synthesis of [^{18}F]4-fluoroantipyrine using ^{18}F] acetylhypofluorite. Int J Appl Radiat Isot 36:643–645

Diksic M, Jolly D (1986) Remotely operated synthesis of 2-deoxy-2-[^{18}F]-fluoro-D-glucose. Int J Appl Radiat Isot 37:1159–1161

Diksic M, Jolly D, Farrokhzad S (1982) An on-line synthesis of "no-carrier-added" [^{11}C]-phosgene. Int J Nucl Med Biol 9:283–285

Diraddo P, Diksic M (1985) Mild and regiospecific synthesis of ^{18}F-labelled vinyl fluoride using [^{18}F]fluorine reacted with silane. Int J Appl Radiat Isot 36:953–956

Dischino DD, Welch MJ, Kilbourn MR, Raichle ME (1983) Relationship between lipophilicity and brain extraction of C-11-labeled radiopharmaceuticals. J Nucl Med 24:1030–1038

Dougan H, Lyster DM, Vincent JS (1985) Macrocyclic lactones as a source for radiohalogenated fatty acid analogs and their precursors. J Radioanal Nucl Chem 89:71–78

Dougan H, Lyster DM, Vincent JS (1986) Efficient production of 15-(p-[^{123}I]iodphenyl)pentadecanoic acid. Int J Appl Radiat Isot 37:919–921

Dudczak R (1983) Myokardszintigraphie mit Iod-123-markierten Fettsäuren. Wien Klin Wochenschr [Suppl 143] 95:Heft 17

Eckelman WC (1982) Receptor-specific radiopharmaceuticals. In: Ell PJ, Holman BL (eds) Computed emission tomography. Oxford University Press, Oxford, pp 263–284

Eckelman WC, Reba RC, Gibson RE, Rzeszotarski WJ, Vieras F, Mazaitis JK, Francis B (1979) Receptor binding radiotracers: a class of potential radiopharmaceuticals. J Nucl Med 20:350–357

Eckelman WC, Reba RC, Rzeszotarski WJ, Gibson RE, Hill Th, Holman BL, Budinger Th, Conklin JJ, Eng R, Grissom MP (1984) External imaging of cerebral muscarinic acetylcholine receptors. Science 223:291–292

Ehrenkaufer RE, MacGregor RR, Wolf AP, Fowler JS, Ruth TJ, Schlyer DJ, Wieland BW (1983) Production of $H^{18}F$ by deuteron irradiation of a neon-hydrogen target. Radiochimica Acta 33:49–56

Ehrenkaufer RE, Potocki JF, Jewett DM (1984) Simple synthesis of F-18-labeled 2-fluoro-2-deoxy-D-glucose. J Nucl Med 25:333–337

Ehrin E, Westman E, Nilsson SO, Nilsson JLG, Larson C-M, Tillberg JE, Malmborg P (1980) A convenient method for production of ^{11}C labeled glucose. J Label Comp Radiopharm 17:453–461

Ehrin E, Farde L, Depaulis T, Eriksson L, Greitz T, Johnström P, Litton JE, Nilsson JLG, Sedvall G, Stone-Elander Sh, Ögren S-O (1985) Preparation of ^{11}C-labelled raclopride, a new potent dopamine receptor antagonist: preliminary PET studies of cerebral dopamine receptors in monkey. Int J Appl Radiat Isot 36:269–273

Ehrin E, Luthra SK, Crouzel C, Pike VW (1986) Preparation of carbon-11 labelled prazosin, a potent and selective α1-adrenoreceptor antagonist. J Label Comp Radiopharm 23:1410–1411

Eisenhut M (1982) Simple labeling of ω-phenylfatty acids by iodine isotope exchange. Int J Appl Radiat Isot 33:499–504

El-Garhy M, Stöcklin G (1974) A novel method of labelling biomolecules with ^{123}I and ^{125}I. Radiochem Radioanal Letters 18:281–290

Elias H, Lotterhos HF (1976) Notiz über eine Radiojod-Markierung durch Halogen-Austausch in Acetamid-Schmelzen. Chem Ber 109:1580–1583

Elmaleh DR, Hnatowich DJ, Kulprathipanja S (1979) A novel synthesis of ^{13}N-L-asparagine. J Label Comp Radiopharm 16:92–93

Eng RR, Spitznagle LA, Trager WF (1983) Preparation of radiolabeled pregnenolone analogs. 21-Fluoropregnenolone-21-^{18}F, 21-fluoropregnenolone-3-acetate-21-^{18}F, 21-fluoropregnenolone-7-^{3}H, and 21-fluoropregnenolone-3-acetate-7-^{3}H. J Label Comp Radiopharm 20:63–72

Europäisches Arzneibuch, Bd 3, Deutscher Apotheker Verlag, Stuttgart 1978, S 378 "Injectabilia" und Europäisches Arzneibuch, Bd 1–3, Erster Nachtrag 1980. Deutscher Apotheker Verlag, Stuttgart 1980

European Community Task Groups: Reports on the methodology of the production and standardization of oxygen-15 gases, [^{11}C]-methyliodide and [2-^{18}F]-fluoro-2-deoxy-D-glucose. Int J Appl Radiat Isot (in press)

Evans JR, Gunton RW, Baker RG, Beanlands DS, Spears JC (1965) Use of radioiodinated fatty acid for photoscans of the heart. Circ Res 16:1–10

Farde L, Ehrin E, Eriksson L, Greitz T, Hall H, Hedström C-G, Litton J-E, Sedvall G (1985) Substituted benzamides as ligands for visualization of dopamine rezeptor binding in the human brain by positron emission tomography. Proc Natl Acad Sci USA 82:3863–3867

Farde L, Hall H, Ehrin E, Sedvall G (1986) Quantitative analysis of D2 dopamine receptor binding in the living human brain by PET. Science 231:258–261

Feinendegen LE, Herzog H, Wieler H, Patton DD, Schmid A (1986) Glucose transport and utilization in the human brain: model using carbon-11 methylglucose and positron emission tomography. J Nucl Med 27:1867–1877

Ferrieri RA, Wolf AP (1983) The chemistry of positron emitting nucleogenic atoms with regard to preparation of labelled compounds of practical utility. Radiochimica Acta 34:69–83

Finn RD, Christman DR, Ache HJ, Wolf AP (1971) The preparation of cyanide-^{11}C for use in the synthesis of organic radiopharmaceuticals II. Int J Appl Radiat Isot 22:735–744

Firnau G, Chirakal R, Sood S, Garnett ES (1980) Aromatic fluorination with xenon difluoride: L-3,4-dihydroxy-6-fluorophenylalanine. Can J Chem 58:1449–1450

Firnau G, Chirakal R, Sood S, Garnett ES (1981) Radiofluorination with xenon difluoride: L-6-(^{18}F)fluoro-DOPA. J Label Comp Radiopharm 18:7–8

Flanagan RJ, Lentle BC, McGowan DG, Wiebe LI (1981) α-Halostilbenes related to diethylstilbestrol. J Radioanal Chem 65:81–94

Flanagan RJ, Wilson JS, Wiebe LI (1986a) A high speed, no-carrier-added radiochemical reactor for the synthesis of halogenated radiopharmaceuticals. J Label Comp Radiopharm 23:1242–1243

Flanagan RJ, Vijayalaksmi K, Somayji VV, Wiebe LI (1986b) Radiolabelling with organomercury compounds. III. High specific activity synthesis of [^{131}I]6-iodo-androsten-5-enes and [^{131}I]6-iodo-pregnen-5-enes. Int J Appl Radiat Isot 37:893–899

Foster NI, Dannals R, Burns HD, Heindel ND (1981) A condition variation study for radioiodination via triazene intermediates. J Radioanal Chem 65:95–105

Fowler JS, Ansari AN, Atkins HL, Bradley-Moore PR, MacGregor RR, Wolf AP (1973a) Synthesis and preliminary evaluation in animals of carrier-free ^{11}C-dopamine hydrochloride. J Nucl Med 14:867–869

Fowler JS, Finn RD, Lambrecht RM, Wolf AP (1973b) The synthesis of ^{18}F-5-fluorouracil. J Nucl Med 14:63–64

Fowler JS, MacGregor RR, Ansari AN, Atkins HL, Wolf AP (1974) Radiopharmaceuticals XII. A new rapid synthesis of carbon-11 labeled norepinephrine hydrochloride. J Med Chem 17:246–248

Fowler JS, Gallagher BM, MacGregor RR, Wolf AP, Ansari AN, Atkins HL, Slatkin DN (1976) Radiopharmaceuticals XIX: ^{11}C-labeled acetylamine, a potential diagnostic agent for lung structure and function. J Nucl Med 17:752–754

Fowler JS, Gallagher BM, MacGregor RR, Wolf AP (1977) ^{11}C-serotonin: a tracer for the pulmonary endothelial extraction of serotonin. J Label Comp Radiopharm 13:194–195

Fowler JS, Lade RE, MacGregor RR, Shiue C, Wan C-N, Wolf AP (1979) Agents for the armamentarium of regional metabolic measurement in vivo via metabolic trapping: ^{11}C-2-deoxy-D-glucose and halogenated deoxyglucose. J Label Comp Radiopharm 16:7–9

Fowler JS, MacGregor RR, Wolf AP, Farrell AA, Karlstroh KI, Ruth TJ (1981) A shielded synthesis system for production of 2-deoxy-2-[^{18}F]fluoro-D-glucose. J Nucl Med 22:376–380

Fowler JS, Arnett CD, Wolf AP, MacGregor RR, Norton EF, Findley AM (1982a) ^{11}C-Spiroperidol: synthesis, specific activity determination, and biodistribution in mice. J Nucl Med 23:437–445

Fowler JS, Shiue C-Y, Wolf AP, Salvadori PA, MacGregor RR (1982b) Synthesis of ^{18}F-labeled acetyl hypofluorite for radiotracer synthesis. J Label Comp Radiopharm 19:1634–1636

Fowler JS, MacGregor RR, Wolf AP, Tesoro A (1986) An improved synthesis of [1-^{11}C]putrescine. J Label Comp Radiopharm 23:1091

Franken K (1987) Entwicklung und Optimierung von Verfahren zur Radiofluorierung aromatischer Verbindungen mit Fluor-18 hoher spezifischer Aktivität. Dissertation Universität zu Köln, Juel-Report JUEL 2137

Freundlieb C, Hoeck A, Vyska K, Machulla HJ, Stöcklin G (1980) Myocardial imaging and metabolic studies with [17-^{123}I]iodo-heptadecanoic acid. J Nucl Med 21:1043–1050

Friedman AM, Huang CC, Kumala HA, Dinerstein R, Navone J, Brunsden B, Gawlas D, Cooper M (1982) The use of radiobrominated p-bromospiroperidol for γ-ray imaging of dopamine receptors. Int J Nucl Med Biol 9:57–61

Fritzberg AR, Eshima D (1982) Iodophenylsulfonamide fatty acid analogs as potential myocardial imaging agents. Int J Appl Radiat Isot 33:451–453

Fukuda H, Matsuzawa T, Tada M, Takahashi T, Ishiwata K, Yamada K, Abe Y, Yoshioka S, Sato T, Ido T (1986) 2-Deoxy-2[^{18}F]fluoro-D-galactose: A new tracer for the measurement of galactose metabolism in the liver by positron emission tomography. Eur J Nucl Med 11:444–448

Gallagher BM, Ansari A, Atkins H, Casella V, Christman DR, Fowler JS, Ido T, MacGregor RR, Som P, Wan CN, Wolf AP, Kuhl DE, Reivich M (1977) Radiopharmaceuticals XXVII.

^{18}F-Labeled 2-deoxy-2-fluoro-D-glucose as a radiopharmaceutical for measuring regional myocardial glucose metabolism in vivo: tissue distribution and imaging studies in animals. J Nucl Med 18:990–996

Gallagher BM, Fowler JS, Gutterson NI, MacGregor RR, Wan C-N, Wolf AP (1978) Metabolic trapping as a principle of radiopharmaceutical design: some factors responsible for the biodistribution of [^{18}F]-2-deoxy-2-fluoro-D-glucose. J Nucl Med 19:1154–1161

Garnett ES, Firnau G, Nahmias C (1983) Dopamine visualized in the basal ganglia of living man. Nature 305:137–138

Gatley SJ, Hichiwa RD, Shangruny WJ, Nickles RJ (1981) ^{18}F-labeled lower fluoroalkanes: Reactor-produced gaseous physiological tracers. Int J Appl Radiat Isot 32:211–214

Gelbard AS (1981) Biosynthetic methods for incorporating positronemitting radionuclides into compounds of biomedical interest. J Label Comp Radiopharm 18:933–945

Gelbard AS, Cooper AJL (1979) Synthesis of [^{13}N]-labeled aromatic L-amino acids by enzymatic transamination of [^{13}N]-L-glutamic acid. J Label Comp Radiopharm 16:94

Gelbard AS, Cooper AJL, Reiman RE, Benua RS (1981) Synthesis of N-13-labeled monocarboxylic amino acids, suitable for patient studies, with immobilized glutamate dehydrogenase. J Nucl Med 22:P74–P75

Gibson RE, Weckstein DJ, Jagoda EM, Rzeszotarski WJ, Reba RC, Eckelman WC (1984) The characteristics of I-125 4-QNB and H-3 QNB in vivo and in vitro. J Nucl Med 25:214–222

Gil-Av E, Tishbee A, Hare PE (1980) Resolution of underivatized amino acids by reversed-phase chromatography. J Am Chem Soc 102:5115–5117

Ginos JZ, Tilbury RS, Haber MT, Rottenberg DA (1982) Synthesis of (2-^{11}C)5,5-dimethyl-2,4-oxazolidinedione for studies with positron tomography. J Nucl Med 23:255–258

Gnade BE, Schwaiger GP, Liotta CL, Fink RW (1981) Preparation of reactor-produced carrier-free ^{18}F-fluoride as the potassium 18-crown-6 complex for synthesis of labelled organic compounds. Int J Appl Radiat Isot 32:91–95

Goldstein L, Katchalski-Katzir F (1976) Immobilized enzymes: A survey. In: Wingard LB, Katchalski-Katzir E, Goldstein L (eds) Applied biochemistry and bioengineering, immobilized enzyme principles, vol I. Academic, New York, pp 1–22

Goodman MM, Knapp FF, Richards P, Mausner LF (1983) A new rapid regiospecific synthesis of ^{123}I-labeled 15-(p-iodophenyl)pentadecanoic acid. J Nucl Med 24:P43

Goodman MM, Callaham AP, Knapp FF (1986) Design, synthesis and evaluation of 2-deoxy-2-iodovinyl-branched carbohydrates as potential brain imaging agents. J Label Comp Radiopharm 23:1209–1210

Goulding RW (1979) The application of HPLC to labelling with short-lived nuclides. J Label Comp Radiopharm 16:210–212

Goulding RW, Palmer AJ (1972) The preparation of fluorine-18 labeled p-fluorophenylalanine for clinical use. Int J Appl Radiat Isot 23:133–137

Goulding RW, Palmer AJ (1973) Aspects of the preparation of carbon-11 labeled glucose. Int J Appl Radiat Isot 24:7–12

Greenwood FC, Hunter WM (1963) The preparation of ^{131}I-labeled human growth hormone of high specific radioactivity. Biochem J 89:114–123

Halldin C, Langström B (1984a) Synthesis of racemic [3-^{11}C]phenylalanine and [3-^{11}C]-DOPA. Int J Appl Radiat Isot 35:779–782

Halldin C, Langström B (1984b) Asymmetric synthesis of L-[3-^{11}C]-phenylalanine using chiral hydrogenation catalysts. Int J Appl Radiat Isot 35:945–948

Halldin C, Langström B (1985) Synthesis of racemic [2-^{11}C]phenylglycine. J Label Comp Radiopharm 22:631–640

Halldin C, Langström B (1986) Synthesis of [3-^{11}C]-phenylpyruvic acid and its use in an enzymatic transamination to [3-^{11}C]-phenylalanine. J Label Comp Radiopharm 23:715–722

Halldin C, Stone-Elander S, Farde L, Ehrin E, Fasth K-J, Langström B, Sedvall G (1986a) Preparation of ^{11}C-labelled SCH 23390 for the in vivo study of dopamine D-1 receptors using positron emission tomography. Int J Appl Radiat Isot 37:1039–1043

Halldin C, Fowler JS, Bjurling P, MacGregor RR, Arnett C, Wolf AP, Langström B (1986b) Synthesis of ^{11}C-labelled tracers for studies of functional MAO activity in brain using PET. J Label Comp Radiopharm 23:1400–1401

Hamacher K, Blessing G (1987) Institut für Chemie, KFA Jülich GmbH, unveröffentlichte Ergebnisse

Hamacher K, Coenen HH, Stöcklin G (1986a) Efficient stereospecific synthesis of no-carrier-added 2-[^{18}F]-fluoro-2-deoxy-D-glucose using aminopolyether supported nucleophilic substitution. J Nucl Med 27:235–238

Hamacher K, Coenen HH, Stöcklin G (1986b) Nca radiofluorination of spiperone and N-methylspiperone via aminopolyether supported direct nucleophilic substitution. J Label Comp Radiopharm 23:1047

Hamacher K, Coenen HH, Stöcklin G (1986c) Stereospecific synthesis of nca 2-[^{18}F]-fluoro-2-deoxy-D-mannose and 2-[^{18}F]-fluoro-2-deoxy-D-glucose and the influence of added carrier (KF) on FDG-synthesis. J Label Comp Radiopharm 23:1095

Hara T, Taylor C, Lembares N, Lathrop KA, Harper PV (1971) L-aspartic acid-4-^{11}C as a tumor scanning agent. J Nucl Med 12:361–362

Hara T, Iio M, Izuchi R, Tsukiyama T, Yokoi F (1985) Synthesis of pyruvate-1-^{11}C as a radiopharmaceutical for tumor imaging. Eur J Nucl Med 11:275–278

Haradahira T, Maeda M, Kai Y, Kojima M (1985) A new, high yield synthesis of 2-deoxy-2-fluoro-D-glucose. J Chem Soc Chem Comm 364–365

Harper PV, Schwartz JMD, Beck RN et al (1973) Clinical myocardial imaging with nitrogen-13 ammonia. Radiology 108:613–617

Helus F, Maier-Borst W, Sahm U, Wiebe LI (1979) F-18 cyclotron production methods. Radiochem Radioanal Letters 38:395–440

Helus F, Maier-Borst W, Oberdorfer F, Silvester DJ (1982) The synthesis of [1-^{11}C]-butanol. J Label Comp Radiopharm 19:1501–1503

Henze E, Schelbert HR, Barrio JR, Egbert JE, Hansen HW, MacDonald NS, Phelps ME (1982) Evaluation of myocardial metabolism with N-13 and C-11 labeled amino acids and positron emission tomography. J Nucl Med 23:671–681

He Youfeng, Coenen HH, Petzold G, Stöcklin G (1982) A comparative study of radioiodination of simple aromatic compounds via N-halosuccinimides and chloramine-T in TFAA. J Label Comp Radiopharm 19:807–819

Hochberg RB (1979) Iodine-125-labeled estradiol: a gamma-emitting analog of estradiol that binds to the estrogen receptor. Science 205:1138–1140

Holden JE, Gatley SJ, Hichawa RD, Ip WR, Shaughnessy WJ, Nickles RJ, Polcyn RE (1981) Cerebral blood flow using PET measurements of fluoromethane kinetics. J Nucl Med 22:1084–1088

Holden JE, Gatley SJ, Koeppe RA, Halama JR, Polcyn RA (1983) Tomographic measurement of unidirectional transport rate of glucose across the blood-brain barrier. J Cereb Blood Flow Metab [Suppl 1] 3:476–477

Hoyte RM, Lin SS, Christman DR, Atkins HL, Hauser W, Wolf AP (1971) Organic radiopharmaceuticals labeled with short lived nuclides III. ^{18}F-labeled phenylalanines. J Nucl Med 12:280–286

Hübner KF, Andrews GA, Buonocore E, Hayes RL, Washburn LC, Collmann IR, Gibbs WD (1979) Carbon-11-labeled amino acids for rectilinear and positron tomographic imaging of the human pancreas. J Nucl Med 20:507–513

Hübner KF, King P, Gibbs WD, Partain CL, Washburn LC, Hayes RL, Holloway E (1980) Clinical investigation with carbon-11-labelled amino acids using positron emission computerized tomography in patients with neoplastic diseases. Medical radionuclide imaging, vol II., IAEA-Vienna, SM-247/90, pp 515–529

Hübner KF, Purvis JT, Mahaley SM, Robertson JT, Rogers S, Gibbs WD, King P, Partain CL (1982) Brain tumor imaging by positron emission computed tomography using ^{11}C-labeled amino acids. J Comput Assist Tomogr 6:544–550

Hunter WM, Greenwood FC (1962) Preparation of iodine-131 labelled human growth hormone of high specific activity. Nature 194:495–496

Ido T, Wan C-N, Casella V, Fowler JS, Wolf AP, Reivich M, Kuhl DE (1978) Labeled 2-deoxy-D-glucose analogs. ^{18}F-labeled 2-deoxy-2-fluoro-D-glucose, 2-deoxy-2-fluoro-D-mannose, and ^{14}C-2-deoxy-2-fluoro-D-glucose. J Label Comp Radiopharm 14:175–183

Imahori Y, Ido T, Ishiwata K, Takahashi T, Yanai K, Miura Y, Iwata R (1986) 2-Deoxy-2-[^{18}F]fluoro-L-fucose; a new tracer of glucoprotein metabolism. J Nucl Med 27:983

Irie T, Fukushi K, Ido T (1982) Synthesis of ^{18}F-6-fluoropurine and ^{18}F-6-fluoro-9-β-D-ribofuranosyl purine. Int J Appl Radiat Isot 33:445–448

Ishiwata K, Monma M, Iwata R, Ido T (1982) Automated photosynthesis of ^{11}C-glucose. J Label Comp Radiopharm 19:1347–1349

Ishiwata K, Ido T, Kawashima K, Murakami M, Takahashi T (1984) Studies on ^{18}F-labeled pyrimidines. II. Metabolic investigation of ^{18}F-5-fluorouracil, ^{18}F-5-fluoro-2′-deoxyuridine and ^{18}F-5-fluorouridine in rats. Eur J Nucl Med 9:185

Ishiwata K, Ido T, Yanai K, Kawashima K, Mura Y, Monma M, Watanuki S, Takahashi T, Iwata R (1985) Biodistribution of a positron-emitting suicide inactivator of monoamine oxidase, carbon-11 pargyline, in mice and a rabbit. J Nucl Med 24:630–636

Iwata R, Ido T, Saji H, Suzuki K, Yoshikawa K, Tamate K, Kasida Y (1979) A remote-controlled synthesis of ^{11}C-iodomethane for the practical preparation of ^{11}C-labeled radiopharmaceuticals. Int J Appl Radiat Isot 30:194–196

Iwata R, Ido T, Tominaga T (1981) The production of ^{11}C-guanidine by proton irradiation of liquid ammonia-nitrous oxide systems and its use in the synthesis of ^{11}C-pyrimidines. Int J Appl Radiat Isot 32:303–308

Iwata R, Ido T, Takahashi T, Monna M (1984) Automated synthesis system for production of 2-deoxy-2-[^{18}F]-fluoro-D-glucose with computer control. Int J Appl Radiat Isot 35:445–454

Jones SC, Bucelewicz WM, Brissette RA, Subramanyam R, Hoop B (1977) Production of ^{13}N-molecular nitrogen for pulmonary positron scintigraphy. Int J Appl Radiat Isot 28:25–28

Jones T, Chesler DA, Ter-Pogossian MM (1976) The continuous inhalation of oxygen-15 for assessing regional oxygen extraction in the brain of man. Br J Radiol 49:339–343

Kabalka GW, Gooch EE, Otto ChA (1981) Rapid synthesis of radioiodinated ω-iodofatty acids. J Radioanal Chem 65:115–121

Kabalka GW, Sastry KAR, Pagni PG (1982a) Rapid incorporation of radiobromine via the reaction of labeled sodium bromide with organoboranes. J Radioanal Chem 74:315–321

Kabalka GW, Gooch EE, Smith TL, Sells MA (1982b) Rapid incorporation of iodine-123 via the reaction of ^{123}I-sodium iodide with organoboranes. Int J Appl Radiat Isot 33:223–224

Kabalka GW, Sastry KAR, Gooch EE (1982c) Synthesis of very high specific activity radioiodinated and radiobrominated materials via organoborane chemistry. J Label Comp Radiopharm 19:1506

Katzenellenbogen JA, Senderoff SG, McElvany KD, O'Brien HA, Welch MJ (1981) 16α-[^{77}Br]Bromoestradiol-17β: a high specific-activity, gamma-emitting tracer with uptake in rat uterus and induced mammary tumors. J Nucl Med 22:42–47

Kiesewetter DO, Kilbourn MR, Landvatter SW, Heiman DF, Katzenellenbogen JA, Welch MJ (1984) Preparation of four fluorine-18-labeled estrogens and their selective uptakes in target tissues of immature rats. J Nucl Med 25:1212–1221

Kiesewetter DO, Eckelman WC, Cohen RM, Finn RD, Larson SM (1986) Synthesis and D$_2$-receptor affinities of derivatives of spiperone containing alipathic halogens. Int J Appl Radiat Isot 37:1181–1188

Kilbourn MR, Welch MJ (1982) New reactions for carbon-11 labeling. J Label Comp Radiopharm 19:1273–1274

Kilbourn MR, Hood JT, Welch MJ, Dence CS, Tewson TJ, Saji H, Maeda M (1984) Carrier-added and no-carrier-added synthesis of [^{18}F]spiroperidol and [^{18}F]haloperidol. Int J Appl Radiat Isot 35:591–598

Klein MS, Goldstein RA, Welch MJ, Sobel BE (1979) External assessment of myocardial metabolism with (^{11}C)-palmitate in rabbit hearts. Am J Physiol 237:H51–H57

Kloster G, Laufer P (1980) Enzymatic synthesis and chromatographic purification of L-3-[^{11}C]-lactic acid via D,L-3-[^{11}C]-alanine. J Label Comp Radiopharm 17:889–894

Kloster G, Stöcklin G (1982) Determination of the rate-determining step in halofatty acid turnover in the heart. Radioaktive Isotope in Klinik und Forschung 15:235–241

Kloster G, Röder E, Machulla H-J (1979) Synthesis, chromatography and tissue distribution of methyl-^{11}C-morphine and methyl-^{11}C-heroin. J Label Comp Radiopharm 16:441–448

Kloster G, Müller-Platz C, Laufer P (1980) 3-[^{11}C]-Methyl-D-glucose, a potential agent for regional cerebral glucose utilization studies: synthesis, chromatography and tissue distribution in mice. J Label Comp Radiopharm 18:855–863

Kloster G, Coenen HH, Szabo Z, Ritzl F, Stöcklin G (1982) Radiohalogenated L-α-methyltyrosines as potential pancreas imaging agents for PECT and SPECT. In: Cox PC (ed) Progress in radiopharmacology, vol 3. Nijhoff, Den Haag, pp 97–107

Kloster G, Laufer P, Stöcklin G (1983a) D-Glucose derivatives labelled with ^{75,77}Br and ^{123}I. J Label Comp Radiopharm 20:391–415

Kloster G, Laufer P, Wutz W, Stöcklin G (1983b) ^{75,77}Br- and ^{123}I-Analogues of D-glucose as potential tracers for glucose utilization in heart and brain. Eur J Nucl Med 8:237–241

Knapp FF, Goodman MM, Callaham AP, Kirsch G (1986) Radioiodinated 15-(p-iodophenyl)-3,3-dimethylpentadecanoic acid: a useful new agent to evaluate myocardial fatty acid uptake. J Nucl Med 27:521–531

Knust EJ, Kupfernagel Ch, Stöcklin G (1979) Long chain F-18 fatty acids for the study of regional metabolism in heart and liver; odd-even effects of metabolism in mice. J Nucl Med 20:1170–1175

Knust EJ, Müller-Platz C, Schüller M (1982) Synthesis, quality control and tissue distribution of 2-[^{18}F]-nicotinic acid diethylamide, a potential agent for regional cerebral function studies. J Radioanal Chem 74:283–291

Koeppe RA, Holden JE, Polcyn RE, Nickles RJ, Gutchins GD, Weese JL (1985) Quantitation of local cerebral blood flow and partition coefficient without arterial sampling: Theory and validation. J Cereb Blood Flow Metab 5:214–223

Kondo K, Lambrecht RM, Wolf AP (1977) Iodine-123 production for radiopharmaceuticals XX. Excitation functions of the ^{124}Te(p,2n)^{123}I and ^{124}Te(p,n)^{124}I reactions and the effect of target enrichment on radionuclidic purity. Int J Appl Radiat Isot 28:395–401

Kothari PJ, Finn RD, Vora MM, Boothe TE, Emran AM, Kabalka GW (1985) [1-^{11}C]Butanol: Synthesis and development as a radiopharmaceutical for blood flow measurements. Int J Appl Radiat Isot 36:412–413

Krizek H, Lembares N, Dinwoodie R, Gloria I (1973) Production of radiochemically pure ^{13}NH$_3$ for biomedical studies using the ^{16}O(p,α)^{13}N reaction. J Nucl Med 14:629

Krohn KA, Mathis ChA (1981) The use of isotopic nitrogen as a biochemical tracer. In: [Root JW, Krohn KA (eds)] Short-lived radionuclides in chemistry and biology. Advances in Chemistry Series 197, American Chemical Society, Washington DC, pp 234–249

Kulkarni PV, Parkey RW (1982) A new radioiodination method utilizing organothallium intermediate: radioiodination of phenyl pentadecanoic acid (PPA) for potential applications in myocardial imaging. J Nucl Med 23:P105

Kulmala HK, Huang CC, Dinerstein RJ, Friedman AM (1981) Specific in-vivo binding of ^{77}Br-p-bromospiroperidol in rat brain: a potential tool for gamma ray imaging. Life Sci 28:1911–1916

Lambrecht RM, Mantescu C, Redvanly C, Wolf AP (1972) Preparation of high-purity carrier-free ^{123}I-iodine monochloride as iodination reagent for synthesis of radiopharmaceuticals IV. J Nucl Med 13:266–273

Lambrecht RM, Neirinckx R, Wolf AP (1978) Cyclotron isotopes and radiopharmaceuticals XXIII. Novel anhydrous ^{18}F-fluorinating intermediates. Int J Appl Radiat Isot 29:175–183

Landvatter SW (1985) Preparation and purification of ^{125}I-iodo-spiroperidol. J Label Comp Radiopharm 22:273–278

Landvatter SW, Kiesewetter DO, Kilbourn MR, Katzenellenbogen JA, Welch MJ (1983) (2R,3S)-1-[^{18}F]fluoro-2,3-bis(4-hydroxyphenyl)pentane ([^{18}F]fluoronorhexestrol), a positron-emitting estrogen that shows highly-selective, receptor-mediated uptake by target tissue in vivo. Life Sci 33:1933–1938

Langston JW, Ballard P, Tetrud JW, Irvin I (1983) Chronic parkinsonism in humans due to a product of meperidineanalogue synthesis. Science 219:979–980

Langström B, Lundquist H (1976) The preparation of ^{11}C-methyliodide and its use in the synthesis of (^{11}C-methyl)-L-methionine. Int J Appl Radiat Isot 27:357

Langström B, Sjöberg S, Ragnarsson U (1981a) A rapid and convenient method for specific ^{11}C-labelling of synthetic polypeptides containing methionine. J Label Comp Radiopharm 18:479–487

Langström B, Sjoberg S, Bergson G, Lundquist H, Malmborg P, Stalnocke CG, Larson B (1981b) [^{11}C]-Methyliodide in the synthesis of ^{11}C-compounds. J Label Comp Radiopharm 18:17

Langström B, Antoni G, Gullberg P, Halldin C, Nägren K, Rimland A, Svärd H (1986) The synthesis of 1-^{11}C-labelled ethyl, propyl, butyl and isobutyl iodides and examples of alkylation reactions. Int J Appl Radiat Isot 37:1141–1145

Lathrop KA, Harper PV, Rich BH, Dinwoodie R, Krizek H, Lembares N, Gloria I (1973) Rapid incorporation of short-lived cyclotron-produced radionuclides into radiopharmaceuticals. In: Radiopharmaceuticals and labelled compounds, vol 1. IAEA Vienna (IAEA-SM-171/46), pp 471–481

Laufer P, Kloster G (1982) Remote control synthesis of 3-[^{11}C]-methyl-D-glucose. Int J Appl Radiat Isot 33:775–776

Laufer P, Machulla H-J, Michael H, Coenen HH, El-Wetery AS, Kloster G, Stöcklin G (1981) Preparation of ω-^{123}I-labelled fatty acids by ^{123}I-for-Br exchange: comparison of three methods. J Label Comp Radiopharm 18:1205–1214

Lemaire C, Guillaume M, Christiaens L, Cantineau R (1986) A new route for the synthesis of ^{18}F-fluoroaromatic substituted amino acids such as p-fluorphenylalanine. J Label Comp Radiopharm 23:1109–1110

Lerman O, Tor Y, Rozen S (1981) Acetyl hypofluorite as a taming carrier of elemental fluorine for novel electrophilic fluorination of activated aromatic rings. J Org Chem 46:4629–4631

Levy S, Elmaleh DR, Livni E (1982) A new method using anhydrous [^{18}F]fluoride to radiolabel 2-[^{18}F]fluoro-2-deoxy-D-glucose. J Nucl Med 23:918–922

Lieser KH (1980) Einführung in die Kernchemie, 3. Aufl. Chemie, Weinheim

Lifton JF, Welch MJ (1971) Preparation of glucose labeled with 20-minute half-lived carbon-11. Radiat Res 45:35–40

Livni E, Elmaleh DR, Levi S, Brownell GL, Strauss WH (1982) Beta-methyl[^{11}C]heptadecanoic acid: A new myocardial metabolic tracer for positron emission tomography. J Nucl Med 23:169–175

Luthra SK, Pike VW, Brady F (1985) The preparation of carbon-11 labelled diprenorphine: a new radioligand for the study of the opiate receptor system in vivo. J Chem Soc Chem Comm 1423–1425

Luxen A, Barrio JR, Bida GT, Satyamurthy N (1986) Regioselective radiofluoro-demercuration: a simple high yield synthesis of 6-[^{18}F]fluorodopa. J Label Comp Radiopharm 23:1066–1067

MacGregor RR, Fowler JS, Wolf AP, Shiue C-Y, Lade RE, Wan C-N (1981) A synthesis of 2-deoxy-D-[1-^{11}C]-glucose for regional metabolic studies: concise communication. J Nucl Med 22:800–803

MacGregor RR, Halldin C, Fowler JS, Wolf AP, Arnett CD, Langström B, Alexoff D (1985) Selective, irreversible in vivo binding of [^{11}C]clorgyline and [^{11}C]-L-deprenyl in mice: potential for measurement of functional monoamine oxidase activity in brain using positron emission tomography. Biochem Pharmacology 34:3207–3210

Machulla H-J, Shanshal A, Stöcklin G (1977) $^{123(125)}$Xe-exposed KIO$_3$, a reagent for iodination with high specific activity. Radiochimica Acta 24:42–46

Machulla H-J, Stöcklin G, Kupfernagel Ch, Freundlieb Ch, Höck A, Vyska K, Feinendegen LE (1978) Comparative evaluation of fatty acids labeled with C-11, Cl-34m, Br-77, I-123 for metabolic studies of the myocardium: concise communication. J Nucl Med 19:298–302

Machulla H-J, Marsmann M, Dutschka K (1980) Radiopharmaceuticals I. Synthesis of radioiodinated phenylfatty acids for studying myocardial metabolism. J Radioanal Chem 56:253–261

Machulla H-J, Knust EJ, Vyska K (1986) Radioiodinated fatty acids for cardiological diagnosis. Int J Appl Radiat Isot 37:777–788

Mangner TJ, Wu J-L, Wieland DM (1982) Solid-phase exchange radioiodination of aryliodides. Facilitation by ammonium sulfate. J Org Chem 47:1484–1488

Marazano C, Maziere M, Berger G, Comar D (1977) Synthesis of methyl iodide-^{11}C and formaldehyde-^{11}C. Int J Appl Radiat Isot 28:49–52

Maziere B, Todd-Pokropek AE, Berger G, Comar D (1977) Carbon-11 labeled compounds in dynamic studies of the brain. Medical Radionuclide Imaging, vol 2. IAEA, Vienna (SM 210/155), pp 21–23

Maziere M, Godot JM, Berger G, Prenant Ch, Comar D (1980) High specific activity carbon-11 labeling of benzodiazepines: diazepam and flunitrazepam. J Radioanal Chem 56:229–235

Maziere M, Comar D, Godot JM, Collard P, Cepeda C, Naquet R (1981) In vivo characterization of muscarinic receptors by positron emission tomography. Life Sci 29:2391–2397

Maziere B, Loc'h C, Hantraye P, Guillon R, Duquesnoy N, Soussaline F, Naquet R, Comar D, Maziere M (1984a) ^{76}Br-Bromospiroperidol: A new tool for quantitative in-vivo imaging of neuroleptic receptors. Life Sci 35:1349–1356

Maziere M, Hantraye P, Prenant C, Sastre J, Comar D (1984b) Synthesis of ethyl 8-fluoro-5,6-dihydro-5-[^{11}C]methyl-6-oxo-4H-imidazol(1,5-a)[1,4]benzodiazepine-3-carboxylate (RO 15.1788-^{11}C): a specific radioligand for the in vivo study of central benzodiazepine receptors by positron emission tomography. Int J Appl Radiat Isot 35:973–976

Mazziotta JC, Phelps ME (1986) Positron emission tomography studies of the brain. In: Phelps ME, Maziotta JC, Schelbert HR (eds) Positron emission tomography and autoradiography. Raven, New York

McAuley RJ, Ice RD, Curtis EG (1974) The limulus test for in vitro pyrogen detection. Am J Hosp Pharm 31:688–691

McElvany KD, Welch MJ (1980) Characterization of bromine-77-labeled proteins prepared using bromoperoxidase. J Nucl Med 21:953–960

McElvany KD, Barnes JW, Welch MJ (1980) Characterization of bromine-77-labeled proteins prepared using myeloperoxidase. Int J Appl Radiat Isot 31:679–688

McElvany KD, Katzenellenbogen JA, Shafer KE, Siegel BA, Senderoff SG, Welch MJ (1982) 16α-[^{77}Br]Bromoestradiol: dosimetry and preliminary clinical studies. J Nucl Med 23:425–430

McEwan AJ, Wyeth P, Ackery D (1986) Radioiodinated iodobenzylguanidines for diagnosis and therapy. Int J Appl Radiat Isot 37:765–775

McPherson DW, Fowler JS, Wolf AP, Arnett CD, Brodie JD, Volkow N (1985) Synthesis and biodistribution of no-carrier-added [1-^{11}C]putrescine. J Nucl Med 26:1186–1189

Mertens J, Vanryckeghem W, Bassuyt A (1985) Fast quantitative labelling of N-isopropyl-para-iodoamphetamine (AMP) with ^{123}I in the presence of Cu(I) and ascorbic acid, allowing kit-form preparation. Radiopharmaceutical and Labelled Compounds. IAEA, Vienna (STI/DUB 672)

Mertens J, Eersels J, Vanryckeghem W, Robbins MS (1986) Fast high yield Cu(I) assisted preparation of ^{123}I-15(4-I-phenyl)-9methylpentadecanoic acid. J Label Comp Radiopharm 23:1255–1256

Mestelan G, Aubert F, Beaucourt JP, Comar D, Pichat L (1979) Rapid synthesis of 2-deoxy-D(1-^{14}C)-glucose suitable for labelling with ^{11}C. J Label Comp Radiopharm 16:661–668

Metwally SAM, Coenen HH, Stöcklin G (1987) Protection of functional group and stannylation of phenylalanine. Bull Chem Soc Jpn, in press

Meyer G-J (1982) Some aspects of radioanalytical quality control of cyclotron-produced short-lived radiopharmaceuticals. Radiochimica Acta 30:175–184

Meyer G-J (1984) Die Herstellung und methodische Anwendung ^{11}C und ^{15}O markierter Verbindungen der physiologischen Stoffwechselindikatoren für die nuklearmedizinische Funktionsdiagnostik. Habilitationsschrift Medizinische Hochschule Hannover

Meyer G-J, Schober O, Hundeshagen H (1985) Uptake of C-11-L- and D-methionine in brain tumors. Eur J Nucl Med 10:373–376

Meyer G-J, Osterholz A, Hundeshagen H (1986) ^{15}O-Water constant infusion system for clinical routine application. J Label Comp Radiopharm 23:1209–1210

Moerlein SM, Coenen HH (1985) Regiospecific no-carrier-added radiobromination and radioiodination of aryltrimethyl group IVb organometallics. J Chem Soc Perkin Trans 1941–1947

Moerlein SM, Stöcklin G (1984) Radiosynthesis of no-carrier-added ^{75,77}Br-brombenperidol. J Label Comp Radiopharm 21:875–887

Moerlein SM, Stöcklin G (1985) Synthesis of high specific activity [^{75}Br]- and [^{77}Br]-bromperidol and tissue distribution studies in the rat. J Med Chem 28:1319–1324

Moerlein SM, Beyer W, Stöcklin G (1986a) Acetic acid-hydrogen peroxide as an in-situ oxidant for no-carrier-added aromatic bromination and iodination. In: Muccino RR (ed) Proc 2nd Int Symp Synthesis and Application of Isotopically Labelled Compounds

Moerlein SM, Laufer P, Stöcklin G, Pawlik G, Wienhard K, Heiss W-D (1986b) Evaluation of ^{75}Br-labelled butyrophenone neuroleptics for imaging cerebral dopaminergic receptor areas using positron emission tomography. Eur J Nucl Med 12:211–216

Moerlein SM, Stöcklin G, Pawlik G, Wienhard K, Heiss W-D (1986c) Regional cerebral pharmacokinetics of the dopaminergic neurotoxin MPTP as examined by positron emission tomography in a baboon is altered by tranylcypromine. Neurosci Lett 66:205–209

Moerlein SM, Mathis ChA, Brennan KM, Budinger ThF (1987) Synthesis and in vivo evaluation of ^{122}I- and ^{131}I-labelled iodoperidol, a potential agens for the tomographic assessment of cerebral perfusion. J Nucl Med Biol 14:91–98

Müller-Platz CM, Kloster G, Stöcklin G (1982) Fluoroacetylaction of urokinase, a new method

of labelling proteins with no-carrier-added ^{18}F. In: Nuclear medicine and biology, proceedings of the Third World Congress of Nuclear Medicine and Biology, vol. II. Pergamon, New York, pp 2112–2115; see also J Label Comp Radiopharm 19:1645–1646

Myers WG (1972) ^{11}C-Acetylen. J Nucl Med 13:699–701

Nägren K, Ragnarsson U, Langström B (1986) The synthesis of the neuropeptide met-enkephalin and two metabolic fragments labelled with ^{11}C in the methionine methyl group. Int J Appl Radiat Isot 37:537–539

Neirinckx RD, Lambrecht RM, Wolf AP (1978) Cyclotron isotopes and radiopharmaceuticals XXV: an anhydrous ^{18}F-fluorinating intermediate: Trifluoromethyl hypofluorite. Int J Appl Radiat Isot 29:323–327

Nickles RJ, Hichwa RD, Daube ME, Hutchins GD, Congdon DD (1983) An ^{18}O$_2$-target for the high yield production of ^{18}F$^-$-fluoride. Int J Appl Radiat Isot 34:625–629

Nickoloff EL (1978) Quality control for commercial and developmental radiopharmaceuticals. In: Heindel ND, Burns HD, Houda T, Brady LW (eds) The chemistry of radiopharmaceuticals. Masson, New York, pp 75–85

Nozaki T, Tanaka Y, Shimamora A, Karasawa T (1968) The preparation of anhydrous H^{18}F. Int J Appl Radiat Isot 19:27

Oberdorfer F, Crouzel C, Comar D (1984) Detailed study of nucleophilic aromatic substitution using carrier-free fluorine-18. J Label Comp Radiopharm 21:1194–1195

Otto CA, Brown LE, Wieland PM, Beierwaltes WH (1981) Radioiodinated fatty acids for myocardial imaging: effect of chain length. J Nucl Med 22:613–618

Otto CA, Lee H, Mangner TJ, Wieland DM (1986) ω-Iodophenyl fatty acids: a convenient method of radioiodination. Int J Appl Radiat Isot 37:205–210

Palmer AJ, Widdowson DA (1979) The preparation of ^{18}F-labelled 4-fluoroestrone and 4-fluorestradiol. J Label Comp Radiopharm 16:14–16

Palmer AJ, Clark JC, Goulding RW (1977) The preparation of fluorine-18 labelled radiopharmaceuticals. Int J Appl Radiat Isot 28:53–65

Pardridge WM, Oldendorf WH (1975) Kinetics of blood-brain-barrier transport of hexoses. Biochim Biophys Acta 382:377–392

Parks NJ, Krohn KA (1978) The synthesis of ^{13}N-labeled ammonia, dinitrogen, nitrite, and nitrate using a single cyclotron target system. Int J Appl Radiat Isot 29:754–756

Parks NJ, Peek NF, Goldstein E (1975) The synthesis of ^{13}N labeled atmospheric gases via proton irradiation of a high pressure oxygen target. Int J Appl Radiat Isot 26:683–687

Petzold G, Coenen HH (1981) Chloramine-T for

"no-carrier-added" labelling of aromatic biomolecules with bromine-75, 77. J Label Comp Radiopharm 18:1319–1336

Phelps ME, Huang SC, Hoffman EJ, Selin CE, Sokoloff L, Kuhl DE (1979) Tomographic measurement of local cerebral glucose metabolic rate in humans with (^{18}F) 2-fluoro-2-deoxy-D-glucose: validation of method. Ann Neurol 6:371–388

Phelps ME, Barrio JR, Huang SC, Keen RE, Chugani H, Mazziotta JC (1984) Criteria for the tracer kinetic measurement of cerebral protein synthesis in humans with positron emission tomography. Ann Neurol 15:5192–5202

Phillips L, Wray V (1971) Stereospecific electro effects, Part I. The ^{19}F nuclear magnetic resonance spectra of deoxyfluoro-D-glucopyranoses. J Chem Soc [B] 1618–1624

Pike VW, Eakins MN, Allan RM, Selwyn AP (1982) Preparation of [1-^{11}C]-acetate – An agent for the study of myocardial metabolism by positron emission tomography. Int J Appl Radiat Isot 33:505–512

Pike VW, Horlock PL, Brown C, Clark JC (1984) The remotely controlled preparation of a ^{11}C-labelled radiopharmaceutical – [1-^{11}C]acetate. Int J Appl Radiat Isot 35:623–627

Plenevaux A, Cantineau R, Guillaume M, Christians L, Tihange G (1987) Fast chemical synthesis of [^{75}Se]-L-seleno-methionine. Int J Appl Radiat Isot 38:59–61

Poe ND, Robinson GD, MacDonald NS (1975) Myocardial extraction of labeled long-chain fatty acid analogs. Proc Soc Exp Biol Med 148:215–218

Poe ND, Robinson GD, Graham LS, MacDonald NS (1976) Experimental basis for myocardial imaging with ^{123}I-labeled hexadecenoic acid. J Nucl Med 17:1077–1082

Qaim SM (1982) Nuclear data relevant to cyclotron produced short-lived medical radioisotopes. Radiochimica Acta 30:147–162

Qaim SM, Stöcklin G (1983) Production of some medically important short-lived neutron-deficient radioisotopes of halogens. Radiochimica Acta 34:25–40

Raichle ME, Eichling JO, Straatman MG, Welch MJ, Larson KB, Ter-Pogossian MM (1976) Blood brain barrier permeability of ^{11}C-labeled alcohols and ^{15}O-labeled water. Am J Physiol 230:543–552

Raichle ME, Welch MJ, Grubb RL Jr, Higgins CS, Ter-Pogossian MM, Larson KB (1978) Measurement of regional substrate utilization rates by emission tomography. Science 199:986–987

Reiffers S, Beerling-van der Molen HD, Vaalburg W, Ten Hoeve W, Paans AMJ, Korf J, Woldring MG, Wynberg H (1977) Rapid synthesis and purification of carbon-11 labelled DOPA: a potential agent for brain studies. Int J Appl Radiat Isot 28:955–958

Reiffers S, Vaalburg W, Wiegman T, Wynberg H, Woldring MG (1980) Carbon-11 labeled methyllithium as methyl donating agent: the addition to 17-keto steroids. Int J Appl Radiat Isot 31:535–539

Reivich M, Kuhl D, Wolf A, Greenberg J, Phelps M, Ido T, Casella V, Fowler J, Hoffman E, Alavi A, Som P, Sokoloff L (1979) The [^{18}F]fluorodeoxyglucose method for the measurement of local cerebral glucose utilization in man. Circ Res 44:127–137

Ritzl F, Kloster G, Coenen HH, Tisljar U, Stöcklin G (1981) L-3-^{123}I-α-Methyltyrosine and L-3-^{75}Br-α-methyltyrosine for tomographic pancreas imaging. J Nucl Med 22:P87

Roberts TR (1978) Radiochromatography. Journal of Chromatography Library, vol 14. Elsevier Scientific Publishing Company, Amsterdam

Robinson GD (1977) Synthesis of ^{123}I-16-iodo-9-hexadecenoic acid and derivatives for use as myocardial perfusion imaging agents. Int J Appl Radiat Isot 28:149–156

Robinson GD, Lee AW (1975) Radioiodinated fatty acids for heart imaging: iodine monochloride addition compared with iodide replacement labeling. J Nucl Med 16:17–21

Roeda D, Westera G (1981) A u.v.-induced on-line synthesis of ^{11}C-phosgene and the preparation of some of its derivatives. Int J Appl Radiat Isot 32:931–932

Roeda D, Crouzel C, Van Zanten B (1978) The production of ^{11}C-phosgene without added carrier. Radiochem Radioanalyt Letters 33:175–178

Rössler K (1986) Chemical modification of insulators by ion implantation, fundamental mechanisms and astrophysical implications. Rad Eff 99:21–70

Rössler K, Vogt M, Stöcklin G (1981) Production of ^{11}C precursors via the ^{14}N (p,α)^{11}C reaction in solid ammonium halides at higher doses. J Label Comp Radiopharm 18:190

Rössler K, Lattke H, Mathias C, Al Shukri LM, Vogt M (1982) In-target production of ^{11}C-precursors in nitrogen containing solids. J Label Comp Radiopharm 19:1618–1619

Rottenberg DA, Ginos JZ, Kearfott KJ (1985) Assessment of regional cerebral acid-base status in man using ^{11}C-dimethyloxazolidinedione and positron emission tomography. In: Greitz T, Ingvar DH, Widen L (eds) The metabolism of the human brain studied with positron emission tomography. Raven, New York, pp 279–284

Rozen S, Lerman O, Kol M (1981) Acetyl hypofluorite, the first member of a new family of organic compounds. J Chem Soc Chem Comm 443–444

Ruiz HV, Wolf AP (1978) Direct synthesis of oxygen-15 labelled water at high specific activities. J Label Comp Radiopharm 15:185–189

Ruth TJ, Wolf AP (1979) Absolute cross section for the production of ^{18}F via the ^{18}O(p,n)^{18}F reaction. Radiochimica Acta 26:21–24

Saji H, Nakatsuka I, Tokui T, Kuge Y, Saig A, Yokoyama A, Torizuda K, Okuno M, Yoshitake A (1986) 2′-Iodospiroperidol: studies of the dopamine receptor. J Nucl Med 27:973

Sargent T III, Budinger TF, Braun G, Shulgin AT, Braun U (1978) An iodinated catecholamine congener for brain imaging and metabolic studies. J Nucl Med 19:71–76

Satyamurthy N, Bida GT, Luxen A, Barrio JR (1986) Syntheses of 3-(2′-[^{18}F]fluoroethyl)spiperone, a dopamine receptor-binding radiopharmaceutical for positron emission tomography. J Label Comp Radiopharm 23:1045–1046

Schelbert HR (1982) The heart. In: Ell PJ, Holman BL (eds) Computed emission tomography. Oxford University Press, Oxford, pp 91–133

Schelbert HR, Schwaiger M (1986) PET studies of the heart. In: Phelps ME, Mazziotta JC, Schelbert HR (eds) Positron emission tomography and autoradiography. Raven, New York

Schober O, Meyer GJ, Gaab MR, Müller JA, Becker H, Schwarzroch R, Hundeshagen H (1986) 11-C-L-Methionine PET in lesions of the brain. Radioaktive Isotope in Klinik und Forschung 17:13–20

Schön RH, Senekowitsch R, Berg D, Schneidereit M, Reidel G, Kriegel H, Pabst HW, Blömer H (1986) Measurement of myocardial fatty acid metabolism: Kinetics of iodine-123 heptadecanoic acid in normal dog hearts. J Nucl Med 27:1449–1455

Scholl H, Kloster G, Stöcklin G (1983) Bromine-75-labeled 1,4-benzodiazepines: potential agents for the mapping of benzodiazepine receptors in vivo: concise communication. J Nucl Med 24:417–422

Schrobilgen G, Firnau G, Chirakal R, Garnett ES (1981) Synthesis of [^{18}F]XeF$_2$, a novel agent for the preparation of ^{18}F-radiopharmaceuticals. J Chem Soc Chem Comm 198–199

Schüller M, Blessing G (1987) Institut für Chemie, KFA Jülich GmbH, unveröffentlichte Ergebnisse

Seevers RH, Counsell RE (1982) Radioiodination techniques for small organic molecules. Chem Rev 82:575–590

Senderoff SG, McElvany KD, Carlson KE, Heiman DF, Katzenellenbogen JA, Welch MJ (1982) Methodology for the synthesis and specific activity determination of 16α-[^{77}Br]-bromoestradiol-17β and 16α-[^{77}Br]-11β-methoxyestradiol-17β, two estrogen receptor-binding radiopharmaceuticals. Int J Appl Radiat Isot 33:545–551

Servian JL (1977) Report of an International Atomic Energy Agency Meeting on Quality Control of Radiopharmaceuticals. Int J Appl Radiat Isot 28:653–658

Shaugnessy WJ, Gatley SJ, Hichwa RO, Lieberman LM, Nickles RJ (1981) Aspects of the production of ^{18}F-2-deoxy-2-fluoro-D-glucose via ^{18}F$_2$ with a Tandem Van de Graaf accelerator. Int J Appl Radiat Isot 32:23–29

Shiue CY, Wolf AP (1981) The synthesis of 1-[C-11]-D-glucose for the measurement of brain glucose metabolism. J Nucl Med 22:P58

Shiue CY, MacGregor RR, Lade RE, Wan C-N, Wolf AP (1979) A new synthesis of 2-deoxy-D-arabinose-hexose. Carbohydr Res 74:323–326

Shiue CY, Kutzman R, Wolf AP (1981) The synthesis of 4-fluoro-2,3-dimethyl-1-phenyl-3pyrazoline-5-one(4-fluoroantipyrine) and ^{18}F-labeled analog by direct fluorination of antipyrine with molecular fluorine. J Label Comp Radiopharm 18:1059–1066

Shiue CY, Salvadori PA, Wolf AP, Fowler JS, MacGregor RR (1982) A new improved synthesis of 2-deoxy-2-[^{18}F]fluoro-D-glucose from ^{18}F-labeled acetyl hypofluorite. J Nucl Med 23:899–903

Shiue CY, To KC, Wolf AP (1983) A rapid synthesis of 2-deoxy-2-fluoro-D-glucose from xenon difluoride suitable for labelling with ^{18}F. J Label Comp Radiopharm 20:157–162

Shiue CY, Watanabe M, Wolf AP, Fowler JS, Salvadori P (1984a) Application of nucleophilic substitution reaction to the synthesis of no-carrier-added [^{18}F]fluorobenzene and other ^{18}F-labeled arylfluorides. J Label Comp Radiopharm 21:533–547

Shiue CY, Wolf AP, Friedkin M (1984b) Syntheses of 5′-deoxy-5-[^{18}F]fluorouridine and related compounds as probes for measuring tissue proliferation in-vivo. J Label Comp Radiopharm 21:865–873

Shiue CY, Fowler JS, Wolf AP, Alexoff D, MacGregor RR (1985a) Gas-liquid chromatographic determination of relative amounts of 2-deoxy-2-fluoro-D-glucose and 2-deoxy-2-fluoro-D-mannose synthesized from various methods. J Label Comp Radiopharm 22:503–508

Shiue CY, Fowler JS, Wolf AP, Watanabe M, Arnett CD (1985b) Synthesis and specific activity determinations of no-carrier-added ^{18}F-labeled butyrophenone neuroleptics – benperidol, haloperidol, spiroperidol, and pipamperone. J Nucl Med 26:181–186

Shiue CY, Bai L-Q, Teng R-R, Wolf AP (1987) Syntheses of no-carrier-added [^{18}F]fluoroalkylhalides and their application in the syntheses of [^{18}F]fluoroalkyl derivatives of neurotransmitter receptor compounds. J Label Comp Radiopharm 24:55–64

Simon H (Hrsg) (1974) Messung von radioaktiven und stabilen Isotopen. Springer, Berlin Heidelberg New York

Sisson J, Wieland DM (1986) Radiolabeled meta-iodobenzylguanidine: pharmacology and clinical studies. Am J Physiol Imag 1:96–103

Smith CB, Davidsen L, Deibler G, Patlak C, Pettigrew K, Sokoloff L (1980) A method for determination of local protein synthesis in brain. Trans Am Soc Neurochem 11:94

Sokoloff L (1986) Cerebral circulation, energy metabolism, and protein synthesis. General characteristics and principles of measurement. In: Phelps ME, Mazziotta JC, Schelbert HR (eds) Positron emission tomography and autoradiography. Raven, New York

Sokoloff L, Reivich M, Kennedy C, Des Rosiers MH, Patlak CS, Pettigrew KD, Sakurada O, Shinohara M (1977) The [^{14}C]deoxyglucose method for the measurement of local cerebral glucose utilization: theory, procedure, and normal values in conscious and anesthetized albino rat. J Neurochem 28:897–916

Sood S, Firnau G, Garnett EX (1983) Radiofluorination with xenon difluoride: a new high yield synthesis of ^{18}F-2-FDG. Int J Appl Radiat Isot 34:743–745

Spitznagle LA, Marino CA (1977) Synthesis of fluorine-18 labeled 21-fluoroprogestesterone. Steroids 30:435–438

Stewart GW, Dymerski PP, Hower CO (1974) Reactions of recoil ^{13}N atoms in the gas phase. J Chem Phys 61:483–490

Stöcklin G (1969) Chemie heißer Atome. Chemie, Weinheim

Stöcklin G (1972) Chimie des atomes chauds. Masson, Paris

Stöcklin G (1977) Bromine-77 and iodine-123 radiopharmaceuticals. Int J Appl Radiat Isot 28:131–147

Stöcklin G (1982) Evaluation of radiohalogen-labelled fatty acids for heart studies. Nucl Med 19:299–304

Stöcklin G, Kloster G (1982) Metabolic analogue tracers. In: Ell PJ, Holman BL (eds) Computed emission tomography. Oxford University Press, Oxford, pp 229–338

Stöcklin G, Coenen HH, Harmand MF, Kloster G, Knust EJ, Kupfernagel Ch, Machulla H-J, Weinreich R, Feinendegen LE, Vyska K, Höck A, Freundlieb C (1980) Comparative evaluation of radiohalogenated fatty acids for myocardial and heptacellular function analysis. Radioaktive Isotope in Klinik und Forschung 14:151–163

Stöcklin G, Moerlein SM, Kloster G, Voges F, Schuier FJ, Wienhard K, Pawlik G, Feinendegen LE, Heiss W-D (1986) Noninvasive measurement of regional cerebral pharmacokinetics of some centrally active agents with PET. Radioaktive Isotope in Klinik und Forschung 17:75–82

Straatman MG (1977) A look at ^{13}N and ^{15}O in radiopharmaceuticals. Int J Appl Radiat Isot 28:13–20

Straatman M, Welch MJ (1973a) The liquid chromatographic purification of carbon-11 labeled glucose. Int J Appl Radiat Isot 24:234–236

Straatman MG, Welch MJ (1973b) Enzymatic synthesis of nitrogen-13 labeled amino acids. Radiat Res 56:48–56

Straatman MG, Welch MJ (1975) A general method for labeling proteins with ^{11}C. J Nucl Med 16:425–428

Straatman MG, Welch MJ (1977) Fluorine-18-labeled diethylaminosulfur trifluoride (DAST): an F-for-OH fluorinating agent. J Nucl Med 18:151–158

Subramanyam R, Bucelewicz WM, Hoop B, Jones SC (1977) A system for oxygen-15 labeled blood for medical applications. Int J Appl Radiat Isot 28:21–24

Sundoro-Wu BM, Schmall B, Conti PS, Dahl JR, Drumm P, Jacobsen JK (1984) Selective alkylation of pyrimidyldianions: Synthesis and purification of ^{11}C-labeled thymidine for tumor visualization using positron emission tomography. Int J Appl Radiat Isot 35:705–708

Suzuki K, Iwata R (1977) A novel method for the production of ^{13}NN proton irradiation of aqueous solution of ammonia. Radiochem Radioanal Letters 28:263–268

Suzuki K, Inoue O, Hashimuto K, Yamasaki T, Kuchiki M, Tamate K (1985) Computer-controlled large scale production of high specific activity [^{11}C]RO 15-1788 for PET studies of benzodiazepine receptors. Int J Appl Radiat Isot 36:971–976

Svärd H, Nägren K, Malmborg P, Sohn D, Sjöberg S, Langström B (1982) The synthesis of various N-[^{11}C-methyl]-pharmaceuticals using ^{11}C-methyliodide. J Label Comp Radiopharm 19:1519–1520

Syrota A, Comar D, Cerf M, Plummer D, Maziere M, Kellersohn C (1979) [^{11}C]-Methionine pancreatic scanning with positron emission computed tomography. J Nucl Med 20:778–781

Syrota A, Dop-Ngassa M, Cerf M, Paraf A (1981) [^{11}C]-L-Methionine for evaluation of pancreatic exocrine function. Gut 22:907–915

Syrota A, Duquesnoy N, Paraf A, Kellershohn C (1982) The role of positron emission tomography in the detection of pancreatic disease. Radiology 143:249–253

Syrota A, Paillotin G, Davy JM, Aumont MC (1984) Kinetics of in vivo binding of antagonist to muscarinic cholinergic receptor in the human heart studied by positron emission tomography. Life Sci 35:937–945

Syrota A, Castaing M, Rougemont D, Berridge M, Maziere B, Baron JC, Bousser MG, Pocidalo JJ (1985) Regional tissue pH and oxygen metabolism in human cerebral infarction studied with positron emission tomography. In: Greitz T, Ingvar DH, Widen L (eds) The metabolism of the human brain studied with positron emission tomography. Raven, New York, pp 285–303

Tada M, Matsuzawa T, Ohrui H, Fukuda H, Ido T, Takahashi T, Shinohara M, Komatsu K (1984) Synthesis of some 2-deoxy-2-fluoro[^{18}F]-hexopyranoses, potential diagnostic imaging agents. Heterocycles 22:565–568

Tang DY, Lipman A, Meyer GJ (1979) ^{11}C-Labeled octanal and benzaldehyde. J Label Comp Radiopharm 16:435–440

Tarle M, Padovan R, Spaventi S (1978) Radioiodination of iodinated estradiol-17-diphosphates. J Label Comp Radiopharm 15:7–21

Tarle M, Padovan R, Spaventi S (1979) Preparation of 2α-^{125}I-dihydrotestosterone by exchange labelling and direct iodination. J Label Comp Radiopharm 16:177–178

Tewson TJ (1983) Synthesis of nca fluorine-18 2-fluoro-2-deoxy-D-glucose. J Nucl Med 24:718–721

Tewson TJ, Welch MJ, Raichle ME (1978) [^{18}F]-Labeled 3-deoxy-3-fluoro-D-glucose: synthesis and preliminary biodistribution data. J Nucl Med 19:1339–1345

Tewson TJ, Raichle ME, Welch MJ (1986) Preliminary studies with [^{18}F]haloperidol: a radioligand for in vivo studies of the dopamine receptors. Brain Res 192:291–295

Thakur ML, Chauser BM, Hudson RF (1975) The preparation of iodine-123 labelled sodium ortho-iodo hippurate and its clearance by the rat kidney. Int J Appl Radiat Isot 26:319–320

Tilbury RS (1981) The chemical forms of ^{13}N produced in various nuclear reactions and chemical environments: a review. In: Root JW, Krohn KA (eds) Short-lived radionuclides in chemistry and biology. Advances in Chemistry Series 197. American Chemical Society, Washington/DC pp 261–267

Tilbury RS, Dahl JR, Mamacos JP, Laughlin JS (1970) Fluorine-18 production for medical use by helium-3 bombardment of water. Int J Appl Radiat Isot 21:277–281

Tilbury RS, Dahl JR, Monaham WG, Laughlin JS (1971) The production of ^{13}N-labeled ammonia for medical use. Radiochem Radioanal Letters 8:317–323

Tisljar U, Kloster G, Ritzl F, Stöcklin G (1979) Accumulation of radioiodinated L-α-methyltyrosine in pancreas of mice: concise communication. J Nucl Med 20:973–976

Tominaga T, Tachikawa E (1981) Modern hot atom chemistry and its applications. Springer, Berlin Heidelberg New York

Tramposch K, Kung H, Blau M (1980) New brain imaging agents: radioiodine labeled tertiary diamines. J Nucl Med 21:P68

Vaalburg W, Kamphuis JAA, Beerling-van der Molen HD, Reiffers S, Rijskamp A, Woldring MG (1975) An improved method for the cyclotron production of ^{13}N-labelled ammonia. Int J Appl Radiat Isot 26:316–318

Vaalburg W, Beerling-van der Molen HD, Reiffers S, Rijskamp A, Woldring MG, Wynberg H (1976) Preparation of carbon-11 labeled phenylalanine and phenylglycine by a new amino acid synthesis. Int J Appl Radiat Isot 27:153–157

Vaalburg W, Reiffers S, Beerling E, Pratt JJ, Woldring MG, Wynberg H (1977) The preparation of carbon-11 labelled 17α-ethynylestradiol. J Label Comp Radiopharm 13:200–201

Vaalburg W, Feenstra A, Wiegman T, Beerling E, Reiffers S, Talma A, Woldring MG, Wynberg H (1981) Carbon-11 labelled moxestrol and 17α-methylestradiol as receptor binding radiopharmaceuticals. J Label Comp Radiopharm 18:100–101

Van Havar D, Rabi NA, Vandewalle M, Goethals P, Vandecasteele C (1985) Routine production of 2-deoxy-D-[1-^{11}C]-glucose: an alternative. J Label Comp Radiopharm 22:657–666

Van Rijn CJS, Herscheid JDM, Visser GWM, Hoekstra A (1985) On the stereoselectivity of the reaction of [^{18}F]-acetylhypofluorite with glucals. Int J Appl Radiat Isot 36:111–115

Vine EN, Young D, Vine WH, Wolf W (1979) An improved synthesis of ^{18}F-5-fluorouracil. Int J Appl Radiat Isot 30:401–504

Visser FC (ed) (1985a) Workshop on radiolabeled free fatty acids, Eur Heart J [Suppl B] 6:1–106

Visser FC, Hachiel J, Van Eenige MJ, Westera G, Den Hollander W, Duwel CMB, van der Wall EE, Heidendal GAK, Roos JP (1985b) Metabolic fate of radioiodinated heptadecanoic acid in the normal canine heart. Circulation 72:565–571

Visser GWM, Halteren BW, Herscheid JDM, Brinkman GA, Hoekstra A (1984) Reaction of acetyl hypofluorite with aromatic mercury compounds: A new selective fluorination method. J Chem Soc Chem Comm 655–656

Visser GWM, Noordhuis P, Zwaagstra O, Aersched JM, Hoekstra A (1986) A simplified synthesis of ^{18}F-labelled cytosine- and uracil-nucleosides. Int J Appl Radiat Isot 37:1074–1076

Volkow N, Goldman SS, Flamm ES, Craviotto H, Wolf AP (1983) Labeled putrescine as a probe in brain tumors. Science 221:673–675

Vora MM, Boothe TE, Finn RD, Kothari PJ, Emram AM, Carroll ST, Gilson AJ (1985) Multi-Curie preparation of 2-[^{18}F]-fluoro-2-deoxy-D-glucose via nucleophilic displacement with fluorine-18 labelled fluoride. J Label Comp Radiopharm 22:953–960

Vyska K, Freundlieb C, Höck A, Becker V, Schmid A, Feinendegen LE, Kloster G, Stöcklin G, Heiss WD (1982) Analysis of local perfusion rate (LPR) and local glucose transport rate (LGTR) in brain and heart in man by means of C-11-methyl-D-glucose (CMG) and dynamic positron emission tomography (dPET). Radioaktive Isotope in Klinik und Forschung 15:129–142

Wagner H jr (1986) Images of the brain: past as prologue. J Nucl Med 27:1929–1937

Wagner HN, Burns H, Dannals RF, Wong DF, Langström B, Duelfer T, Frost JJ, Haxden TR, Links JM, Rosenbloom SB, Lukas SE (1983) Imaging dopamine receptors in the human brain by positron tomography. Science 221:1264–1266

Wagner R (1984) A fast synthesis of ^{18}F-fluoromethane from ^{18}F-F$_2$. J Label Comp Radiopharm 21:1229–1230

Wagner R (1986) Synthesis of ^{18}F-labeled 4-fluoro-antipyrine via gaseous acetylhypofluorite: Optimization of reaction parameters and remote controlled production. J Label Comp Radiopharm 23:1100

Wagner R, Stöcklin G, Schaack W (1981) Production of carbon-11 labelled methyl iodide by direct recoil synthesis. J Label Comp Radiopharm 18:1557–1566

Wanek PM (1981) Notes on the radioiodination of hippuric acid. Radiochem Radioanal Letters 46:401–404

Washburn LC, Wieland BW, Sun TT, Hayes RL, Butler TA (1978) [1-^{11}C]D,L-Valine, a potential pancreas imaging agent. J Nucl Med 19:77–83

Washburn LC, Sun TT, Byrd BL, Callahan AP (1982) Production of L-[1-^{11}C]valine by HPLC resolution. J Nucl Med 23:29–33

Weiss ES, Hoffman EJ, Phelps ME, Welch MJ, Henry PD, Ter-Pogossian MM, Sobel BE (1976) External detection and visualization of myocardial ischemia with ^{11}C-substrates in vitro and in vivo. Circ Res 39:24–32

Welch MJ, Lifton JF, Ter-Pogossian MM (1969) Preparation of millicurie quantities of oxygen-15-labeled water. J Label Comp Radiopharm 5:168–172

Welch MJ, Wittmer SL, Dence CS, Tewson TJ (1981) Radiopharmaceuticals labeled with ^{11}C and ^{18}F. Considerations related to the preparation of ^{11}C-palmitate. In: Root JW, Krohn KA (eds) Short-lived radionuclides in chemistry and biology. Advances in chemistry series. American Chemical Society, Washington/DC, pp 407–417

Welch MJ, Kilbourn MR, Mathias CJ, Mintun MA, Raichle ME (1983) Comparison in animal models of ^{18}F-spiroperidol and ^{18}F-haloperidol: potential agents for imaging the dopamine receptor. Life Sci 33:1687–1693

West JB, Dollery CT (1961) Absorption of inhaled radioactive water vapor. Nature 189:588

Westera G (1981) Labelled fatty acids. Synthesis and biological behaviour. A review. In: Cox PH (ed) Progress in radiopharmacology, vol 2. Biomedical, Elsevier/North Holland

Westera G, Gijlswijk HJM (1979) Radioiodination of aromatic compounds with ^{123}I and ^{131}I by exchange. J Label Comp Radiopharm 16:174

Wilbur DS, Anderson KW, Stone WE, O'Brien HA (1982) Radiohalogenation of non-activated aromatic compounds via aryltrimethylsilyl intermediates. J Label Comp Radiopharm 19:1171–1188

Winchell HS, Baldwin RM, Lin TH (1980) Development of I-123 labeled amines for brain studies: localization of I-123 iodophenylalkyl amines in rat brain. J Nucl Med 21:940–946

Wolf AP, Redvanly CS (1987) Carbon-11 and radiopharmaceuticals. Int J Appl Radiat Isot 28:29–48

Wolf AP, Christman DR, Fowler JS, Lambrecht RM (1973) Synthesis of radiopharmaceuticals and labelled compounds using short-lived isotopes. In: Radiopharmaceuticals and labelled compounds. IAEA, Vienna, (IAEA-SM-171/92) pp 345–381

Wu JHC, Harper PV, Lathrop KA (1981) Separation of racemic tryptophan. J Nucl Med 22:P74

Yamamoto YL, Hakim AM, Diksic M, Pokrupa RP, Meyer E, Tyler J, Evans AC, Worsley K, Thompson CJ, Feindel WH (1985) Focal flow disturbances in acute strokes: Effects on regional metabolism and tissue pH. In: Heiss W-D (ed) Functional mapping of the brain in vascular disorders. Springer, Berlin Heidelberg New York Tokyo

Yin ET, Galanos E, Kinsky S, Bradshaw RA, Wesser S, Cuderitz O, Sarmiento ME (1972) Picogram sensitive assay for endotoxin gelation of limulus polyphemus blood cell lysate, induced by purified polysacharides and lipid A from gram-negative bacteria. Biochem Biophys Acta 261:284

Zalutsky MR, Wu J, Harper PV, Wickland T (1981) Synthesis of ^{11}C-D,L-tryptophan and its purification using high pressure liquid chromatography. Int J Appl Radiat Isot 32:182–184

1.3 Spezielle Probleme des Strahlenschutzes

Von

D. Junker und J. Fitschen

Mit 9 Abbildungen und 4 Tabellen

A. Allgemeiner Überblick

Am Zyklotron werden überwiegend Radionuklide mit Neutronenunterbesetzung der Atomkerne produziert. Dies bedeutet, daß die erzeugten Radionuklide durch einen Betaprozeß unter Emission von Positronen (β^+) oder durch einen Elektroneneinfangprozeß (EC) zerfallen. Beide Zerfallsreaktionen sind konkurrierende Prozesse. Im unteren Ordnungszahlbereich überwiegen die β^+-Strahler, im oberen Ordnungszahlbereich die Elektroneneinfang-Strahler. Es gibt deshalb zwei verschiedene zyklotron-produzierte Radionuklidarten: Im unteren Ordnungszahlbereich die reinen Positronenstrahler wie ^{11}C, ^{13}N, ^{15}O und ^{18}F, im mittleren und oberen Ordnungszahlbereich die EC- oder Gemischtstrahler wie ^{123}J, ^{201}Tl bzw. ^{52}Fe, ^{68}Ga.

Von den physiologisch wichtigen Elementen wie Kohlenstoff, Stickstoff, Sauerstoff und auch Fluor existieren keine gammastrahlenden Radionuklide, die eine relevante Halbwertszeit haben. Die Bedeutung des klinisch vollintegrierten Zyklotrons liegt nun gerade darin, daß radioaktive Isotope dieser Elemente nur von einem Zyklotron als Positronenstrahler kurzer Halbwertszeit erzeugt werden können. Während längerlebige zyklotron-produzierte Radionuklide ohne weiteres käuflich erworben werden können, ist dies bei den kurzlebigen Radionukliden nicht möglich, da die Halbwertszeiten zu kurz sind (2 bis 100 min). Sie müssen deshalb in unmittelbarer Nähe der Klinik produziert und aufgearbeitet werden.

Positronenstrahler emittieren eine 511 keV-Gammastrahlung und sind deshalb schwieriger abzuschirmen als die meisten in der Nuklearmedizin eingesetzten Radionuklide. Wegen der Kurzlebigkeit der Radionuklide muß außerdem eine deutlich höhere Anfangsaktivität hergestellt werden, um am Ende des radiochemischen Aufarbeitungsprozesses eine genügend hohe Applikationsaktivität zu erhalten.

Produktion, Markierung und medizinische Anwendung kurzlebiger, zyklotron-produzierter Radionuklide bilden deshalb im Sinne des Strahlenschutzes eine arbeitstechnische Einheit.

Bei allen Produktions- und Verarbeitungsschritten kann es zu einer Strahlenexposition des Personals und unter Umständen auch der Umwelt kommen. Von Störfällen abgesehen ist die Strahlenexposition abhängig von der baulichen und administrativen Konzeption des Produktionsprozesses, der Höhe der produzierten und verarbeiteten Aktivität sowie der Häufigkeit der Untersuchungen. Ökologisch und ökonomisch sinnvoller Strahlenschutz bedeutet: Messung und Bilanzierung der während des gesamten Betriebsablaufes abgeleiteten Radioaktivitäten sowie der auftretenden Dosen und der Versuch, durch strahlenschutzgerechte Planung der Anlage, durch Abschirmung und durch Organisation der Arbeitsabläufe die Strahlenexposition nach dem von der ICRP konzipierten ALARA-Prinzip (As low as reasonable achievable) zu minimalisieren.

Spezielle Gesichtspunkte des Strahlenschutzes eines medizinisch genutzten Zyklotrons sind: Anlagenstrahlenschutz, Personalstrahlenschutz, Umweltschutz und Patientenstrahlenschutz.

B. Anlagenstrahlenschutz

Die Produktion von Radionukliden am Zyklotron erfolgt durch Beschuß der Gas- und Feststofftargets mit elektrisch geladenen und auf hohe Energie beschleunigten Teilchen. Bei vielen Reaktionsprozessen werden dabei hochenergetische Neutronen freigesetzt, die ihrerseits durch Wechselwirkung mit der Umgebung und den Betonwänden des Zyklotronbunkers sekundär Gammastrahlung auslösen. Auf diese Weise ist die Beschaffenheit der Abschirmung unmittelbar abhängig von der Maximalenergie der beschleunigten Teilchen und damit auch direkt abhängig von der Größe der Maschine. Alle äußeren Strahlenschutzmaßnahmen müssen deshalb auf den Maschinentyp und die Bedingungen des Strahlbetriebes so zugeschnitten sein, daß die Dosisgrenzwerte der Strahlenschutzverordnung für die verschiedenen Strahlenschutzbereiche nicht nur eingehalten, sondern möglichst unterschritten werden.

Bei der Neuplanung von Zyklotronanlagen bestehen normalerweise hinsichtlich der Strahlenschutzkonzeption keine wesentlichen Probleme. Die Einhaltung bzw. Unterschreitung der vorgegebenen Grenzwerte der Strahlenschutzverordnung kann in diesem Fall durch ausreichende Dimensionierung der Abschirmwände nach oben und seitlich im allgemeinen leicht erreicht werden. Zusätzlich hat man die Möglichkeit, durch entsprechende Planung der zum Zyklotron gehörenden Betriebsräume die Ortsdosisleistung der frei zugänglichen Bereiche zu minimieren.

Grundregeln des Strahlenschutzes beim Zyklotron-Neubau sind:

- Die Hauptstrahlrichtung des Zyklotrons (beam) sollte entweder in das Erdreich oder in Richtung der Zyklotronversorgungsräume gewählt werden.
- Allgemein zugängliche Räume, die außerbetriebliche Überwachungsbereiche sind (maximal 1,5 mSv/Jahr bzw. 150 mrem/Jahr) sollten nicht unmittelbar an Kontroll- oder Sperrbereiche angrenzen.
- Eine ausreichende Deckenabschirmung ist für den Fall zu fordern, daß die über der Anlage liegenden Bereiche frei genutzt werden sollen. Liegt die Anlage außerhalb – aber in engster Nähe eines frei genutzten Gebäudes, ist es vorteilhaft, die Abschirmung auch gegen die sekundäre Gammastrahlung durch Erdaufschüttung auf dem Zyklotronbau zu gewährleisten.
- Durch Einrichtung von Schleusen und u.U. durch Einschränkung der Zugangsberechtigung zu bestimmten Räumen innerhalb des Zyklotronbereichs kann die Einhaltung des Minimalprinzips der Strahlenschutzverordnung erreicht werden.

Ein Zyklotron ist in der Lage, Neutronenstrahlung mit hoher Dosisleistung zu erzeugen. Sie entsteht, wenn der Primärstrahl auf das zu bestrahlende Material (Target) auftrifft und die beschleunigten Ionen aus den Atomkernen Neutronen freisetzen. Aber nicht nur in den Targets können Neutronen ausgelöst werden, sie entstehen auch ungewollt durch einen nicht exakt fokussierten Primärstrahl in den Rohrwandungen des Strahlführungssystems. Desgleichen wird ein hoher Neutronenpegel erzeugt, wenn der Primärstrahl in den Strahlpausen auf den Hauptstrahlstopp trifft.

20 MeV-Deuteronen, dies entspricht ungefähr der maximalen Deuteronenenergie der meisten medizinisch genutzten Kompaktzyklotrons, liefern auf Beryllium geschossen nach Jean u. Fauchet (1978) im Abstand von 1,25 m vom Target ca. 1 Gy/min. Nach Meißner (1978)

mißt man bei einem Deuteronenstrahl der Energie von 14,03 MeV auf Beryllium und einem Deuteronenstrom von 100 µA extern im Abstand von 1,25 m vom Target frei in Luft eine Energiedosisleistung von 0,34 Gy/Minute. Das Neutronenbündel breitet sich dabei vorzugsweise in einem kleinen Winkelbereich um die Richtung des einfallenden Deuterons aus (Vorwärtsstreuung). Die Ortsdosisleistung variiert mit dem Abstand vom Target. In einer Entfernung von 4 m vom Target in Strahlrichtung (bei 90°-Stellung des Strahlerkopfes) beträgt die Dosisleistung 0,033 Gy/min. Mit dem effektiven Qualitätsfaktor für schnelle Neutronen nicht bekannter Energie (durch Wechselwirkung mit der Umgebung verändert sich die Energie der Neutronen) von ca. 10 entsprechend der Strahlenschutzverordnung, Anhang XIV, Tabelle XIV,2 (1976), ergibt dies eine Äquivalentdosisleistung von 20 Sv/h bzw. 2000 rem/h vor der Bunkerwand. In 5,5 m Entfernung vom Target ergibt sich nach MEISSNER (1978) eine Dosisleistung von ca. 10,6 Sv/h bzw 1060 rem/h. Soll an der Außenseite einer an dieser Stelle liegenden Abschirmwand ein außerbetrieblicher Überwachungsbereich anschließen, so darf die Dosis für nicht beruflich strahlenexponierte Personen 1,5 mSv (150 mrem) im Jahr nicht überschreiten (Strahlenschutzverordnung, § 44). Soll der erforderliche Reduktionsfaktor abgeschätzt werden, muß man berücksichtigen, daß dieser in starkem Maße beeinflußt wird durch die geplante Betriebsstundenzahl des Zyklotrons pro Jahr und den Aufenthaltsfaktor T, der die zu erwartende Aufenthaltsdauer von Personen im zu schützenden Bereich angibt (in Anlehnung an DIN 6812 und 54113, Teil 3). Für einen Aufenthaltsfaktor von $T = 0,1/1$ und eine Betriebsstundenzahl von 1000 h pro Jahr/2000 h pro Jahr ergeben sich notwendige Schwächungsfaktoren von $0,7 \cdot 10^6$ bis $1,4 \cdot 10^7$ für Neutronenstrahlung.

Die Einhaltung der Strahlenschutzgrenzwerte in verschiedenen Strahlenschutzbereichen setzt deshalb eine ausreichende Dimensionierung und Materialbeschaffenheit der Abschirmwände voraus. Die Dicke der Wände ist abhängig von der Neutronenquellstärke des Zyklotrons und wird somit direkt von der Teilchenart, der Energie der Teilchen und der externen Stromstärke des Strahls bestimmt. Ebenso von Bedeutung für die Neutronenausbeute ist die Wahl des Targetmaterials. Untersuchungen haben ergeben, daß dicke Berylliumtargets die höchsten Neutronenausbeuten liefern. Dies ist auch aus dem Verlauf der Neutronenausbeutefunktion für verschiedene Reaktionen nach PATTERSON u. THOMAS (1973) ersichtlich (s. Abb. 1).

Nach Messungen von HELMEKE u. JUNKER (1978), SAUERMANN et al. (1978) und SAUERMANN (1985) können die Reaktionen

$$^9\text{Be (p,n) } ^9\text{B}$$

$$^9\text{Be (d,n) } ^{10}\text{B}$$

bezogen auf die Neutronenausbeute als "worst case"-Reaktionen angesehen werden. Bei der Abschätzung der Neutronenfreisetzungsrate eines Kompaktzyklotrons muß allerdings beachtet werden, daß aus physikalischen Gründen die maximal mögliche Protonenenergie doppelt so hoch sein kann wie die maximal mögliche Deuteronenenergie.

Die bei diesen Reaktionen im Target freigesetzen Neutronen sind sehr energiereich und haben im Gegensatz zu den Neutronen von Neutronengeneratoren, die überwiegend monoenergetische Neutronen z.B. von 14 MeV emittieren, ein kontinuierliches Neutronenspektrum. Abbildung 2 zeigt verschiedene Neutronenenergiespektren von (d,n)-Reaktionen auf Beryllium für drei Deuteronenenergien.

Zur Abschirmung schneller Neutronen mit Energien zwischen 100 keV und 10 MeV sind Materialien geeignet, die einen hohen Anteil an Elementen mit niedrigem Atomgewicht haben. Diese Stoffe moderieren die schnellen Neutronen überwiegend durch elastische Stöße. Wasser, Polyäthylen, Paraffin und Kunststoffe eignen sich deshalb besonders als Abschirmmaterialien für Neutronen in diesem Energiebereich.

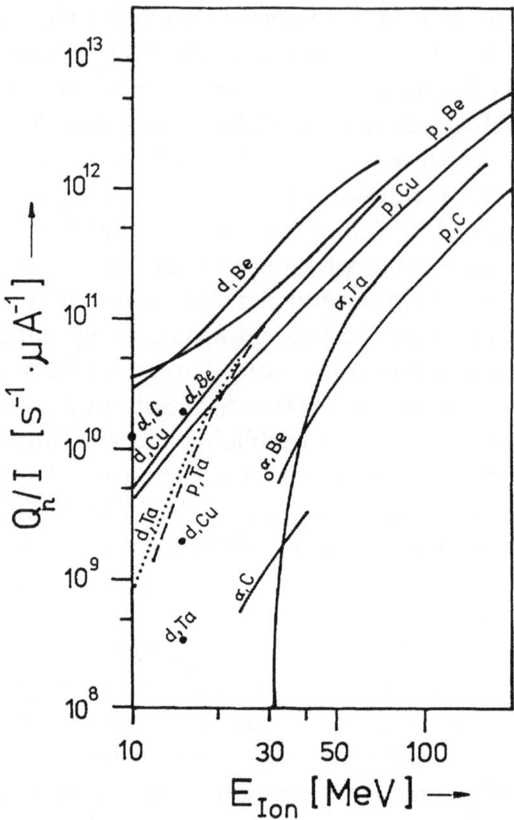

Abb. 1. Totale Neutronenausbeute bezogen auf den Targetstrom verschiedener Reaktionen in Abhängigkeit von der Energie der einfallenden Teilchen nach Patterson u. Thomas (1973)

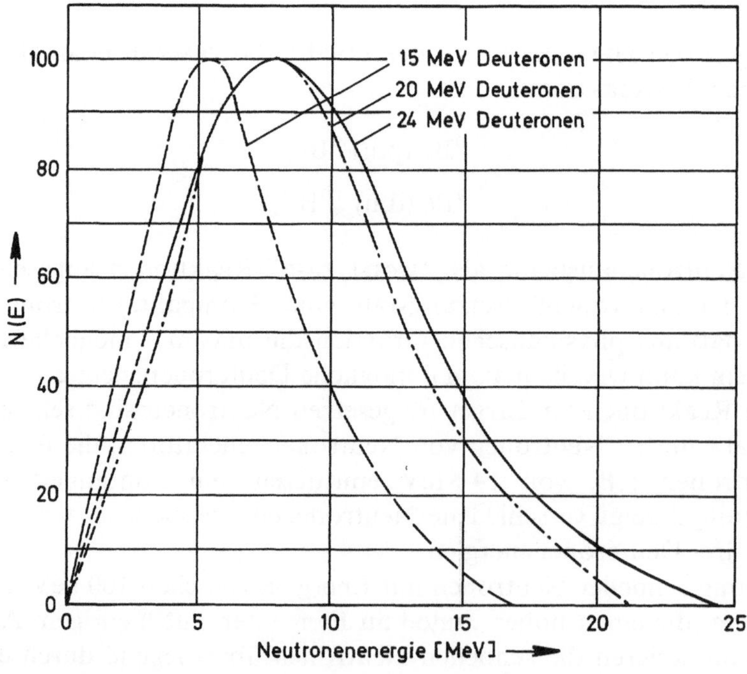

Abb. 2. Neutronen-Energiespektren von Beryllium-Targets für verschiedene Deuterium-Energien. (Nach Tochilin u. Kohler 1958 und Cohen u. Falk 1951)

Für Neutronenenergien oberhalb 10 MeV überwiegt der Wirkungsquerschnitt für unelastischen Stoß und verschiedene Kernreaktionen im Vergleich zu dem des elastischen Stoßes. Dies gilt besonders für schwere Kerne. Deshalb ist z.B. Eisen gut als Moderator für schnelle Neutronen geeignet.

Als häufigstes Abschirmmaterial für Neutronenstrahlung wird in der Praxis Beton verwendet. Beton ist ein Gemisch aus Zement, Kies, Sand und Wasser. Er hat also einen hohen Anteil an Elementen mit geringem Atomgewicht wie Sauerstoff, Silizium, Aluminium und Kalzium und ist deshalb für Neutronenenergien unterhalb 10 MeV besonders gut geeignet. Die Abschirmwirkung läßt sich durch stark wasserhaltigen Beton erhöhen.

Das Wasser des Betons muß jedoch als Kristallwasser gebunden sein, weil es sich andernfalls verflüchtigen würde. Dies läßt sich z.B. durch Zusatz von Limonit (Zusammensetzung $2Fe_2O_3 \cdot 3\,H_2O$) erreichen. Der Kristallwassergehalt des Limonits liegt bei 9–11%, der Eisenanteil zwischen 55 und 58%. Wegen des hohen Eisenanteils ist limonithaltiger Beton auch gleichzeitig gut für die Abschirmung von Neutronen oberhalb von 10 MeV geeignet. Limonitbeton läßt sich aber schwer verarbeiten und ist zudem teuer. Deshalb werden häufig nur die inneren Wände der Abschirmung aus Limonitbetonsteinen gemauert. Die restliche notwendige Abschirmung wird dann oft in Normalbeton ausgeführt.

Verschiedene Betonarten wurden von SAUERMANN (1971) in ihrer Abschirmwirkung für monoenergetische 14 MeV-Neutronen untersucht (s. Tabelle 1). Man erkennt, daß die beste Reduktion der 14 MeV-Neutronen durch eine Abschirmung aus Wasser oder Limonitbeton erreicht wird.

Tabelle 1. Abhängigkeit des Transmissionsfaktors Tr für 14 MeV-Neutronen von der Wandstärke des Abschirmmaterials nach SAUERMANN (1971) für Wasser, Normalbeton (NB, Dichte $\rho = 2,33\ \mathrm{g \cdot cm^{-3}}$), Limonitbeton (LB, $\rho = 2,97\ \mathrm{g \cdot cm^{-3}}$), Limonitbeton mit Eisenzusatz (LS, $\rho = 4,26\ \mathrm{g \cdot cm^{-3}}$) und Eisen

Transmissions-faktor Tr	Wandstärke cm				
	H_2O	NB	LB	LS	Fe
$5 \cdot 10^{-1}$	8,4	12,9	10,1	10,4	12,9
$2 \cdot 10^{-1}$	19,5	30	23,4	24,2	28
$1 \cdot 10^{-1}$	28	43	33,5	34,6	40
$5 \cdot 10^{-2}$	36	56	44	45	52
$2 \cdot 10^{-2}$	47	73	67	59	68
$1 \cdot 10^{-2}$	56	86	67	69	80
$5 \cdot 10^{-3}$	64	99	77	80	92
$2 \cdot 10^{-3}$	75	116	91	94	108
$1 \cdot 10^{-3}$	84	129	101	104	120
$5 \cdot 10^{-4}$	92	142	111	114	132
$2 \cdot 10^{-4}$	103	159	124	128	147
$1 \cdot 10^{-4}$	112	172	134	139	159
$5 \cdot 10^{-5}$	120	185	144	149	171
$2 \cdot 10^{-5}$	131	202	158	163	187
$1 \cdot 10^{-5}$	140	215	168	173	199
$5 \cdot 10^{-6}$	148	228	178	184	211
$2 \cdot 10^{-6}$	159	245	191	198	227
$1 \cdot 10^{-6}$	167	258	201	208	239

Ferner wurde die Abschirmwirkung von Normalbeton bezüglich der Neutronen, die durch verschiedene Teilchenarten und Teilchenenergien im Zyklotron freigesetzt werden, untersucht (s. Tabelle 2).

Tabelle 2. Abhängigkeit des Transmissionsfaktors Tr von der Wandstärke des Abschirmmaterials (Normalbeton) nach Sauermann et al. (1980). Neutronen aus Reaktionen verschiedener Teilchenarten mit Beryllium am Kompaktzyklotron

Transmissions-faktor Tr	Wandstärke cm			
	d 14 MeV	p 24 MeV	^{3}He 35 MeV	^{4}He 28 MeV
$5 \cdot 10^{-1}$	9,2	9,8	10,2	11,7
$2 \cdot 10^{-1}$	21,4	22,7	23,6	27,3
$1 \cdot 10^{-1}$	30,6	32,5	33,8	39,0
$5 \cdot 10^{-2}$	39,8	42,3	44,0	50,7
$2 \cdot 10^{-2}$	52,0	55,2	57,4	66,3
$1 \cdot 10^{-2}$	61,2	65,0	76,6	78,0
$5 \cdot 10^{-3}$	70,4	74,8	77,8	89,7
$2 \cdot 10^{-3}$	82,6	87,7	91,2	105,3
$1 \cdot 10^{-3}$	91,8	97,5	101,4	117,0
$5 \cdot 10^{-4}$	101,0	107,3	111,6	128,7
$2 \cdot 10^{-4}$	113,2	120,2	125,0	144,3
$1 \cdot 10^{-4}$	122,4	130,0	135,2	156,0
$5 \cdot 10^{-5}$	131,6	139,8	145,4	167,7
$2 \cdot 10^{-5}$	143,8	152,7	158,8	183,3
$1 \cdot 10^{-5}$	153,0	162,5	169,0	195,0
$5 \cdot 10^{-6}$	162,2	172,3	179,2	206,7
$2 \cdot 10^{-6}$	174,4	185,2	192,6	222,3
$1 \cdot 10^{-6}$	183,6	195,0	202,8	234,0

Neben der Neutronenstrahlung muß auch die Gammastrahlung bei den Abschirmmaßnahmen berücksichtigt werden. Ein Teil der Gammastrahlung entsteht als prompte γ-Strahlung im Target, ein weiterer Anteil stammt aus den Abschirmwänden selbst. Er entsteht durch (n,γ)-Reaktion der auf thermische Energie moderierten Neutronen mit den aktivierbaren Elementen des Betons. Diese intensive und energiereiche γ-Strahlung muß ebenfalls außerhalb des Target-Zyklotronbunkers auf Werte unterhalb der zulässigen Grenzwerte der einzelnen Strahlenschutzbereiche entsprechend der Strahlenschutzverordnung reduziert werden. Untersuchungen zeigen, daß zumindest bei kleineren Zyklotrons, wie sie in der Klinik installiert werden, die für die Abschirmung der γ-Strahlen notwendigen Wandstärken geringer oder zumindest nicht wesentlich größer sind, als die notwendigen Wandstärken zur Abschirmung der Neutronenstrahlung. Das geht auch aus Abb. 3 hervor, wo die Äquivalentdosisleistung der Gammastrahlung deutlich geringer als die der Neutronenstrahlung im Fall der (d,n)-Reaktionen ist.

Für den Fall der (p,n)-Reaktionen haben Waterman et al. (1979) und Johnsen (1977, 1978, 1979) die Dosistransmissionsfaktoren in Abhängigkeit von dem Streuwinkel ψ (Winkel zwischen Primärstrahl und gestreuten Neutronen) und der Wandstärke der Normalbetonabschirmung gemessen (s. Abb. 4, 5).

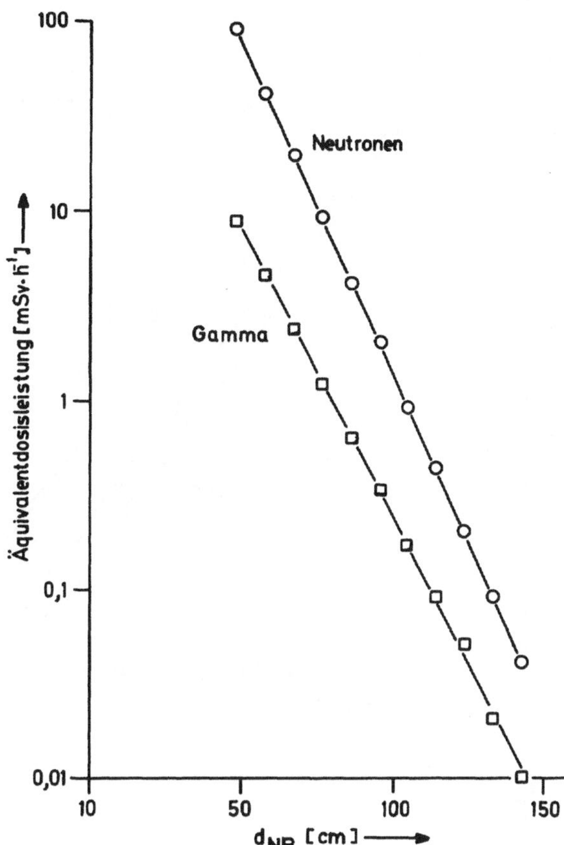

Abb. 3. Äquivalentdosisleistung von Neutronen und Gammastrahlung bei der ^{9}Be $(d,n)^{10}$B – Reaktion, $E_d = 14$ MeV, $I_d = 10$ μA, als Funktion der Abschirmdicke d_{NB} aus Normalbeton. (Nach SAUERMANN et al. 1978)

Als Beispiel für eine Neukonzeption einer Zyklotronanlage sei die Anlage im Universitätsklinikum Essen angeführt, die der Neutronentherapie und Radionuklidproduktion dient (Abb. 6 nach RASSOW 1982). Es handelt sich dabei um die Installation eines TCC-Kompakt-Isochron-Zyklotrons CV 28 mit maximaler Protonenenergie von 24 MeV und maximaler Deuteronenenergie von 14 MeV. Der externe Strahlstrom beträgt dabei 79 bzw. 110 μA. MEIßNER (1978) berichtet, daß an der Zyklotronanlage außerhalb der Bunker keine größeren Ortsdosisleistungen hinter den Betonwänden als 1 μSv/h auftraten, typisch waren 0,3 μSv/h. Die Reduktion der Dosisleistung wurde erreicht durch eine 180 cm dicke Abschirmwand aus Limonitbeton in Richtung der Arbeitsplätze und Räume ohne Beschränkung der Aufenthaltsdauer. Die innenliegenden Trennwände zwischen den einzelnen Bestrahlungsräumen bestehen aus 150 cm Limonitbeton.

Ähnlich sind die Abschirmwände des Jülicher Kompaktzyklotrons dimensioniert. Die Außenwände des Beschleunigerraums bestehen aus 180 cm Normalbeton (Dichte 2,4 g/cm³) mit einer Wasserbindung von 140 ltr/m³ zur Neutronenabschirmung nach HEMMERICH et al. (1977). Beim Beschuß von dicken Berylliumtargets mit 14 MeV-Deuteronen, 50 μA Strahlstrom, lagen die Dosisleistungen außerhalb der Abschirmung in der Größenordnung von 10^{-3} mGy/h.

Als Beispiel für ein in eine bestehende Klinik integriertes Zyklotron, das ausschließlich für die Produktion von kurzlebigen Radionukliden genutzt wird, sei das Zyklotron MC 35 der Fa. Scanditronix in der Abt. für Nuklearmedizin der Medizinischen Hochschule

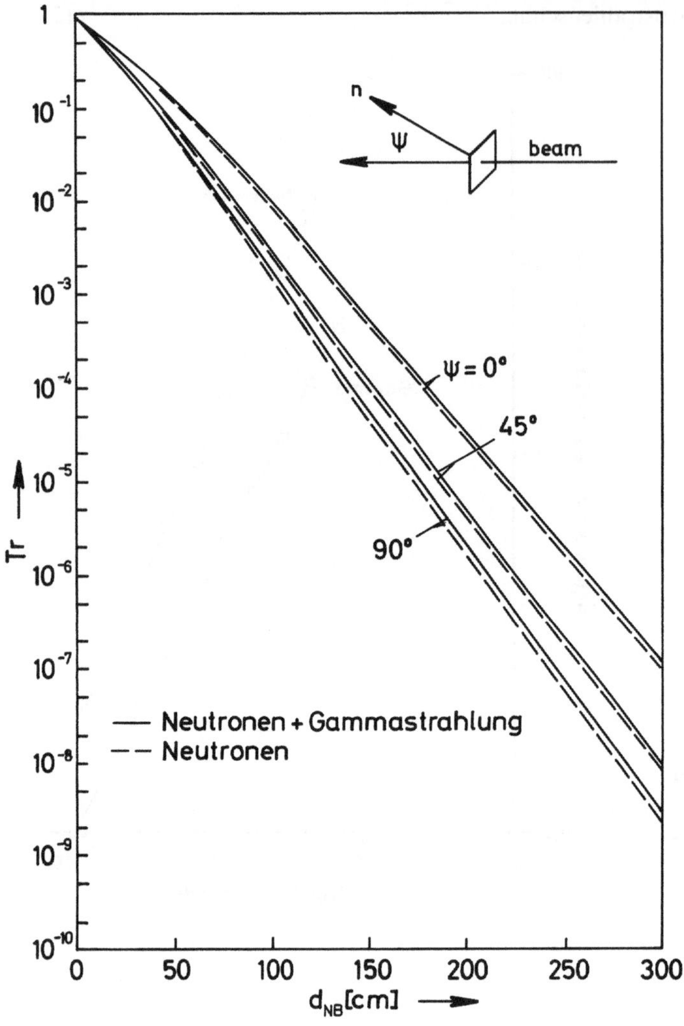

Abb. 4. Effektiver Transmissionsfaktor Tr von Normalbeton für Neutronen aus der Reaktion 35 MeV-Protonen auf dickes Berylliumtarget. Neutronenspektrum nach WATERMAN. Sicherheitsbericht Kompaktzyklotron Med. Hochschule Hannover (1985).

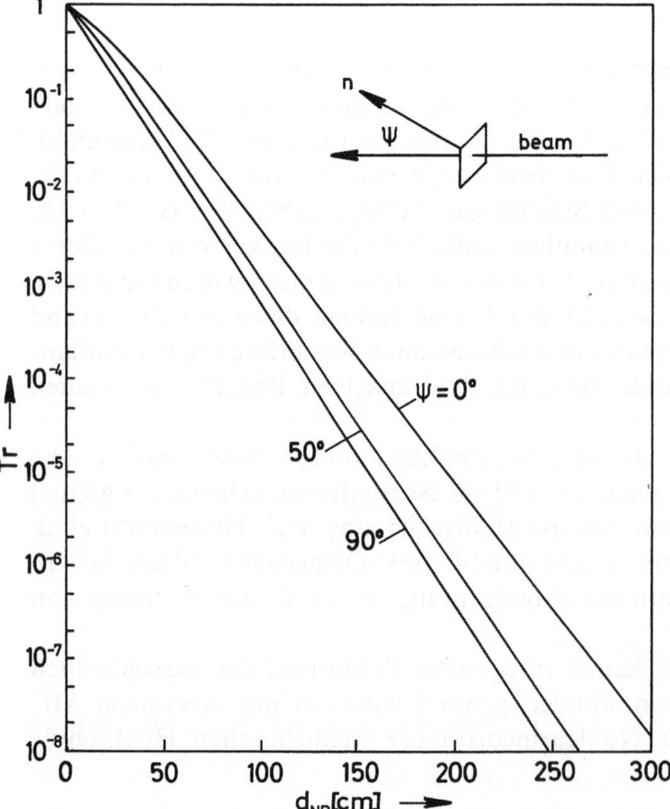

Abb. 5. Effektiver Transmissionsfaktor Tr für Neutronen aus der Reaktion 35 MeV-Protonen auf dickes Beryllium-Target (nur Neutronenkomponente). Neutronenspektrum nach JOHNSEN. Sicherheitsbericht Kompaktzyklotron Med. Hochschule Hannover (1985)

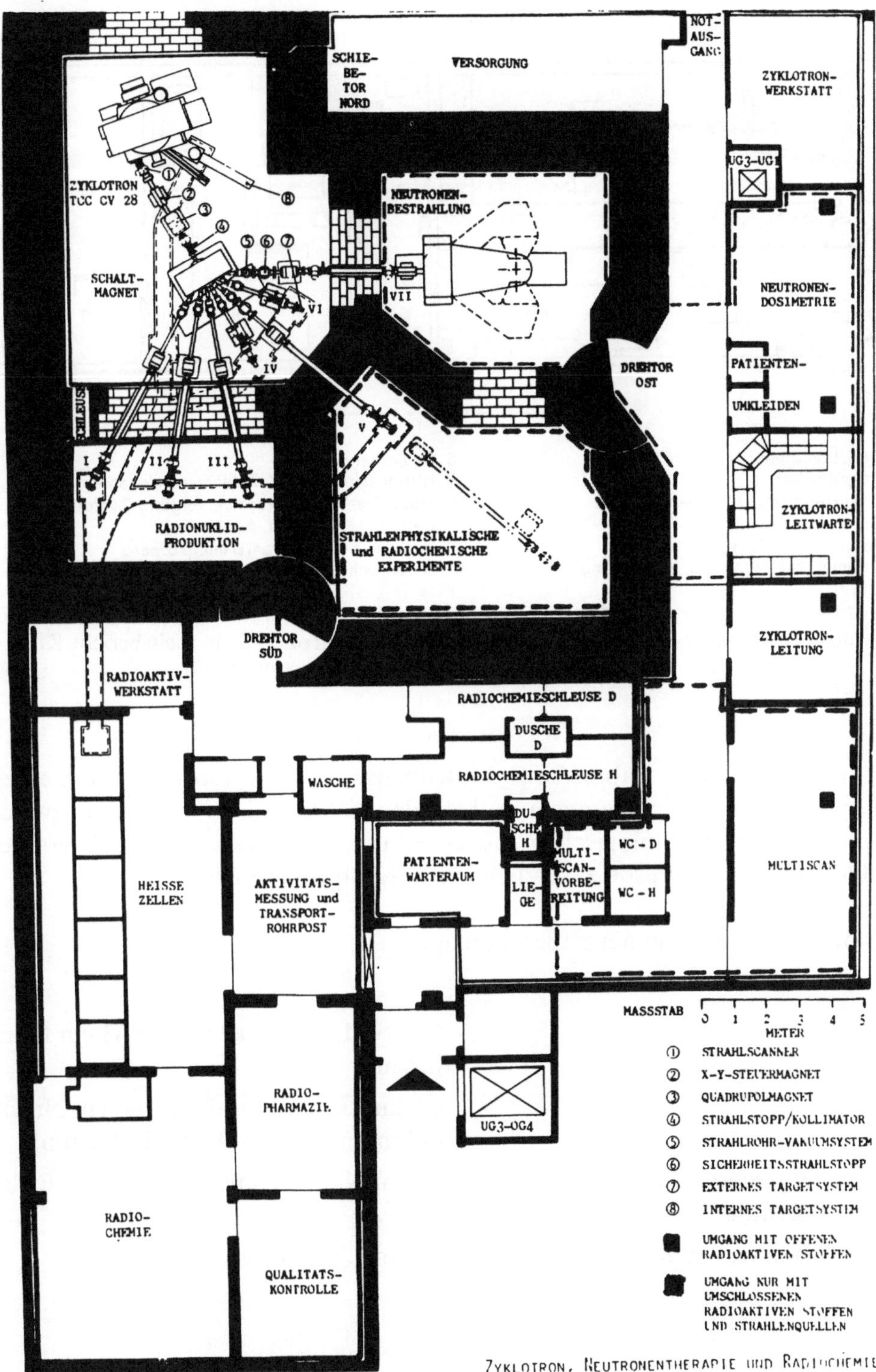

Abb. 6. Grundriß des TCC-Kompaktzyklotrons CV 28 des Universitätsklinikum Essen, Abt. Medizinische Strahlenphysik. (Nach RASSOW 1982)

in Hannover angeführt (Abb. 7). Die Anlage wurde nachträglich in einem schon vorhandenen Raum installiert. Die Energie der Teilchen, die im Kompaktzyklotron erzeugt werden können, ist variabel. Die maximale Protonenenergie des Zyklotrons beträgt 35 MeV, der größte Strahlstrom 60 μA extern.

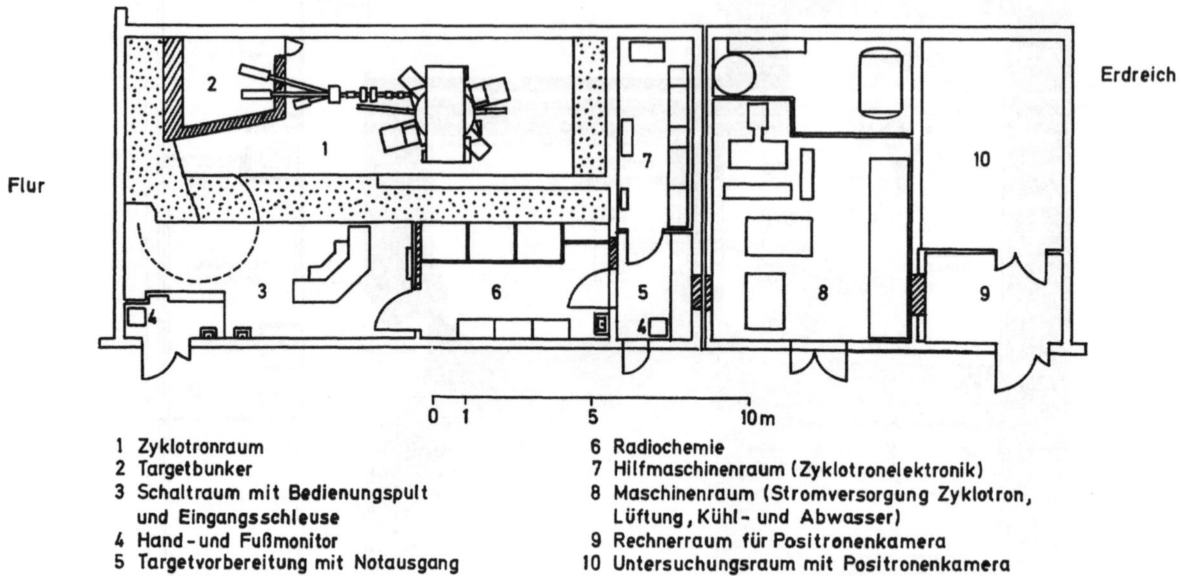

Abb. 7. Grundriß der klinisch integrierten Zyklotronanlage der Medizinischen Hochschule Hannover, Abt. für Nuklearmedizin. Kompaktzyklotron MC 35 der Firma Scanditronix. Sicherheitsbericht Kompaktzyklotron der Medizinischen Hochschule Hannover (1985)

Das Zyklotron, das Heiße Labor der Zyklotronchemie, die Versorgungsräume des Zyklotrons und der Patientenuntersuchungsraum befinden sich auf der Kellerebene zwischen den Gebäudekomplexen des Radiologischen Institutes und der Physikalischen Therapie. Innerhalb des Zyklotronbunkers wurde zusätzlich ein Targetbunker installiert.

Die Abschirmung wurde folgendermaßen konzipiert:

Targetbunker:

in Strahlrichtung	185 cm Limonitbeton und 53 cm Normalbeton.
Decke	63 cm Limonitbeton und 80 cm Normalbeton und 120 cm Erdaufschüttung.
Wände zum Kellergeschoß der Physikalischen Therapie	74 cm Normalbeton und 193 cm Erdreich
Wand des Targetbunkers zum Zyklotronraum	30 cm Limonitbeton

Zyklotronraum:

Wand zum Schaltraum	150 cm Limonitbeton
Wand zum Kellergeschoß der Physikalischen Therapie	74 cm Normalbeton und 193 cm Erdreich
Wand zwischen Zyklotron und Radiochemie	100 cm Limonitbeton und 50 cm Normalbeton
Decke	80 cm Normalbeton und 120 cm Erdreich
Wand zu den Versorgungsräumen (entgegen der Strahlrichtung)	100 cm Limonitbeton und 45 cm Normalbeton

Die Dichten der verwendeten Materialien betragen: Normalbeton 2,3 g/cm^3, Limonitbeton 2,97 g/cm^3, Erdschüttung 1,6 g/cm^3.

Zur Prüfung der Abschirmung wurden 35 MeV-Protonen mit einem Strahlstrom von 30 µA extern auf ein Beryllium-Target geschossen. Die dabei außerhalb der Anlage ermittelte Äquivalentdosisleistung betrug maximal:

Neutronenstrahlung:	$\dot{H} =\ \ 1$ µSv/h
Gammastrahlung:	$\dot{H} = 0{,}1$ µSv/h
Gammastrahlung direkt oberhalb des Zyklotrons:	$\dot{H} =\ \ 1$ µSv/h

C. Personalstrahlenschutz

Der Betrieb eines Beschleunigers und die Anwendung der produzierten kurzlebigen Radionuklide am Menschen kann zu einer Strahlenexposition des Personals führen. Folgende Berufsgruppen sind davon betroffen:

- Zyklotronpersonal (Physiker, Ingenieure, Operateure).
- Zyklotronradiochemie (Chemiker, chemisch-technische Assistenten).
- Medizinische Applikation (Ärzte, medizinisch-technische Assistenten).

I. Strahlenexposition des Zyklotronpersonals bei Betriebs- und Wartungsarbeiten

Jeder Teilchenbeschleuniger stellt während des Strahlbetriebes eine sehr intensive Strahlenquelle dar. Aber nicht nur während des Betriebes, sondern auch nach Abschalten des Beams können etliche Anlagenteile noch sehr radioaktiv sein. Durch Streuung des Primärstrahls innerhalb der Maschine und im Strahlführungssystem kommt es zu einer Aktivierung der Anlagenteile. Die Aktivierung selbst ist abhängig von der Betriebsart des Zyklotrons, z.B. Strahlzeit, Teilchenart, Energie der Teilchen und Stromstärke. Besonders radioaktiv werden die Targets und Teile des Extraktionssystems, vor allem Septum und Deflektor.

Der Betrieb eines Zyklotrons erfordert in gewissen Abständen Wartungsarbeiten. Ist dabei ein Öffnen der Maschine notwendig, so sollten unbedingt vorher die Ortsdosisleistungen an der Maschine und an den heißen Bereichen gemessen werden. MEIßNER (1978) berichtet, daß am Essener Zyklotron kurz nach Abschalten der Maschine am Deflektor Dosisleistungen bis zu 0,1 Sv/h aufgetreten sind. Eigene Messungen und Messungen von HELMEKE (1982) am Zyklotron Hannover bestätigen im Prinzip die Messungen von MEIßNER. Wartungsarbeiten im Innern der Maschine sollten deshalb grundsätzlich erst nach einer Abklingzeit von mindestens 2–3 Tagen durchgeführt werden, um kurzlebige Aktivitätsanteile abklingen zu lassen. Die nach dieser Abklingzeit gemessenen Dosisleistungen betragen je nach Betriebszeit des Zyklotrons am Preseptum 0,80–2,00 mSv/h, an den Deflektorsonden 0,25–0,30 mSv/h und am Antiseptum 0,30–0,50 mSv/h. Diese Werte treten bei monatlichen Strahlzeiten zwischen 25 und 40 h auf. Die eigentliche Wartungszeit beträgt bei offener Maschine im Mittel ca. 40–60 min, wobei die Arbeiten an extrem heißen Bauelementen auf wenige Minuten zu beschränken sind. Die jährlich akkumulierte Ganzkörperdosis liegt nach unseren Messungen im Mittel zwischen 2 und 3,60 mSv/a. Die Exposition der Hände läßt sich durch Verwendung von Greifwerkzeugen deutlich reduzieren und liegt dann nur maximal 2–3mal höher als die Ganzkörperdosis. Die pro Person und Wartung gemessene Ganzkörperexposition liegt im Mittel bei 0,20–0,40 mSv.

Eine Überwachung des Personals mit neutronenempfindlichen Kernspurfilmen ergab bisher keinen Hinweis auf eine relevante Neutronenexposition beim Betrieb des Zyklotrons.

Bonnett u. Bell (1982) berichten, daß die Ganzkörperdosis des Zyklotronpersonals in Edinburgh für den Überwachungszeitraum 1982 4 mSv/a (Bereich 3–5 mSv/a) und die korrespondierende mittlere Fingerdosis 34 mSv/a (Bereich 10–60 mSv/a) beträgt.

Ein besonderes Problem stellen die dünnen Folien dar, die das Strahlrohr vom Targetsystem abtrennen. Wird eine solche Folie zu stark vom Strahl erhitzt, so brennt sie durch. Das Strahlrohr wird durch eine Schnellschlußvorrichtung vom eigentlichen Zyklotron abgetrennt, so daß die Folie, ohne das Zyklotron abschalten zu müssen, ausgetauscht werden kann. Der Austausch kann beim $^{11}C/^{15}O$-Target nach ca. 1 h vorgenommen werden, beim Kryptontarget sind hingegen mindestens 12–15 h Wartezeit notwendig. Dann liegt die Dosisleistung im Arbeitsbereich je nach vorangegangener Betriebsart des Zyklotrons und nach Abklingen der kurzlebigen Aktivitätsanteile bei 0,60 bis 0,80 mSv/h. Durch sorgfältiges Planen aller Arbeitsschritte kann die Personalexposition auf weniger als 0,10 bis 0,20 mSv pro Folientausch beschränkt werden. Voraussetzung dazu ist allerdings, daß bei längerlebigen Radionukliden das gesamte Aktivitätsinventar der Targets entfernt wurde oder durch physikalischen Zerfall abgeklungen ist. Die gesamte Arbeitszeit beim Wechseln der Folie liegt erfahrungsgemäß bei 30–40 min, die Arbeitszeit zum Entfernen der alten heißen Folie kann auf einige Minuten begrenzt werden.

II. Strahlenexposition des Radiochemie-Personals

Die am Zyklotron in den Targets produzierten Radionuklide werden durch ein Transportsystem in die Verarbeitungsboxen der Zyklotronchemie geleitet. Die aktiven Gase können meistens durch Teflon- oder Stahlleitungen vom Zyklotronbunker direkt in die Verarbeitungsboxen befördert werden, wo sie dann zur Weiterverarbeitung zur Verfügung stehen. Ist bei extrem kurzlebigen Radionukliden, z.B. ^{15}O, eine „constant infusion"-Methode erforderlich, müssen auch die Verbindungsleitungen zum Applikationsraum ausreichend abgeschirmt sein. Für Feststofftargets sind separate Transportsysteme erforderlich, da ein manueller Zugriff wegen der hohen Dosisleistungen nicht möglich ist.

Kurzlebige zyklotronproduzierte Radionuklide sind häufig Positronenstrahler, die bekanntlich eine 511 keV-Photonenstrahlung emittieren. Da zusätzlich die meisten reinen Positronenstrahler auch eine sehr hohe Photonenemissionsrate von fast 200% haben, ist auch die Gammadosisleistungsrate relativ hoch (ca. 0,15 $\mu Gy \cdot m^2/MBq \cdot h$), etwa das 10fache der ^{99m}Tc-Dosisleistungskonstante. Wegen der Kurzlebigkeit der Radionuklide müssen außerdem relativ hohe Anfangsaktivitäten eingesetzt werden, die häufig schon im Bereich von hundert GBq liegen. Diese Randbedingungen beeinflussen in einem hohen Maße den gesamten Arbeitsablauf in der Radiochemie. Sämtliche Verarbeitungsschritte müssen deshalb hinter einer mindestens 5 cm dicken Bleiabschirmung erfolgen. Wegen möglicher Freisetzungen von Radioaktivitäten sind alle Markierungsarbeiten in geschlossenen Boxen mit separater Be- und Entlüftung durchzuführen. Das Ausmessen der Aktivitäten sollte ebenfalls halbautomatisch mit Greifwerkzeugen in der Verarbeitungsbox erfolgen.

Die Verarbeitungsboxen der Radiochemie müssen ausreichend abgeschirmt sein. Dabei ist es nicht nur notwendig, die Primärstrahlung nach vorn zu berücksichtigen, sondern auch für die Boxendecken und -wände eine ausreichende Abschirmung vorzusehen. Andernfalls wird die ausgelöste Sekundärstrahlung erhebliche Dosisleistungen im Arbeits- und Verkehrsbereich erzeugen. Auch die Abschirmungen der inneren Arbeitsflächen nach unten sowie Durchführungen für Versorgungsleitungen sind sorgfältig zu planen und zu überprüfen. Notfalls müssen innerhalb der Verarbeitungsbox zusätzliche bewegliche Abschirmwände installiert werden.

Als Beispiel sei die Verarbeitung einer 74 GBq ^{11}C-Aktivität genannt. Die Dosisleistung in einer Verarbeitungsbox mit 5 cm Bleiwandstärke beträgt in Höhe der Greifer direkt hinter der Abschirmwand 60 µSv/h. Unter der Annahme eines störungsfreien Ablaufs der Verarbeitung beträgt die durchschnittliche Ganzkörperexposition der Chemiker nach JUNKER (1982) für eine 40minütige Aufarbeitungszeit 20–50 µSv/Charge. Da die Spritzen automatisch in der Verarbeitungsbox aufgezogen werden, liegt die Exposition der Hände für diesen Verarbeitungsschritt in der gleichen Größenordnung. Die durchschnittliche Strahlenexposition eines Radiochemikers in den letzten Jahren erreichte am Hannover Zyklotron ca. 3,7 mSv/a, die Exposition der entsprechenden CTA ca. 1,1 mSv/a. Die produzierte Aktivität schwankte dabei zwischen 1000 und 1850 GBq/Monat, wovon im Mittel 30–70% vom Target extrahiert werden konnten und sich in den Verarbeitungsboxen befanden.

SAUERMANN et al. (1982) berichtet, daß durch den stetigen Anstieg der zu verarbeitenden Aktivität bedingt auch die Personaldosen angestiegen sind. Durch zusätzliche Abschirmmaßnahmen, Verbesserung der experimentiellen Einrichtungen und Einführung automatisch arbeitender Bedienungselemente konnte 1981 die Einzeldosis der Ganzkörperbelastung im Mittel auf 3,66 mSv/Jahr (höchste Einzeldosis 10,6 mSv/Jahr) begrenzt werden. Die Handdosis lag für den gleichen Zeitraum im Mittel bei 20 mSv/Jahr, die höchste Einzeldosis lag bei 62 mSv/Jahr.

III. Strahlenexposition des medizinischen Personals

Die in der Zyklotronchemie produzierten und in Spritzen aufgezogenen Radiopharmaka sollten zum Applikationsort entweder mittels einer separaten Rohrpostanlage oder im Abschirmbehälter transportiert werden (bei 2 cm Bleiwand Reduktion der Dosisleistung auf ca. 3%). Im Untersuchungsraum ist eine Vorratsbox mit Abschirmung aus mindestens 5 cm Blei vorzusehen.

Die zu erwartende Strahlenexposition bei der Injektion sei am Beispiel einer 555 MBq ^{11}C-Aktivität (Palmitinsäure oder Methionin) in einer 2 bzw. 5 ml-Spritze dargestellt. Diese Ergebnisse sind, bezogen auf den Applikationszeitpunkt, weitgehend auch auf alle anderen Positronenstrahler mit einer ca. 100%-Positronenemissionsrate und annähernd gleichen Dosisleistungskonstanten übertragbar, wie ^{13}N, ^{15}O und ^{18}F. Betrachtet werden die Expositionen des Ganzkörpers und die Belastung der Finger des untersuchenden Arztes. Zum Zweck der genauen Bestimmung der Fingerdosen wurden von JUNKER (1982) die Dosisleistungen an den applikationsfertigen Spritzen ermittelt (s. Abbildungen 8 und 9).

Die gemessenen Werte sind Richtwerte, im Einzelfall können die tatsächlichen Werte je nach Positionierung der Finger an den verschiedenen Expositionsorten z.T. stark abweichen. Ferner ist zu berücksichtigen, daß auch die Wandstärke des Spritzenmaterials bei der Beurteilung der Hautdosen eingeht, da durch unterschiedliche Wandstärken die Absorption der Positronen im Wandmaterial verschieden ist. Die Gesamtbelastung der Finger ergibt sich durch Multiplikation der Dosisleistungen mit den mittleren Expositionszeiten. Es stellt sich heraus, daß bei der Applikation hohe Fingerdosen auftreten, so daß zusätzliche Strahlenschutzmaßnahmen erforderlich werden. Die handelsüblichen Spritzenabschirmungen aus Bleiglas der Dichte 6,2 g/cm^3 reduzieren die Dosen nicht wesentlich (Reduktionsfaktor für 511 keV ca. 1,4 gegenüber 70 für 140 keV des ^{99m}Tc). Aus diesem Grunde muß die Injektion von Positronenstrahlern höherer Aktivität grundsätzlich mit einem Perfusionsbesteck erfolgen.

Die Strahlenexposition des Arztes bei der Injektion einer 555 MBq ^{11}C-Aktivität mittels Perfusionsbesteck wurde folgendermaßen gemessen: Der Abstand des Arztes vom Perfusionsbesteck betrug ca. 50 cm, die Dosisleistung der aktiven butterfly-Spritze vor der Injektion

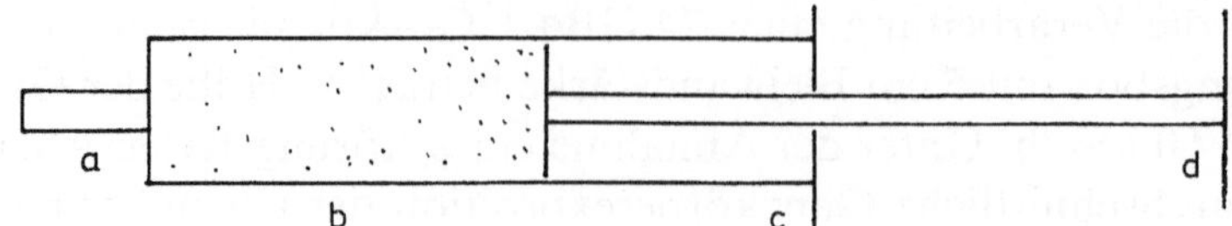

Meßpunkt	a	b	c	d
Dosisleistung cGy/min	0,62	1,8	0,07	0,01

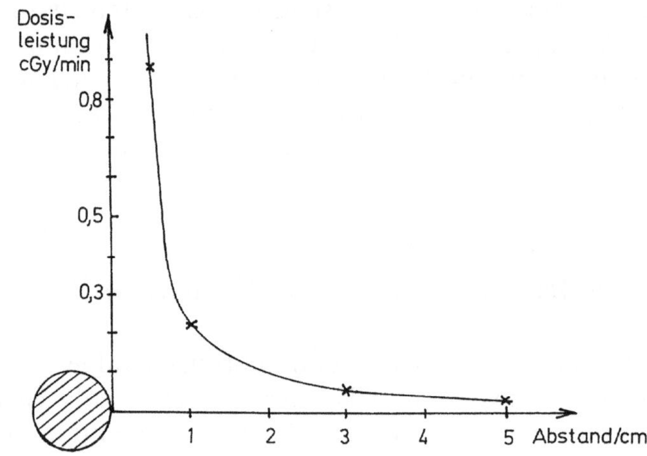

Abb. 8. Axialer und radialer Dosisleistungsverlauf einer 555 MBq ^{11}C-Aktivität in einer 2 ml-Spritze. Gemessen mit TLD 100 Dosimetern, kalibriert mit geeichten TOL/E-Kammern der Fa. Berthold bei 511 keV

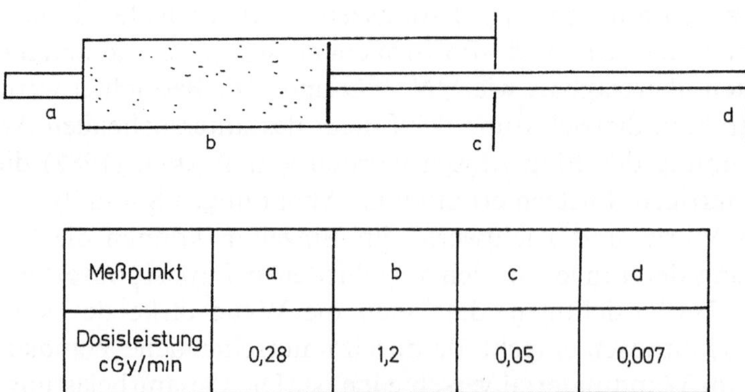

Meßpunkt	a	b	c	d
Dosisleistung cGy/min	0,28	1,2	0,05	0,007

Abb. 9. Axialer Dosisleistungsverlauf einer 555 MBq ^{11}C-Aktivität in einer 5 ml-Spritze. Gemessen mit TLD 100 Dosimetern, kalibriert mit geeichten TOL/E-Kammern der Fa. Berthold bei 511 keV

ca. 0,30 mSv/h, die Dosisleistung des Patienten nach der Injektion im Abstand von 1 m ca. 0,08 mSv/h. Die gesamte Strahlenexposition des Arztes für Applikation und Untersuchung ergibt bei strahlenbewußtem Verhalten ca. 0,02–0,03 mSv pro Untersuchung. Die Exposition der Finger beträgt bei Injektion einer 2 ml-Spritze unter Benutzung des Perfusionsbestecks: Zeige-/Mittelfinger je ca. 0,20–0,40 mSv pro Applikation, Daumen 0,03–0,05 mSv.

D. Schutz der Umwelt und Genehmigungsfragen

I. Genehmigungsfragen

Bei der Konzeption einer Zyklotronanlage sind nach der Strahlenschutzverordnung vorher die radioökologischen Verhältnisse des Standortes zu klären. Darunter ist die Untersuchung der radiologischen Vorbelastung der Umgebung zu verstehen, die entweder durch Langzeitmessungen oder Überwachung des Umgangs zu bestimmen oder durch Rechnungen abzuschätzen ist. Für den endgültigen Betrieb eines Kompaktzyklotrons in einer Klinik ist i. allg. die Vorlage eines Sicherheitsberichtes bei den Behörden erforderlich. Dieser enthält u.a. die Betrachtung folgender sicherheitsrelevanter Angaben:

- Jahresabgabe radioaktiver Stoffe mit der Luft und dem Wasser durch andere, dem Antragsteller bereits genehmigte Tätigkeiten.
- Vorbelastung der Umgebung durch Ableitung radioaktiver Stoffe aus anderen Anlagen und Einrichtungen gemäß Angaben der zuständigen Behörden.
- Betrachtungen der meteorologischen Bedingungen des Standortes der Anlage, insbesondere das Auftreten von Inversionswetterlagen.
- Hydrologie des Oberflächen- und Grundwassers.
- Zukünftige Ableitung radioaktiver Stoffe über den Abluft- und Abwasserpfad und daraus resultierende Strahlenexpositionen von Personen, die nicht beruflich strahlenexponiert sind und in der Nähe der Anlage wohnen.
- Störfallbetrachtung beim Betrieb der Anlage.
- Entsorgung radioaktiver Stoffe (längerlebige Radionuklide).

Die Konzeption der Anlage mit dem vorläufigen Sicherheitsbericht ist der zuständigen Behörde zur Prüfung vorzulegen. Die Behörde wird im Einzelfall über den Antrag entscheiden und die Randbedingungen für den Betrieb der Anlage festlegen. Für die Antragstellung ist es hilfreich, den einzelnen Punkten der Genehmigungsanträge die „Merkpostenliste" zu Genehmigungsfragen für Anlagen zur Erzeugung ionisierender Strahlen, Gemeinsames Ministerialblatt (1978), zugrunde zu legen.

II. Umweltschutz

1. Luftaktivierung durch Neutronen im Target- und Beschleunigerraum

Da der Primärionenstrahl bis zum Target oder Ionenstopp im Vakuum geführt wird, ist eine Aktivierung der Luft im Zyklotronraum nur durch sekundäre Neutronen möglich, wie sie z.B. durch (p,n)- oder (d,n)-Reaktionen entstehen. Dabei sind zwei Reaktionen möglich:
- Aktivierung durch schnelle Neutronen, die direkt vom Target kommen, und
- Einfangreaktionen langsamer Neutronen, die durch Streuung an der Abschirmung moderiert worden sind.

Die wichtigsten Kernreaktionen, die zur Luftaktivierung in der Umgebung von Kompaktzyklotronen beitragen, sind:

$$^{14}N\,(n, 2n)\,^{13}N \qquad (T_p = 9,96\ min)$$
$$^{16}O\,(n, 2n)\,^{15}O \qquad (T_p = 2,03\ min)$$
$$^{16}O\,(n, p)\,^{16}N \qquad (T_p = 7,13\ sec)$$
$$^{40}Ar\,(n, \gamma)\,^{41}Ar \qquad (T_p = 1,83\ h)$$

Die ersten drei Reaktionen werden durch schnelle, die letzte Reaktion wird durch Einfang thermischer Neutronen ausgelöst. Bis auf ^{41}Ar haben alle erzeugten Radionuklide eine relativ kurze physikalische Halbwertszeit T_p. Meißner (1978) berichtet, daß am Zyklotron in Essen keine relevante Luftaktivierung beobachtet worden ist. Die gemessene spezifische Aktivität lag bei 16fachem Luftwechsel im Bestrahlungsraum unterhalb 11 kBq/m^3. Am Hannoverschen Zyklotron konnte ^{41}Ar in geringen Mengen nachgewiesen werden; jedoch führt diese Aktivitätsableitung zu keiner relevanten Strahlenexposition der Umgebung.

2. Abgeleitete Radioaktivität während des Zyklotronbetriebs und der Untersuchung der Patienten

Bei der Produktion von Radiopharmaka können radioaktive Stoffe aus dem Target der Radiochemie und dem Untersuchungsraum freigesetzt werden, die zum Teil gasförmig sind und über das Lüftungssystem nach außen abgegeben werden. Sind diese Freisetzungen durch Filter zu binden, so können die üblicherweise im Lüftungssystem vorhandenen Filteranlagen den größten Teil der radioaktiven Stoffe zurückbehalten. Wegen der Kurzlebigkeit der meisten Positronenstrahler stellt deren Kontamination kein besonderes Problem dar. Häufig werden auch Kombinationsfilter mit Aktivkohle oder anderen Sorptionsmitteln eingesetzt. Die Filter müssen möglichst nahe am Freisetzungsort installiert werden, damit zur Verlängerung der Standzeit der Luftdurchsatz klein gehalten werden kann.

Eine weitere sehr vorteilhafte Möglichkeit bei kurzlebigen radioaktiven Gasen besteht darin, Verzögerungs- oder Puffersysteme in die Abluftleitung einzuschalten. Dadurch wird erreicht, daß ein großer Teil der Aktivität bereits vor der Abgabe in die Umwelt abgeklungen ist. Im Hannoverschen Zyklotron MC 35 ist es auf diese Weise möglich, die Gesamtabgabe einschließlich der abgeatmeten Radioaktivität des Patienten auf maximal 4% der hergestellten Radioaktivität zu beschränken (Junker 1982; Helmeke 1985). Allerdings muß berücksichtigt werden, daß im Störfall (undichte Transportleitungen, Zerstörung eines Umsetzungsgefäßes aus Glas in der Radiochemie, u.a.) bei einer bolusförmigen Freisetzung der Aktivität der durch Verzögerung erreichte Reduktionsfaktor nicht ausreicht und unter Umständen ein hoher Anteil der produzierten Aktivität austreten kann.

Allgemein gilt, daß nicht nur beim Produktionsprozeß, sondern auch bei der Aufarbeitung darauf zu achten ist, daß keine Aktivitäten unkontrolliert freigesetzt werden. Alle Verarbeitungsschritte dürfen deshalb grundsätzlich nur in einer geschlossenen Heißen Zelle mit einer separaten Be- und Entlüftung – wie oben beschrieben – durchgeführt werden. Bei Radionukliden längerer Halbwertszeit oder höherer Radiotoxizität (z.B. ^{123}J) muß besonders auf absolute Dichtheit der Targetsysteme und der Heißen Zelle geachtet werden.

3. Kontamination und Inkorporation

Die klinische Verwendung von Radiopharmaka, die mit kurzlebigen Positronenstrahlern markiert worden sind, erfordert im Gegensatz zu den üblicherweise in der Nuklearmedizin eingesetzten Radionukliden in allen Phasen der Verarbeitung und Anwendung wesentlich höhere Aktivitätsmengen. Treten dabei Kontaminationen auf, so werden erfahrungsgemäß fast immer die Grenzwerte für Flächenkontaminationen nach der Strahlenschutzverordnung, Anlage IX (1976) überschritten. Andererseits sind wegen der Kurzlebigkeit der meisten im Zyklotron erzeugten Positronenstrahler Kontaminationen bis auf wenige Ausnahmen schon nach relativ kurzer Zeit durch Abklingen der Radioaktivität nicht mehr vorhanden. Wenn der Betriebsablauf es zuläßt, ist deshalb in den meisten Fällen Abwarten die beste Dekontaminationsmethode.

Kontaminationen durch längerlebige Radionuklide (z.B. Verunreinigungen beim Produktionsprozeß) sind durch allgemein bekannte konventionelle Dekontaminationsmaßnahmen zu beseitigen. Diese sind von SCHIEFERDECKER (1985) eingehend behandelt worden.

Bei kurzlebigen Radionukliden ist eine direkte Überwachung der Personen auf Inkorporation nur bedingt möglich. Sie erfolgt indirekt durch Überwachung der in die Raumluft freigesetzten Aktivitätsmengen mittels Installation von Raumluftmonitoren.

E. Patientenstrahlenschutz

I. Überlegungen zur Dosierung von kurzlebigen Radiopharmaka

Jede Untersuchung des Patienten mit einem Radioparmakon bedeutet für diesen eine Strahlenexposition, die i. allg. über den eigentlichen Untersuchungszeitraum weit hinausreicht. Bei kurzlebigen Positronenstrahlern wirken dagegen wegen der geringen Halbwertszeiten der Radionuklide diese jedoch nur eine kurze Zeit auf den menschlichen Körper ein. Selbst bei Untersuchungen mit ^{18}F-Verbindungen ($T_p = 110$ min) wird man einige Stunden nach der Untersuchung nur noch Bruchteile der ursprünglichen Radioaktivität im Körper des Patienten feststellen können. Andererseits ist bei diesen Radionukliden, z.B. ^{15}O ($T_p = 2$ min), der Anreichungsfaktor des Radiopharmakons bei bolusförmiger Applikation im interessierenden Organ, wie theoretische Überlegungen zeigen, von vornherein sehr klein. Zur genauen Untersuchung des Organs ist aber eine Mindestaktivität bzw. eine Mindestimpulsrate notwendig. Deshalb wird häufig entweder die zu applizierende Aktivität erhöht oder die Untersuchungsmethode wird geändert, indem auf eine „constant infusion" des Radiopharmakons übergegangen wird. Beide Möglichkeiten bedeuten jedoch eine Erhöhung der Strahlenexposition des Patienten. Andererseits muß deutlich hervorgehoben werden, daß zur Gewinnung klinisch aussagekräftiger Ergebnisse die statistische Absicherung des Untersuchungsergebnisses (Qualität der Aufnahme) gewährleistet sein muß. Die Dosierung kurzlebiger Radiopharmaka stellt deshalb in der Praxis einen Kompromiß dar, der beiden Zielen gerecht werden muß. Die Dosierung kann dabei von Untersuchungsmethode zu Untersuchungsmethode und von Kamera zu Kamera verschieden sein.

Grundvoraussetzung jeder Untersuchung ist jedoch die Qualitätssicherung aller wichtigen Funktionsgrößen der Kamera wie Homogenität, Auflösungsvermögen, Linearität und Empfindlichkeit des bildgebenden Verfahrens. An dieser Stelle sei auf die grundlegenden Arbeiten von STIEVE (1986), KARLSSON et al. (1982), SKRETTING et al (1984), ROEDLER (1986) sowie BÖRNER u. REINER (1982) verwiesen.

II. Bestimmung der Organdosen (Erwachsenenalter) nach dem MIRD-Konzept

1. Vorbemerkung

Die durch die Untersuchung bedingte Strahlenexposition des Patienten kann im Einzelfall nach dem bekannten MIRD-Konzept des absorbierten Bruchteils (Literatur bei JUNKER und FITSCHEN 1980, S. 425) ermittelt werden – s. unten und Tabelle 3 – oder soweit bekannt der Tabelle 4 entnommen werden. Die meisten in der Tabelle 4 angegebenen Dosiswerte basieren jedoch auf der Ermittlung biokinetischer Daten durch Tierversuche. Diese Daten werden auf den Standardmenschen nach ICRP 23 angewandt und die Personendosen nach dem bekannten MIRD-Konzept ermittelt. Diese so abgeschätzten Patientendosen gelten daher nur für einen normal arbeitenden Organismus. Da die für die Dosimetrie maßgebenden biologischen Faktoren selbst für den Normalfall streuen, sind die abgeschätzten Strahlendosen nur als Mittelwerte zu verstehen. Unter pathologischen Bedingungen können sich stark abweichende Verteilungen ergeben, woraus erhebliche Veränderungen der Energiedosen resultieren. Sollen die Dosiswerte im Individualfall genau bestimmt werden, müssen die biologischen Parameter direkt am Patienten ermittelt werden. Wegen der Kurzlebigkeit der hier diskutierten Positronenstrahler ist jedoch eine genauere Bestimmung der einzelnen Verteilungsfaktoren und damit auch der Individualdosen mit großem meßtechnischem Aufwand verbunden.

2. Dosisberechnung nach dem MIRD-Konzept

Die Dosisberechnung erfolgt im allgemeinen nach dem Konzept des absorbierten Bruchteils (MIRD-Konzept). Es wird zwischen dem Source-Organ σ (Speicherorgan der Radioaktivität) und dem Target-Organ τ (Organ, für das die Dosis berechnet werden soll) unterschieden. Die mittlere Dosis im Target-Organ eines Standardmenschen ergibt sich zu:

$$\bar{D}_\tau = \sum_\sigma \tilde{A}_\sigma \cdot S_{\tau \leftarrow \sigma}$$

Dabei ist $\tilde{A}_\sigma = \int_{t_1}^{t_2} A_\sigma(t)dt$ die akkumulierte Aktivität (Aktivitätszeitintegral) im Source-Organ σ. Bei einer monoexponentiellen Ausscheidungsfunktion kann in erster Näherung für $\tilde{A}_\sigma$ abgeschätzt werden (mit $t_1 = 0$, $t_2 = \infty$):

$$\tilde{A}_\sigma = \frac{A_0 \cdot F_\sigma \cdot T_\sigma}{\ln 2} = 1,44 \cdot A_0 \cdot F_\sigma \cdot T_\sigma$$

Hierbei ist:

A_0 = applizierte Aktivität in MBq

F_σ = Verteilungsfaktor des Radionuklids im Organismus für das Source-Organ σ $(0 \leq F_\sigma < 1)$ zurückextrapoliert auf den Applikationszeitpunkt.

T_σ = effektive Halbwertszeit des Radiopharmakons im Source-Organ σ in h

$S_{\tau \leftarrow \sigma}$ = Dosiskonstante in μGy/MBq·h bzw. rd/μCi·h nach Tabelle 3 oder Handbuch der Radiologie, Bd XV/1A, S. 447–463, Tabelle 1

Eine genaue Bestimmung biokinetischer Daten für bolusförmige Applikationen ist mit einem großen meßtechnischen Aufwand verbunden. Einige Autoren haben biokinetische Daten in Tierversuchen ermittelt und diese durch Umrechnung und Berücksichtigung der unterschiedlichen Massen auf den Standardmenschen übertragen. Andere Autoren haben die Verteilungsfaktoren direkt aus Untersuchungen am Menschen gewonnen. Die Ergebnisse der Dosisabschätzungen sind in der Tabelle 4 aufgetragen. Die Wiedergabe der gewonnenen Daten erfolgt ohne Bewertung der einzelnen Meßmethoden zur Ermittlung der biokinetischen Daten.

Tabelle 3. S-Werte für ausgewählte Radionuklide und Organe zur Bestimmung der Dosis nach dem MIRD-Konzept.

Hinweise zum Gebrauch der Tabellen der S-Werte.

1. Radionuklidangabe: Die Massenzahl steht hinter dem chemischen Symbol. Beispiel: C 11 statt ^{11}C.

2. Ziffern in den Tabellen: xy–z bedeutet $xy \cdot 10^{-z}$ und u–vw bedeutet $u \cdot 10^{-vw}$ Beispiele: $12–3 = 12 \cdot 10^{-3}$ $07–9 = 7 \cdot 10^{-9}$
Werte $\leq 9{,}9 \cdot 10^{-9}$ wurden gerundet, Werte $< 1 \cdot 10^{-20}$ sind gleich Null gesetzt.

3. Die S-Werte sind in mGy pro 1 MBq·h des entsprechenden Nuklids angegeben, ausgenommen
Br 77: Summe der S-Werte in mGy pro 1 MBq·h von Br 77 und 0,0219 MBq·h von Se 77m (Aktivitität im rad. Gleichgewicht).
Rb 81: Summe der S-Werte in mGy pro 1 MBq·h von Rb 81 und 0,96 MBq·h von Kr 81m (Aktivität im rad. Gleichgewicht). Soll allein Rb 81 berücksichtigt werden, erhält man den richtigen S-Wert aus der Differenz der S-Werte von Rb 81 und Kr 81m.

4. Umrechnung: $\dfrac{mGy}{MBq \cdot h} = \dfrac{1}{270{,}27} \cdot \dfrac{rd}{\mu Ci \cdot h}$

5. Die Werte sind berechnet für Organe des Standardmenschen mit Massen, die im folgenden angegeben sind. Die S-Werte wurden aus MIRD-Pamphlet No. 10 entnommen. Die S-Werte für HW stammen aus COFFEY u. WATSON (1981) oder wurden selbst errechnet anhand MIRD-Pamphlet No. 10 und No. 13.

6. Abkürzungen und Massen der berücksichtigten Organe.

Abkür-zung	Organ als Target	Masse (g)	Organ als Source	Masse (g)
BL	Blasenwand	45	Inhalt der Blase	200
OD	Wand des oberen Dickdarms (Colon asc. u. transv.)	209	Inhalt des oberen Dickdarms	220
UD	Wand des unteren Dickdarms (Colon desc. u. sigm.)	160	Inhalt des unteren Dickdarms	137
DD	Wand des Dünndarms	644	Inhalt des Dünndarms	400
HI	Gehirn		–	
HW	Herzwand	299	–	
KG	Knochen, gesamtes Skelett	10470	–	
KC	–		Knochen, Cortex	4000
KT	–		Knochen, Trabekel	1000
KM	rotes Knochenmark	1500	rotes Knochenmark	1500
LE	Leber	1809	Leber	1809
LG	Lunge (gesamt, mit Blut)	999	Lunge (gesamt, mit Blut)	999
MG	Magenwand	150	Inhalt des Magens	247
MZ	Milz	174	Milz	174
NI	Nieren (beide)	284	Nieren (beide)	284
OV	Ovarien (beide)	8	–	
PA	Pankreas	60	Pankreas	60
TE	Testes (beide)	37	–	
UT	Uterus, nicht gravid	65	–	
GK	Ganzkörper	69880	Ganzkörper	69880

Tabelle 3 (Fortsetzung)

Source:	BL	OD	UD	DD	KC	KM	LE	LG	MG	MZ	NI	PA	HW	GK
Target: BL – Wand der Blase [mGy/MBq·h]														
C 11	73–2	38–4	11–3	68–4	13–4	14–4	70–5	15–5	92–5	27–5	78–5	41–5	23–5	70–4
N 13	86–2	38–4	11–3	68–4	13–4	14–4	70–5	15–5	92–5	27–5	78–5	41–5	23–5	76–4
O 15	12–1	38–4	11–3	68–4	13–4	14–4	70–5	15–5	92–5	27–5	78–5	41–5	23–5	97–4
F 18	49–2	38–4	11–3	68–4	13–4	14–4	68–5	15–5	89–5	27–5	76–5	38–5	23–5	57–4
Br 77	65–3	13–4	38–4	19–4	38–5	49–5	18–5	46–6	25–5	11–5	24–5	11–5	68–6	13–4
Kr 81m	11–2	57–5	17–4	68–5	13–5	21–5	41–6	13–6	59–6	43–6	81–6	41–6	10–6	97–5
Rb 81	38–2	24–4	70–4	38–4	73–5	89–5	35–5	84–6	49–5	19–5	46–5	22–5	12–5	38–4
Rb 82	20–1	41–4	12–3	70–4	14–4	15–4	73–5	16–5	10–4	32–5	84–5	41–5	26–5	15–3
Tl 201	78–3	41–5	15–4	49–5	89–6	19–5	21–6	46–7	41–6	16–6	35–6	18–6	58–7	76–4
Target: OD – Wand des oberen Dickdarms [mGy/MBq·h]														
C 11	49–4	59–2	84–4	46–3	14–4	41–4	51–4	78–5	68–4	27–4	57–4	43–4	10–4	73–4
N 13	49–4	73–2	86–4	46–3	14–4	41–4	51–4	78–5	68–4	27–4	59–4	43–4	10–4	81–4
O 15	49–4	10–1	86–4	46–3	14–4	41–4	51–4	78–5	68–4	27–4	59–4	43–4	10–4	10–3
F 18	46–4	41–2	84–4	46–3	14–4	41–4	51–4	76–5	65–4	27–4	57–4	43–4	10–4	59–4
Br 77	15–4	41–3	27–4	16–3	46–5	13–4	16–4	22–5	21–4	86–5	18–4	14–4	29–5	14–4
Kr 81m	62–5	92–3	11–4	65–4	19–5	57–5	65–5	62–6	92–5	32–5	76–5	59–5	90–6	10–4
Rb 81	30–4	32–2	51–4	30–3	86–5	25–4	30–4	43–5	41–4	17–4	35–4	26–4	57–5	41–4
Rb 82	51–4	18–1	89–4	49–3	15–4	43–4	54–4	84–5	70–4	30–4	62–4	46–4	11–4	15–3
Tl 201	41–5	65–3	95–5	68–4	13–5	41–5	51–5	35–6	78–5	30–5	57–5	41–5	62–8	78–5
Target: UD – Wand des unteren Dickdarms [mGy/MBq·h]														
C 11	14–3	59–4	95–2	14–3	19–4	62–4	65–5	16–5	26–4	14–4	18–4	11–4	25–5	73–4
N 13	14–3	59–4	11–1	14–3	19–4	62–4	65–5	16–5	26–4	14–4	18–4	11–4	25–5	81–4
O 15	14–3	59–4	16–1	14–3	19–4	62–4	65–5	16–5	26–4	14–4	18–4	11–4	25–5	10–3
F 18	14–3	59–4	62–2	13–3	19–4	59–4	65–5	15–5	25–4	14–4	17–4	11–4	24–5	59–4
Br 77	46–4	19–4	57–3	46–4	65–5	19–4	19–5	57–6	81–5	43–5	57–5	35–5	81–6	13–4
Kr 81m	19–4	78–5	15–2	19–4	27–5	76–5	62–6	27–6	35–5	17–5	22–5	15–5	23–6	97–5
Rb 81	86–4	38–4	49–2	84–4	12–4	38–4	38–5	11–5	16–4	84–5	11–4	68–5	14–5	41–4
Rb 82	15–3	65–4	30–1	14–3	20–4	65–4	70–5	17–5	27–4	15–4	19–4	12–4	28–5	15–3
Tl 201	17–4	68–5	10–2	18–4	20–5	59–5	32–6	81–7	23–5	11–5	11–5	97–6	12–6	78–5
Target: DD – Wand des Dünndarms [mGy/MBq·h]														
C 11	51–4	32–3	18–3	35–2	16–4	54–4	32–4	57–5	54–4	27–4	54–4	35–4	80–5	73–4
N 13	54–4	32–3	18–3	41–2	16–4	54–4	32–4	57–5	54–4	27–4	57–4	35–4	80–5	81–4
O 15	54–4	32–3	18–3	59–2	16–4	54–4	32–4	57–5	54–4	27–4	54–4	35–4	80–5	10–3
F 18	51–4	32–3	18–3	24–2	16–4	54–4	30–4	54–5	51–4	27–4	54–4	35–4	78–5	59–4
Br 77	17–4	11–3	57–4	30–3	51–5	17–4	10–4	17–5	17–4	89–5	18–4	11–4	24–5	14–4
Kr 81m	76–5	43–4	25–4	54–3	20–5	68–5	43–5	51–6	68–5	38–5	76–5	49–5	83–6	11–4
Rb 81	32–4	20–3	11–3	18–2	97–5	32–4	20–4	32–5	32–4	17–4	35–4	22–4	46–5	41–4
Rb 82	57–4	35–3	19–3	10–1	17–4	57–4	35–4	59–5	57–4	30–4	59–4	38–4	85–5	15–3
Tl 201	59–5	41–4	22–4	38–3	14–5	51–5	30–5	27–6	54–5	26–5	57–5	32–5	45–6	78–5
Target: KG – Knochen, gesamtes Skelett [mGy/MBq·h]														
C 11	12–4	15–4	21–4	16–4	51–3	16–3	15–4	20–4	12–4	15–4	20–4	19–4	17–4	62–4
N 13	12–4	15–4	21–4	16–4	62–3	20–3	15–4	20–4	12–4	16–4	20–4	19–4	17–4	70–4
O 15	12–4	15–4	21–4	16–4	89–3	30–3	15–4	20–4	12–4	16–4	20–4	19–4	17–4	89–4
F 18	12–4	14–4	21–4	15–4	35–3	11–3	14–4	20–4	12–4	15–4	19–4	18–4	17–4	49–4
Br 77	41–5	49–5	70–5	54–5	38–4	18–4	49–5	68–5	41–5	51–5	65–5	62–5	58–5	11–4
Kr 81m	21–5	25–5	35–5	27–5	81–4	22–4	24–5	32–5	20–5	25–5	32–5	30–5	29–5	97–5
Rb 81	78–5	95–5	14–4	10–4	27–3	86–4	95–5	13–4	78–5	10–4	13–4	12–4	11–4	35–4
Rb 82	12–4	15–4	22–4	17–4	16–2	49–3	16–4	21–4	13–4	16–4	21–4	20–4	18–4	14–3
Tl 201	20–5	30–5	46–5	32–5	62–4	14–4	30–5	43–5	22–5	30–5	38–5	38–5	36–5	92–5

Tabelle 3 (Fortsetzung)

Source:	BL	OD	UD	DD	KC	KM	LE	LG	MG	MZ	NI	PA	HW	GK
Target: KM – Rotes Knochenmark [mGy/MBq·h]														
C 11	25–4	43–4	62–4	51–4	78–4	12–2	22–4	25–4	21–4	23–4	51–4	35–4	24–4	65–4
N 13	25–4	43–4	62–4	51–4	86–4	15–2	22–4	26–4	21–4	23–4	51–4	35–4	24–4	73–4
O 15	25–4	43–4	62–4	51–4	12–3	19–2	22–4	26–4	21–4	23–4	51–4	35–4	24–4	92–4
F 18	25–4	43–4	62–4	49–4	68–4	84–3	21–4	25–4	21–4	22–4	49–4	35–4	24–4	51–4
Br 77	89–5	15–4	21–4	17–4	23–4	89–4	73–5	84–5	70–5	78–5	17–4	12–4	81–5	12–4
Kr 81m	46–5	78–5	11–4	89–5	11–4	21–3	35–5	41–5	35–5	38–5	81–5	59–5	40–5	10–4
Rb 81	17–4	30–4	41–4	32–4	49–4	68–3	14–4	16–4	14–4	15–4	32–4	23–4	15–4	38–4
Rb 82	27–4	46–4	68–4	54–4	19–3	35–2	23–4	27–4	22–4	24–4	54–4	38–4	26–4	14–3
Tl 201	51–5	97–5	16–4	11–4	15–4	18–3	38–5	51–5	35–5	41–5	10–4	70–5	48–5	11–4
Target: LE – Leber [mGy/MBq·h]														
C 11	57–5	49–4	70–5	35–4	14–4	21–4	18–2	49–4	41–4	22–4	81–4	84–4	57–4	68–4
N 13	57–5	49–4	70–5	35–4	14–4	21–4	21–2	49–4	41–4	22–4	81–4	84–4	57–4	76–4
O 15	57–5	49–4	70–5	35–4	14–4	21–4	27–2	49–4	41–4	22–4	81–4	84–4	57–4	95–4
F 18	57–5	49–4	68–5	35–4	14–4	20–4	13–2	46–4	41–4	21–4	78–4	81–4	56–4	54–4
Br 77	17–5	16–4	21–5	12–4	46–5	65–5	21–3	15–4	13–4	68–5	25–4	26–4	18–4	12–4
Kr 81m	54–6	68–5	73–6	49–5	18–5	26–5	27–3	65–5	51–5	27–5	10–4	12–4	77–5	95–5
Rb 81	32–5	30–4	41–5	22–4	86–5	12–4	97–3	30–4	25–4	13–4	49–4	51–4	34–4	38–4
Rb 82	62–5	51–4	76–5	38–4	15–4	22–4	46–2	51–4	43–4	23–4	84–4	86–4	61–4	14–3
Tl 201	23–6	51–5	35–6	35–5	12–5	16–5	20–3	54–5	41–5	17–5	84–5	95–5	68–5	73–5
Target: LG – Lunge [mGy/MBq·h]														
C 11	10–5	70–5	21–5	68–5	20–4	24–4	49–4	26–2	38–4	43–4	19–4	49–4	11–3	65–4
N 13	10–5	70–5	21–5	68–5	20–4	24–4	49–4	30–2	38–4	43–4	19–4	49–4	11–3	70–4
O 15	10–5	70–5	21–5	68–5	20–4	24–4	49–4	43–2	38–4	43–4	19–4	49–4	11–3	92–4
F 18	97–6	68–5	20–5	65–5	19–4	24–4	46–4	17–2	38–4	43–4	19–4	46–4	11–3	51–4
Br 77	30–6	21–5	68–6	20–5	62–5	78–5	15–4	18–3	12–4	14–4	59–5	15–4	35–4	11–4
Kr 81m	68–7	73–6	23–6	65–6	26–5	32–5	65–5	41–3	43–5	59–5	22–5	65–5	15–4	89–5
Rb 81	54–6	41–5	12–5	38–5	12–4	15–4	30–4	14–2	22–4	27–4	11–4	30–4	67–4	35–4
Rb 82	11–5	73–5	23–5	73–5	21–4	26–4	51–4	78–2	41–4	46–4	21–4	51–4	12–3	14–3
Tl 201	27–7	41–6	11–6	32–6	19–5	23–5	57–5	30–3	38–5	51–5	16–5	54–5	15–4	70–5
Target: MG – Wand des Magens [mGy/MBq·h]														
C 11	65–5	73–4	35–4	68–4	12–4	20–4	38–4	38–4	57–2	20–3	68–4	35–3	64–4	68–4
N 13	65–5	73–4	38–4	68–4	12–4	20–4	38–4	38–4	68–2	20–3	68–4	35–3	64–4	76–4
O 15	65–5	73–4	38–4	68–4	12–4	20–4	38–4	38–4	95–2	20–3	68–4	35–3	64–4	95–4
F 18	65–5	70–4	35–4	68–4	12–4	19–4	38–4	35–4	38–2	19–3	65–4	32–3	62–4	54–4
Br 77	22–5	23–4	11–4	22–4	38–5	68–5	12–4	12–4	46–3	62–4	21–4	11–3	21–4	13–4
Kr 81m	76–6	97–5	46–5	97–5	15–5	30–5	51–5	49–5	84–3	25–4	89–5	49–4	90–5	10–4
Rb 81	41–5	43–4	22–4	43–4	70–5	12–4	23–4	22–4	30–2	12–3	41–4	21–3	39–4	38–4
Rb 82	73–5	76–4	38–4	73–4	12–4	22–4	41–4	41–4	16–1	21–3	70–4	35–3	67–4	15–3
Tl 201	38–6	84–5	35–5	78–5	95–6	17–5	38–5	41–5	59–3	24–4	73–5	43–4	77–5	73–5
Target: MZ – Milz [mGy/MBq·h]														
C 11	46–5	25–4	19–4	32–4	17–4	16–4	20–4	43–4	19–3	15–1	17–3	38–3	46–4	68–4
N 13	46–5	25–4	19–4	32–4	17–4	16–4	20–4	43–4	19–3	18–1	17–3	38–3	46–4	76–4
O 15	46–5	25–4	19–4	32–4	17–4	16–4	20–4	43–4	19–3	26–1	17–3	38–3	46–4	95–4
F 18	46–5	24–4	19–4	30–4	16–4	16–4	20–4	41–4	19–3	10–1	16–3	38–3	45–4	54–4
Br 77	14–5	84–5	59–5	10–4	51–5	57–5	65–5	14–4	62–4	13–2	54–4	12–3	14–4	13–4
Kr 81m	59–6	38–5	21–5	41–5	17–5	24–5	25–5	59–5	26–4	24–2	23–4	49–4	57–5	97–5
Rb 81	27–5	16–4	11–4	19–4	97–5	10–4	12–4	26–4	12–3	81–2	10–3	23–3	27–4	38–4
Rb 82	49–5	26–4	20–4	32–4	18–4	18–4	22–4	46–4	20–3	43–1	18–3	41–3	48–4	15–3
Tl 201	92–6	30–5	15–5	27–5	12–5	17–5	16–5	49–5	24–4	17–2	21–4	49–4	45–5	73–5

Tabelle 3 (Fortsetzung)

Source:	BL	OD	UD	DD	KC	KM	LE	LG	MG	MZ	NI	PA	HW	GK
Target: NI – Nieren [mGy/MBq·h]														
C 11	78–5	54–4	17–4	65–4	18–4	49–4	76–4	21–4	68–4	17–3	89–2	12–3	24–4	68–4
N 13	78–5	54–4	17–4	65–4	18–4	49–4	76–4	21–4	68–4	17–3	11–2	12–3	24–4	76–4
O 15	78–5	54–4	17–4	65–4	18–4	49–4	76–4	21–4	68–4	17–3	15–1	12–3	24–4	95–4
F 18	76–5	54–4	16–4	62–4	18–4	46–4	73–4	21–4	65–4	17–3	59–2	12–3	23–4	54–4
Br 77	23–5	18–4	57–5	20–4	59–5	15–4	24–4	65–5	21–4	54–4	76–3	41–4	75–5	12–4
Kr 81m	73–6	73–5	25–5	81–5	24–5	59–5	10–4	23–5	92–5	23–4	14–2	17–4	30–5	97–5
Rb 81	43–5	32–4	11–4	38–4	11–4	30–4	46–4	12–4	41–4	11–3	46–2	76–4	14–4	38–4
Rb 82	84–5	59–4	18–4	68–4	20–4	51–4	81–4	22–4	70–4	18–3	26–1	13–3	25–4	15–3
Tl 201	38–6	57–5	14–5	62–5	16–5	43–5	84–5	15–5	73–5	21–4	10–2	14–4	19–5	73–5
Target: OV – Ovarien [mGy/MBq·h]														
C11	13–3	25–3	32–3	18–3	22–4	73–4	41–5	30–5	11–4	21–4	24–4	78–5	46–5	68–4
N 13	13–3	26–3	32–3	18–3	22–4	73–4	41–5	32–5	11–4	22–4	24–4	78–5	46–5	73–4
O 15	13–3	26–3	32–3	18–3	22–4	73–4	41–5	32–5	11–4	22–4	24–4	78–5	46–5	95–4
F 18	12–3	25–3	30–3	17–3	21–4	70–4	41–5	30–5	10–4	21–4	23–4	76–5	45–5	54–4
Br 77	41–4	76–4	11–3	59–4	62–5	20–4	22–5	95–6	38–5	57–5	78–5	27–5	14–5	12–4
Kr 81m	20–4	30–4	51–4	27–4	18–5	62–5	13–5	32–6	12–5	14–5	32–5	86–6	49–6	10–4
Rb 81	78–4	15–3	21–3	11–3	12–4	41–4	35–5	18–5	65–5	11–4	15–4	49–5	26–5	38–4
Rb 82	13–3	26–3	35–3	19–3	23–4	76–4	51–5	32–5	12–4	22–4	25–4	92–5	49–5	14–3
Tl 201	15–4	25–4	41–4	26–4	14–5	73–5	78–6	14–6	11–5	62–6	19–5	73–6	19–6	76–5
Target: PA – Pankreas [mGy/MBq·h]														
C 11	51–5	35–4	15–4	43–4	18–4	35–4	97–4	57–4	35–3	41–3	13–3	27–1	91–4	68–4
N 13	51–5	35–4	15–4	43–4	18–4	35–4	97–4	57–4	35–3	41–3	13–3	32–1	91–4	76–4
O 15	51–5	35–4	15–4	43–4	18–4	35–4	97–4	57–4	35–3	41–3	13–3	46–1	91–4	95–4
F 18	51–5	35–4	15–4	41–4	18–4	32–4	95–4	54–4	35–3	38–3	13–3	18–1	89–4	54–4
Br 77	18–5	13–4	46–5	13–4	62–5	11–4	30–4	17–4	11–3	12–3	41–4	24–2	29–4	13–4
Kr 81m	78–6	65–5	19–5	54–5	27–5	43–5	10–4	68–5	46–4	49–4	17–4	43–2	13–4	11–4
Rb 81	32–5	24–4	89–5	25–4	12–4	21–4	57–4	32–4	21–3	24–3	78–4	15–1	55–4	41–4
Rb 82	57–5	38–4	16–4	43–4	19–4	35–4	10–3	59–4	38–3	41–3	14–3	78–1	96–4	14–3
Tl 201	30–6	43–5	12–5	38–5	15–5	32–5	95–5	54–5	43–4	46–4	14–4	32–2	10–4	81–5
Target: TE – Testes [mGy/MBq·h]														
C 11	10–3	11–4	41–4	73–5	12–4	86–5	24–5	49–6	54–6	19–5	30–5	13–5	77–6	70–4
N 13	10–3	11–4	41–4	73–5	12–4	86–5	24–5	51–6	54–6	19–5	30–5	13–5	77–6	78–4
O 15	10–3	11–4	41–4	73–5	12–4	86–5	24–5	51–6	54–6	19–5	30–5	13–5	77–6	97–4
F 18	10–3	10–4	41–4	70–5	11–4	86–5	23–5	49–6	51–6	19–5	30–5	12–5	75–6	57–4
Br 77	32–4	30–5	13–4	24–5	38–5	26–5	78–6	15–6	32–6	57–6	92–6	46–6	22–6	12–4
Kr 81m	12–4	84–6	51–5	92–6	16–5	86–6	22–6	32–7	17–6	17–6	30–6	19–6	53–7	81–5
Rb 81	59–4	57–5	25–4	46–5	73–5	49–5	14–5	27–6	49–6	11–5	18–5	84–6	41–6	38–4
Rb 82	11–3	11–4	43–4	81–5	12–4	92–5	27–5	54–6	76–6	21–5	32–5	15–5	84–6	15–3
Tl 201	11–4	38–6	35–5	43–6	11–5	73–6	68–7	81–8	62–7	51–7	97–7	59–7	14–7	62–5
Target: UT – Uterus, nicht gravid [mGy/MBq·h]														
C 11	30–3	89–4	11–3	18–3	12–4	38–4	89–5	19–5	18–4	95–5	17–4	13–4	27–5	68–4
N 13	30–3	89–4	11–3	18–3	12–4	38–4	89–5	19–5	18–4	95–5	17–4	13–4	27–5	76–4
O 15	30–3	89–4	11–3	18–3	12–4	38–4	89–5	19–5	18–4	95–5	17–4	13–4	27–5	95–4
F 18	30–3	86–4	11–3	17–3	11–4	38–4	86–5	19–5	18–4	92–5	16–4	12–4	26–5	54–4
Br 77	95–4	30–4	38–4	57–4	41–5	13–4	27–5	65–6	57–5	30–5	57–5	41–5	97–6	14–4
Kr 81m	41–4	13–4	19–4	25–4	16–5	59–5	10–5	25–6	22–5	11–5	27–5	16–5	29–6	11–4
Rb 81	18–3	57–4	73–4	11–3	73–5	24–4	51–5	12–5	11–4	57–5	11–4	76–5	16–5	41–4
Rb 82	32–3	95–4	12–3	18–3	13–4	41–4	95–5	21–5	19–4	10–4	18–4	14–4	31–5	15–3
Tl 201	49–5	62–5	68–5	76–5	95–6	41–5	76–5	73–5	54–5	59–6	73–5	76–6	93–7	81–5

Tabelle 3 (Fortsetzung)

Source:	BL	OD	UD	DD	KC	KM	LE	LG	MG	MZ	NI	PA	HW	GK
Target: GK – Ganzkörper [mGy/MBq·h]														
C 11	41–4	54–4	57–4	65–4	62–4	65–4	68–4	62–4	46–4	68–4	68–4	73–4	66–4	62–4
N 13	43–4	57–4	62–4	73–4	70–4	73–4	76–4	70–4	49–4	76–4	76–4	81–4	75–4	70–4
O 15	43–4	68–4	73–4	86–4	89–4	92–4	95–4	89–4	54–4	95–4	95–4	10–3	95–4	89–4
F 18	38–4	46–4	49–4	54–4	49–4	51–4	54–4	49–4	41–4	54–4	54–4	59–4	53–4	49–4
Br 77	12–4	13–4	13–4	14–4	11–4	11–4	12–4	11–4	12–4	12–4	12–4	14–4	12–4	11–4
Kr 81m	57–5	76–5	81–5	95–5	89–5	95–5	97–5	89–5	62–5	97–5	97–5	11–4	96–5	89–5
Rb 81	25–4	32–4	32–4	38–4	35–4	35–4	38–4	35–4	27–4	38–4	38–4	41–4	37–4	35–4
Rb 82	51–4	92–4	10–3	13–3	14–3	14–3	14–3	14–3	70–4	14–3	14–3	15–3	14–3	14–3
Tl 201	49–5	62–5	68–5	76–5	73–5	76–5	76–5	73–5	54–5	76–5	73–5	84–5	75–5	70–5

Source: HW	Target: HW – Wand des Herzens [mGy/MBq·h]
C 11	86–2
N 13	11–1
O 15	15–1
F 18	58–2
Br 77	64–3
Kr 81m	14–2
Rb 81	46–2
Rb 82	26–1
Tl 201	93–3

Tabelle 4. Strahlenexposition durch zyklotronproduzierte Radiodiagnostika (ausgewählte Beispiele). Abkürzungen s. Erläuterungen zu Tabelle 3.

Untersuchungs-methode	Radionuklid-verbindung	Applikations-art	Strahlenexposition [μGy/MBq]							
Regionaler pH-Wert im Hirngewebe	[^{11}C]-Di-methyloxazo-lidinedione (DMO)	i.v.	BL	3,8	KG	2,4	NI	4,6	UT	6,2
			DD	6,2	LE	5,1	OD	5,1		
			GK	3,0	LG	5,1	OV	5,1		
			HI	3,0	MG	2,7	TE	2,7		
			HW	5,7	MZ	4,3	UD	5,1		
Pankreas-Darstellung	[^{11}C]-L-Tryptophan	i.v.	DD	11	MZ	5,4				
			GK	3,0	NI	6,2				
			KM	4,6	OV	5,1				
			LE	9,5	PA	68				
			LG	4,6	TE	2,7				
Pankreas-Darstellung	[^{11}C]-L-Valin	i.v.	DD	2,4	MZ	6,0				
			GK	3,0	NI	5,1				
			KM	5,7	OV	3,0				
			LE	7,6	PA	51				
			LG	3,8	TE	1,9				
Lungenfunktion, Hirndurchblutung	^{11}CO	inhal. "single breath" und i.v. als Bolus	BL	3,8	KG	2,4	MZ	24,6	UD	17
			DD	23,2	KM	2,7	NI	7,6	UT	4,3
			GK	5,1	LE	5,7	OD	16,8		
			HI	1,2	LG	14,9	OV	7,3		
			HW	8,9	MG	4,1	TE	2,3		

Tabelle 4 (Fortsetzung)

Untersuchungs-methode	Radionuklid-verbindung	Applikations-art	Strahlenexposition [µGy/MBq]
Ammonium-metabolismus im Hirn	$^{13}NH_3$	i.v.	BL 13,8 NI 1,5 GK 1,5 OV 2,7 HI 4,3 TE 2,7 KM 1,5 LE 4,6
Hirndurchblutung, Lungenfunktion *(s. Fußn. b)*	$CO^{15}O$	inhal. kontinuierlich (1 h)	BL 0,32 KG 0,21 MZ 0,57/0,53 UD 0,54 DD 0,57 KM 0,32 NI 0,57/0,53 UT 0,51 GK 0,43/0,30 LE 0,54/0,49 OD 0,54 Trachea- HI 0,16/0,60 LG 1,7/0,86 OV 0,57/0,44 Mucosa HW 0,59/0,59 MG 0,51 TE 0,57/0,49 6,2
Hirndurchblutung, Lungenfunktion	$CO^{15}O$	inhal. "single breath"	BL 0,32 KG 0,21 MZ 0,57 UD 0,57 DD 0,59 KM 0,32 NI 0,57 UT 0,51 GK 0,43 LE 0,54 OD 0,57 HI 0,16 LG 1,3 OV 0,57 HW 0,59 MG 0,51 TE 0,57
Hirndurchblutung, Lungenfunktion	$CO^{15}O$	i.v. kontinuierlich (1 h) und i.v. als Bolus	BL 0,35 KG 0,21 MZ 0,57 UD 0,59 DD 0,59 KM 0,32 NI 0,57 UT 0,51 GK 0,43 LE 0,54 OD 0,59 HI 0,16 LG 0,54 OV 0,57 HW 0,57 MG 0,57 TE 0,59
Hirndurchblutung, Lungenfunktion *(s. Fußn. b)*	$C^{15}O$	inhal. kontinuierlich	BL 0,41 KG 0,30 MZ 4,1/1,2 UD 2,7 DD 3,8 KM 0,41 NI 1,2/0,59 UT 0,57 GK 0,43/0,24 LE 0,81/0,41 OD 2,5 HI 0,16/0,06 LG 3,5/2,1 OV 1,1/0,68 HW 1,2/0,66 MG 0,49 TE 0,27/0,13
Hirndurchblutung, Lungenfunktion	$C^{15}O$	inhal. "single breath"	BL 0,43 KG 0,30 MZ 4,1 UD 2,7 DD 3,8 KM 0,41 NI 1,2 UT 0,57 GK 0,43 LE 0,81 OD 2,5 HI 0,16 LG 3,0 OV 1,1 HW 1,2 MG 0,49 TE 0,27
Hirndurchblutung, Lungenfunktion	$C^{15}O$	i.v. kontinuierlich und i.v. als Bolus	BL 0,49 KG 0,30 MZ 4,1 UD 2,7 DD 3,8 KM 0,41 NI 1,2 UT 0,57 GK 0,43 LE 0,81 OD 2,5 HI 0,16 LG 2,3 OV 1,1 HW 1,2 MG 0,54 TE 0,30
Lungenfunktion *(s. Fußn. b)*	$O^{15}O$	inhal. kontinuierlich	GK 0,23 LG 2,7 TE 0,22 HI 0,32 MZ 0,71 HW 0,50 NI 0,44 LE 0,35 OV 0,44
Glukosemetabolismus im Hirn *(s. Fußn. a, c)*	2-[^{18}F]-Fluoro-2-Deoxy-D-Glukose (2-FDG)	i.v. als Bolus	BL 60/68 LE 16/18 TE 14,6 GK 10,5/11,6 LG 16/18 HI 18/22 MZ 39/50 HW 40/43 NI 19/21 KM 11,4 OV 15/17

Tabelle 4 (Fortsetzung)

Untersuchungs-methode	Radionuklid-verbindung	Applikations-art	Strahlenexposition [µGy/MBq]			
Glukosemetabolis-mus im Hirn	3-[^{18}F]-Fluoro-3-Deoxy-D-Glukose (3-FDG)	i.v.	GK 19,2 HI 4,3 HW 17 KG 14,3 LE 36,5	LG 25,4 MG 24,9 MZ 19,7 NI 45,4 OV 14,1	PA 26,8 SD 49,2 UT 14,1	
Dopamin-Metabo-lismus im Hirn	6-[^{18}F]-Fluoro-L-Dopa	i.v.	BL 695 DD 11,4 GK 8,9 KG 7,0 KM 8,4	LE 8,7 LG 6,2 MG 7,3 MZ 8,4 NI 7,3	OD 11,1 OV 16,8 TE 15,1 UD 18,7 UT 30,5	
Herz-Durch-blutung (Myokard)	^{38}K-Chlorid	i.v.	BL 1,7 DD 5,4 GK 3,2 HI 0,4	HW 11,4 KG 1,4 KM 1,7 LE 4,3	LG 5,1 MG 3,8 MZ 3,5 NI 15,1	OD 4,3 TE 1,1 UD 4,3
Darstellung von Tumoren	^{64}Cu-Citrat	i.v.	GK 26,5 KG 23 KM 49 LE 119 LG 32	MZ 38 NI 378 OV 30 TE 32		
Darstellung von Mamma-Tumoren *(s. Fußn. c)*	16 α-[^{77}Br]-Bromo-estradiol	i.v.	BL 20 DD 67,6 GK 8,1 LE 18,9 LG 2,7	MZ 8,1 NI 13,5 OD 91,9 OV 5,4 UD 116	UT 46	
Herz-Durch-blutung (Myokard)	^{81}Rb-Chlorid	i.v.	BL 32,4 DD 29,7 GK 23,2 HI 1,0 HW 14,6	KG 29,7 KM 32,4 LE 29,7 LG 22,2 MG 29,7	MZ 32,4 NI 32,4 OD 29,7 TE 16,0 UD 27,0	
Herz-Durch-blutung (Myokard) *(s. Fußn. a)*	^{82}Rb-Chlorid	i.v.	BL 0,46 DD 1,3 GK 0,43/0,35 HI 0,07 HW 3,5/2,0	KG 0,43 KM 0,46/0,35 LE 0,73/0,81 LG 1,9/1,6 MG 0,57	MZ 0,49 NI 5,1/8,4 OD 0,68 OV –/0,32 TE 0,16/0,54	UD 0,70
Herz-Durch-blutung (Myokard)	^{130}Cs-Chlorid	i.v.	BL 1,0 DD 19,5 GK 3,2 HI 1,0 HW 18,4	KG 3,8 KM 5,4 LE 8,4 LG 8,7 MG 4,9	MZ 5,1 NI 40,5 OD 8,1 TE 1,4 UD 10,0	

[a] Schrägstrich: Werte verschiedener Autoren

[b] Angabe der Werte verschiedener Autoren. Die 2. Werte, die ursprünglich in rad/h erfolgten, sind dabei mit Hilfe weiterer Daten aus der Originalarbeit umgerechnet worden.

[c] Strahlenexposition der Blase nach 1 h Entleerung

Beziehungen zwischen SI Einheiten und älteren Maßeinheiten

$1\,\mu\mathrm{Ci} = 37\,\mathrm{kBq} = 0{,}037\,\mathrm{MBq}$	$1\,\mathrm{mrd} = 10\,\mu\mathrm{Gy}$	$1\,\mathrm{mrd}/\mu\mathrm{Ci} = 270\,\mu\mathrm{Gy}/\mathrm{MBq}$
$1\,\mathrm{mCi} = 37\,\mathrm{MBq}$	$1\,\mathrm{rd} = 1\,\mathrm{cGy}$	$1\,\mathrm{mrd}/\mathrm{mCi} = 0{,}270\,\mu\mathrm{Gy}/\mathrm{MBq}$
$1\,\mathrm{Ci} = 37\,\mathrm{GBq}$	$1\,\mathrm{mrem} = 10\,\mu\mathrm{Sv}$	$1\,\mathrm{rd}\cdot\mathrm{m}^2/\mathrm{Ci}\cdot\mathrm{h} = 0{,}270\,\mu\mathrm{Gy}\cdot\mathrm{m}^2/\mathrm{MBq}\cdot\mathrm{h}$
	$1\,\mathrm{rem} = 1\,\mathrm{cSv}$	

Literatur

Allgemeine Berechnungsgrundlage für die Strahlenexposition bei radioaktiven Ableitungen mit der Abluft oder in Oberflächengewässer (Richtlinie zu § 45 StrlSchV) (1979) GMBL No. 21

Amols HI, Dicello JF, Awschalom M, Coulson L, Johnsen SW, Theus RB (1977) Physical characterisation of neutron beams produced by protons and deuterons of various energies bombarding beryllium and lithium targets of several thicknesses. Med Phys 4:6

Bonnett DE, Bell K (1982) Radiation protection, Edinburgh cyclotron, in medical research council cyclotron unit, annual research and development report. Western General Hospital Edinburgh, p 98

Börner W, Reiner Chr (1982) Gesichtspunkte zum Ablauf nuklearmedizinischer Untersuchungen im Hinblick auf die Strahlenexposition. In: Börner W, Messerschmidt O, Seyss R, Holeczke F (Hrsg) Strahlenschutz in Forschung und Praxis, Bd XXIV. Thieme, Stuttgart New York, S 40–49

Bruninx E, Crombeen J (1969) Thick target neutron yields and neutron spectra produced by 20 MeV Helium-3 ions, 14 MeV Protons and 7.5 MeV Deuterons on a Beryllium Target. Int Journal Radiation Isotopes 20:255–264

Burrill EA (1970) Shielding of nucleon accelerators, direct nucleon accelerators. In: Jaeger RG (ed) Shield design and engineering. Springer, Berlin Heidelberg New York (Engineering compendium on radiation shielding, Vol III

Butler HM et al (1973) Half-value thicknesses of ordinary concrete for neutrons from cyclotron targets. Health Phys 24/4:438–439

Cohen BL, Falk CE (1951) (d,n) Reactions with 15-Mev Deuterons. II. Neutron energy spectra and yields. Physical Review 84/2:October 15

Deutsches Institut für Normung eV (1977) Dekontamination von radioaktiv kontaminierten Oberflächen-Bestimmung der Oberflächenkontamination, DIN 25415, Teil 2

Deutsches Institut für Normung eV (1978) Nuklearmedizinische Betriebe, Regeln für die Errichtung und Ausstattung, DIN 6844

Deutsches Institut für Normung eV (1980) Strahlenschutzregeln für die technische Anwendung von Röntgenanlagen bis 500 kV-Formeln und Diagramme für die Strahlenschutzberechnung, DIN 54113, Teil 3

Deutsches Institut für Normung eV (1981) Strahlenschutzregeln für den Umgang mit offenen radioaktiven Stoffen in der Medizin, DIN 6843

Deutsches Institut für Normung eV (1985) Medizinische Röntgenanlagen bis 300 kV-Strahlenschutzregeln für die Errichtung, DIN 6812

Deutsches Institut für Normung eV (1986) Dekontamination von radioaktiv kontaminierten Oberflächen-Verfahren zur Prüfung und Bewertung der Dekontaminierbarkeit, DIN 25415, Teil 1, Entwurf

Friedrich W, Knieper J, Printz H, Sauermann PF (1974) Untersuchungen über die Ableitung radioaktiver Gase in der Umgebung von niederenergetischen Teilchenbeschleunigern, Jahrestagung 1974 des Fachverbandes für Strahlenschutz 23.–29. Sept 1974 in Helgoland

Gelbard AS, Hard T, Tilbury RS, Laughlin JS (1973) Recent aspects of cyclotrons production of medically useful radionuclides, in radiopharmaceuticals and labelled Compounds, (Vol I.) IAEA, Vienna

Goodhead DT, Berry RJ, Bance DA, Gray P, Stedeford JBH (1977) High energy fast neutrons from the Harwell variable energy cyclotron. I. Physical characteristics. Am Roentgenol 129:709–716

Handbook on Nuclear Activation Cross-Sections (1974) IAEA Technical Report Series, No 156. International Atomic Agency, Vienna

Harrison GH (1975) Preliminary study of the neutron beam from 70 MeV deuterons on thick beryllium at the University of Maryland cyclotron. Eur J Cancer 10/4:261–262

Hartmann G, Konovalczyk W, Wolber G (1976) Compact-Cyclotron, Statusbericht 1975/1976. Deutsches Krebsforschungszentrum, Institut für Nuklearmedizin, Heidelberg

Helmeke H-J (1982) Abt für Nuklearmed der Med Hochschule, Hannover. Private Mitteilung

Helmeke H-J (1985) Abt für Nuklearmed der Medizinischen Hochschule Hannover. Private Mitteilung

Helmeke H-J, Junker D (1985) Messungen der Neutronenausbeuten am Beryllium-Target 1978. In: Sicherheitsbericht Kompaktzyklotron. Abt für Nuklearmedizin der Medizinischen Hochschule Hannover

Hemmerich J, Hölzle R, Kogler W (1977) Das Jülicher Kompaktzyklotron – eine vielseitig einsetzbare Bestrahlungsanlage. Kerntechnik. 19. Jahrgang, No 2

Höver KH, Engenhart R, Lorenz WJ, Maier-Borst W (1978) Comparison of dose data for the two neutron therapy facilities at the german cancer research center in Heidelberg. Proceedings Third Symposium on Neutron Dosimetry in Biology and Medicine, Neuherberg, 23–27 May, 1977. Kommission der Europäischen Gemeinschaften, Euratom, EUR 5848 De/EN/FR

Ihnen E, Jensen JM (1982) Neue Untersuchungen zur Luftaktivierung durch die 42-MeV-Bremsstrahlung eines Betatrons. Strahlentherapie 158/1:30–33

Jean R, Fauchet M (1978) Die medizinischen Anwendungen des Zyklotrons. Strahlentherapie 154/8:526–536

Johnsen SW (1977) Proton-Beryllium neutron production at 25 to 55 MeV. Med Phys 4/3:255

Johnsen SW (1978) Polyethylene filtration of 30 and 40 MeV p-Be neutron beams. Phys Med Biol 23/3:499

Johnson DL, Mann FM, Watson JW, Ullmann J, Wyckoff WG (1979) Measurements of neutron spectra from 35 MeV deuterons on thick lithium for the FMIT facility. International Conference on Nuclear Cross-Sections for Technology, Knoxville, Tennessee, Oct 22–26, HEDL – S/A – 1905 – FP

Junker D (1982) Die Strahlenexposition des Personals bei der Anwendung von Zyklotron-produzierten Radionukliden. Aus: Strahlenschutz für Patienten und Personal in Diagnostik und Therapie mit offenen Radionukliden, 23. Jahrestagung der Vereinigung Dtsch Strahlenschutzärzte eV. 8. Jahrestagung des Verbandes für medizinischen Strahlenschutz in Österreich. Strahlenschutz Forsch Prax XXIV:111–119

Junker D, Fitschen J (1980) Dosimetrie inkorporierter Strahler. In: Hundeshagen H. (Hrsg) Nuklearmedizin: Radiopharmaka, Gerätetechnik, Strahlenschutz. Springer, Berlin Heidelberg New York (Handbuch der medizinischen Radiologie, Bd XV, Teil 1 A, S 425–482)

Karlsson H-E, Pöyhönen L, Saukkonen H, Vauramo E, Virjo A (1982) A field survey of gamma cameras in Finnland – A comprehensive national study. NucCompact 13:228–234

Kuhn H (1975) Dosimetry of fast neutrons for radiotherapy at the DKFZ cyclotron in Heidelberg. Eur J Cancer 10/5:320–321

Langmann HJ (1961) Die Abschirmung gegen die energiereichen Neutronen des Karlsruher Zyklotrons. Kernforschungsanlage Karlsruhe, Zyklotronbereich, Arbeitsbericht 1. Kernreaktor Bau- und Betriebsgesellschaft, Karlsruhe

Laughlin JS, Tilbury RS, Dahl JR (1971) The cyclotron: source of short-lived radionuclides and positron emitters for medicine. Prog Atomic Medicine 3:39–62

Laughlin JS, Canada TR, Simpson LD, McDonald JC, Kuo TYT, Mittelman A (1973) Compact cyclotron neutron dosimetry. In: Breit A, Kärcher KH (Hrsg) Gemeinsamer Kongreß der Deutschen und der Österreichischen Röntgengesellschaft 1973 (Fortsetzung von Deutscher Röntgenkongreß). Thieme, Stuttgart, S 352–353

Lederer CM, Shirley VS (1978) Table of isotopes, 7th edn. Wiley, New York Chichester Brisbane Toronto

Lone MA, Bigham CB, Fraser JS, Schneider HR, Alexander TK, Ferguson AJ, Mc Donald AB (1977) Thick target neutron yields and spectral distributions from the Li-7(d/p,n) and Be-9(d/p,n) reactions. Nucl Instr Meth 143:331

MacDonald NS (1978) The UCLA biomedical cyclotron facility. Prog Nucl Med 4:23–27

Medical Research Council Cyclotron Unit: Annual Research and Development Report (1982); Medical Research Council Unit, Hammersmith Hospital London W 12 OHS and Western General Hospital Edinburgh, EH4 2XU

Meißner P (1978) Strahlenschutzprobleme bei der Neutronentherapie mit einer Zyklotronanlage. In: Messerschmidt O, Scherer E (Hrsg) Risiken und Nutzen der Strahlentherapie bösartiger Tumoren. Thieme, Stuttgart

Merkposten zu Antragsunterlagen in den Genehmigungsverfahren für Anlagen zur Erzeugung ionisierender Strahlen.-Reaktorsicherheit (1978) Sicherheit sonstiger kerntechnischer Anlagen, Strahlenschutz Gemeinsames Ministerialblatt, 29. Jahrgang, Nr 4, S 51–55

NCRP Report No 51 (1977) Radiation protection design guidelines for 0.1–100 MeV particle accelerator facilities. National Council on Radiation and Measurements, Washington

Patterson HW, Thomas RH (1973) Accelerator Health Physics. Academic, New York London

Rassow J (1978) Strahlenschutzprobleme bei der Tumortherapie mit schnellen Neutronen – Methodische Grundlagen der Tumortherapie mit schnellen Neutronen und apparative und bauliche Erfordernisse zur Realisierung der isozentrischen Neutronentherapie mit Neutronengenerator- und Zyklotronanlagen. In: Messerschmidt O, Scherer E (Hrsg) Risiken und Nutzen der Strahlentherapie bösartiger Tumoren. Thieme, Stuttgart, S 32–48

Rassow J (1979) Die Zyklotronanlage im Universitätsklinikum Essen CIRCE + PARCE – Cyclotron Isocentric Neutron Therapy Facility Radiation Physics Essen – Production Facilities for Activaded Materials. Biotechnische Umschau 3:2

Rassow J (1982) Medical cyclotron facilities – useful tools for clinical therapy, diagnosis and analysis. Proceeding of the International Symposium on

Applications and Technology of Ionizing Radiations, Riyadh, Vol 1, pp 47–100

Rassow J, Hüdepohl G, Maier E, Meißner P (1978) CIRCE – cyclotron isocentric neutron therapy facility, radiation physics Essen. Proceedings Third Symposium on Neutron Dosimetry in Biology and Medicine, Neuherberg, 23–27 May, 1977. Kommission der Europäischen Gemeinschaften, Euratom, EUR De/EN/FR, pp 327–337

Richtlinie für die physikalische Strahlenschutzkontrolle (§§ 62 und 63 StrschV) (1979) verabschiedet vom Länderausschuß für Atomkernenergie am 22. Febr 1978, Nds MBl Nr 36

Roedler HD (1986) Qualitätssicherung in der Nuklearmedizin, Inst für Strahlenhygiene des BGA, 8042 Neuherberg. In: Holeczke F, Seyss R, Börner W, Messerschmidt O (Hrsg) Qualitätskontrolle in der Radiologie und Nuklearmedizin unter dem Aspekt des Strahlenschutzes, Strahlenschutzes in Forschung und Praxis, Bd XXVII. Thieme, Stuttgart

Salvadori PA, Bottigli U, Guzzardi R, Crouzel C, Comar D (1982) Cyclotrons for medical use: Characteristics and installation aspects. J Nucl Med Allied Sci 26:1

Sauermann PF (1971) Abschirmung der schnellen Neutronen von Zyklotrons für die medizinisch-biologische Forschung. (Kompaktzyklotron), Report Jül-751-PC (April 1971)

Sauermann PF (1985) Abschirmungspraxis – Aus 25 Jahren Erfahrung – (1960–1985), KFA Kernforschungsanlage, Jülich GmbH, Institut für Chemie – Strahlenschutz (Aug 1985)

Sauermann PF, Friedrich W, Knieper J, Komnick K, Printz H (1978) Versuchseinrichtung zur Ermittlung der Abschirmungserfordernisse für Kompaktzyklotrons zur Neutronentherapie und Radionuklid-Erzeugung. In: Messerschmidt O, Scherer E (Hrsg) Risiken und Nutzen der Strahlentherapie bösartiger Tumoren. Thieme, Stuttgart

Sauermann PF, Friedrich W, Knieper J, Komnick K, Printz H (1980) Radiation protection problems at compact cyclotrons for medical and other use. Proc 5th Congress of the International Radiation Protection Association (IRPA), Jerusalem

Sauermann PF, Knieper J, Printz H (1982) Die Strahlenexposition des Personals bei der Erzeugung und Verarbeitung kurzlebiger Radionuklide mit dem Kompakt-Zyklotron der Kernforschungsanlage Jülich. In: Börner W, Messerschmidt O, Seyss R, Holeczke F (Hrsg) Strahlenschutz für Patienten und Personal in Diagnostik und Therapie mit offenen Radionukliden, Strahlenschutz in Forschung und Praxis, Bd XXIV. Thieme, Stuttgart, S 120–121

Schieferdecker H (1985) Dekontaminationsmaßnahmen. In: Kriegel H (Hrsg) Handbuch der Nuklearmedizin, Bd 1/1. Grundlagen der Nuklearmedizin. Fischer, Stuttgart, S 421–430

Shima Y, Alsmiller RG Jr (1970) Calculation of the photon-production spectrum from proton-nucleus collisions in the energy range 15 to 150 MeV and comparison with experiment. Nucl Science Eng 41:47

Sicherheitshauptbericht Kompaktzyklotron (1985) Medizinische Hochschule Hannover

Skretting A, Rootwelt K, Berthelsen T, Hertzenberg L, Bjornerud T, Boye E, Nerdrum H-J, Falch D, Bremer PO (1984) A Norwegian nationwide quality assurance project in nuclear medicine. In: Schmidt HAE, Vauramo E (eds) Nuklearmedizin – Nuklearmedizin in Forschung und Praxis. Schattauer, Stuttgart New York, S 110–113

Stephens LD, Miller AJ (1969) Radiation studies at a medium energy accelerator. In: Proceedings of the Second International Conference on Accelerator Dosimetry and Experience, Stanford, California, Nov 5–7 (CONF-691101)

Stieve FE (1986) Qualitätssicherung in der Radiologie: Entwicklung Erfordernis, Folgerungen. In: Holeczke F, Seyss R, Börner W, Messerschmidt O (Hrsg) Qualitätskontrolle in der Radiologie und Nuklearmedizin unter dem Aspekt des Strahlenschutzes. Strahlenschutz in Forschung und Praxis, Bd XXVII. Thieme, Stuttgart

Strahlenschutz in der Medizin (1979) Richtlinie für den Strahlenschutz bei Verwendung radioaktiver Stoffe und beim Betrieb von Anlagen zur Erzeugung ionisierender Strahlen und Bestrahlungseinrichtungen mit radioaktiven Quellen in der Medizin. (Richtlinie Strahlenschutz in der Medizin). Hoffmann, Berlin 38

Technischer Überwachungsverein Hannover (1978) 6. Bericht über die sicherheitstechnische Überprüfung (Abnahmeprüfung) des Zyklotrons der Medizinischen Hochschule Hannover vom 11.01.1978

Tochilin E, Kohler GD (1958) Neutron beam characteristics from the University of California 60 inch Cyclotron. In: Marley WG (ed) Health Physics, vol 1. Pergamon, New York, pp 332–339

Verordnung über den Schutz vor Schäden durch ionisierende Strahlen. (1976) Strahlenschutzverordnung. Bundesgesetzblatt Teil 1, Nr 125, 2905–3000

Wallace R (1970) Shielding of nucleon accelerators, cyclotrons: neutron emission and attenuation. In: Jaeger RG (ed) Shield design and engineering. Springer, Berlin Heidelberg New York (Engineering compendium on radiation shielding, vol III)

Waterman FM, Kuchnir FT, Skaggs LS, Kouzes RT, Moore WH (1979) Neutron spectra from 35 and 46 MeV protons, 16 and 28 MeV Deuterons, and 44 MeV He-3. Ions on thick Beryllium. Med Phys 6/5:432

Wolber G (1980) Medizinische Zyklotrons heute,

Statusbericht 1980. Deutsches Krebsforschungszentrum, Institut für Nuklearmedizin, Arbeitsgruppe Zyklotron, Heidelberg
Zobel W, Maienschein FC, Todd JH, Chapman GT (1968) Gamma rays from bombardment of light and intermediate weight nuclei by 16-to 160-MeV protons and 59-MeV alpha particles. Nucl Science Eng 32:392

Literatur zu Tabellen 3 und 4

Bigler RE, Sgouros G (1983) Biological analysis and dosimetry for ^{15}O-labeled O_2, CO_2 and CO gases administered continuously by inhalation. J Nucl Med 24:431

Bigler RE, Sgouros G, Zanzonico PB, Cosma M, Leonard RW, Dahl JR (1985) Radiation dose to the respiratory airway linings from inhalation of ^{15}O-carbon dioxide. J Nucl Med 26:P 62

Chen CT, Harper PV, Lathrop KA (1984) Radiation absorbed dose to the bladder from 2-FDG and other radiopharmaceuticals. J Nucl Med 25:P 93

Coffey JL, Cristy M, Warner GG (1981) Specific absorbed fractions for photon sources uniformly distributed in the heart chambers and heart wall of a heterogeneous phantom. MIRD Pamphlet No. 13. J Nucl Med 22:65–71

Coffey JL, Watson EE (1981) S values for selected radionuclides and organs with the heart wall and heart contents as source organs. Third Int. Radiopharmaceutical Dosim. Sympos. (FDA-81-8166), Oak Ridge, pp 563–594

Crook JE, Carlton JE, Stabin M, Watson E (1985) Radiation dose estimates for copper-64 citrate in man. Fourth Int. Radiopharmaceutical Dosim. Sympos. (CONF-851113). Oak Ridge, pp 212–215

Dillman LT, Von der Lage FC (1975) Radionuclide decay schemes and nuclear parameters for use in radiation-dose estimation. MIRD Pamphlet No. 10. J Nucl Med 16

Feller PA, Sodd VJ (1975) Dosimetry of four heart-imaging radionuclides: K-43, Rb-81, Cs-129 and Tl-201. J Nucl Med 16:1070

Goodman MM, Elmaleh DR, Kearfott KJ, Ackerman RH et al (1981) F-18-labeled 3-deoxy-3-fluoro-D-glucose for the study of regional metabolism in the brain and heart. J Nucl Med 22:138

Harvey J, Firnau G, Garnett ES (1985) Estimation of the radiation dose in man due to 6-[^{18}F]-fluoro-L-dopa. J Nucl Med 26:931

Jones SC, Alavi A, Christman D, Montanez I, Wolf AP, Reivich M (1982) The radiation dosimetry of 2-[^{18}F] fluoro-2-deoxy-D-Glucose in man. J Nucl Med 23:613; und (1983) J Nucl Med 24:447

Kearfott KJ (1982) Absorbed dose estimates for positron emission tomography (PET): C^{15}O, ^{11}CO and CO^{15}O. J Nucl Med 23:1031

Kearfott KJ (1982) Radiation absorbed dose estimates for positron emission tomography (PET): K-38, RB-81, Rb-82 and Cs-130. J Nucl Med 23:1128

Kearfott KJ, Junck L, Rottenberg DA (1983) C-11 dimethyloxazolidinedione (DMO): biodistribution, radiation absorbed dose, and potential for PET measurement of regional brain pH: concise communication. J Nucl Med 24:805

Lockwood AH (1980) Absorbed doses of radiation after an intravenous injection of N-13 ammonia in man: Concise communication. J Nucl Med 21:276

Mc Elvany KD, Katzenellenbogen JA, Shafer KE, Siegel BA, Senderoff SG, Welch MJ (1982) $16\alpha-$[^{77}Br] Bromoestradiol: dosimetry and preliminary clinical studies. J Nucl Med 23:425

Meyer E, Yamamoto YL, Evans AC, Tyler J, Diksic M, Feindel W (1985) Radiation dose to trachea from inhaled oxygen-15 labelled carbon dioxide. J Nucl Med 26:P 62

Powell GF, Schuchard RA, Reft CS, Harper PV (1984) Radiation absorbed dose to tracheal mucosa from inhaled oxygen-15-labelled carbon dioxide. Ann Neurol (Suppl) 15:S 107

Powell GF, Harper PV, Reft CS, Chen CT, Lathrop KA (1985) Problems in radiation absorbed dose estimation from positron emitters. Fourth Int. Radiopharmaceutical Dosim. Sympos. (CONF-851113) Oak Ridge, pp 194–211

Reivich M, Kuhl D, Wolf A, Greenberg J, Phelps M, Ido T et al (1979) The [^{18}F]-fluorodeoxyglucose method for the measurement of local cerebral glucose utilisation in man. Circ Res 44:127

Ryan JW, Harper PV, Stark VS, Peterson EL, Lathrop KA (1985) Radiation absorbed dose estimate for rubidium-82 determined from in vivo measurements in human subjects. Fourth Int. Radiopharmaceutical Dosim. Sympos. (CONF-851113) Oak Ridge, pp 346–357

Tilbury RS, Myers WG, Chandra R, Dahl JR, Lee R (1980) Production of 7.6-minute potassium-38 for medical use. J Nucl Med 21:867

Washburn LC, Byrd BL, Sun TT, Crook JE, Hubner KF, Coffey JL, Watson EE (1985) Dosimetry of D- and L-enantiomers of ^{11}C-labelled tryptophan and valine. Fourth Int. Radiopharmaceutical Dosim. Sympos. (CONF-851113) Oak Ridge, pp 239–244

2. Meßtechnik in der Emissions-Computertomographie

Von

K. Jordan unter Mitarbeit von B. Knoop

Mit 111 Abbildungen und 6 Tabellen

A. Einleitung

Der Begriff Emissions-Tomographie bedarf einer Erläuterung, da nicht eindeutig festliegt, wo die flächige Szintigraphie aufhört und die Tomographie beginnt. Man könnte annehmen, daß mit Einführung des fokussierenden Vielloch-Kollimators beim szintigraphischen Scanner durch Newell et al. (1952) die Tomographie ihren Anfang genommen hat, denn in der Tat hat dieser Kollimator tomographische Eigenschaften. Er bildet eine bestimmte Objektschicht (Fokusebene) scharf ab, während die davor und dahinter liegenden Schichten mehr oder weniger unscharf abgebildet werden. Dieser Effekt war anfänglich bei den damals üblichen NaJ(Tl)-Szintillationskristallen mit 2 Zoll Durchmesser relativ gering, wurde dann aber bei den gebräuchlichen 5 Zoll Kristallen und besonders bei kürzeren Fokusabständen doch merklich. Trotzdem möchte ich diesen Scannern keine tomographischen Eigenschaften zuerkennen, denn diese Kollimatoren wurden entwickelt, um die Ausbeute gegenüber der einzelnen zylindrischen Bohrung ganz erheblich zu erhöhen und nicht, um damit Tomographie zu betreiben. Im Gegenteil, diese fokussierende Eigenschaft störte eher bei der flächigen Szintigraphie, da sie dazu zwang, den Kollimator-Objekt-Abstand möglichst exakt zu wählen. Auch wurde die räumliche Auflösung in den nicht fokussierten Schichten unnötigerweise schlecht.

Ich möchte im folgenden Beitrag als Emissions-Tomographie solche Verfahren diskutieren, deren gezielte Aufgabe es ist, die Aktivitätsverteilung in ausgewählten Objektschichten bildlich darzustellen. Nur Geräte dieser Art sollen als Tomographen bezeichnet werden. Interessant ist in diesem Zusammenhang, daß einer der ersten Tomographen genau solch ein Scanner mit einem fokussierenden Kollimator war, nämlich der „Tomographic Gamma-Ray Scanner" von Anger (1968).

Allerdings wird hier eine wesentliche zusätzliche Information benutzt, um echt tomographische Eigenschaften gegenüber dem einfachen Scanner zu erreichen, nämlich die Kenntnis, durch welche der vielen Kollimatorbohrungen das jeweils registrierte Gammaquant den Kristall erreicht hat. Die einzelne Bohrung des fokussierenden Vielloch-Kollimators legt ein sehr eng begrenztes empfindliches Meßvolumen im Objekt fest, welches im Idealfall die Form einer Stricknadel hat. Es wird ein „Meßstrahl" durch das Objekt gelegt *unter verschiedenen Winkeln*. Dies ist der entscheidende Schritt, der von der flächigen Szintigraphie zur Tomographie geführt hat, s. auch Abb. 56.

Die tomographischen Verfahren lassen sich von der verfahrenstechnischen Seite her in zwei Kategorien einteilen, die transversale und die longitudinale Tomographie. Diese schon 1963 von Kuhl getroffene Unterscheidung hat auch heute noch volle Gültigkeit (s. Abb. 1).

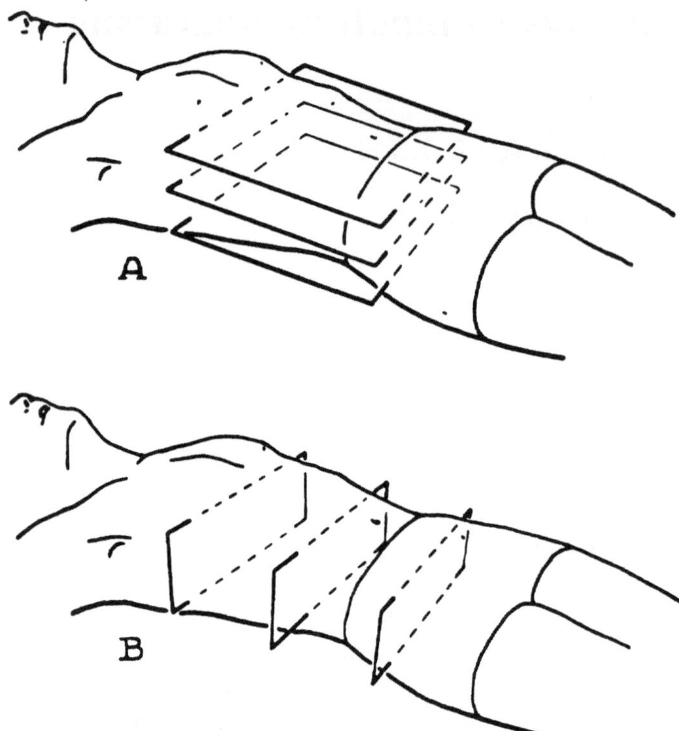

Abb. 1. Longitudinale Tomographie **A** und transversale Tomographie **B**. (Aus Kuhl u. Edwards 1963)

Der grundlegende Unterschied beider Verfahren besteht darin, daß

1. bei der transversalen Tomographie schon bei der Informationsgewinnung eine zweidimensionale Schicht im Objekt selektiv ausgewählt wird, zum Beispiel durch entsprechende Kollimation und Abtastung (s. Abb. 2), während bei der longitudinalen Tomographie die Information stets aus dem dreidimensionalen Objektbereich gewonnen wird, woraus dann durch geeignete Umverteilung zweidimensionale Schichtbilder berechnet werden (s. Abb. 3);
2. bei der transversalen Tomographie der Meßstrahl stets in der gewählten Schichtebene liegt (s. Abb. 2), während er bei der longitudinalen Tomographie senkrecht bis schräg durch die berechneten Schichtebenen verläuft (s. Abb. 3);
3. bei der transversalen Tomographie der Winkelbereich, unter dem die Schicht „betrachtet" wird, meist 360° beträgt (s. Abb. 2), während bei der longitudinalen Tomographie das Objekt nur unter einem begrenzten Raumwinkel gesehen wird (s. Abb. 3).

Der Einsatz von Einzelphotonen-Strahlern, im Folgenden generell Gamma-Strahler genannt, und von Positronen-Strahlern macht eine weitere Unterteilung möglich und notwendig. Wichtig ist hierbei, daß der Unterschied im wesentlichen nur in der Art der Kollimation besteht, nämlich durch Einsatz von Kollimatoren bei den Gamma-Strahlern und der elektronischen Kollimation (Koinzidenzabfrage) bei den Positronen-Strahlern.

Ich will versuchen, mit dieser Einteilung in transversale und longitudinale Tomographie jeweils mit Gamma- beziehungsweise mit Positronen-Strahlern die Emissions-Tomographie abzuhandeln. Wie bei jeder solchen Klassifizierung wird es den einen oder anderen Grenzfall geben, der eine eindeutige Zuordnung nicht zuläßt.

Noch ein Wort zum Begriff „Computertomographie". Dieser Begriff wurde Anfang der siebziger Jahre zusammen mit der Röntgen-Computertomographie eingeführt. Heute spricht

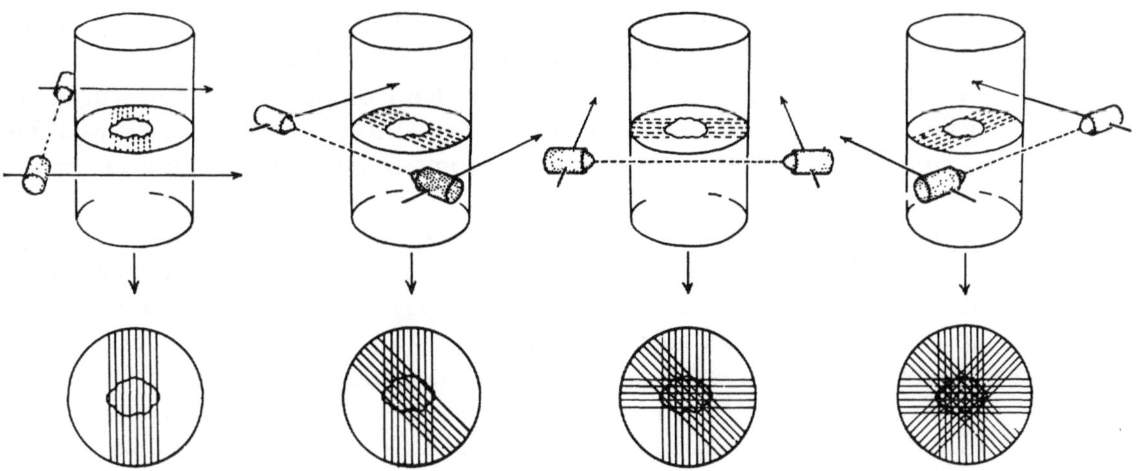

Abb. 2. Aufnahme einer transversalen Schicht mit kollimierten Detektoren. (Aus KUHL u. EDWARDS 1963)

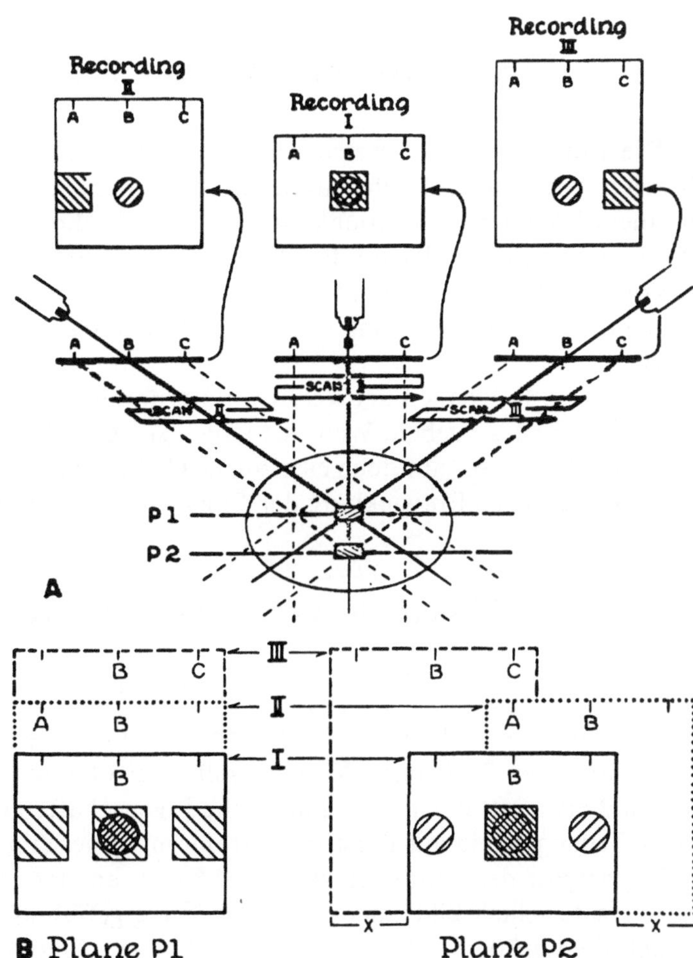

Abb. 3. Aufnahme von longitudinalen Schichten unter verschiedenen Sichtwinkeln. (Aus KUHL u. EDWARDS 1963)

man exakter von der Transmissions-Computertomographie (TCT) und der hier zu besprechenden Emissions-Computertomographie (ECT).

Die Ergänzung durch den Begriff „Computer" hat sicher ihre Berechtigung, denn obwohl der Computer mit dem tomographischen Meßverfahren unmittelbar nichts zu tun hat, so ist dennoch die notwendige Informationsverarbeitung und Darstellung ohne seine Mithilfe heute schlechterdings unmöglich. Man muß sich aber darüber im klaren sein, daß bis gegen Ende der sechziger Jahre Emissions-Tomographie ohne den Computer betrieben wurde und auch kommerzielle Tomographen (z.B. Pho/Con von Searle Radiographics) noch weit darüber hinaus bis zum heutigen Tage ohne Computer tomographische Abbildungen ermöglichen.

Dennoch hat der Computer eine entscheidende Wende herbeigeführt, indem er durch Einsatz mathematischer Hilfsmittel eine echte Rekonstruktion der in der dargestellten Schicht vorhandenen Aktivitätsverteilung ermöglichte. Dies war gegenüber der bis dahin möglichen einfachen Rückprojektionen, d.h. der lagegerechten Summation aller Meßwerte der einzelnen Meßstrahlen, der entscheidende Fortschritt, der sich in dem Begriff Computertomographie ausdrückt.

Ein eigenes Kapitel „Mathematische Grundlagen der Rekonstruktion und quantitativen Aktivitätsbestimmung in vivo" befaßt sich mit diesem computergestützten Verfahren der Rekonstruktion. Es wurde dankenswerterweise von Herrn Dr.-Ing. B. Knoop bearbeitet.

B. Historische Entwicklung der Emissions-Tomographie

Die Frage nach dem ersten Emissions-Tomographen bzw. nach dem ersten Schichtbild läßt sich, wie häufig in solchen Situationen, nicht exakt beantworten, es lag gewissermaßen zu einem bestimmten Zeitpunkt in der Luft. Mehrere Gruppen arbeiteten gleichzeitig und unabhängig voneinander an der Realisierung. Eines ist aber erstaunlich, es wurden alle vier im Vorwort festgelegten Möglichkeiten fast gleichzeitig realisiert bzw. Vorschläge dazu veröffentlicht, für transversale und longitudinale Tomographie mit Gamma- und Positronenstrahlern.

Es soll im Folgenden der Versuch unternommen werden, einen nach Jahreszahlen geordneten Rückblick zu geben. Wenn sich auch einzelne Stationen nicht immer ganz exakt zeitlich einordnen lassen, so gibt doch eine solche Ordnung einen, wie ich meine, sehr eindrucksvollen Überblick über die Entwicklung der Emissions-Tomographie.

I. Historische Entwicklung unterteilt nach Jahreszahlen

Das Jahr 1959:

Anfang dieses Jahres macht Anger auf einem Seminar der IAEA, Anger (1959), den Vorschlag einer Positronen-Kamera mit zwei Gamma-Kameraköpfen in Koinzidenzschaltung und erwähnt deren tomographische Eigenschaften (s. Abb. 4). Es wird hier eine longitudinale Tomographie mit Positronenstrahlern vorgeschlagen.

Im August des Jahres entsteht bei Kuhl an der University of Pennsylvania das erste transversale Schichtbild einer mit ^{131}J-Lösung gefüllten Plastikflasche, die in einem mit Wasser gefüllten größeren Becherglas stand. Dieses „Phantom" stand auf einem Drehteller, der in Abb. 5 vorne rechts zu erkennen ist. Es wurde von einem Szintillationszähler mit fokussierendem Kollimator (links hinter dem Becherglas zu erkennen) in einer horizontalen Zeile abgetastet. Die Abtastbewegung besorgte der Vorschub einer Fräsmaschine. Nach jeder Abtastung wurde das Phantom um 15° gedreht. Auf diese Weise wurden 24 unterschiedliche Aktivitätsprofile des Phantoms aufgenommen und nacheinander auf einem Oszillographenschirm sichtbar gemacht, wobei die Helligkeit von der Impulsrate gesteuert wurde. Eine

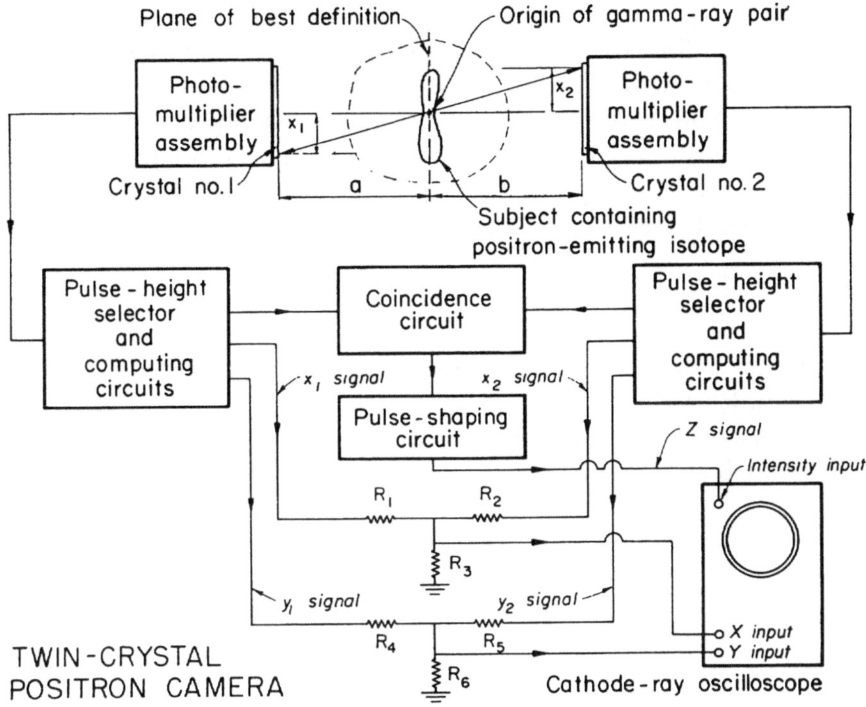

Abb. 4. Prinzipbild einer Positronen-Kamera. (Aus ANGER 1959)

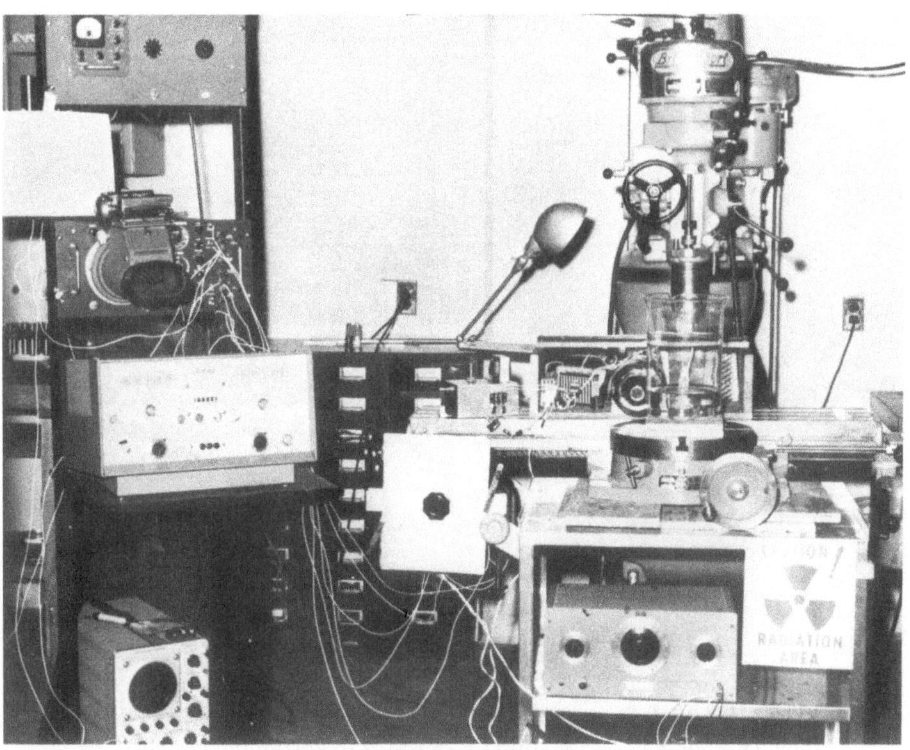

Abb. 5. Der erste „transversale Tomograph" für Gamma-Strahler, 1959. (Freundlicherweise von D.E. KUHL zur Verfügung gestellt)

Kamera mit geöffnetem Verschluß vor dem Oszillographenschirm (links im Bild) hat alle Profile auf einem Film aufintegriert, wobei die Richtung der Strahlauslenkung synchron mit der Phantomdrehung verstellt wurde, nach dem Prinzip der Abb. 2.

Das Ergebnis ist in Abb. 6 dargestellt, eine einfache Rückprojektion ohne Computer. Man kann dies sicher als die Geburtsstunde der Emissions-Tomographie ansehen, zumal sich an dem grundsätzlichen Prinzip der Informationsgewinnung bis heute nichts geändert hat. Kuhl trägt Ende des Jahres erstmalig darüber öffentlich vor.

Das Jahr 1962:

Kuhl stellt auf dem Jahreskongreß der Society of Nuclear Medicine seinen „Mark II Scanner" vor (Kuhl u. Edwards 1962). Ein transversaler Tomograph mit zwei kollimierten Sonden nach dem Prinzip der Abb. 2, der sowohl die lineare Bewegung wie die Drehbewegung um den Patienten ermöglicht (s. Abb. 7).

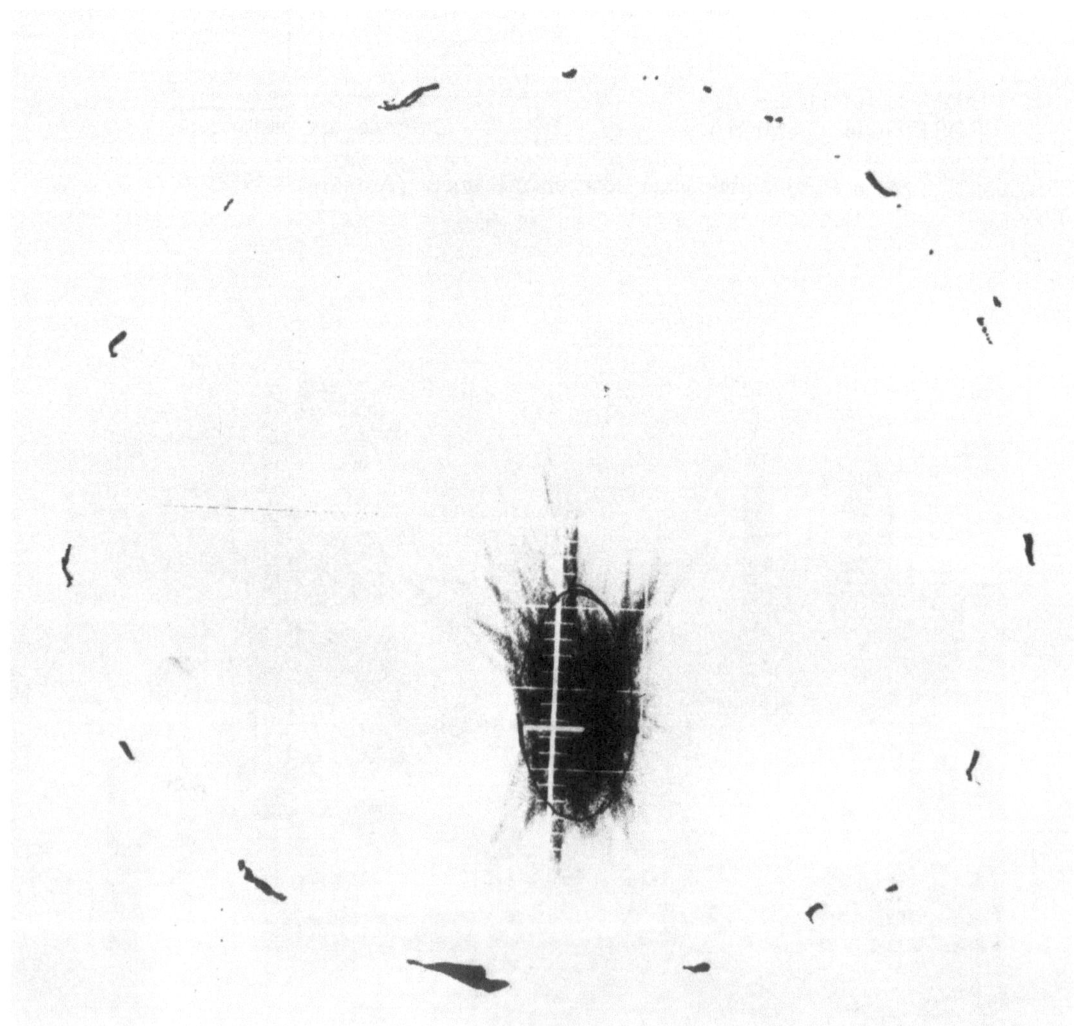

Abb. 6. Das erste transversale Schichtbild einer mit ^{131}I gefüllten Flasche ovalen Querschnitts, aufgenommen 1959. (Freundlicherweise von D.E. Kuhl zur Verfügung gestellt)

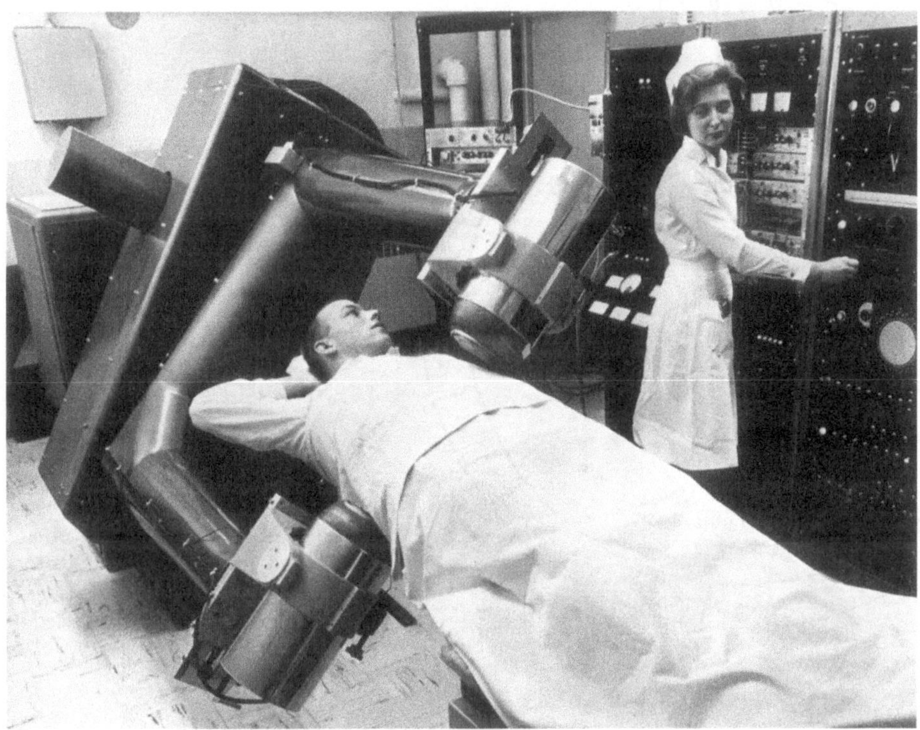

Abb. 7. Der transversale Schichtscanner Mark II, 1962. (Freundlicherweise von D.E. KUHL zur Verfügung gestellt)

RANKOWITZ vom Brookhaven National Laboratory beschreibt die erste stationäre ringförmige Detektoranordnung mit 32 Szintillationssonden im Koinzidenzbetrieb zur transversalen Positronentomographie (RANKOWITZ et al. 1962). In Abb. 8 ist das Prinzip der Anordnung zur Herstellung von Schichtaufnahmen des Hirns dargestellt. Die Möglichkeiten der Informationsverarbeitung und bildlichen Darstellung mit dem Computer waren damals leider noch nicht gegeben. RANKOWITZ speicherte die koinzidenten Ereignisse im Speicher eines zweidimensionalen Impulshöhenanalysators. Wenn auch seiner Zeit etwas vorauseilend, kann man dies als die Geburtsstunde der transversalen Positronen-Tomographen ansehen (s. auch ROBERTSON et al. 1973).

Das Jahr 1963:

Schon in diesem Jahr weist CORMACK (1963) auf die Möglichkeiten hin, bei der Positronen-Koinzidenzmessung eine echte quantitative Rekonstruktion durchführen zu können, einschließlich Absorptionskorrektur.

Der Bericht über den Mark II Scanner wird veröffentlicht (KUHL u. EDWARDS 1963).

Das Jahr 1964:

Die ersten transversalen Schichtbilder von Leber und Hirn werden von KUHL u. EDWARDS (1964) veröffentlicht, aufgenommen mit dem Mark II und ^{198}Au bzw. ^{197}Hg.

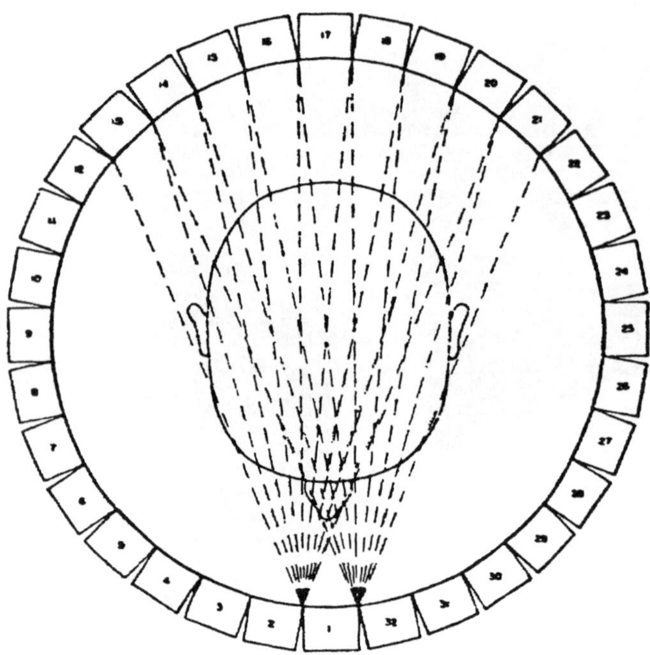

Abb. 8. Erste Darstellung einer ringförmigen Anordnung von Detektoren zur transversalen Tomographie mit Positronen-Strahlern. (Aus Rankowitz et al. 1962)

Das Jahr 1965:

Kuhl zeigt das erste Transmissions-Schichtbild eines menschlichen Thorax auf der Jahrestagung der Society of Nuclear Medicine (Kuhl u. Hale 1965). Es wurde aufgenommen mit einer kollimierten ^{241}Am Quelle als Strahlenquelle (60 keV Gammastrahlung), die eine der beiden Sonden des Mark II ersetzte. Dieses erste Transmissions-Schichtbild hatte eine für damalige Verhältnisse überraschend gute Qualität (Kuhl et al. 1966).

Harper et al. (1965) schlagen vor, den Patienten vor einer Kamera zu drehen und so z.B. 48 Einzelaufnahmen unter verschiedenen Blickwinkeln zu gewinnen, die sie auf einzelne Filmbilder speichern. Über ein geeignetes Spiegelsystem (Abb. 9), kann dann ein dreidimensionales Bild der Objektverteilung erzeugt werden.

Das Jahr 1966:

Auf der Jahrestagung der Gesellschaft für Nuklearmedizin in Heidelberg schlägt Anger vor, einen Patienten vor einer Kamera rotieren zu lassen und gibt wiederum ein photographisches Verfahren an, um transversale Schichtbilder zu erzeugen (Anger 1967).

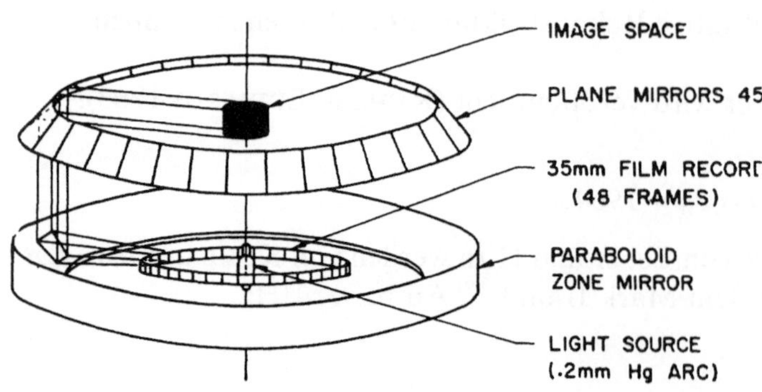

Abb. 9. Vorschlag zur dreidimensionalen Darstellung einer Objektverteilung mit Hilfe von 48 einzelnen Kamera-Aufnahmen eines Patienten unter verschiedenen Winkeln mit 7,5° Abstand. (Aus Harper 1968)

Man muß sich hier vergegenwärtigen, daß in diesem Jahr gerade die ersten Magnetkernspeicher Eingang in die Szintigraphie fanden, eine sinnvolle Computerverarbeitung tomographischer Daten war noch nicht möglich.

ANGER berichtet erstmalig über seinen Tomographic Gamma-Ray Scanner (ANGER 1966). Eine Weiterentwicklung der KUHLschen Idee der longitudinalen Tomographie, die zum ersten praktisch anwendbaren longitudinalen Tomographen führt (s. auch ANGER 1968, 1969). Abb. 10 zeigt das Prinzip. Die Quelle 2, die in der Fokusebene C liegt, wird nur in einer einzigen Meßkopfposition (Mitte der Zeile 3) erfaßt und erzeugt ein homogenes Bild über den vollen Kristalldurchmesser.

Die Punktquellen 1 und 3 außerhalb der Fokusebene erzeugen kleinere Teilbilder unterschiedlicher Lage, wie in Abb. 10c dargestellt. Sie werden unscharf und verschmiert abgebildet. Um auch diese Quellen scharf abzubilden, muß eine Refokussierung durchgeführt werden. ANGER löste diese Aufgabe in genialer Weise mit einem optischen Registriersystem (Abb. 11). Der Schirm der Kathodenstrahlröhre der Kamera wird durch ein feststehendes Linsensystem gleichzeitig auf fünf Filmabschnitte abgebildet und zwar mit unterschiedlicher Vergrößerung und Invertierung der Abbildungen A und B gegenüber D und E.

Durch diesen Trick wird z.B. der Tatsache Rechnung getragen, daß das Bild von Quellen oberhalb der Fokusebene (Quelle 1) auf dem Kamerabildschirm entgegen der Scanrichtung läuft, während es bei Quellen unterhalb der Fokusebene in Scanrichtung über den Bildschirm wandert (s. Abb. 10c).

Die zur Refokussierung der Ebenen außerhalb der Fokusebene notwendige Verschiebung des Registrierfilms gegenüber den Lichtstrahlen wird durch eine zeilenförmige Verschiebung des Films streng synchron mit der Meßkopfbewegung erzielt. Abb. 12 zeigt die Abbildung der drei Punktquellen auf den Ebenen A bis E zugeordneten Filmabschnitten. Man kann zwei wesentliche Dinge erkennen. Die Punktquellen in den Schichten A, C und E werden

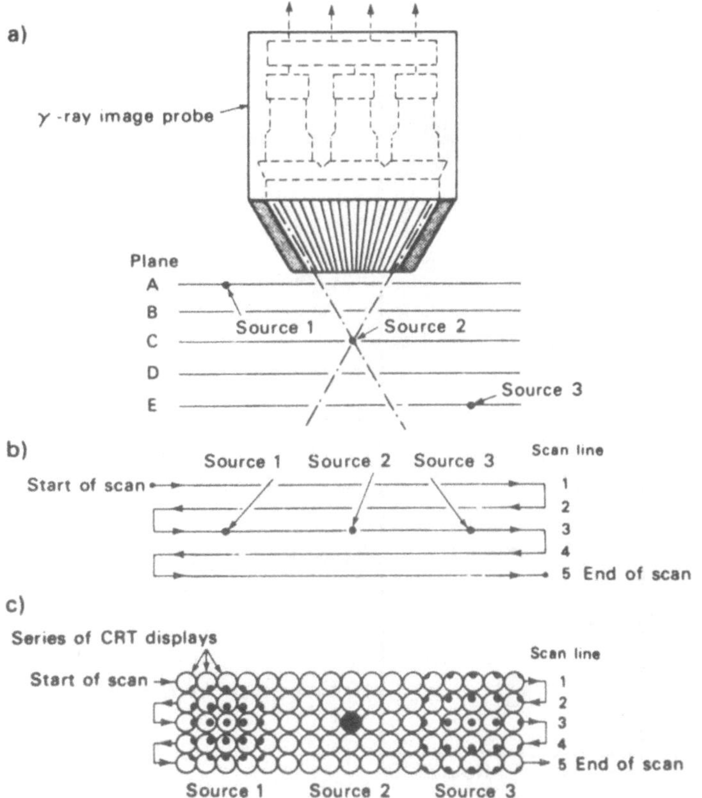

Abb. 10a–c. Der Multiplane Tomographic Scanner. Eine Anger-Kamera mit fokussierendem Kollimator bewegt sich zeilenförmig über dem Objekt, wie der übliche szintigraphische Scanner. Ein Objekt bestehend aus drei Punktquellen, die in einer Ebene senkrecht zur Kollimatoroberfläche in drei verschiedenen Tiefen liegen (**a**), erzeugen beim zeilenförmigen Abtasten (**b**) auf dem Kamerabildschirm unterschiedliche Abbildungen (**c**). (Aus ANGER 1969)

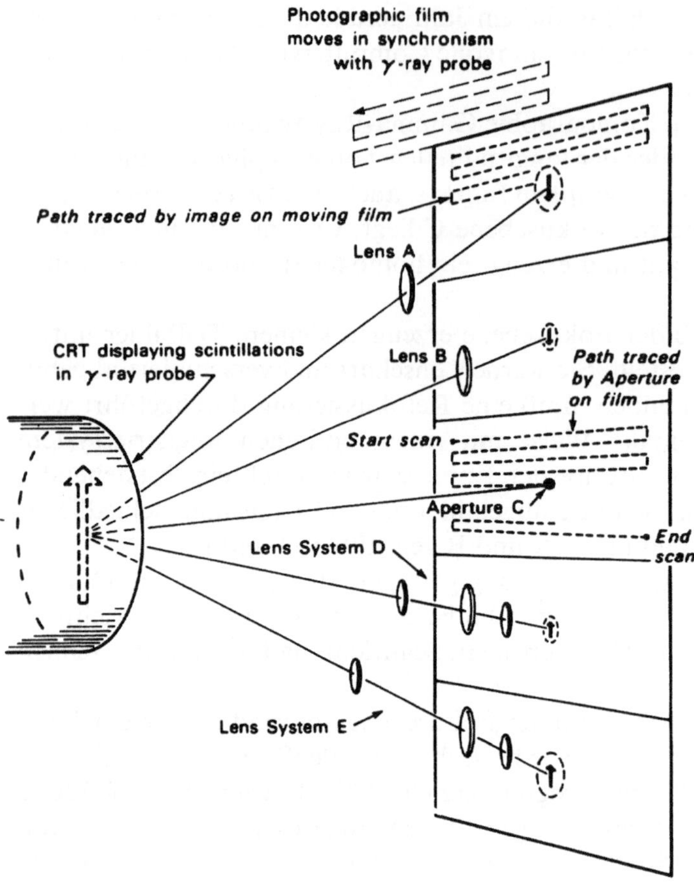

Abb. 11. Optisches Registriersystem des Tomographic Scanner. Die einzelnen Lichtpunkte auf dem Kamerabildschirm werden über ein Linsensystem simultan auf fünf verschiedene Filmabschnitte projiziert, entsprechend den fünf angenommenen Schichten A bis E. Dabei wird der Gesamtfilm zeilenförmig verschoben synchron mit der Bewegung des Meßkopfes. (Aus ANGER 1969)

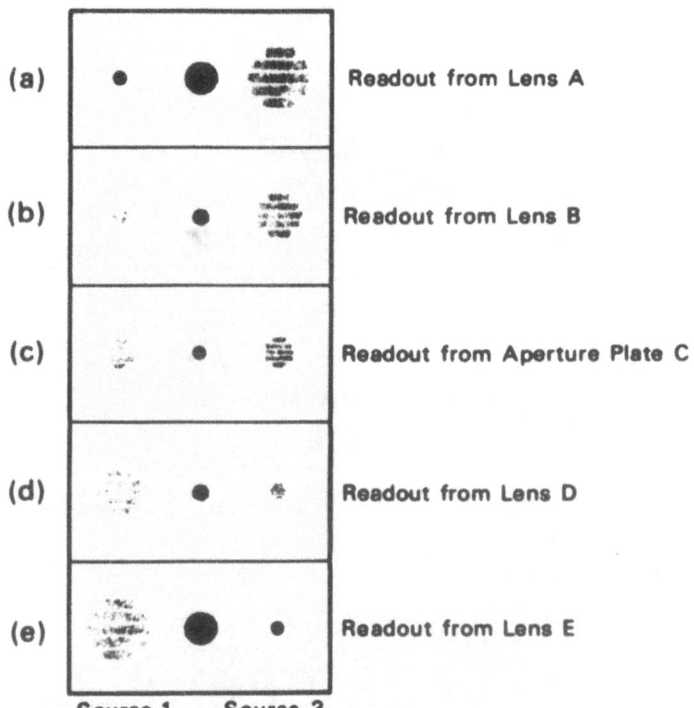

Abb. 12. Abbildung der drei Punktquellen auf den fünf verschiedenen Filmabschnitten. (Aus ANGER 1969)

in den zugehörigen Schichtdarstellungen a, c und e jeweils scharf abgebildet, die Refokussierung funktioniert. Gleichzeitig werden aber in allen Schichtbildern a bis e die jeweils anderen Quellen mehr oder weniger verschmiert abgebildet. Diese Verwischungsbilder erscheinen auch in den Schichtbildern b und d, in denen eigentlich gar keine Abbildung erfolgen dürfte, da in den Schichten B und D keine Punktquellen lagen. Dies ist die typische Eigenschaft der einfachen Rückprojektion. Scharfe, d.h. refokussierte Abbildungen einer Schicht, aber gleichzeitige Überlagerung mit den Verwischungsbildern der darüber bzw. darunter liegenden Aktivitätsverteilung. Das gleiche gilt auch für transversale Schichtbilder, nur sind hier die Aktivitätsverteilungen in Nachbarschichten ohne Einfluß, dafür erzeugen die Aktivitätsanreicherungen innerhalb der dargestellten Schicht ihre eigenen Verwischungsbilder, die der Schichtdarstellung überlagert sind.

Das Jahr 1967:

BRACEWELL u. RIDDLE (1967) setzen erstmals in der Radioastronomie die Rückprojektion von gefilterten Projektionen ein. Sie verwenden ein Rampenfilter und die Berechnung erfolgt im Ortsbereich durch Faltung. Auch die Frage der optimalen Winkelabtastung wird diskutiert.

Das Jahr 1968:

KUHL u. EDWARDS (1968) verwenden erstmals die digitale anstelle der photographischen Summation der Projektionen. Die auf Lochstreifen gesammelten Daten werden auf einen magnetischen Trommelspeicher übertragen und von dort per Programm in eine Matrix von 100×100 Bildelementen einsortiert. Die Bildmatrix wird auf dem Oszillographenschirm mit Helligkeitssteuerung dargestellt oder mit einem Drucker als Zahlenmatrix ausgedruckt.

Ferner berichten sie auf dem IAEA Symposium (KUHL u. EDWARDS 1969) über den Bau und die Eigenschaften vom Mark III Scanner, ein Hirntomograph mit vier Meßsonden.

BROWNELL et al. (1969) beschreiben auf dem IAEA Symposium in Salzburg erstmals die geplante Positronenkamera mit zwei gegenüberstehenden Multikristall-Blöcken (s. auch Abb. 37).

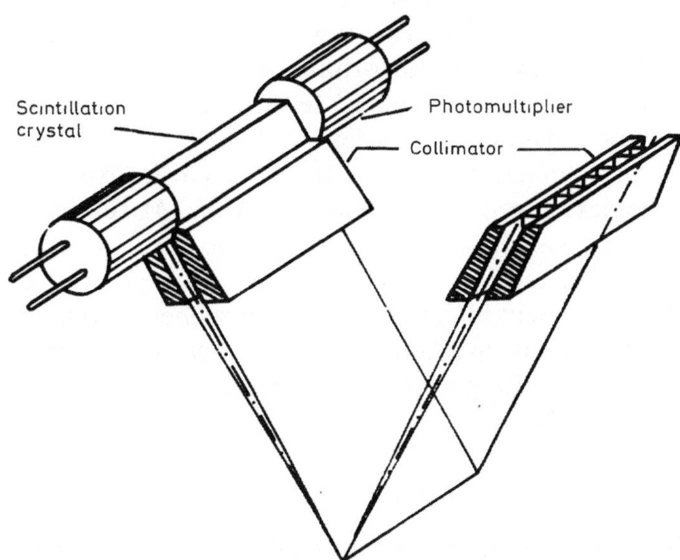

Abb. 13. Prinzip des Tomoscanners mit „slit-hybrid collimator". Stabförmige NaJ(Tl)-Kristalle mit schlitzförmigen Kollimatoren. Die Ortung des Absorptionsortes im Kristall erfolgte durch Amplitudenvergleich der beiden Photomultiplier an den Stirnflächen. (Aus MIRALDI u. DI CHIRO 1970)

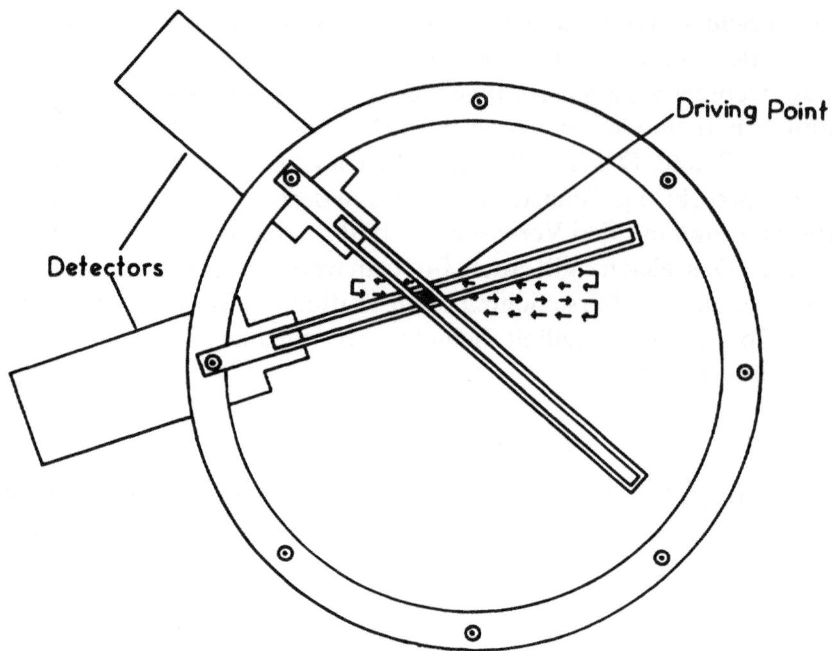

Abb. 14. Tomoscanner für Hirnaufnahmen mit acht Sonden in ringförmiger Anordnung, wobei die Neigung der Sonden automatisch verändert wird. (Aus Patton et al. 1973)

Bozzo et al. (1968) setzen einen Rechner beim Positronenring mit 32 Sonden ein. Die in einem zweidimensionalen Impulshöhenanalysator zwischengespeicherten Daten werden auf Lochstreifen gestanzt und auf ein IBM-kompatibles Band umgesetzt und mit Hilfe des Rechners als Bild dargestellt.

Das Jahr 1969:

Miraldi et al. (1969) berichten auf der Jahrestagung der Society of Nuclear Medicine über ihren Tomoscanner mit „slit-hybrid collimator", eine Variation des Tomographic Scanners von Anger (Abb. 13). Siehe auch Miraldi u. Di Chiro (1970).

Cassen (1969) schlägt ein Verfahren vor, um die Verschiebung der Filmebene, wie sie z.B. Anger bei seinem Tomographic Scanner durchführt, zu umgehen, indem die auf Bandspuren aufgenommenen Signale der einzelnen Meßstrahlen mit unterschiedlicher zeitlicher Verzögerung abgespielt und aufsummiert werden.

Eine Sondenanordnung ähnlich der von Kuhl schlagen Patton et al. (1969) vor. Acht auf einem Ring um das Objekt angeordnete Sonden (s. Abb. 14), führen keine lineare Scanbewegung mehr aus und rotieren auch nicht mehr um das Objekt. Die Achsen ihrer Kollimatoren werden mit einer simplen mechanischen Vorrichtung so geneigt, daß sie sich stets in einem bestimmten Volumenelement in der Objektschicht schneiden. Dieser Schnittpunkt wird zeilenförmig in einem Feld von 20 cm × 20 cm innerhalb der Schicht verschoben.

Der rotierende Slanthole-Kollimator vor der Angerkamera wird erstmalig von McAffee et al. (1969) beschrieben (s. Abb. 15).

Das Jahr 1970:

Mit Beginn der 70er Jahre beginnt eine entscheidende zweite Phase der Tomographie, die sogenannte Computer-Tomographie. Der Computer übernimmt die Datenverarbeitung und Darstellung, und er ermöglicht eine echte Rekonstruktion der gemessenen Objektverteilung, weitgehend frei von Verwischungsbildern.

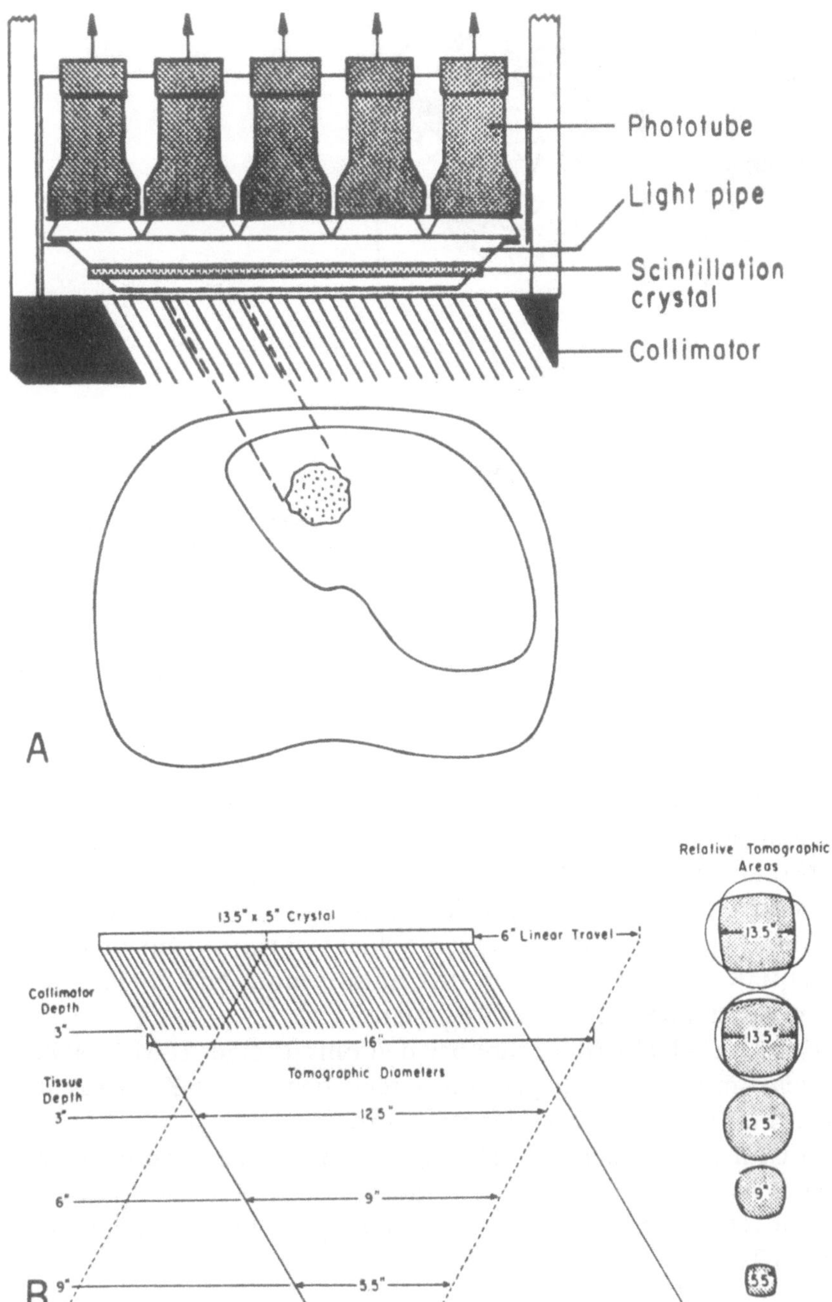

Abb. 15. Der Slanthole-Kollimator. Ein Parallelloch-Kollimator mit gleichmäßig um 30° geneigten Bohrungen drehbar vor einer Anger-Kamera zur longitudinalen Tomographie (Aus McAffee u. Mozley 1969)

Unabhängig von den bereits vielfach geleisteten Vorarbeiten auf dem Gebiet der Radioastronomie (Bracewell 1956), oder auf dem Gebiet der Elektronenmikroskopie (De Rosier u. Klug 1968), kann man doch den Beginn der echten Rekonstruktion bei der Emissions-Tomographie in dieses Jahr verlegen, als Gordon et al. (1970) ihre Arbeit über iterative „Algebraic Reconstruction Technique (ART)" veröffentlichen.

Auch der generelle Einsatz des Rechners zur Datenerfassung und Darstellung setzt sich durch. So stellen Kuhl u. Edwards (1970) ihren Mark III Kopfscanner vor, der mit vier Meßsonden eine transversale Schicht aufzunehmen gestattet (s. Abb. 16). Die Bildzusammen-

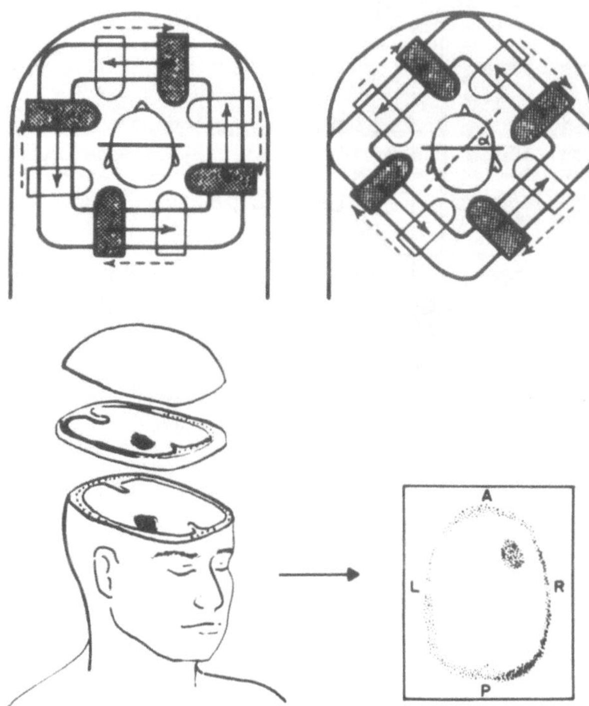

Abb. 16. Der Mark III-Scanner zur Erzeugung transversaler Schichtbilder des Schädels. Da gleichzeitig vier Sonden eine Projektion aufnehmen, sind nur noch 6 verschiedene Stellungen mit einem jeweiligen Drehwinkel von $\alpha = 15°$ notwendig. (Aus Kuhl u. Edwards 1970)

setzung durch Rückprojektion erfolgt durch einen Computer, auf dessen Bildschirm das Bild auch dargestellt wird.

Während Muehllehner (1970, 1971) über die Anwendung eines rotierenden Slanthole-Kollimators berichtet, wobei die Registrierung noch über das Kamerascope erfolgt, indem die Strahlposition der jeweils dargestellten Schicht entsprechend analog verschoben wird, berichtet Freedman (1970) bereits über den Einsatz eines ND 50/50 Computers in Verbindung mit einem rotierenden Slanthole-Kollimator.

Auch Monahan et al. (1970) beschreiben den Einsatz einer IBM 1800 bei der Realisierung einer Positronenkamera mit zwei gegenüberstehenden Anger-Kameras in Koinzidenz, wie sie von Anger (1959) bereits vorgeschlagen wurde.

Interessant ist hier auch der erste Hinweis auf die großen Probleme mit den sehr hohen Impulsraten, der nicht durch Kollimatoren abgeschirmten Kameras. Sie nennen eine Maximalaktivität von 100 µCi im Meßfeld, was für damalige Verhältnisse wohl noch optimistisch gewesen sein dürfte.

Das Jahr 1971:

Die Drehung des Objektes vor einer Kamera mit Parallelloch-Kollimator ermöglicht es Muehllehner u. Wetzel (1971) acht Kamera-Aufnahmen von Patienten unter jeweils um 45° gedrehter Aufnahmerichtung anzufertigen. Die Einzelaufnahmen werden in einem 1600-Kanal Analysator für zwei Parameter digitalisiert (40×40 Matrix) und auf ein Magnetband übertragen, welches in eine IBM 360/30 eingelesen wird. Hier werden nicht nur die Rückprojektionen für die einzelnen Schichten senkrecht zur Kollimatoreintrittsfläche berechnet, sondern ein einfacher iterativer Vergleich zwischen rückprojizierter Verteilung und den gemessenen acht Projektionen mit einer Differenzbildungs-Rechenvorschrift führt zu einer Rekonstruktion der Aktivitätsverteilung in der Schicht, wenn auch noch mit erheblichen Einschränkungen, allein auch schon wegen der sehr geringen Anzahl von Projektionen. Doch der Schritt zur echten Rekonstruktion war gegeben.

Einen anderen Weg beschreitet CHESLER unter Einsatz der Positronen-Koinzidenzmessung. Mit einem Detektorpaar nimmt er nacheinander Projektionen einer Objektschicht auf und rekonstruiert die Schichtverteilung durch Rückprojektion, wobei die Projektionen vorher im Computer gefiltert werden (CHESLER 1971). Gleichzeitig werden mit einem externen Positronenstrahler unter gleichen Winkeln Projektionen der Transmission durch das Objekt bestimmt und damit eine Absorptionskorrektur durchgeführt (s. auch CHESLER 1973).

Das Jahr 1972:

Dieses Jahr ist für die Tomographie im allgemeinen von ganz besonderer Bedeutung. Der erste von HOUNSFIELD entwickelte EMI-Kopfscanner Mark I wird vorgestellt (HOUNSFIELD 1973).

Die Transmissions-Computertomographie tritt damit ihren Siegeszug an, der sich ohne Zweifel auch auf die weitere Entwicklung der Emissions-Computertomographie positiv auswirkt. Der Erfolg des ersten EMI-Scanners ist unter anderem dadurch begründet, daß er von Anfang an echte rekonstruierte transversale Schichten darstellte, die mit einem iterativen Rechenalgorithmus berechnet wurden.

Unabhängig davon beschreibt SCHMIDLIN (1972) einen iterativen Rekonstruktionsalgorithmus ISS für den Fall der longitudinalen Positronen-Tomographie mit zwei gegenüberstehenden Gammakameras (s. Abb. 17). Die einfach rückprojizierten Schichten zeigen keine Details, die Aktivitätsanteile in den einzelnen Objektschichten sind in allen Schichtbildern überlagert. Die rekonstruierten Schichten zeigen die echte Aktivitätsverteilung. SCHMIDLIN trägt darüber bereits 1971 vor (s. SCHMIDLIN 1973).

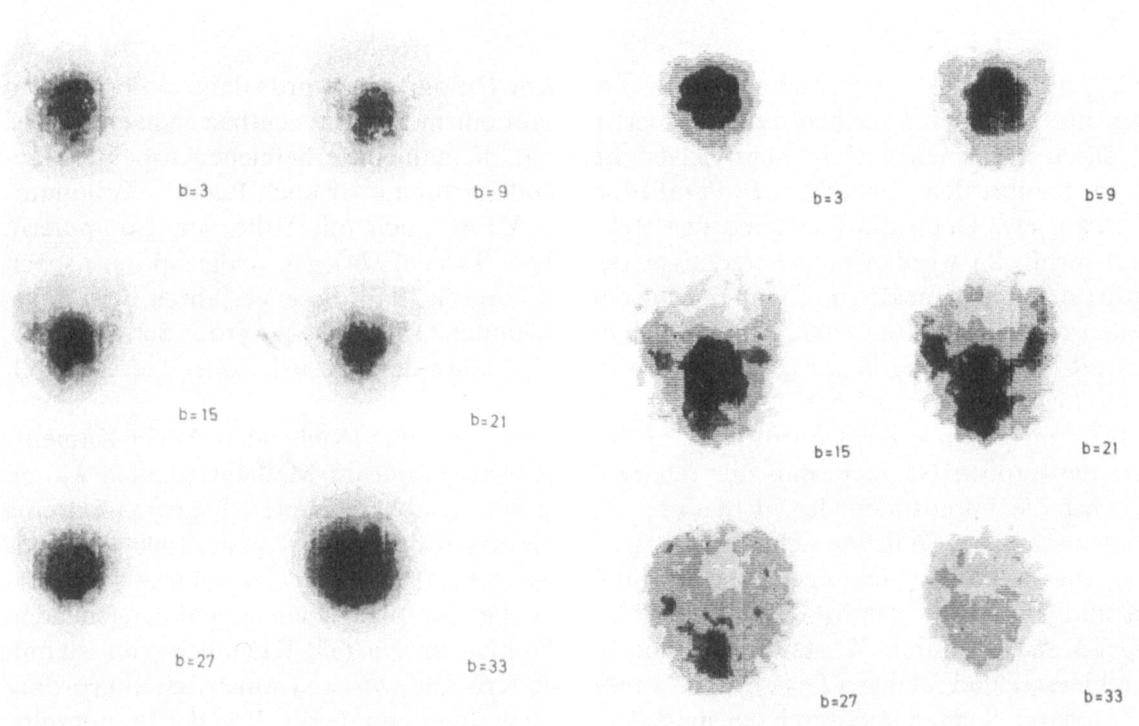

Abb. 17a, b. Darstellung von sechs longitudinalen Schichten durch den Schädel, aufgenommen mit dem Positronenstrahler ^{18}F und zwei gegenüberstehenden Gamma-Kameras in Koinzidenz. **a** sechs Schichten mit einfacher Rückprojektion, **b** mit iterativer Rekonstruktion errechnet. (Aus SCHMIDLIN 1972)

Neben weiteren Arbeiten, Gilbert (1972), Goitein (1972), über iterative Rekonstruktion von transversalen Schichten, werden auch den Nebeneffekten wie Absorption und unterschiedliche Auflösung je nach Abstand vom Kollimator erhöhte Aufmerksamkeit gewidmet. So befassen sich Muehllehner u. Hashmi (1972) erstmals mit der Frage der räumlichen Auflösung in den Schichten bei verschiedenen tomographischen Systemen.

Die Anwendung holographischer Abbildungsmethoden der Optik auf die Nuklearmedizin werden erstmals beschrieben, Barrett (1972) und Rogers et al. (1972). Zwischen Objekt und Kamera-Kristall befindet sich eine Bleimaske mit dünnen ringförmigen konzentrischen Schlitzen unterschiedlichen Durchmesssers, die Nachbildung einer Fresnel-Linse für Gammastrahlung von ^{99m}Tc (s. Abb. 18).

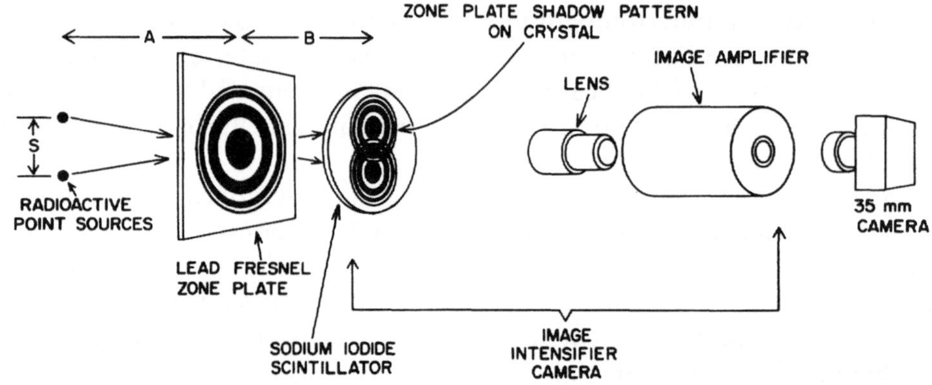

Abb. 18. Vorrichtung zur Aufnahme eines Hologramms mit Hilfe einer Fresnel-Zonenplatte aus Blei und einer Anger-Gamma-Kamera oder Bildverstärker-Kamera. (Aus Rogers et al. 1972)

Das auf einem transparenten Film aufgenommene Hologramm wurde dann auf optischem Wege mit Hilfe von Laserlicht rekonstruiert und auf einem Schirm sichtbar gemacht. Diese Verfahren erschienen zunächst sehr vielversprechend, da man eine erhebliche Ausbeutesteigerung gegenüber den sonst üblichen Parallelloch-Kollimatoren oder auch Pinhole-Kollimatoren erwartete. Doch die Probleme der Rekonstruktion, auch mit Hilfe von Computern, waren groß. So wurden bald berechtigte Bedenken (Levy 1974) gegen die optimistischen Erwartungen angemeldet mit dem entscheidenden Hinweis, daß diese Verfahren bei Punktquellen zwar gut funktionieren, bei räumlich ausgedehnten Objekten aber große Schwierigkeiten auftreten. Und so ist es geblieben, auch nach Ersatz der Fresnel Zone Platten durch unterschiedlich kodierte Lochblenden.

Die longitudinale Positronentomographie mit zwei gegenüberstehenden Anger-Kameras hatte den großen Nachteil, daß nur relativ kleine Aktivitäten im Meßfeld zulässig waren, da sonst die Impulsraten der nicht durch Kollimatoren abgeschirmten Kameras extreme Werte annahmen. So ließen sich auch nur maximale Koinzidenzraten von ca. 1000 s^{-1} erreichen. Dieses Problem umgingen Burnham u. Brownell (1972) vom Massachusetts General Hospital durch Bau der MGH Positronenkamera, bei der die beiden gegenüberstehenden Anger-Kameras durch Kristallblöcke von je 127 kleinen NaJ(Tl)-Kristallen von 20 mm Durchmesser und 38 mm Länge ersetzt waren. Die Kristalle waren symmetrisch angeordnet in Zeilen und Spalten und durch ein spezielles Kodiersystem konnte die Zahl der Photomultiplier für die 127 Kristalle auf 72 Stück begrenzt werden (Abb. 19). Das empfindliche Meßfeld betrug 30×27 cm^2 mit einer räumlichen Auflösung von kleiner 1 cm FWHM in der mittleren Ebene zwischen den Detektorblöcken. Jeder Kristall eines Meßkopfes arbeitete in Koinzidenz

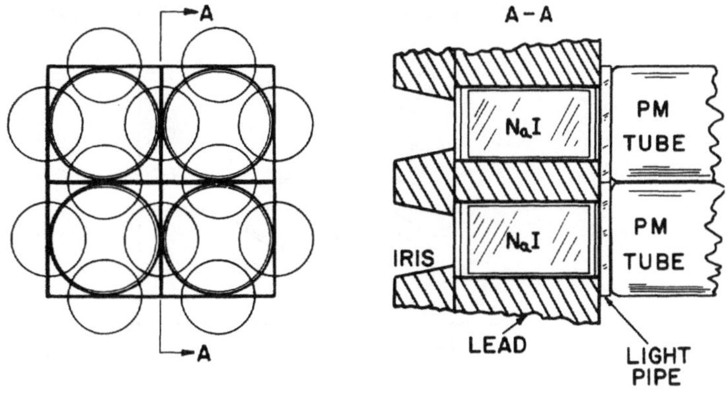

Abb. 19. Anordnung der Kristalle und Photomultiplier in der MGH Positronen-Kamera. Jeder Kristall wird von zwei Photomultipliern gesehen und jeder Photomultiplier sieht gleichzeitig vier Kristalle. (Aus BURNHAM u. BROWNELL 1972)

mit dem direkt gegenüberliegenden Kristall und seinen unmittelbaren 24 Nachbarkristallen. So wurden 2549 unterschiedliche Meßstrahlen durch das Objekt gelegt. Diese PC-I genannte Kamera ermöglichte durch einfache Rückprojektion die Fokussierung mehrerer Schichten zwischen und parallel zu den Meßköpfen. Um die räumliche Auflösung zu optimieren, war es möglich, während der Messung die Detektorblöcke gegenüber dem Objekt geringfügig zu bewegen, wobei unterschiedliche Bewegungsabläufe möglich waren (BROWNELL u. BURNHAM 1973).

Der entscheidende Vorteil dieser Kamera lag in der Fähigkeit sehr hohe Impulsraten zu verarbeiten. Eine nutzbare Koinzidenzrate von $50\,000\ \mathrm{s}^{-1}$ war möglich.

Die Tomographie mit Gammastrahlern erhält einen neuen Impuls von KUHL et al. (1973a), die auf dem IAEA-Kongreß über die Rekonstruktion mit der „Orthogonal Tangent Correction (OTC)" vortragen und damit nicht nur eine recht gute Rekonstruktion ihrer transversalen Schicht erreichen, sondern auch eine quantitative Aktivitätsbestimmung innerhalb der Schicht ermöglichen (KUHL et al. 1973b).

Das Jahr 1973:

BOWLEY et al. (1973) beschreiben den ASS – Aberdeen Section Scanner, ein universeller Scanner mit zwei Meßköpfen und vier unterschiedlichen Abtastarten (s. Abb. 20). Wenn auch die transversale Tomographie das Hauptanliegen war, so war es auch möglich, longitudinale Tomographie durchzuführen, indem nacheinander fünf Scans durchgeführt wurden mit jeweils anderer Stellung der Kollimatorachse, Positionen O, A, B, C und D in Abb. 20.

Die Daten wurden auf Lochstreifen gestanzt und eine PDP 8/I führte die einfache Rückprojektion durch. Man muß den ASS als Vorläufer der kommerziellen J & P Tomogscanner ansehen.

BUDINGER et al. (1973, 1974) setzen sich für den Fall der transversalen Tomographie mit den iterativen Rekonstruktionsmethoden auseinander und vergleichen verschiedene Algorithmen mit Hilfe von Phantomen.

Die longitudinale Tomographie mit einfacher Rückprojektion wird ausführlich diskutiert in Bezug auf die auftretenden Strukturen in den Verwischungsbildern der jeweils nicht fokussierten Schichten. So setzt sich ANGER (1973) mit der Frage der linienförmigen, kreuzförmigen, ringförmigen Verwischung bei seinem Tomographic Scanner auseinander (Abb. 21). FREEDMAN (1973) untersucht die Verwischungsbilder unabhängig von der Anzahl der Meßpositionen beim rotierenden slant hole Kollimator vor der Anger-Kamera. Auch MUEHLLEHNER (1973) setzt sich mit dieser Frage auseinander, und besonders die Diskussion zu diesem Vortrag macht deutlich, daß die Strukturen in den Verwischungsbildern häufig überbewertet

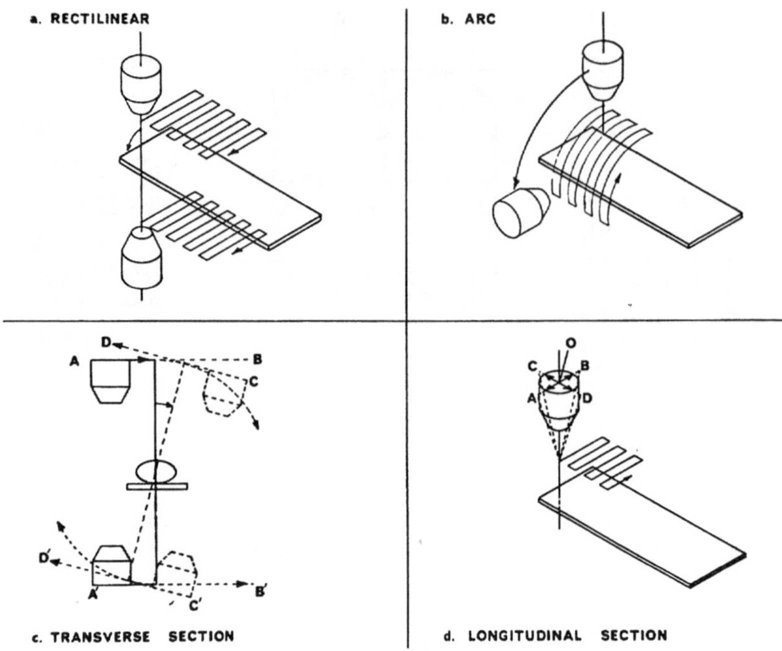

Abb. 20. Die vier verschiedenen Bewegungsabläufe des ASS – Aberdeen Section Scanner. (Aus Bowley et al. 1973)

wurden, da sie bei räumlich ausgedehnten und mehr oder weniger homogenen Objekten eine viel geringere Rolle spielten als bei den meist verwendeten Phantomen mit sehr hohem Kontrast.

Für die Positronentomographie schlagen Kaplan et al. (1973) erstmals den Einsatz von zwei gegenüberstehenden gasgefüllten Vieldraht-Proportionalkammern vor, die über eine Verzögerungsleitung zur Ortsbestimmung der Absorption ausgelesen werden.

An dieser Stelle sei noch daran erinnert, daß Lauterbur (1973) erstmals über die Messung der räumlichen Verteilung der NMR Relaxationszeiten innerhalb inhomogener Proben berichtet, und damit den Beginn der NMR-Tomographie markiert.

Das Jahr 1974:

Die longitudinale Tomographie ist nach wie vor aktuell. So realisieren Mathieu u. Budinger (1974) einen Tomoscanner, indem sie den Patienten unter einer Gammakamera mit Pinhole-Kollimator in 36 verschiedene Positionen relativ zur Kollimatorachse verschieben, wobei die Positionen auf einem rechtswinkligen Netz mit 2 cm Maschenweite liegen. Ein kleiner Computer HP-5407 ermöglichte die Rückprojektion der Einzelaufnahmen (Abb. 22).

Jordan et al. (1974) stellen ihren Longitudinalen Emissions Multikristall Tomoscanner LEMT vor, der ähnlich dem Prinzip des Tomographic Scanner von Anger einen Meßkopf mit fokussierenden Eigenschaften aufweist. 60 einzelne Szintillationsmeßsonden mit je einem austauschbaren fokussierenden Kollimator (s. Abb. 23b), sind so angeordnet, daß sich die Achsen der 60 Einzelkollimatoren in einem Fokus schneiden (s. Abb. 23a). Dieser Meßkopf wird wie üblich in zeilenförmiger Scanbewegung über dem Objekt verschoben. Die Rückprojektion der einzelnen longitudinalen Schichten erfolgt im Computer, die Darstellung mit einem schnellen Plotter (Jordan u. Geisler 1972). Die Konstanz der 60 Sonden wurde ebenfalls per Rechner überwacht, der auch das automatische Setzen der Energieschwelle durchführte (Jordan u. Gettner 1977).

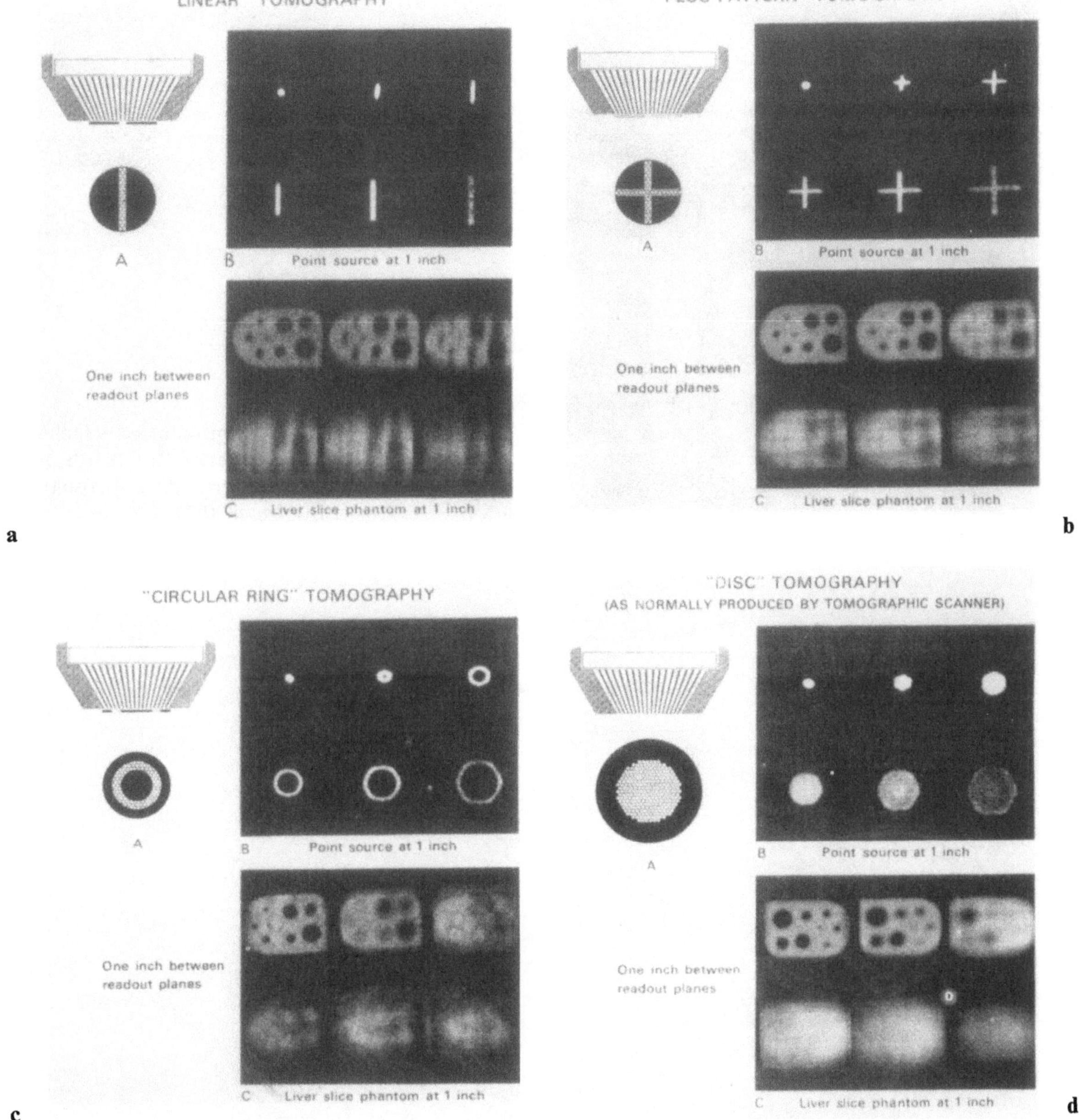

Abb. 21a–d. Die Struktur von Verwischungsbildern beim Tomographic-Scanner, bei **a** linienförmiger, **b** kreuzförmiger, **c** ringförmiger und **d** scheibenförmiger Verwischung. Sie wurde realisiert durch entsprechende Teilabdeckung des fokussierenden Kamerakollimators. (Aus ANGER 1973)

Da gegenüber dem Tomographic Scanner von ANGER keinerlei Ortungsfehler in der Kamera auftreten konnten, war die räumliche Auflösung sehr gut, z.B. für 10 cm Kollimatorabstand 5,4 mm, 7 mm bzw. 11 mm FWHM bei Bestückung mit Fein-, Mittel- bzw. Grobfokus-Kollimatoren. Der Einfluß der Sondenanordnung auf die Struktur der Verwischungsbilder ließ sich nach dieser Anordnung besonders einfach untersuchen, da jeweils entweder alle oder beliebige Anordnungen von Sonden an der Messung bzw. Rückprojektion beteiligt werden konnten.

Auch die Abbildung über kodierte Aperturen wurde weiter verfolgt, wobei die während der Messung zeitlich veränderliche Apertur erstmals vorgeschlagen wurde. So berichten TANAKA u. IINUMA (1974, 1976) über eine rotierende Schlitzapertur (Abb. 24).

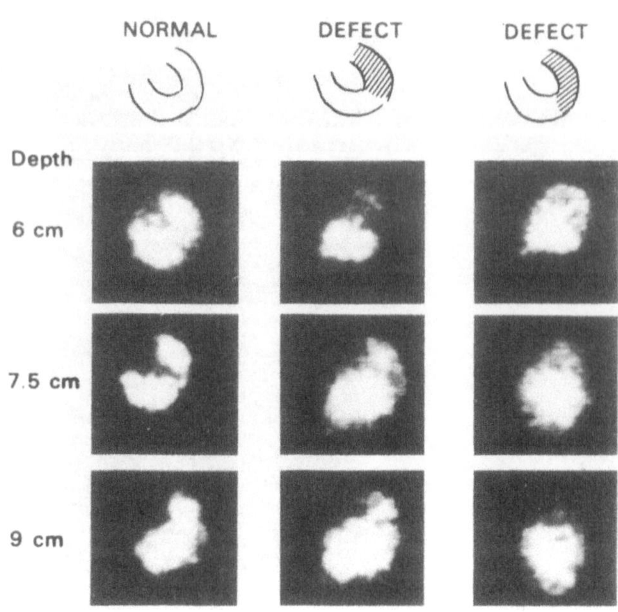

Abb. 22. Darstellung longitudinaler Schichten des mit ^{81}Rb angereicherten Myokards mit Hilfe einer Pinhole-Kamera. (Aus Mathieu u. Budinger 1974)

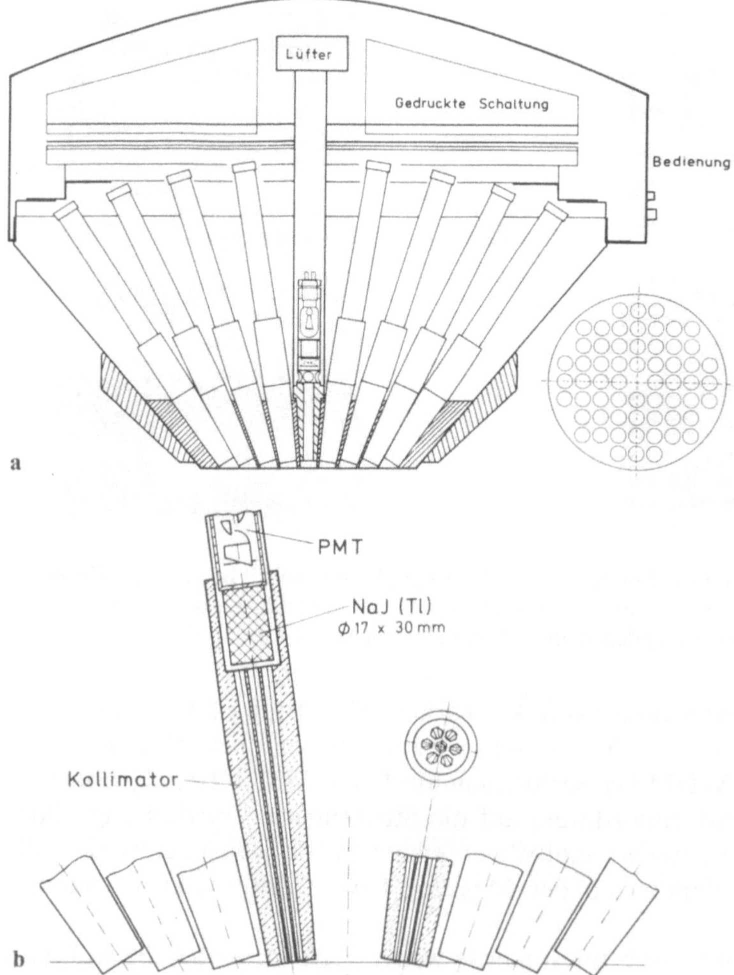

Abb. 23a, b. Longitudinaler Emissions Multikristall Tomoscanner LEMT. **a** Schnitt durch den Meßkopf in einer Hauptachse zeigt die Anordnung von 8 der insgesamt 60 kollimierten Meßsonden, deren Achsen sich alle in einem Fokus schneiden; **b** Schnitt durch die Kollimatoren der einzelnen Meßsonden

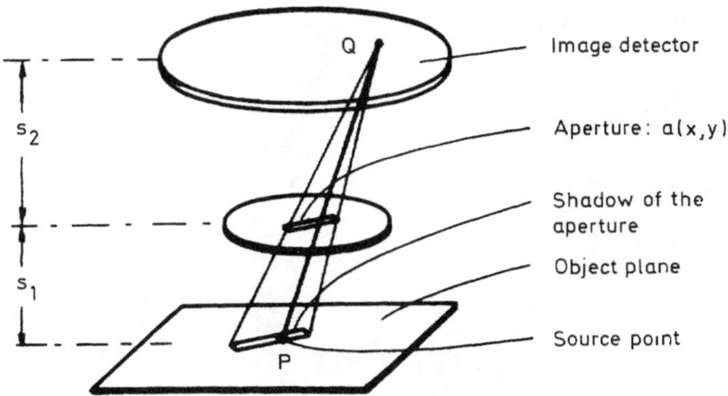

Abb. 24. Abbildung mit einer kodierten Aperture in Form eines Schlitzes, wobei der Schlitz um seinen Mittelpunkt in einer Ebene parallel zur Detektorebene rotiert. (Aus TANAKA u. IINUMA 1974)

Interessant ist hier auch die Arbeit von BARRETT u. DE MEESTER (1974), die schon sehr deutlich auf die Probleme der Abbildung mit kodierten Aperturen bei räumlich ausgedehnten Objekten hinweisen, während bei einzelnen Punktquellen diese Verfahren gute Ergebnisse liefern.

Die dreidimensionale Rekonstruktion per Computer nimmt immer konkretere Formen an, wobei allerdings die iterativen Methoden noch bevorzugt werden, und die Anwendung auf transversale Tomographie beschränkt bleibt (BUDINGER u. GULLBERG 1974a, b).

Die Einbeziehung der Absorptionskorrektur in die Rekonstruktion sowie der Hinweis, daß nur die iterativen Methoden dies ermöglichen, ist hier interessant.

In diesem Jahr stellen auch NESTOR u. HUANG (1975) auf dem 21st Nuclear Science Symposium die guten Eigenschaften von $Bi_4Ge_3O_{12}$-Kristallen (BGO) im Vergleich zu NaJ(Tl) heraus. Diese BGO-Kristalle lösen in den Folgejahren besonders bei ringförmigen Positronen-Kameras die NaJ(Tl)-Kristalle weitgehend ab.

Das Jahr 1975:

Die Versuche, mit Hilfe kodierter Aperturen tomographische Abbildungen zu erzeugen, dauern an. So schlagen KORAL et al. (1975) vor, anstelle eines Pinhole-Kollimators eine Bleiplatte mit vielen unregelmäßig angeordneten Löchern während der Messung zwischen Objekt und Kamerakristall zu verschieben (s. Abb. 25). Sie erzielen ein verbessertes Signal zu Rauschverhältnis, vertreten aber auch die Meinung, daß ein echter Gewinn nur bei punktförmigen Aktivitätsanreicherungen zu erzielen ist.

Eine Anwendung der Apertur-Abbildung auf die transversale Tomographie schlägt erstmals PRICE (1975) vor. In seinem CCA-System (cylindrically shaped coded aperture) befinden sich zwischen Objekt und dem umgebenden Detektorring zwei zylindrische Bleimasken mit abwechselnd für die Gammastrahlung transparenten und undurchlässigen Abschnitten (s. Abb. 26). Dieses nur auf dem Computer simulierte System versprach zunächst enorme Vorteile gegenüber bestehenden Systemen, die dann von ihm selbst relativiert wurden (PRICE 1978, 1979). Auch wurde die Doppelmaske durch eine einfache Ringmaske ersetzt. Hauptvorteile sollen die hohe Nachweiswahrscheinlichkeit und die absolute Aktivitätsbestimmung im Objekt sein. Das System wurde noch nicht realisiert.

Für die tomographische Abbildung mit einer Fresnel-Zonen-Platte geben BUDINGER u. MACDONALD (1975) einen digitalen Rekonstruktionsalgorithmus, mit gutem Ergebnis für punktförmige Quellen.

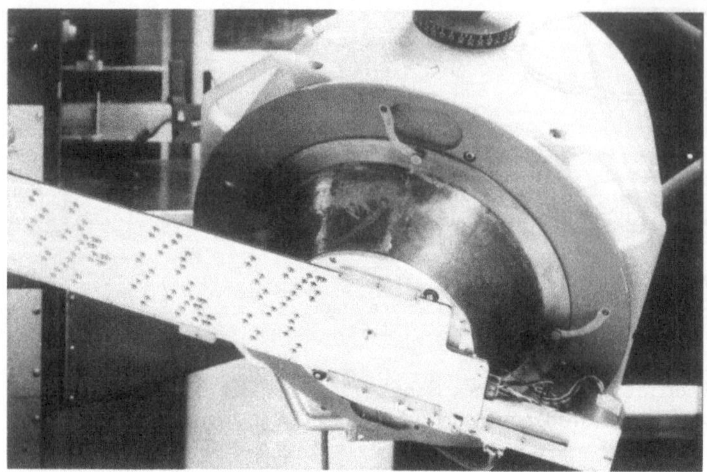

Abb. 25. Tomographische Kamera mit einer zeitlich veränderlichen statistisch verteilten Lochanordnung. Die längliche Bleiplatte von 2 mm Dicke mit Löchern von 3,6 mm Durchmesser wurde während der Messung vor dem Kamerakristall verschoben. (Freundlicherweise von J.W. Keyes, Jr. zur Verfügung gestellt)

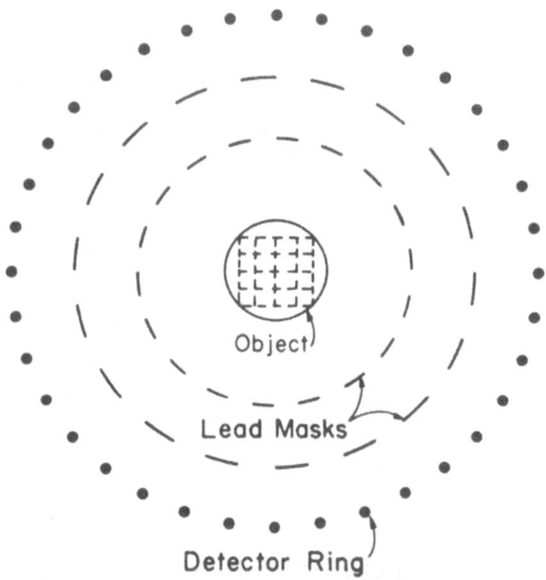

Abb. 26. Das CCA – System. Die Aktivitätsverteilung des Objektes wird über zwei zylindrische Bleimasken mit entsprechenden Schlitzen auf einen äußeren Ring vom Gamma-Detektoren abgebildet. (Aus Price 1975)

Die transversale Positronentomographie in Form ringförmiger Detektoranordnungen beginnt nach den ersten Anfängen im Jahre 1972 endgültig Gestalt anzunehmen. Ter-Pogossian et al. (1975) und Phelps et al. (1975a) beschreiben erstmals den PETT (Positron Emission Transaxial Tomograph). 24 Szintillationsdetektoren in sechs Blöcken á 4 Sonden in hexagonaler Ringform angeordnet umgeben das Objekt (Abb. 27). Jeweils sich exakt gegenüber stehende Sonden wurden in Koinzidenz betrieben, so daß 12 Meßstrahlen simultan durch das Objekt gelegt wurden, welches in 7,5° Schritten um 180° bzw. 360° gedreht wurde. Die Rekonstruktion erfolgte über gefilterte Rückprojektion in einem Interdata 70 Minicomputer.

Parallel zur hexagonalen Anordnung des PETT werden erstmals die Möglichkeiten einer gleichmäßigen Ringanordnung hoher räumlicher Auflösung mit sehr vielen Sonden untersucht (Derenzo et al. 1975). Eine Studie über einen Ring mit 288 NaJ(Tl)-Kristallen von 8 mm Breite führt zu einer Auflösung von 4–7 mm in einer Schicht von 30 cm Durchmesser. Jeder Kristall wird mit 62 gegenüberstehenden in Koinzidenz betrieben, das ergibt 8928

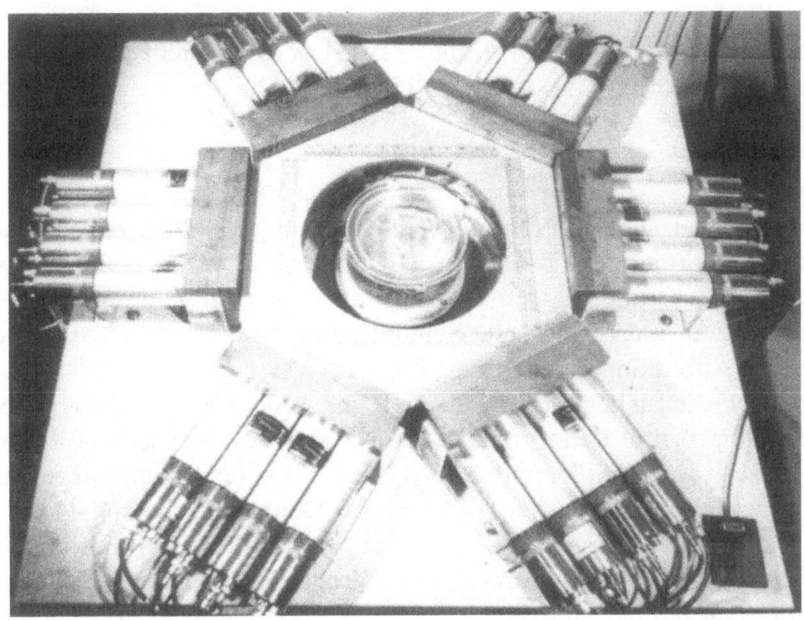

Abb. 27. Prototyp des PETT. 24 Szintillationssonden mit 2″ × 2″ NaJ(Tl)-Kristallen, in sechs Blöcken hexagonal angeordnet, umgeben das Objekt, welches drehbar im Zentrum angeordnet ist. (Aus Ter-Pogossian et al. 1975)

Meßstrahlen durch das Objekt. Eine spezielle Kodierung mit Hilfe von jeweils zwei getrennten Lichtleitern pro Kristall, die zu verschiedenen Photomultipliern führten, ermöglichte den Betrieb mit insgesamt nur 72 Photomultipliern und 12 Koinzidenzstufen. Diese Einsparung ist übrigens später beim realisierten Donner-Ring wieder fallengelassen worden.

Cho et al. (1976) berichten auf dem 22nd Nuclear Science Symposium über das Konzept ihrer Circular Ring Transverse Axial Positron Camera (CRTAPC) mit 72 NaJ(Tl)-Kristallen von 2 cm Durchmesser und 3,8 cm Höhe. Jeder Detektor war mit seinen 23 gegenüberliegenden Detektoren in Koinzidenz geschaltet.

Für die gasgefüllten Vieldrahtkammern schlagen Jeavons et al. (1975) einen Konverter vor, der die Nachweiswahrscheinlichkeit auf 5% erhöht für 662 keV Gammaquanten. Chu et al. (1976) berichten noch im gleichen Jahr über eine Positronenkamera mit zwei gegenüberstehenden Kammern von 25 × 25 cm² Fläche (s. auch Chu et al. 1977).

Das große Problem der extrem hohen Impulsraten bei Realisierung eines Positronentomographen mit Hilfe von zwei gegenüberstehenden Anger-Kameras ohne Kollimatoren, versucht Muehllehner (1975) mit Hilfe von speziell abgestuften Strahlenfiltern vor den Kameras zu verringern. Ihre Aufgabe war es, die Primärstrahlung von 511 keV möglichst wenig, die niederenergetische Streustrahlung aus dem Objekt aber möglichst stark zu schwächen.

Kuhl et al. (1975) bestimmen erstmals mit Hilfe ihres Mark III Scanners das lokale zerebrale Blutvolumen, indem sie ^{99m}Tc markierte rote Blutkörperchen i.v. injizieren.

Die Frage der Reichweite von Positronen im Gewebe und ihr Einfluß auf die erzielbare räumliche Auflösung wird diskutiert (Phelps et al. 1975b; Cho et al. 1975). Während dieser Effekt als gering eingestuft wird, weist Muehllehner (1976) in einer Stellungnahme hierzu auf die Tatsache hin, daß der Winkel von 180° zwischen den beiden Emissionsrichtungen der 511 keV-Quanten nicht konstant ist, sondern nach einer Gauß-Verteilung mit 0,6° Halbwertsbreite streut. Diese Tatsache sei kritischer bezüglich der räumlichen Auflösung als die endliche Reichweite der Positronen.

Eine ausführliche Übersicht über die Theorie der Rekonstruktion bei der transversalen Tomographie wird von BROOKS u. DI CHIRO (1975) veröffentlicht und im folgenden Jahr in erweiterter Form wiederholt (BROOKS u. DI CHIRO 1976).

Das Jahr 1976:

Dieses Jahr wird beherrscht von der Weiterentwicklung der Positronentomographie. Die transversale Positronenkamera CRTAPC an der Universität von Californien wird optimiert (ERIKSSON u. CHO (1976)) und im Herbst des Jahres tragen CHO et al. (1977a, b) über die 64-Kristallversion vor und zeigen erste Schichtaufnahmen von Pankreas, Herz und Leber mit N-13-L-alamine. Abbildung 28 zeigt das CRTAPC System.

HOFFMAN et al. (1976) stellen den PETT III vor, eine hexagonale Anordnung von 48 NaJ(Tl)-Kristallen von 51 mm Durchmesser und 76 mm Länge in sechs Blöcken á 8 Kristallen. Abbildung 29 zeigt die ringförmige Anordnung mit einer Patientenöffnung von 51 cm. Der Abstand von gegenüber stehenden Blöcken von Detektoren betrug 111 cm. Das größte Meßfeld hatte 48 cm Durchmesser und die räumliche Auflösung innerhalb dieser Schicht betrug 14 mm FWHM. Erste Aufnahmen von Hirn, Herz (getriggert), Leber und Nieren werden gezeigt, bei Aufnahmezeiten von 10–15 min und Injektion von ^{13}NH$_3$ bzw. Einatmung von ^{11}CO (Abb. 30). Über weitere Beispiele berichten PHELPS et al. (1976) und PHELPS et al. (1977) auf dem IAEA-Symposium, sowie TER-POGOSSIAN et al. (1977).

Auf dem 23nd Nuclear Science Symposium geben DERENZO et al. (1977) eine detaillierte Beschreibung des 280-Kristall Donner-Ringes mit NaJ(Tl)-Kristallen von 8 mm × 30 mm Eintrittsfläche und 50 mm Dicke. Die Ankoppelung an die einzelnen Photomultiplier erfolgt über speziell geformte Quarz-Lichtleiter. Als räumliche Auflösung in der Schicht werden 7,5 mm FWHM im Zentrum genannt. Nutzimpulsraten bis 10000 s^{-1} sind möglich.

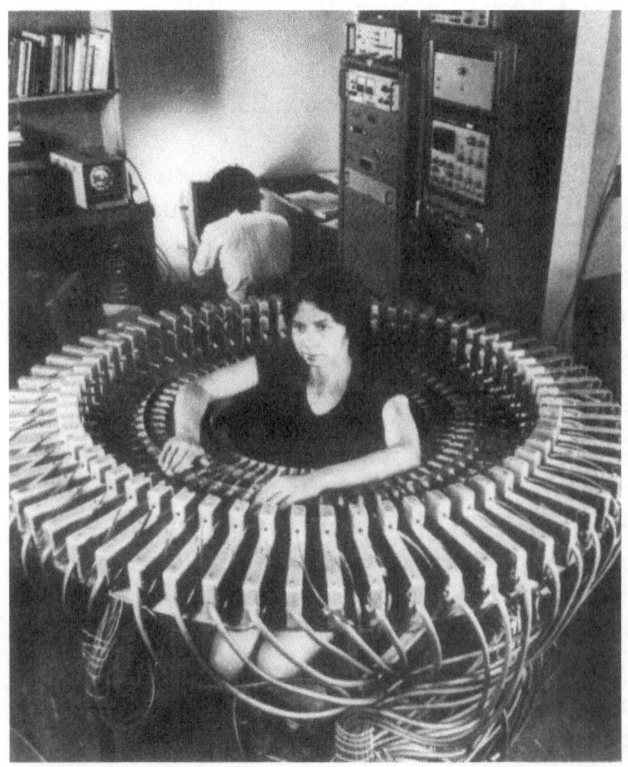

Abb. 28. Gesamtansicht der CRTAPC Positronen-Kamera der UCLA mit 64 NaJ(Tl)-Kristallen. (Aus CHO et al. 1977a)

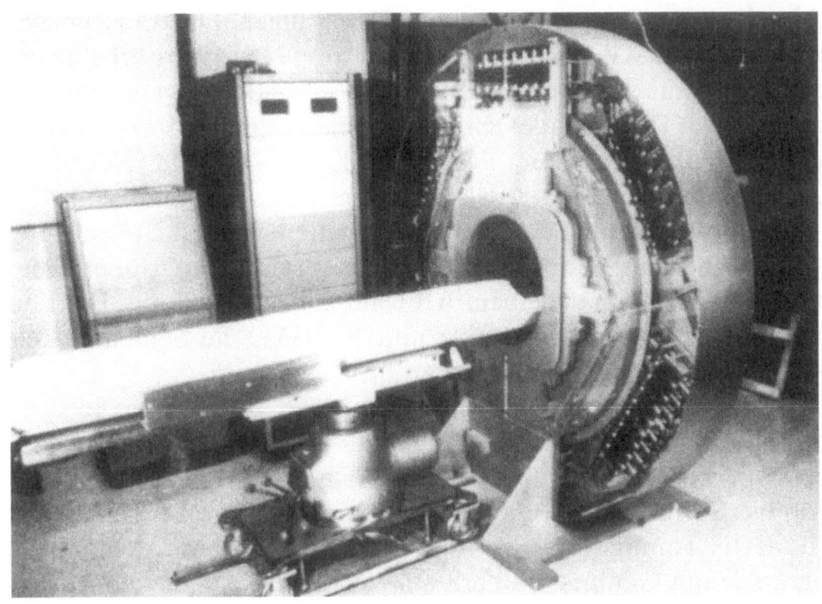

Abb. 29. Der PETT III. Ein Ganzkörper-Positronen-Tomograph zur Aufnahme und Darstellung einer transversalen Schicht. (Aus HOFFMAN et al. 1976)

MUEHLLEHNER et al. (1976, 1977) stellen die Positronenkamera mit zwei gegenüberstehenden Kameraköpfen in Koinzidenz vor, die sowohl statisch longitudinale Schichten als auch, um den Patienten rotierend, transversale Schichten erzeugt. Zwei Großfeldkameras mit 39 cm Meßfelddurchmesser und 25 mm Kristalldicke ergeben eine hohe Empfindlichkeit von 200 Imp/sec/µCi. Durch die Anwendung von Strahlenfiltern (s. MUEHLLEHNER 1975) und einer speziellen schnellen Impulselektronik konnten klinisch nutzbare Impulsraten von 8000 s^{-1} erreicht werden.

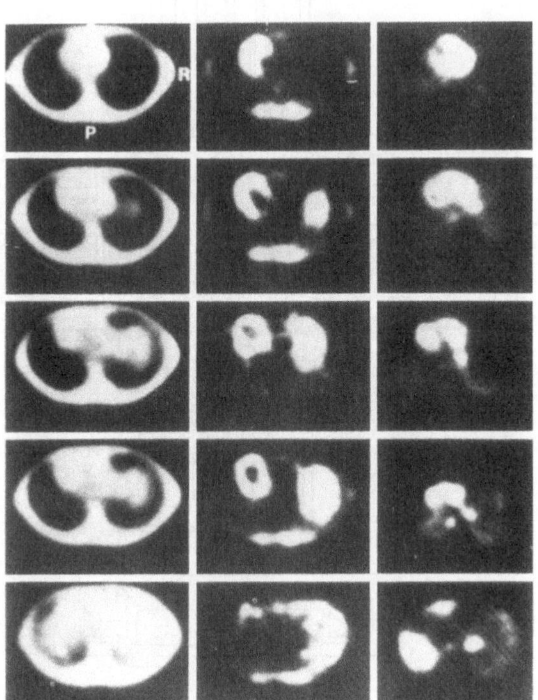

Abb. 30. Schichtaufnahmen des Herzens mit dem PETT III. Linke Spalte Transmissions-Schichtbilder, mittlere Spalte Perfusionsstudie mit $^{13}NH_3$, rechte Spalte blood pool, Darstellung mit ^{11}CO. Schichtabstand 1,5 cm. (Aus PHELPS et al. 1976)

Auf dem Gebiet der SPECT zeigen sich einige Neuerungen. Die transversale Tomographie wird durch den neuen Mark IV Scanner (Kuhl et al. 1976, 1977) erheblich verbessert. Er ist jetzt mit 32 Sonden bestückt, die in vier Blöcken à 8 Sonden angeordnet sind (s. Abb. 31). Es wurden eckige NaJ(Tl)-Kristalle eingesetzt mit einer Strahleneintrittsfläche von 75×25 mm^2 und einer Höhe von 25 mm. Vor jedem Kristall war ein fokussierender Kollimator angeordnet. Gegenüber stehende Kristalle hatten einen Abstand von 47 cm. Es wurde nur noch eine Rotationsbewegung um 360° in Schritten von 2,5° durchgeführt innerhalb von 50 sec, wobei üblicherweise fünf Umdrehungen zu einem Bild überlagert wurden. Die Rekonstruktion erfolgte iterativ nach einem ART ähnlichen Verfahren. Die räumliche Auflösung in der Schicht lag zwischen 16 und 18 mm FWHM, die Schichtdicken zwischen 17 und 20 mm FWHM.

Kuhl et al. (1977) berichten erstmals auf dem IAEA Symposium in diesem Jahr über den Einsatz von F-18-Fluorodeoxyglucose (FDG) zur lokalen Bestimmung des Glukosestoffwechsels im Hirn in Verbindung mit ihrem Mark IV.

Der Tomographic Scanner von Anger ist inzwischen kommerziell lieferbar unter der Bezeichnung PHO/CON Tomographic Multi-Plane Scanner. Damit steht ein Gerät zur longitudinalen Tomographie mit Gammastrahlern zur Verfügung. Da die Schichtbilder nur durch einfache Rückprojektion auf photographischem Wege gewonnen werden, ist der damit erzielbare klinische Fortschritt begrenzt (s. Turner et al. 1976a,b).

Erstmals wird über eine iterative Rekonstruktion bei der longitudinalen Tomographie mit Gammastrahlern von Lottes u. Jordan (1978a) berichtet, die bei ihrem Tomoscanner LEMT das ART-Verfahren anwenden.

Über den Einsatz der Fourier-Transformation zur Rekonstruktion bei der longitudinalen Tomographie berichten Chang et al. (1976). Doch hier sind die Probleme wegen des begrenzten Raumwinkels groß.

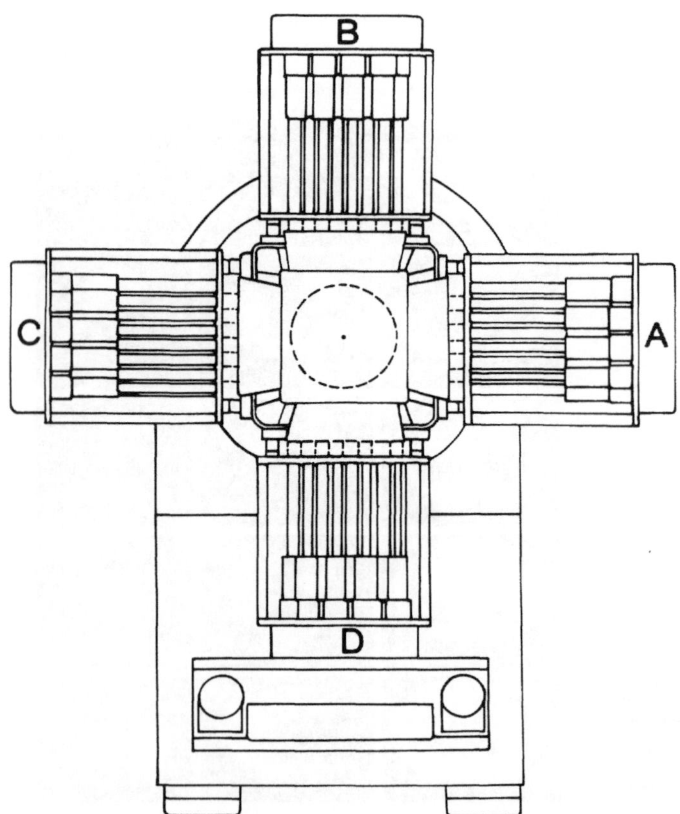

Abb. 31. Der Mark IV-Scanner mit 32 kollimierten Einzelsonden zur Aufnahme von transversalen Hirnschichten mit Gamma-Strahlern. (Freundlicherweise von D.E. Kuhl zur Verfügung gestellt)

Halbleiterdetektoren finden erstmals Anwendung in einem Tomoscanner. PATTON et al. (1977) berichten auf dem IAEA Symposium über einen longitudinalen Tomoscanner mit 9 Germanium-Detektoren von je 35 mm Durchmesser und 10 mm Dicke (Abb. 32). Die Ausbeute ist niedrig und der tomographische Effekt ist gering wegen des kleinen Neigungswinkels der Meßstrahlen und der einfachen Rückprojektion (s. auch PATTON et al. 1978).

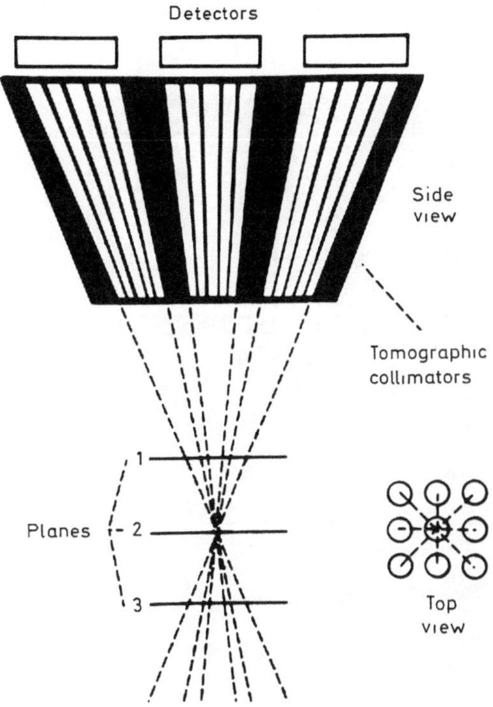

Abb. 32. Tomoscanner mit neun Germanium-Detektoren und einem fokussierenden Kollimator. (Aus PATTON et al. 1977)

Das Jahr 1977:

In diesem Jahr erscheinen einige bemerkenswerte Übersichtsarbeiten, die sich sowohl mit der Beschreibung des Standes der apparativen Entwicklung, als auch mit der Frage des Nutzens der ECT befassen. BUDINGER et al. (1977a) stellen die Tomographie mit Gammastrahlern und Positronenstrahlern gegenüber. Interessant ist hier unter anderem die Aussage, daß zum Beispiel bei Einsatz einer Positronen-Ringkamera nur 20% aller auftretenden 511 keV-Photonenpaare aus einem mit Wasser gefüllten Zylinder von 20 cm Durchmesser ohne Streuung und Absorption austreten. Zum Vergleich treten die viel niederenergetischeren Gammaquanten von ^{99m}Tc unter gleichen Bedingungen zu 40% aus (s. auch Abb. 73).

PHELPS (1977b) setzt sich mit der Emissions-Computertomographie allgemein auseinander und stellt die Unterschiede von SPECT und PCT heraus. TER-POGOSSIAN (1977) faßt die Prinzipien der transversalen Computertomographie zusammen und stellt dabei erstmals das Konzept einer sehr wesentlichen Weiterentwicklung des PETT III zum PETT IV vor.

Dieser Ringtomograph bot erstmals die Möglichkeit der simultanen Aufnahme mehrerer nebeneinander liegender Schichten, ohne daß sich der materielle Aufwand wesentlich erhöhte (s. auch TER-POGOSSIAN et al. 1978a und Abb. 36).

PHELPS (1977a) fragt in einer weiteren Übersicht ganz generell nach dem Wert der ECT für die Nuklearmedizin. Die Aussagen, daß SPECT den Vorteil hat, daß es mit einer großen Zahl von Radiopharmaka, meist mit ^{99m}Tc markiert, arbeiten kann, während die PCT die bessere Auflösung besonders bei großen Organen (Ganzkörperaufnahmen) und die exaktere Absorptionskorrektur ermöglicht, haben auch heute noch Gültigkeit.

Bei der transversalen Tomographie mit Gammastrahlern (SPECT) setzt sich die rotierende Gammakamera durch. KEYES Jr. et al. (1977) berichten über ihr Humongotron. Ein Pho/Gamma HP Kamerakopf rotiert mit Hilfe eines speziell konstruierten Statives 360° um den Patienten mit wählbaren Geschwindigkeiten bis max. eine Umdrehung pro min. Das Inkrement für die Datensammlung lag meist zwischen 6° und 12° (s. Abb. 33). Weitere klinische Beispiele finden sich bei BROWN et al. (1977).

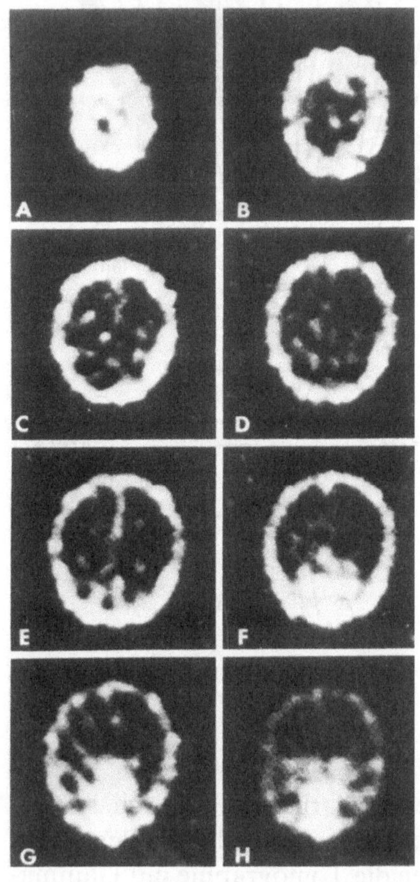

Abb. 33. Verschiedene Schichtaufnahmen des Hirns, aufgenommen mit dem Humongotron bei Gabe von 15 mCi ^{99m}Tc Pertechnetat bei einem gesunden Patienten. (Aus KEYES Jr. et al. 1977)

JASZCZAK et al. (1977) konstruieren eine ähnliche rotierende Kamera speziell für Hirnaufnahmen. Sie sammeln Daten in 4° Inkrementen. Das Problem der Absorption und Streuung verringern sie teilweise, indem sie das geometrische Mittel jeweils gegenüber liegender Ansichten bilden (s. Abb. 34).

Die tomographische Aufnahme des Herzens mit rotierender Kamera und EKG-Triggering beschreiben BUDINGER et al. (1977b). Der Patient rotiert in sitzender Stellung vor der Kamera (Abb. 35) und es werden 72 Einzelaufnahmen mit 5° Inkrement aufgenommen. Jede Einzelaufnahme wird in acht Zeitintervalle á 100 ms Dauer gerastet. Obwohl bis zu 10 mCi appliziert werden, sind Aufnahmedauern von 60 min und mehr notwendig.

Auch mit Hilfe der Fresnel Zonenplatte und eines Röntgenfilms als Strahlungsdetektor wurden Schichtaufnahmen von Hundeherzen aufgenommen (HOLMAN et al. 1977).

Auf der 15. Jahrestagung der Gesellschaft für Nuklearmedizin wird der Tomoscanner MS 425-CAT der Firma J & P vorgestellt (BERNARD et al. 1978). Es handelt sich um einen

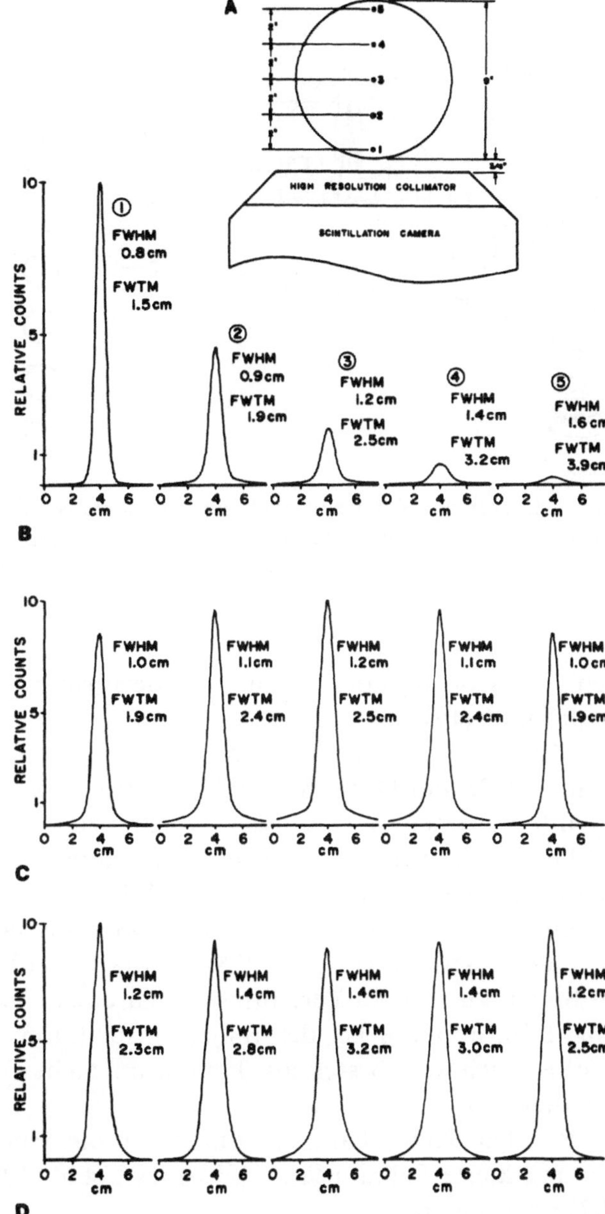

Abb. 34. A Anordnung einer ^{99m}Tc Linienquelle in fünf verschiedenen Positionen in einem Wassertank von 23 cm Durchmesser. **B** Linienbildfunktionen mit FWHM und FWTM aus einer einzelnen Meßposition gewonnen. **C** Geometrisches Mittel von jeweils genau gegenüberliegenden Meßpositionen. **D** Rekonstruktionen der Linienquellen mit Fouriertransformation. (Aus JASZCZAK et al. 1977)

transversalen Scanner mit 2 kollimierten Sonden, nach dem Prinzip von KUHL u. EDWARDS (1963) bzw. BOWLEY et al. (1973). FEINE et al. (1977) berichten über erste klinische Erfahrungen an 81 Patienten mit diesem Tomoscanner.

LOTTES u. JORDAN (1978b, c) setzen sich auf der gleichen Tagung mit dem Einfluß des Rauschens bei der dreidimensionalen iterativen Rekonstruktion nach dem ART und SIRT Verfahren auseinander und demonstrieren rekonstruierte Schichtbilder von Phantomen, aufgenommen mit dem Tomoscanner LEMT.

Schließlich stellen noch BRUNOL et al. (1978) den direkten Vorläufer des 7-pinhole-Kollimators vor. Sie verwenden 8 Pinholes auf einem Kreis von 18 cm Durchmesser in Verbindung mit einer LFOV Anger-Kamera zur Tomographie des Herzens.

Die longitudinale Abbildung über zeitlich modulierte Multi-pinhole Aperturen üblicher Art (ROSENFELD u. MACOVSKI 1977) führt bei KNOLL u. WILLIAMS (1977) zu dem Vorschlag eines transversalen ringförmigen Tomographen, wobei zwischen Patient und einem umgeben-

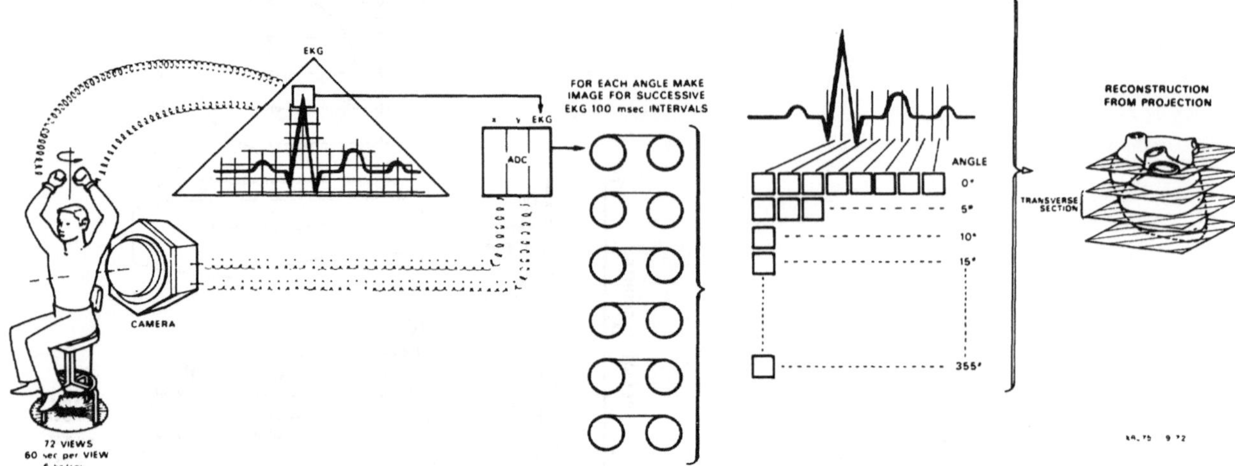

Abb. 35. Tomographische Darstellung des Herzens eines vor der Kamera rotierenden Patienten. Für jede Ansicht im 5° Abstand werden die im List-Mode gespeicherten Daten von der R-Zacke ausgehend in acht Zeitintervallen à 100 ms unterteilt und dann rekonstruiert. (Aus Budinger et al. 1977 b)

den Detektorring koaxial eine zylinderförmig kodierte Apertur gedreht wird. Siehe hierzu auch Price (1975).

Mit den Rekonstruktionsproblemen der transversalen Tomographie setzen sich Keyes et al. (1977) und Huesman (1977) auseinander, wobei letzterer besonders die Probleme bei unvollkommener Datenerfassung (begrenzter Raumwinkel etc.) bespricht.

Die transversale Positronen-Tomographie wird bezüglich der Geräteentwicklung durch den Ersatz der NaJ(Tl)-Kristalle durch BGO-Kristalle geprägt. Cho u. Farukhi (1977) geben nochmals eine ausführliche Analyse beider Kristalle und stellen die Vorteile von BGO heraus (s. auch Nestor u. Huang 1975). Budinger (1977) prophezeit erstmals den großen Gewinn an Signal zu Rausch-Verhältnis bis zu einem Faktor 10 durch Einbeziehung der Time-of-Flight Information bei der Bildrekonstruktion. Dabei geht er davon aus, daß sich TOF-Auflösungen von besser als 3 cm wohl nicht realisieren lassen, womit er bis heute recht behalten hat.

Bei den Radiopharmaka findet für die Herzdarstellung ^{82}Rb (Yano et al. 1977), die ^{11}C markierte Palmitinsäure (Hoffman et al. 1977) und ^{13}N Ammoniak (Brownell et al. 1977) Anwendung.

Yamamoto et al. (1977) berichten über zerebrale Messungen an über 120 Patienten mit dem 32 Kristall Positronenring des Brookhaven National Laboratory (s. Robertson et al. 1973). Sie injizieren ^{68}Ga-EDTA zur Messung der Transit Time und für Verteilungsstudien, und lassen ^{77}Kr inhalieren für quantitative rCBF Studien.

Die Frage der exakten quantitativen Bestimmung der Aktivitätskonzentration in vivo gewinnt immer mehr an Bedeutung, und mit der transversalen Positronentomographie gelingt dies mit erstaunlicher Genauigkeit, wie z.B. Eichling et al. (1977) mit Phantommessungen am PETT beweisen.

Auf dem 24th Nuclear Science Symposium stellen Bohm et al. (1978) ihren Positronen-Ring-Tomographen PC-95 vor, mit 95 NaJ(Tl)-Kristallen von 8 mm × 20 mm Eintrittsfläche und 50 mm Dicke und 1900 simultanen Koinzidenzabfragen. Neu ist hier eine wobbelartige Bewegung des Ringes um sein Zentrum, so daß alle Kristalle gleichzeitig eine Bewegung auf dem Umfang eines kleinen Kreises ausführen. Damit wird eine sehr gleichmäßige Abtastung der Objektschicht erreicht. Eine Auflösung von 6,5 mm FWHM innerhalb der Schicht wurde gemessen (s. auch Ter-Pogossian et al. 1978 b).

Das Jahr 1978:

Die Erkenntnis, daß die Zukunft der Nuklearmedizin nicht in der bildlichen Darstellung der Morphe, sondern in der Diagnostik funktioneller Abläufe in vivo liegt, setzt sich immer mehr durch (WAGNER Jr. 1978; ELL et al. 1978; HUNDESHAGEN 1979). Entsprechend verläuft auch die Weiterentwicklung der Tomographie.

Die ringförmigen Positronen-Tomographen erhalten immer mehr Einzelkristalle, um Ausbeute und Auflösung ohne Ringbewegung zu erhöhen und die gleichzeitige Aufnahme mehrerer Schichten wird realisiert. TER-POGOSSIAN et al. (1978a) und MULLANI et al. (1978) stellen den PETT IV, eine Weiterentwicklung des PETT III, vor. Die simultane Aufnahme von sieben Schichten wird dadurch erreicht, daß die einzelnen NaJ(Tl)-Kristalle jetzt in Zylinderform mit 5 cm ∅ und 17,5 cm Länge so angeordnet werden, daß sie quer zur Schichtebene orientiert sind und an ihren Stirnflächen je einen Photomultiplier tragen (s. Abb. 36). Dadurch wird es möglich, jeder Absorption im Kristall einem bestimmten der vier Kristallbereiche zuzuordnen (lineare Anger-Ortung). Durch geeignete Bleiblenden, als auch durch Koinzidenzabfrage direkt gegenüberliegender Kristallbereiche (Linie b in Abb. 36) werden vier Hauptschichten festgelegt. Durch zusätzliche Schrägabfrage (Linie a und c in Abb. 36) zwischen benachbarten Adressenbereichen werden noch drei Zwischenschichten erfaßt. Die vier Hauptschichten haben eine Dicke von 16 mm FWHM im Zentrum und 17 mm in 10 cm Entfernung vom Zentrum. Für die Zwischenschichten betragen die entsprechenden Werte 12 mm und 17,5 mm FWHM. Die räumliche Auflösung innerhalb der Schicht lag bei 15 mm FWHM bzw. 12 mm mit zusätzlichen Kollimatoren. Neben den transversalen Schichten konnte der Rechner auch koronare oder sagittale Schichten berechnen mit einer Pixelgröße von $4,8 \times 4,8$ mm^2.

Neben diesem Ganzkörpertomograph entstand noch im selben Jahre der PETT V, ein spezieller Hirntomograph (TER-POGOSSIAN et al. 1978b). Die konsequente Verkleinerung des Meßfeldes auf 25 cm Durchmesser und die symmetrische Anordnung der 48 Meßsonden

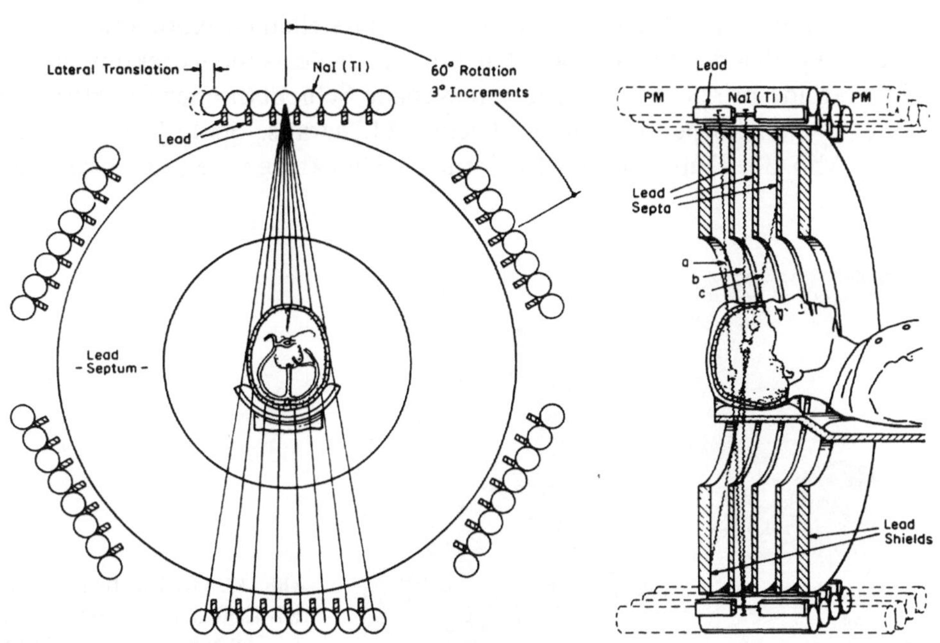

Abb. 36. Die Anordnung der Meßsonden und der Bleiblenden beim PETT IV. Mit Hilfe von zwei Photomultipliern (*PM*) an den jeweiligen Stirnflächen der zylinderförmigen Kristalle, wird der Absorptionsort längs des Kristallzylinders bestimmt. (Aus TER-POGOSSIAN et al. 1978a)

auf einem Ring von 60 cm Durchmesser zeichnen dieses Gerät aus. Es werden nach dem gleichen Prinzip wie beim PETT IV simultan sieben Schichten gemessen, wobei der Ring nur noch eine kleine Rotationsbewegung und zusätzlich eine Wobbelbewegung um sein Zentrum ausführt (s. auch BOHM et al. 1978). Die kürzeste Aufnahmezeit beträgt 1 s. Die Empfindlichkeit wird mit einer Impulsrate von $50\,000\ \mathrm{s}^{-1}$ für eine Aktivitätskonzentration von $1\ \mu\mathrm{Ci/cm}^3$ in einem Phantom mit 20 cm Durchmesser angegeben. Mit dem PETT IV werden nur $40\,000\ \mathrm{s}^{-1}$ unter gleichen Bedingungen erreicht.

CHO et al. (1978) greifen das Mehrschicht-Prinzip des PETT IV auf, ersetzen NaJ(Tl)-Kristalle durch BGO und stellen in einer Entwurf-Studie ein Ringkonzept vor, das sowohl für Positronen-Emmissionstomographie, als auch in Verbindung mit einer rotierenden Röntgenröhre für Transmissionstomographie geeignet ist.

Die kommerzielle Ausführung des PETT III der ECAT der Fa. Ortec Inc., Oak Ridge, wird von PHELPS et al. (1978) ausführlich beschrieben. Gegenüber dem PETT III werden hier 66 NaJ(Tl)-Kristalle mit 3,8 cm $\varnothing$ und 7,5 cm Dicke in sechs Blöcken á 11 Detektoren angeordnet, mit insgesamt 363 Koinzidenzabfragen. Das Meßfeld hat 50 cm Durchmesser und die Kristalle haben einen Abstand von 100 cm. Drei verschiedene Auflösungen sind wählbar. Neben der tomographischen Schichtdarstellung können auch übliche zweidimensionale Scans angefertigt werden, indem der Patient per Liege durch den Ring geschoben wird, und jeweils direkt gegenüberstehende Detektorblöcke in Koinzidenz betrieben werden. So entstehen drei Scans unter verschiedenen Ansichten, und zwar eine ventral-dorsal und zwei dazu um 60° geneigte Ansichten.

Von der Cyclotron Corporation wird die Positronen Kamera Model 4200 angeboten (CARROLL 1978). Es ist die kommerzielle Ausführung der MGH Positronen Kamera PC II von BROWNELL et al. (1978). Zwei gegenüberstehende Detektorblöcke von je 140 NaJ(Tl)-Kristallen, die auf einem rechteckigen Gitter mit einer Maschenweite von 28 mm angeordnet sind. Die Anordnung der Photomultiplier ist ähnlich wie bei der PC I (s. Abb. 19). Im Rotationsbetrieb beider Köpfe können bis zu 23 transversale Schichten simultan aufgenommen werden, mit einer Schichtdicke von 14 mm FWHM. Die Rekonstruktion erfolgt durch Rückprojektion gefilterter Projektionen. Im Stillstand lassen sich vier longitudinale Schichten zwischen den Köpfen durch einfache Rückprojektion darstellen (s. Abb. 37).

Auch auf dem Gebiet der SPECT werden kommerzielle Neuentwicklungen vorgestellt. Die Fa. Union Carbide bringt interessante transversale Schichtscanner für Hirnaufnahmen, Cleon 710, und für Ganzkörperaufnahmen, Cleon 711, heraus. Beide Geräte arbeiten nach dem Prinzip der Abb. 38. Durch die großvolumigen Detektoren wird eine verhältnismäßig

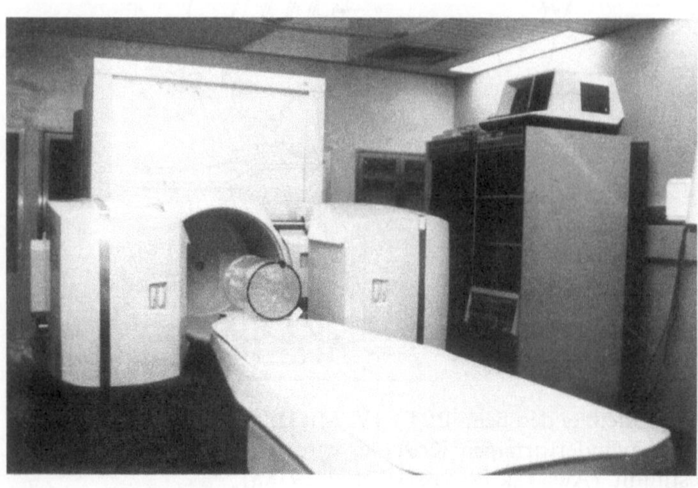

Abb. 37. Die Positronen-Kamera Model 4200 der Cyclotron Corporation, in Betrieb an der Medizinischen Hochschule Hannover. Sie entspricht der PC II vom Massachusetts General Hospital

hohe Meßempfindlichkeit und durch die Verschiebung des Fokus der Kollimatoren durch die Objektschicht hindurch eine große Gleichmäßigkeit an Auflösung und Schichtdicke erreicht. Über erste klinische Erfahrungen berichten HILL et al. (1978) unter Anwendung von ^{99m}Tc-DPTA bei Hirnaufnahmen, und HOLMAN et al. (1979) unter Verwendung von ^{201}Tl bei Herzaufnahmen.

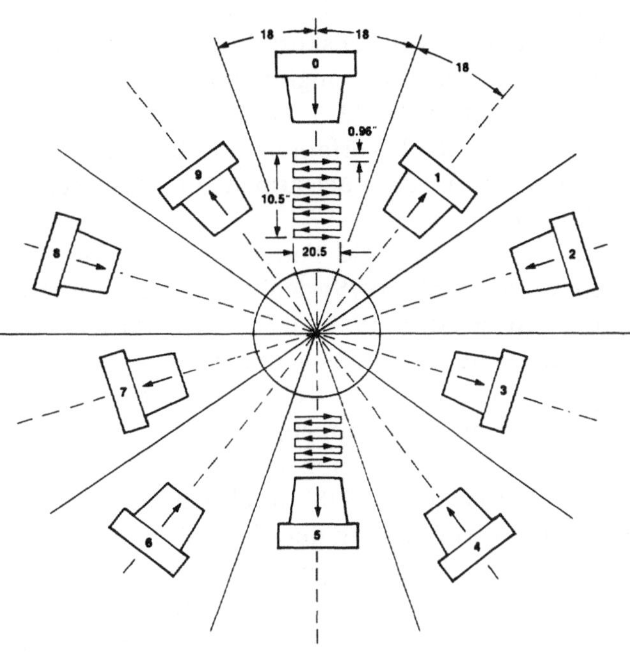

Abb. 38. Prinzip der Detektoranordnung beim Cleon 710/711. Die einzelnen Meßsonden (10 Stück beim Cleon 711, 12 Stück beim Cleon 710) mit großen 20 cm × 13 cm NaJ(Tl)-Kristallen von 2,5 cm Dicke haben fokussierende Kollimatoren. Sie sind in der Schichtebene ringförmig angeordnet und führen neben der Drehbewegung mit 18° Inkrement eine zeilenförmige Scanbewegung in der Schichtebene durch, wobei sich gegenüberstehende Sonden wechselseitig auf das Objekt zu bzw. davon weg bewegen. (Aus Firmenprospekt der Fa. Union Carbide)

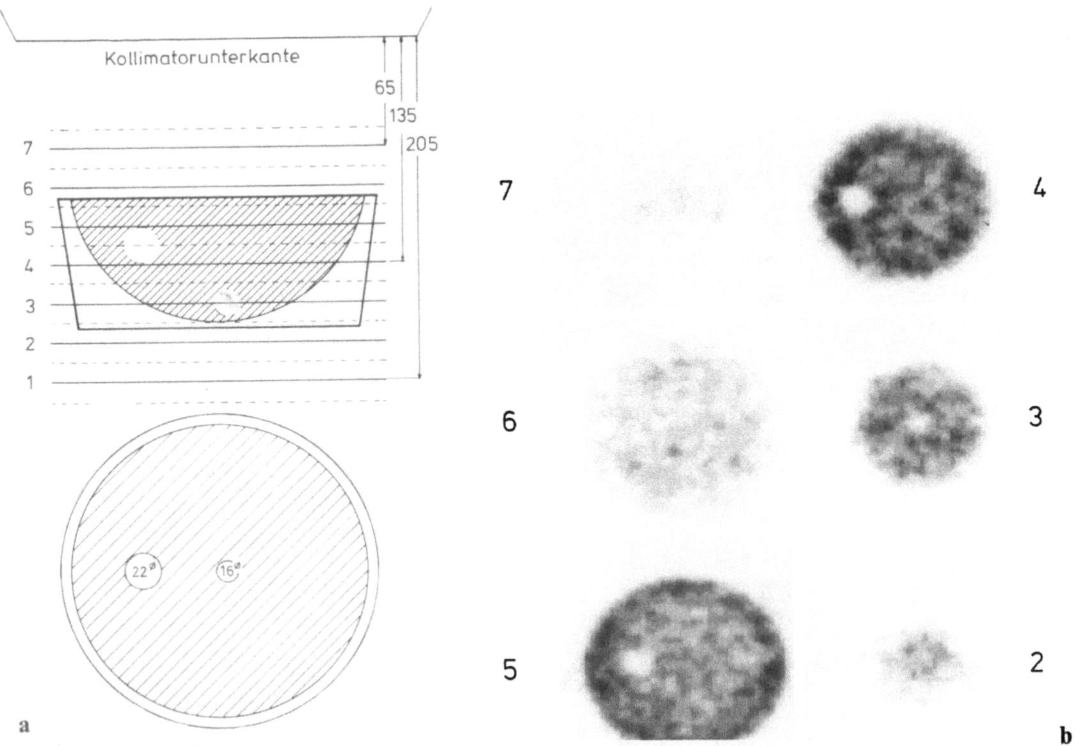

Abb. 39a, b. Schichtaufnahmen mit dem LEMT bei iterativer Rekonstruktion nach dem SIRT-Verfahren. **a** großvolumiges aktives Phantom in Form einer Kugelkalotte mit zwei „kalten Knoten". **b** rekonstruierte longitudinale Schichten, deren Lagen im linken Bild eingezeichnet sind

Der Tomogscanner II der Firma J & P löst als Weiterentwicklung mit grundsätzlich gleichem Konzept den Tomoscanner MS 425-CAT ab.

Über den erfolgreichen Einsatz der rotierenden Gamma-Kamera zur Myokarddarstellung mit ^{99m}Tc Pyrophosphat bzw. ^{201}Tl berichten Keyes Jr. et al. (1978a, b).

Mit den Problemen des Rauschens bei quantitativen Aktivitätsbestimmungen in transversalen Schichten setzten sich Budinger et al. (1978) und Tsui u. Budinger (1978) auseinander. Probleme der Absorptionskorrektur bei SPECT bespricht Chang (1978).

Auf dem Gebiet der longitudinalen Tomographie mit Gamma-Strahlern Untersuchungen Lottes u. Jordan (1979a) die dreidimensionalen iterativen Rekonstruktionsverfahren und bewerten das SIRT-Verfahren am besten, und demonstrieren auf der 16. Jahrestagung der Gesellschaft für Nuclearmedizin entsprechende Beispiele (Lottes u. Jordan 1979b) (s. Abb. 39).

Für die longitudinale Tomographie kleiner Objekte, etwa bis zur Größe eines Herzens, stellen Vogel et al. (1978) den 7-pinhole-Kollimator vor. Bei diesem Verfahren, ebenso wie auch schon bei Brunol et al. (1978), werden über mehrere Lochaperturen separate Bilder des Objektes auf dem Kristall einer Großfeld-Kamera erzeugt und zwar unter verschiedenen Sichtwinkeln. Die Rekonstruktion mehrerer longitudinaler Schichten erfolgt nach einem iterativen Verfahren (s. Abb. 40).

Mit der Rekonstruktion bei der longitudinalen Tomographie mit Positronen-Strahlern setzen sich Tam et al. (1978) durch Anwendung einer Dekonvolutionsmethode und Lim et al. (1978) durch Anwendung iterativer Methoden auseinander.

Eine ebenfalls neuartige Meßanordnung für eine dreidimensionale Positronen-Kamera schlagen Nickels u. Meyer (1978) vor. Sie gehen davon aus, in langen zylindrischen stabförmigen Szintillatoren mit je einem schnellen Photomultiplier an den beiden Stirnflächen durch Flugzeitmessung den Absorptionsort im Szintillator ausreichend genau bestimmen zu können. Läßt sich dann noch durch Flugzeitmessung zwischen zwei solchen Szintillatorstäben

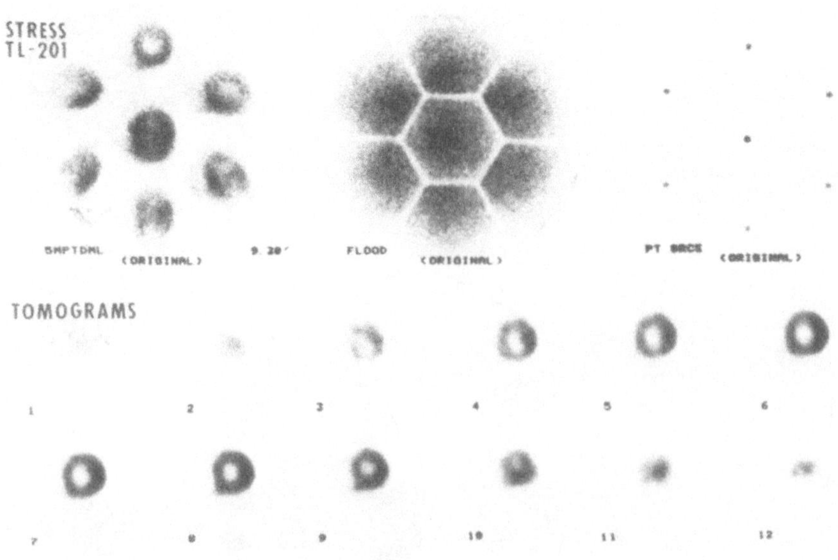

Abb. 40. Abbildungen mit dem 7-Pinhole-Kollimator. *Oben links:* Abbildung des Myokards durch die 7 Pinholes. *Oben Mitte* bzw. *rechts:* Abbildung einer Flächenquelle bzw. einer Punktquelle. *Unterer Bildteil:* 12 rekonstruierte Schichten von je 11 mm Dicke durch das Myokard. (Freundlicherweise von R. Vogel zur Verfügung gestellt)

der Emissionsort bestimmen, so wird eine dreidimensionale Ortung im Raum unmittelbar möglich, d.h., ohne jegliche Rekonstruktion. Diese zunächst bestechende Methode ist praktisch nicht realisierbar, da durch die großen Laufzeitstreuungen der Lichtquanten innerhalb der langen Szintillatoren die erzielbare räumliche Auflösung sehr schlecht ist, wie umfangreiche Messungen von JORDAN u. GETTNER (1982) und JORDAN et al. (1982) bewiesen haben.

RUSINEK et al. (1978) kommen in einer theoretischen Studie zu dem Schluß, daß für die Rekonstruktion der ^{133}Xe-Verteilung im Hirn eine sphärische Anordnung von 200 Detektoren rund um den Kopf am optimalsten sei, wobei Aktivitätskonzentrationen von 1 μCi/cm^3 völlig ausreichen.

Das Jahr 1979:

Die transversale Tomographie mit zwei rotierenden Gamma-Kameras findet mehr und mehr Anwendung (JASZCZAK et al. 1979a; MURPHY et al. 1979; BURDINE et al. 1979). Interessant ist hier auch der Einsatz eines speziellen ‚fan beam' Kollimators, an Stelle des Parallellochkollimators, (JASZCZAK et al. 1979b). Abbildung 41 zeigt die Charakteristik dieses Kollimators. Eine Verbesserung der Auflösung auf 11,5 mm FWHM gegenüber einem hochauflösenden Parallellochkollimator mit 14 mm FWHM und gleiche bis leicht erhöhte Ausbeute sind die Vorteile.

Von Erfolgen beim Einsatz der Cleon-Schichtscanner (STODDART u. STODDART 1979) wird sowohl beim Herzen (HOLMAN et al. 1979) als auch beim Hirn berichtet (JARRITT et al. 1979).

FIRUSIAN u. SCHMIDT (1979) setzen den Tomoscanner 425-CAT der Firma J & P bei 113 Leberpatienten ein und berichten von einer Verbesserung, während die Leistungen des Vorläufermodells, des Aberdeen Section Scanner (BOWLEY et al. 1973), in einer Studie über 512 Hirnpatienten unter Beweis gestellt werden (CARRIL et al. 1979).

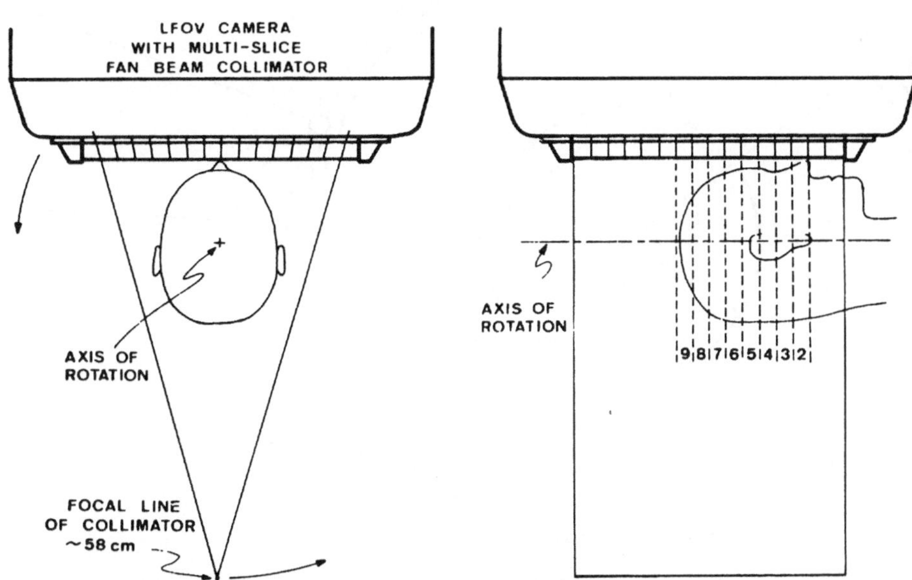

Abb. 41. Der fan beam-Kollimator bei der rotierenden Anger-Kamera. Konvergierendes Verhalten innerhalb jeder transversalen Schicht (*links*), übliche Parallellochkollimatoren längs der Rotationsachse (*rechts*). (Aus JASZCZAK et al. 1979b)

Vogel et al. (1979) berichten über die Leistung des 7-pinhole-Kollimators an einer Gruppe von 65 Herzpatienten. Die Aufnahmedauer einschließlich Rekonstruktion beträgt 15 Minuten.

Die Idee von Price (1975, 1978, 1979) und Knoll u. Williams (1977) nimmt immer mehr Gestalt an, nämlich einen ringförmigen Tomographen für Gammastrahler mit Hilfe der codierten Apertur-Abbildung zu realisieren. Während Price bis jetzt die Anordnung nur auf einem Rechner simuliert hat, beginnen Williams et al. (1979) bzw. Williams u. Knoll (1979) einen ersten Prototyp aufzubauen und nennen ihn SPRINT (Single Photon Ring Tomograph) (s. Abb. 42).

Erste Rekonstruktionen von Punktquellen erscheinen Erfolg versprechend, wie sich räumlich ausgedehnte Quellen verhalten bleibt abzuwarten. Zur Rekonstruktion bietet sich das iterative ART-Verfahren an (Koral u. Rogers 1979). Die Rechnersimulation von Price (1979) ergibt eine gute Darstellung auch von kalten Knoten, allerdings unter der Annahme von hochauflösenden Detektoren ($<1\%$ Energieauflösung) zur Ausschaltung von Streustrahlung.

Auf dem Gebiet der Positronenmeßtechnik wird neben der Beschreibung von Aufbau und Leistung bekannter Geräte Brownell et al. (1979) für die MGH Positron Camera PC II, Derenzo et al. (1979) für den Donner Ring Tomographen, Williams CW et al. (1979) für den ECAT-II, das Positome-II von Thompson et al. (1979) vorgestellt. Es handelt sich um die Weiterentwicklung zu einem 2-Ring System mit je 64 BGO-Kristallen, mit einer Eintrittsfläche von 18×30 mm^2 und 30 mm Dicke. Der Meßfelddurchmesser beträgt 30 cm bei 20 mm Schichtdicke. Drei Schichten werden simultan gemessen. Das Gerät wird von der Atomic Energy of Canada Ltd unter der Bezeichnung „Therascan 3128" zum Kauf angeboten.

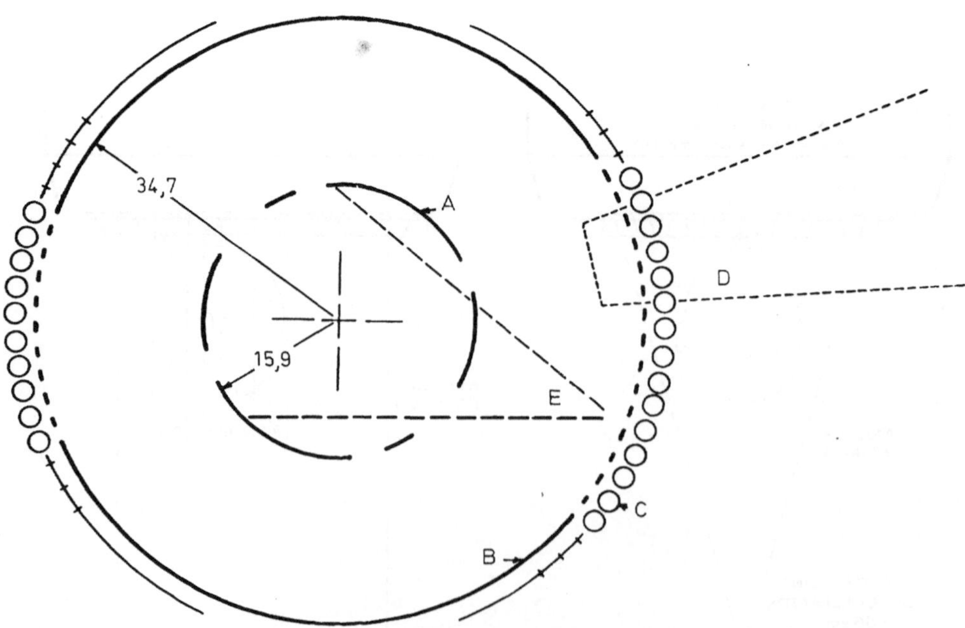

Abb. 42. Die ringförmige Anordnung des SPRINT. *A* ringförmige Bleiblende mit schlitzförmigen Aperturen. Rotiert um das Objekt im Inneren; *B* Bleiblenden vor den fest stehenden NaJ(Tl)-Kristallen, zur Festlegung der Schicht; *C* Detektoren; *D* gedruckte Schaltung für je 5 Detektoren *E* ungefährer Sichtwinkel eines einzelnen Detektors. (Aus Williams et al. 1979)

Über mehrere interessante Anwendungen der Positronen-Tomographie wird berichtet. PHELPS et al. (1979) setzen den ECAT ein zur quantitativen Bestimmung des zerebralen Blutvolumens mit ^{11}C markierten roten Blutkörperchen und HOFFMAN et al. (1979b) berichten über die getriggerte Herzaufnahme zur Herzinnenraum- und Myokard-Darstellung mit dem ECAT. SYROTA et al. (1979) verwenden den ECAT bei 32 Pankreaspatienten in Verbindung mit ^{11}C-Methionin.

Mit der MGH Positron Camera PC-II wird der regionale pulmonale Blutfluß durch Einatmung von ^{15}O markiertem Kohlendioxyd bestimmt (NICHOLS et al. 1979) und die regionale myokardiale Durchblutung mit ^{68}Ga markiertem Albumin Mikrosphären abgeschätzt (BELLER et al. 1979).

Ganz allgemein wird in diesem Jahr besonders der quantitativen Aktivitätsbestimmung in vivo starke Beachtung geschenkt. Die Einflüsse der Absorption im Gewebe und Möglichkeiten zu deren Korrektur werden untersucht sowohl für Gammastrahler (CHANG 1979; GULLBERG 1979; KEYES 1979; LOTTES u. JORDAN 1980) als auch für Positronenstrahler (HOFFMAN et al. 1979a; HUANG et al. 1979).

Der Einfluß des Raumwinkels, unter dem das Objekt gemessen wird (CHANG 1979; INOUYE 1979; NALCIOGLU et al. 1979; TAM et al. 1979; WOOD et al. 1979), und der begrenzten Anzahl von Meßstrahlen auf quantitative Messungen wird analysiert (HUANG et al. 1980; HOFFMAN et al. 1979c; LLACER 1979).

Einen umfassenden Überblick über den Stand der Emissions-Computertomographie geben BUDINGER et al. (1979a). Hier werden sowohl die bekannten Verfahren beschrieben, als auch ihre individuellen Probleme und Schwächen analysiert.

Das Jahr 1980:

Das Jahr 1980 kann man als den Beginn einer neuen Ära der Positronen-Tomographie ansehen. Der Einsatz der Flugzeitmessung zur Bestimmung des Emissionsortes von Positronenstrahlern im dreidimensionalen Raum beginnt möglich zu werden durch einen sehr schnellen Szintillator hoher Dichte, das Cäsiumfluorid CsF, mit ca. 10facher Koinzidenzausbeute wie vergleichbare schnelle Plastikszintillatoren. Obwohl CsF schon von VAN SCIVER u. HOFSTAEDTER (1952) beschrieben wird, berichten erst in diesem Jahr drei Gruppen unabhängig voneinander über den möglichen Einsatz in der Positronenmeßtechnik (ALLEMAND et al. 1980; JORDAN u. GETTNER 1981; MULLANI et al. 1980a, b).

Durch Messung des Zeitunterschiedes zwischen dem Eintreffen der beiden Gammaquanten der Vernichtungsstrahlung in den gegenüberstehenden Detektoren, kann der Emissionsort auf der Verbindungslinie beider Detektoren bestimmt werden. Dies gelingt unter realistischen Meßbedingungen zunächst mit Ortsauflösungen von kleiner 5 cm FWHM (s. JORDAN u. GETTNER 1981) (Abb. 75).

Auch mit HP Ge Halbleiterdetektoren lassen sich Auflösungen von 10 cm FWHM erreichen (KAUFMAN et al. 1980).

Interessant bei der Weiterentwicklung der Positronenkameras sind auch die Bemühungen, die Unterteilung in eine immer größer werdende Zahl kleinster Kristalle zu umgehen durch Einsatz langer stabförmiger Kristalle und elektronischer Bestimmung des Absorptionsortes durch eindimensionale Angerortung. MUEHLLEHNER u. COLSHER (1980) schlagen einen hexagonalen Ring vor, der aus sechs NaJ(Tl)-Stäben von 5×5 cm^2 Querschnitt und 40 cm Länge gebildet wird (s. Abb. 43). Die großen Probleme der hohen Impulsraten pro Detektor werden durch spezielle Impulsverkürzung und kurze Koinzidenzzeiten gemildert.

Der Einsatz von großflächigen Vieldraht-Proportionalkammern als Positronenkamera wird stetig weiter verfolgt. So berichten TOWNSEND u. ZANELLA (1980) und JEAVONS et al. (1981) über eine Positronenkamera mit zwei gegenüberstehenden 20×20 cm^2 Kammern mit

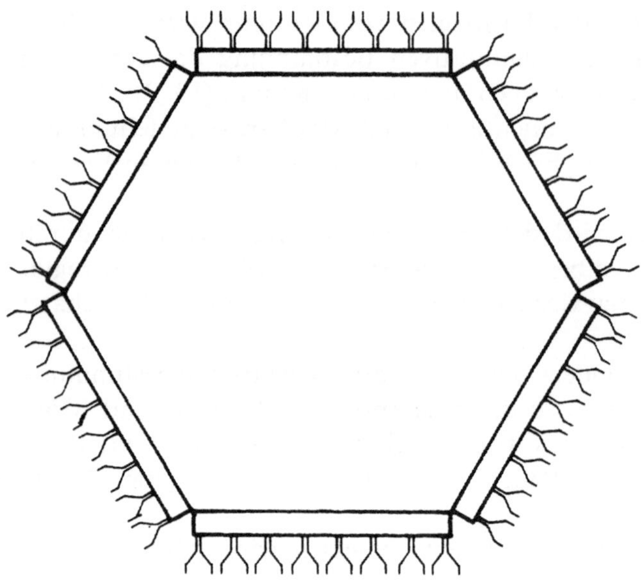

Abb. 43. Hexagonale Anordnung von 6 stabförmigen NaJ(Tl)-Kristallen von 40 cm Länge bei einer Positronen-Kamera. Jeder Kristall ist mit 7 Photomultipliern zur Bestimmung des Absorptionsortes bestückt. (Aus Muehllehner u. Colsher 1980)

30 cm Abstand. Die Nachweiswahrscheinlichkeit der Kammer für 511 keV-Quanten wurde durch spezielle Konverter (Jeavons et al. 1975) auf 8,5% verbessert. Die Koinzidenzzeit liegt bei 20 ns und die räumliche Auflösung bei 2–3 mm. 16 longitudinale Schichten von 1 cm Dicke werden rekonstruiert. Eine interessante Kammerkonstruktion schlagen Bateman et al. (1980) vor. Sie schichten viele dünne MWPC-Kammern übereinander, wobei die trennenden Kathodenflächen aus 0,125 mm dicken und 3 mm breiten Bleistreifen bestehen, die mit 0,8 mm Abstand auf eine dünne Kunststoffolie geklebt sind. Die einzelnen Kammern mit einer Fläche von 30×30 cm^2 sind ca. 5 mm dick und 20 Kammern werden übereinander geschichtet. Sie erreichen eine Nachweiswahrscheinlichkeit von über 10% bei einer räumlichen Auflösung von 6 mm FWHM. Zwei Kammerblocks stehen sich gegenüber und Koinzidenzraten zwischen 5000 und 10000 s^{-1} werden erwartet.

Fast schon revolutionär muten die Vorschläge von McIntyre (1980a, b, c) an, eine Positronen-Ring-Kamera auf der Basis von NE 102 Plastikszintillatoren zu realisieren mit einer räumlichen Auflösung von 2,4 mm FWHM. Abbildung 44 zeigt die prinzipielle Anordnung. Die notwendige Absorptionswahrscheinlichkeit wird durch eine große Szintillatordicke von 163 mm in radialer Richtung r erreicht. Um die zwangsläufigen großen Paralaxenfehler zu vermeiden, wird diese Dicke aus 16 Einzelszintillatoren von je einer Höhe $L \approx 10$ mm zusammengesetzt, wobei jeder einzelne Szintillator über insgesamt nur 200 Photomultiplier bei total 10 Detektorringen (entspricht 163840 Szintillatoren) individuell angesprochen werden kann. Die Breite der Einzeldetektoren beträgt $W = 2$ mm am inneren, $W = 3$ mm am äußeren Durchmesser. Die Dicke $s = 4,8$ mm ergibt eine Schichtdicke von ca. 2,4 mm FWHM. Die Empfindlichkeit bei 10 Schichten und einer Ausdehnung in z-Richtung von ca. 9 cm ist vergleichbar mit der des Donner-Ringes (Derenzo et al. 1979) bei besserer räumlicher Auflösung und geringeren Kosten. Der ideale Tomograph? Man muß einer Realisierung mit Interesse entgegensehen, obwohl die Probleme der Lichtleitung sehr groß sein dürften.

Weitgehend realisiert ist der „Neuro-PET", der von Brooks et al. (1980) vorgestellt wird. Neben dem Positom-II (Thompson et al. 1979) ist es der zweite Tomograph mit BGO-Kristallen. 4 Ringe mit je 128 Kristallen, einer Eintrittsfläche von $8,25 \times 20$ mm^2 und einer Höhe von 35 mm ermöglichen die simultane Aufnahme von sieben Schichten einer Dicke von 10 mm FWHM im Zentrum, bei einer geometrischen Auflösung von 4,5 mm im Zentrum

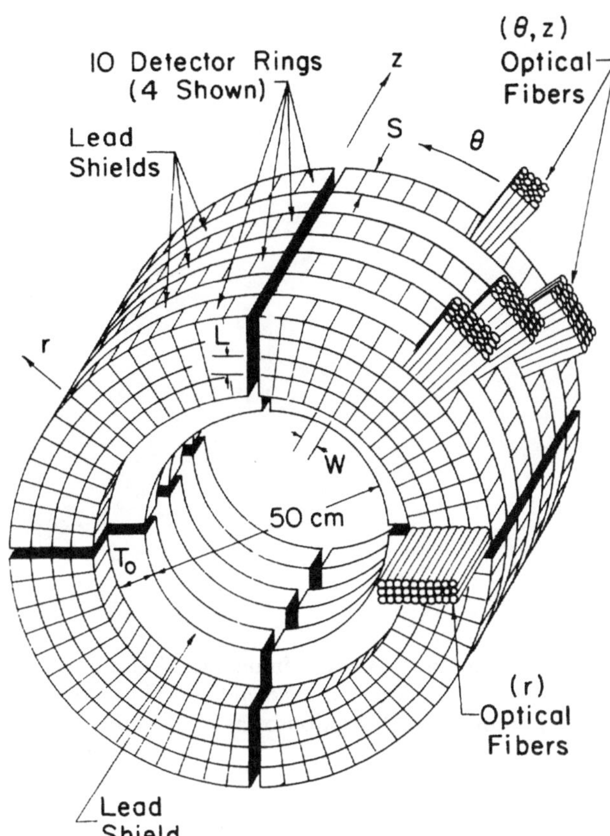

Abb. 44. Vorschlag einer Positronen-Kamera mit mehreren Detektorringen, die aus je 16 384 kleinen Plastikszintillatoren gebildet werden, deren Licht durch Lichtleitung innerhalb einer Szintillatorreihe und durch Fiberoptiken zu Photomultipliern geführt werden. (Aus McIntyre 1980b)

und 7 mm auf einen 10 cm Radius. Die Patientenöffnung ist mit 25 cm so knapp wie möglich für Hirnaufnahmen gehalten. Die gemessene Auflösung im Zentrum beträgt 6,3 mm FWHM (Brooks et al. 1982).

Ebenfalls mit BGO-Kristallen bestückt ist der Positronen-Hirntomograph „Positologica" von Nohara et al. (1980). Interessant ist hier die unregelmäßig verteilte Anordnung der 64 Kristalle auf einem Ring von 88 cm Durchmesser, der kontinuierlich mit bis zu einer Umdrehung pro sec rotiert. Dies ergibt eine sehr gute Sampling-Charakteristik. Die Kristalle haben eine Eintrittsfläche von 12×20 mm^2 bei 26 mm Höhe und die Auflösung in der Schicht wird mit 8–9 mm FWHM angegeben.

Ausführliche Beschreibungen vom Donner-Ring geben Budinger et al. (1980) bzw. Huesman u. Cahoon (1980), und vom PC-95 Ring-Tomographen wird über ein Jahr praktische Erfahrung berichtet (Eriksson et al. 1980).

Die klinische Anwendung der Positronentomographie konzentriert sich besonders auf Herz und Hirn (Schelbert et al. 1980a; Kuhl et al. 1980; Ericson et al. 1980; Frackowiak et al. 1980).

Auf dem Gebiet der transversalen Tomographie mit Gammastrahlern ist besonders die Vorstellung des „DCAT" interessant (Stokely et al. 1980), der von der dänischen Firma medimatic unter dem Namen „Tomomatic 64" vertrieben wird. Es handelt sich bei dem bereits auf dem 1st International Symposium on Positron Emission Tomography, Montreal 1978, von Lassen et al. (1978) vorgestellten Gerät um einen Hirn-Tomographen für niederenergetische Gammastrahler (<200 keV), der simultan drei Schichten mißt. 64 kollimierte NaJ(Tl)-Kristalle in vier Bänken à 16 Kristalle angeordnet (ähnlich dem Mark IV von Kuhl) rotieren in 5 Sek. um 180° um das Objekt (s. Abb. 45). Die erwartete Empfindlichkeit pro Schicht soll 57 000 imp/sec/µCi/ml betragen für ein 20 cm Durchmesser Phantom gefüllt

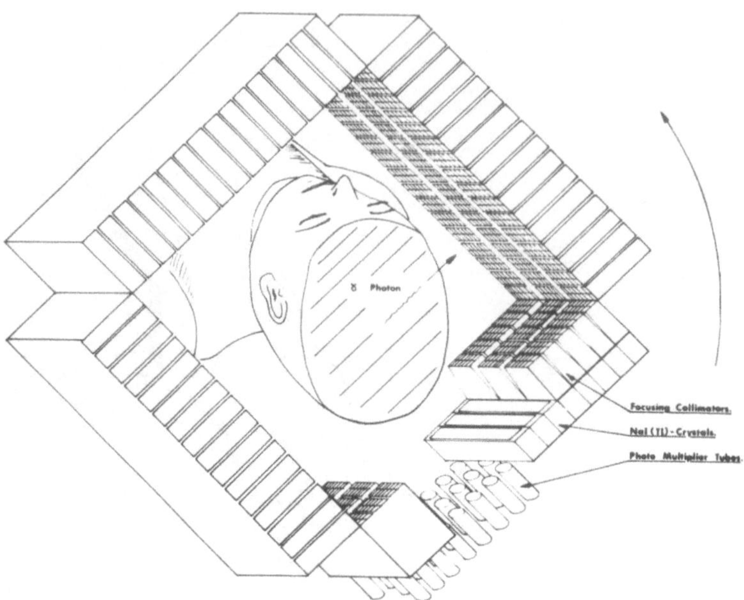

Abb. 45. Hirntomograph zur simultanen Aufnahme von 3 parallelen Schichten. 64 stabförmige NaJ(Tl)-Kristalle sind mit je drei fokussierenden Kollimatoren ausgerüstet und mehrere Photomultiplier sorgen für die Bestimmung des Absorptionsortes im Kristall. (Freundlicherweise von der Fa. Medimatic A/S zur Verfügung gestellt)

mit ^{99m}Tc, bei einer Auflösung von 17 mm im Zentrum und einer Schichtdicke von 23 mm. Über erste Anwendungen bei rCBF-Messungen mit ^{133}Xe Inhalation berichten HENRIKSON et al. (1980).

Über die Leistungen des Cleon 710 Hirn-Tomographen erscheinen mehrere Arbeiten, die sich sowohl mit den physikalischen Leistungsparametern auseinandersetzen (JARRITT et al. 1981; MCCREADY et al. 1980; FLOWER u. PARKER 1980) als auch von sehr erfolgreichem Einsatz bei der Hirnszintigraphie mit ^{99m}Tc Pertechnetat berichten (ELL et al. 1980; MCCREADY et al. 1980).

In die weiterhin positiven Berichte über den 7-pinhole-Kollimator (VOGEL et al. 1980; KIRCH et al. 1980) mischen sich auch bereits die ersten kritischen Stimmen. So weisen WILLIAMS et al. (1980) darauf hin, wie schlecht die überlagerungsfreie Trennung der einzelnen Schichten gelingt, und CHANG u. HENKIN (1980) registrieren einen sehr unterschiedlichen Schichtabstand mit zunehmender Tiefe. Die zum Teil widersprüchlichen Ergebnisse, besonders von Phantommessungen, klärt BUDINGER (1980) mit dem Nachweis, daß die Güte der Rekonstruktion von der geometrischen Form und räumlichen Orientierung des Objektes abhängt.

LOTTES u. JORDAN (1981) weisen darauf hin, daß immer dann, wenn das Rekonstruktionsvolumen in der Tiefe kleiner ist als die räumliche Ausdehnung der Aktivität im Objekt, bei der longitudinalen Tomographie unkorrigierbare Randfehler auftreten. Schließlich weisen ROLLO u. PATTON (1980) noch einmal mit aller Deutlichkeit auf die Schwächen des 7-pinhole-Kollimators hin.

ROGERS et al. (1980) kombinieren ihre Methode der Abbildung mit zeitlich modulierten codierten Aperturen mit einer kleinen portablen Kamera zu Myokardaufnahmen und geben Auflösungen in den Schichten zwischen 4 und 8 mm FWHM an, bei Schichtdicken zwischen 11 und 29 mm FWHM je nach Lage der Schicht.

Die Bemühungen, auch für den Pho/Con-Scanner eine Rekonstruktion der Schichten per Computer zu erreichen, werden besonders von PICKENS et al. (1980, 1981) fortgeführt.

Die von RUSINEK et al. (1978) erwähnte Studie über die Anordnung von 200 Detektoren sphärisch um den Schädel zur Rekonstruktion der ^{133}Xe Verteilung im Hirn hat Gestalt angenommen, und über erste Phantommessungen berichten RUSINEK et al. (1980).

Die Probleme der quantitativen Aktivitätsbestimmung werden weiter intensiv diskutiert (SOUSSALINE et al. 1981a; BERGSTRÖM et al. 1980; BRITTON et al. 1981).

Für die rotierende Kamera weisen LIM et al. (1980) noch einmal detailliert auf die Vorteile des fokussierenden Kollimators in Verbindung mit einer Großfeldkamera hin, JASZCZAK et al. (1980) geben einen ausführlichen allgemeinen Überblick über die Tomographie mit Gamma-Strahlern und LARSSON (1980) analysiert in sehr anschaulicher Weise die Probleme bei der rotierenden Kamera.

Einen ausführlichen Überblick über den Stand der tomographischen Hirnuntersuchungen mit Gamma-Strahlern geben COWAN u. WATSON (1980) und über den Einsatz der Emissions-Tomographie am Herzen SCHELBERT et al. (1980b).

Das Jahr 1981:

Der Trend zur weiteren Optimierung der Positronen-Tomographen hält unvermindert an. Dabei wird sowohl weiterhin der NaJ(Tl)-Kristall durch BGO-Kristalle (MOSZYNSKI et al. 1981; ALKHAFAJI 1981) ersetzt, als auch die Konstruktion bezüglich Ausbeute und Auflösung optimiert, d.h. für Hirnaufnahmen werden ganz spezielle Hirn-Tomographen realisiert. So stellt die Firma EG & G Ortec ihren „Neuro-ECAT" vor (WILLIAMS et al. 1981; HOFFMAN et al. 1981a). Im Gegensatz zum ECAT-II sind nicht sechs Detektorbänke hexagonal, sondern acht Bänke oktagonal angeordnet, während die Scan-Bewegungen die gleichen sind. Jede Bank enthält drei nebeneinander liegende Reihen von je 11 BGO-Kristallen mit 17×21 mm^2 Eintrittsfläche und 29 mm Höhe. Das ergibt 88 Kristalle pro Ring bzw. 264 für die drei Ringe, mit denen fünf Schichten rekonstruiert werden. Abbildung 46 zeigt den Querschnitt durch zwei gegenüberstehende Detektorbänke und die möglichen Betriebsarten. Im Betriebsmodus a beträgt die räumliche Auflösung in der Schicht 10,35 mm FWHM bei einer Empfindlichkeit von 39000 Imp/s/µCi/ml, in der Betriebsart b sind die entsprechenden Werte 8,9 bzw. 16500. Die zugehörigen Schichtdicken sind 15,5 mm bzw. 13,5 mm FWHM. Der Gewinn an Auflösung und Kontrast bei Betriebsart b wird in der Arbeit von HOFFMAN et al. (1981a) eindrucksvoll an Patientenaufnahmen demonstriert.

Die Firma Instrument AB Scanditronix stellt den Positronen-Hirn-Tomographen PC 384-7B vor, der von ERIKSSON et al. (1982) ausführlich beschrieben wird (s. auch das Jahr 1982).

Den Bemühungen von MUEHLLEHNER (s. Abb 43), die Unterteilung in diskrete Einzelkristalle beim Ring zu umgehen, setzen BURNHAM et al. (1981) eine interessante Zwischenlösung entgegen. Sie bauen den Kristallstab aus einer Vielzahl optisch getrennter kleiner Einzelkristalle auf, die eng aneinander gepackt sind und erreichen damit bei Anger-Ortung mit längs aufgesetzten Photomultipliern eine erheblich bessere Ortung, als mit dem homogenen Kristallstab (s. auch Abb. 54).

Eine interessante Lösung für ein hybrides Ringsystem schlagen KANNO et al. (1981) vor, das „Headtome". Eine ringförmige Anordnung von 64 NaJ(Tl)-Kristallen mit einer Eintrittsfläche von 16×28 mm^2 und 70 mm Dicke ermöglicht sowohl übliche Positronen-Tomographie bei einer Rotations- und einer Wobbelbewegung des Detektorringes als auch Tomographie mit niederenergetischen Gammastrahlern wie ^{99m}Tc, ^{81m}Kr und ^{132}Xe. Zu diesem Zweck wird vor die Kristalle ein spezieller Kollimatorring geschoben (s. Abb. 47). Als Auflösung werden 7,5–10 mm FWHM genannt bei 21000 Imp/s/µCi/ml für ein 20 cm Durchmesser

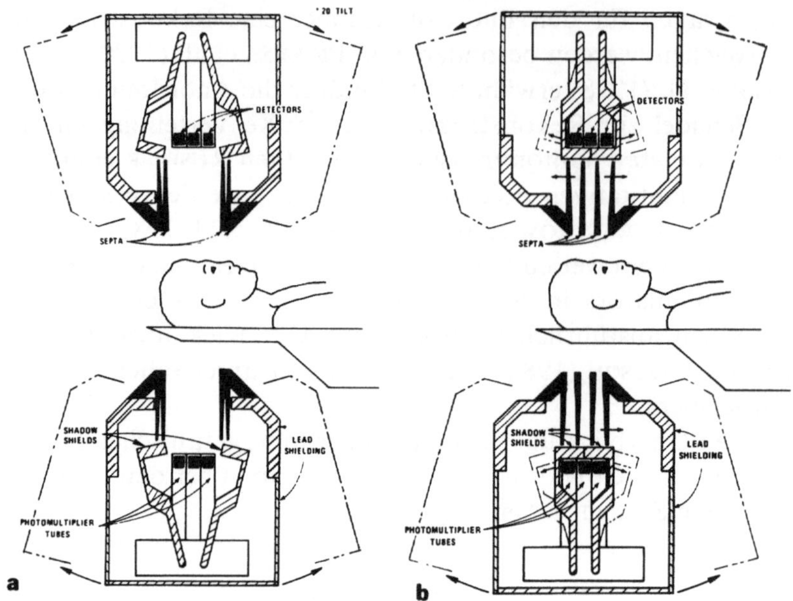

Abb. 46a, b. Zwei unterschiedliche Betriebsarten beim Neuro-ECAT. **a** Die drei Reihen nebeneinander liegender Kristalle sind nicht durch Bleiblenden abgeschirmt (die Shadow Shields sind weggeklappt) und die Bleisepten zwischen den Schichten sind entfernt. Hohe Empfindlichkeit, geringere Auflösung; **b** Bleiblenden vor den Kristallen begrenzen das Eintrittsfeld der einzelnen Detektoren und Bleisepten sorgen für zusätzliche Schichttrennung. Hohe Auflösung und Kontrast, geringere Empfindlichkeit. (Aus Williams et al. 1981)

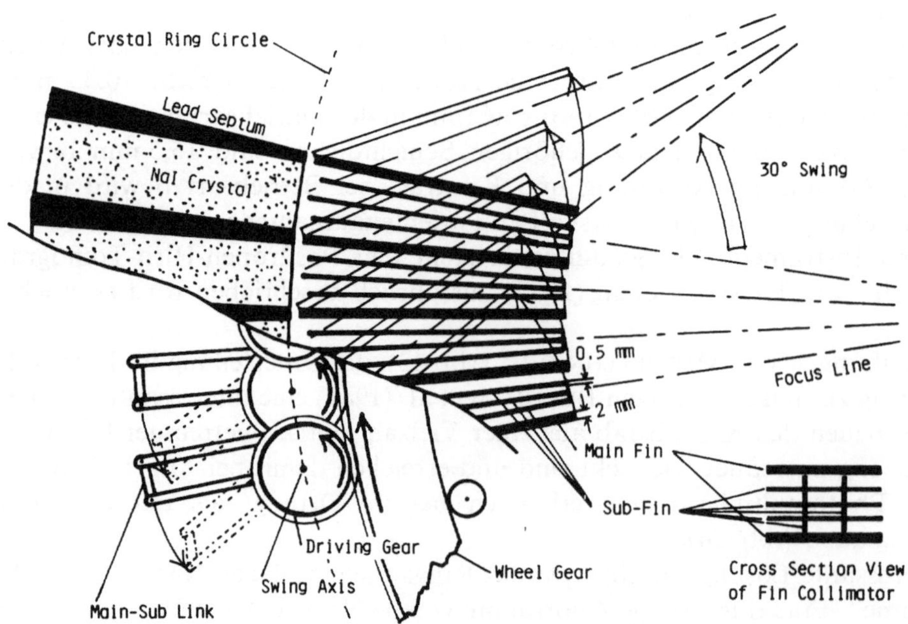

Abb. 47. Anordnung der Kollimatoren für niederenergetische Gammastrahlung beim HEADTOME. Sie bestehen aus Wolframblechen und haben fokussierende Eigenschaften. Die Achsen aller einzelnen Kollimatoren werden synchron um ±30° um ihre Mittellage motorisch bewegt, so daß alle Kollimatorachsen das Meßfeld von 21 cm Durchmesser voll überstreichen. Zusätzlich führt der Ring eine schrittweise rotatorische Bewegung aus. (Aus Kanno et al. 1981)

Phantom. Weitere technische Einzelheiten finden sich bei TANAKA et al. (1981). Es werden hier übrigens NaJ(Tl)-Kristalle eingesetzt wegen der erheblich besseren energetischen Auflösung, die zur Streustrahlungsunterdrückung bei Gamma-Messung wichtig ist.

DERENZO et al. (1981) berichten über die Umrüstung des Donner 280 Kristallringes von NaJ(Tl) auf 280 BGO-Kristalle und steigern die Empfindlichkeit um einen Faktor 2,3 bei gleichbleibender räumlicher Auflösung.

Neben der Rotations- und Wobbelbewegung der Detektorringe wurden immer wieder andere Anordnungen und Bewegungsabläufe vorgeschlagen. Einen interessanten Vorschlag machen CHO et al. (1981) mit ihrem „Dichotomic Ring". Der Ring wird in zwei Hälften aufgeteilt, die im Gegensatz zur zweidimensionalen Wobbelbewegung 4 diskrete Stellungen zueinander einnehmen (s. auch Abb. 81).

COLSHER u. MUEHLLEHNER (1981) setzen sich mit der Wobbelbewegung auseinander, und KOURIS et al. (1981) geben einen allgemeinen Überblick über die Probleme des Datensammelns beim Positronen-Ring.

TER-POGOSSIAN et al. (1981) diskutieren ausführlich die Möglichkeiten der Flugzeitmessung bei der Positronen-Tomographie. Sie rechnen mit einer Zeitauflösung von kleiner als 500 ps bzw. kleiner als 75 mm Ortsauflösung. Damit läßt sich bei der Rekonstruktion das Signal/Rausch Verhältnis um etwa einen Faktor 4 verbessern (s. auch Abb. 77, 78).

Das Problem der langwierigen Aufnahme eines Transmissions-Scans zur Korrektur der Absorption beim Positronen-Tomographen umgehen HUANG et al. (1981) dadurch, daß sie die Transmissionsaufnahme nicht unmittelbar zur Korrektur heranziehen, sondern in einer vergleichsweise statistisch schlechten Transmissionsaufnahme (kürzere Aufnahmezeiten) per Rechner die Grenzen von Gewebebereichen bestimmen lassen, die signifikant unterschiedliche Absorptionskoeffizienten aufweisen. Mit Hilfe dieses Verteilungsbildes werden dann die Korrekturfaktoren berechnet.

Die sehr ausführliche Serie von Arbeiten über die Probleme der quantitativen Aktivitätsbestimmung mit Hilfe der Positronen-Tomographie (HOFFMAN et al. 1979a; HUANG et al. 1979, 1980) wird mit zwei Beiträgen fortgesetzt, HOFFMAN et al. (1981b) und MAZZIOTTA et al. (1981). Von den zahlreichen klinischen Anwendungsbeispielen soll erwähnt werden der Einsatz von ^{82}Rb in Verbindung mit dem Donner-Ring zur Untersuchung von Störungen der Blut-Hirn-Schranke (YEN u. BUDINGER 1981). Es wurden dabei Tumoranreicherungen von ^{82}Rb um den Faktor 10 gegenüber dem normalen Hirngewebe festgestellt.

GOODMAN et al. (1981) setzen neben dem bekannten ^{18}F-2-FDG ein ^{18}F-3-FDG zur Stoffwechseluntersuchung von Hirn und Herz ein in Verbindung mit der MGH Kamera PC II. Mit der gleichen Kamera werden regionale Ventilations- und Perfusionsstudien der Lunge mit ^{13}N durchgeführt (AHLUWALIA et al. 1981), und die quantitative Bestimmung der regionalen extravaskulären Lungendichte gelingt durch Kombination von Emissions-Tomographie mit ^{11}CO und Transmissions-Tomographie (RHODES et al. 1981). ^{11}C markierte Methylglukose wird zur Stoffwechseluntersuchung am Herzen eingesetzt (VYSKA et al. 1981).

Die Tomographie mit Gamma-Strahlern wird bereichert durch die Ergebnisse, die LASSEN mit dem Tomomatic 64 bei Inhalation von ^{133}Xe erzielt (LASSEN et al. 1981; LASSEN 1982; LAURITZEN et al. 1981) (s. auch Abb. 48). Interessant sind nicht nur die Verteilungsbilder der Hirndurchblutung, sondern auch die Möglichkeit der absoluten Berechnung des regionalen Blutflusses (CELSIS et al. 1981).

Bei der Tomographie mit rotierender Gamma-Kamera mehren sich die Bemühungen, neben den gemessenen transversalen Schichten per Computer auch sagittale und frontale Schichten (SOUSSALINE et al. 1981b) bzw. schräg liegende Schichten zu berechnen (BORELLO et al. 1981). MIRELL et al. (1981) rekonstruieren Herzwandtomogramme des linken Ventrikels aus nur zwei statischen Aufnahmen des Herzens, frontal und 45° LAO, während verschiedener Herzphasen.

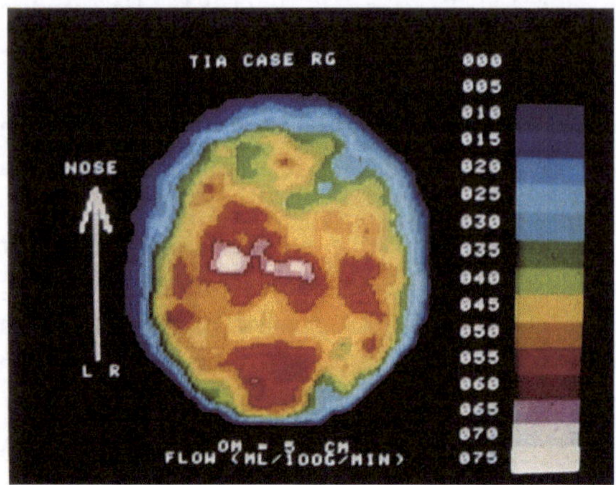
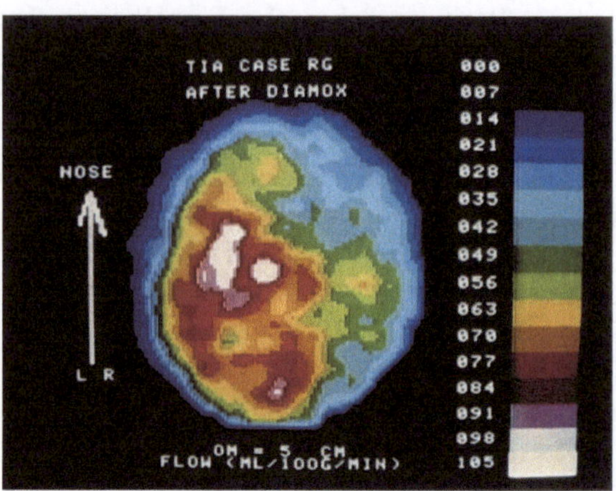

Abb. 48. 63jährige Patientin mit TIA (transitorische ischämische Attacken) nach zwei Episoden rechtsseitiger Blindheit. Im Angiogramm fand sich ein Verschluß der re. A. carotis int., der CT-Befund war unauffällig. Das ^{133}Xe CBF Tomogramm ist in Höhe OM + 5 cm dargestellt. Unter Ruhebedingungen beobachtet man einen diskret verminderten Fluß rechts; 30 min nach Azetazolamid (1 g) (DIAMOX) wächst der Fluß auf der linken, nicht so auf der rechten Seite. (Freundlicherweise von N.A. Lassen zur Verfügung gestellt)

Ein interessantes Korrekturverfahren für die Absorption auf iterativer Basis geben Walters et al. (1981) an, wobei sie sich Transmissionsmessungen ersparen.

Eine große Zahl von Arbeiten befassen sich mit der 7-pinhole-Tomographie, wobei die meisten kritisch urteilen. Stellvertretend soll hier eine Diskussion der geistigen Väter dieser Methode genannt werden, Le Free et al. (1981). Vergleiche zwischen 7-pinhole- und rotierender Kamera, fallen eindeutig zu Gunsten der letzteren aus (Tamaki et al. 1981; Mullani et al. 1981). Auch dem rotierenden Slanthole-Kollimator wird eine Überlegenheit über den 7-pinhole-Kollimator bescheinigt (Lewis et al. 1981).

Eine elektronische Kollimierung für Gamma-Strahler schlagen Singh u. Doria (1981) vor. Das Objekt wird beobachtet von zwei planen-flächigen Detektoren, die in festem Abstand parallel zueinander angeordnet sind. So kann der Eintrittsdetektor (1) eine rechteckige Matrize von vielen kleinen Halbleiterkristallen sein, während dahinter eine Gamma-Kamera (2) angeordnet ist (s. Abb. 49). Durch Koinzidenzabfrage kann die Richtung des von Detektor 1 ausgehenden Streuquants bestimmt werden. Aus der absorbierten Energie ΔE im ersten Detektor läßt sich der Streuwinkel θ berechnen. Die Einfallsrichtung des primären Gammaquants E muß also auf der Mantelfläche eines Kegels mit dem Öffnungswinkel $2\,\theta$ liegen, dessen Spitze mit dem Detektorelement 1 identisch ist. Die Einfallsrichtung kann nicht eindeutig festgelegt werden, die Rückprojektion einer Punktquelle in eine oder mehrere Bildebenen besteht also aus der Überlagerung von vielen Kreisen bzw. Ellipsen. Es handelt sich auch um eine Art codierter Apertur-Abbildung und nur durch iterative Rekonstruktion (Doria u. Singh 1982) lassen sich daraus Schichtverteilungen berechnen. Obwohl das Verfahren für niedrige Energien (141 keV) eine sehr hohe Empfindlichkeit aufweist, da kein Kollimator vorhanden ist, ist zu befürchten, daß wie bei allen codierten Apertur-Abbildungen der hohe Informationsgewinn durch die extreme Rauschverstärkung bei der Rekonstruktion verloren geht.

Eine Reihe umfangreicher Übersichtsarbeiten setzen sich mit den Möglichkeiten sowohl der Positronen-Tomographie (Phelps 1981; Ter-Pogossian 1981; Wolf 1981) wie auch der Tomographie mit Gamma-Strahlern auseinander (Ell u. Khan 1981; Budinger 1981). Budinger spricht dabei sogar von einer Wiedergeburt der Hirnszintigraphie und beruft sich dabei auf die Leistungen von Cleon 710, Mark IV, Tomomatic 64 und Headtome.

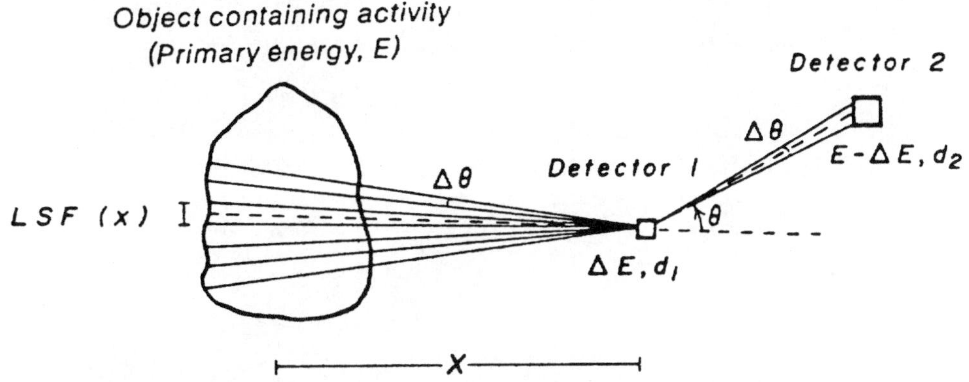

Abb. 49. Prinzip der elektronischen Kollimierung von Gammastrahlung. In einem Detektorelement des Detektors 1 findet eine Comptonabsorption statt. Das koinzident auftretende Streuquant wird von einem Detektorelement des Detektors 2 absorbiert. Durch Bestimmung der absorbierten Energie ΔE im Detektor 1 ist die Energie des Streuquants $E - \Delta E$ bekannt und damit nach den Regeln der Comptonstreuung der Streuwinkel θ. (Aus Singh u. Doria 1981)

Allgemeine Übersichten über die apparative Seite der Tomographie geben Jordan (1981) und speziell für die Positronen-Tomographie Brooks et al. (1981) sowie für die Gammastrahlen-Tomographie Muehllehner u. Colsher (1981).

Das Jahr 1982:

Eine größere Zahl von Veröffentlichungen befaßt sich mit der Anwendung der Flugzeitmessung (TOF) bei der Positronen-Tomographie. Stellvertretend sollen hier genannt werden zwei Arbeiten zum Super PETT I, Ter-Pogossian et al. (1982a) und Yamamoto et al. (1982a), und zwei Arbeiten zum LETI TTV.01 Tomograph aus Grenoble, Laval et al. (1982) und Gariod et al. (1982).

Der Super PETT I ist ein Vier-Ring-Tomograph mit 4×96 CsF-Kristallen von 25 mm $\varnothing$ und 45 mm Höhe, und einem Meßfeld von 45 cm Durchmesser. Die Ringe führen eine Wobbelbewegung auf einem 3 cm $\varnothing$ Kreis, eine Rotationsbewegung um 20° und eine lineare Bewegung von 7,5 mm längs der Patientenhauptachse durch. Sieben Schichten werden simultan registriert, mit einem Schichtabstand von 1,5 cm. Minimale Scanzeit eine Sekunde. Die Auflösung innerhalb der Schicht beträgt 8 mm FWHM im High Resolution Mode (Kristall-Eintrittsöffnung 10×25 mm²) und 12 mm FWHM im Low Resolution Mode (Eintrittsöffnung 25 mm $\varnothing$). In longitudinaler Richtung werden 11,4 mm FWHM genannt. Abbildung 50 zeigt Beispiele von Hirn und Herz.

Der LETI Tomograph ist sehr ähnlich aufgebaut, mit vier Ringen à 96 CsF-Kristallen von 24 mm Durchmesser und 40 mm Höhe. Der Ring wobbelt auf einem Kreis von 28 mm $\varnothing$ und rotiert zusätzlich. Als erreichte Zeitauflösung werden ca. 350 ps entsprechend 5,25 cm FWHM genannt. Die Möglichkeit der Verbesserung durch Ersatz der CsF- durch BaF_2-Kristalle wird erstmals erwähnt, und von 300 ps FWHM Zeitauflösung berichtet, entsprechend 45 mm FWHM.

Kleinere CsF-Kristalle mit 18 mm Durchmesser und 45 mm Länge verwenden Mullani et al. (1982) in ihrem TOF PET. Fünf Ringe mit je 144 Detektoren erlauben die simultane Aufnahme von 20 Schichten mit einem Schichtabstand von 5,4 mm, wenn während der Aufnahme eine lineare Scanbewegung in z-Richtung (senkrecht zur Schichtebene) durchgeführt wird. Die Auflösung in der Schichtebene wird mit 7–13 mm FWHM erwartet.

WASHINGTON UNIVERSITY
M.I.R. RAD. SCIENCES
SUPER PETT I
SUBJECT ID: P8
C-11 CO INHALATION

a

WASHINGTON UNIVERSITY
M.I.R. RAD. SCIENCES
SUPER PETT I
SUBJECT ID: P5
C-11 PALMITATE INJECTION
MYOCARDIAL INFARCT
TOF

b

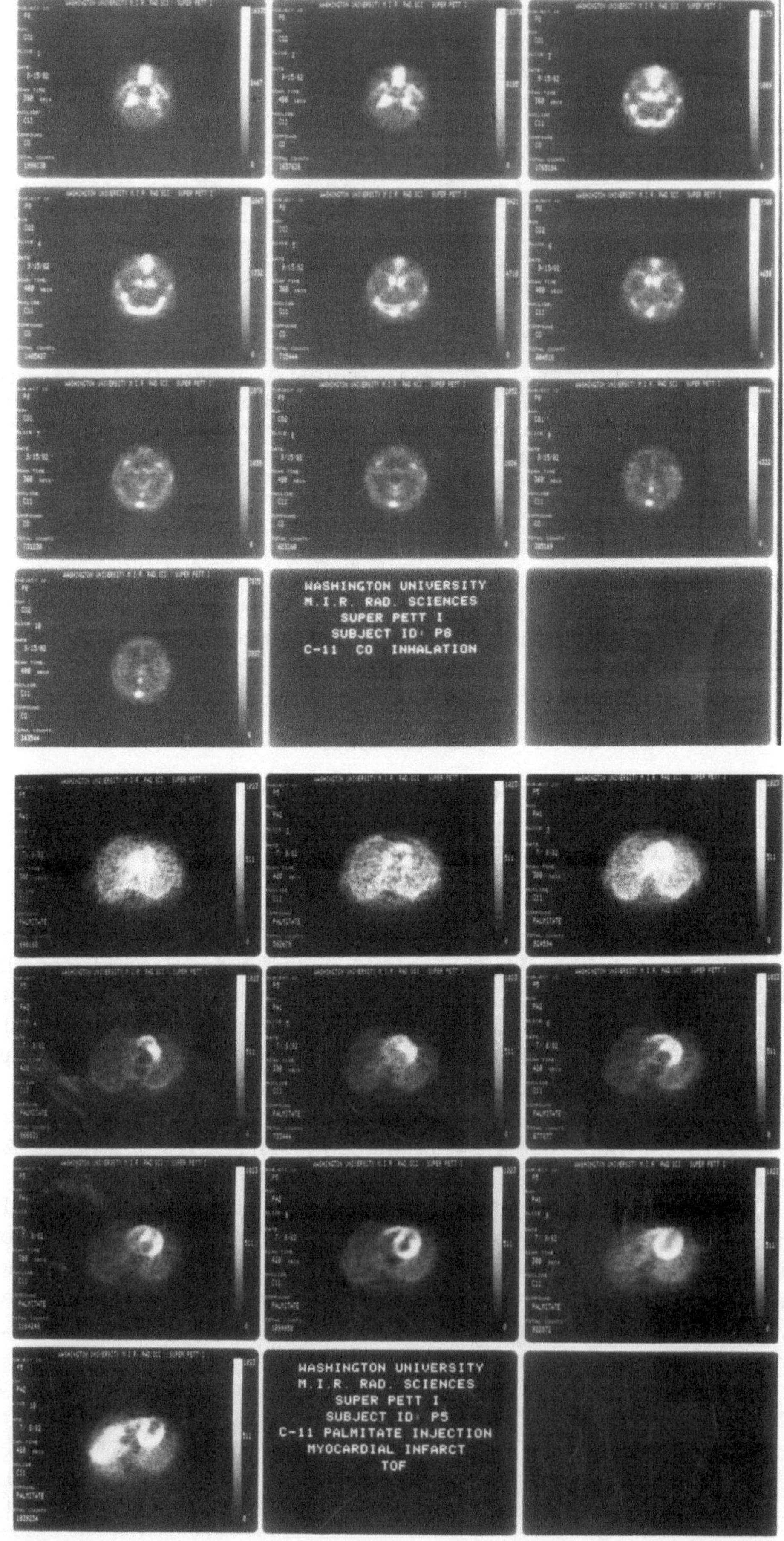

JORDAN u. GETTNER (1982) und JORDAN et al. (1982) weisen nach, daß sich in längeren stabförmigen Kristallen mit der TOF-Methode Ortsauflösungen bei der Bestimmung des Absorptionsortes von nur 40 mm FWHM unter realistischen Meßbedingungen erreichen lassen.

McINTYRE (1982) variiert den Vorschlag seiner Positronen-Kamera mit Plastik-Szintillatoren (s. Abb. 44), indem er Photomultiplier radial außen an den Kristallringen aufsetzt und so zusätzlich TOF-Messungen durchführt.

LLACER et al. (1982) kommen in einer theoretischen Studie zu dem Ergebnis, daß sich mit HP Ge-Halbleiterdetektoren Zeitauflösungen vergleichbar mit denen von CsF erreichen lassen müssen.

Eine interessante Neuentwicklung, der PETT VI, verwendet ebenfalls CsF-Kristalle, aber ohne Flugzeitmessung, nur mit extrem kurzer Koinzidenzauflösungszeit des Systems von 5,9 ns, auf Grund der sehr kurzen Abklingzeitkonstante der Kristalle mit 1,5 ns FWHM Zeitauflösung für das einzelne Detektorpaar (TER-POGOSSIAN et al. 1982b; YAMAMOTO et al. 1982b). Damit läßt sich die Anzahl der zufälligen Koinzidenzen erheblich verringern und hohe Impulsraten verarbeiten.

Der PETT VI hat vier Detektorringe mit je 72 CsF-Kristallen einer Eintrittsfläche von 20×24 mm^2 und 65 mm Höhe. Das Meßfeld hat 27 cm $\varnothing$ und sieben Schichten mit einem Abstand von 1,44 cm werden registriert. Im Low Resolution Mode ist die volle Kristallfläche wirksam, im High Resolution Mode reduzieren Bleiblenden auf 10×24 mm^2 Eintrittsfläche. Die entsprechenden Auflösungen in den Schichten liegen zwischen 11,6 und 13,9 mm bzw. 6,8 und 7,8 mm FWHM. Niedrigste Scanzeit ist eine Sekunde.

Die Instrument AB Scanditronix bietet an den „PETT 600", der dem PETT VI entspricht und den „SUPERPETT 2000", der dem Super PETT I entspricht.

Der Trend zu immer kleineren Kristallbreiten hält an. NAHMIAS et al. (1982) stellen einen Ring mit 160 BGO-Kristallen auf einem Durchmesser von 52 cm vor. Die Kristalle mit 10×25 mm^2 Eintrittsfläche und 45 mm Höhe sind eng aneinander gepackt, ohne jegliche Zwischenabschirmung. Jeder Kristall hat seinen eigenen Photomultiplier. Sie geben 6,4 mm FWHM als Auflösung an, ohne jegliche Bewegung des Ringes.

Noch kleinere BGO-Kristalle mit 4,5 mm Breite schlagen RICCI et al. (1982) vor, die sie ebenfalls eng aneinander packen und nur mit der optischen Reflexionsfarbe als Zwischenschicht. Bei 100 cm Detektorringdurchmesser und einer ^{64}Cu Linienquelle erreichen sie Auflösungen von < 5 mm FWHM und < 11 mm FWTM.

Eine neue Hirn-Positronenkamera mit vier Ringen von je 96 BGO-Kristallen auf einem Durchmesser von 48 cm stellen ERIKSSON et al. (1982) vor. Es werden sieben Schichten mit einer Auflösung von 7,7 mm FWHM bei Schichtdicken um die 12 mm gemessen (s. Abb. 51).

Die Weiterentwicklung der Positronenkamera „Positologica" (siehe 1980) zur „Positologica II" bringt eine Erweiterung auf drei Ringe von je 160 BGO-Kristallen (YAMAMOTO u. KAWAGUCHI 1982). Dabei sind jeweils vier Kristalle mit zwei Photomultipliern zu einem sog. Quad-Detektor zusammengefaßt (MURAYAMA et al. 1982) (s. auch Abb. 52). Auf jedem Ring sind 40 Quad-Detektoren wieder ungleichmäßig verteilt angeordnet. Eine sehr gute analytische Untersuchung mit Anwendung auf diesen Tomographen geben TANAKA et al. (1982).

Ebenfalls weiterentwickelt zu einer Drei-Ring-Anordnung wurde das hybride System Headtome II, s. auch 1981. HIROSE et al. (1982) geben eine Beschreibung des Gerätes, welches dem Headtome sehr ähnlich ist und UEMURA et al. (1982) zeigen eindrucksvolle rCBF Auf-

---

Abb. 50a, b. Jeweils 10 Schnitte durch das menschliche Hirn nach ^{11}CO-Inhalation (**a**) und durch das menschliche Herz mit Infarkt nach i.v. Injektion von ^{11}C markierter Palmitinsäure (**b**) (Freundlicherweise von M.M. TER-POGOSSIAN zur Verfügung gestellt)

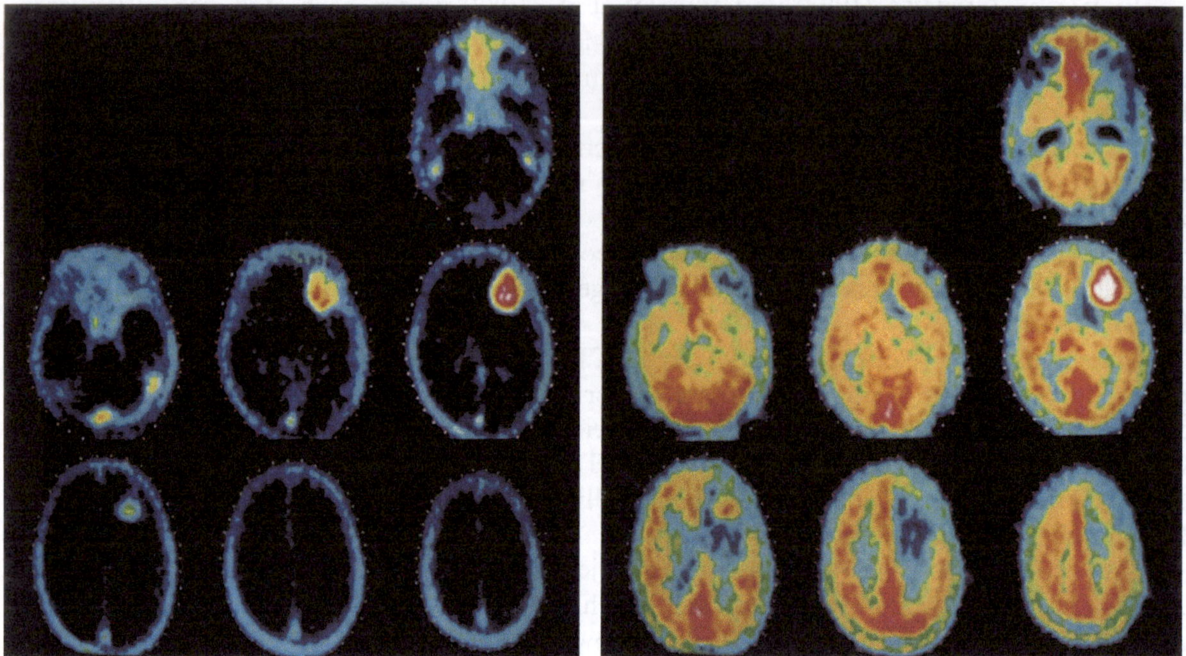

Abb. 51. Meningiom nach Applikation von ^{68}Ga EDTA (**a**) bzw. ^{11}C markierter Glukose (**b**). Aufgenommen im Karolinska Hospital, Stockholm, mit der PC 384-7B Positronen-Kamera. (Freundlicherweise von L. ERIKSSON zur Verfügung gestellt)

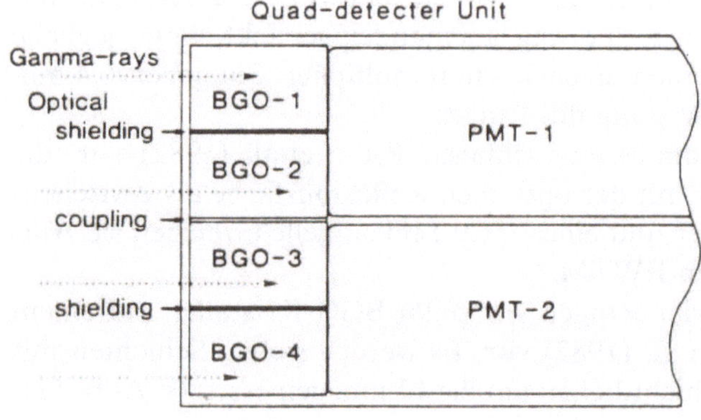

Abb. 52. Anordnung von 4 BGO-Kristallen mit 2 Photomultipliern zu einem Quad-Detector. Die beiden äußeren Kristalle 1 und 4 sind optisch abgeschirmt gegen die beiden Kristalle 2 und 3, die optisch gekoppelt sind. Damit läßt sich eine eindeutige Zuordnung zu jedem einzelnen Kristall finden. (Aus YAMAMOTO u. KAWAGUCHI 1982)

nahmen mit ^{81m}Kr als Beispiel für den Betrieb mit Gamma-Strahlern, hier noch mit dem Headtome aufgenommen.

HUESMAN et al. (1982) stellen für ringförmige Tomographen ein neues Sampling-Schema vor, nach Art der Bewegung von Muschelschalen, und nennen es Clamshell-Sampling. Es kennt nur zwei mechanische Stellungen, die eng beieinander liegen (s. auch Abb. 80).

Den Aufbau einer Mehrschicht-Positronenkamera höchster Auflösung, mit Hilfe von 6 hexagonal angeordneten Vieldraht-Proportionalkammern, schlagen DEL GUERRA et al. (1982a) vor. Sie nennen 3 mm FWHM für die Auflösung in der Schicht, bei 3 mm Schichtdicke. Die Empfindlichkeit liegt ca. um einen Faktor 4,5 niedriger als bei großen BGO-Kristall-Systemen. Die Koinzidenzauflösungszeit des Systems beträgt 200 ns.

Für eine longitudinale Positronenkamera mit zwei gegenüberstehenden Vieldraht-Proportionalkammern von 25×25 cm^2 Fläche, zur Untersuchung kleinerer Objekte, werden Auflösungen von 4 mm FWHM genannt. Über dieses „SHARP" genannte System berichtet McKee (1982).

Stellvertretend für die große Anzahl von Arbeiten, die sich mit den Einflüssen der verschiedenen Parameter (Sampling, Kristallgröße, Zeitverhalten, Kollimation usw.) auf die Leistung eines Positronen-Tomographen befassen, sei hier die Übersicht von Derenzo et al. (1982) genannt, die auch ein umfangreiches Literaturverzeichnis enthält. Hoffman et al. (1982) setzen sich mit dem Einfluß der nicht über das ganze Meßfeld gleichmäßigen räumlichen Auflösung auseinander, und Ter-Pogossian et al. (1982) diskutieren den Einfluß der Organbewegung bei quantitativen Herzuntersuchungen. Schließlich analysieren Phelps et al. (1982), welchen Vorteil immer kleinere Kristalle für die Auflösungsverbesserung ohne unerträgliche Rauschverstärkung haben. Sie nennen dies Verfahren SAT (Signal-Amplification Technique) und es beruht auf der Verwendung von Kristallen mit so kleiner Eintrittsbreite, daß die resultierenden Meßstrahlen dünner sind als die räumliche Auflösung in der rekonstruierten Schicht. Diskutiert wird dieses Verfahren erstmals von Phelps et al. (1981).

Auf der Anwendungsseite der Positronen-Tomographie sind zunächst die Überlegungen von Huang et al. (1982a) zu erwähnen, die versuchen, die Doppel-Tracer-Technik auch für Positronenstrahler zu realisieren. Da die Energie immer gleich ist (511 keV), werden hier die unterschiedlichen Zerfallszeiten ausgenutzt, um zwischen zwei simultan vorhandenen Strahlern zu unterscheiden. Dies könnte auch dazu dienen, die Messung der Absorptionskoeffizienten mit äußerer Strahlenquelle und die Messung der Aktivitätskonzentration im Objekt simultan durchzuführen. Die Probleme, besonders mit der Rauschverstärkung, sind allerdings noch groß.

Stoffwechsel und Durchblutung von Herz und Hirn bestimmen die Anwendung der Positronen-Tomographie (Goldstein 1982; Baron et al. 1982; Vyska et al. 1982; Huang et al. 1982b). Budinger et al. (1982) geben allgemeine Kriterien zur notwendigen Leistung eines Positronen-Tomographen bei Herzuntersuchungen. Über den Einsatz von ^{11}C markiertem Methionin zur Pankreasuntersuchung berichten Meyer et al. (1982). Dosisabschätzungen für gebräuchliche Positronenstrahler gibt Kearfott (1982a, b).

Die Tomographie mit Gammastrahlern wird von der rotierenden Gamma-Kamera beherrscht. 10 verschiedene Systeme kommerzieller Bauart werden in einer ausführlichen Übersicht bezüglich ihrer physikalischen Daten und Leistungsparameter verglichen (Jaszczak 1982). Zusätzlich wurde das inzwischen von der Shimadzu Corp. gelieferte Headtome SET-230 in den Vergleich mit aufgenommen, welches dem Headtome II entspricht. Auch die rotierende Kamera „Omega 500" von der Firma Technicare ist in der Übersicht enthalten, die erstmals die Möglichkeit einer elliptischen Bewegungsbahn um den Patienten bietet, neben der üblichen Kreisbewegung (Gottschalk u. Salem 1982). Damit werden Verbesserungen der räumlichen Auflösung und der Homogenität erzielt.

Eine Beschreibung des Standes der Technik gibt Budinger (1982a) und die Perspektiven der SPECT beschreiben Keyes Jr. (1982) und Ell et al. (1982). Coleman et al. (1982b) brechen eine Lanze für die Hirn-Tomographie mit Gammastrahlern. Eine Vielzahl von Arbeiten setzt sich mit den äußeren Einflüssen auf die Leistung von SPECT Systemen auseinander. So berichten u.a. Soussaline et al. (1982) und Moore (1982) den Einfluß der Absorption, Beck et al. (1982) den Einfluß der Streustrahlung, Rogers et al. (1982a) den Einfluß des Rauschens und Jaszczak et al. (1982a) den Einfluß der Organbewegung. Eine Zusammenfassung geben Larsson u. Israelson (1982).

Auf dem Gebiet der dringend notwendigen Qualitätskontrolle nehmen die Bestrebungen zu, einheitliche Richtlinien zu erstellen (Keyes Jr. 1982; Todd-Pokropek 1982).

Fast zu einer Weltanschauung entwickelt sich die Frage, ob man bei Aufnahmen des Herzens 180° oder 360° um den Patienten mit dem Kamerakopf rotieren soll (Tamaki et al. 1982; Coleman et al. 1982a; MacIntyre et al. 1982). Dabei wird stets ^{201}Tl eingesetzt und die 68–83 keV Photonen gemessen. In diesem speziellen Fall erreicht man bei 180° Rotation in der Tat etwas kontrastreichere Bilder, wenn man auf Absorptionskorrektur und auf jegliche quantitative Aussagen völlig verzichtet. Hoffman (1982) analysiert die Frage sehr sachlich und kommt zu der Meinung, daß die 180°-SPECT nur deshalb brauchbar ist, weil ein Radionuklid (^{201}Tl) verwendet wird, dessen Gamma-Energien besonders ungeeignet sind in Bezug auf das Meßinstrument und die Abtasttechnik.

Quantitative Aktivitätsbestimmung in vivo auch mit Gammastrahlern gelingt mit speziellen Tomographen. So setzen Kuhl et al. (1982) ihren Mark IV Scanner ein, um nach i.v. Injektion von ^{123}I markiertem IMP quantitative rCBF Messungen durchzuführen. Über Erfahrungen mit dem Tomomatic 64 und ^{133}Xe Inhalation berichten Hedde et al. (1982).

Die großen Abstände zwischen den 3 gemessenen Schichten des Tomomatic 64 sollen mit Hilfe eines neuen Kollimators beseitigt werden und 6 eng aneinandergrenzende Schichten simultan gemessen werden (Stokely 1982).

Ein System, ähnlich dem Tomomatic 64 oder Mark IV, mit einer Detektorebene stellen Cho et al. (1982) vor. Das „Gammatom-1" genannte Gerät hat vier Blöcke mit je neun NaJ(Tl)-Szintillationssonden, die einzeln konvergierende Kollimatoren haben. Die vier Blöcke sind auf den Seiten eines Quadrates ringförmig angeordnet, welches eine Rotation um 360° und zusätzlich laterale Bewegungen ausführt. Auflösungen von 7 mm FWHM in der Schicht und eine Empfindlichkeit von 10 000 Imp/s/µCi/cm^3 werden angegeben.

Ebenfalls vier Blöcke à 6 NaJ(Tl)-Kristalle quadratisch angeordnet hat der „Aberdeen Section Scanner Mark II" (Smith et al. 1982). Auch hier rotiert der Ring und die Sondenblöcke werden in der Schichtebene linear bewegt. 8 mm FWHM Auflösung werden angestrebt.

Bei der Realisierung des SPRINT (s. Abb. 42) zu einem klinisch anwendbaren Gerät ist interessant, daß die ursprünglich vorgesehene rotierende Schlitzblende mit unregelmäßig angeordneten Schlitzen ersetzt wurde durch eine Schlitzblende mit acht regelmäßig angeordneten Schlitzen von 3,2 mm Breite und 15 mm Länge (Rogers et al. 1982b). Dabei ist wichtig, daß jeder einzelne Schlitz das volle Meßfeld auf jeweils den achten Teil des Detektorringes abbildet, so daß *keine* Überlappung der einzelnen Teilbilder mehr auftritt. Damit dürften die großen Probleme der Rauschverstärkung bei der Rekonstruktion bedeutend vermindert sein. Die gleiche Anordnung wird auch von Genna et al. (1982) vorgeschlagen, die lediglich anstelle der diskreten Detektoren auf dem Ring, einen kontinuierlichen Kristall mit radial aufgesetzten Photomultipliern und einer sehr schnellen digitalen Ortselektronik vorschlagen.

Bei der longitudinalen Tomographie gesellt sich zum 7-pinhole Kollimator ein 3-pinhole Kollimator (Webb et al. 1982) und ein 12-pinhole Kollimator (Hasegawa et al. 1982). Beide können die grundsätzlichen Probleme der 7-pinhole Abbildung nicht lösen, wenn sie auch beide eine geringe Vergrößerung des Meßfeldes ermöglichen.

Eine Lösung zwischen dem 7-pinhole Kollimator und dem rotierenden Slanthole-Kollimator (Ratib et al. 1982) stellt der Quadrant Slanthole-Kollimator dar (Chang et al. 1982). Der Kollimator ist in vier gleiche Kuchenstücke aufgeteilt, die je einen Slanthole-Kollimator bilden. Die um 40° geneigten Achsen der vier Kollimatorabschnitte sind in Richtung auf die Kollimator-Mittelachse gerichtet. Der Kollimator kann um 45° gedreht werden, so daß acht verschiedene Ansichten des Objektes gewonnen werden (s. Abb. 53). Das Meßfeld hat ca. 15 cm Durchmesser und Tiefe. Der Vorteil liegt darin, daß man den Kamera-Meßkopf vor der Aufnahme exakt ausrichten kann, da man die vier bzw. acht Teilbilder auf dem Bildschirm beobachten kann.

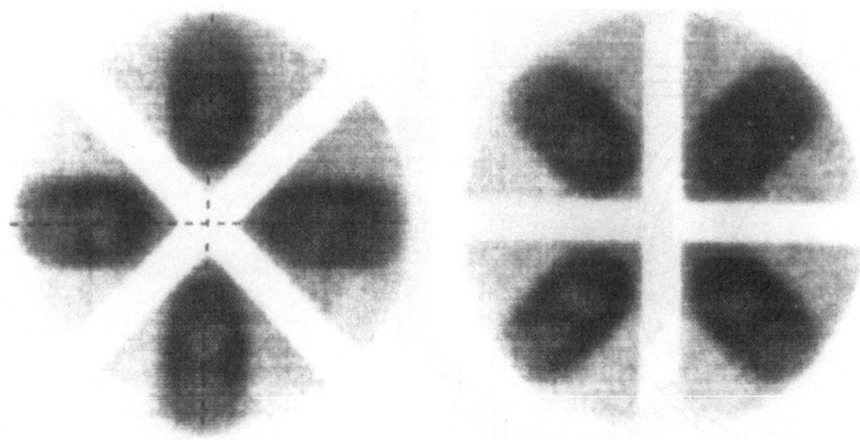

Abb. 53. Abbildung eines Herzphantoms auf dem Scope mit Hilfe eines Quadrant-Slant-Hole-Kollimators. Rechte Seite nach Drehung des Kollimators um 45°. Man kann exakt vor der Messung die Hauptachse des linken Ventrikels mit den X, Y-Achsen der Kamera zur Deckung bringen. (Aus CHANG et al. 1982)

Als Abbildungsverfahren mit codierten Aperturen greifen GINDI et al. (1982) den rotierenden Schlitzkollimator von TANAKA u. IINUMA (1974) wieder auf und kombinieren ihn mit einem Pinhole. Sie beschreiben im Detail die Probleme der codierten Abbildung und gehen auch auf das Problem der Rauschverstärkung bei der Rekonstruktion ein.

Großes Gewicht wird in diesem Jahr der dreidimensionalen Darstellung von tomographischen Meßwerten beigemessen. So werden alleine beim 3. Weltkongreß für Nuklearmedizin in Paris über 10 Vorträge zu diesem Thema gehalten. Stellvertretend soll hier die Übersichtsarbeit mit kritischer Wertung von BUDINGER (1982b) genannt werden. Er befaßt sich sowohl mit den Methoden der Computer-Graphik, also der dreidimensionalen Darstellung auf dem Bildschirm, als auch mit den optischen Methoden wie Holographie, Stereoskopie und schnell wechselnder Einzelbilder.

Das Jahr 1983:

Der Trend zu immer kleineren Kristallen bei den Positronen-Ring-Tomographen hält unvermindert an. Beim ECAT III werden 512 BGO Kristalle $5{,}6 \times 30 \times 30$ mm^3 auf einem Ring mit 100 cm Durchmesser angeordnet. Dies ergibt eine Packungsdichte von über 90% und eine Auflösung zwischen 4,4 und 9 mm FWHM, je nach verwendetem Rekonstruktionsfilter (HOFFMAN et al. 1983b). Jeder einzelne Kristall ist an einen Miniatur-Photomultiplier mit 10 mm Durchmesser angekoppelt.

BURNHAM et al. (1983) lösen das Problem der Kristall-PMT Kopplung, wie sie es schon 1981 vorgeschlagen haben. 360 BGO Kristalle, deren Breite konisch von 4 auf 4,5 mm zunimmt, bei 20 mm Höhe und 30 mm Dicke, sind auf einem Ring mit 45 cm Durchmesser angeordnet. Der Zwischenraum zwischen den Kristallen beträgt 0,125 mm und dient der optischen Trennung. Damit ergibt sich eine Packungsdichte von nahezu 100%. Über einen ringförmigen Lichtleiter sind 90 Photomultiplier mit je 20 mm Durchmesser angekoppelt (s. Abb. 54). Die inhärente Auflösung bei der Ortsbestimmung im Ring beträgt max. 4 mm FWHM.

Der 1980 von NOHARA vorgestellte Ringtomograph Positologica hat eine Nachfolgeversion Positologica II bekommen mit drei Ringen von je 160 rechteckigen BGO Kristallen von 15 mm Breite (TAKAMI et al. 1983). Das Prinzip der Quad-Detectors (Abb. 52) und die unregelmäßige Anordnung der Detektoren auf den Ringen ist beibehalten worden. Auflösungen um die 10 mm FWHM in der Schicht werden erreicht.

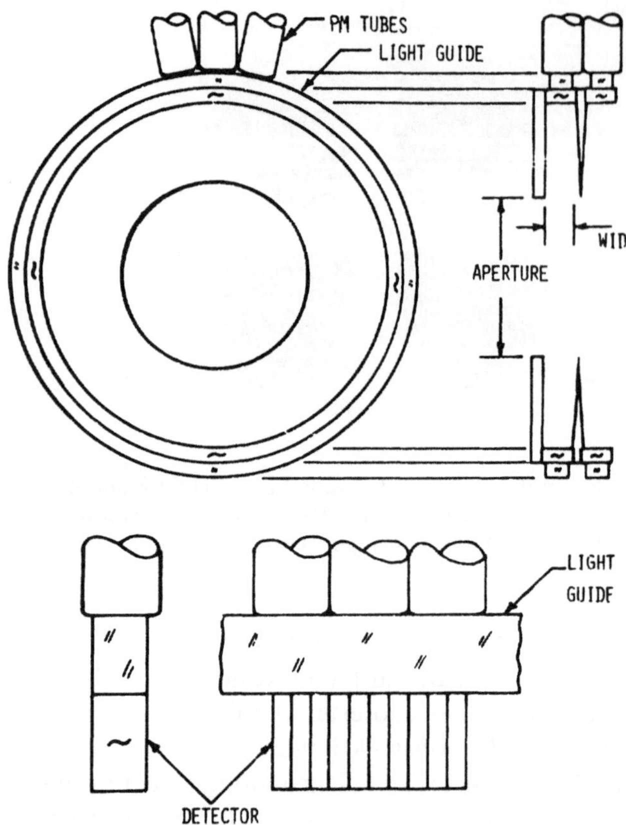

Abb. 54. Anordnung von 360 kleinen rechtekkigen Kristallen beim MGH Positronen-Tomograph, die über einen Lichtleiter an 90 Photomultiplier angekoppelt sind. (Aus Burnham et al. 1982)

Das Problem der Ankopplung der immer kleiner werdenden Kristalle an die vergleichweise großen Photomultiplier veranlassen Derenzo et al. (1983) zu einer Untersuchung über mögliche Kristall-Photomultiplier-Kombinationen, wobei auch der Einsatz von HgI_2-Photodetektoren zur Kodierung der einzelnen Kristalle angesprochen wird.

Ein ausführlicher Bericht von Hoffman et al. (1983a) befaßt sich mit den Leistungen des Neuro-ECAT (s. auch Abb. 46). Durch detaillierte Korrekturverfahren für zufällige und gestreute Koinzidenzen sowie Totzeitverluste wird eine hohe Abbildungsgüte erreicht (s. Abb. 55).

Über die Leistungen des Neuro-PET Scanners, siehe das Jahr 1980, wird von Sank et al. (1983) berichtet. Die Schichtauflösung wird mit 6–7 mm FWHM angegeben.

Für die von Bateman et al. (1980) vorgestellte Positronenkamera auf der Basis von Vieldraht-Proportional-Kammern (MWPC) werden erste klinische Ergebnisse mitgeteilt (Ott et al. 1983a). Sie erreichen eine Auflösung in der Schicht von 8 mm FWHM bei einer max. Koinzidenzrate von $10\,000\ \mathrm{s}^{-1}$. Verbesserungen werden für die von Del Guerra et al. (1982) vorgestellte Positronenkamera mit 6 auf einem hexagonalen Ring angeordnete MWPC's berichtet (Perez-Mendez et al. 1983). Bei einer räumlichen Auflösung von 4,5 mm FWHM und einer Koinzidenzauflösungszeit von 100 ns wird eine echte Koinzidenzrate pro Kammerpaar von $84\,000\ \mathrm{s}^{-1}$ erreicht.

Ein möglicher Ersatzszintillator für BGO wird von Kobayashi et al. (1983) vorgestellt. Es handelt sich um Wismutsilikat BSO ($Bi_4Si_3O_{12}$), welches im Gegensatz zu BGO ($Bi_4Ge_3O_{12}$) zwar nur 20% Lichtausbeute hat, aber eine um einen Faktor 3 kleinere Abklingzeitkonstante. Bei vergleichbarer Dichte ist BSO erheblich billiger als BGO.

Carroll et al. (1983) ersetzen die ringförmige Strahlenquelle zur Aufnahme eines Transmissionsbildes zwecks optimaler Absorptionskorrektur bei PET durch eine rotierende Punktquelle. Da jeweils nur die Sonden abgefragt werden, die der Quelle gegenüber stehen, wird

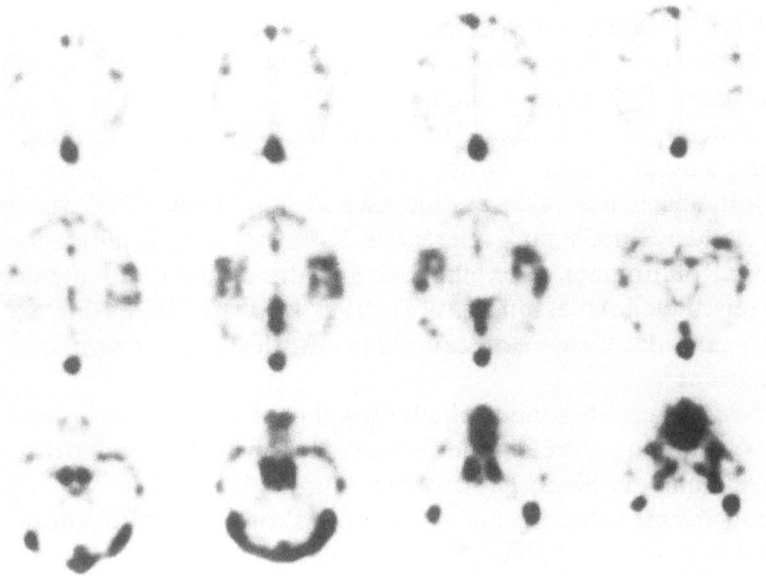

Abb. 55. ^{11}C-Monoxyd Hirnstudie zur Darstellung des Blutvolumens. Aufgenommen mit dem Neuro-ECAT. (Aus HOFFMAN et al. 1983a)

die Zahl der registrierten Quanten, die das Objekt nicht durchdrungen haben, erheblich reduziert.

Auf dem Gebiet der Time-of-Flight Tomographen berichten MULLANI et al. (1983) über die drei verschiedenen Betriebsarten ihres TOFPET, der mit seinen 5 Ringen simultan 9 Schichten aufnimmt, und durch eine zusätzliche Scanbewegung in z-Richtung (senkrecht zur Schichtebene) 20 parallele Schichten rekonstruieren kann. Die Auflösung in der Schicht liegt hierbei zwischen 9 und 14 mm FWHM. In einer dritten Betriebsweise wird eine sehr hohe Empfindlichkeit für dynamische Studien bei einer Auflösung von 22 mm FWHM erreicht.

BUDINGER (1983a) stellt in einer allgemeinen Betrachtung die Möglichkeiten von TOF-PET gegenüber konventioneller PET zusammen. Die Vorteile liegen neben einem indirekten Empfindlichkeitsgewinn (besseres Signal/Rauschverhältnis), vor allem auch in der Schnelligkeit solcher Systeme. Es können sehr hohe Impulsraten verarbeitet werden und die Zahl der zufälligen Koinzidenzen läßt sich merklich reduzieren.

Aus der klinischen Anwendung der PET berichten MEYERS WG et al. (1983) über den Einsatz von ^{13}N-L-Glutamat und beobachten hohe Anreicherungen von ^{13}N in Herz, Pankreas und Leber.

Eine Übersicht über die Grundlagen der quantitativen Bestimmungen von Stoffwechsel, Durchblutung und Funktion des Herzens geben SCHÖN et al. (1983).

Zur Messung der regionalen Hirnfunktion schlägt OSAMU (1983) den Einsatz von ^{14}C-N-Methylphenylethylamine (MPEA) vor und berichtet über erfolgreiche Versuche an Mäusehirnen. Über die Möglichkeit der regionalen pH-Messung im Hirn mit ^{11}C Dimethyloxazolidinedione (DMO) berichten KEARFOTT et al. (1983), rCBF-Messungen mit $H_2{}^{15}O$ analysieren HERSCOVITCH et al. (1983) und RAICHLE et al. (1983).

Über regionale Blutflußmessungen in Weichteiltumoren mit $C^{15}O_2$ berichten KAIRENTO et al. (1983) und die quantitative Bestimmung des regionalen extravaskulären Lungenwassers mit $H_2{}^{15}O$ führen MEYER et al. (1983) und SCHOBER et al. (1983) durch.

Der regionale Hirnstoffwechsel mit ^{18}F-Deoxyglucose wird von Di Chiro et al. (1983), Friedland et al. (1983) und Brownell et al. (1983) untersucht. Als Ersatz für ^{11}C-Deoxyglukose schlagen Kloster et al. (1983) mit ^{75}Br markierte 3-deoxy-3-bromo-D-glukose vor und weisen signifikante Speicherung nach.

Einen allgemeinen Überblick über den Stand der Positronen-Tomographie gibt Wagner Jr. (1983) in seiner Zusammenfassung über zwei PET-Tagungen in diesem Jahre, und Budinger (1983 b) faßt hauptsächlich die physiologischen Aspekte der PET zusammen.

Auf dem Gebiet der SPECT mit rotierenden Kameras setzt sich immer mehr die Erkenntnis durch, daß die Rotation auf einer elliptischen Bahn um den Patienten erhebliche Vorteile gegenüber der kreisrunden Abtastung hat (Todd-Pokropek 1983 a; Gottschalk et al. 1983; Blum 1983). Nicht nur der Gewinn an räumlicher Auflösung, sondern auch an Homogenität ist hier von Bedeutung.

Weitere Verbesserungen, besonders auch bezüglich der großen Probleme bei der quantitativen Aktivitätsbestimmung, durch immer bessere Rekonstruktionsalgorithmen kennzeichnen die weitere Entwicklung der SPECT (Soussaline u. Le Coq 1983).

Die Bemühungen, eine befriedigende Absorptionskorrektur durchzuführen, werden weiter verfolgt (Gullberg et al. 1983; Webb et al. 1983).

Wesentliche Beiträge zur Qualitätskontrolle von rotierenden Kameras liefern Jaszczak et al. (1983) und Areeda et al. (1983).

Die beim Herzen heiß diskutierte Frage einer 180° oder 360° Rotation der Kamera wird jetzt auch auf Leber und Milz ausgedehnt. Ott et al. (1983 b) untersuchen die Frage und kommen zu dem Schluß, daß der Kontrast nicht speichernder Bezirke bei 180° Abtastung besser sei, aber je nach Lage des 180°-Bogens bestimmte Teile von Leber und Milz nur schlecht dargestellt würden.

Übersichtsarbeiten über SPECT behandeln das Thema sowohl aus der mathematisch-physikalischen Sicht (Todd-Pokropek 1983 b), aus apparativer Sicht (Beck 1983) und aus klinischer Sicht (Büll et al. 1983 a). Bei der ^{201}Tl-Herzdiagnostik in Ruhe bescheinigen Kirsch et al. (1983) der SPECT eine Sensitivität von 93% gegenüber der üblichen planaren Szintigraphie mit Computerauswertung von 68%, wobei die Spezifität beider Verfahren gleich ist. Biersack et al. (1983 b) berichten über ein Verfahren zur parametrischen Darstellung der linksventrikulären Wandbewegung mittels SPECT.

Die Frage rotierender Slanthole-Kollimator oder 7-pinhole Kollimator zur Tomographie des Herzens wird weiter diskutiert. Condon et al. (1983) kommen zu dem Schluß, daß der rotierende Slanthole in seinen Abbildungseigenschaften überlegen ist, der 7-pinhole Kollimator aber die bessere Ausbeute aufweist.

Auf dem Gebiet der ringförmigen SPECT-Systeme bringt die Fa. Medimatic den Tomomatic 32 heraus. Eine preiswerte einfachere Version des Tomomatic 64, die mit 32 NaJ(Tl) Szintillationssonden eine einzelne Schicht zu messen gestattet.

Zu der von Singh u. Doria (1981) vorgeschlagenen elektronischen Kollimierung (s. Abb. 49) werden ausführliche Abschätzungen zur Realisierung eines entsprechenden SPECT-Systems vorgestellt (Singh 1983), und erste experimentelle Ergebnisse mit einem simplen Aufbau aus Gamma-Kamera und einem kleinen HP-Ge-Detektor ergeben für Punktquellen von ^{99m}Tc erste Darstellungsergebnisse (Singh u. Doria 1983). Das große Rauschproblem bei kodierten Abbildungsverfahren mit räumlich ausgedehnten Quellen ist damit noch keineswegs gelöst.

II. Tabellarische Auflistung der historischen Entwicklung

Die wesentlichen Ereignisse besonders der apparativen Entwicklung der Emissions-Tomographie, wie sie in Abschnitt A.I. besprochen wurden, werden in einer kurzen Tabelle aufgelistet.

1959 (S. 152)

1. ANGER schlägt eine Positronen-Kamera mit zwei gegenüberstehenden Kameras vor.
2. KUHL realisiert das erste transversale Schichtbild mit ^{131}I.

1962 (S. 154)

1. KUHL stellt seinen transversalen Tomographen „Mark II Scanner" vor.
2. RANKOWITZ stellt die erste ringförmige Positronen-Kamera vor.

1963 (S. 155)

CORMACK schlägt quantitative Rekonstruktion beim Positronen-Tomograph vor, einschließlich Absorptionskorrektur.

1964 (S. 155)

KUHL veröffentlicht die ersten transversalen Schichtbilder, aufgenommen mit dem Mark II.

1965 (S. 156)

1. KUHL erzeugt das erste Transmissions-Schichtbild eines menschlichen Thorax mit 60 keV-Gammastrahlung.
2. HARPER schlägt vor, den Patienten vor einer Kamera zu drehen und die 48 Einzelaufnahmen über ein Spiegelsystem dreidimensional darzustellen.

1966 (S. 156)

1. ANGER schlägt vor, den Patienten vor einer Kamera zu drehen und führt eine Rückprojektion aus den Einzelaufnahmen auf optischem Wege durch.
2. ANGER stellt seinen longitudinalen Tomographic Gamma-Ray Scanner vor.

1967 (S. 159)

1. BRACEWELL u. RIDDLE berichten über die Rückprojektion gefilterter Projektionen in der Radioastronomie.

1968 (S. 159)

1. KUHL stellt den Mark III Scanner vor.
2. BROWNELL beschreibt die geplante Positronen-Kamera mit zwei Multi-Kristall-Blöcken.
3. BOZZO beschreibt die Datenverarbeitung per Rechner bei einem 32-Sonden Positronen-Ring.

1969 (S. 160)

1. MIRALDI beschreibt den Tomoscanner mit „Slit-Hybrid Collimator".
2. PATTON beschreibt einen transversalen Tomographen für Gammastrahler in Ringform mit 8 Sonden.
3. MCAFFEE beschreibt den rotierenden Slant-Hole Collimator.

1970 (S. 160)

1. GORDON stellt den iterativen Rekonstruktionsalgorithmus „ART" vor.
2. MUEHLLEHNER und FREEDMAN berichten über den Einsatz des Slant-Hole Kollimators, letzterer in Verbindung mit einem Computer.
3. MONAHAN beschreibt den Einsatz eines Computers bei der Positronen-Kamera mit zwei Kameraköpfen.

1971 (S. 162)

1. MUEHLLEHNER dreht Patienten vor der Kamera und rekonstruiert Schichten mit einer Differenzbildungs-Rechenvorschrift.
2. CHESLER setzt die gefilterte Rückprojektion bei der Positronen-Kamera ein.

1972 (S. 163)

1. HOUNSFIELD stellt den Transmissions-Computer-Tomographen EMI Kopfscanner Mark I vor.
2. SCHMIDLIN beschreibt ein iteratives Rekonstruktionsverfahren für die longitudinale Positronen-Tomographie.
3. GILBERT und GOITEIN beschreiben die iterative Rekonstruktion für transversale Schichten.
4. BARRETT und ROGERS beschreiben die tomographische Abbildung mit Fresnel Zonen Platten.
5. BURNHAM beschreibt die MGH Positronen-Kamera PC-I.
6. KUHL führt die „Orthogonal Tangent Correction" beim Mark III Scanner ein.

1973 (S. 165)

1. BOWLEY beschreibt den „Aberdeen Section Scanner – ASS"
2. BUDINGER setzt sich mit iterativen Rekonstruktionsmethoden für transversale Schichten auseinander.
3. KAPLAN schlägt eine Positronen-Kamera mit Vieldraht-Proportionalkammern (MWPC) vor.

1974 (S. 166)

1. MATHIEU schlägt die longitudinale Tomographie mit einem Pinhole-Kollimator vor.
2. JORDAN stellt den Longitudinalen Emissions Multikristall Tomoscanner LEMT vor.
3. TANAKA schlägt rotierende Schlitzapertur als zeitlich modulierte Apertur vor.
4. NESTOR stellt die Eigenschaften von BGO-Kristallen heraus.

1975 (S. 169)

1. TER-POGOSSIAN und PHELPS beschreiben den PETT.
2. DERENZO schlägt einen Positronen-Ring-Tomographen mit 288 Kristallen vor.
3. CHO stellt den Positronenring CRTAPC vor.
4. KORAL stellt die zeitmodulierte codierte Abbildung mit einer Vielzahl von Pinholes vor.
5. PRICE schlägt einen transversalen Ring-Tomographen mit codierter Apertur vor.
6. JEAVONS schlägt Konverter vor MWPC's vor zur Erhöhung der Absorption.
7. MUEHLLEHNER beschreibt spezielle Strahlenfilter bei der Positronen-Tomographie.

1976 (S. 172)

1. HOFFMAN stellt den PETT III vor.
2. DERENZO beschreibt den 280-Kristall Donner Ring.
3. MUEHLLEHNER stellt seine Positronen-Kamera mit zwei Kameraköpfen vor.
4. KUHL stellt den Mark IV Scanner vor.
5. PATTON setzt Germanium Halbleiterdetektoren bei einem longitudinalen Tomoscanner ein.
6. LOTTES führt die iterative Rekonstruktion beim LEMT ein.
7. Der Pho/Con Tomographic Multi-Plane Scanner kommt auf den Markt.

1977 (S. 175)

1. TER-POGOSSIAN stellt das Konzept des PETT IV vor.
2. BOHM beschreibt den Positronen-Ring-Tomographen PC-95.
3. KEYES Jr. beschreibt das Humongotron.
4. JASZCZAK beschreibt rotierende Kamera speziell für Hirnaufnahmen.
5. BUDINGER berichtet über EKG-Triggerung bei rotierender Kamera.
6. BRUNOL stellt den 8-pinhole-Kollimator vor.
7. KNOLL schlägt das Konzept vom Single Photon Ring Tomograph SPRINT vor.
8. Der Tomoscanner MS 425-CAT der Firma J & P ist lieferbar.
9. Firma Ortec Inc. liefert den ECAT.

1978 (S. 179)

1. TER-POGOSSIAN beschreibt den PETT IV und PETT V.
2. BROWNELL stellt die Positronen-Kamera PC-II vor.
3. VOGEL stellt den 7-pinhole-Kollimator vor.
4. NICKELS schlägt eine Positronen-Kamera mit Stabszintillatoren und Flugzeitmessung vor.
5. Firma Ortec Inc. stellt den ECAT-II vor.
6. Firma Cyclotron Corp. stellt die Positronen-Kamera Modell 4200 vor.
7. Firma Union Carbide stellt den Cleon 710 und 711 vor.
8. Firma J & P stellt den Tomogscanner II vor.

1979 (S. 183)

1. JASZCZAK beschreibt seine Doppel-Kopf-Tomo-Kamera mit Fan Beam Kollimatoren.
2. WILLIAMS stellt den Prototyp des SPRINT vor.
3. THOMPSON beschreibt das Positome-II.
4. HOFFMAN führt getriggerte Herzaufnahmen mit dem ECAT durch.

5. Firma Ortec Inc. kündigt den „Neuro-ECAT" an.
6. Atomic Energy of Canada Ltd. stellt den Ringtomographen „Therascan 3128" vor.

1980 (S. 185)

1. Allemand, Mullani und Jordan kündigen den Einsatz der Flugzeitmessung in der Positronen-Meßtechnik an.
2. Muehllehner schlägt hexagonale Ringkamera aus langen NaJ(Tl)-Stäben vor.
3. MacIntyre stellt das Konzept einer Positronen-Ringkamera mit über 160000 kleinen Plastikszintillatoren vor.
4. Brooks stellt den „Neuro-PET" vor.
5. Nohara beschreibt den Hirn-Tomographen „Positologica".
6. Stokely stellt den Hirn-Tomographen „DCAT" für niederenergetische Gammastrahler vor.
7. Die Firma Medimatic bietet den Hirn-Tomographen „Tomomatic 64" an.

1981 (S. 189)

1. Kanno beschreibt das hybride Ringsystem „Headtome".
2. Derenzo berichtet über die BGO-Version des 280-Kristall Donner Ringes.
3. Cho stellt den „Dichotomic Ring" vor.
4. Burnham schlägt quasi homogenen Kristallring mit Anger-Ortung vor.
5. Singh schlägt eine Art codierte Apertur-Abbildung mit Hilfe der Compton-Kollimierung vor.
6. Die Firma Instrument AB Scanditronix stellt den Positronen-Hirn-Tomographen PC 384-7B vor.

1982 (S. 193)

1. Ter-Pogossian beschreibt den Super PETT I mit TOF und den PETT VI.
2. Laval beschreibt den Ringtomographen LETI TTV.01 mit TOF.
3. Mullani stellt den TOF PET vor.
4. Yamamoto stellt den „Positologica II" mit Quad-Detektoren vor.
5. Nahmias beschreibt einen Hirn-Positronen-Ring mit 160 BGO-Kristallen.
6. Del Guerra schlägt einen Ringtomographen mit sechs MWPC vor.
7. McKee beschreibt die longitudinale Positronen-Kamera „SHARP" mit MWPC's.
8. Hirose beschreibt das hybride System „HEADTOME II".
9. Cho stellt das „Gammatom-1" vor.
10. Smith beschreibt den „Aberdeen Section Scanner Mark II".
11. Rogers beschreibt die neue Version des „SPRINT".
12. Chang stellt den Quadrant Slant-Hole Kollimator vor.
13. Jordan beschreibt die TOF-Ortung in stabförmigen Szintillatoren.
14. Die Shimadzu Corp. liefert das Headtome SET-230.

1983 (S. 199)

1. Hoffman stellt den ECAT III vor.
2. Burnham beschreibt den MGH Positronenring.
3. Takami stellt die 3-Ringversion Positologica-II vor.
4. Fa. Medimatic bietet den Hirn-Tomographen „Tomomatic 32" an.

5. KOBAYASHI stellt „BSO" als möglichen Ersatz für BGO-Kristalle vor.
6. CARROLL schlägt die rotierende Punktquelle als Ersatz für die ringförmigen Quellen zur Transmissionsmessung bei PET vor.

C. Grundlagen der Emissionstomographie

I. Allgemeine Vorbemerkungen

Obwohl die Anfänge der Emissions-Computer-Tomographie (ECT) auf den Beginn der 60er Jahre zurückgehen, wurde die ECT von der viel später (1972) realisierten Transmissions-Computer-Tomographie (TCT) in der Anwendungshäufigkeit und klinischen Bedeutung bei weitem übertroffen. Dies hat seinen Grund darin, daß die prinzipiellen physikalisch-meßtechnischen Bedingungen bei der ECT viel schwieriger sind als bei der TCT. Ein Vergleich beider Verfahren zeigt die grundlegenden Probleme auf. Bei der ECT versucht man, die räumliche Lage und Intensität einer Radionuklidverteilung innerhalb eines unterschiedlich absorbierenden Mediums darzustellen, während bei der TCT lediglich die Verteilung der unterschiedlichen Absorptionseigenschaften des Mediums dargestellt wird. Daraus wird sofort die ungleich schwierigere Aufgabe der ECT ersichtlich, die noch zusätzlich ganz wesentlich dadurch erschwert wird, daß der Informationsfluß bzw. die Zahl der registrierten Photonen bis zu einem Faktor 10^4 kleiner ist als bei der TCT.

Die Probleme mit dem statistisch bedingten Rauschen sind also unvergleichlich größer. Durch längere Untersuchungszeiten läßt sich bei der ECT nur vereinzelt eine kleine Verbesserung erzielen, da physiologisch bedingte schnelle Umverteilungen der markierten Testsubstanz in vivo oder deren schneller radioaktiver Zerfall dies verhindern, ganz abgesehen von der maximal zumutbaren Untersuchungszeit für den Patienten. Wenn trotzdem heute Emissions-Tomographen mit erstaunlicher Leistung zur Verfügung stehen, räumliche Auflösungen in den dargestellten Schichten von wenigen mm FWHM erreicht werden und Aufnahmedauern im Sekundenbereich möglich sind, so zeugt dies von einer konsequenten und variantenreichen Forschung und Entwicklung in den 25 zurückliegenden Jahren. Abschnitt B gibt hierüber einen ausführlichen Überblick.

II. Gewinnung der tomographischen Information

Gegeben ist eine räumliche Verteilung unterschiedlicher Aktivitätskonzentrationen im Objekt, die im folgenden kurz Objektverteilung genannt werden soll. Die notwendige meßtechnische Information gewinnt man ganz generell, indem man mit möglichst dünnen (hohe räumliche Auflösung) Meßstrahlen das Objekt unter den verschiedensten Winkeln abtastet, und die zu jeder Lage des Meßstrahles gehörige Strahlsumme registriert. Diese Strahlsumme mit der Dimension einer Impulsrate ist ein Maß für die Summe aller Aktivitätskonzentrationen, die in dem vom Meßstrahl erfaßten Teilvolumen des Objektes vorhanden sind (s. Abb. 56a). Verschiebt man die Meßsonde in der Schichtebene zum Beispiel so, daß viele parallel liegende Meßstrahlen durch die Objektschicht verlaufen, so ergibt sich eine eindimensionale Projektion durch das Objekt (s. Abb. 56b). Nimmt man viele solcher Projektionen unter verschiedenen Winkeln auf, entsprechend Abb. 56c, und addiert sie lagegerecht, so erhält man eine einfache Rückprojektion der gemessenen Objektschicht. Dies ist die denkbar einfachste Darstellung einer Aktivitätsverteilung bei der transversalen Tomographie.

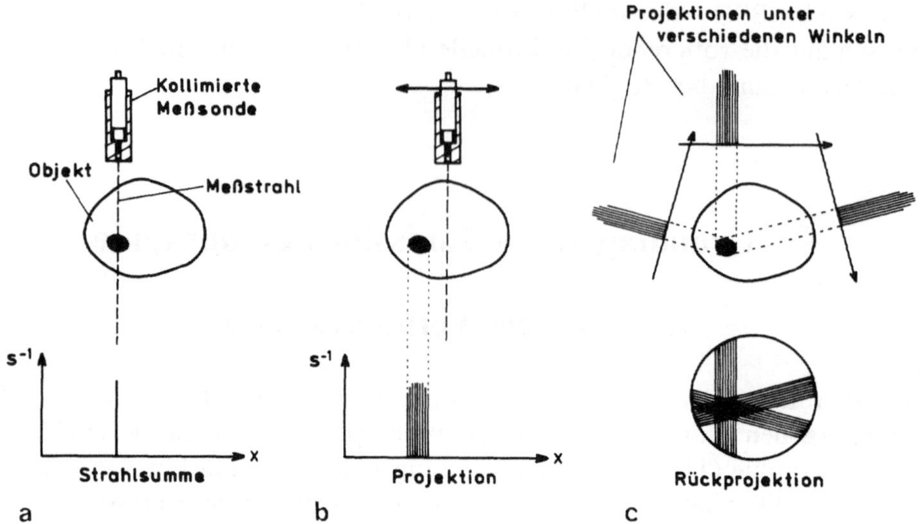

Abb. 56a–c. Zur Definition von **a** Meßstrahl und Strahlsumme, **b** Projektion und **c** Rückprojektion

Die *transversale Tomographie* zeichnet sich dadurch aus, daß der einzelne Meßstrahl während des Abtastvorganges oder während der tomographischen Messung sich stets in ein und derselben Ebene bewegt und daß die gemessenen Projektionen eindimensional sind, es sind Profile. Für Anordnungen mit vielen Sonden, z.B. Ringanordnungen, liegen sinngemäß alle Meßstrahlen in derselben Ebene. Dies gilt z.B. auch für die um das Objekt rotierende Gammakamera. Auch wenn man hier pro Winkelstellung eine zweidimensionale Projektion des Objektes erhält, so muß man sich darüber im klaren sein, daß sich diese nur aus einer Aneinanderreihung von vielen parallel liegenden eindimensionalen Projektionen zusammensetzt, und in diesem Sinne auch die Weiterverarbeitung der Informationen erfolgt bei der Rekonstruktion der einzelnen parallelen Schichten. Das dreidimensionale Objekt wird in einen Stapel von zweidimensionalen Schichten unterteilt, wobei jede Schicht und ihr zugehöriger Datensatz von den übrigen Schichten *unabhängig* ist. Ein weiteres Merkmal der transversalen Tomographie, welches in der Regel erfüllt ist, besteht darin, daß die Projektionen über einen vollen Winkelbereich von 180° gemessen werden. In diesem Fall ist jeder Datensatz *vollständig* bezüglich der Beschreibung der zugehörigen Schicht. Im speziellen Fall der SPECT ist wegen der ortsvarianten Abbildungseigenschaften dazu approximativ der Bereich von 360° sowie die Zusammenfassung opponierender Projektionen erforderlich.

Die *longitudinale Tomographie* zeichnet sich dagegen dadurch aus, daß die einzelnen Meßstrahlen während des Meßvorganges nicht in einer bestimmten Ebene liegen und die gemessenen Projektionen zweidimensional sind. Die Meßstrahlen können jede Orientierung im Raum annehmen, wobei aus praktischen Gründen meist nur eingeengte Raumwinkelbereiche möglich sind. Im englischen Sprachraum wird daher auch von „limited-angle tomography" gesprochen. Ein typisches Beispiel ist der „Seven Pinhole Kollimator" in Verbindung mit einer Gammakamera (s. Abb. 40). Sieben zweidimensionale Projektionen des Objekts werden über je eine Pinhole-Aperture auf den Kamerakristall projiziert, u. zw. unter verschiedenen Raumwinkeln. Aus diesen zweidimensionalen Projektionen werden dann longitudinale Schichten in verschiedener Tiefe berechnet. Diese longitudinalen Schichten sind voneinander *abhängig*, da sie nicht auf unabhängigen Datensätzen beruhen. Ferner sind die Datensätze *unvollständig* auf Grund des eingeschränkten Raumwinkels. Lottes (1982) gibt eine tabellarische Gegenüberstellung beider Verfahren (Tabelle 1).

Tabelle 1. Unterschiede zwischen transversalen und longitudinalen ECT-Systemen. (Aus LOTTES 1982)

	Transversale ECT	Longitudinale ECT
Dimensionen der Projektionen	Eindimensional (Profil)	Zweidimensional (Bild)
Dimensionen des rekonstruierten Objekts	Primär zweidimensional, Rekonstruktion des dreidimensionalen Objekts sukzessive Schicht für Schicht	Dreidimensional, Rekonstruktion aller Schichten gleichzeitig notwendig
Speicherbedarf im Rechner	Relativ gering	Sehr groß
Rechenzeit	Abhängig vom Algorithmus	Abhängig vom Algorithmus
Einfluß von Randfehlern	Gering	Groß
Absorptionskorrektur	Schwierig	Sehr schwierig
Meßdaten nur aus begrenztem Winkelbereich	Nein	Ja
Geometrische Lage der Schichten des Objekts	Festgelegt bei der Aufnahme, üblicherweise senkrecht zur Längsachse des Patienten	Wird erst bei der Rekonstruktion festgelegt, üblicherweise parallel zur Längsachse des Patienten

In neuerer Zeit werden auch mathematische Verfahren für die direkte *dreidimensionale Tomographie* diskutiert. Zu nennen ist hier der Ansatz für den spherischen Detektor von PELC u. CHESLER (1979) sowie die Untersuchungen von COLSHER (1980), RA u. CHO (1981), RA et al. (1982) und CHO et al. (1983b) für einen Detektor in Form einer Kugelschicht (truncated sphere). Eine solche Anordnung wird näherungsweise von Positronenkameras mit gegenüberstehenden planaren Meßköpfen bei vollständiger transversaler Rotation oder von Mehrfach-Ringtomographen realisiert. Dabei ist es notwendig zusätzlich schräg zur Rotationsachse liegende Meßstrahlen zu verwerten, d.h. Meßstrahlen, die durch mehrere transversale Schichten verlaufen. Neben den vollständigen und unabhängigen Daten der transversalen Schichten werden auch unvollständige und abhängige Datensätze als Zusatzinformation mit einbezogen. Für den (nur theoretisch realisierbaren) vollständigen spherischen Detektor weisen PELC u. CHESLER (1979) darauf hin, daß unter der Voraussetzung einer gleichen Anzahl registrierter Zerfälle der rein mathematische Gewinn an Signal/Rausch-Verhältnis gering sei. Da bei der Positronentomographie aber die Anzahl der registrierten Koinzidenzen erheblich zunimmt, ergibt sich ein merklicher Gewinn, der allerdings mit einem verstärkten Streustrahlungsanteil auf Grund des vergrößerten Öffnungswinkels erkauft werden muß.

III. Rekonstruktion der Objektverteilung

Die Rekonstruktionsverfahren werden ausführlich in Abschnitt G.IV. behandelt. Hier soll nur eine kurze Übersicht gegeben werden. Man kann die Verfahren in drei Hauptklassen einteilen:
1. Rekonstruktion mit Hilfe der linearen Superposition oder auch Rückprojektion genannt.
2. Analytische Rekonstruktion.
3. Algebraische Rekonstruktion.

1. Rekonstruktion mit Hilfe der linearen Superposition oder auch Rückprojektion genannt

Es ist häufig darüber diskutiert worden, ob die einfache Rückprojektion überhaupt eine Rekonstruktionsmethode sei, ich meine ja. Wenn aus einzelnen Projektionen durch lagegerechte Addition eine bildliche Darstellung der Objektverteilung erzeugt wird (s. Abb. 2), dann ist dies eine Rekonstruktion. Es spielt dabei zunächst keine Rolle, wie gut oder schlecht das so rekonstruierte Bild ist. Selbstverständlich kann man auf diese Weise nicht die wahre Objektverteilung rekonstruieren, da bei der endlichen Anzahl der Projektionen jede in der dargestellten Objektschicht vorhandene Aktivitätskonzentration ein sternförmiges Verwischungsmuster erzeugt, das mit der wahren Objektverteilung nichts gemein hat. Dies deutet sich auch in Abb. 56c an. Im dreidimensionalen Fall der longitudinalen Tomographie erscheint eine in einer rekonstruierten Objektschicht vorhandene Aktivitätskonzentration auch in allen anderen rekonstruierten Schichten in mehr oder weniger verwischter Form, wobei diese Verwischungsbilder noch unterschiedliche Strukturen aufweisen, je nach Art der Informationsgewinnung (s. Abb. 21). So kann eine Punktquelle in den benachbarten Schichten als Strich, Ring, Kreuz oder auch mehr oder weniger homogene Fläche erscheinen.

Die Aufgabe der analytischen und algebraischen Rekonstruktion ist es nun, diese Verwischungsbilder möglichst vollständig zu eliminieren.

2. Analytische Rekonstruktion

Bei der analytischen Rekonstruktion versucht man, durch die mathematische Operation der Filterung der einzelnen Projektionen die wahre Objektverteilung zu rekonstruieren. Zwei prinzipielle Wege stehen dabei offen, wie es in Abb. 57 dargestellt ist. Im linken Zweig wird die einfache Rückprojektion in geeigneter Weise gefiltert, im rechten Zweig wird eine Rückprojektion aus gefilterten Projektionen durchgeführt, was fälschlicherweise häufig gefilterte Rückprojektion genannt wird. Abbildung 58 zeigt rein schematisch den Vorgang der Filterung der Projektionen von Abb. 56. Faltet man die Projektionen mit einem geeigneten Filter, so erhält man eine gefilterte Projektion, die auch negative Strahlsummen enthält. Bildet man aus einer großen Anzahl solcher gefilterter Projektionen eine Rückprojektion, so sorgen die negativen Anteile der Projektionen dafür, daß bei geeigneter Form, d.h. bei richtiger Wahl des Filters, und einer ausreichenden Anzahl von Projektionen die strahlförmigen Verwischungsbilder verschwinden und nur das Bild der wahren Objektverteilung übrig bleibt. Abbildung 59 zeigt dies in anschaulicher Weise. Weitere Einzelheiten sind in Abschnitt G.IV.1. nachzulesen.

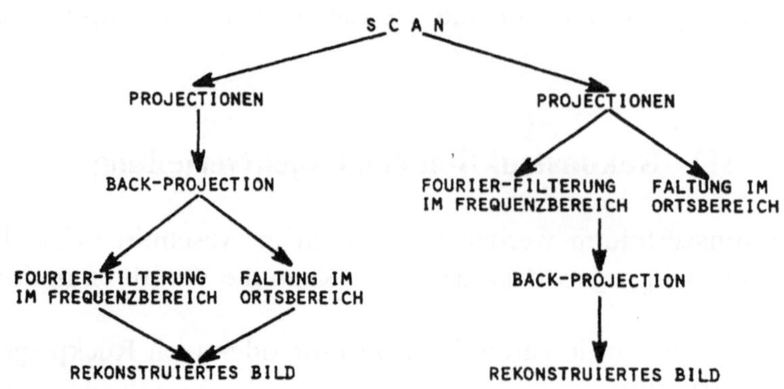

Abb. 57. Prinzipielle Möglichkeiten der analytischen Rekonstruktion. (Aus Lottes 1982)

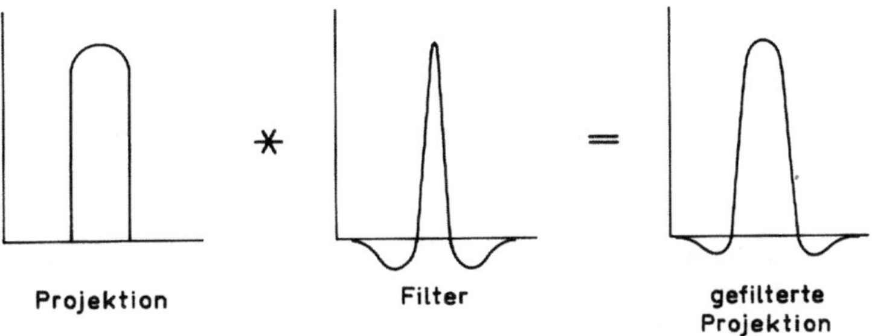

Abb. 58. Die Filterung einer Projektion. Die Projektion wird im Ortsbereich mit einem Filter gefaltet. Das Ergebnis ist die gefilterte Projektion mit negativen Anteilen

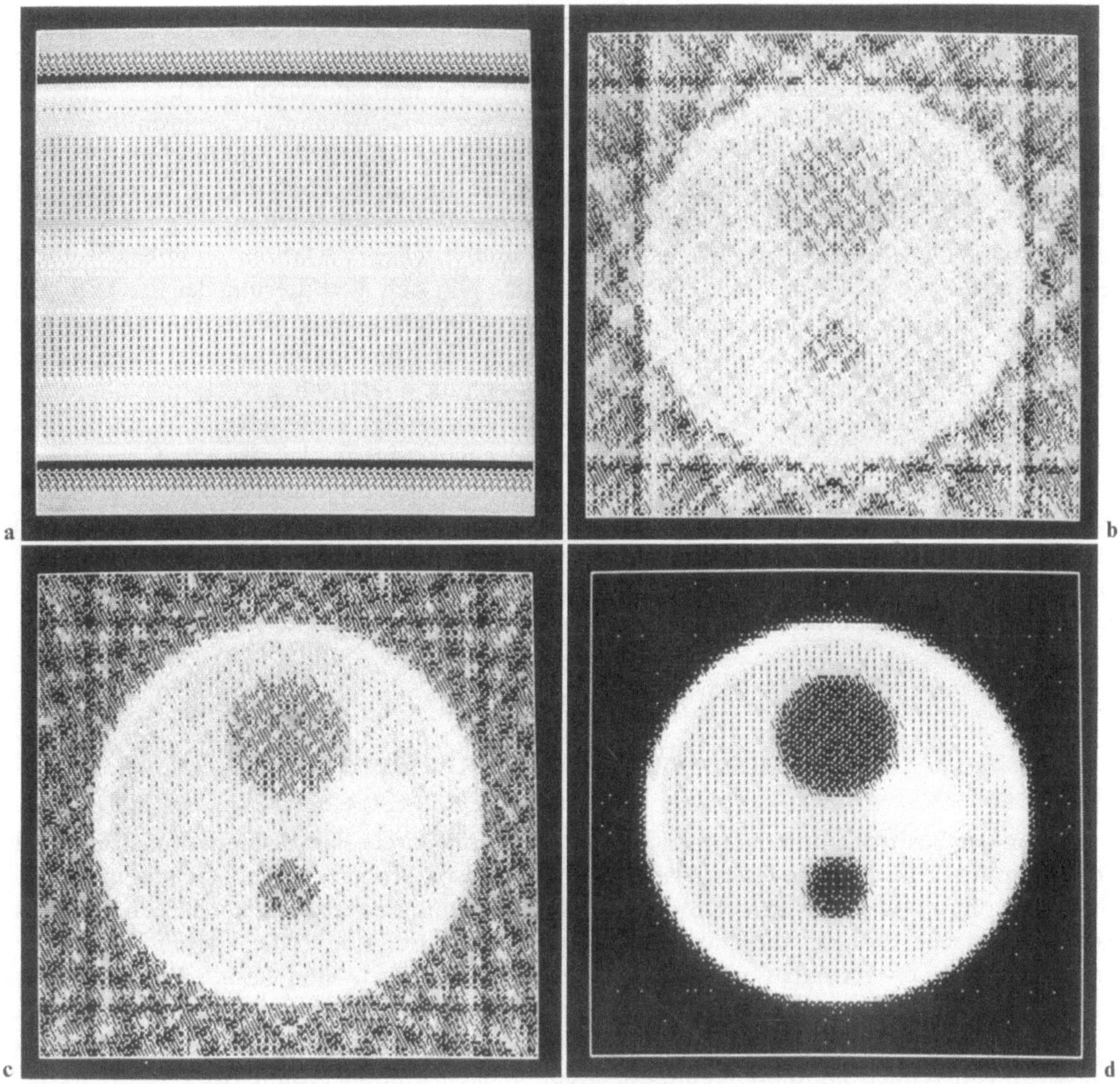

Abb. 59a–d. Überlagerung gefilterter Projektionen eines im Rechner simulierten Phantoms. **a** einzelne gefilterte Projektion. **b** 8, **c** 16 und **d** 101 gefilterte Projektionen überlagert. Bei der verwendeten 64 × 64 Matrix werden vom Abtasttheorem 101 Projektionen gefordert (s. auch Abschn. G.V.1.a)

3. Algebraische Rekonstruktion

Digitalisiert man das Bild der Rückprojektion in Abb. 56c, indem man es in eine Matrix von kleinen Bildelementen (pixel) entsprechenden Inhaltes aufteilt, so kann man es per Rechner in der gleichen Weise abtasten, wie dies bei der Bestimmung der gemessenen Projektionen beim Objekt geschehen ist. Man bildet also die Summe aller pixel-Inhalte, die längs eines „Meßstrahles" liegen und erhält so errechnete Strahlsummen bzw. errechnete Projektionen. Diese werden sich von den gemessenen Strahlsummen bzw. Projektionen mehr oder weniger unterscheiden. Durch Vergleich der gemessenen mit den aus dem Bild errechneten Strahlsummen wird ein Korrekturfaktor bestimmt, z.B. Differenz oder Quotient der Werte. Mit diesem Faktor werden nun alle pixel-Inhalte längs des Meßstrahles im Bild korrigiert. Ist diese Korrektur für alle Meßstrahlen durchgeführt, ist die erste Iteration beendet. Aus dieser neuen Bildmatrix werden nun wieder genauso errechnete Strahlsummen gebildet und mit den ursprünglich gemessenen Strahlsummen verglichen, und die Bildmatrix entsprechend erneut korrigiert. Nach jeder Iteration werden die Abweichungen zwischen gemessenen und errechneten Strahlsummen geringer werden, und man setzt die einzelnen Iterationsschritte solange fort, bis diese Abweichungen einen gewünschten Minimalwert erreicht haben. Für den theoretischen Fall, daß die Abweichungen zu Null werden, entspricht das so rekonstruierte Bild exakt der Objektverteilung, wenn man hier zunächst einmal die vielen Randprobleme wie statistische Streuung, Absorption, Streuung, endliche Meßstrahldurchmesser usw. unberücksichtig läßt. Eine vergleichende Wertung der beiden Rekonstruktionsverfahren ist nicht einfach, da sie stark vom jeweiligen Anwendungsfall und den gegebenen Randbedingungen abhängt. Generell kann man sagen, daß die analytischen Verfahren erheblich weniger rechenintensiv sind als die iterativen Verfahren. Auch läßt sich die Filterung der Projektionen bereits unmittelbar nach ihrer Messung durchführen (kürzere Rekonstruktionszeiten). Die Theorie der Signalverarbeitung läßt sich anwenden, so daß die Optimierung der Filter schon theoretisch möglich wird. Optimal einsetzen lassen sich die analytischen Verfahren allerdings nur, wenn die Abtastung über den vollen Winkelbereich erfolgt (transversale Tomographie), das sampling theorem erfüllt ist, die Absorption vernachlässigbar klein ist, das Objekt nicht größer ist als das rekonstruierte Volumen (Randfehler) und die Meßdaten nicht allzusehr verrauscht sind. Sind eine oder mehrere dieser Randbedingungen nicht erfüllt, so sind auch bei der transversalen Tomographie die algebraischen Verfahren vorzuziehen und bei der longitudinalen Tomographie immer anzuwenden, schon wegen des hier sehr begrenzten Raumwinkels bei der Abtastung.

D. Tomographie mit Gammastrahlern (SPECT)

Neben der Positronentomographie (PET) hat sich die Single Photon Emission Computed Tomography (SPECT) einen festen Platz in der Diagnostik erobert, obwohl sie rein meßtechnisch und physiologisch (kein C,O,N) der Positronentomographie weit unterlegen ist. Dies hat zwei einfache Gründe: die Gammastrahler wie zum Beispiel ^{99m}Tc, ^{123}I, ^{201}Tl, ^{133}Xe sind relativ einfach verfügbar und die notwendigen Meßgeräte sind häufig koventioneller Art, wie die rotierende Kamera. Die Mehrkosten für einen tomographischen Meßplatz halten sich daher in Grenzen. Dies gilt genauso für die nachträgliche Ausrüstung einer Kamera mit einem rotierenden slanthole-Kollimator oder einem 7-pinhole-Kollimator.

Man muß andererseits aber auch in Kauf nehmen, daß mit diesen Systemen der große Durchbruch der ECT in der Nuklearmedizin nicht realisiert werden konnte. Der echte klinische Gewinn an diagnostischer Treffsicherheit bei vergleichbaren Untersuchungszeiten gegenüber einfacher flächiger Kameraaufnahme ist nicht so spektakulär wie ursprünglich erhofft. Wenn auch eine größere Zahl von Arbeiten der SPECT eine Überlegenheit gegenüber normaler planarer Szintigraphie bescheinigen, z.B. BÜLL et al. (1983a), KIRSCH et al. (1983), MAUBLANT et al. (1982), STRAUSS et al. (1982), BIERSACK et al. (1983), so gibt es doch auch eine Reihe von Berichten, die sich kritisch mit der SPECT auseinandersetzen (SMALLING 1983; MULLANI et al. 1981; RIZI et al. 1981).

KEYES Jr. (1982) sagt in seiner Übersichtsarbeit, wie ich meine, sehr richtig: „SPECT trägt weder zur Wiedergeburt der Nuklearmedizin bei noch ist es eine unsinnige Methode. Es ist eine Technik, die manches in der Nuklearmedizin verbessern wird, die aber sicher nicht ähnlich revolutionär verlaufen wird wie die TCT in der Röntgendiagnostik. Andererseits ist über diese neue Technologie ein beachtlicher Unsinn geschrieben und gesprochen worden, sowohl im optimistischen wie pessimistischen Sinne."

Besonders die Hoffnungen auf eine quantitative Aktivitätsbestimmung in vivo mit Hilfe der SPECT haben sich bisher nicht erfüllt, wenn man vom Hirn absieht. In seiner ausführlichen Übersichtsarbeit vertritt BUDINGER (1980) klar die Meinung, daß wegen der großen Absorptionsprobleme und der schlechten Statistik wohl nur beim Hirn quantitative Bestimmungen mit SPECT durchführbar sein werden, und äußert diese Meinung auch 2 Jahre später (BUDINGER 1982a).

I. Rotierende Gamma-Kamera

Die rotierende Kamera ist der transversalen Tomographie zuzuordnen. Heutige kommerzielle Bauformen zeigen beispielhaft die Abb. 60–64. Der Kamerakopf rotiert üblicherweise auf einer Kreisbahn um den Patienten, wobei die Rotationsachse mit der Körperlängsachse zusammenfällt.

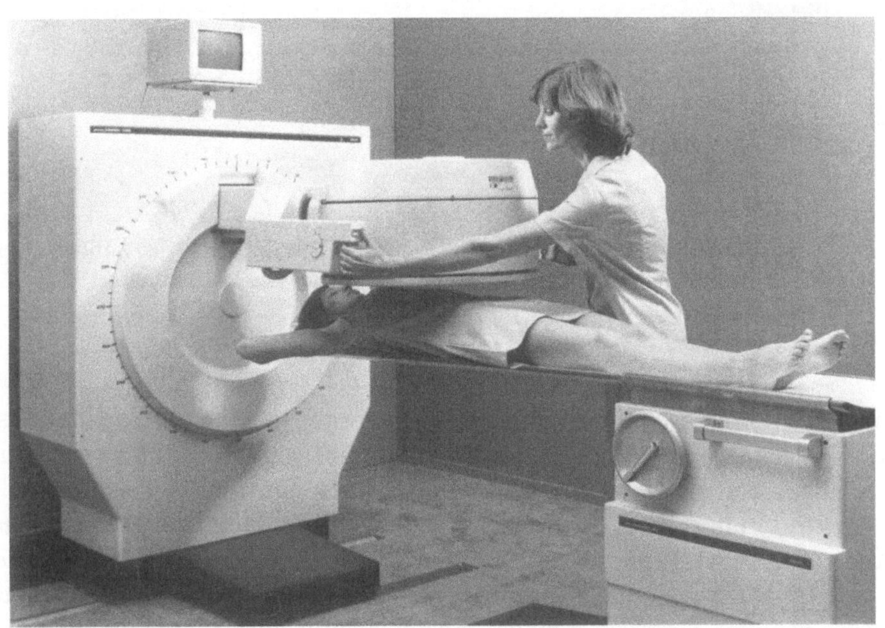

Abb. 60. Moderne Tomo-Kamera „Gamma Diagnost" mit Rotationsstativ und vollem Gewichtsausgleich des Meßkopfes. (Freundlicherweise von Fa. Philips zur Verfügung gestellt)

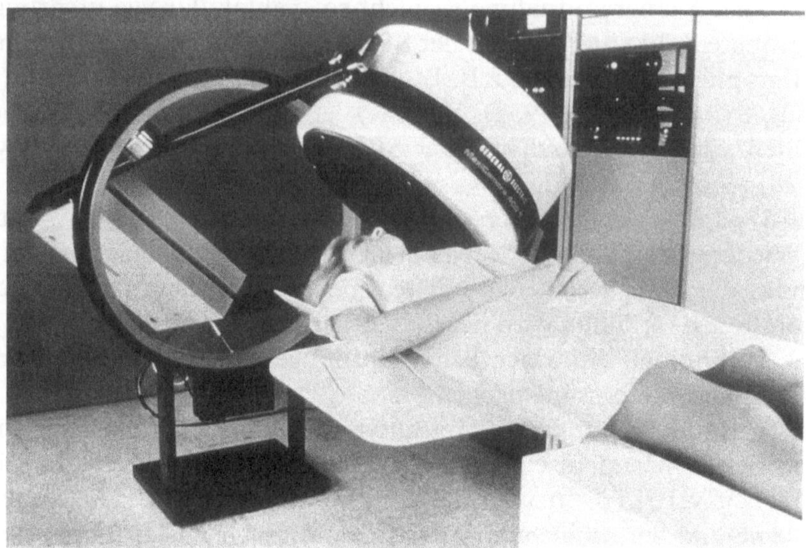

Abb. 61. Eine der ersten rotierenden Kameras „Maxicamera 400 T". (Freundlicherweise von Fa. General Electric zur Verfügung gestellt)

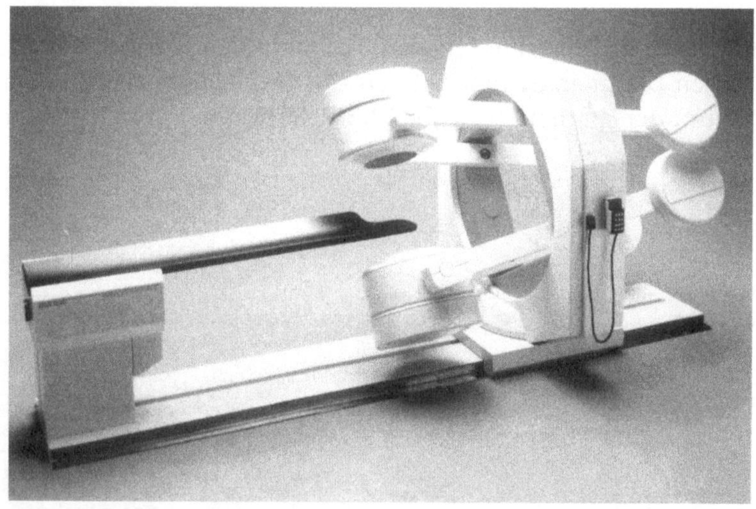

Abb. 62. Moderne Tomo-Kamera mit Rotationsstativ und Gewichtsausgleich für wahlweise ein oder zwei Kamerameßköpfe. (Freundlicherweise von Fa. Picker zur Verfügung gestellt)

Die physikalischen Eigenschaften von 10 Systemen sind tabellarisch in einer ausführlichen Übersicht von Jaszczak (1982) zusammengestellt. Die Meßfelddurchmesser der Kameras liegen in der Regel bei 38–40 cm, mit Ausnahme der Omega 500 von Fa. Technicare (s. Abb. 63), die mit ihrem rechteckigen Meßfeld in Richtung längs zur Rotationsachse 51 cm erfaßt. Die Kristalldicke schwankt zwischen 6,4 und 12,7 mm, die Anzahl der Photomultiplier zwischen 37 und 75. Der maximale Rotationsdurchmesser, der ja eine Art Patientenaperture festlegt, läßt sich bei allen Geräten ≥ 60 cm einstellen und die Art der Rotation ist meistens wählbar zwischen kontinuierlicher und schrittweiser Bewegung. Die Rotationszeit liegt minimal bei 30 s und maximal zwischen 6 min und ∞.

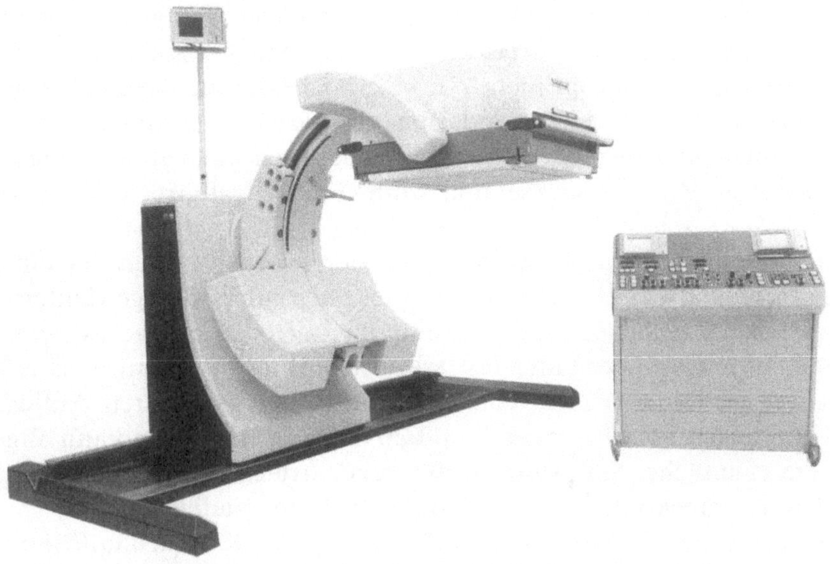

Abb. 63. Moderne Rotations-Kamera OMEGA 500 mit rechteckigem Meßfeld. (Freundlicherweise von Fa. Technicare zur Verfügung gestellt)

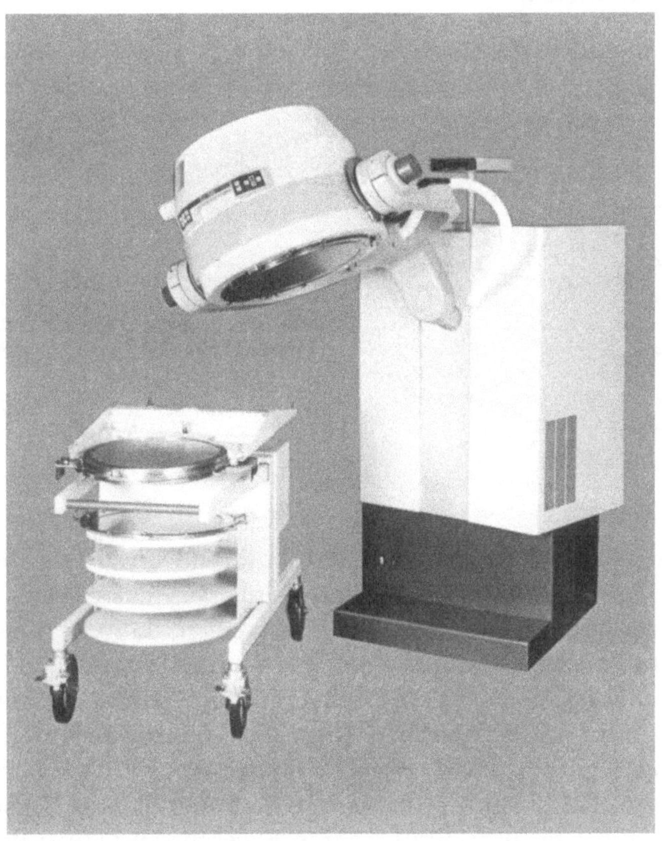

Abb. 64. Moderne rotierende Gamma-Kamera mit Gewichtsausgleich des Meßkopfes. (Freundlicherweise von Fa. Siemens zur Verfügung gestellt)

Die Rotation erfolgte ursprünglich ausschließlich auf einem Kreisbogen, was keine optimale Anpassung an den elliptischen Querschnitt des liegenden Patienten darstellte. In zunehmendem Maße werden auch nicht kreisrunde Umlaufbahnen realisiert, wie z.B. bei der OMEGA 500 (Abb. 63). Dies bringt nicht nur eine Verbesserung der räumlichen Auflösung um 1–3 mm (Gottschalk et al. 1983), sondern auch eine Verringerung der Homogenitätsartefakte, wenn die nicht kreisförmige Umlaufbahn dadurch erzeugt wird, daß eine laterale Verschiebung zwischen Rotationsachse und Objekt durchgeführt wird (Todd-Pokropek 1983 a).

Die erzielbare räumliche Auflösung innerhalb der rekonstruierten Schicht ist abhängig vom Auflösungsvermögen des Kamera-Meßkopfes, besonders des gewählten Kollimators, vom Abstand zwischen Kamera-Kollimator und Objekt (Rotationsradius), von der Position innerhalb der Schicht und von der Güte des Rekonstruktionsprogrammes. Hier ist besonders die Eigenschaft des gewählten Filters von Bedeutung. Die erzielbaren Auflösungen liegen je nach Randbedingungen zwischen etwa 9 und 20 mm FWHM. Man kann allgemein davon ausgehen, daß die räumliche Auflösung in der rekonstruierten Schicht etwa gleich ist der Auflösung des Kamerameßkopfes im Abstand des Rotationsradius.

Entscheidend bei SPECT ist aber die Verbesserung der Kontrastauflösung von kleinen kalten oder heißen Bereichen innerhalb eines ausgedehnten Organs, z.B. der Leber. Hier macht sich die mehr oder weniger überlagerungsfreie Darstellung der Aktivitätsverteilungen innerhalb der gemessenen Objektschichten sehr positiv bemerkbar. Abbildung 65 zeigt ein Leberphantom und Abb. 66 jeweils vier Schichten in transversaler bzw. koronaler Richtung und die konventionelle planare Kameraaufnahme. Man erkennt den deutlich besseren Kontrast in den tomographischen Schichten. Allerdings wurden die Schichten auch mit je einer Million Impulsen aufgenommen.

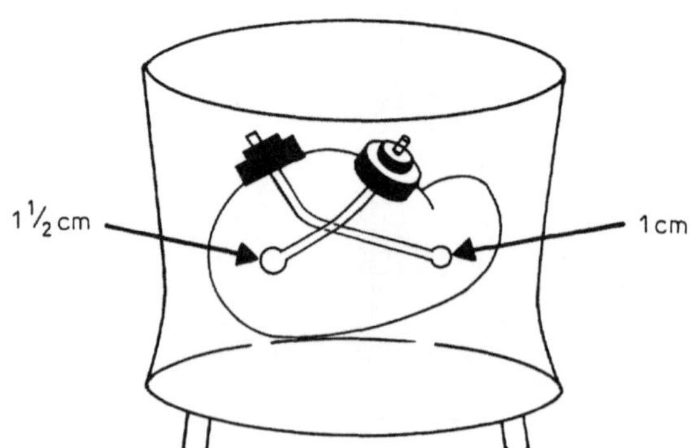

Abb. 65. Leberförmiges Phantom mit zwei „kalten Knoten" von 1,5 bzw. 1 cm Durchmesser, homogen mit Aktivität gefüllt. Diese Leber befand sich in einem mit Wasser gefüllten Alderson Körperphantom. (Aus Jaszczak et al. 1982b)

Nicht vergessen darf man die Tatsache, daß während der 26 min dauernden SPECT-Aufnahme keinerlei Organbewegungen aufgetreten sind, was in der Praxis zu einer merklichen Kontrastverschlechterung führt, und man darf unterstellen, daß vor diesen Aufnahmen eine exakte Qualitätskontrolle des Systems durchgeführt wurde.

SPECT mit rotierender Kamera ist ein Meßverfahren, welches nur dann zu brauchbaren Ergebnissen führt, wenn es mit Akribie betrieben wird, d.h. wenn durch *ständige* Qualitätskontrolle *alle* Randbedingungen und Parameter überprüft und korrigiert werden. Eine Kamera-Inhomogenität von 10% mag für die planare Aufnahme unter Umständen noch akzeptabel sein, bei SPECT führt sie zu unbrauchbaren Ergebnissen (Todd-Pokropek u. Soussaline 1982; Jaszczak u. Coleman 1980). Weitere Vorschläge zur Qualitätskontrolle bei SPECT findet man bei Lonn et al. (1983) und Jarritt u. Cullum (1983).

Spect   Conventional

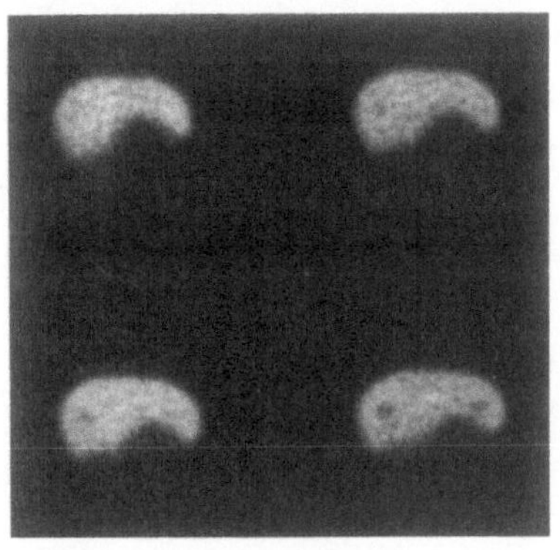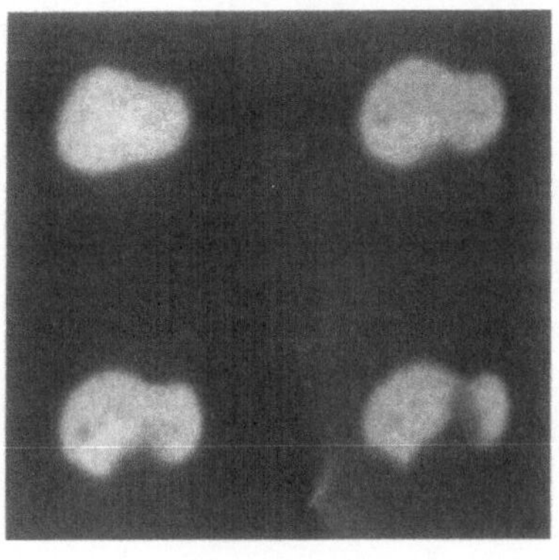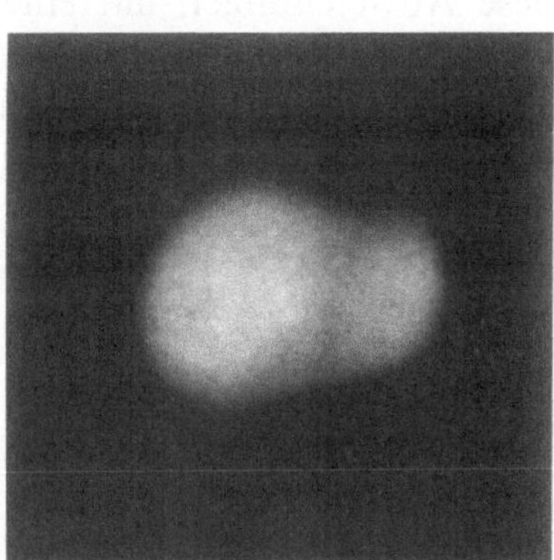

Transverse   Coronal

Abb. 66. Transversale und koronale Schichten durch das Phantom von Abb. 65, aufgenommen mit einer rotierenden Doppelkopfkamera. Rechts eine planare Kamera-Aufnahme mit 1 Mill. Impulsen zum Vergleich. In der koronalen Schicht rechts unten ist die Halterung mit 6 mm $\varnothing$ der 1 cm Kugel sichtbar. (Aus JASZCZAK et al. 1982b)

Wesentliche Einflüsse auf die Bildqualität haben:

1. Fehler bezüglich des Rotationszentrums;
2. die Inhomogenität der Kamera, und zwar sowohl die Inhomogenität bei stillstehendem Kamerakopf als auch die Homogenitätsänderungen bedingt durch unterschiedliche räumliche Lage des Kamerakopfes (z.B. Einfluß des Magnetfeldes);
3. Variationen des Streustrahlanteils abhängig von der Kopfstellung.

Zu 1.: Befindet sich eine Punktquelle auf der Rotationsachse des Systems, so muß das Maximum der Punktbildfunktion, z.B. bei einer 128er Matrix, genau zwischen Pixel 64 und 65 liegen (s. Abb. 67). Im rekonstruierten Bild erscheint die Punktquelle dann scharf abgebildet. Wenn durch Verstärkungsänderung eine Verschiebung des elektronischen Koordinatensystems der Kamera eingetreten ist oder der Kamerakopf nicht exakt parallel zur Rotationsachse ausgerichtet ist, kommt es zu ringförmigen Artefaktbildungen, wie in Abb. 67b zu sehen. Beträgt wie hier angedeutet die Verschiebung nur 1,5 Pixel bei einer typischen Pixelbreite von 3 mm, so beträgt der Durchmesser des Artefaktringes schon 9 mm. Entsprechend verschlechtert sich auch die räumliche Auflösung, nämlich um 4,5 mm.

Zu 2: Die Inhomogenität der Kamera äußert sich normalerweise auch in der Form von ringförmigen Artefakten. Abbildung 68 gibt eine schematische Darstellung der Entstehung solcher „Ringe", wenn die Kamera an einer bestimmten Stelle eine erhöhte Empfindlichkeit aufweist.

Abbildung 69 zeigt deutlich an einem praktischen Beispiel, wie groß der Einfluß der Inhomogenität ist. Die häufig geäußerte Ansicht, daß solche Inhomogenitäten im routinemäßigen klinischen Einsatz ohne große Bedeutung seien, ist gefährlich und eigentlich nicht zu verantworten. Das Beispiel eines klinischen Lebertomogramms in Abb. 69 untere Zeile zeigt deutlich, daß solche Artefakte sehr wohl die Befundung erheblich beeinflussen können. Die beste Homogenitätskorrektur nützt nichts, wenn die Homogenität der Kamera sich während der Rotation ändert, zum Beispiel durch den Einfluß des Erdmagnetfeldes (JAHANGIR et al. 1983). Wenn dieser Einfluß bei modernen Kameras mit automatischer PM-Stabilisierung auch weitgehend eliminiert ist, so geben neuere Messungen von JOHNSON et al. (1983)

sehr zu denken, die bei modernen Kameratypen zwischen zwei um 180° verschiedenen Kopfstellungen Abweichungen der Ortskoordinaten um bis zu 1,7 mm gemessen haben, wobei diese Abweichungen mit einer Zeitkonstanten von etwa einer Stunde exponentiell kleiner werden. Als Ursache scheidet also das Erdmagnetfeld hier aus. Thermische Einflüsse oder Änderungen der Multiplier-Kristall-Kopplung werden vermutet.

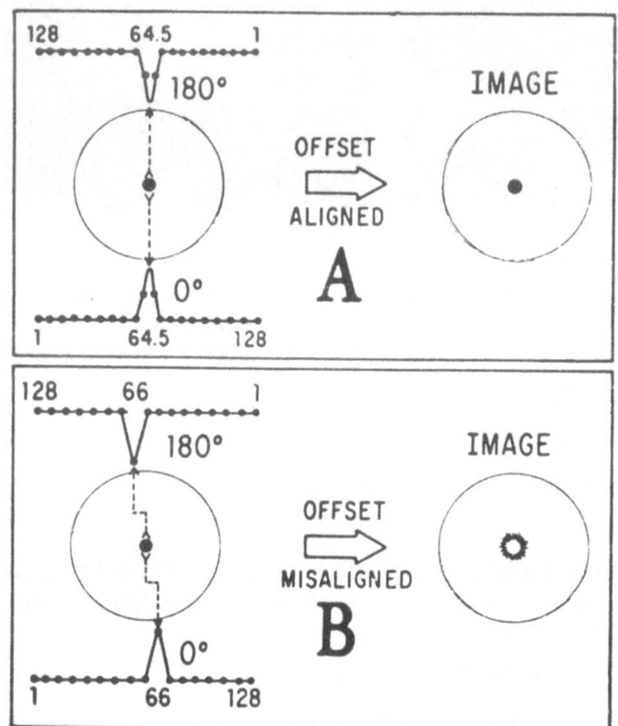

Abb. 67. Ringförmige Artefaktbildung bei nicht exakt abgeglichener Kamera bezüglich des Rotationszentrums. (Aus Jaszczak et al. 1980)

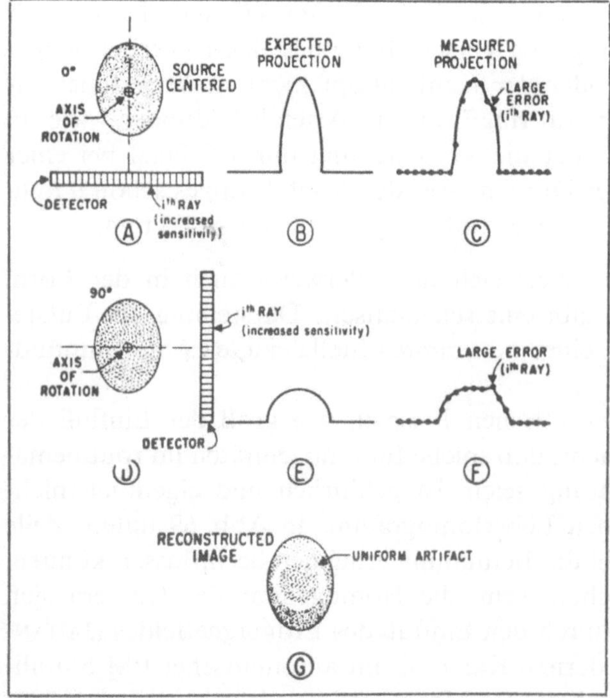

Abb. 68. Ringförmige Artefakte bei einer inhomogenen Kamera. (Aus Jaszczak et al. 1980)

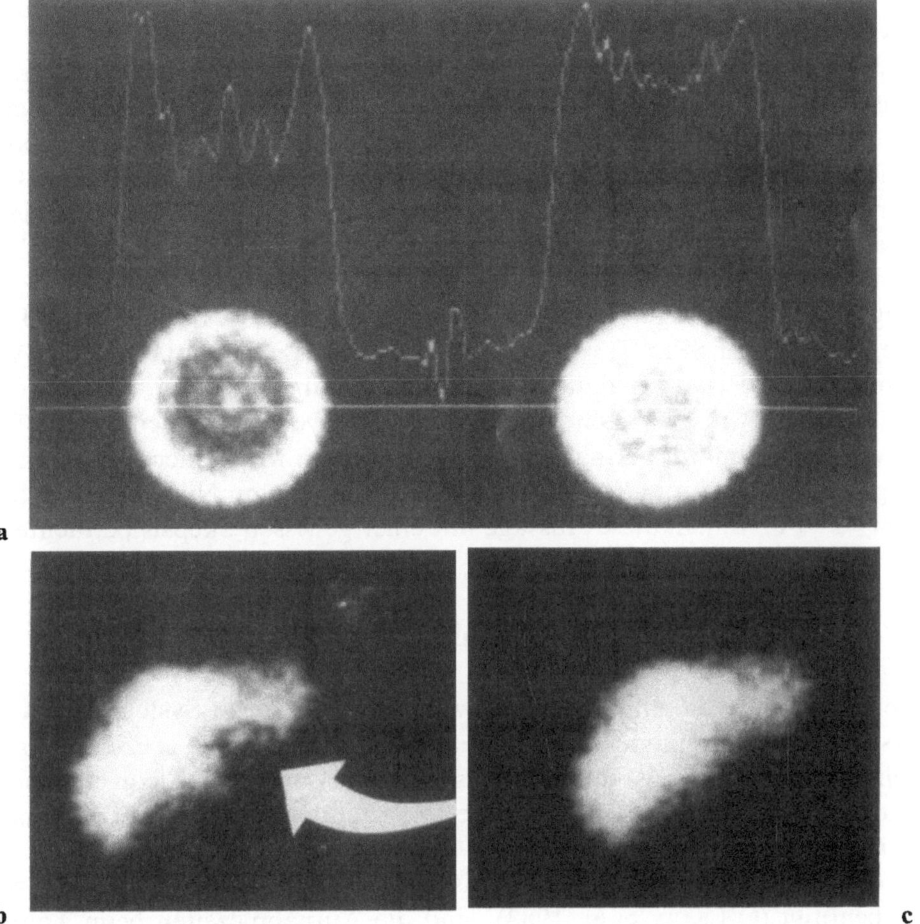

Abb. 69. a Rekonstruierte Schicht eines homogen mit Aktivität gefüllten Zylinders. *Links* ohne Homogenitäts-korrektur der Kamera, *rechts* mit Korrektur (aus TODD-POKROPEK 1983b). **b, c** Rekonstruierte Schicht durch eine Leber. **b** mit Artefakt, hervorgerufen durch Inhomogenität (*Pfeil*). **c** der gleiche Leberschnitt nach Homogenitätskorrektur (aus TODD-POKROPEK u. JARRIT 1982)

Zu 3: Der Einfluß der Streustrahlung und deren Korrektur stellt eines der schwierigsten Kapitel bei SPECT dar (PANG u. GENNA 1979). Der Anteil an Streustrahlung ist extrem abhängig von der Einstellung des Energiefensters und damit auch von einer eventuellen Änderung der Fensterlage während der Rotation. Ferner ist der Streustrahlanteil abhängig von der Beschaffenheit des Objektes und dem Betrachtungswinkel, unter dem das Objekt gesehen wird. Man muß also versuchen, durch exakte Fenstereinstellung den Anteil an Streustrahlung schon bei der Messung so gering wie möglich zu halten. Diesem eventuellen Anheben der unteren Schwelle des Energiefensters wird aber durch die Homogenitätsforderung sehr schnell eine Grenze gesetzt, da unsymmetrische Fenstereinstellungen starke Inhomogenitäten hervorrufen und außerdem auch die Empfindlichkeit des Systems stark herabsetzen.

Dies sind einige Gründe, warum SPECT nur dann befriedigende Ergebnisse liefern kann, wenn eine exakte und häufige Qualitätskontrolle durchgeführt wird. Damit wird zum Teil auch verständlich, warum sehr unterschiedliche Meinungen über den Wert der Methode geäußert werden (s. auch Abschnitt B, das Jahr 1982).

Eine ganz wesentliche Aufgabe fällt hier der Software eines Systems zu. Wenn vom Rechner keine geeigneten und umfassenden Qualitätskontroll-Routinen zur Verfügung gestellt werden, hat das beste SPECT-System für die routinemäßige Anwendung nur einen begrenzten Wert.

Unabhängig von all diesen Qualitätskontroll-Probleme wird über den erfolgreichen Einsatz der rotierenden Kamera berichtet in Verbindung mit ^{123}J-Amphetamin bei Epilepsie (Biersack et al. 1983a) oder ^{123}J-HIPDm bei Gliomen und zerebralem Infarkt (Drayer et al. 1983). Dagegen scheinen Versuche, den Stoffwechsel mit ^{123}J markierter Glukose zu messen, vorerst wenig Erfolg zu versprechen (Kloster et al. 1983). Über eine selektive arterielle Infusion von ^{81m}Kr zur Messung des zerebralen Blutflusses durch SPECT in Verbindung mit Röntgen-CT Aufnahmen berichten Higa et al. (1983).

Die häufig diskutierte Frage, welcher Kollimator bei der Messung von ^{123}J verwendet werden sollte, ist auch bei SPECT von besonderem Interesse. Coleman et al. (1983) stellen in einer Phantom- und Patientenstudie fest, daß bei „sauberem" ^{123}J, z.B. gewonnen über ^{127}J→^{123}Xe, niederenergetische Kollimatoren eingesetzt werden können, und daß ein hochauflösender LEHR-Kollimator geringfügig besser ist als ein Mittelenergie-Kollimator. Nach Untersuchungen von Döring et al. (1983) über das Verhalten von Niederenergiekollimatoren bei „sauberem" ^{123}J muß man diese Aussage mit einer gewissen Skepsis betrachten.

II. Ringförmige Systeme

Neben der rotierenden Gammakamera gewinnen ringförmige Systeme zur Darstellung von transversalen Schichten immer mehr Bedeutung, besonders als spezielle Hirntomographen. Ausgehend vom Mark IV von Kuhl (s. Abb. 31) über die Cleon Scanner von Fa. Union Carbide (s. Abb. 38), ist besonders die Weiterentwicklung zum Tomomatic 64 der Fa. Medimatic von Interesse (s. Abb. 45).

Während der Cleon 710 noch eine verhältnismäßig hohe Scanzeit pro Schicht von mehreren Minuten benötigt (O'Leary et al. 1983), sind die Aufnahmezeiten beim Tomomatic 64 auf 5 s geschrumpft, d.h. genauer, in 5 s wird eine Rotation um 180° durchgeführt, so daß alle möglichen und notwendigen Projektionen der betrachteten drei Schichten gemessen wurden. Dies bedeutet nicht, daß nach 5 s Schichtaufnahmen mit brauchbarer Qualität vorliegen, aber nach einem kontinuierlichen Untersuchungsgang von z.B. 5 min liegen eine große Zahl von abgeschlossenen Projektionssätzen vor, die beliebig addiert und nach Rekonstruktion zur Berechnung und bildlichen Darstellung dynamischer Flußwerte dienen (Lassen et al. 1983; Büll et al. 1983b; Bonte et al. 1983) (s. auch Abb. 48). Diese Methode bewährt sich für dynamische Hirnuntersuchungen mit ^{133}Xe und ^{123}J-Amphetamin in zunehmendem Maße (s. Hedde et al. 1984). Spezielle für ^{133}Xe Inhalationsmessungen liefert die Fa. Medimatic auch eine preiswerte Ein-Schichtversion mit 32 NaJ(Tl) Szintillationsdetektoren, den Tomomatic 32. Die Kristalle sind ebenfalls auf den Seiten eines Quadrates zu je 8 angeordnet. Ein Computer mit Farbmonitor zur Rekonstruktion und Darstellung der Schichtaufnahme sowie eine zusätzliche Meßsonde über der Lunge des Patienten vervollständigen den Meßplatz.

Ähnlich konzipierte Geräte sind das „Gammatom-1" mit 36 NaJ(Tl)-Kristallen (Cho et al. 1982) und der „Aberdeen Section Scanner Mark II" mit 24 NaJ(Tl)-Kristallen (Smith et al. 1982). Das Headtome (s. Abb. 47) wurde zu einem Drei-Ringsystem Headtome II weiterentwickelt (Hirose et al. 1982) und wird von der Shimadzu Corp. unter dem Namen Headtome SET-230 vertrieben.

III. Slanthole-Pinhole-Kollimatoren

Auf dem Gebiet der longitudinalen SPECT behaupten sich nach wie vor der rotierenden Slanthole-Kollimator und die mehrfach Pinhole-Kollimatoren (s. Abb. 15, 40, 53).

Da bei modernen Gamma-Kameras mit Datenverarbeitung der Mehrpreis für eine SPECT Ausführung in der gleichen Größenordnung liegt wie die zusätzliche Ausrüstung mit Slanthole- oder Pinhole-Kollimatoren, gewinnt die Frage nach der Leistungsfähigkeit der verschiedenen Verfahren eine besondere Bedeutung.

Neben den in Abschnitt B (Jahre 1981/82) zitierten Arbeiten über die longitudinalen Verfahren gibt es wenige Arbeiten, die über einen direkten Vergleich der drei Methoden berichten. MYERS MJ et al. (1983) vergleichen an einem relativ realistischen Herzmodell und ^{201}Tl direkt die rotierende Kamera mit dem rotierenden Slanthole-Kollimator und bringen die Ergebnisse in Relation mit früheren Ergebnissen von WILLIAMS et al. (1980) über den 7-Pinhole-Kollimator. Obwohl die erzielbare räumliche Auflösung beim rotierenden Slanthole-Kollimator innerhalb der Schicht am besten ist, bedingt die schlechte Schichttrennung bei den longitudinalen Verfahren, daß der Kontrast bei der rotierenden Kamera weitaus am besten ist, und auf den kommt es im wesentlichen an. Als besten Ersatz für die rotierende Kamera kann man speziell bei Herzmessungen, und nur dafür kommt er praktisch in Frage, den rotierenden Slanthole-Kollimator ansehen, während am wenigsten der 7-Pinhole-Kollimator geeignet erscheint. Das deckt sich auch mit Untersuchungen von CONDON et al. (1983). Interessant ist noch die Entwicklung eines Slanthole-Kollimators mit variabler Neigungseinstellung der Bohrungen zwischen 0 und 40° zur Kollimatorachse. Durch Verwendung einer Vielzahl nur 0,125 mm dicker Wolframbleche werden relativ hohe Auflösung und Ausbeute gegenüber konventionellen Kamera-Kollimatoren erreicht (MOORE et al. 1983). Diese Variabilität gestattet eine Anpassung an das Objektvolumen bzw. die Wahl eines möglichst großen Neigungswinkels zur Verbesserung der Schichtrennung.

Eine Zusammenfassung der Einsatzmöglichkeiten von SPECT in der Diagnostik vermittelt die von BÜLL et al. (1983) aufgestellte Tabelle 2. Sie leitet gleichzeitig über zu dem folgenden Kapitel über Positronen-Tomographie PET, deren Anwendungsmöglichkeiten ebenfalls aufgelistet sind.

E. Tomographie mit Positronenstrahlern (PET)

Die Positronentomographie ist sowohl in physiologischer wie auch meßtechnischer Sicht die optimale Methode der ECT. Die körpereigenen und am Stoffwechsel unmittelbar beteiligten Elemente Kohlenstoff, Stickstoff und Sauerstoff kommen in der Natur leider nur in einer einzigen isotopen Form vor, die sich für Messungen in vivo eignet, u. zw. ^{11}C, ^{13}N und ^{15}O, und dies sind Positronenstrahler. Mit ihren sehr kurzen Halbwertszeiten von abgerundet 20, 10 und 2 min sind sie leider nur in der Nähe von geeigneten Generatoren, meist Zyklotrons, verfügbar.

Dies ist der Hauptgrund, warum die Positronentomographie bis heute nur wenig Verbreitung finden konnte, obwohl sie auch meßtechnisch der SPECT erheblich überlegen ist.

Die größten Erfolge kann die PET auf dem Gebiet der Messung der lokalen Hirnfunktion verzeichnen. KUHL (1984) gibt hierüber einen zusammenfassenden Bericht. Speziell mit der Sauerstoffverwertung des Hirns setzen sich MINTUN et al. (1984) auseinander.

Die meßtechnischen Vorteile sind darin begründet, daß beim Positronenzerfall (β^+-Zerfall) nicht nur ein γ-Quant emittiert wird, sondern stets gleichzeitig ein Paar gleicher γ-Quanten mit je 511 keV Energie. Zusätzlich ist eine strenge Winkelbeziehung zwischen beiden

Tabelle 2. Emissionstomographie: Einsatzmöglichkeiten, Radiopharmazeutika, Tracerwege und Ziele. (Aus Büll et al. 1983a)

Gehirn	SPECT (D-ECT)	^{99m}Tc-Chelate	Blut-Hirn-Schranke
		^{123}J-Amphetamin	Regionale Durchblutung
		^{133}Xe-Gas	Regionale Durchblutung
	PET	^{11}CO	Regionales Blutvolumen
		$C^{15}O_2$	Regionale Durchblutung
		^{18}F-DOG	Regionaler Glukosestoffwechsel
Herz	PET	^{18}F-DOG	Myokardialer Glukosestoffwechsel
		^{11}C-Palmitat	Myokardialer Fettsäurestoffwechsel
		^{13}NH$_4$	Regionale Myokarddurchblutung
	SPECT	^{201}Tl	Regionale Myokard-„perfusion"
		^{123}J-Fettsäuren	Myokardialer Fettsäurestoffwechsel
		^{99m}Tc-Erys	Regionale LV-Pumpfunktion
Leber	SPECT	^{99m}Tc-Kolloide	Regionale RES-Funktion
Pankreas	PET	^{11}C-Aminosäuren	Regionaler Aminosäurestoffwechsel
Knochen	SPECT	^{99m}Tc-Dipp	Regionale Chemisorption (Perfusion)
Lunge	SPECT	^{99m}Tc-Mikrosph.	Regionale Blutverteilung
	PET	$C^{15}O_2$, ^{13}N	Regionale Belüftung, Durchblutung

Quanten gegeben, sie werden genau diametral gerichtet zueinander emittiert beim Zerfallsprozeß. Diese Zusatzinformation gegenüber einfachen Gammastrahlern (single photon emitter) läßt sich physikalisch hervorragend nutzen zur „elektronischen" Kollimierung, so daß die üblichen Bleikollimatoren mit ihren meist unzureichenden Eigenschaften entfallen können.

I. Räumliche Auflösung

Die Vorteile der Positronen-Koinzidenzmessung zeigt in überzeugender Weise Abb. 70. Drei Linienquellen von 2 mm Durchmesser in einem zylindrischen mit Wasser gefüllten Phantom von 18 cm Durchmesser wurden mit einer Anger-Kamera mit üblichem Parallellochkollimator betrachtet, wobei die 3 Quellen einen Abstand von 2, 9 bzw. 16 cm von der Kollimatoroberfläche hatten und mit ^{99m}Tc gefüllt waren.

Im linken Bildteil ist in der Mitte die Kameraaufnahme zu sehen und unten die zugehörigen Linienbildfunktionen. Die Halbwertsbreiten variieren zwischen 11 und 19 mm, die Ausbeute nimmt mit größerem Abstand stark ab. Im rechten Bildteil wurden die mit dem Positronenstrahler ^{64}Cu gefüllten Quellen mit ringförmig angeordneten unkollimierten Detektoren gemessen, wobei jeweils gegenüberliegende Sonden in Koinzidenz betrieben wurden und eine Schicht des Phantoms rekonstruiert wurde. Die Halbwertsbreiten und die Ausbeute bleiben praktisch konstant, leichte Abweichungen sind nur bei Messungen mit niedriger Energieschwelle feststellbar.

Die Halbwertsbreite des Meßstrahles zwischen zwei in Koinzidenz betriebenen Sonden ist abhängig vom Durchmesser d der Kristalle bzw. dem Durchmesser d der Blendenöffnung,

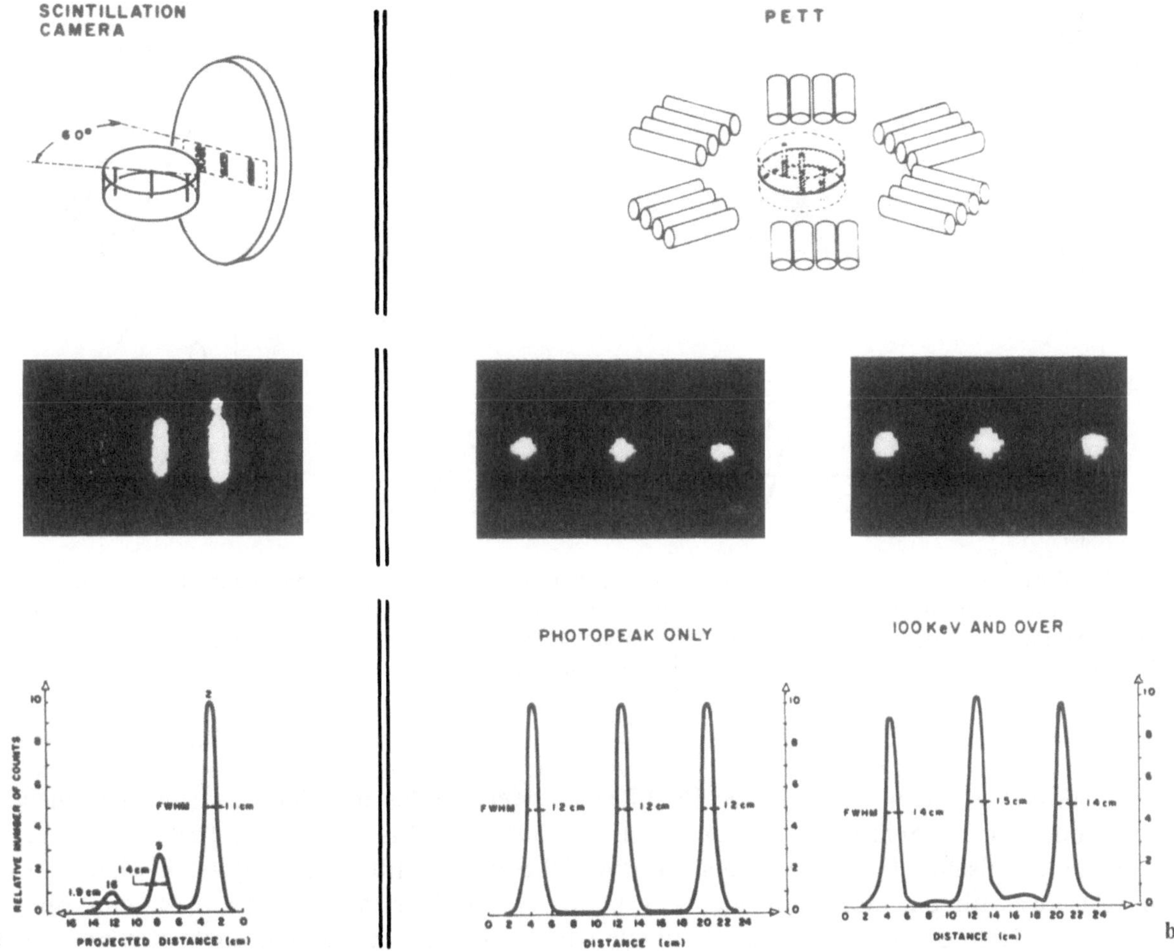

Abb. 70. a 3 Linienquellen ^{99m}Tc aufgenommen mit der Gamma-Kamera und Parallelloch-Kollimator. **b** 3 Linienquellen ^{64}Cu aufgenommen mit einer ringförmigen Anordnung von nicht kollimierten Meßsonden in Koinzidenz betrieben und eine Schicht rekonstruiert. (Aus PHELPS et al. 1975a)

wenn die Kristalle in ihrer Randzone mit einer Bleiblende abgeschirmt sind. Die Halbwertsbreite in der Mitte zwischen beiden Detektoren beträgt dann etwa (BROWNELL et al. 1978) $\text{FWHM} \approx 0,42 \cdot d$.

Für rechteckige Kristalle mit einer Breite b ergibt sich $\text{FWHM} \approx 0,5 \cdot b$. Hierbei handelt es sich um die geometrische Auflösung. Die praktisch auftretenden Werte sind abhängig von dem Kristallmaterial, den Abmessungen und der Energieschwelle beim Messen. PHELPS et al. (1982) geben in tabellarischer Form für rechteckige BGO Kristalle mit einer Höhe und Tiefe von etwa 30 mm und einer Breite b gemessene Halbwertsbreiten und Zehntelwertsbreiten an, die sich in der Form

$$\text{FWHM} = 0,55 \cdot b + 0,6$$

(Maße in mm)

$$\text{FWTM} = b + 0,6$$

ausdrücken lassen, u. zw. für eine Energieschwelle 100 keV und eine Strahlerposition in der Mitte zwischen den beiden Kristallen. Genaue Messungen über die Abhängigkeit dieser Werte von der Lage der Quelle zwischen den Detektoren bzw. innerhalb der dargestellten Schicht findet man bei HOFFMAN et al. (1982).

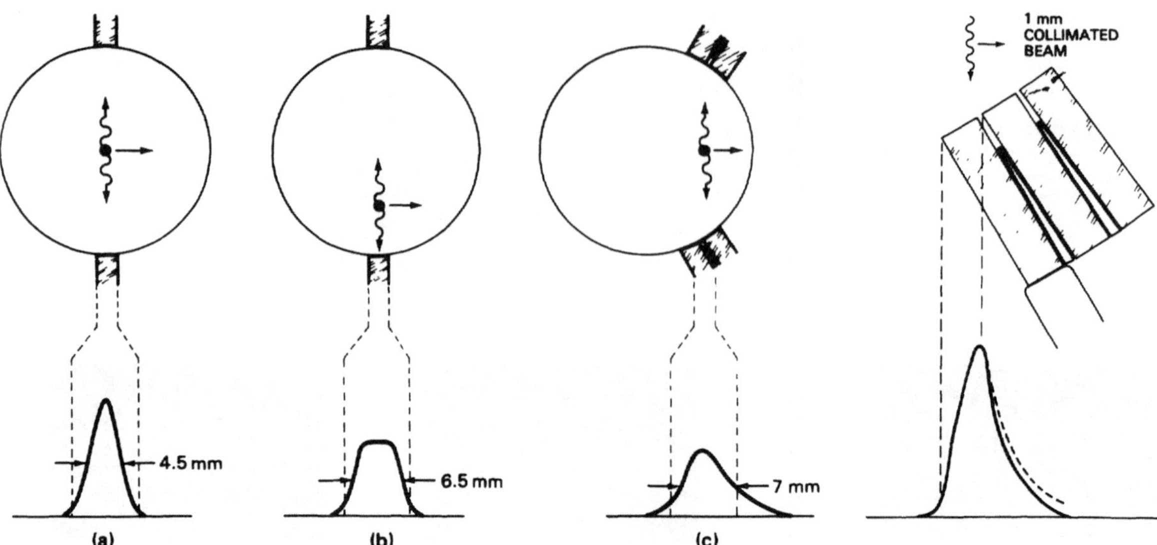

Abb. 71. *Links:* Änderung des Profils eines Meßstrahles zwischen zwei Sonden, wenn der Strahler sich **a** in der Mitte **b** auf einem Radius von 10 cm und **c** auf einem Radius von 10 cm befindet und von einem äußeren Sondenpaar gemessen wird. *Rechts:* Unsymmetrische Verbreiterung durch Schrägeinstrahlung. (Aus BROOKS et al. 1980)

Abbildung 71 zeigt wie sich das Profil eines Meßstrahles mit der Position der Quelle ändert und wie bei Schrägeinstrahlung von hier 30° eine Unsymmetrie auftritt. An diesen von einer Gaußschen Glockenkurve stark abweichenden Profilformen zeigt sich wieder einmal klar, was für ein unzureichender Parameter die Halbwertsbreite ist zur Beschreibung der Profile. Hier ist tatsächlich die Äquivalenzbreite weitaus besser geeignet (KNOOP et al. 1984a, b).

Die erreichbare räumliche Auflösung ist zusätzlich von verschiedenen Faktoren abhängig. Zwei physikalische Effekte setzen eine untere Grenze, die endliche Reichweite der Positronen im Gewebe bevor sie zerstrahlen und Abweichungen der Winkelbeziehung zwischen beiden Gammaquanten vom 180°-Winkel. Beide Effekte sind nur bei hochauflösenden Systemen von Interesse. PHELPS et al. (1975b) berichten für ein Sonden-Paar von einer Vergrößerung der Halbwertsbreite von 2,4 mm auf 3,3 mm beim Wechsel vom niederenergetischen ^{64}Cu ($E_{max} = 0,656$ MeV) zum hochenergetischen ^{15}O ($E_{max} = 1,72$ MeV), JEAVONS (1979) gibt 2,0 mm für ^{22}Na ($E_{max} = 0,5$ MeV) und 3,5 mm für ^{68}Ga ($E_{max} = 1,9$ MeV) als Halbwertsbreite bei seiner Positronenkamera mit Multi-Wire-Chambers an. Genaue Messungen führt DERENZO (1979) durch und kommt zu noch kleineren Variationen.

Einen Effekt ähnlicher Größenordnung muß man der Tatsache zuschreiben, daß der Emissionswinkel von 180° nach einer Gaußverteilung mit einer Halbwertsbreite von etwa 0,5° streut (die Angaben schwanken zwischen 0,2° und 0,7°). Dies ergibt für den Mittelpunkt der Schicht einen Verlust an räumlicher Auflösung von 1,3 mm bei 60 cm und 2,2 mm bei 100 cm Ringdurchmesser (MUEHLLEHNER u. COLSHER 1982).

Ein weiterer physikalischer Effekt, nämlich die simultane Aussendung von drei Gammaquanten pro Zerstrahlungsprozeß, kommt nur in 0,27% aller Fälle vor (ORE u. POWELL 1949). Da die Summe der emittierten Gammaquanten auch hier der doppelten Ruhemasse (1,022 MeV) entsprechen muß, haben die Quanten auch nicht mehr ihre Nennenergie. Der Einfluß auf die räumliche Auflösung ist zu vernachlässigen.

II. Ausbeute

Da Positronen-Meßsysteme keine Bleikollimatoren mehr benutzen, erwartet man zunächst eine um Größenordnungen höhere Ausbeute, Der Positronenstrahler befindet sich in einem absorbierenden Medium mit einem totalen Absorptionskoeffizienten μ (s. Abb. 72).

Die beiden γ-Quanten haben die individuellen Wahrscheinlichkeiten $e^{-\mu l}$ bzw. $e^{-\mu r}$ die Detektoren L bzw. R zu erreichen. Die Wahrscheinlichkeit, daß beide Quanten die Detektoren erreichen, ist dann das Produkt $e^{-\mu l} \cdot e^{-\mu r} = e^{-\mu(l+r)}$.

Die Ausbeute wird unabhängig von der Position der Quelle im Objekt, sie ist nur noch abhängig von der Objektdicke $(l+r)$ und dem Absorptionskoeffizienten μ. Das Produkt $\mu \cdot (l+r)$ läßt sich durch eine einfache Transmissionsmessung mit 511 keV-Quanten abhängig von allen Richtungen durch das Objekt bestimmen. Damit wird eine quantitative Aktivitätsbestimmung in vivo möglich.

Die Tatsache, daß immer ein Paar von γ-Quanten ungestreut aus dem Objekt austreten muß, um ein Koinzidenzsignal zu erzeugen, führt zu einer erheblichen Reduzierung der Ausbeute. Abbildung 73 zeigt, daß bei 20 cm Objektdurchmesser zwar 40% aller 140 keV-γ-Quanten ungestreut austreten, aber nur 20% der Positronen-Vernichtungsstrahlung. Dies bedeutet einen Empfindlichkeitsverlust um einen Faktor 2 gegenüber dem niederenergetischen $^{99\mathrm{m}}$Tc. Die Absorptionswahrscheinlichkeit der Szintillatoren ist für 511 keV z.B. nur 50%. Die Koinzidenzausbeute beträgt dann nur 25% (Quadrat der Einzelausbeuten) gegenüber 100% bei 140 keV. Der hohe Gewinn an Empfindlichkeit durch Wegfall der Kollimatoren von etwa zwei Größenordnungen wird also wieder reduziert zu etwa einer Größenordnung.

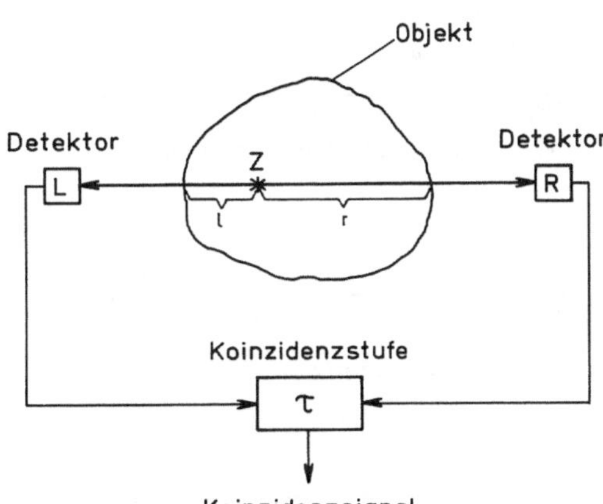

Abb. 72. Positronen-Messung. Die Koinzidenzstufe hat eine Auflösungszeit τ. Signale von L und R, deren zeitlicher Abstand $\leq \tau$ ist, werden als Koinzidenzsignal registriert

III. Unerwünschte Koinzidenzsignale

Neben den echten Koinzidenzen treten noch Streukoinzidenzen und zufällige Koinzidenzen auf (s. Abb. 74). Obwohl die gestreute Koinzidenz im zeitlichen Sinne eine echte Koinzidenz ist, führt sie doch stets zu einer Fehlortung und damit zu einer Bildverschlechterung. Da kleine Streuwinkel (Vorwärtsstreuung) bevorzugt auftreten bei 511 keV, sind die Fehlortungen um die wahre Lage herum konzentriert. Hohe Energieschwellen beim Messen können den Anteil an Streukoinzidenzen ein wenig verringern, verringern aber auch die Ausbeute. Abschätzungen über das Verhältnis Streukoinzidenzen/echte Koinzidenzen geben DERENZO et al. (1975). Dieses Verhältnis ist unabhängig von der Rate der echten Koinzidenzen.

Ganz anders verhalten sich die zufälligen Koinzidenzen, die immer dann auftreten, wenn zufällig zwei unabhängige Absorptionsprozesse in beiden Detektoren zu einer Koinzidenz führen (Abb. 74c). Die Rate der zufälligen Koinzidenzen ist proportional dem Produkt der Einzelraten n_L und n_R beider Detektoren

$$K_{Zuf} = n_L \cdot n_R \cdot \tau.$$

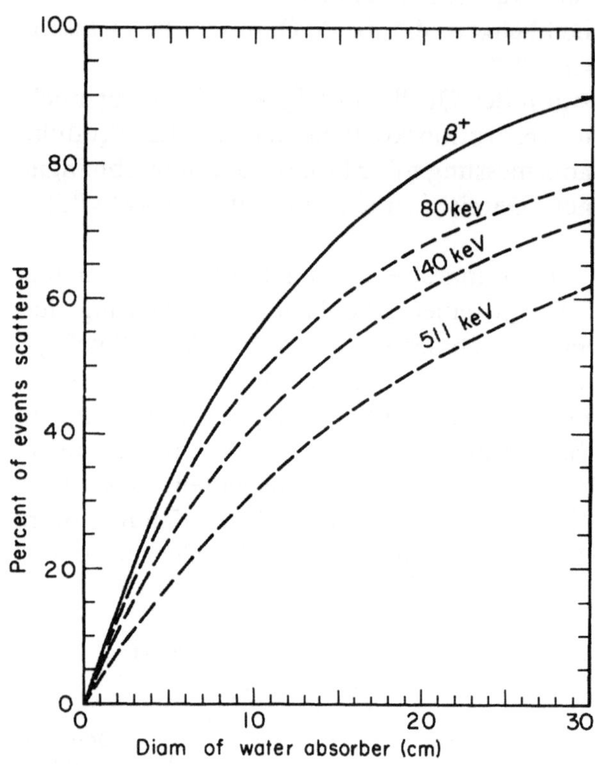

Abb. 73. Prozentsatz der Zerfallsprozesse bei denen die emittierten γ-Quanten bzw. Quanten-Paare (β^+) mindestens einen Streuprozeß erleiden in einem gleichmäßig mit Aktivität gefüllten Zylinder eines auf der Abszisse angegebenen Durchmessers. (Aus BUDINGER et al. 1979a)

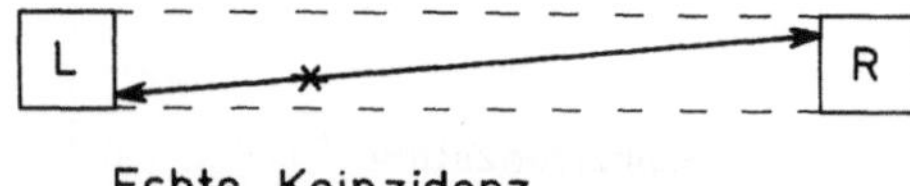

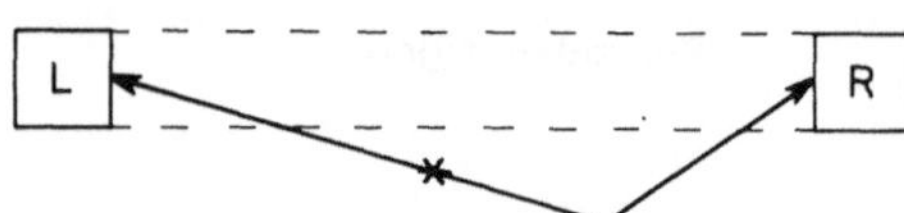

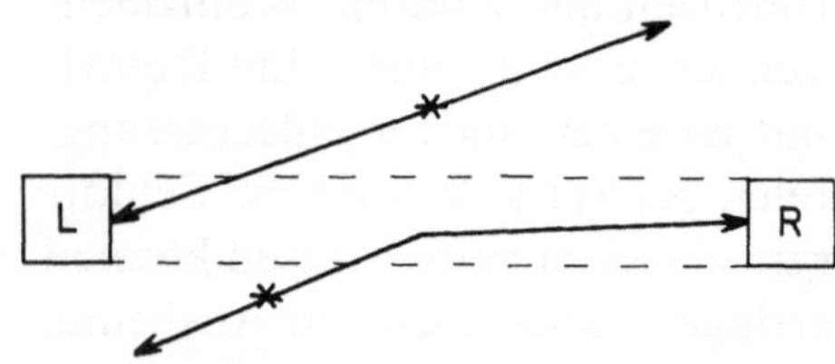

Abb. 74. Echte und zufällige Koinzidenzen bei der Positronen-Messung

Die zufällige Koinzidenzrate ist auch proportional dem Quadrat der Rate der echten Koinzidenz. Eine Verringerung der Koinzidenzauflösungszeit τ ist ein wesentliches Mittel zur Reduzierung der zufälligen Koinzidenzrate. Die Breite des bei der Messung benutzten Koinzidenzfensters ist $\pm\tau$, das heißt 2τ. Man wählt das Koinzidenzfenster so schmal wie möglich, ohne die Ausbeute nennenswert zu reduzieren. Ein guter Kompromiß ist Fensterbreite gleich Zehntelwertsbreite des Zeitspektrums, d.h. der Häufigkeitsverteilung der koinzidenten Impulse aufgetragen über dem zeitlichen Abstand zwischen beiden Impulsen. Minimale Fensterbreiten von 10 ns für BGO-Kristalle sind heute üblich.

Die zufälligen Koinzidenzen enthalten wenig ortsabhängige Information, sie sind mehr oder weniger gleichmäßig im Bild verteilt. Da sie zahlenmäßig über die echte Koinzidenzrate ansteigen können, verschlechtern sie den Bildkontrast erheblich. Detaillierte Untersuchungen findet man bei HOFFMAN et al. (1981 b), siehe auch Abschnitt G.V.4.

IV. Time-of-Flight Informationen

Die Einführung der Flugzeitmessung im Jahre 1980 als zusätzliche Information über die Lage des jeweiligen Emissionsortes brachte neue Möglichkeiten zur Verbesserung der Leistung von Positronen-Tomographen. Das Prinzip der Flugzeitmessung ist in Abb. 75 dargestellt. Von den Ausgangssignalen der beiden Photomultiplier werden schnelle Zeitsignale abgeleitet, deren zeitlicher Abstand zueinander in eine proportionale Impulsamplitude umgewandelt wird. Ein üblicher Amplitudenanalysator liefert dann ein Zeitspektrum. Die Lage des Peaks auf der Zeitachse entspricht der Lage der Quelle zwischen beiden Detektoren, die Breite des Peaks entspricht der erreichbaren Zeitauflösung. Die dreidimensionale Ortung der Punktquelle wird damit möglich. Da die erreichbaren Zeitauflösungen unter realistischen Meßbedingungen heute noch bei mehr als 270 ps FWHM liegen, was einer Verschiebung der Punktquelle um mehr als 40 mm entspricht, ist eine unmittelbare tomographische Abbildung mit der erforderlichen Auflösung nicht möglich. Als zusätzliche Information bei der Rekonstruktion ist die TOF-Information aber äußerst nützlich, siehe auch Abschnitt G.IV.1.d.

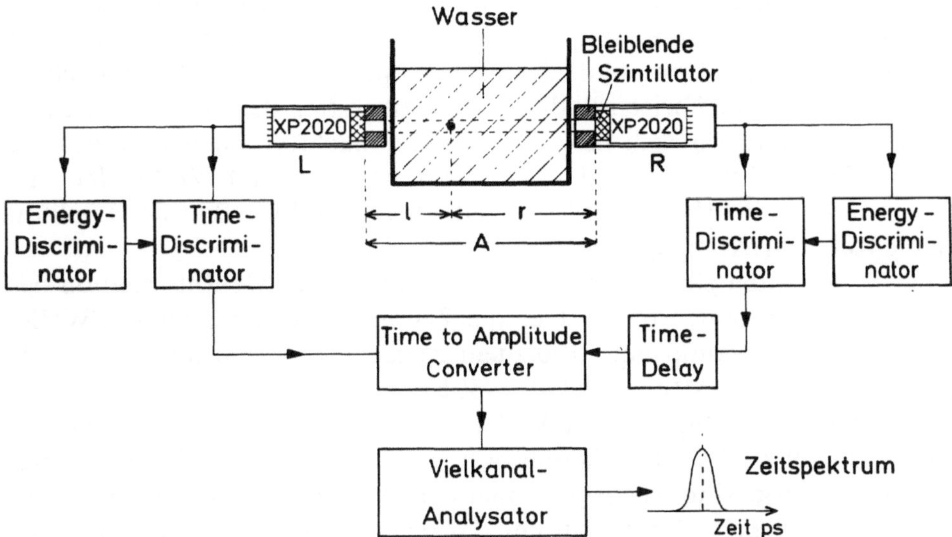

Abb. 75. Prinzip der Ortung einer Punktquelle durch Einsatz der Flugzeitmessung. (Aus JORDAN u. GETTNER 1981)

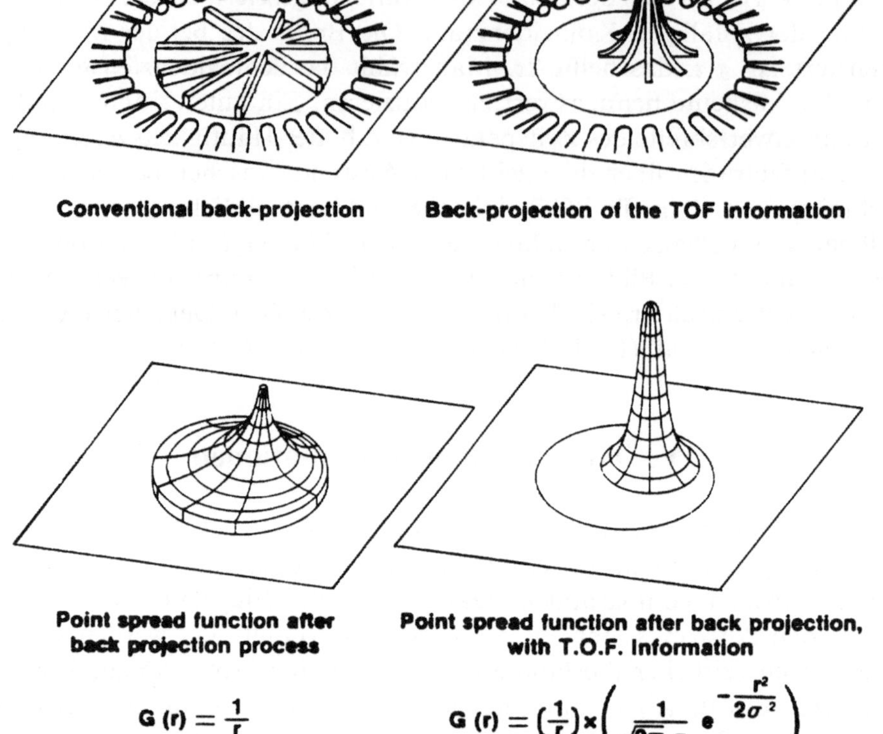

$$G(r) = \frac{1}{r}$$

$$G(r) = \left(\frac{1}{r}\right) \times \left(\frac{1}{\sqrt{2\pi}\,\sigma}\ e^{-\frac{r^2}{2\sigma^2}} \right)$$

Abb. 76. Zur Wirkung der zusätzlichen TOF-Information bei der einfachen Rückprojektion. (Aus LAVAL et al. 1982)

In Abb. 76 ist im linken Bildteil die übliche Rückprojektion einer Punktquelle zu sehen, wenn, wie hier bei einem Positronen Ringtomographen, die einzelnen Meßstrahlen überlagert werden. Die Information, die die Punktquelle liefert, wird gleichmäßig über den vollen Bilddurchmesser längs der einzelnen Meßstrahlen verteilt. Es ergibt sich die übliche Informationsverstärkung im Bildbereich der Punktquelle. In Abb. 76 rechts sorgt die zusätzliche TOF-Information dafür, daß die Information, die die Punktquelle liefert, im Bildbereich der Punktquelle konzentriert wird. Die übrigen Bildbereiche bleiben frei, das Signal/Rausch-Verhältnis wird erheblich verbessert, was sich besonders bei der nachfolgenden Rekonstruktion auswirkt. Wäre die Zeitauflösung gut genug, z.B. nur wenige mm FWHM, dann hätte man mit der Rückprojektion in Abb. 76 rechts bereits das endgültige Bild der Punktquelle und könnte sich die Rekonstruktion sparen.

Abbildung 77 vermittelt eindrucksvoll den Gewinn durch TOF-Information bei der Rekonstruktion eines Phantoms, obwohl hier die Zeitauflösung nur 800 ps FWHM betrug, entsprechend 12 cm TOF-Auflösung. Trotzdem zeigen die Profile im oberen Bildteil den erheblichen Gewinn (s. auch MULLANI et al. 1980b).

Die Verbesserung des Signal/Rausch-Verhältnisses führt zu einem indirekten Empfindlichkeitsgewinn, da für die gleiche Bildgüte weniger Information gesammelt werden muß. Dieser Empfindlichkeitsgewinn ist proportional dem Verhältnis vom Durchmesser des Rekonstruktionsfeldes zur Zeitauflösung in cm FWHM (s. Abb. 78). Die Angaben einzelner Autoren differieren ein wenig (BUDINGER 1983a; SNYDER 1982; WONG et al. 1983; TOMITANI 1982; GARIOD et al. 1982).

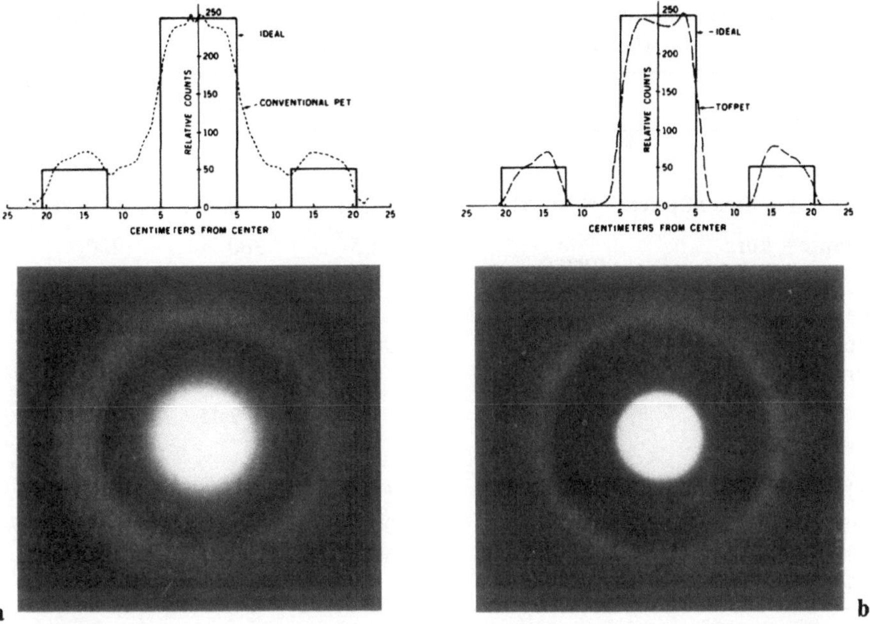

Abb. 77a, b. Konventionelle (**a**) und TOF-unterstützte (**b**) Rekonstruktion eines homogen gefüllten Phantoms, bestehend aus einem 10 cm $\varnothing$ Zylinder mit spez. Aktivität 5 und einem umgebenden Ring mit den Durchmessern 25 bzw. 42 cm und der spez. Aktivität 1. (Aus Ter-Pogossian et al. 1981)

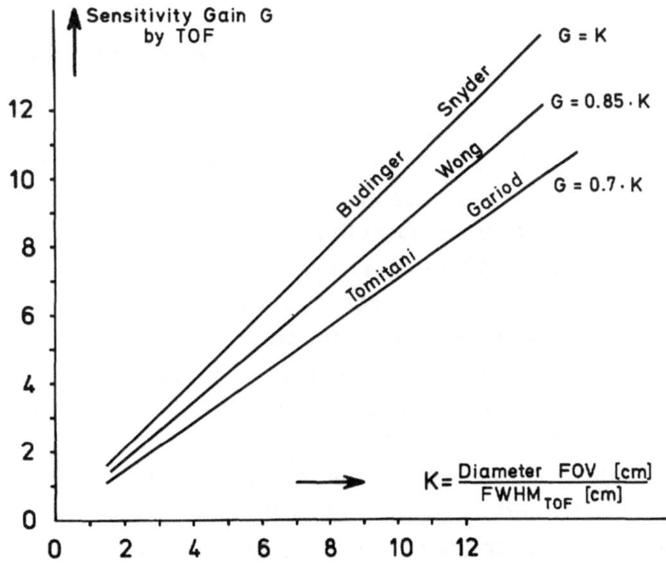

Abb. 78. Indirekter Empfindlichkeitsgewinn durch TOF-Information in Abhängigkeit vom Durchmesser des Rekonstruktionsfeldes und der Zeitauflösung nach den Angaben verschiedener Autoren. (Aus Jordan et al. 1984a)

Der Nachteil der TOF-Messung liegt in der Forderung nach Szintillatoren mit möglichst extrem kleiner Abklingzeitkonstante der Lichtemission. Hier bietet sich z.Zt. nur Bariumfluorid BaF_2 (Laval et al. 1983) und Cäsiumfluorid CsF (Moszynski et al. 1983) an. Beide Kristalle haben zwar eine höhere Absorptionswahrscheinlichkeit als NaJ(Tl), aber dennoch eine wesentlich kleinere als BGO (s. Tabelle 3). BaF_2 hat im Vergleich zu CsF den großen Vorteil der höheren Dichte, es ist nicht hygroskopisch und noch schneller. Als Nachteil muß man die extrem kurze Wellenlänge von 225 nm des Szintillationslichtes ansehen, zumindest bei der wichtigen schnellen Komponente. Trotzdem ist BaF_2 von allen z.Zt. bekannten Szintillatoren der geeignetste für TOF-Systeme (Judas et al. 1984).

Tabelle 3. Physikalische Eigenschaften einiger wesentlicher Szintillatoren für die Positronen-Tomographie. (Nach Werten aus Gariod et al. 1982)

	CsF	BGO	NaJ(Tl)	BaF$_2$
Dichte (g/cm^3)	4,64	7,13	3,67	4,89
Linearer Absorptionskoeffizient μ (cm^{-1}) für 511 keV	0,44	0,92	0,34	0,47
Abklingzeitkonstante – kurz	2,5	300	250	0,8
– lang	–	–	–	620
Lichtwellenlänge (nm)				
schnelle Komponente	390	480	410	225
langsame Komponente	–	–	–	310
Brechungsindex	1,48	2,15	1,85	1,57
				1,55
Energieauflösung bei 511 keV	25%	20%	9%	13%[a]
Zeitauflösung für Positronenstrahler, 150 keV Energieschwelle, Kristall 20 mm $\varnothing$ × 40 mm	400 ps 60 mm	2,5 ns 375 mm	1 ns 150 mm	300 ps 45 mm

[a] Bei totaler Lichtintegration

V. Abtastung (Sampling)

Die Halbwertsbreite FWHM eines Meßstrahles zwischen zwei gegenüberstehenden Detektoren ist grob halb so groß wie der Kristalldurchmesser beziehungsweise die Kristallbreite (s. Abschnitt E.I.). Der Abstand a nebeneinander liegender Meßstrahlen im Meßfeld (üblicherweise mit einem Durchmesser etwa halb so groß wie der Detektorringdurchmesser) ist $\leq$ dem Kristallabstand A, also dem Abstand benachbarter Kristallmitten. Damit ist a etwa doppelt so groß wie die Strahlbreite, wenn die Kristalle entsprechend Abb. 79 dicht gepackt sind. Nach dem sampling theorem (s. Abschnitt G.V.1.a) darf aber a höchstens halb so groß wie die Strahlbreite sein, d.h. die Abtastung muß mindestens viermal feiner erfolgen als es mit dem still stehenden Ring möglich ist. Man kann den Abstand a halbieren, indem man den Ring um ein Winkelinkrement entsprechend dem halben Detektorabstand A rotieren läßt und erneut mißt, der Abstand a ist dann $\leq A/2$. Die notwendige weitere Halbierung dieses Abstandes ist nur mit Hilfe von speziellen Ringbewegungen möglich. Abbildung 80 gibt einen Überblick über heute angewendete Verfahren. b) zeigt den typischen Bewegungsablauf bei 6- oder 8eckigen Systemen (z.B. PETT III, IV, ECAT II), c) verdeutlicht die Wobbelbewegung (z.B. PC-95, TOF-PET, ECAT III), d) zeigt das Abtastschema bei der Positologica, e) zeigt die Aufteilung in zwei Ringhälften beim Dichotom-I und f) deutet die „Clamshell" – Anordnung an, die nur zwei mechanische Stellungen kennt, nämlich geschlossener Ring und um einen Detektorabstand A geöffneter Ring (Derenzo et al. 1982; Huesman et al. 1982).

Abbildung 81 zeigt wie sich ein Abtastabstand A/4 erreichen läßt am Beispiel der „dichotomic"-Abtastung. Die beiden Ringhälften nehmen vier unterschiedliche Positionen zueinander ein.

Diese lineare Abtastung wird ergänzt durch die zirkulare Abtastung. Entscheidend ist hier die Frage nach der Anzahl M der Projektionen bzw. nach dem Winkelinkrement $\Delta\theta$, um das sich benachbarte Projektionsrichtungen unterscheiden. Mit dem Meßfelddurchmesser D und $a \approx A/4$ wird

$$M \approx \frac{2 \cdot \pi \cdot D}{A} \approx \frac{\pi \cdot D}{2 \cdot a}$$

$$\Delta\theta \approx \frac{180°}{M} \approx 2 \cdot \frac{a}{D}$$

(s. auch SNYDER u. COX 1977; HUESMAN 1977).

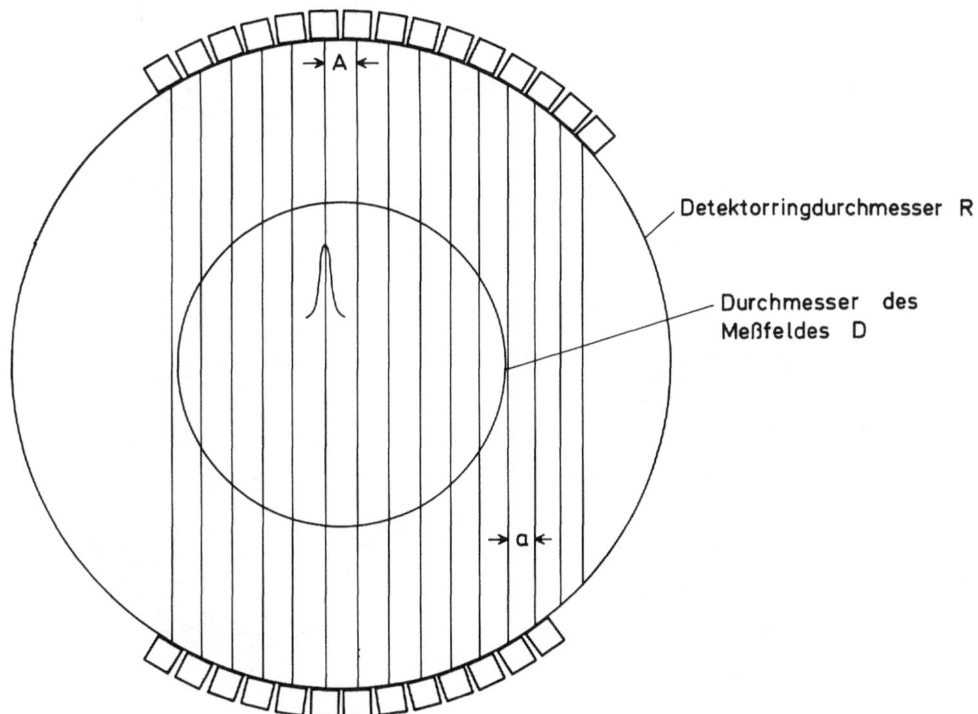

Abb. 79. Positronen-Ring mit regelmäßiger Kristallanordnung. Parallelprojektion durch Koinzidenzabfrage gegenüberstehender Detektoren

VI. Realisierte Systeme

Die Entwicklung der Positronen-Tomographen ist fast ausschließlich von ringförmigen Konfigurationen geprägt. Um den Patienten rotierende, sich gegenüberstehende Kameras haben praktisch keine Bedeutung erlangt. Abbildung 82a–h gibt einen Überblick über realisierte Systeme.

Die Ein-Ringsysteme haben entweder eine 6- oder auch 8eckige blockweise Sondenanordnung, a) und b), oder eine streng ringförmige gleichmäßige Sondenanordnung, c) und d). Um das Abtast-Theorem zu erfüllen (s. Abschnitt E.V.), führen die Systeme a) und b) sowohl eine Rotationsbewegung als auch eine lineare Bewegung der einzelnen Kristallblöcke während der Aufnahme durch. Bei den Systemen c), d) und h) wird eine Rotation und eine Wobbelbewegung oder auch allein eine Wobbelbewegung durchgeführt. Bei Verzicht auf höchste räumliche Auflösung kann auch bei Stillstand des Ringes gemessen werden.

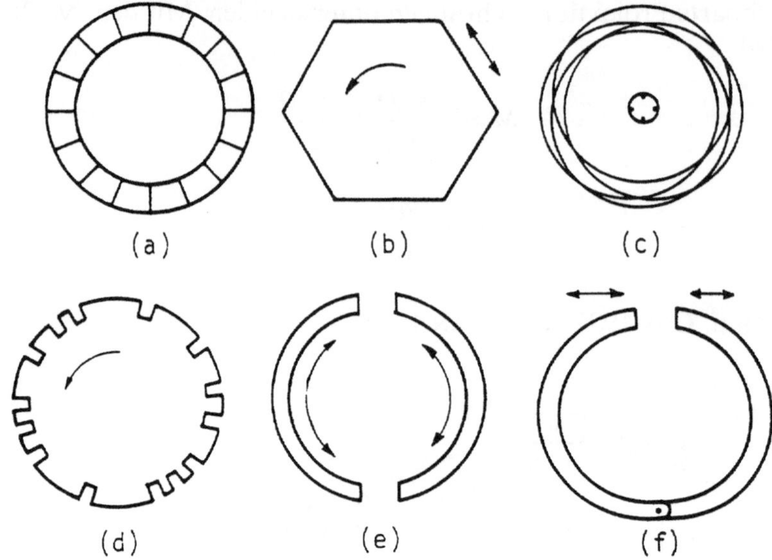

Abb. 80 a–f. Verschiedene Möglichkeiten der Abtastung: **a** stationärer Ring, **b** lineare und rotatorische Bewegung, **c** Wobbelbewegung, **d** 360°-Rotation mit unregelmäßiger Kristallanordnung, **e** „dichotomic", **f** „clamshell". (Aus DERENZO et al. 1982)

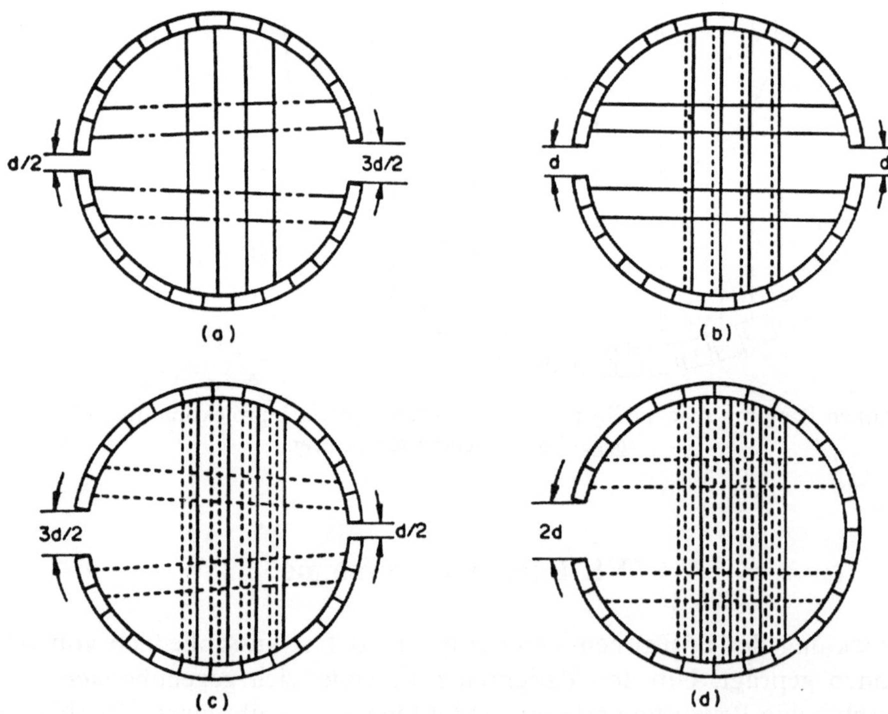

Abb. 81 a–d. „Dichotomic"-Abtastung durch vier diskrete Stellungen der beiden Ringhälften zueinander. (Aus CHO et al. 1981)

Letzteres ist von Bedeutung bei schnellen dynamischen Vorgängen. Die Systeme g) und h) sind Mehr-Ringsysteme, die entweder durch parallele Anordnung von Einzelringen entstehen, was heute die Regel ist, oder sie entstehen wie im Falle von PETT IV und V durch Anordnung von stabförmigen Kristallen längs zur Ringachse, die in vier separate Adressenbe-

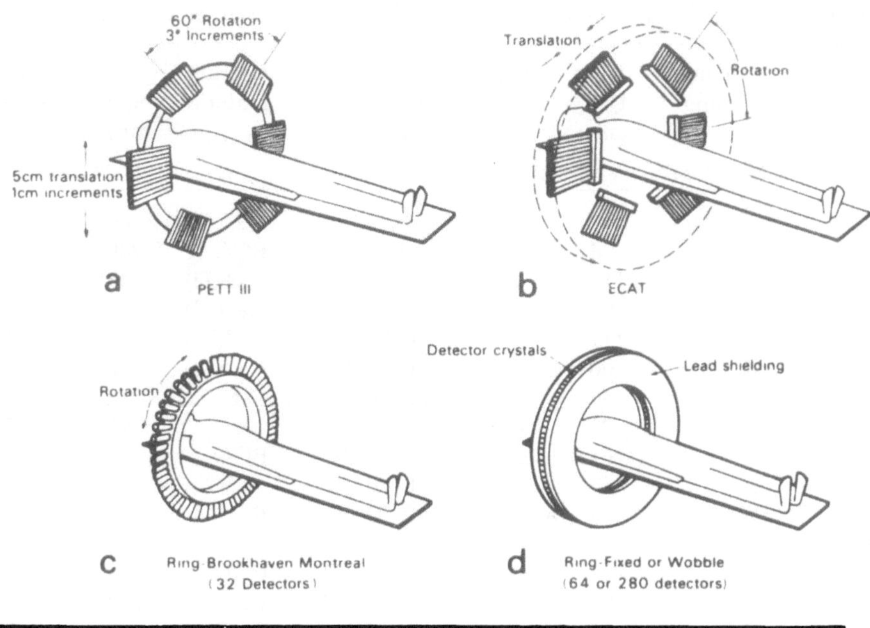

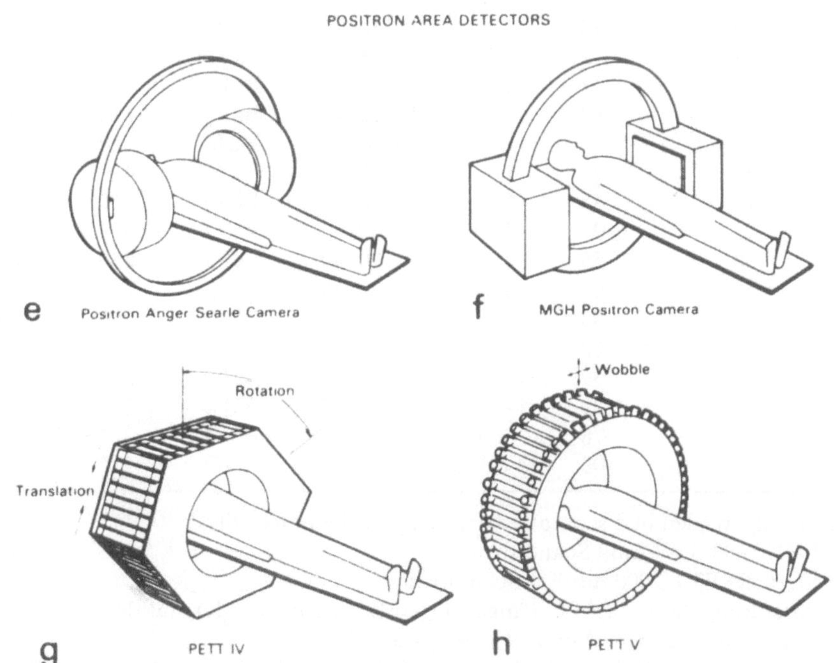

Abb. 82a–h. Verschiedene Ausführungsformen von Positronen-Tomographen. (Aus Budinger et al. 1979b)

reiche unterteilt sind und so vier eng nebeneinander angeordnete Ringe bilden (s. auch Abb. 36).

Eine völlig andere Betriebsweise ergibt sich durch Rotation von zwei Angerkameras in Koinzidenzbetrieb, System e), oder wie bei System f) durch Rotation von zwei „Kameras", die aus je einem Block von vielen Einzelsonden bestehen (s. auch Abb. 19, 37).

Diese Betriebsart ist unmittelbar vergleichbar mit der rotierenden Kamera bei der SPECT. Es wird eine Vielzahl paralleler transversaler Schichten gleichzeitig gemessen, die Information steht aber erst nach einer Rotation um mindestens 180° zur Verfügung. Auf die einzelne Schicht bezogen ist die Aufnahmedauer relativ hoch, da nur wenig Detektorfläche pro Einzel-

Tabelle 4. Neuere Positronen-Tomographen, die sich in Betrieb bzw. Aufbau befinden.

	Patienten-öffnung $\varnothing$ cm	Ring $\varnothing$ cm	Anzahl Ringe	Kristall-größe mm	Kristall-material	Kri-stalle pro Ring	Packungs-dichte %	Photo-multipl. pro Ring
CRTAPC	–	47	1	$20\,\varnothing\cdot38$	NaJ(Tl)	64	≈68	64
Donner-Ring	50	94	1	$9{,}5\cdot32\cdot32$	BGO	280	90	280
PETT III	51	111	1	$51\,\varnothing\cdot76$	NaJ(Tl)	48	≈55	48
Ortec ECAT II	50	100	1	$38\,\varnothing\cdot76$	NaJ(Tl)	66	≈63	66
PETT IV[a]	52	111	4	$50\,\varnothing\cdot175$	NaJ(Tl)	48	≈54	24
PETT V[a]	30	60	4	$30\cdot70\cdot140$	NaJ(Tl)	48	76	24
PETT VI[b]	29	57	4	$20\cdot24\cdot65$	CsF	72	80	72
Super PETT I[c]	46,5	90	4	$25\,\varnothing\cdot45$	CsF	96	≈67	96
Ortec Neuro ECAT	30	65	3	$17\cdot27\cdot29$	BGO	88	73	88
PC-95 Karolinska	23–30	47	1	$8\cdot20\cdot50$	NaJ(Tl)	95	51	95
PC 384-7B	27	48	4	$12\cdot20\cdot30$	BGO	96	76	96
TOF PET	60	99	5	$18\,\varnothing\cdot45$	CsF	144	≈66	144
Neuro-PET	25	38	4	$8{,}25\cdot20\cdot35$	BGO	128	88	128
ECAT-III	65	100	1–4	$5{,}6\cdot30\cdot30$	BGO	512	91	512
Positologica-II	56	85	3	$15\cdot24\cdot24$	BGO	160	90	80
Dichotom-I[d]		54	1	$20\,\varnothing\cdot38$	NaJ(Tl)	63	19 bzw. 41	63
Positome-II[e]	24·28	42	2	$18\cdot30\cdot30$	BGO	64	86	64
Headtome-II[f]	24	42	3	$16\cdot28\cdot70$	NaJ(Tl)	64	78	64
LETI TTV-01	48	92	4	$24\cdot24\cdot40$	BaF$_2$	96	80	96
SATOF-I[g]	50	80	1	$10\cdot25\cdot40$	BaF$_2$	234	93	78+234
MGH PC-II[h]	22–74	50–90	12	$20\,\varnothing\cdot38$	NaJ(Tl)	24	≈24–13	≈14
MGH Ringtomograph	50	90	1	$6{,}7\cdot22\cdot50$	NaJ(Tl)	420	99,9	84
MGH Ringtomograph	28	45	1	$4\cdot20\cdot30$	BGO	360	99,9	90
PC 2048-7WB	55	107	4	$6\cdot20\cdot30$	BGO/GSO	512	91,4	256
PC 1024-7B	30	55	4	$6\cdot20\cdot30$	BGO/GSO	256	88,9	128
PC 1024-7WB	55	107	4	$12\cdot20\cdot30$	BGO	256	91,4	256
McMaster Univ.	32	53,5	1	$10\cdot25\cdot45$	BGO	160	95	160
PC 4600	28.5	60	5	$19\,\varnothing\cdot38$	BGO	96	≈76	96
LETI TTV-13	33	59	1–6	$7\cdot18\cdot45$	BaF$_2$	216	81,6	216
LETI TTV-03	54	89	1–6	$7\cdot18\cdot45$	BaF$_2$	324	81,1	324
POSICAM Camera[i]	57	78	3–6	$9\cdot20\cdot30$	BGO	224	82,3	112
PT 931 ECAT[j]	65	100	4 od. 8	$5{,}6\cdot16\cdot30$	BGO	512	88	64

[a] Stabförmige Kristalle werden in 4 separate Adressenbereiche unterteilt
[b] Baugleich mit PETT 600 der Firma Scanditronix
[c] Baugleich mit SUPERPETT 2000 der Fa. Scanditronix
[d] Auflösungs-Verbesserung des CRTAPC-Ringes durch Einengung der Kristallfläche
[e] Baugleich mit Therascan 3128 von AECL (Cooke et al. 1984)
[f] Hybrides System, mit spez. Wolfram-Kollimator auch für SPECT. Baugleich mit Headtome SET-230 der Shimadzu Corp.
[g] 234 kleine Photomultiplier zur Kristallkodierung
[h] Rotierende Doppelkopf-Kamera, baugleich mit Modell 4200 der Cyclotron Corp.
[i] Wahlweise auch mit $8\cdot20\cdot45$ BaF$_2$ Kristallen lieferbar, dann Packungsdichte 73% und TOF-Messung möglich
[j] Die Kristallänge 16 mm ist auch mit 12,5 oder 20 mm lieferbar

schicht zur Verfügung steht, was einer niedrigen Packungsdichte entspricht (s. auch Tabelle 4). Beide Systeme konnten sich nicht durchsetzen, wobei bei der rotierenden Gammakamera, System e), noch das Problem der extrem hohen Impulsraten der nicht durch Kollimatoren abgeschirmten Kameraköpfe die Anwendung höherer Aktivitäten unmöglich machte (Muehllehner et al. 1976).

TOF- Techn. FWHM mm	Länge der Bleiblenden cm	Ring- bewegung	Räumliche Auflösung mm	Rekonstruk- tionsfeld $\varnothing$	Literatur	Abb. Nr.
–	bis 12	–	17–20	–	CHO et al. (1977a, b)	28
–	22	–	7–12	50	DERENZO et al. (1981)	–
–	25,5	rot., lin.	14	–	HOFFMAN et al. (1976)	29, 30
–	20	rot., lin.	11–17	50	WILLIAMS CW et al. (1979)	–
–	25	rot., lin.	15	–	TER-POGOSSIAN et al. (1978a)	36
–	15	rot., wobble	7–15	25	TER-POGOSSIAN et al. (1978b)	–
–	12	rot., wobble	7–13,5	27	TER-POGOSSIAN et al. (1982b)	–
75	21,5	rot., wobble	8–12	45	TER-POGOSSIAN et al. (1982a)	50
–	17	rot., wobble	8,4–11,2	25	HOFFMAN et al. (1983a)	46, 55
–	8,5–12	rot., wobble	7	25	BOHM et al. (1978)	–
–	10,5	wobble	7–12	26	Firma Scanditronix	51
90	12	wobble	9–14	45	MULLANI et al. (1983)	–
–	6,5	wobble	6–7	25	BROOKS et al. (1981)	–
–	17	wobble	4,4–9	50	HOFFMAN et al. (1983b)	–
–	14,5	rot.	9–12	51	TAKAMI et al. (1983)	52
–	–	dichotomic	6,5–10	–	CHO et al. (1983a)	–
–	6–9	rot., wobble	8–15	–	THOMPSON et al. (1979)	–
–	8	rot., wobble	8–11,5	21	HIROSE et al. (1982)	47
50–60	–	rot., wobble	7–11	46	GAROID et al. (1982)	–
50–60	14	wobble	6–10	40	JORDAN et al. (1984a, b)	–
–	8	rot., lin.	10–15	36	BROWNELL et al. (1979)	19, 37
–	20	–	7–15	–	BURNHAM et al. (1982)	–
–	10	–	4,5–6,5	–	BURNHAM et al. (1983, 1984)	54
–	–	wobble	6	52	Firma Scanditronix	–
–	12	wobble	6	26	Firma Scanditronix	–
–	–	wobble	8–8,5	52	Firma Scanditronix	–
–	10	–	8–10	–	NAHMIAS et al. (1984)	–
–	16	rot., wobble	11	24	KEARFOTT u. CARROLL (1984)	–
90	10	wobble	6–7	30	LETI Grenoble (1985)	–
90	10	wobble	6–7	45	LETI Grenoble (1985)	–
–	16	wobble	6–8,5	40	Positron Corp., Houston (1984)	–
–	17	wobble	5–6,8	55	Firma CTI, Knoxville (1985)	–

Einen Überblick über die heute in Betrieb oder im Aufbau befindlichen Positronen-Tomographen vermittelt Tabelle 4. Zunächst einmal kann man unterscheiden Systeme für Ganzkörperanwendung mit Detektorring-Durchmessern zwischen 80 und 111 cm und Kristallzahlen zwischen 48 und 512 Kristallen pro Ring. Daneben Systeme speziell für die Hirndiagnostik mit Ringdurchmessern zwischen 38 und 65 cm und Kristallzahlen zwischen 48 und 360. Das spezielle System PC-II vom Massachusetts General Hospital (MGH) mit rotierenden gegenüberstehenden Kristallblöcken fällt mit seinen 24 Kristallen pro „Ring" aus dem Rahmen, bietet dafür aber 12 „Ringe" simultan.

Die Entwicklung der Ringsysteme wird eindrucksvoll durch Abb. 83 wiedergegeben, die einen direkten Größenvergleich ermöglicht.

Der Trend zu immer mehr und kleineren Kristallen bei modernen Systemen ist unverkennbar. Ebenso der Übergang von NaJ(Tl) zu BGO. Dies hat zwei Gründe: Höhere Packungsdichte und höhere räumliche Auflösung bei der Messung. Die Packungsdichte schwankt zwischen 19% beim Dichotom-I und praktisch 100% bei dem neuen MGH-Ringtomographen. Da das Quadrat der Packungsdichte ein Maß für die geometrische Ausbeute darstellt,

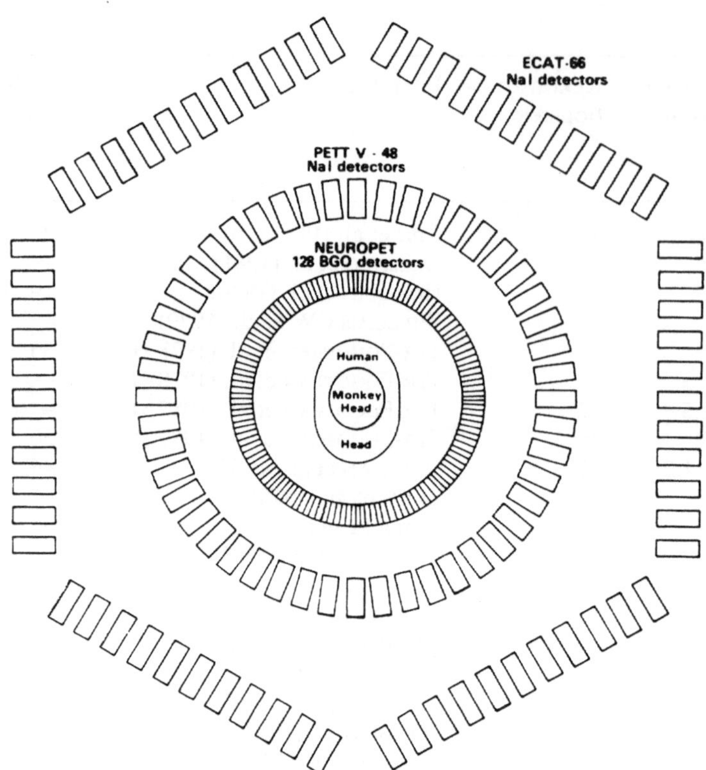

Abb. 83. Zur Entwicklung der Positronen-Ringsysteme, am Beispiel ECAT II, PETT V und Neuro-PET. (Aus Brooks et al. 1981)

stehen sich hier Ausbeuten von 3,6% bzw. 100% gegenüber, was einem Faktor 28 entspricht. Hohe Packungsdichten sind also ein geeignetes Mittel, um die Empfindlichkeit der Systeme zu erhöhen.

Wenn man bei der Messung mit höherer räumlicher Auflösung (entsprechend dünne Meßstrahlen) abtastet als es der später im rekonstruierten Bild gegebenen Auflösung entspricht, kann man das Signal/Rausch-Verhältnis merklich verbessern, was einer indirekten Empfindlichkeitssteigerung gleich kommt, ähnlich wie bei der zusätzlichen TOF-Information (s. Abschnitt E.IV.). Diese bekannte Tatsache, die besonders von Phelps et al. (1982) unter dem Namen Signal Amplification Technique (SAT) propagiert wird, erfordert schmale Kristalle, siehe Abschnitt G.V.2.

TOF-Information setzen 7 Systeme ein, wobei zwei mit runden CsF-Kristallen und 5 mit rechteckigen BaF_2-Kristallen arbeiten. Extrem schmale Kristalle verschlechtern die TOF-Auflösung merklich, da die Lichtübertragung auf die Photokathode große Probleme aufwirft. Ein Kompromiß von 8–10 mm breiten Kristallen ergibt noch eine gute TOF-Auflösung von 50–60 mm FWHM und gleichzeitig einen SAT-Gewinn (Jordan et al. 1984a, b). Der Empfindlichkeitsgewinn bei größeren Rekonstruktionsfeldern von 40 cm Durchmesser und nicht extrem hoher Bildauflösung ist erheblich (s. Abb. 84).

Der Einsatz immer schmalerer rechteckiger Kristalle wirft Probleme auf bezüglich der Kristall-Photomultiplier Kopplung. Entweder es werden sehr kleine Photomultiplier mit Außendurchmessern bis herunter zu 10 mm auf die schmalen Kristallseiten aufgesetzt (z.B. ECAT-III, LETI TTV-03, PC 1024-7WB, McMaster Univers.) oder mehrere Kristalle werden parallel auf entsprechend großflächige Photomultiplier aufgesetzt (z.B. SATOF-I, PC 1024-7B, PC 2048-7WB, Positologica-II). Die erstere Methode hat den Nachteil, daß sich nur ein kleiner Teil des Szintillationslichtes auskoppeln läßt, was zu schlechter spektraler Auflösung bzw. TOF-Auflösung führt. Die letztere Methode erfordert zusätzliche Maßnah-

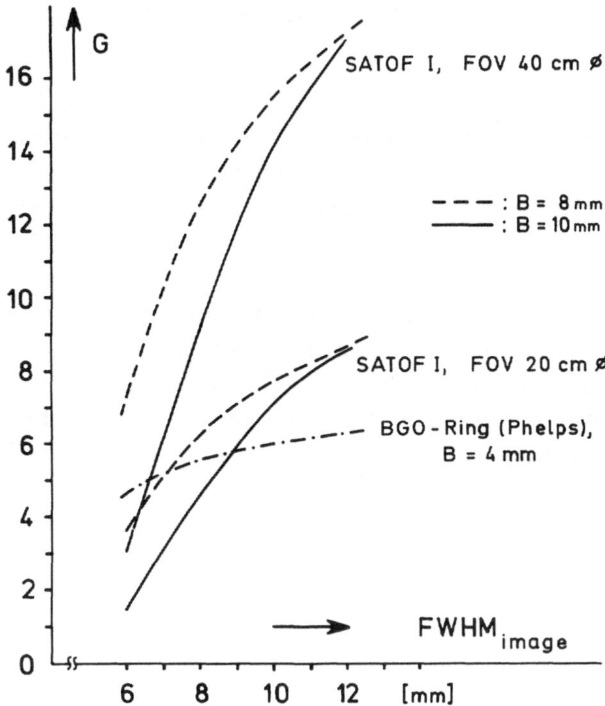

Abb. 84. Indirekter Empfindlichkeitsgewinn *G* aufgetragen über der Auflösung im rekonstruierten Bild beim SATOF I mit 40 cm ∅ bzw. 20 cm ∅-Rekonstruktionsfeld und bei einem Vergleichsring mit BGO-Kristallen und B = 4 mm Kristallbreite. Die geringere Ausbeute von BaF$_2$ gegenüber BGO ist voll berücksichtigt. (Aus JORDAN et al. 1984a)

men, um zu erkennen, welcher Kristall jeweils aktiv war. Hier bietet sich an das zusätzliche Aufsetzen kleiner Photomultiplier zur Erzeugung eines Kodiersignals (z.B. SATOF-I) oder die Verknüpfung von 4 Kristallen mit 2 Photomultipliern nach Art des Quad-Detektors (s. Abb. 52) oder das Aufsetzen eines Kristall-Paares auf einen Photomultiplier, wobei verschiedene Kristalle mit unterschiedlicher Abklingzeitkonstante Verwendung finden, so daß aus der Impulsform auf den jeweils aktiven Kristall geschlossen werden kann (z.B. PC-1024-7B, 2048-7WB). Hier sind jeweils ein BGO-Kristall mit einem GSO-Kristall gepaart. Die Abklingzeitkonstanten betragen 300 bzw. 600 ns. Beim GSO-Kristall handelt es sich um Gadoliniumorthosilikat Gd$_3$SiO$_5$(Ce), welches mit Cer dotiert ist. Der nicht hygroskopische Kristall hat eine Dichte von 6,71 und ist damit geringfügig leichter als BGO (s. Tabelle 3).

Allgemeine Überlegungen zur Kristall-Photomultiplier Kopplung, auch mit eckigen Photokatoden, stellen YAMASHITA et al. (1984) an.

Eine gewisse Sonderstellung nimmt die Kamera PT 931 ECAT der CTI (Computer, Technology & Imaging, Inc., USA) ein. 64 rechteckige kleine „Gammakameras" mit je 8 × 4 = 32 rechteckigen BGO Kristallen bilden ein Ringsystem. Das ergibt 8 × 64 = 512 Kristalle pro Ring bei insgesamt 4 parallelen Ringen. Die einzelnen Blöcke von 8 × 4 Kristallen werden von je 4 Photomultipliern nach Art der Angerortung abgefragt. Diese Positronenkamera bildet einen Kompromiß zwischen zwei Extremen. Das eine Extrem sind zwei gegenüberstehende planare Kameras, die um den Patienten rotieren. Die Realisierung einer PET-Kamera durch nur 2 unabhängige Detektoren ermöglicht nur extrem niedrige Raten an echten Koinzidenzen und damit keine schnellen Studien. Die Realisierung eines Ringsystems durch eine große Anzahl von untereinander unabhängigen Einzelsonden (z.B. LETI TTV-03) stellt das andere Extrem dar. Hier sind die max. möglichen Impulsraten nur noch durch das Registriersystem und den Rechner limitiert. Die Anordnung von 64 „Kameras" bei der PT 931 stellt einen guten Kompromiß dar, wenn auch kurze Aufnahmezeiten pro Schicht bei vertretbarem Zählverlust Probleme bereiten dürften.

F. Spezielle Verfahren der Emissionstomographie

Neben den bekannten Verfahren der SPECT und PET hat es immer wieder Bemühungen gegeben, andere physikalische Phänomene für die Emissionstomographie einzusetzen. Hierzu gehören der γ-γ-Kaskadenzerfall einiger weniger geeigneter Gammastrahler und die Möglichkeit der Fluoreszenzanregung von Elementen höherer Stellenzahl in vivo durch von außen eingestrahlte Röntgen- bzw. Gammastrahlung.

Die verschiedenen Varianten der Compton-Streutomographie (Compton Tomography, Compton Scatter Imaging) sollen hier nicht besprochen werden. Hierbei wird Röntgen- oder Gammastrahlung in kollimierter Form in den darzustellenden Körperbereich eingestrahlt und die in vivo entstehende Streustrahlung von außen gemessen, mit speziellen Detektoren oder auch mit Gammakameras. Ich möchte diese Verfahren der Transmissionstomographie zuordnen, zumal auch eine morphologische Darstellung erfolgt, die mit der funktionellen Darstellung der Emissionstomographie in der Nuklearmedizin wenig gemein hat. Stellvertretend seien einige wenige, jüngere Arbeiten zitiert: Harding (1982), Aurich u. Stange (1982), Del Guerra et al. (1982b), Leichter et al. (1984).

I. γ-γ-Koinzidenz Tomographie

Eine Reihe von Gammastrahlern sendet beim Zerfall praktisch gleichzeitig zwei oder auch mehrere Gammaquanten aus. Dabei geht häufig der angeregte Energiezustand über angeregte Zwischenenergieniveaus in Kaskade in den Grundzustand über. Ist die Lebensdauer dieser Zwischenzustände ($\tau_{1/2}$ in Tabelle 5) entsprechend kurz, kann man von Gleichzeitigkeit sprechen und mit Hilfe geeigneter Koinzidenzmessungen eine Ortung des Zerfallsortes unmittelbar erreichen, d.h. tomographische Messungen durchführen. Der grundlegende Unterschied zum Positronenzerfall besteht darin, daß beim γ-Kaskadenzerfall die beiden Gammaquanten unter beliebigen Winkeln zueinander emittiert werden, während beim Positronenzerfall die 180° Beziehung gilt. Tabelle 5 führt einige für die medizinische Anwendung evtl. in Frage kommende Radionuklide an. Das Problem besteht darin, daß beide Gammaquanten in einem meßtechnisch günstigen Energiebereich liegen müssen, daß diese Zerfallsart mit hoher Wahrscheinlichkeit auftreten muß, und daß die Gleichzeitigkeit gegeben sein muß. Zerfallsverzögerung zwischen beiden Quanten von $\tau_{1/2} = 85$ ns wie z.B. beim ^{111}In, machen die sonst günstigen Eigenschaften zunichte, da das erforderliche sehr breite Koinzidenzfenster bei der Messung große Probleme mit zufälligen Koinzidenzen bringt.

Schmitz-Feuerhake (1970) hat als erste eine geeignete Meßanordnung beschreiben (Abb. 85). Der übliche Meßkopf eines Scanners tastet das Objekt ab. Zusätzlich wird mit Hilfe von großen rechteckigen Plastikdetektoren und fokussierenden Schlitzkollimatoren eine Objektschicht parallel zur Scanebene ausgeblendet. Durch Koinzidenzmessung wird dafür gesorgt, daß vom Scanner nur Ereignisse registriert werden, die ihren Ursprung in der ausgeblendeten Schicht haben. Später wurde der Scanner durch eine Kamera ersetzt, wobei die Verwendung eines Pinhole-Kollimators einen zusätzlichen Empfindlichkeitsgewinn brachte (von Boetticher et al. 1982). Auch zwei Kameras unter 90° zueinander angeordnet wurden vorgeschlagen (Monahan et al. 1973).

Mehrere Einzelsonden in unterschiedlicher räumlicher Anordnung schlagen Hart u. Rudin (1977) sowie Helmers et al. (1982) vor. Einen Überblick über bestehende Systeme vermitteln Chung et al. (1980).

So bestechend diese Verfahren der unmittelbaren dreidimensionalen Aufnahmetechnik sind, so wenig haben sie bisher Einzug in die klinische Routine finden können. Die äußerst geringe Ausbeute und die geringe Variabilität bei der Radionuklidwahl setzen hier Grenzen.

Tabelle 5. Gamma-Kaskaden Strahler für medizinische Anwendungen. n ist die Anzahl der mit einer Wahrscheinlichkeit p gleichzeitig emittierten Gammaquanten pro Zerfall, E ist deren Energie. Ein * vor der Energieangabe weist auf eine charakteristische Röntgenstrahlung nach einem Elektroneneinfang (EC) hin. $\tau_{1/2}$ ist die Halbwertzeit des angeregten Zustandes mit dessen Energieniveau in Klammern (Aus VON BOETTICHER et al. 1982).

Isotope	$T_{1/2}$	Decay	n	p (%)	E (keV)	$\tau_{1/2}$
^{43}K	22.3 h	β^-	2	79	618/373	
^{48}Cr	22.96 h	EC/β^+	2	95	113/308	7 ns (308)
^{52}Fe	8.3 h	β^+/EC	3	58	169/511/511	
^{73}Se	7.1 h	β^+/EC	4	45	361/67/511/511	5 ns (67)
			3	19	361/511/511	
			2	23	361/67	
^{75}Se	120.4 d	EC	2	55	136/264	
			2	16	121/279	
			2	3	96/303	
^{75}Br	1.63 h	β^+/EC	3	49	287/511/511	30 ns (293)
			2–5	20	141–573	
^{111}In	2.83 d	EC	2	86	171/245	85 ns (245)
^{123}J	13.2 h	EC	2	70	*29/159	
^{127}Xe	36.4 d	EC	2–3	23	*31/172/203	
^{169}Yb	30.7 d	EC	2	16	198/109	
			2	11	177/131	
			2	45	*54/63	
^{179}Hf^{m2}	25.1 d	IT	3–6	80	123–454	
^{180}Hf^{m}	5.5 h	IT	3	64	443/332/215	
			3	11	501/332/215	
^{178}Ta	2.4 h	EC	3–6	97	*60–426	1.5 ns (93)
^{192}Ir	74.0 d	β^-/EC	3	23	308/296/317	
			2	7	604/317	
			2	40	468/317	
^{196}Au	6.18 d	EC/β^-	3	23	*71/333/356	
			2	68	*71/356	
^{202}Tl	12.2 d	EC	2	80	*76/440	

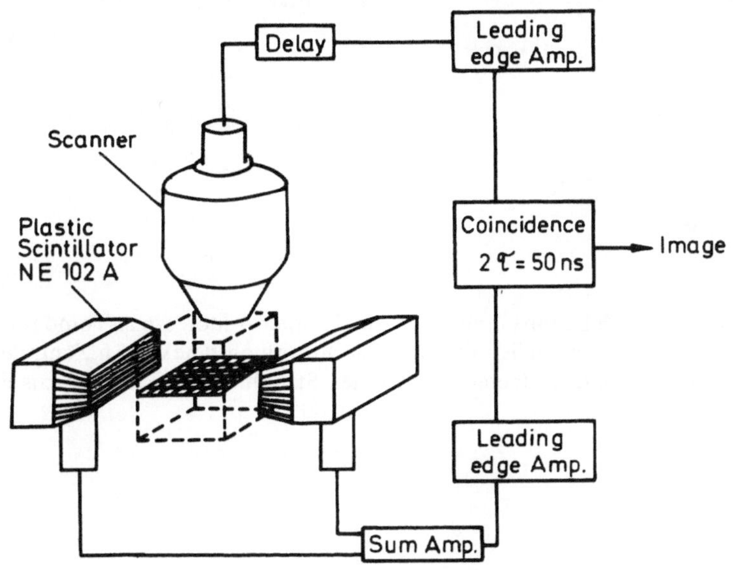

Abb. 85. Meßanordnung für ein γ-γ Koinzidenz-Tomographie-System. (Aus SCHMITZ-FEUERHAKE 1970)

II. Röntgen-Fluoreszenz-Tomographie

Im Gegensatz zur γ-γ-Koinzidenz Tomographie handelt es sich bei der Fluoreszenz-Tomographie um einen Grenzfall zwischen Transmissions- und Emissionstomographie. Da hierbei aber die Konzentration bestimmter natürlicher Nuklide im Körper dargestellt wird, z.B. ^{127}J in der Schilddrüse, ist der Bezug zur Nuklearmedizin gegeben. Bei diesem Verfahren wird kollimiert eine Gammastrahlung oder Röntgenstrahlung von außen in den Körper eingestrahlt und die nach Photoabsorption in der K-Schale des betreffenden Elementes auftretende Röntgen-Fluoreszenz-Strahlung (K-Strahlung) von außen gemessen.

In Abb. 86a wird durch kollimierte Gammastrahlung von 60 keV des ^{241}Am das natürliche Jod in der Schilddrüse in einer bestimmten Schichttiefe angeregt, und die emittierte Fluoreszenzstrahlung (K-Strahlung) von 28,5 keV mit einem kollimierten Halbleiterdetektor gemessen. Der gesamte Meßkopf tastet das Organ zeilenförmig ab. In Abb. 86b ist die Position von Strahlenquelle und Detektor vertauscht. Die zentrale ^{241}Am Quelle regt gleichzeitig alle Schichten in der Tiefe an, aber mit 8 kollimierten Halbleiterdetektoren wird eine grobe Schichtausblendung erzielt (longitudinale Tomographie) (s. auch Abb. 32).

Die klinische Anwendung der Fluoreszenz-Tomographie ist sehr beschränkt. Es lassen sich nur schwere Elemente darstellen ($Z > 50$), da einerseits die relativ niedrige Energie der Fluoreszenzstrahlung mit der Stellenzahl Z wächst und andererseits auch die Ausbeute an Fluoreszenzstrahlung gegenüber der Aussendung von Augerelektronen mit Z größer wird (Jordan 1980). Es lassen sich nur sehr oberflächennahe Körperbereiche abbilden wegen der hohen Absorption der niederenergetischen K-Strahlung, so daß die Anwendung auf das Jod der Schilddrüse und gegebenenfalls noch auf zerebrale Flußmessungen mit Xe ($Z = 54$) beschränkt bleibt.

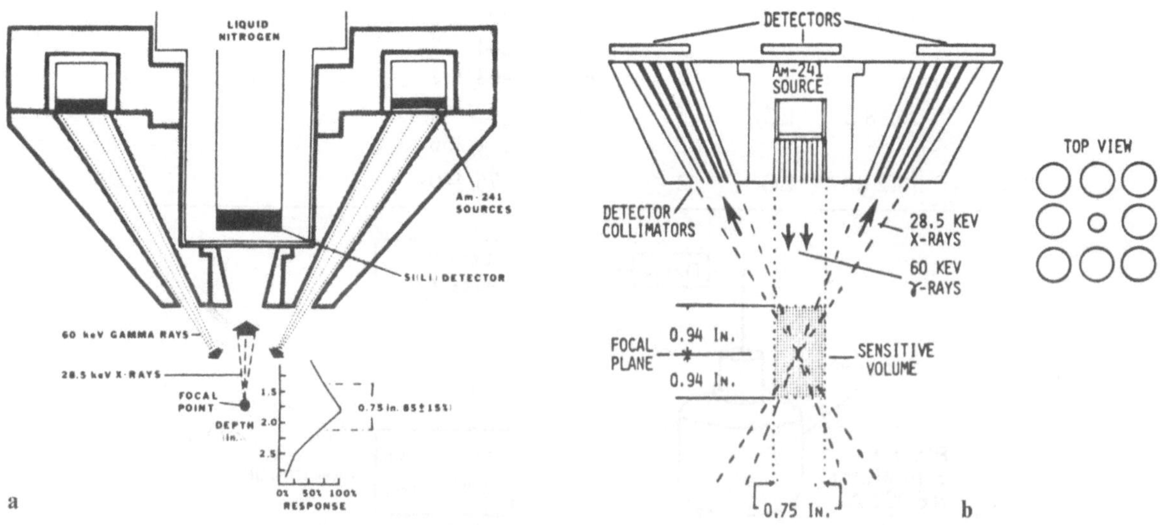

Abb. 86a, b. Zwei verschiedene Meßanordnungen für die Röntgen-Fluoreszenz-Tomographie. **a** Ringförmige Anordnung der kollimierten Strahlenquelle mit zentralem Strahlungsdetektor. **b** Zentrale Strahlenquelle mit 8 auf den Seiten eines Quadrats angeordneten fokussierten Strahlungsdetektoren. (Aus Patton et al. 1980)

G. Mathematische Grundlagen der Rekonstruktion und quantitativen Aktivitätsbestimmung in vivo

I. Einleitung

Das Gebiet der Rekonstruktion eines n-dimensionalen Objektes aus seinen $(n-1)$-dimensionalen Projektionen übergreift viele Bereiche der wissenschaftlichen Forschung; Anwendungen finden sich z.B. in der Kristallographie, Radioastronomie, Elektronenmikroskopie, Röntgendiagnostik und Röntgentherapie, Nuklearmedizin, Ultraschall und Kernspinresonanz. Lange Zeit fanden die Verfahren der Bildrekonstruktion (image reconstruction), die in enger Verwandtschaft zur Bildrefokussierung (image restoration) stehen, in der Medizin wenig Beachtung. Charakteristisch für diese Anfangszeit ist vielleicht die folgende Aussage CORMACKs bezüglich der Resonanz auf seine 1963 publizierte echt rekonstruktive Transmissionstomographie in der radiologischen Anwendung, in der auch bereits die Anwendung des Verfahrens für PET angesprochen wird: „Es gab kaum eine Resonanz. Die interessanteste Nachfrage nach einem Sonderdruck kam vom Schweizer Zentrum für Lawinenforschung. Die Methode wäre für die Bestimmung der Schneehöhen auf Bergen geeignet, falls man entweder den Detektor oder die Quelle in das Gestein unter den Schnee bringen könnte!" (CORMACK 1980, p. 660).

Erst mit der Einführung des EMI-Scanners durch HOUNSFIELD nahm das Interesse sprunghaft zu sowohl in der Radiologie als auch in der Nuklearmedizin. Es folgte eine explosionsartige Zunahme von wissenschaftlichen Publikationen, und bis heute hat die Literatur zu diesem Thema in den unterschiedlichsten Fachgebieten einen Umfang erreicht, der in diesem Artikel nur auszugsweise wiedergegeben werden kann. Diese Tendenz wurde sicherlich auch unterstützt durch die Entwicklung auf dem Gebiet der Rechnertechnologie.

Die mathematische Problematik der Bildrekonstruktion und der Vergleich unterschiedlicher mathematischer Ansätze wird in zahlreichen Übersichtsarbeiten behandelt. So vergleichen z.B. HERMAN u. ROWLAND (1973) analytische und algebraische Verfahren, ebenso GORDON u. HERMAN (1974) sowie BUDINGER u. GULLBERG (1974a, b), die gleichzeitig das Absorptionsproblem mit berücksichtigen. BARRETT et al. (1976) weisen die Äquivalenz aller analytischen Verfahren bezüglich des Signal-Rauschverhältnisses nach, MERSEREAU (1976) gibt eine ausführliche Diskussion der Interpolations- und Abtastprobleme, PHELPS et al. (1977) fassen die mathematischen Anforderungen an ein ECT-System zusammen. BUDINGER (1980) diskutiert ausführlich die Problematik der longitudinalen Tomographie. Weitere sehr umfassende Übersichten geben BROOKS u. DI CHIRO (1975, 1976), PHELPS (1977b), BUDINGER et al. (1979a), JASZCZAK et al. (1980), KOURIS et al. (1982b) und TODD-POKROPEK (1983b); eine rein mathematisch orientierte Zusammenstellung findet sich bei ROWLAND (1979).

Die mathematische Theorie zur Rekonstruktion eines Objektes aus seinen Projektionen (vgl. Abb. 56) und die erforderlichen Voraussetzungen sind allgemein gültig und unabhängig von der jeweiligen physikalischen Realisierung. Spezifisch für jedes Anwendungsgebiet dagegen ist, wie gut die idealisierten mathematischen Voraussetzungen approximiert werden können. Wie bereits in Abschnitt C.I. dargestellt, treten bei der ECT durch die Verknüpfung von Radionuklidverteilung und Verteilung der Absorptionskoeffizienten Schwierigkeiten dadurch auf, daß die gemessene Strahlsumme nur eine relativ schwache Approximation des mathematisch vorausgesetzten Linienintegrals der Objektgröße „Radionuklidverteilung" ergibt. Eine ähnliche Aussage resultiert aus den statistischen Fehlern der Meßgröße aufgrund des niedrigen Photonenflusses, aus dem Auftreten von Streustrahlung, von zufälligen Koinzidenzen (PET) und Abbildungsfehlern des Meßsystems (vgl. Abschnitt D.I.). Weitere Probleme ergeben sich speziell für die longitudinale Tomographie durch den eingeschränkten Winkelbereich der Abtastung. Aus Gründen der besseren Verständlichkeit soll auf diese Effekte in gesonderten Abschnitten näher eingegangen werden, nachdem zuvor unter mehr idealisierten Voraussetzungen die mathematischen Grundlagen und die wichtigsten Rekonstruktionsverfahren erläutert werden.

II. Problemstellung

Das Problem der Rekonstruktion eines dreidimensionalen Objekts (Radionuklidverteilung) reduziert sich erheblich, wenn das Objekt wie bei der transversalen Tomographie in einen Stapel zweidimensionaler Schichten zerlegt werden kann, die unabhängig voneinander gemessen und berechnet werden. Wegen der weiten Verbreitung der transversalen Tomographie und aus Gründen der Übersichtlichkeit soll in den folgenden Abschnitten nach dieser Methode verfahren werden, die speziellen Probleme der longitudinalen Tomographie werden in Abschnitt G.V.1.b behandelt. Unter dieser Voraussetzung ergibt sich das Problem der tomographischen Bildrekonstruktion wie folgt.

Die unbekannte Objektverteilung ist zweidimensional und wird mit $f(x, y)$ bezeichnet. Bekannt sind lediglich die eindimensionalen Projektionen von $f(x, y)$ unter einer begrenzten Anzahl von Winkeln θ. Die Aufgabe ist dann die Berechnung von $f(x, y)$ aus den gemessenen Projektionen $p(l, \theta)$. Dieses Problem ist schlecht konditioniert, d.h. kleine Fehler der gemessenen Projektionen rufen große Fehler in der Berechnung von $f(x, y)$ hervor. So ist eine Rekonstruktion des Objekts nur in eingeschränkter Form möglich, die unterschiedlichen Algorithmen zur Lösung des Rekonstruktionsproblems unterscheiden sich in diesen Beschränkungen und in dem eingebrachten a priori Wissen zur Stabilisierung der Lösung. Allgemein gesprochen existiert kein optimales Verfahren, eine Optimierung – auch im Hinblick auf den Rechenaufwand – kann nur in enger Relation zum jeweiligen Anwendungsfall gefunden werden. Darauf weisen bereits Herman u. Rowland (1973) hin, ebenso Gordon (1974) und Phelps et al. (1977).

Eine ähnliche Aussage gilt auch für die verwandte Problematik der Bildrefokussierung, wie der ausführliche Überblick von Frieden (1975) zeigt; wie denn auch zahlreiche Verfahrensweisen in beiden Problemkreisen parallel verlaufen.

III. Radontransformation und Projection-Slice-Theorem

Für integrierbare Funktionen, um die es sich in physikalisch realistischen Fällen immer handelt, wird eine Projektion des Objekts mathematisch durch einen Satz von Linienintegralen dargestellt, wie es in Abb. 87a für die übliche Parallelgeometrie gezeigt ist. Mit den Bezeichnungen nach Abb. 87b gilt für die Gesamtheit aller Projektionen bei einer Darstellung des Objekts in Polarkoordinaten

$$p(l, \theta) = \int\limits_{L(l, \theta)} f(r, \phi)\, ds \tag{1}$$

Für $\theta = $ const. ergibt sich damit eine Projektion des Objekts unter dem Winkel θ als eindimensionale Funktion der linearen Variablen l mit dem Parameter θ.

Im vertrauteren Kartesischen Koordinatensystem führt Gl. (1) auf die Darstellung

$$p(l, \theta) = \iint\limits_{-\infty}^{+\infty} f(x, y) \cdot \delta(l - x \cos\theta - y \sin\theta)\, dx\, dy \tag{2}$$

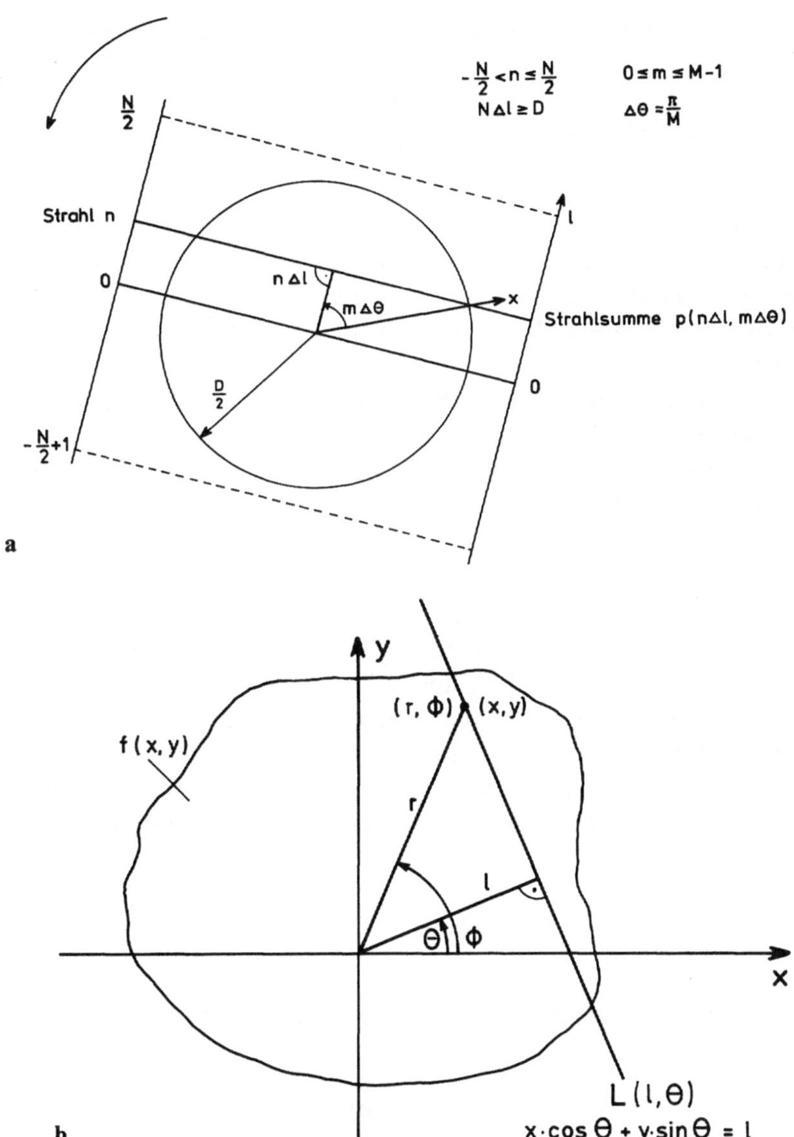

Abb. 87a, b. Projektionsgeometrie. **a** Jede parallel organisierte Projektion besteht aus Strahlsummen, die durch die laterale Koordinate $l = n\,\Delta l$ und den allen gemeinsamen Projektionswinkel $\theta = m\,\Delta\theta$ gekennzeichnet werden. Der Gesichtsfelddurchmesser ist D. **b** Eine Strahlsumme repräsentiert das Linienintegral von $f(x, y)$ längs der Geraden $L(l, \theta)$ und wird gekennzeichnet durch den Abstand l vom Ursprung und den Winkel θ

wobei die Integrationslinie beschrieben wird durch die Geradengleichung

$$l - x \cos\theta - y \sin\theta = 0$$

Die Gln. (1) und (2) für die Parallelgeometrie stellen die Verknüpfung zwischen $p(l, \theta)$ und $f(x, y)$ durch eine Integraltransformation dar, die inverse Transformation ermöglicht die Rekonstruktion des Objekts aus seinen Projektionen. Zu Ehren von Johann RADON, der dieses Problem zuerst löste (RADON 1917), wird diese spezielle Integraltransformation auch Radontransformation genannt. Unabhängig vom gewählten Verfahren ist eine Invertierung der Gln. (1) und (2) nur möglich, wenn $f(x, y)$ stetig und von endlicher örtlicher Ausdehnung ist sowie im Funktionswert eine endliche obere Grenze hat, vgl. auch z.B. TODD-POKROPEK

(1983b). Für die Parallelgeometrie führt Radons Problemlösung auf folgende Darstellung

$$f(x, y) = \frac{1}{2\pi^2} \int\limits_0^\pi \left[\int\limits_{-\infty}^{+\infty} \frac{\partial p(l, \theta)}{\partial l} \cdot \frac{1}{l' - l} \, dl \right] d\theta \tag{3}$$

Dieses Faltungsintegral konvergiert wegen der Unstetigkeitsstelle für $l' = l$ nicht, der Faltungskern l^{-1} muß durch eine Regularisierungsfunktion approximiert werden, welche die Unstetigkeitsstelle behebt. Bei der Darstellung der Rekonstruktion im Fourierraum führt diese Regularisierung auf eine bandbegrenzte Rekonstruktion durch Einführung einer Fensterfunktion (vgl. Abschnitt G.IV.1.c.α).

Das Problem der Regularisierung wird näher ausgeführt zum Beispiel von Todd-Pokropek (1983b) und Kouris et al. (1982b).

Eine ausführliche, streng mathematisch orientierte Ableitung findet der interessierte Leser bei Herman u. Naparstek (1977).

Die Anwendung von Radons Lösung in ihrer direkten Form nach Gl. (3) hat wenig Verbreitung gefunden, nicht zuletzt wegen der Schwierigkeit der numerischen Approximation des partiellen Differentials. Einen der wenigen Ansätze in dieser Richtung gibt Cormack (1973). Obwohl, wie Barrett et al. (1976) zeigen, alle analytischen Verfahren einschließlich Radons Inversionsformel äquivalent sind, bestehen Unterschiede in der diskretisierten Implementierung, welche zur weiten Verbreitung der in Abschnitt G.IV.1.c dargestellten Methoden führen. Unabhängig von Rekonstruktionsverfahren, ob analytisch oder algebraisch, läßt sich die über das unbekannte Objekt in einer oder einem Satz von bekannten Projektionen enthaltene Information anschaulich mit Hilfe der Fouriertransformation darstellen.

Für

$$F(k_x, k_y) = \int\limits_{-\infty}^{+\infty} \int\limits_{-\infty}^{+\infty} f(x, y) \exp[-j(x k_x + y k_y)] \, dx \, dy$$

als Frequenzspektrum oder Frequenzraumdarstellung des Objekts $f(x, y)$ und

$$P(k, \theta) = \int\limits_{-\infty}^{+\infty} p(l, \theta) \exp(-j l k) \, dl$$

als Frequenzspektrum der Projektion unter dem Winkel θ gilt

$$P(k, \theta) = F(k_x, k_y) \Big|_{\substack{k_x = k \cos\theta \\ k_y = k \sin\theta}} \tag{4}$$

Das heißt, die eindimensionale Fouriertransformierte einer Projektion $p(l, \theta = \text{const})$ ist gleich dem Schnitt oder Profil durch die zweidimensionale Fouriertransformierte des Objekts unter dem Winkel θ entlang der Geraden durch den Koordinatenursprung.

Diese von Bracewell (1956) angegebene Beziehung wird als „projection-slice"-Theorem bezeichnet und ist von grundsätzlicher Bedeutung für die tomographische Rekonstruktion. Wegen der umkehrbar eindeutigen Verknüpfung zwischen einer Funktion und ihrer Fouriertransformierten bedeutet die vollständige Kenntnis von $f(x, y)$ auch die vollständige Kenntnis von $F(k_x, k_y)$ und umgekehrt.

In Verbindung mit dem Abtasttheorem (z.B. Bracewell 1978) gibt daher Gl. (4) unabhängig vom gewählten Rekonstruktionsverfahren an, inwieweit durch die gemessenen Projektionen das Objekt $f(x, y)$ bestimmt ist. Zur Veranschaulichung ist in Abb. 88a dargestellt, für welche Funktionsargumente im Fourierbereich die Funktion $F(k_x, k_y)$ bei acht kontinuierlichen, im Winkel äquidistanten Projektionen bekannt ist. Unterliegt die Bildauflösung keinen Beschränkungen, so zeigt das „projection-slice"-Theorem, daß zur exakten Festlegung von $f(x, y)$ unendlich viele kontinuierliche Projektionen in einem Winkelbereich von 180° erforderlich sind.

Bei Durchführung der Rekonstruktion mit dem Digitalrechner und in der üblichen Meßpraxis kann nur eine begrenzte Anzahl M von Projektionen verarbeitet werden, die zudem in Richtung der l-Koordinate nur an N diskreten Punkten über eine Länge D bekannt sind. Durch diese Digitalisierung, d.h. die Einführung von Abtastintervallen im Winkel und in der linearen Koordinate, wird von vornherein die Bildauflösung begrenzt, es ergibt sich nach dem Abtasttheorem eine maximal auflösbare Ortsfrequenz $k_{\max}$. Das resultierende Abtastmuster im Frequenzbereich zeigt Abb. 88b.

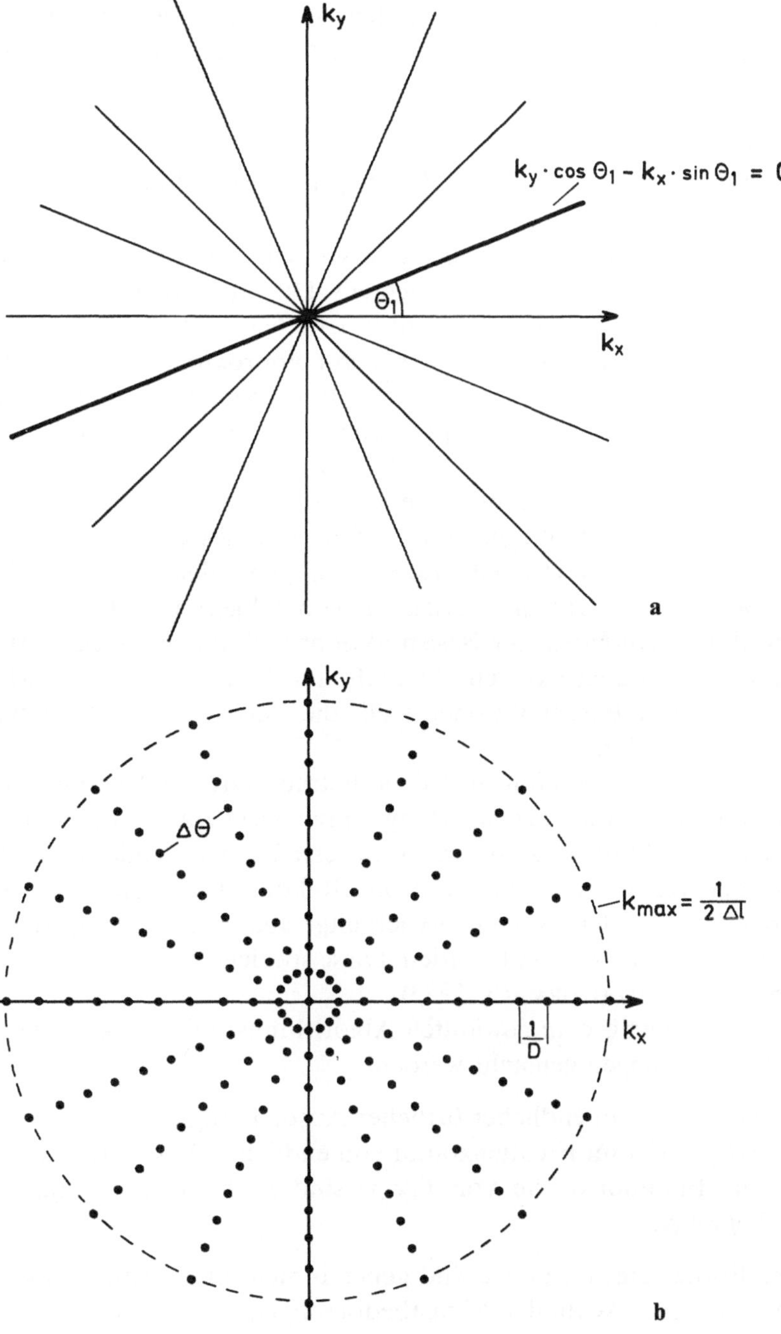

Abb. 88a, b. Abtastmuster im Frequenzbereich. **a** Die Fouriertransformierte des Objekts $f(x, y)$ ist bei kontinuierlichen Projektionen, aber einer endlichen Anzahl von Projektionswinkeln ($M=8$) an den durch die Geraden bezeichneten Stützstellen bekannt. Hervorgehoben ist die Schnittgerade durch die zweidimensionale Funktion $F(k_x, k_y)$ für die Projektion unter dem Winkel θ_1 **b** Bei zusätzlich auch in lateraler Richtung diskretisierter Abtastung resultiert die Einführung einer Nyquistfrequenz $k_{\max}$ und ein lateraler Stützstellenabstand von D^{-1}

Die Gl. (4) lautet dann

$$P(q\Delta k, m\Delta\theta) = F(q\Delta k\,\cos(m\Delta\theta), q\Delta k\,\sin(m\Delta\theta))$$
$$\text{für } |q\Delta k| \leq k_{\max} \tag{4'}$$

Es wird also eine Funktion rekonstruiert, die mit dem Objekt nur innerhalb der erzielten Bildauflösung übereinstimmt. Wegen der erwähnten schlechten Konditionierung des Rekonstruktionsproblems ist eine solche Beschränkung zur Stabilisierung der Lösung erforderlich und wird als Regularisierung bezeichnet (Todd-Pokropek 1983 b). Eine weitere Einschränkung der Bildauflösung wird durch die realen Meßbedingungen verursacht, da das Linienintegral durch eine Strahlsumme approximiert wird, die mit endlicher örtlicher Auflösung bestimmt wird (bei Positronen-Ringen die inhärente Detektorauflösung, bei SPECT-Kameras die Systemauflösung). Das Problem wird von Bracewell (1956) diskutiert. Er zeigt den Einfluß dieser Meßauflösung auf die resultierende Bildauflösung und die Abtastbedingungen.

IV. Verfahren zur Bildrekonstruktion

Üblicherweise werden die unterschiedlichen Rekonstruktionsalgorithmen in analytische und algebraische Verfahren eingeteilt. Die analytischen Verfahren bemühen sich um die Lösung der Gln. (1) und (2) im kontinuierlichen Fall, die dann für die tatsächliche Implementierung in digitaler Form möglichst gut approximiert werden müssen. Diese Verfahren sind in der Regel nicht iterativ. Die algebraischen Ansätze gehen direkt von der digitalisierten Form des Rekonstruktionsproblems aus, sowohl Objekt als auch Bild und Projektionen liegen in gerasterter Form vor. Dieser Ansatz erfordert die Lösung eines in der Regel sehr umfangreichen Gleichungssystems und kann auch als Inversion einer Matrixgleichung betrachtet werden. Wegen des Umfanges dieses Gleichungssystems ist die Lösung üblicherweise nur iterativ möglich. Eine mehr generalisierte Form der Betrachtung algebraischer Verfahren führt auf die Zerlegung von Objekt und Projektionen in einen Satz sorgfältig gewählter orthonormaler Basisfunktionen (Reihenentwicklung), die Bestimmung der zugehörigen Bewichtungsfaktoren führt z.B. auf die oben erwähnte Matrixinversion. Eine mögliche Wahl solcher Basisfunktionen stellt die Zerlegung des Objekts in die Pixel der Digitalisierungsmatrix dar.

Aber auch eine kontinuierliche Betrachtung des Rekonstruktionsproblems kann zu einer Lösung durch Reihenentwicklung führen, wie Cormack (1963) zeigt. Er entwickelt den gemessenen Projektionssatz in eine Fourierreihe der Winkelvariablen. Dann ist das Objekt in gleicher Weise darstellbar und das Rekonstruktionsproblem kann durch Bestimmung der Koeffizienten der Reihenentwicklung aus der Lösung des resultierenden Integralgleichungssystems bestimmt werden. Diese spezielle Methode beinhaltet ebenfalls Radons direkte Problemlösung (Cormack 1973).

Unabhängig vom gewählten Algorithmus müssen bezüglich der Objektfunktion folgende Einschränkungen gemacht werden:

1. $f(x, y)$ ist von endlicher örtlicher Ausdehnung.
2. $F(k_x, k_y)$ ist im Frequenzraum von endlicher Ausdehnung.
3. Die Funktionswerte von $f(x, y)$ sind nach oben hin auf einen endlichen Maximalwert begrenzt.

Die Forderungen 1 und 2 sind generell nicht gleichzeitig exakt erfüllbar, können aber durch entsprechende Wahl der Abtastbedingungen gut approximiert werden.

1. Analytische Verfahren

In diesem Abschnitt sollen die hauptsächlichen Rekonstruktionsverfahren besprochen werden, und zwar für die Geometrie der Projektion längs paralleler Strahlen. Diese Geometrie tritt z.B. bei rotierenden Gammakameras auf. Die divergierenden Strahlen von Positronen-Ringen (fan-beam) können entweder durch „rebinning" in die Parallelgeometrie umsortiert werden oder erfordern spezielle Modifikationen der Algorithmen, auf die dann explizit hingewiesen wird.

a) Direkte 2D-Fouriersynthese

Die direkte Fourierrücktransformation der entsprechend dem „projection-slice"-Theorem abgetasteten Funktion $F(k_x, k_y)$ liefert als Objektrekonstruktion die zweidimensionale Faltung des Objekts $f(x, y)$ mit der Punktbildfunktion $s(x, y)$ der Abtastfunktion $S(k_x, k_y)$ nach Abb. 88, wie dies generell für jede Form der Digitalisierung gilt (BRACEWELL 1978)

$$\hat{f}(x, y) = f(x, y) * * s(x, y) \tag{5}$$

Diese Abtastfunktion hat die Eigenschaft, daß die Abtastwerte auf konzentrischen Kreisen liegen und daher für niedrige Ortsfrequenzen k sehr viel dichter beieinander sind als für höhere Frequenzen – die Flächendichte der Abtastpunkte ist umgekehrt proportional zum Betrag der Ortsfrequenz. KLUG u. CROWTHER (1972) demonstrieren, daß dieses Faltungsintegral im wesentlichen die einfache Rückprojektion ergibt. Der sich natürlicherweise anbietende Weg zur Rekonstruktion von $f(x, y)$ ist, das Objektspektrum $F(k_x, k_y)$, ausgehend von den radialen Abtastwerten, auf ein regelmäßiges Raster in kartesischen Koordinaten zu interpolieren. Anschließend kann das Objekt $f(x, y)$ aus seinem Spektrum durch eine diskrete 2D-Fourierrücktransformation gewonnen werden. Bei einer Wahl des kartesischen Rasters entsprechend dem Abtasttheorem führt dann die neue Abtastfunktion $S'(k_x, k_y)$ nach Gl. (5) nur zu einer periodischen Wiederholung der Objektfunktion ohne störende Überlagerungen. Dieses Verfahren der direkten 2D-Fouriersynthese ist schematisch in Abb. 89 dargestellt und erfordert die folgenden Rechenschritte:

1. Berechnung der transformierten Projektionen $P(k, \theta)$ durch eindimensionale diskrete Fouriertransformation.
2. Berechnung von $F(k_x, k_y)$ im kartesischen Abtastraster durch zweidimensionale Interpolation im Frequenzbereich.
3. Berechnung $f(x, y)$ durch zweidimensionale diskrete Fourierrücktransformation von $F(k_x, k_y)$.

Dieser Algorithmus wurde erstmals von DE ROSIER u. KLUG (1968) in der Elektronenmikroskopie eingesetzt. Anwendungen in der Nuklearmedizin finden sich bei KAY et al. (1974) sowie bei MERSEREAU (1973). Eine Relation zu anderen Rekonstruktionsverfahren stellen z.B. GORDON u. HERMAN (1974), BROOKS u. DI CHIRO (1976), MERSEREAU (1976) und BARRETT et al. (1976) her.

Die Hauptschwierigkeit und der anteilig größte Rechenaufwand der Methode liegt in der erforderlichen zweidimensionalen Interpolation, die, wie BRACEWELL (1979) zeigt, auch unter Annahme der Existenz einer maximalen Grenzfrequenz des Objekts nicht mathematisch exakt durchführbar ist. Das von ihm vorgeschlagene bestmögliche Interpolationsschema durch exakte sinc-Interpolation in radialer Richtung und approximativer Interpolation in Winkelrichtung ist als globales Schema sehr rechenaufwendig. Ein ähnliches Verfahren in Verbindung mit einer ausführlichen mathematischen Diskussion der Abtastproblematik schlagen STARK et al. (1981) vor. Ebenfalls eine ausführliche Untersuchung betreffs unter-

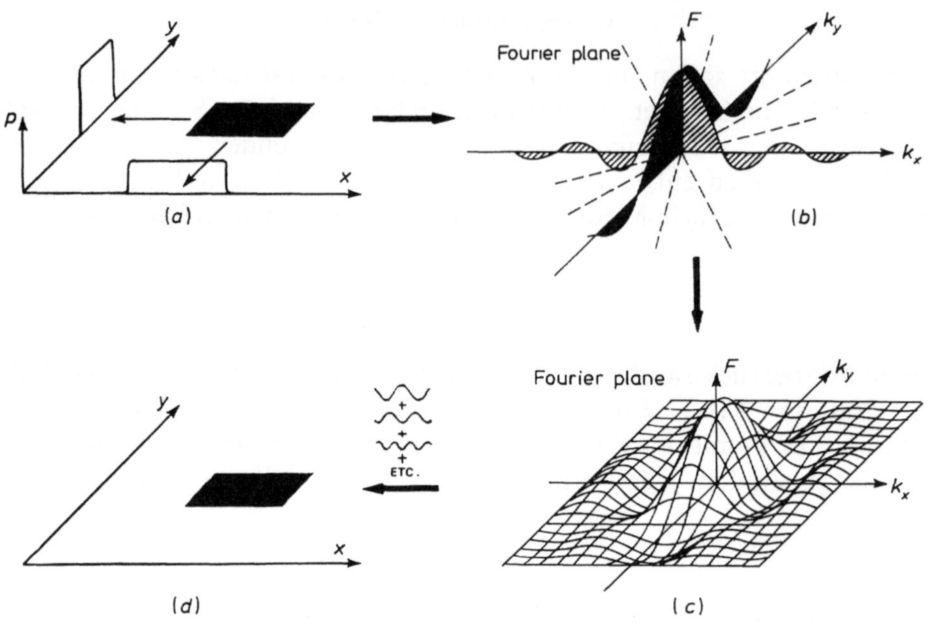

Abb. 89a–d. Graphische Verdeutlichung der Fouriersynthese (aus Brooks u. Di Chiro 1976). **a** Projektionen. **b** Transformierte Projektionen als Schnitte des zweidimensionalen Objekts (vgl. Abb. 88a), **c** Interpolation im Frequenzraum, **d** Rekonstruiertes Objekt durch 2D-Fourier-Rücktransformation

schiedlicher globaler und lokaler Interpolationsschemata führt Mersereau (1976) durch. Durch diese Problematik der $2D$-Interpolation bezüglich Genauigkeit, Rechenaufwand und Fehlerfortpflanzung hat das Verfahren der direkten $2D$-Fouriersynthese an Bedeutung gegen die im folgenden dargestellte Convolution-Methode verloren. Daran ändert auch nichts die von Mersereau (1976) vorgeschlagene Vereinfachung durch Abtasten der Projektionen mit einem je nach Winkelstellung variablen linearen Abtastintervall. Diese Methode führt im Frequenzbereich zu einem Abtastmuster in Form konzentrischer Quadrate anstelle der Kreise und erfordert nur noch eindimensionale Interpolation. Diesem Vorteil steht dann allerdings der Nachteil eines mit dem Winkel variablen Abtastintervalls entgegen, welches z.B. bei allen Ringanordnungen prinzipiell nicht erfüllbar ist.

b) Rückprojektion und gefilterte Rückprojektion

Das wohl älteste „Rekonstruktionsverfahren" ist die bereits in Abschnitt C.III.1. besprochene Rückprojektion (Backprojection). Auch heute noch ist die einfache Rückprojektion von erheblicher Bedeutung, da dieses Verfahren implizit oder explizit in nahezu allen analytischen und algebraischen Verfahren enthalten ist. Eine frühe nuklearmedizinische Anwendung findet sich z.B. bei Kuhl u. Edwards (1963, 1964, 1968). Mathematisch läßt sich die Rückprojektion beschreiben zu

$$b(x, y) = \int\limits_0^\pi p(x \cos \theta + y \sin \theta, \theta) \, d\theta \tag{6}$$

Die Gleichung läßt sich auf zwei Arten lesen:

1. Für einen punktweisen Aufbau des Bildes $b(x, y)$ wird für ein festes (x_0, y_0) in jeder Projektion der Projektionswert an der entsprechenden Stelle entnommen und aufsummiert, d.h.

der Wert $b(x_0, y_0)$ wird direkt gebildet als Summe aller Strahlsummen, die durch diesen Punkt gehen. Der Vorgang wird dann für alle x, y wiederholt.

2. Für einen projektionsweisen Aufbau von $b(x, y)$ werden für jede Projektion alle Punkte des Bildes, die auf der Geraden $l = x \cos\theta_0 + y \sin\theta_0$ liegen, um den Projektionswert an der jeweiligen Stelle l erhöht und der Vorgang für alle Projektionen wiederholt.

Dies entspricht der graphischen Darstellung in Abb. 2.

In digitalisierter Form wird Gl. (6) approximiert durch

$$b(i\Delta x, j\Delta y) = \Delta\theta \sum_{m=0}^{M-1} p[i\Delta x \cos(m\Delta\theta) + j\Delta y \sin(m\Delta\theta), m\Delta\theta] \tag{6'}$$

Nach dieser Beziehung wird der Projektionswert an der Stelle

$$l^* = i\Delta x \cos(m\Delta\theta) + j\Delta y \sin(m\Delta\theta)$$

benötigt, liegt aber nur an den Punkten $l = n\Delta l$ vor. Da diese Werte im allgemeinen nicht übereinstimmen, ist eine eindimensionale Interpolation der gerasterten Projektion in l-Richtung erforderlich.

Diese einfache Rückprojektion bewirkt einen Verwischungseffekt, der z.B. für ein punktförmiges Objekt und eine geringe Projektionsanzahl den bekannten Sternartefakt erzeugt. Durch iterative Subtraktion dieses Artefakts an markanten Bildpunkten versuchen MUEHL-LEHNER u. WETZEL (1971) die Qualität der Rückprojektionsmethode zu verbessern.

Der exakte Zusammenhang zwischen der durch Rückprojektion erzeugten Rekonstruktion $b(x, y)$ und dem Objekt $f(x, y)$ wurde erstmals explizit von BATES u. PETERS (1971) angegeben und zu einer echten Rekonstruktionsmethode ausgebaut.

Im Fourierraum ergibt sich

$$B(k_x, k_y) = F(k_x, k_y) \cdot |k|^{-1}$$
$$\text{mit } k = \sqrt{k_x^2 + k_y^2} \tag{7}$$

Das heißt, die Fouriertransformierte der Rückprojektion ist gleich der Fouriertransformation des Objekts, dividiert durch den Betrag der Ortsfrequenz. In Bezug auf die Aussagen in Abschnitt G.IV.1.a ist die äquivalente Aussage, daß $B(k_x, k_y)$ aus $F(k_x, k_y)$ entsteht durch Multiplikation mit der Dichteverteilung der Abtastwerte. Diese Aussagen gelten exakt für unendlich viele Projektionen.

Im Ortsbereich gilt dann

$$b(x, y) = f(x, y) * r^{-1}$$
$$\text{mit } r = \sqrt{x^2 + y^2} \tag{8}$$

Der Rekonstruktionsalgorithmus von BATES u. PETERS beruht auf der direkten Invertierung von Gl. (7) und wird als Gefilterte Rückprojektion (rho-filtered layergram) bezeichnet.

$$F(k_x, k_y) = B(k_x, k_y) \cdot |k|$$
$$\text{für } |k| \leq k_{\max} \tag{9}$$

Folgende Schritte sind erforderlich:

1. Berechnung der einfachen Rückprojektion $b(x, y)$ aus den gemessenen Projektionen (Gl. 6).
2. Zweidimensionale Fouriertransformation.

3. Filterung durch Multiplikation mit dem Betrag der Ortsfrequenz bis zu einer Frequenz k_{max}.

4. Berechnung von $f(x, y)$ durch Inverse Fouriertransformation.

Gerade an dieser Darstellung wird die unmittelbare Verwandtschaft zwischen Bildrefokussie-rung und Bildrekonstruktion deutlich. Das Bild entsteht aus dem Objekt durch Faltung mit einer nivellierenden Funktion. In dieser Nomenklatur entspricht das Verfahren der gefil-terten Rückprojektion direkt dem Begriff des „Inversen Filters mit begrenzter Bandbreite". Obwohl das Verfahren von Bates u. Peters (1971) auf optischem Wege ohne Einsatz eines Computers realisiert wurde, wird man entsprechend dem heutigen Stand eine digitale Imple-mentierung wählen. Vorteilhaft im Vergleich zur Fouriersynthese ist, daß lediglich eindimen-sionale Interpolation in Richtung der linearen Koordinate erforderlich ist. Im Vergleich zur Methode der Rückprojektion gefilterter Projektionen bestehen die Nachteile darin, daß zum einen vor Beginn der Rechnung bereits alle Projektionen vorliegen müssen, zum anderen zur Vermeidung von Randfehlern die Berechnung in einer Matrix durchzuführen ist, die etwa die vierfache Größe des Datenfeldes hat.

c) Rückprojektion gefilterter Projektionen

Die Methode der Rückprojektion gefilterter Projektionen, auch Convolution-Algorithmus genannt, stellt heute bei Anwendung analytischer Verfahren wegen ihrer rechentechnischen Eleganz die Methode der Wahl dar. Zum einen können alle wesentlichen Rechenschritte eindimensional ausgeführt werden, zum anderen kann die Berechnung schon nach Vorliegen der ersten Projektion begonnen werden. Die Convolution-Methode wird abgeleitet aus der gefilterten Rückprojektion durch eine vertauschte Reihenfolge der Rechenoperationen. Diese Vertauschung ist wegen der Linearität des Verfahrens und der Existenz des „Projection-slice"-Theorems zulässig und führt auf folgenden Algorithmus:

1. Berechnung von $P(k, \theta)$ durch eindimensionale Fouriertransformation.

2. Berechnung von modifizierten, gefilterten Projektionen $P'(k, \theta)$.

3. Eindimensionale Fourierrücktransformation von $P'(k, \theta)$.

4. Rückprojektion von $p'(l, \theta)$ inklusive eindimensionaler Interpolation.

Es gilt

$$f(x, y) = \int_0^\pi p'(x \cos \theta + y \sin \theta, \theta)\, d\theta \tag{10}$$

$$P'(k, \theta) = P(k, \theta) \cdot G(k) \tag{11}$$

$$G(k) = |k| \quad \text{für } |k| \leq k_{max} \tag{12}$$

Diese Schreibweise drückt die Modifikation der Projektion durch Anwendung eines Filters $G(k)$ aus, in diesem Fall die bandbegrenzte Version des Rampenfilters. Die Bandbegrenzung ist zur Regularisierung erforderlich und bewirkt bei einem auf k_{max} bandbegrenzten Objekt keine Approximationsfehler.

Wegen des Faltungstheorems der Fouriertransformation kann gleichwertig im Ortsbereich geschrieben werden

$$p'(l, \theta) = p(l, \theta) * g(l) \tag{13}$$

Durch Verknüpfung der Gln. (10), (11) und (12) kann das Rekonstruktionsverfahren im Fre-quenzbereich oder, äquivalent über Gln. (10) und (13), im Ortsbereich durchgeführt werden. Die dann erforderliche Berechnung von Faltungsintegralen in Gl. (13) begründet die alterna-tive Bezeichnung der Methode als Convolution-Verfahren.

Die erste Anwendung der Methode wird von BRACEWELL u. RIDDLE (1967) beschrieben, unabhängig davon erfolgte die Neuentdeckung des Verfahrens durch RAMACHANDRAN u. LAKSHMINARAYANAN (1971), den ersten klinischen Einsatz im ACTA-Scanner geben LEDLEY et al. (1974) an. Beide Autoren verwenden das Filter nach Gl. (12) als Faltungsfilter aufgrund seiner besonders einfachen diskretisierten Form

$$k_{\text{max}} = \frac{1}{2\,\Delta l} \tag{14}$$

$$g(n\Delta l) = \begin{cases} \dfrac{1}{4\,\Delta l} & n = 0 \\[2ex] -\dfrac{1}{\pi^2 n^2\,\Delta l} & n \text{ ungerade} \\[2ex] 0 & n \text{ gerade} \end{cases} \tag{15}$$

Die Rauschverstärkung und besonders die Neigung zu Rekonstruktionsartefakten an scharfen Objektkanten führten zur Modifikation von SHEPP u. LOGAN (1974)

$$G_{SL}(k) = |k| \cdot \text{sinc}\left(\frac{k}{2\,k_{\text{max}}}\right) \quad \text{für } |k| \leq k_{\text{max}} \tag{16}$$

$$g_{SL}(n\Delta l) = \frac{2}{\pi^2\,\Delta l(1 - 4n^2)} \tag{17}$$

Die gleichen Autoren geben noch eine weitere Modifikation für stärker verrauschte Daten an.

In Gl. (16) wird der Einbezug einer Regularisierungsfunktion in das Rekonstruktionsfilter explizit erkennbar, die auch in Gl. (12) bereits implizit durch die Begrenzung der Maximalfrequenz vorhanden ist. Durch die geschickte Wahl dieser theoretisch erforderlichen Regularisierungsfunktion, die auch Fensterfunktion (window-function) genannt wird, kann das Rekonstruktionsergebnis im Hinblick auf Rauschverstärkung, Artefaktneigung und Auflösung beeinflußt werden, wie auch aus der Theorie der Bildrefokussierung hinlänglich bekannt ist. Interessant ist in diesem Zusammenhang auch, daß bei Einbezug der notwendigen Regularisierungsfunktion die direkte RADON-Inversionsformel und die Convolution-Methode unmittelbar auseinander hervorgehen, wie z.B. BARRETT et al. (1976) und TODD-POKROPEK (1983b) ableiten.

α) Fensterfunktion

Wie bereits gezeigt, wird das Rekonstruktionsfilter aus der erforderlichen Rampenfunktion $|k|$ und einer Fensterfunktion $W(k)$ mit Tiefpaßcharakteristik zusammengesetzt, in direkter Analogie zum Verfahren des „windowed estimate" der Bildrefokussierung.

$$G(k) = |k| \cdot W(k) \tag{18}$$

Generell erweist es sich als vorteilhaft, zur Unterdrückung von Rekonstruktionsartefakten aufgrund des Gibbschen Phänomens einen weichen Übergang des Rekonstruktionsfilters von seinem Maximalwert hin zum Wert Null an der Filtergrenzfrequenz zu erzeugen. Das gleiche Verhalten ist ebenfalls zur Begrenzung der Rauschverstärkung anzustreben, d.h. eine exakte Annäherung an das erforderliche Rampenfilter für niedrige Frequenzen mit gutem Signal-Rauschverhältnis sowie eine Dämpfung der Verstärkung bei höheren Frequenzen. Gleichzeitig wird durch diese Maßnahme die resultierende Bildauflösung verschlechtert, die sich aus der Ortsbereichsdarstellung der Fensterfunktion und der inhärenten Meßauflösung ergibt. So zeigen Chesler u. Riederer (1975) die Unterdrückung von oszillatorischen Rekonstruktionsartefakten durch Verwendung eines Hamming-Fensters, weisen aber gleichzeitig darauf hin, daß zur Erzielung einer konstanten Bildauflösung die Grenzfrequenz des Hamming-Fensters doppelt so hoch wie bei der Verwendung des Rechteckfensters nach Gl. (12) sein müßte. Ebenfalls ein Hamming-Fenster mit einstellbarer Grenzfrequenz verwendet Carroll (1978).

Die Punktbildfunktion $h(r)$ der Rekonstruktion, unbeschadet der inhärenten Auflösung des Meßinstruments, ergibt sich aus dem Rekonstruktionsfilter durch Rückprojektion (vgl. z.B. Barrett u. Swindell 1977).

$$h(r) = \int\limits_0^\pi g(r \cos \theta)\, d\theta \tag{19}$$

Andere Formen der Charakterisierung ergeben sich aus der Hankeltransformation der Fensterfunktion $W(k)$ – die Linienbildfunktion der Rekonstruktion wird charakterisiert durch die Fensterfunktion $w(l)$. Ersetzt man in Gl. (19) die Filterfunktion $g(l)$ durch das Faltungsintegral von Filter und Linienbildfunktion des Meßsystems, ergibt sich die Punktbildfunktion des Systems. In gleicher Weise läßt sich auch der Einfluß der Interpolation berücksichtigen.

Kwoh et al. (1977) schlagen eine Klasse von Fensterfunktionen der Form $\exp(-c \cdot k)^n$ vor, die durch Variation von n und c in weiten Grenzen variiert werden kann. Einen zusätzlichen rauschabhängigen Tiefpaßanteil des Rekonstruktionsfilters verwenden Chu u. Tam (1977). Das Verfahren entspricht der aus dem Gebiet „image restoration" stammenden Methode der „constrained deconvolution" nach Phillips (vgl. Frieden 1975). Huesman et al. (1977) implementieren Butterworth-, Hann-, Hamming-, Parzen- und Rechteckfenster; Budinger et al. (1979a) diskutieren ebenfalls Vor- und Nachteile dieser Funktionen. Eine graphische Darstellung sowohl der Fenster- als auch der zugehörigen Filterfunktionen gibt Abb. 90a, b. Einen umfassenden Überblick über die Eigenschaften von Fensterfunktionen auf dem Gebiet der Spektralanalyse periodischer Zeitvorgänge (Anwendung im Zeitbereich) gibt Harris (1978). Diese Zusammenstellung wird auszugsweise auf das Gebiet der Bildrefokussierung (Anwendung im Frequenzbereich) übertragen von Knoop (1982), verbunden mit Kriterien zur Auswahl des Fensters unter Berücksichtigung von Rauschverstärkung und -textur, Artefaktneigung, örtlicher Auflösung und Filterlänge. Diese Ergebnisse sind unmittelbar auf das Rekonstruktionsproblem übertragbar. Die gebräuchlichsten Fensterfunktionen sind in Tabelle 6 zusammengestellt.

Tabelle 6. Gebräuchliche Fensterfunktionen. Für alle Fenster gilt: $a = \dfrac{k}{k_g}$; $W(k) = 0$ für $|k| > k_g$

Name	$W(k)$
Rechteck	1
Shepp-Logan	$\mathrm{sinc}(0{,}5a)$
Hann	$0{,}5 + 0{,}5 \cos(\pi a)$
Hamming	$0{,}54 + 0{,}46 \cos(\pi a)$
Butterworth	$(1 + a^{2n})^{-1}$

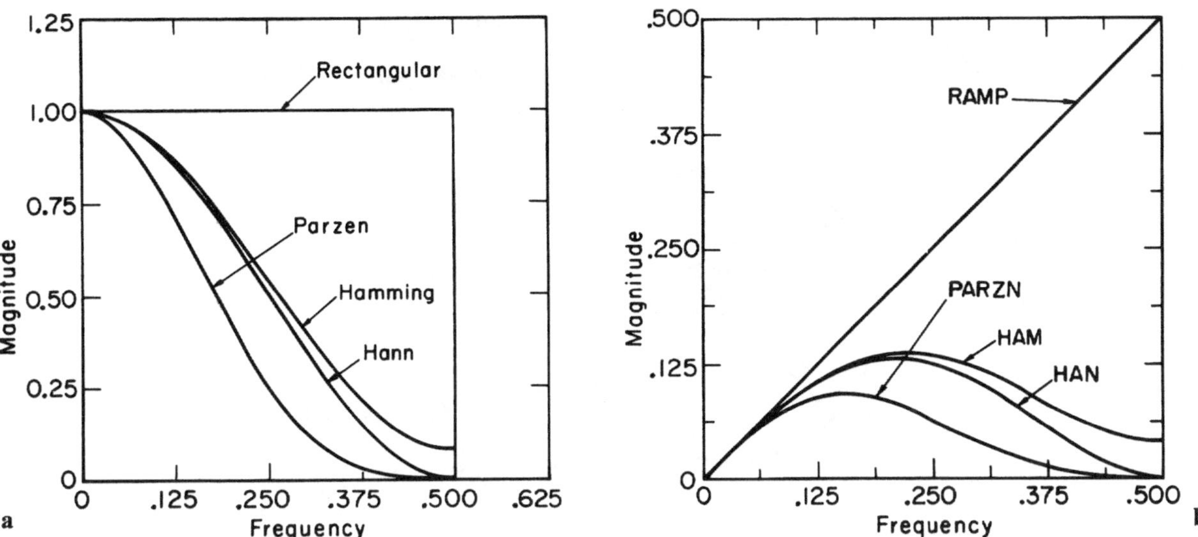

Abb. 90a, b. Rekonstruktionsfilter im Frequenzbereich (aus BUDINGER et al. 1979a). **a** gebräuchliche Fensterfunktionen ($k_g = 0,5$), **b** zugehörige Filterfunktionen als Produkt von Fenster- und Rampenfunktion

β) Interpolation

Eine exakte Interpolation der abgetasteten Projektionswerte kann durch die sinc-Interpolation (vgl. BRACEWELL 1978) durchgeführt werden. Dieser globale Interpolator ist sehr rechenaufwendig. Da die Rechenzeit eines Rekonstruktionsverfahrens wesentlich von der Interpolation bestimmt wird, beschäftigen sich zahlreiche Autoren mit der Eignung einfacherer Interpolationsfunktionen. Untersucht werden hauptsächlich Lagrangesche Polynome unterschiedlicher Ordnung, deren bekannteste Vertreter die "Methode des nächsten Nachbarn" (0. Ordnung) und die lineare Interpolation (1. Ordnung) sind. Beispielhaft seien genannt OPPENHEIM (1975) und HERMAN et al. (1979), die sich mit linearer und spline-Interpolation sowie deren Frequenzgang in Verbindung mit dem Rekonstruktionsfilter beschäftigen, MERSEREAU (1976) mit einer gründlichen Diskussion der Interpolationsproblematik sowie die ausführliche Studie von ROWLAND (1979), der auch für Lagrange-Interpolatoren höherer Ordnung in Verbindung mit einer Vielzahl von Fensterfunktionen die resultierende Auflösung und das Auftreten oszillatorischer Artefakte vergleicht. Zusammenfassend läßt sich sagen, daß nach heutigem Stand immer noch die lineare Interpolation die Methode der Wahl ist.

γ) Convolution-Methode für Fächergeometrie

Bei Positronen-Ringdetektoren ist die inhärente Projektionsgeometrie nach Abb. 91 als Fächergeometrie (fan-beam) darstellbar, eine Projektion wird in der Form $p(\gamma, \beta)$ gemessen, wobei der Winkel β den jeweiligen Scheitelpunkt des Fächers angibt, der Winkel γ den Projektionsstrahl innerhalb des Fächers auswählt und der Öffnungswinkel des gesamten Fächers 2δ beträgt. Der Abstand des Fächerscheitels vom Rotationszentrum wird mit R bezeichnet. Diese Projektionen müssen über den vollen Winkelbereich von 360° gemessen werden.

Prinzipiell ist es möglich und auch üblich, den vollständigen Satz $p(\gamma, \beta)$ in die vertraute Parallelgeometrie umzusortieren, gegebenenfalls werden zur Verbesserung des linearen Abtastintervalls Δl jeweils zwei Projektionsstrahlen in geeigneter Weise durch Interpolation zu einem zusammengefaßt. Nach diesem „rebinning" genannten Verfahren folgt dann die übliche Rekonstruktion in Parallelgeometrie.

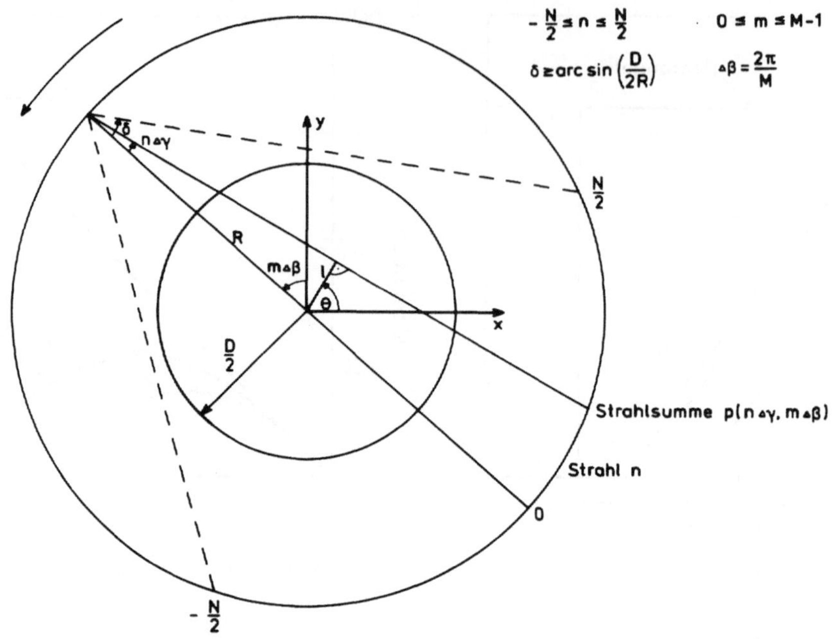

Abb. 91. Kennzeichnung von Projektionen in Fächergeometrie. Jede Fächerprojektion besteht aus $N+1$ Strahlsummen, die durch den Winkel $\gamma = n\,\Delta\gamma$ innerhalb des Fächers und durch den allen gemeinsamen Winkel $\beta = m\,\Delta\beta$ gekennzeichnet werden. Der Winkel 2δ bezeichnet den Öffnungswinkel des Fächers, seine Mindestgröße wird durch den Gesichtsfelddurchmesser D und den Bahnradius R des Fächerscheitels festgelegt

Es ist aber auch möglich, die Rekonstruktion direkt aus den divergierenden Projektionen durchzuführen. Erforderlich ist dann eine Modifikation der Rückprojektion (Gl. 6) sowie bei Anwendung der Convolution-Methode eine veränderte Form des Rekonstruktionsfilters beziehungsweise des Faltungskerns g. Für das Rechteckfenster wird die Methode erstmals von HERMAN et al. (1976) sowie HERMAN u. NAPARSTEK (1977) beschrieben. Die exakte mathematische Ableitung beinhaltet implizit auch die Verwendung alternativer Regularisierungs- bzw. Fensterfunktionen.

Die Rekonstruktionsformeln lauten dann:

$$f(r,\phi) = \frac{1}{4\pi^2} \int_0^{2\pi} \frac{R}{W^2} \int_{-\delta}^{+\delta} \left[g_1(\gamma' - \gamma)\cos\gamma + g_2(\gamma' - \gamma)\cos\gamma' \right] \cdot p(\gamma, \beta)\, d\gamma\, d\beta \tag{20}$$

mit

$$g_1(u) = \begin{cases} -2\pi^2 k_g^2 & \text{für } u = 0 \\ \dfrac{\cos(2\pi u k_g) - 1}{\sin^2 u} & \text{für } u \neq 0 \end{cases} \tag{21a}$$

$$g_2(u) = \begin{cases} 4\pi^2 k_g^2 & \text{für } u = 0 \\ \dfrac{2\pi k_g \sin(2\pi u k_g)}{\sin u} & \text{für } u \neq 0 \end{cases} \tag{21b}$$

$$W = \sqrt{[r\cos(\beta - \phi)]^2 + [R + r\sin(\beta - \phi)]^2} \tag{22}$$

$$\gamma' = \arctan \frac{r\cos(\beta - \phi)}{R + r\sin(\beta - \phi)} \tag{23}$$

Das innere Integral in Gl. (20) ist ein Faltungsintegral und beinhaltet die Modifikation der gemessenen Projektionen $p(\gamma, \beta)$ durch das Rekonstruktionsfilter. Diese Faltung enthält zwei Schritte: die Faltung der mit $\cos \gamma$ bewichteten Projektion mit g_1 und die Faltung der gleichen Projektion mit g_2, multipliziert mit dem jeweils konstanten Faktor $\cos \gamma'$. Das äußere Integral stellt die bewichtete Rückprojektion der gefilterten Projektionen dar, wobei das Gewicht W den Abstand des Punktes (r, ϕ) vom Fächerscheitel angibt. Die Größe γ' kennzeichnet den Projektionsstrahl, der durch den Punkt (r, ϕ) geht und der aus der gefilterten Projektion gegebenenfalls durch Interpolation berechnet werden muß.

HERMAN u. NAPARSTEK (1977) vergleichen diesen Algorithmus mit der üblichen Parallelmethode und geben gleichzeitig Beispiele für Fehler, die dann entstehen, wenn divergente Projektionen ohne rebinning als Parallelprojektionen verarbeitet werden. Auch HUESMAN et al. (1977) implementieren die Convolution-Methode für Fächergeometrie. Das Verfahren wird ferner in den Reviews von BUDINGER et al. (1979a) und KOURIS et al. (1982b) besprochen. Eine Modifikation des in Gln. (20–23) beschriebenen Algorithmus schlagen TRUONG et al. (1983) vor. Sie verwenden anstelle des Rechteckfensters die von KWOH et al. (1977) vorgeschlagene Klasse von Exponentialfenstern.

Zu erwähnen ist an dieser Stelle auch der von MARR (1974) entwickelte Algorithmus speziell für Ringanordnungen, der auch von HUESMAN et al. (1977) implementiert wurde. Dieses Verfahren beruht nicht auf der Convolution-Methode, sondern geht von einer Reihenentwicklung von orthogonalen Polynomen für Objekt und Projektion aus und löst das entstehende Gleichungssystem. Eine genauere Beschreibung der Methode geben auch BUDINGER et al. (1979a).

d) Rekonstruktion für TOF-Systeme

Durch die zusätzliche Ortungsinformation längs des Projektionsstrahles aufgrund der Flugzeitmessung (TOF) ergibt sich eine wesentliche Verbesserung der Bildrekonstruktion, auch wenn die Flugzeitauflösung erheblich schlechter ist als die angestrebte Bildauflösung. Im – allen Rekonstruktionsverfahren gemeinsamen – Schritt der Rückprojektion wird die gemessene Information nicht mehr wie in der konventionellen Tomographie längs des gesamten Meßstrahles verteilt, sondern in Relation zur Flugzeitauflösung um den tatsächlichen Emissionsort konzentriert.

Wie aus Abb. 76 ersichtlich, ergibt diese Methode der Rückprojektion eine wesentlich kompaktere Form der aus der einfachen Rückprojektion resultierenden Punktbildfunktion, so daß der nachfolgende Rekonstruktionsalgorithmus von wesentlich besseren Ausgangsdaten (pre-image) ausgehen kann. Bereits 1977 schätzte BUDINGER ab, daß dadurch bei gleicher statistischer Güte der Meßdaten für eine Flugzeitauflösung von 3 cm FWHM eine um den Faktor 10 geringere Verstärkung der Rauschvarianz durch den Rekonstruktionsalgorithmus möglich ist. Diese verminderte Rauschverstärkung entspricht einer virtuellen Steigerung der Systemempfindlichkeit, so daß in Analysen von TOF-Systemen die Verbesserung häufig in Form eines "sensitivity gain" ausgedrückt wird. Eine alternative Betrachtungsweise findet sich bei TANAKA (1982), der darauf hinweist, daß mit Flugzeitortung eine geringere Anzahl von Winkelprojektionen für die adäquate Rekonstruktion des Objekts erforderlich ist. Speziell dieser Punkt wird auch von TOMITANI (1982) untersucht. Das Simulationsergebnis zeigt für rauschfreie Daten, daß bei 6 cm Flugzeitauflösung eine 128×128 Matrix ($\Delta x = 0{,}5$ cm) aus nur 16 Winkelprojektionen rekonstruiert werden kann.

Mehrere Autoren beschreiben die erforderlichen Modifikationen des Rekonstruktionsalgorithmus der gefilterten Rückprojektion (ALLEMAND et al. 1980; TOMITANI 1981; SNYDER et al. 1981; SNYDER 1982; POLITTE u. SNYDER 1982; CHESLER 1982; TANAKA 1982). Erheblichen Raum nimmt die Diskussion des geeigneten Algorithmus der Rückprojektion ein. Zum ersten kann jedes nachgewiesene Ereignis in Projektionsrichtung, also senkrecht zur Koordinate *l*, an der Stelle einsortiert werden, an der es mit der TOF-Information geortet wurde. Das resultierende Zwischenbild wird als „most likely position array (MLP)" bezeichnet, die in Abb. 76 angegebene Gaußfunktion entspricht der TOF-Auflösung. Beim zweiten Verfahren wird jedes Ereignis in Strahlrichtung mit einer Bewichtungsfunktion zurückprojiziert (line writing function $w_l(t)$), die im Sinne des „matched filters" gleich der TOF-Auflösungsfunktion ist. Das so entstehende Zwischenbild wird als „confidence weighted array (CW)" bezeichnet, die resultierende Punktbildfunktion entspricht der Faltung von TOF-Abbildung $g(t)$ und Bewichtungsfunktion $w_l(t)$. Nach der Formierung des Zwischenbildes folgt der eigentliche Rekonstruktionsschritt durch Filterung mit der inversen Übertragungsfunktion der Rückprojektion.

Durch die Art der Rückprojektion kann das Signal-Rauschverhältnis bzw. der „sensitivity gain" beeinflußt werden. Die Überlegenheit der Methode des „confidence weighted array" wurde zuerst von TOMITANI (1981) angegeben und von SNYDER et al. (1981), SNYDER (1982) und POLITTE u. SNYDER (1982) aufgrund ausführlicher mathematischer Analysen und Simulationsrechnungen bestätigt. TANAKA (1982) untersucht den Einfluß unterschiedlicher Formen der Bewichtungsfunktion. So resultiert aus der Approximation der optimalen Gaußfunktion durch die einfachere Dreieckfunktion nur eine Varianzerhöhung von 0,4%. Daneben bezieht TANAKA auch den Einfluß der Absorptionskorrektur mit ein, die Ergebnisse für eine homogene Scheibe sind in Abb. 92 dargestellt. Nach neueren Untersuchungen von CHEN u. METZ (1984) besitzt allerdings die CW-Methode gegenüber dem MLP-Verfahren bei gleicher Rekonstruktionsauflösung keine Vorteile im Signal-Rauschverhältnis, begrenzt aber die maximal rekonstruierbare Auflösung. Die gleichen Autoren schlagen die Verwendung des aus der Bildrefokussierung bekannten Metz-Filters vor.

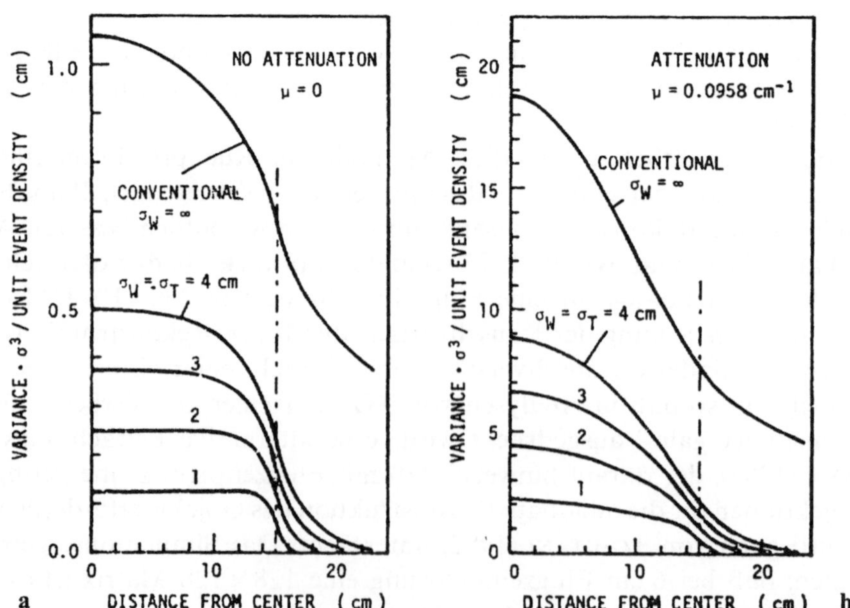

Abb. 92a, b. Virtueller Empfindlichkeitsgewinn eines TOF-Tomographen in Abhängigkeit von der Flugzeitauflösung (FWHM = 2,355 σ_T). Das Objekt ist eine homogene Scheibe von 30 cm Durchmesser, die Rekonstruktion wurde nach der Methode des „confidence weighted array" durchgeführt. Die mit „conventional" bezeichnete Kurve gilt für einen Positronen-Tomographen ohne Flugzeitortung (aus TANAKA 1982). Bemerkenswert ist, daß die Rauschvarianz auch außerhalb der physikalischen Dimensionen der Scheibe verschieden von Null ist. **a** Objekt ohne Absorption, **b** Objekt mit Absorption

TANAKA (1982) modifiziert auch das Rekonstruktionsverfahren der Rückprojektion gefilterter Projektionen für die TOF-Anwendung. Jede Winkelprojektion ist jetzt zweidimensional, abgetastet in der gewohnten linearen l-Koordinate der Projektion sowie in der t-Koordinate in Strahlrichtung (TOF-Information). Die Vorteile dieses Verfahrens liegen zum einen darin, daß die Erzeugung des CW-Zwischenbildes nicht mehr die speicher- und zeitaufwendige Datenakquisition im list-mode erfordert, sondern aus dem MLP-Zwischenbild durch einfache eindimensionale Faltung erzeugt werden kann. Hinzu kommen die auch aus der konventionellen Tomographie bekannten Vorteile des nur eindimensionalen Rekonstruktionsfilters. Dieses Filter ergibt sich für ein TOF-System aus jedem konventionellen Filter $f_0(l)$ zu

$$f(l) = g_E(l) \cdot f_0(l)$$

oder

$$F(k) = G_E(k) * F_0(k) \tag{24}$$

Die Funktion $g_E(t)$ ist das eindimensionale Faltungsintegral zwischen TOF-Abbildung und Bewichtungsfunktion in t-Richtung, und wird dann als $g_E(l)$ in Richtung der linearen Koordinate l angewendet.

$$g_E(t) = w(t) * g(t)$$

In Abb. 93 sind Rekonstruktionsfilter für unterschiedliche TOF-Auflösungen dargestellt.

In letzter Zeit untersuchen SNYDER u. POLITTE (1983) sowie POLITTE u. SNYDER (1984) verbesserte TOF-Rekonstruktionen mit Hilfe eines iterativen Algorithmus aus der Klasse der „Maximum-Likelihood"-Verfahren (EM-Algorithmus) anhand von Simulationsrechnungen und realen Daten des Super PETT I. CHEN u. METZ (1984) diskutieren eine rechentechnisch wesentlich weniger aufwendige Modifikation des vorstehend genannten Verfahrens.

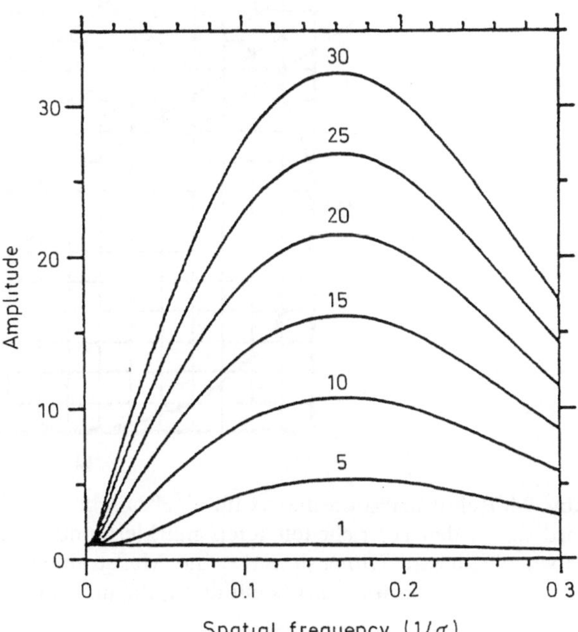

Abb. 93. Rekonstruktionsfilter für unterschiedliche TOF-Auflösungen (aus TOMITANI 1981). Parameter ist das Verhältnis von Flugzeit- zur Bildauflösung

2. Algebraische Rekonstruktionsverfahren

Beim algebraischen Ansatz werden sowohl das rekonstruierte Objekt als auch die gemessenen Projektionen von vornherein als diskrete Funktionen aufgefaßt. Wie in Abb. 94 dargestellt, besteht das Objekt z.B. aus $S = a \times a$ Bildelementen der Fläche Δx^2. Es kann also durch S Zahlenwerte f_i charakterisiert werden, wobei der Wert f_i den Mittelwert der Funktion $f(x, y)$ über die Fläche eines Bildelementes darstellt. Jede der M Winkelprojektionen besteht aus N Projektionsstrahlen der Breite Δl, so daß insgesamt $T = M \times N$ Projektionsstrahlen gemessen werden. Bezeichnet man mit w_{ij} den Anteil, den das Bildelement i zum Projektionsstrahl j liefert (w_{ij} entspricht häufig der in Abb. 94 markierten Teilfläche), so läßt sich Gl. (1) im algebraischen Ansatz ersetzen durch

$$p_j = \sum_{i=1}^{S} w_{ij} f_i \qquad j = 1, 2, \dots T \tag{25}$$

wobei nur die Werte w_{ij} verschieden von Null sind, die zum Projektionsstrahl j gehören. Dieses lineare Gleichungssystem, welches T Gleichungen zur Bestimmung der S Unbekannten beinhaltet, läßt sich auch in Matrixform schreiben

$$\mathbf{P} = \mathbf{W} \cdot \mathbf{F} \tag{26}$$

Die Objektrekonstruktion ist dann gegeben durch die Invertierung der Bewichtungsmatrix $\mathbf{W}$

$$\mathbf{F} = \mathbf{W}^{-1} \cdot \mathbf{P} \tag{27}$$

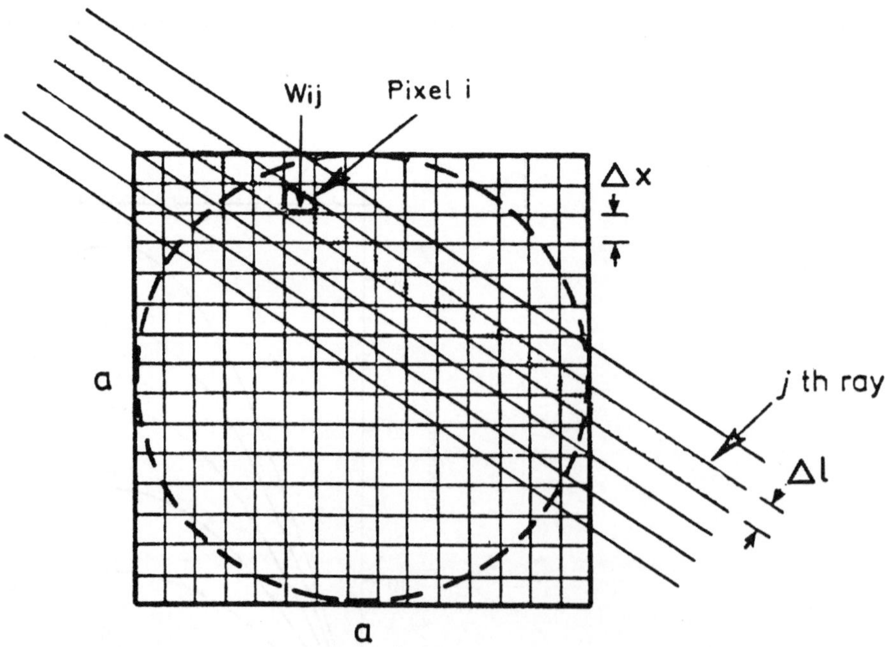

Abb. 94. Rekonstruktionsmatrix für algebraische Verfahren (aus Brooks u. Di Chiro 1976). Das Gesichtsfeld wird durch den gestrichelten Kreis markiert und ist in a Pixel auf den Durchmesser aufgeteilt. Die Pixel haben die lineare Dimension Δx, die Meßstrahlen die Breite Δl. Der Beitrag des i-ten Pixels zum j-ten Strahl, dargestellt durch die umrahmte Fläche, ist der Bewichtungsfaktor w_{ij}

Diese direkte Lösung ist nicht praktikabel. Zum einen ist die Matrix $\mathbf{W}$ schlecht konditioniert, so daß eine Invertierung zu einer hyperrauschempfindlichen Lösung führt. Daneben ist die Größe der Matrix $\mathbf{W}$ $(T \times S)$ enorm, so daß sich rechentechnische Probleme ergeben. Auch existiert keine eindeutige Lösung für ein unterbestimmtes System, d.h. $T < S$.

Eine Lösungsmöglichkeit ist das Verfahren von LLACER (1982). Bei diesem, auch aus dem Gebiet „image restoration" bekannten Ansatz (FRIEDEN 1975), wird die Matrixinverse durch die „Moore-Penrose" Pseudoinverse approximiert. Es ergibt sich eine Eigenwertzerlegung, bei der Auflösung und Rauschverstärkung von der Anzahl der verwendeten Eigenwerte und deren Konditionierung abhängen. Aber auch hier ergeben sich bereits für $S = 169$ schwere numerische Probleme, die die Lösung inpraktikabel machen. Erst der Zusatz der TOF-Information ergibt eine wesentlich verbesserte Konditionierung, was ja auch für die analytischen Verfahren gilt.

Wegen der skizzierten Schwierigkeiten verfolgen alle tatsächlich angewendeten algebraischen Verfahren die Strategie, die Gln. (25) und (26) auf iterativem Wege zu invertieren. Ausgehend von einer Anfangsschätzung f_i^0 wird versucht, diese Schätzung schrittweise zu verbessern. Grundlage ist dabei stets der Vergleich zwischen den gemessenen Strahlsummen p_j und den aus der Schätzung der Objektverteilung f_i^q resultierenden, theoretischen Strahlsummen r_j^q, die nach Gl. (28) berechnet werden. Aus diesem Vergleich, z.B. in Form von Differenzen (additive Korrektur) oder Quotienten (multiplikative Korrektur) oder aber auch in Form von Gütekriterien (z.B. minimale Summe der quadratischen Abweichungen oder Maximum Likelihood), werden Korrekturterme abgeleitet, die zur neuen Schätzung f_i^{q+1} führen.

Da in der Regel nicht alle Werte f_i in einem Schritt so korrigiert werden können, daß das gesamte Gleichungssystem (Gln. 25, 26) gleichzeitig erfüllt ist, muß das ganze Verfahren zyklisch wiederholt werden.

Problematisch ist die Entscheidung, nach wie vielen solchen Iterationsschritten das Verfahren beendet werden soll, denn eine möglichst weitgehende Übereinstimmung zwischen gemessenen und berechneten Strahlsummen gewährleistet noch nicht eine gute Übereinstimmung zwischen Objektschätzung und Objekt, da die Verknüpfungsgleichung einen mittelnden Charakter hat. Häufig wird aufgrund von Simulationsuntersuchungen die Zahl der Iterationen festgelegt, andere Autoren verwenden die Änderung eines Gütekriteriums, welches in seiner Wahl wiederum problematisch ist. Diskutiert werden der Quotient der quadratischen Abweichung von Rekonstruktionsergebnis und wahrem Objekt zur Varianz des Objekts (z.B. GILBERT 1972; OPPENHEIM 1980; HERMAN u. ROWLAND 1973), die Entropie (GORDON et al. 1970), die maximale Abweichung zwischen Objektschätzung und Objekt (HERMAN u. ROWLAND 1973) sowie die Likelihood-Funktion (SHEPP u. VARDI 1982). Eine visuelle Beurteilung schlägt GORDON (1974) vor, der auch betont, daß der Zusammenhang zwischen visueller Güte einer Rekonstruktion und einem der vorstehend erwähnten Gütekriterien mehr oder weniger heuristisch ist.

Auch HERMAN u. ROWLAND (1973) favorisieren die visuelle Beurteilung und stellen anhand ihrer umfangreichen, vergleichenden Simulationsuntersuchungen heraus, daß das Verhalten eines Rekonstruktionsverfahrens entscheidend von der Art der Objektverteilung, z.B. Punktquellen oder ausgedehnte Quellen, abhängig ist. Ferner ist das Ergebnis abhängig von der Meßgeometrie (Winkelbereich), dem Abtastmuster und den Datenfehlern, so daß eine Verfahrensauswahl und -beurteilung anwendungsspezifisch anhand von Simulationsmodellen durchgeführt werden sollte. GORDON u. HERMAN (1974) diskutieren ebenfalls, welche Einflußgrößen experimentell zur Beurteilung eines Algorithmus herangezogen werden sollten.

Folgend der Klassifizierung von BROOKS u. DI CHIRO (1976) lassen sich die iterativen Verfahren entsprechend der Korrektursequenz in drei Gruppen einteilen:

1. Gleichzeitige Korrektur aller Objektpixel. Ausgehend von der aus dem vorhergehenden Iterationsschritt resultierenden Objektschätzung werden alle theoretischen Strahlsummen berechnet und mit den gemessenen Werten zur Bestimmung der Korrekturterme verknüpft. Die Aufdatierung der Objektschätzung erfolgt für alle Pixel gleichzeitig am Ende des Iterationsschrittes. Vertreter dieser Methode sind die „Iterative Least Squares (ILST)"-Verfahren, zuerst in der Emissionstomographie angewendet von GOITEIN (1972), und der EM-Algorithmus, der von SHEPP u. VARDI (1982) auf tomographischem Gebiet eingesetzt wurde. Da bei dieser Korrektursequenz die gesamte, ein Objektelement betreffende Information zur Berechnung des Korrekturterms benutzt wird, zeigen diese Verfahren eine gute Stabilität gegen Fehler in den Meßdaten und ein stetiges, aber relativ langsames Konvergenzverhalten. Für den ILST-Algorithmus weist allerdings bereits GOITEIN (1972) darauf hin, daß diese Konvergenz nur durch Einführung eines Dämpfungsfaktors erreicht werden kann, da die verwendete Korrektursequenz eine Tendenz zur Überkompensation beinhaltet. Auch BRACE-WELL (1956) erkennt bei seinem Lösungsvorschlag nach der Methode „peeling the onion" dieses Konvergenzproblem.

2. Punktweise Korrektur. Für jedes Pixel der Objektmatrix wird der Korrekturterm aus dem Vergleich aller durch diesen Punkt laufenden gemessenen und berechneten Strahlsummen gebildet, d.h. im wesentlichen aus dem Vergleich von gemessener und berechneter Rückprojektion. Innerhalb des laufenden Iterationsschrittes werden die bereits korrigierten Pixel zur Korrektur für die noch nicht bearbeiteten Pixel benutzt, so daß die berechneten Strahlsummen während eines Iterationsschrittes viele Male neu gebildet werden müssen. Dadurch wird die Methode zwar wesentlich rechenaufwendiger, verliert aber die Tendenz zur Überkompensation. Auch hier zeigt sich eine gute Stabilität gegen Datenfehler und eine relativ langsame Konvergenz. Hauptvertreter ist die „Simultaneous Iterative Reconstruction Technique (SIRT)", eingeführt von GILBERT (1972).

3. Projektionsweise Korrektur. Für jeden Projektionsstrahl einer Winkelprojektion wird aus dem Vergleich von gemessener und berechneter Strahlsumme ein Korrekturterm bestimmt, der dann gleichzeitig auf alle Objektpixel längs dieses Strahles angewendet wird. Beim Übergang zum nächsten Projektionswinkel werden dann die bereits korrigierten Objektpunkte bei der Berechnung der Strahlsummen verwendet. Bedeutendste Vertreter dieser Modelle sind die „Algebraic Reconstruction Technique (ART)" von GORDON et al. (1970) sowie deren Modifikationen. Der Rechenaufwand ist wesentlich geringer als beim SIRT-Verfahren, da während eines Iterationsschrittes alle Strahlsummen nur einmal berechnet werden. Jedes Objektpixel wird während eines Iterationsschrittes entsprechend der Anzahl der Winkelprojektionen M-fach korrigiert, so daß bei geschickter Vorgehensweise eine rasche Anfangskonvergenz erreicht werden kann (vgl. OPPENHEIM (1980), welcher über Konvergenz in nur zwei Iterationen berichtet). Da die Pixelinhalte f_i im wesentlichen durch die Daten der zuletzt verwendeten Winkelprojektionen beeinflußt werden, sollten in der Reihenfolge möglichst voneinander unabhängige Winkelprojektionen verarbeitet werden, d.h. Projektionen im Abstand von jeweils 40°–60° (vgl. OPPENHEIM 1980; HOUNSFIELD 1972).

Da die angebrachten Korrekturterme jeweils nur auf einer einzigen gemessenen Strahlsumme beruhen, sind die ART-Verfahren empfindlich gegen Rauschstörungen und Approximationsfehler bei der Berechnung der Strahlsummen (vgl. GILBERT 1972; HERMAN u. ROWLAND 1973; LOTTES 1982).

Im folgenden soll kurz auf die vorstehend genannten, wesentlichen Iterationsverfahren eingegangen werden. Andere Methoden wie die „Orthogonal Tangent Correction" von KUHL et al. (1973a, b) und der „Iterative Section Separation"-Algorithmus von SCHMIDLIN (1972) seien hier nur der Vollständigkeit halber erwähnt. Für alle Verfahren gilt für die berechneten Strahlsummen

$$r_j^q = \sum_{i=1}^{s} w_{ij} f_i^q \tag{28}$$

Der ART-Algorithmus wurde von GORDON et al. (1970) publiziert und lautet in seiner multiplikativen Originalform (partially constrained ART)

$$f_i^{q+1} = \frac{p_j}{r_j^q} w_{ij} f_i^q \tag{29}$$

Die additive Form ist

$$f_i^{q+1} = \max\left[f_i^q + \frac{p_j - r_j^q}{N_j}, 0 \right]$$

$$\text{für alle } i \text{ im Projektionsstrahl } j. \tag{30}$$

In der Originalfassung werden die Bewichtungsfaktoren so gewählt, daß $w_{ij}=1$ ist, wenn das Pixel i im Projektionsstrahl j liegt, und Null sonst. Dann ist die Größe N_j die Anzahl der Pixel im Projektionsstrahl. Diese rechentechnische Vereinfachung führt beim ART-Verfahren zur Divergenz (vgl. GILBERT 1972). Im allgemeinen Fall wird der Faktor N_j durch den für jedes Pixel im Strahl variablen Faktor N_{ij} ersetzt. Dann gibt der Kehrwert von N_{ij} an, mit welchem Anteil das Pixel i am gesamten Strahl j beteiligt ist.

$$N_{ij} = \frac{\sum w_{ij}}{w_{ij}} \quad \text{für alle } i \text{ im Strahl } j \tag{31}$$

Das ART-Verfahren ist vielfach modifiziert worden, ein erschöpfender Überblick findet sich bei GORDON (1974) und umfaßt z.B. „partially" und „fully constrained" ART, ART2 sowie das rauschmodifizierte ART3. Die Diskussion umfaßt ferner die Problematik der Berechnung der Werte w_{ij} sowie ihrer Approximation. Unter der Voraussetzung der Konsistenz der Projektionsgleichungen, d.h. der Existenz einer Lösung, die allerdings durch Rauschen, ungeeignete Meßgeometrie sowie zu wenig Projektionsstrahlen, eingeschränkten Winkelbereich oder Randfehler verloren gehen kann, beschreibt GORDON auch das Konvergenzverhalten der unterschiedlichen ART-Verfahren.

Das von GILBERT (1972) publizierte SIRT-Verfahren lautet in seiner additiven bzw. multiplikativen Form

$$f_i^{q+1} = \max\left[f_i^q + \frac{\displaystyle\sum_j p_j}{\displaystyle\sum_j L_j} - \frac{\displaystyle\sum_j r_j^q}{\displaystyle\sum_j N_j}, 0 \right] \tag{32}$$

$$f_i^{q+1} = \max\left[\frac{\displaystyle\sum_j p_j}{\displaystyle\sum_j r_j^q} \cdot \frac{\displaystyle\sum_j N_j}{\displaystyle\sum_j L_j} \cdot f_i^q, 0 \right] \tag{33}$$

Die Summationen sind für alle Projektionsstrahlen j durchzuführen, die durch das Pixel i verlaufen. In der angegebenen Form sind wiederum die w_{ij} im Strahlengang durch den Wert 1 approximiert, so daß N_j die Anzahl der Pixel im Strahl und L_j die Strahllänge darstellen. Das SIRT-Verfahren ist wesentlich unempfindlicher gegen diese Approximation als das ART-Verfahren. In der Tat stellen die erwähnten Summen das Ergebnis der Rückprojektion im Pixel i dar, so daß die Korrekturterme im SIRT-Verfahren aus dem Vergleich der aus den Meßdaten bestimmten und der aus den mathematischen Projektionen berechneten Rückprojektion bestimmt werden.

Sowohl beim ILST- als auch beim EM-Verfahren werden die Projektionen p_j als Meßwerte einer Funktion angesehen, die durch die theoretischen Projektionen r_j über die Wahl der „Parameter" f_i ausgeglichen werden sollen. Bei ILST-Verfahren wird dazu, wie üblich, das Gütekriterium der mit der Varianz der Meßwerte bewichteten Summe der quadratischen Abweichungen zwischen p_j und r_j minimiert. GOITEIN (1972) führte dieses Verfahren erstmalig in der Tomographie zu einer praktikablen Lösung und gibt als Iterationsgleichung an

$$f_i^{q+1} = f_i^q + \Delta \cdot \frac{\displaystyle\sum_j \frac{w_{ij}(p_j - r_j^q)}{\sigma_j^2}}{\displaystyle\sum_j \frac{w_{ij}}{\sigma_j^2}} \tag{34}$$

Die Summation wird wiederum für alle Strahlen j durch das Pixel i ausgeführt, die Größe σ_j ist die Streuung des Meßwertes p_j und der Faktor Δ ist der bereits erwähnte Dämpfungsfaktor zur Erzielung der Konvergenz. Auch BUDINGER u. GULLBERG (1974a, b) verwenden die Methode der kleinsten Quadrate, BUDINGER et al. (1979a) geben einen Überblick über unterschiedliche iterative Strategien zur Minimierung des erwähnten Gütekriteriums. Anzumerken ist, daß speziell bei poisson-verrauschten Daten das erwähnte bewichtete Gütekriterium gleichbedeutend mit der Maximum-Likelihood-Schätzung der Objektdaten f_i ist (KNOOP 1982).

Explizit von der Likelihood-Funktion als Gütekriterium geht der EM-Algorithmus (Expectation-Maximization), eingeführt in die Emissions-Tomographie von SHEPP u. VARDI (1982), aus. Gesucht wird die Objektrekonstruktion mit der größten bedingten Wahrscheinlichkeit bei gegebenen Projektionen.

$$f_i^{q+1} = f_i^q \cdot \frac{1}{\displaystyle\sum_j w_{ij}} \cdot \sum_j w_{ij} \frac{p_j}{r_j^q} \tag{35}$$

Im Vergleich mit Gl. (34) fällt auf, daß eine ähnliche Verwandtschaft besteht wie zwischen den additiven und multiplikativen Formen des ART- bzw. SIRT-Verfahrens. Aufgrund der Eigenschaften der Likelihood-Schätzung ist, zumindest theoretisch, die strikte Konvergenz des Algorithmus zu erwarten. Dieser Punkt wird ausführlich von LANGE u. CARSON (1984) diskutiert. Speziell auf die TOF-Anwendung zugeschnitten wird das Verfahren von SNYDER u. POLITTE (1983), POLITTE u. SNYDER (1984) sowie SNYDER (1984) angewendet.

Der große Nachteil aller iterativen Verfahren ist die wesentlich längere Rechenzeit im Vergleich zu den analytischen Methoden. Dagegen bieten die iterativen Verfahren den Hauptvorteil einer größeren Flexibilität. Wesentlich ist dabei die Leichtigkeit, mit der Zusatzbedingungen wie z.B. die Positivität der f_i, eine obere Grenze für die f_i oder die endliche örtliche Ausdehnung des Objekts realisiert werden können. Diese „constraints" machen ein Verfahren nichtlinear und bewirken, wie z.B. FRIEDEN (1975) beschreibt, unter Umständen eine Verbesserung der Rekonstruktion bezüglich örtlicher Auflösung und Rauschempfindlichkeit. Dieser Gewinn ist allerdings von der Objektstruktur und der damit verbundenen Wirkungsmöglichkeit der „constraints" abhängig. So greift z.B. die Bedingung der Positivität bei impulsförmigen Objekten sehr viel besser als bei ausgedehnten Quellen. Auch die Anpassung des Rekonstruktionsalgorithmus an ein detailliertes meßtechnisches Modell, z.B. durch Berücksichtigung der örtlichen Verteilung der Absorptionskoeffizienten oder der örtlichen Variation der räumlichen Auflösung und Empfindlichkeit, läßt sich im Prinzip einfach in Form der Bewichtungsfaktoren w_{ij} durchführen (vgl. z.B. Lange u. Carson 1984). Budinger u. Gullberg (1974a, b) führen auf diese Weise für das ILST-Verfahren eine Absorptionskorrektur durch.

Dagegen ist die von verschiedenen Autoren, z.B. Gordon et al. (1970) und Herman u. Rowland (1973) den iterativen Verfahren zugeschriebene Fähigkeit, auch bei unterbestimmten Gleichungssystemen zur Lösung zu führen, nicht unbestritten. So demonstriert Todd-Pokropek (1980) an einem einfachen Beispiel die Mehrdeutigkeit der Lösung für das ART-Verfahren, auch Lange u. Carson (1984) weisen auf die Abhängigkeit der Lösung von den Startwerten im unterbestimmten Fall hin. Auch die Abschätzung von Goitein (1972) deutet in diesem Punkt auf keine Überlegenheit der algebraischen Verfahren hin, Klug u. Crowther (1972) äußern Skepsis gegenüber Aussagen, daß bestimmte Verfahren bei allgemeinen Objekten mit weniger Daten auskommen könnten als andere.

Verschiedene Autoren vergleichen iterative und analytische Verfahren. Herman u. Rowland (1973) stellen ART, SIRT und die Convolution-Methode gegenüber. Oppenheim (1974) vergleicht ART und Convolution-Algorithmus für inkomplette Projektionen, Shepp u. Logan (1974) vergleichen ihr Verfahren mit ART, Budinger u. Gullberg (1974) untersuchen das Verhalten von SIRT, ILST und Convolution, Gilbert (1972) stellt SIRT und ART gegenüber. Koral u. Rogers (1979) sowie Vogel et al. (1978) verwenden das ART-Verfahren für die longitudinale Tomographie, in der gleichen Anwendung entscheidet sich Lottes (1982) aufgrund eines Vergleiches von ART und SIRT für das letztere. Politte u. Snyder (1984) vergleichen analytische Rekonstruktion und EM-Algorithmus für TOF-Systeme. Wegen der Vielfalt der unterschiedlichen Randbedingungen und ihrer Einflußmöglichkeiten hat die Aussage von Herman u. Rowland (1973) wohl noch nicht an Gültigkeit verloren: „Jeder der beabsichtigt, sich mit dem Gebiet der Rekonstruktion aus Projektionen für eine spezielle Anwendung zu beschäftigen, sollte veröffentlichte Aussagen bezüglich der relativen Vorzüge verschiedener Methoden mit extremer Skepsis betrachten".

V. Randbedingungen bei realen Systemen

Reale physikalische Systeme, hier speziell SPECT- und PET-Kameras, weichen von den idealisierten mathematischen Voraussetzungen dahingehend ab, daß die Meßdaten nur in begrenzter Anzahl und möglicherweise nur über einen eingeschränkten Raumwinkel gemessen werden können, daß die Anzahl registrierter Photonen begrenzt ist, daß Absorption und Streustrahlung sowie, bei PET-Systemen, zufällige Koinzidenzen den linearen Zusammenhang zwischen Strahlsumme und Aktivitätsverteilung stören, und daß der Detektor nicht perfekt bezüglich ortsinvarianter Auflösung und Empfindlichkeit ist. Ferner besteht die Möglichkeit von Abgleich- und Justagefehlern. Insgesamt steht also der „perfekten" Rekonstruktion die Einschränkung durch die Daten entgegen.

1. Einfluß einer begrenzten Anzahl von Meßwerten

a) Abtastbedingungen und Auflösung

Sowohl unter physikalisch-meßtechnischen als auch unter rechentechnischen Bedingungen muß das Objekt in diskreter Form abgetastet werden. Daraus folgt die Einführung von Abtastintervallen sowohl in der linearen Koordinate (Δl) als auch im Winkel ($\Delta\theta$).

Für ein bandbegrenztes Signal, welches keine Frequenzkomponenten größer als k_{max} beinhaltet, fordert das Abtasttheorem

$$\Delta l \leqq \frac{1}{2\,k_{\text{max}}} \tag{36}$$

Das Abtastintervall ist also so zu wählen, daß die resultierende Nyquistfrequenz $k_{ny} = (2\,\Delta l)^{-1}$ mindestens so groß wie die maximale Signalfrequenz ist. Andernfalls treten Fehler auf, die als „aliasing" bezeichnet werden und die durch keine spätere Manipulation rückgängig gemacht werden können. Crawford u. Kak (1979) sowie Brooks et al. (1979b) analysieren die durch zu grobes Abtasten entstehenden Bildfehler in Form von Streifen tangential zu scharfen Kanten, wie auch in Abb. 95 dargestellt.

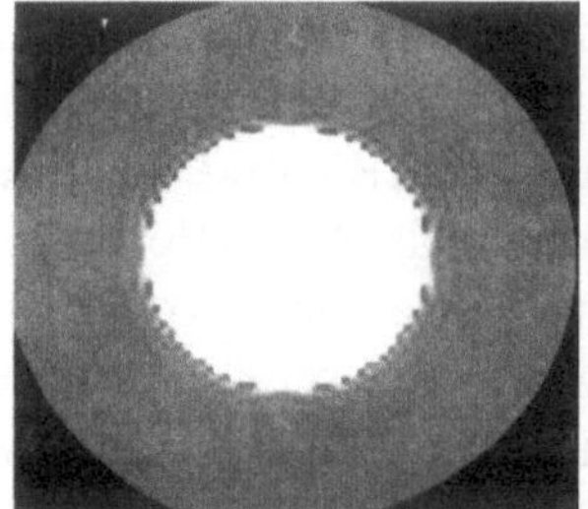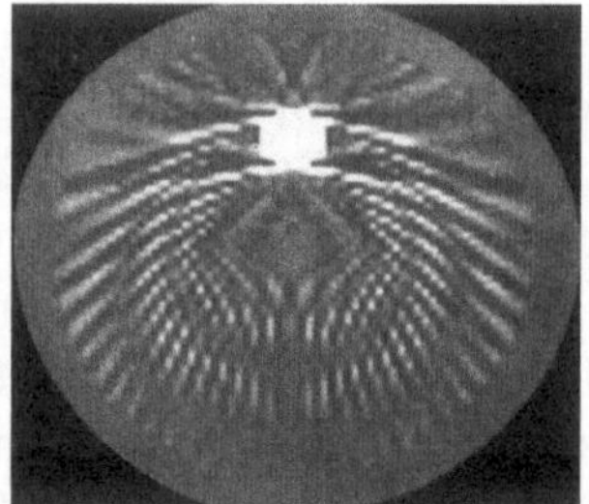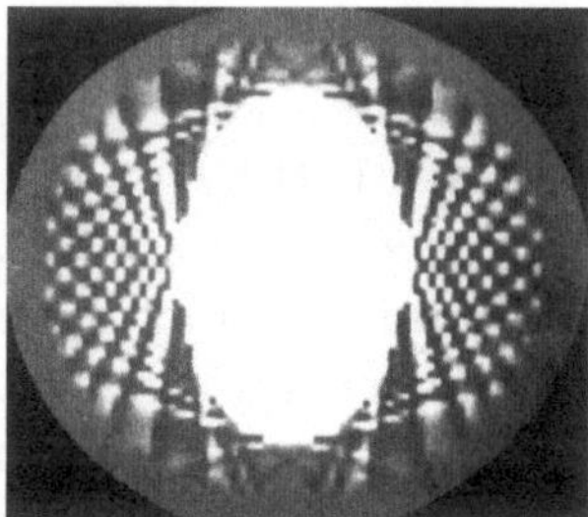

Abb. 95. Simulation von „aliasing"-Artefakten in kontrastverstärkter Darstellung (aus Brooks et al. 1979b). Rekonstruiert wurde eine Matrix von 64 × 64 Pixeln aus 100 Projektionen zu je 64 Abtastwerten bei unbeschränkter Meßauflösung. Die Projektionen enthalten wegen unzureichender lateraler Abtastung Frequenzen oberhalb der Nyquistfrequenz. Typisch für diesen „aliasing"-Fehler sind die tangential zur Objektkante verlaufenden Streifenartefakte, die im mittleren Beispiel noch durch Moiré-Artefakte aufgrund der linearen Interpolation in der Rückprojektion überlagert sind. (Im linken, streng rotationssymmetrischen Beispiel fehlen die tangentialen Streifen, da alle Winkelprojektionen identisch sind und somit auch die entstehenden Artefakte rotationssymmetrisch sein müssen.)

Für ein generalisiertes Objekt ohne Einschränkungen wird die Bandbegrenzung durch die Auflösung des kollimierten Detektors erreicht, so daß das lineare Abtastintervall entsprechend der Linienbildfunktion festgelegt wird.

Unter der Voraussetzung gaußförmiger Linienbildfunktionen schätzt Phelps (1977b) das erforderliche Abtastintervall kleiner als 50% der Halbwertsbreite, Tsui u. Jaszczak (1984) kommen aufgrund einer ausführlichen Untersuchung, die auch die spektralen Effekte der Signalintegration über die Strecke Δl beinhaltet, etwa zum gleichen Ergebnis. Huang et al. (1980) untersuchen den Einfluß der Abtastbedingungen auf die Quantifizierbarkeit des Bildes und fordern $\Delta l \leqq 0,33$ FWHM. Diese Autoren weisen auch darauf hin, daß diese strenge Forderung bei verrauschten Daten etwas abgemildert werden könne. Huesman (1977) sagt aus unter dem Gesichtspunkt der möglichst effizienten Nutzung der Daten bezüglich der Rauschverstärkung, daß die Rasterweite des rekonstruierten Objekts um den Faktor $\sqrt{2}$

grobmaschiger als das Abtastintervall Δl sein sollte. Ausgehend von den Abtastbedingungen diskutiert auch ROWLAND (1979) diese Frage, BROOKS et al. (1978) stellen anhand einer Diskussion der durch die Interpolationsfunktion bewirkten zusätzlichen „aliasing"-Fehler ebenfalls fest, daß zur Abmilderung von Artefakten die Projektionen feinmaschiger als das rekonstruierte Bild gerastert sein sollen.

Aus Abb. 88b ist ersichtlich, daß das Abtastmuster der Projektionen eine kreisförmige Region im Frequenzraum spezifiziert, während die Rekonstruktion in kartesischen Koordinaten eine quadratische durch die Abtastwerte festgelegte Region erfordert. Der erwähnte Faktor $\sqrt{2}$ bezieht sich dann auf das dem Kreis einbeschriebene Quadrat.

Interessant ist in diesem Zusammenhang, daß sowohl das von MERSEREAU (1973) beschriebene „concentric squares raster" als auch das von HERMAN u. ROWLAND (1973) sowie MERSEREAU (1976) vorgeschlagene winkelabhängige Abtastintervall für iterative Verfahren zu den gleichen Ergebnissen führt. Insgesamt ergibt sich also

$$\Delta l \leq 0{,}33 \, \text{FWHM} \ldots 0{,}5 \, \text{FWHM} \tag{37}$$

Die strengere Forderung erlaubt dann, im Zusammenhang mit dem vorstehend genannten grobmaschigeren Raster des rekonstruierten Bildes, auch im Bild die Meßauflösung der Projektionen beizubehalten. Bei zu grobem Abtastmuster hingegen treten sowohl „aliasing"-Fehler als auch eine Einschränkung der Bildauflösung auf.

Für Positronen-Kameras mit diskreten Detektoren, z.B. Ringanordnungen, ergibt sich für einen der Strahlung exponierten Detektordurchmesser d eine Auflösung von $0{,}5d$ bis $0{,}6d$ FWHM, so daß für das lineare Abtastintervall folgt (s. auch BROOKS et al. 1979a; HUANG et al. 1980)

$$\Delta l \leq 0{,}16d \ldots 0{,}3d \tag{38}$$

Gleichzeitig stellt der exponierte Detektordurchmesser d auch den minimal möglichen Detektorabstand dar, so daß die vorstehende Bedingung von keiner rein stationären diskreten Sondenanordnung erfüllbar ist. Zahlreiche Autoren beschäftigen sich daher mit der Möglichkeit, durch geeignete Bewegungen des Ringdetektors das lineare Abtastmuster zu verbessern. So publizieren CHO et al. (1983c) das „dichotomic sampling" für einen zweigeteilten Ringdetektor, dessen Hälften sich relativ zueinander um $0{,}5d$ bewegen. Gebräuchlicher sind die von anderen Autoren vorgeschlagenen Möglichkeiten, den gesamten Ring konzentrisch um den halben Detektorabstand zu drehen oder aber den Ring exzentrisch auf einem Kreis mit kleinem Radius (typischerweise im Bereich $0{,}2d$ bis $0{,}75d$) zu bewegen. Diese letztere, „Wobbeln" genannte Bewegung kann auch noch mit der genannten Halbdrehung verbunden werden.

Während die reine Halbdrehung bei paralleler Datenorganisation das lineare Abtastintervall auf den eigentlich noch zu groben Wert $0{,}5d$ reduziert, erlaubt die Wobbelbewegung bei geschickter Wahl des Wobbelradius und der Wobbelpunkte ein sehr viel feineres lineares Abtastmuster, welches jedoch in der Regel erst durch Interpolation auf exakt äquidistante Werte gebracht werden muß. Eine streng mathematische Optimierungsbetrachtung geeigneter Wobbelparameter gibt HERMAN (1979a), etwas anschaulichere Beschreibungen finden sich z.B. bei HERMAN (1979b), BROOKS et al. (1979a) sowie COLSHER u. MUEHLLEHNER (1981).

Eine weitere Möglichkeit zur Verfeinerung des Abtastmusters schildern TANAKA et al. (1979) und YAMAMOTO u. KAWAGUSHI (1982), welche eine unregelmäßige Detektoranordnung auf dem Kreisumfang verwenden in Verbindung mit einer Rotation des ganzen Ringes im Bereich von 360°. HERMAN u. LUNG (1980) stellen fest, daß divergente Datenorganisation in Verbindung mit einem fan-beam-Algorithmus zu den gleichen Ergebnissen wie die Verfahren für parallele Geometrie, evtl. in Verbindung mit einem „rebinning" Verfahren, führt, wenn für die Abtastbedingungen gilt

$$\Delta l \approx R\Delta\gamma = 0{,}5\,d \tag{39}$$

$$\Delta\beta \approx \Delta\theta \tag{40}$$

Ein Ringdetektor erfordert daher für parallele Organisation die Halbdrehung zur Erzielung eines linearen Abtastinkrements von $0{,}5\,d$, während bei divergenter Organisation des gleichen Datensatzes die Halbdrehung für die Halbierung des Winkelinkrements auf den in der Parallelorganisation erreichten Wert erforderlich ist.

Im Vorgriff auf die im folgenden behandelte Diskussion der Winkelabtastung hat die Einhaltung der linearen Abtastbedingungen dann die Priorität, wenn durch Symmetrie-Eigenschaften des Objekts die erforderliche Winkelabtastung abgeschwächt werden kann. Auf dieser Tatsache beruht vermutlich die von KOURIS et al. (1981) und KOURIS et al. (1982 a, b) betonte Aussage, daß bei Verwendung eines fan-beam-Algorithmus die Halbdrehung zu keiner Verbesserung des Rekonstruktionsergebnisses führe. Die gleichen Autoren (KOURIS et al. 1982 c) stellen fest, daß für den stationären Ring der fan-beam-convolution-Algorithmus wesentlich bessere Ergebnisse produziert als das iterative ART-Verfahren. Abhilfe schafft eine virtuelle Verbesserung des Abtastrasters durch zusätzliche interpolierte Projektionsstrahlen.

Positronenkameras mit linearen Detektorbänken wie die PETT-Typen oder die PC-II erreichen das erforderliche lineare Abtastraster durch einfache translatorische Bewegungen (vgl. CAROLL 1978; HOFFMAN et al. 1983 a).

Über die Größe des maximal zulässigen Winkelintervalls $\Delta\theta$ zwischen benachbarten Projektionen finden sich in der Literatur scheinbar widersprüchliche Angaben. Betrachtet werden soll der Standardfall der transversalen Tomographie über den vollen Winkelbereich von 180° in der parallelen Geometrie. Bei SPECT-Systemen sind wegen der ortsvarianten Abbildungseigenschaften und des Einflusses der Absorption opponierende Projektionen verschieden, so daß sich unter sonst gleichen Bedingungen die Anzahl der Projektionen wegen der erforderlichen Verdoppelung des Winkelbereiches auf 360° ebenfalls verdoppelt. Auch bei divergenter Datenorganisation ist eine Abtastung über 360° erforderlich.

Soll das Objekt mit der gleichen Auflösung, die der Betrachtung über die Größe des zulässigen linearen Abtastintervalles zugrunde liegt, rekonstruiert werden, so darf entsprechend dem Abtasttheorem im Frequenzbereich der Stützstellenabstand bei der Nyquistfrequenz k_{ny} in tangentialer Richtung nicht größer sein als in der radialen Koordinate (vgl. auch Abb. 88 b). Daraus folgt unmittelbar für die erforderliche Projektionsanzahl im Bereich von 180°

$$M = \frac{\pi}{2} \cdot \frac{D}{\Delta l} = \pi D k_{ny} \tag{41}$$

bzw. für das Winkelintervall, ausgedrückt im Bogenmaß

$$\Delta\theta = \frac{\pi}{M} = \frac{2\Delta l}{D} \tag{42}$$

Diese Ableitung findet sich bereits bei BRACEWELL u. RIDDLE (1967), KLUG u. CROWTHER (1972) kommen aufgrund ihrer Eigenwertanalyse zum gleichen Ergebnis, GOITEIN (1972) gelangt für das algebraische ILST-Verfahren zu einer vergleichbaren Abschätzung. MERSEREAU (1976) zeigt, daß bei einer geringeren Anzahl von Projektionen als nach Gl. (41) gefordert die Rekonstruktion anisotrop wird, HUESMAN (1977) gelangt vom Ansatz der möglichst effizienten Nutzung der Daten bezüglich des Signal-Rauschverhältnisses zu diesem Ergebnis. ROWLAND (1979) weist nach, daß aufgrund der Winkelabtastung in der Rekonstruktion oszillatorische Artefakte auf konzentrischen Kreisen auftreten, deren Amplitude – unbeschadet der Beeinflussung durch die Wahl des Rekonstruktionsfilters und der Interpolationsmethode – umgekehrt proportional zur Anzahl der Winkelprojektionen ist. Dies wird auch verdeutlicht in Abb. 96a, b.

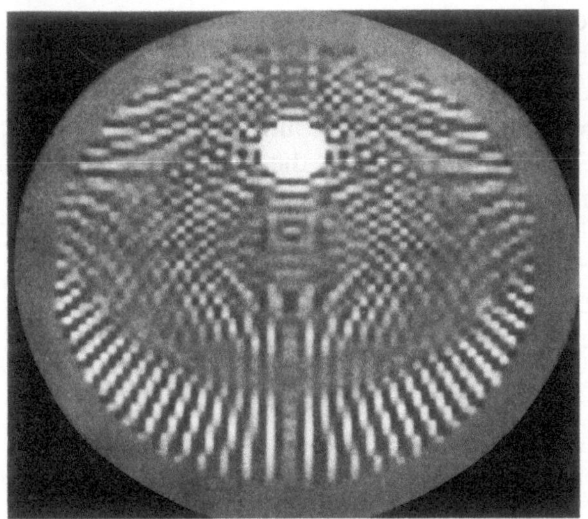 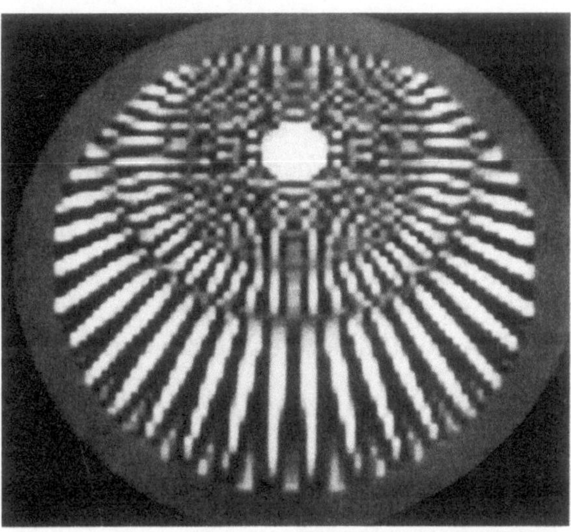

a   b

Abb. 96a, b. Artefakte durch ein zu grobes Winkelinkrement (aus BROOKS et al. 1978). Rechnersimulierte Rekonstruktion einer exzentrisch angeordneten Kreisscheibe in einer Matrix von 64 × 64 Pixeln bei 64 lateralen Abtastwerten pro Projektion und einer unzureichenden Anzahl von Winkelprojektionen. Typisch für diese Art von Abtastfehler ist das radiale Streifenmuster (oszillatorische Artefakte auf konzentrischen Kreisen). Amplitude und Frequenz der Oszillationen stehen in Relation zur Anzahl der Projektionen. **a** 50 Winkelprojektionen pro 180°, **b** 25 Winkelprojektionen pro 180°

BROOKS et al. (1978) kommen durch eine Fehleranalyse für rotationssymmetrische Bilder zu der im Vergleich zu Gl. (41) halbierten Forderung

$$M \gtrsim 1{,}1 \cdot \frac{\pi}{4} \cdot \frac{D}{\Delta l} \tag{43}$$

Ein vergleichbares Ergebnis erhalten auch BRACEWELL u. RIDDLE (1967) bei der Tolerierung gewisser Fehlergrenzen. Für eine Projektionsanzahl geringer als in Gl. (41) spezifiziert schlagen BROOKS et al. (1978) zur Verringerung der Artefakte durch ein zu grobes Winkelinkrement eine Modifikation der Rückprojektion vor, die einer Interpolation nach der Methode des „nächsten Nachbarn" in der Winkelvariablen gleichkommt. WEISS et al. (1982) verfeinern das Verfahren durch Berechnung von Phantom-Projektionen mit Hilfe linearer Interpolation im Winkel. RANGAYAN u. GORDON (1982) versuchen in Verbindung mit dem ART-Verfahren die typischen Streifenartefakte durch nachträgliche adaptive Filterung zu eliminieren.

Allerdings gilt auch hier wie für die lineare Abtastung, daß die durch ein zu grobes Abtastintervall begrenzte Auflösung nicht mehr verbessert sowie die entstehenden „aliasing"-Fehler durch keine nachträgliche Manipulation entfernt, sondern lediglich durch geeignete Tiefpaßfilterung, zu der auch die Interpolation gehört, auf Kosten der Auflösung optisch abgemildert werden können. Weist dagegen das Objekt gewisse Symmetrieeigenschaften auf, so kann die erforderliche Projektionsanzahl durch dieses a priori Wissen deutlich reduziert werden. Auf diese Tatsache weisen schon BRACEWELL u. RIDDLE (1967) hin.

In der SPECT-Anwendung resultiert aus den Eigenschaften des Detektorsystems und der Gammastrahlung eine tiefenabhängige Variation von Auflösung und Absorption, welche den mathematischen Voraussetzungen der Bildrekonstruktion zuwiderläuft. Ein gewisser Ausgleich ist möglich durch die Zusammenfassung opponierender Projektionen, erfordert aber eine Abtastung über volle 360°. Eine detaillierte Diskussion zu dieser Problematik gibt LARSSON (1980). Diese verbesserte Konstanz der Abbildungseigenschaften wird unter Umständen erkauft mit einer durch den Mittelungsprozeß leicht verschlechterten Auflösung. Dieser Effekt wird deutlich in Abb. 97a, b, die einen Transversalschnitt durch ein zylindrisches Phantom mit inaktiven Stäben (Durchmesser von 50 mm bis 16 mm) bei 180° und 360° Abtastung zeigt. In der 180° Studie sieht man einen leicht verbesserten Kontrast für den dünnsten nachgewiesenen Stab, verbunden mit einem deutlich unruhigeren Bild und einem Verlust an Gleichförmigkeit der örtlichen Auflösung. Abhilfe verspricht in dieser Hinsicht die von ISENBERG u. SIMON (1978) vorgeschlagene Technik, opponierende Projektionen nicht zu mitteln, sondern bei der Rückprojektion die Pixel umgekehrt proportional zu ihrem Abstand vom Kollimator zu bewichten und somit der Verschlechterung der Kameraauflösung in z-Richtung Rechnung zu tragen. In neuerer Zeit ist dieses Verfahren aufgegriffen worden und als Algorithmus auch kommerziell erhältlich.

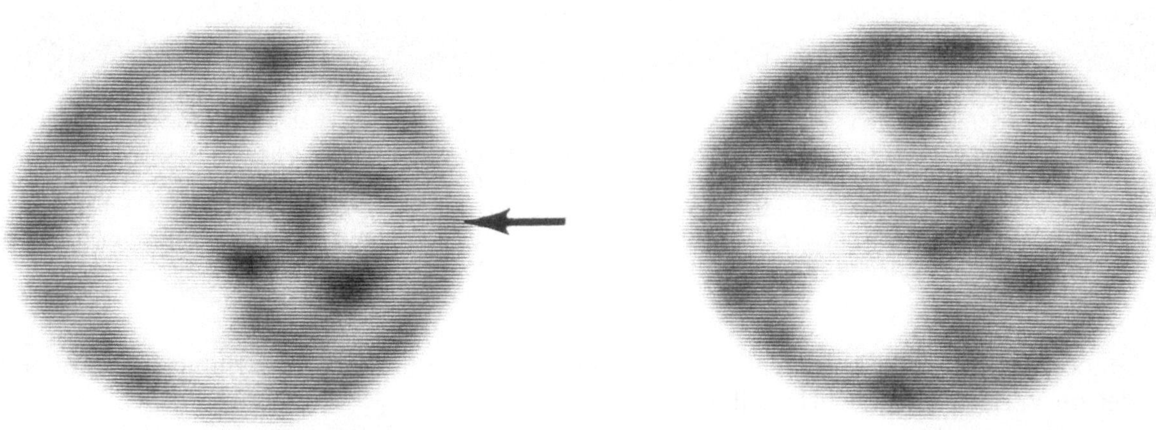

a   b

Abb. 97a, b. Vergleich 180–360° Winkelbereich bei SPECT (aus OTT et al. 1983b). **a** Winkelbereich 180°, zentriert auf die Pfeilmarkierung, **b** Winkelbereich 360°. Der bei genauer Zentrierung des 180°-Bogens auf die abzubildende Struktur (hier kleinster nachgewiesener Stab) zu erreichenden Auflösungsverbesserung steht ein Verlust der Abbildungstreue nach Form und Größe sowie ein statistisch deutlich unruhigeres Bild gegenüber

Speziell für die Myokarddarstellung mit ^{201}Tl wird die Frage der 180° bzw. 360° Abtastung kontrovers diskutiert, z.B. COLEMAN et al. (1982a), TAMAKI et al. (1982), LEWIS et al. (1982) und OTT et al. (1983b). Eine zutreffende Zusammenfassung des Diskussionsstandes gibt HOFFMAN (1982), der zwischen qualitativer (180°) und quantitativer (360°) Anwendung unterscheidet. Den Nutzen der 180°-SPECT bei der Myokarddarstellung charakterisiert er wie bereits auf S. 196 zitiert.

Bei Einhaltung des Abtasttheorems resultiert bei analytischen Verfahren eine Bildauflösung, die objektunabhängig von der Meßgeometrie und den Rekonstruktionsbedingungen bestimmt wird. Werden nichtlineare iterative Verfahren verwendet, kann die Auflösung objektabhängig werden, so daß die anhand von Punktquellen bestimmte Rekonstruktionsauflösung nicht die bei ausgedehnten Objekten erreichbare Auflösung repräsentiert.

b) Begrenztes Gesichtsfeld und eingeschränkter Raumwinkel, longitudinale Tomographie

In den mathematischen Voraussetzungen der tomographischen Rekonstruktion wird gefordert, daß das Objekt von endlicher örtlicher Ausdehnung ist und daß seine Projektionen unter allen Winkelrichtungen vollständig erfaßt werden. Ist nun in allen oder einem Teil der Winkelprojektionen das Objekt, d.h. die vorhandene Aktivitätsverteilung, größer als das Gesichtsfeld, treten auch innerhalb des rekonstruierten wahren Gesichtsfeldes Artefakte auf. So demonstrieren BRACEWELL u. WERNECKE (1975), daß ein vollständig außerhalb des Gesichtsfeldes liegender aktivitätsgefüllter Ring bei der Rekonstruktion Randfehler innerhalb des Gesichtsfeldes verursacht. Wie von OPPENHEIM (1975) beschrieben, zeigt Abb. 98a die bei der Abbildung einer homogenen Scheibe durch ein zu kleines Gesichtsfeld verursachten, beschnittenen Projektionen, während Abb. 98b das Objekt zeigt, welches mit diesen beschnittenen Projektionen unter der Voraussetzung hinreichender Datenlänge konsistent ist. Seine experimentellen Untersuchungen sowohl für den Convolution-Algorithmus als auch für das ART-Verfahren zeigen, daß ohne Korrekturansatz bezüglich der Randartefakte auch in tatsächlichen Rekonstruktionsergebnissen die in Abb. 98b sichtbare typische Überhöhung am Rand des Gesichtsfeldes auftritt. Den gleichen Effekt sagen GORE u. LEEMAN (1980) aufgrund theoretischer Untersuchungen voraus, LOTTES (1982) demonstriert für die longitudinale Tomographie bei Verwendung des SIRT-Algorithmus ein ähnliches Verhalten.

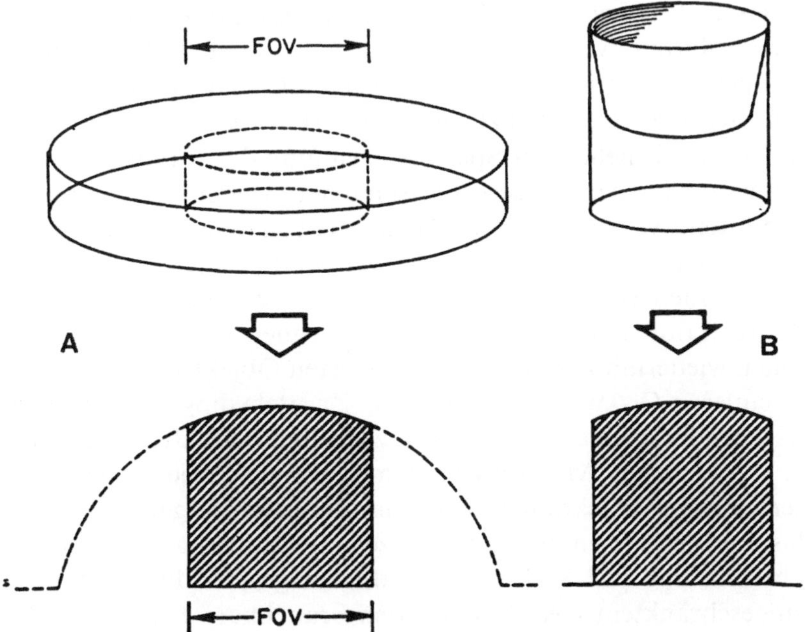

Abb. 98A, B. Begrenztes Gesichtsfeld und Randfehler (aus OPPENHEIM 1975). **A** Objekt (homogene Kreisscheibe) und die durch das zu kleine Gesichtsfeld beschnittenen Projektionen. **B** Objekt, welches bei unbegrenztem Gesichtsfeld die gleichen Projektionen wie unter **A** ergibt

In der transversalen Tomographie werden Randfehler nur durch externe Quellen innerhalb der betrachteten Schicht verursacht, so z.B. durch Raumkontamination oder, speziell bei der rotierenden Gammakamera, durch Reduktion des Gesichtsfeldes für die äußersten Schichten. Weitere Fehlermöglichkeiten entstehen bei Einsatz eines konvergierenden Kollimators zur Verbesserung der räumlichen Auflösung (CHANG 1979) sowie bei Verwendung von Zoom-Einstellungen. Für die longitudinale Tomographie dagegen verschärft sich das Problem durch Einbezug aller drei Raumkoordinaten in die Einflußsphäre sowie durch die Tatsache, daß entsprechend der Detektorkonfiguration häufig die Größe des Gesichtsfeldes mit dem Detektorabstand variiert bzw. daß bei Anordnungen wie dem „Seven-Pinhole"- und dem rotierenden „Slant-Hole"-Kollimator das Rekonstruktionsvolumen von vornherein klein gegen die Abmessungen des menschlichen Körpers ist.

Die Korrektur der Randartefakte innerhalb des Gesichtsfeldes erfordert entweder im Rekonstruktionsprozeß eine Berücksichtigung der Tatsache, daß bestimmte Projektionswerte nicht gemessen wurden, oder aber eine Schätzung der fehlenden Strahlsummen. Während der erstere Ansatz nur für algebraische Verfahren durchführbar ist, ist die zweite Methode gleichermaßen für algebraische und analytische Verfahren anwendbar. So gelingt Lottes (1982) eine Randfehlerkorrektur dadurch, daß im Iterationsprozeß Objektpunkte im Randbereich, durch die eine verminderte Anzahl von Projektionsstrahlen verläuft, bei der Reprojektion entsprechend bewichtet werden. Der gleiche Autor stellt fest, daß dagegen die durch eine im Verhältnis zur Objektausdehnung zu geringe Anzahl longitudinaler Schichten verursachten Randfehler nicht korrigierbar sind. In der transversalen Tomographie untersucht Oppenheim (1975) die Korrekturmöglichkeiten der Datenextrapolation und, für den ART-Algorithmus, die Ignorierung fehlender Strahlsummen im Rechenprozeß. Gleichzeitig weist Oppenheim die deutliche Verbesserung des Korrekturverfahrens durch Einbringen des a priori Wissens der tatsächlichen Objektkontur nach. Dieser „constraint" der bekannten endlichen Objektausdehnung bedingt, wie z.B. Frieden (1975) darstellt, daß das Objektspektrum eine analytische Funktion ist und als solche aus der Wertekenntnis in einem begrenzten Frequenzbereich für die gesamte Frequenzebene berechnet werden kann, z.B. durch Entwicklung in eine Taylor-Reihe. Aufgrund von Rauschstörungen ist diese Extrapolationsmethode, wie aus dem Gebiet „image restoration" hinlänglich bekannt, nicht direkt anwendbar. Sie bildet jedoch die Basis für iterative Strategien zur Randfehlerkorrektur.

So schlägt Chang (1979) neben der Spezialanwendung der Randkorrektur für einen konvergierenden Kollimator aus den Meßergebnissen einer zweiten Aufnahme mit Parallellochkollimator folgende iterative Sequenz vor: Nach einer ersten randfehlerbehafteten Rekonstruktion, z.B. durch ein analytisches Verfahren, werden die fehlerhaft außerhalb der bekannten Objektkontur liegenden Werte bewichtet, aus der so veränderten ersten Objektschätzung werden durch Reprojektion Fehlerprojektionen berechnet, die nach Verknüpfung mit den Originalprojektionen wiederum zur zweiten verbesserten Objektschätzung führen, usw. Noch deutlicher implementieren Ogawa et al. (1984) die Zusatzbedingung der endlichen örtlichen Ausdehnung. Ausgehend von einer Anfangsschätzung innerhalb der bekannten Objektkontur werden über den tatsächlichen Meßbereich hinausgehende Projektionen zur Extrapolation der tatsächlich gemessenen Projektionen berechnet. Nach der folgenden analytischen Rekonstruktion wird das a priori Wissen durch Nullsetzen aller außerhalb der Objektkontur liegenden Werte eingebracht, und das Verfahren iterativ fortgesetzt. Die Autoren demonstrieren auch bei stark eingeschränktem Gesichtsfeld noch brauchbare Ergebnisse. Dennoch führen alle diese Korrekturverfahren nicht zu der Bildqualität, die mit vollständigen Projektionen erreichbar ist, und dürften wegen ihrer Extrapolationseigenschaften zu einer erhöhten Rauschverstärkung führen.

Diese Aussage gilt in noch stärkerem Maße, wenn die einzelnen Projektionen zwar vollständig sind, dafür aber der abgetastete Winkelbereich eingeschränkt ist, also kleiner als 180° bzw. 360° bei der transversalen oder kleiner als 4π Raumwinkel bei der longitudinalen Tomographie. Während in der transversalen Tomographie der eingeschränkte Winkelbereich eigentlich nicht die Norm ist, außer z.B. bei schnellen dynamischen Vorgängen, ist in der longitudinalen Methodik der Raumwinkel durch die Detektoranordnung eigentlich prinzipiell beschränkt, typischerweise auf eine Öffnung von etwa 60°. Aus dem „Projection-Slice"-Theorem folgt, daß bei einem eingeschränkten Winkelbereich der Messung das Frequenzspektrum des Objekts in einem entsprechenden Sektor unbekannt ist. Diese fehlende Information bedingt eine Modifikation des Rekonstruktionsfilters und bewirkt eine Verschlechterung der räumlichen Auflösung senkrecht zum unbekannten Winkelbereich. Diese Anisotropie der räumlichen Auflösung demonstriert Abb. 99 am Beispiel der transversalen Tomographie. Bei der longitudinalen Tomographie drückt sich dieser Effekt in einer deutlich verschlechterten Tiefenauflösung aus. Ferner wird der Rekonstruktionsalgorithmus merklich empfindlicher gegen Rauschstörungen. Beide Effekte werden bereits in der von KLUG u. CROWTHER (1972) veröffentlichten Eigenwertanalyse deutlich.

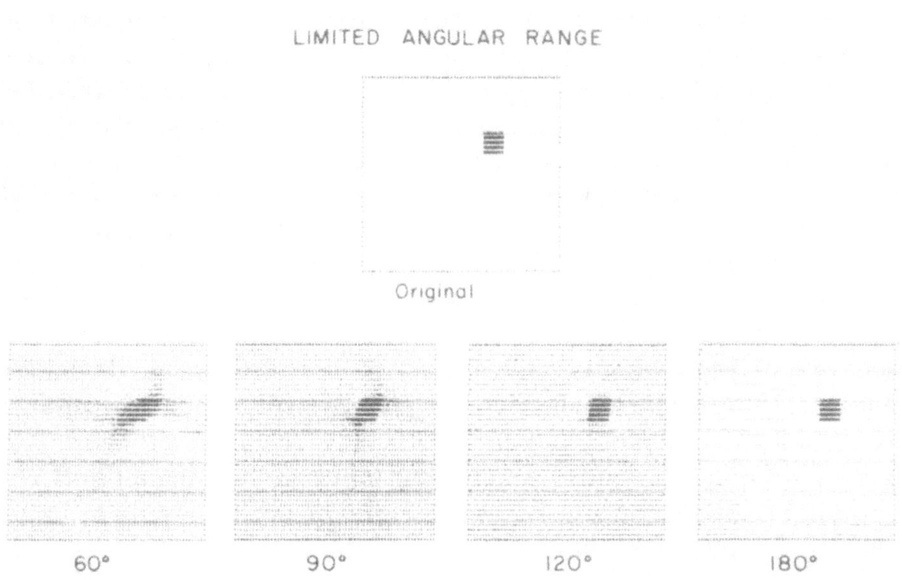

Abb. 99. Bildverzeichnungen durch einen eingeschränkten Winkelbereich (aus BUDINGER 1980). Im dargestellten Beispiel ist die Anisotropie der räumlichen Auflösung durch einen eingeschränkten Raumwinkel für die transversale Tomographie dargestellt. Die Ergebnisse der Rekonstruktion sind abhängig von der Form des Objekts und seiner Orientierung relativ zum Abtastbereich

Methoden zur Rekonstruktion bei eingeschränktem Winkelbereich können eingeteilt werden in Verfahren, welche die fehlenden Projektionen ignorieren und in Algorithmen, die durch Datenextrapolation in den fehlenden Frequenzbereich den Datensatz zu vervollständigen suchen und die sich dabei auf das bereits im anderen Zusammenhang erwähnte a priori Wissen der endlichen örtlichen Ausdehnung stützen. Diese Klassifizierung ist unabhängig davon, ob analytisch oder algebraisch rekonstruiert wird.

Zur ersteren Methode zählen die Lösungsansätze von TOWNSEND et al. (1978) durch Eigenwertzerlegung und Pseudoinverse, TOWNSEND et al. (1980) durch inverses Frequenzfilter mit Fensterfunktion, CHU u. TAM (1977) nach der Methode der „Constrained Deconvolution" sowie die analytische und algebraische Techniken vergleichende Studie von HERMAN u. ROWLAND (1973). Auch der Ansatz von LOTTES (1982) mit der Modifikation des SIRT-Algorithmus für die longitudinale Tomographie sowie der von WOOD et al. (1979) vorgenommene Vergleich eines „Minimum Variance"-Verfahrens mit dem ART-Algorithmus gehören in diese Kategorie, ebenso die Anwendung des SIRT-Verfahrens für den „Seven-Pinhole"-Kollimator (VOGEL et al. 1980). CHANG et al. (1976) versuchen, den Rechenaufwand der longitudinalen Tomographie dadurch zu reduzieren, daß sie nicht eine Entfaltung mit der dreidimensionalen Punktbildfunktion vornehmen, sondern den Abbildungsvorgang gedanklich direkt in die Abbildung eines in Schichten zerlegten Objekts mit den entsprechenden „Schicht zu Schicht"-Übertragungsfunktionen zerlegen. Sie fassen die Bildsummation in der z-Koordinate also als eine Art „Übersprechen" auf und lösen das resultierende Gleichungssystem im Frequenzbereich. Das Verfahren wird auch von PICKENS et al. (1980) für den Pho/Con angewendet.

Zu den Verfahren mit Datenextrapolation gehören die von INOUYE (1979) gewählte Methode der analytischen Fortsetzung im Frequenzbereich sowie die von PERES (1979) beschriebene Momentenmethode samt Extrapolation durch Legendresche Polynome. Beide Autoren stellen fest, daß die Anwendung der Algorithmen stark durch die Rauschempfindlichkeit aufgrund des fehlenden Raumwinkels eingeschränkt wird, PERES weist zusätzlich noch auf die generell resultierende Anisotropie der räumlichen Auflösung hin. In Erweiterung ihrer Deconvolutions-Methode bringen TAM et al. (1979) das a priori Wissen der bekannten örtlichen Ausdehnung in die Rekonstruktion ein. Sie berechnen die analytische Datenfortsetzung in den fehlenden Raumwinkel durch iterative Folge von analytischer Rekonstruktion, Inkorporation des a priori Wissens und Reprojektion der fehlenden Daten, wie schon beim Problem des begrenzten Gesichtsfeldes beschrieben. In einer weiterführenden Veröffentlichung (TAM et al. 1980) folgt der Konvergenzbeweis und quantitative Untersuchungen über die Abhängigkeit der entstehenden Fehler vom Öffnungswinkel und vom Rauschanteil. Auf der Suche nach zusätzlichem a priori Wissen zur weiteren Verbesserung der Lösung finden TAM u. PEREZ-MENDEZ (1981) globale Kriterien wie „Minimum Norm" und „Maximum Entropie" wenig hilfreich. TAM u. PEREZ-MENDEZ (1983) erweitern die Methode auf die Fächergeometrie bei kompletter Durchführung im Ortsbereich, TAM (1983) stellt fest, daß die zusätzliche Inkorporierung der Positivitätsbedingung nur bei „hot spot" Objekten verbessernd wirkt. Einen ebenfalls mit Reprojektion arbeitenden Algorithmus ohne zusätzliches a priori Wissen stellen NASSI et al. (1982) vor, HEFFERNAN u. ROBB (1983) modifizieren diese rein lineare Methode durch Einschluß des a priori Wissens praktisch auf das Verfahren von TAM. Im Vergleich mit der einfachen Rekonstruktion ohne Extrapolation und dem Originalverfahren von NASSI demonstrieren sie die deutliche Verbesserung der Lösung durch die Zusatzbedingung der bekannten endlichen örtlichen Ausdehnung.

Als Versuch, die inhärenten Begrenzungen der „Limited Angle Tomography" zu überwinden, kann der von KORAL et al. (1982) gemachte Vorschlag gewertet werden, die Rekonstruktion durch Addition eines zusätzlichen Satzes orthogonaler Projektionen zu stabilisieren. Diese meßtechnische Lösung ist aber wegen der Größe des resultierenden gemeinsamen Gesichtsfeldes nur für kleine Organe anwendbar.

Die aus dem eingeschränkten Winkelbereich resultierenden Probleme bewirken ganz allgemein, daß longitudinale Systeme in bezug auf die tomographische Abbildungsgüte den transversalen Anordnungen unterlegen sind, vgl. z.B. den Vergleich von rotierendem „Slant-Hole"-Kollimator und der rotierenden Gammakamera von MYERS MJ et al. (1983).

In einer Diskussion longitudinaler Systeme und Algorithmen stellt BUDINGER (1980) fest, daß gegenwärtig die beste Methode zur Lösung des Problems des begrenzten Raumwinkels kein mathematisches Verfahren ist, sondern in der meßtechnischen Komplettierung des Abtastbereiches liegt, wie es auch in der transversalen Tomographie praktiziert wird. Systeme wie der „Seven-Pinhole"-Kollimator oder die kodierten Aperturen führen eher noch zur Problemverstärkung. Beim „Seven-Pinhole"-Kollimator bewirkt das ausgeprägte „undersampling" im Winkel in Verbindung mit den für die Tomographie ungünstigen Abbildungseigenschaften der Lochblende zu der in Abb. 100 von BUDINGER (1980) veranschaulichten extremen Abhängigkeit des Rekonstruktionsergebnisses von der Orientierung der Kollimatorachse relativ zur Symmetrieachse des Herzens. Auch die von anderen Autoren vorgenommenen meßtechnischen Untersuchungen dieses Systems, z.B. WILLIAMS et al. (1980), CONDON et al. (1983) und BROOKEMAN u. MAISEY (1982) zeigen, daß die Ergebnisse eine Quantifizierung in vivo nicht erlauben. Weitere kritische Anmerkungen finden sich im Review von ROLLO

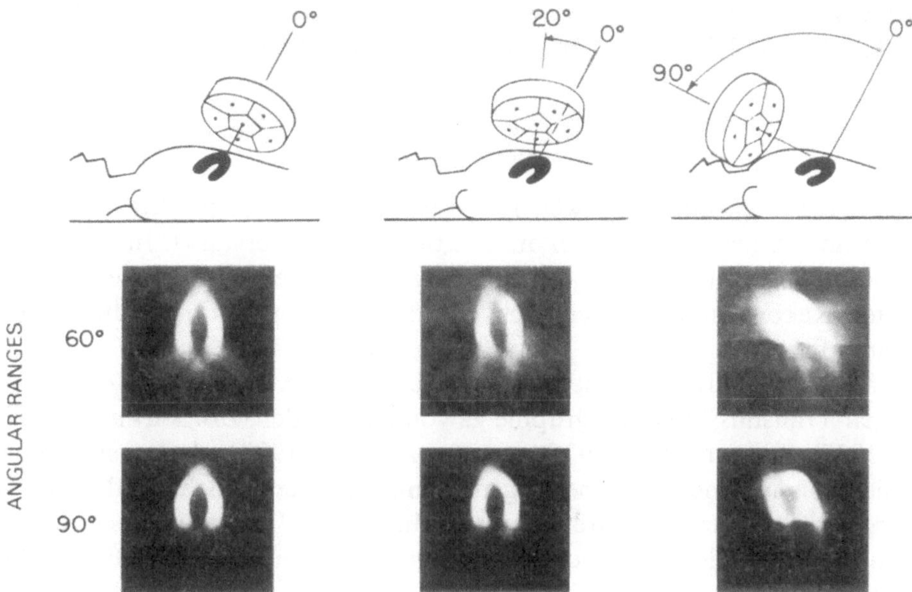

Abb. 100. Auswirkungen des eingeschränkten Winkelbereichs am Beispiel der longitudinalen 7-pinhole Tomographie (aus BUDINGER 1980). Für ein Myokardphantom führt bereits eine Dejustierung der Kollimatorachse relativ zur Herzachse von 20° wegen Verstoßes gegen die vorausgesetzten Symmetriebedingungen zu schweren Verzeichnungen, ein Versatz von 90° ergibt völlig unbrauchbare Bilder. Die Rekonstruktionen wurden unter Idealbedingungen durchgeführt (keine Absorption, kein Rauschen, ILST-Verfahren)

u. PATTON (1980). Auch der von HASEGAWA et al. (1982) vorgeschlagene „12 Pinhole"-Kollimator kann die geometrischen Unzulänglichkeiten des Konzeptes nicht überwinden.

Die Empfindlichkeit longitudinaler Systeme gegen Rauschstörungen führte zu der Idee der kodierten Aperturen. Die Systemempfindlichkeit wird über den Ersatz des Kollimators durch eine Apertur von wesentlich höherer Durchlässigkeit zunächst um Größenordnungen gesteigert. Beispiele sind die Fresnel-Platten von BARRETT et al. (1972), BARRETT u. HORRIGAN (1973), BARRETT et al. (1974), BUDINGER u. MacDONALD (1975), WILSON u. PARKER (1975), HOULE u. JOY (1977), RENAUD et al. (1979); die zeitmodulierten Aperturen von KORAL et al. (1975), KORAL et al. (1979); sowie der rotierende Schlitzkollimator (GINDI et al. 1982). Das Kennzeichen aller kodierten Aperturen ist, daß die Abbildung mehrerer Punkte zu großflächigen Überlagerungen führt, so daß die üblichen Bilder eines Objektes oder seiner Projektionen zunächst durch einen Dekodierprozeß von generell rauschverstärkender Wirkung berechnet werden müssen. Diese Rauschverstärkung ist um so ausgeprägter, je ausgedehnter das Objekt ist, und wirkt dem durch die gesteigerte Systemempfindlichkeit verbesserten Signal-Rauschverhältnis wieder entgegen. So kommen BARRETT u. DE MEESTER (1974) zu der Aussage, daß für ein Objekt mit der Größe von Z Auflösungselementen das Signal-Rauschverhältnis entsprechend $\sqrt{Z}$ absinkt. KORAL et al. (1979) zeigen für ihre zeitmodulierte Apertur eine Abhängigkeit des Signal-Rauschverhältnisses vom Verhältnis der jeweiligen Signalintensität zur mittleren Intensität im gesamten Gesichtsfeld. BUDINGER u. MacDONALD (1975) schließen, daß für die planare Abbildung ausgedehnter Objekte die kodierte Apertur keinen Gewinn im Vergleich zum einfachen pinhole-Kollimator ermöglicht, dafür aber zusätzlich das Gesichtsfeld reduziert. Diese Aussagen verdeutlichen, daß der Einsatz kodierter Aperturen nur bei kleinen Objekten vorteilhaft sein kann. Bezüglich der tomographischen Fähigkeit kodierter Aperturen summiert BUDINGER (1980) als wesentliche Nachteile: die rauschverstärkende und rechenintensive Dekodierung, die komplexe Absorptionskorrektur, die bei pinhole-ähnlichen Systemen auftretenden geometrischen Verzerrungen und eben den begrenzten Raumwinkel. Aus diesen Gründen haben sich die kodierten Aperturen bis heute nicht durchsetzen können.

2. Rauschverstärkung

Die gemessenen Projektionswerte weichen vom vorausgesetzten Ideal ab, diese Abweichungen werden im mathematischen Rekonstruktionsprozeß verstärkt. In diesem Abschnitt soll die Verstärkung der statistischen Rauschstörung besprochen werden, die allerdings neben dem verwendeten Rekonstruktionsfilter auch von den Approximationen durch die diskrete Abtastung beeinflußt wird.

Zahlreiche Autoren analysieren diese Rauschverstärkung. Auch die Ergebnisse, die für die reine Röntgen-Transmissionstomographie gewonnen wurden, z.B. Shepp u. Logan (1974), Chesler et al. (1977), Barrett et al. (1976) und Kouris et al. (1982b), lassen sich ohne Schwierigkeiten auf die Emissionsmessung übertragen, wenn man berücksichtigt, daß im Transmissionsfall die Varianz der einzelnen Strahlsummen durch den Logarithmierschritt umgekehrt proportional zum Meßwert ist, während sie im Emissionsfall durch den Meßwert abgeschätzt werden kann. Da ferner Barrett et al. (1976) die Äquivalenz aller analytischen Verfahren bezüglich der Rauschverstärkung nachweisen und Huesman (1977) zeigt, daß analytische und iterative (Least squares) Verfahren zu vergleichbaren Rauschverstärkungen führen, ist die im folgenden dargestellte Abschätzung für das Verfahren der Rückprojektion gefilterter Projektionen hinreichend.

Bezeichnet man mit σ_p^2 die Varianz einer Strahlsumme in Parallelgeometrie, so ergibt sich, wie für jedes digitale Filter (Metz u. Beck 1974), als Varianz der gefilterten Projektion

$$\sigma_g^2(l, \theta) = \sigma_p^2(l, \theta) * |g(l)|^2 \tag{44}$$

Die Bildvarianz ergibt sich daraus durch Rückprojektion (vgl. Gl. (6)).

$$\sigma_I^2(x, y) = \int_0^\pi \sigma_g^2(x \cos \theta + y \sin \theta, \theta).d\theta \tag{45}$$

Unter der häufig zu findenden Approximation einer näherungsweise im Bereich des Filters konstanten Varianz, die streng genommen nicht einmal für eine homogene Scheibe gilt, vereinfacht sich diese Beziehung zu

$$\sigma_g^2 = \sigma_p^2 \int_{-\infty}^{+\infty} |g(l)|^2 \, dl = \sigma_p^2 \int_{-k_g}^{+k_g} G^2(k) \, dk \tag{46}$$

Unter Berücksichtigung des Rückprojektionsschrittes, mit der Abschätzung der Varianz durch den Meßwert und unter dem in der Emissionstomographie sinnvollen Bezug auf die insgesamt für die ganze Schicht akkumulierten Ereignisse N_{tot}, ergibt sich damit als relative Rauschstreuung des Bildes einer homogenen Scheibe des Durchmessers D die z.B. von Phelps et al. (1982) angegebene Beziehung

$$\frac{\sigma_I}{m} \leq \text{const.} \sqrt{\frac{D^3}{N_{tot}} \int_{-k_g}^{+k_g} G^2(k) \, dk} \tag{47}$$

mit m als mittlerem Bildinhalt/Pixel.

Diese Abhängigkeit der prozentualen Streuung von $D^{3/2}$ bei sonst konstanten Bedingungen findet sich auch bei anderen Autoren, z.B. ALPERT et al. (1982), KOURIS et al. (1982 b) sowie TODD-POKROPEK u. JARRITT (1982). Ferner gilt, daß für das Rampenfilter das Integral in Gl. (47) proportional zu k_g^3 und damit, bei Gleichsetzung von Filtergrenzfrequenz und Nyquistfrequenz, proportional zu Δl^{-3} ist.

Damit gilt für tomographische Rekonstruktionen, daß eine Halbierung der Auflösungsdistanz, ausdrückbar durch die Filtergrenzfrequenz, bei konstanter prozentualer Streuung des Bildrauschens eine Verachtfachung von N_{tot} bedingt, im Gegensatz zum Faktor 4 bei der planaren Szintigraphie. Es ergibt sich die von BUDINGER (1977, 1980) angegebene approximative Beziehung für die relative Rauschstreuung in der Rekonstruktion einer homogenen Scheibe (ohne Absorption)

$$\frac{\sigma_I}{m} = \text{const.} \ \frac{(\text{Anzahl der Auflösungselemente})^{3/4}}{(\text{Anzahl der insgesamt registrierten Ereignisse})^{1/2}} \qquad (48)$$

Für das von BUDINGER untersuchte iterative „Least squares"-Verfahren hat die Konstante den Wert 1,2, wenn das rekonstruierte Pixel um den Faktor 1,5 grober ist als das Abtastintervall. In der gleichen Größenordnung liegen die Werte für das lineare Verfahren mit Rampenfilter (s. auch TODD-POKROPEK u. JARRITT 1982). Zu beachten ist, daß diese Formel nur bei Einhaltung der Abtastbedingungen gilt (BUDINGER et al. 1979 a). Anderenfalls erhöht sich das Rauschen, wie auch die Untersuchungen von HUESMAN (1977) zeigen. Eine graphische Darstellung der Gl. (48) zeigt Abb. 101.

Verwendet man andere Fensterfunktionen, so bleibt die Beziehung weiterhin gültig. Lediglich der Wert der Konstanten verändert sich, vgl. z.B. LIM et al. (1982). In gleicher Weise verringert sich durch Reduktion der Filtergrenzfrequenz entweder die Konstante durch Änderung des bestimmten Integrals in Gl. (47) oder aber die Anzahl der Auflösungselemente, die von der Grenzfrequenz abhängt und nicht unbedingt mit der Anzahl der Pixel übereinstimmt.

Diese Methode, die Rauschverstärkung auf Kosten der Bildauflösung zu begrenzen, bildet auch die Grundlage des von PHELPS et al. (1982) veröffentlichten SAT-Prinzips (signal amplification technique). Durch deutliche Verbesserung der Meßauflösung (Verbesserung des Signal-Rauschverhältnisses bei höheren Frequenzen) resultiert auch bei reduzierter Rekonstruktionsauflösung immer noch eine akzeptable Bildauflösung, da letztere proportional zum Produkt der Übertragungsfunktionen für die Messung und für die digitale Rekonstruktion ist.

Eine weitere Methode zur Begrenzung der Rauschverstärkung ist der bereits in Abschnitt G.IV.1.d diskutierte Einsatz der Flugzeitmessung, der durch eine Ortung in Projektionsrichtung die Rekonstruktion aus einem Datensatz höheren Informationsgehaltes erlaubt.

Eine Erweiterung der Gl. (48) für das Problem der Detektion eines Targets in einem homogenen Background geben BUDINGER et al. (1979 a) an in Form einer „effektiven" Anzahl von Auflösungselementen

$$M_{\text{eff}} = M_t + \frac{M_B}{C} \qquad (49)$$

mit

M_t Anzahl der Auflösungselemente des Targets
M_B Anzahl der Auflösungselemente des Backgrounds
C Bildinhalt Target/Bildinhalt Background.

Die für die Gln. (46–49) verwendete Approximation der konstanten Varianz der Strahlsummen ist streng genommen nicht gültig und führt dazu, daß die Rauschvarianz auch für

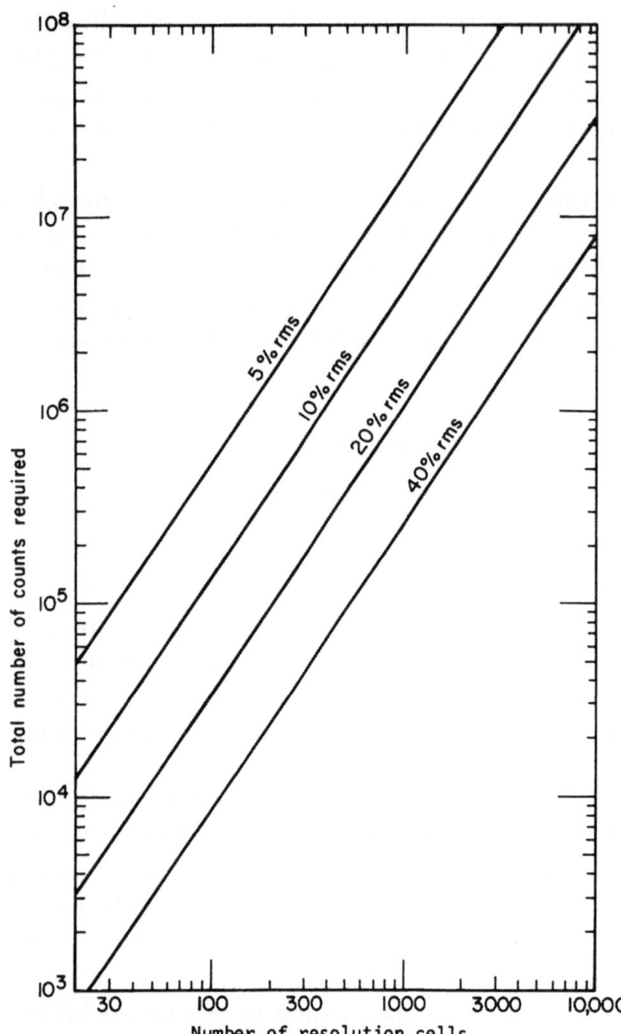

Abb. 101. Rauschverstärkung der tomographischen Rekonstruktion in Abhängigkeit von Auflösung und Anzahl der nachgewiesenen Ereignisse pro Schicht (aus BUDINGER 1980). Die graphische Darstellung von Gl. (48) zeigt die für eine gewünschte relative Rausch-streuung im Bild und für eine gegebene Anzahl von Auflösungselementen (nicht notwendigerweise Anzahl der Pixel) erforderliche Anzahl registrierter Photonen

eine homogene Scheibe örtlich variabel ist mit einem Maximum im Zentrum der Scheibe, und auch über den Rand der Scheibe hinaus reicht, vgl. z.B. ALPERT et al. (1982) sowie Abb. 92. Somit stellt das rekonstruierte Rauschen keinen ergodischen Prozeß dar. BARRETT et al. (1976) zeigen, daß das rekonstruierte Rauschen mit einer Abbildungsfunktion dargestellt wird, die der ungefilterten Rückprojektion entspricht. Ähnliche Ergebnisse finden sich bei ALPERT et al. (1982) und GULLBERG u. BUDINGER (1981).

Durch die erforderliche Absorptionskorrektur tritt eine weitere Rauschverstärkung ein, und zwar um so stärker, je größer der Absorptionskoeffizient und der Durchmesser des Objekts sind sowie je zentraler das betrachtete Pixel im Objekt liegt. So geben z.B. ALPERT et al. (1982) für die Positronentomographie eine Rauschverstärkung um den Faktor 1,5 für eine analytische Absorptionskorrektur an sowie einen weiteren Faktor von 1,5 für die meßtechnische Korrektur. Dieser Faktor ist allerdings abhängig von der statistischen Qualität der Transmissionsmessung. Letzteres Problem wird auch diskutiert von HUANG et al. (1979) und HUANG et al. (1981). In der SPECT-Anwendung wird die mit der Absorptionskorrektur verknüpfte Rauschverstärkung diskutiert u.a. von GULLBERG (1979), GULLBERG u. BUDINGER (1981) sowie LIM et al. (1982).

Weitere, zur Quantifizierung des Rekonstruktionsergebnisses erforderliche Korrekturen wie Streustrahlungskompensation, Subtraktion zufälliger Koinzidenzen und Korrektur von

Empfindlichkeitsvariationen bzw. Inhomogenitäten des Meßgerätes sind ebenfalls von Einfluß auf die statistische Genauigkeit des berechneten Bildes.

3. Absorption

Während in der Transmissionstomographie TCT bei bekannter Position von Quelle und Quellintensität die örtliche Verteilung $\mu(x, y)$ der Absorptionskoeffizienten die Meßgröße darstellt, die durch die logarithmische Transformation der Strahlsummen entsprechend den Rekonstruktionsvoraussetzungen linearisiert wird, stellt eben diese Verteilung der Absorptionskoeffizienten in der Emissionstomographie ECT einen Störfaktor dar, welcher zum einen bekannt sein muß und zum anderen den linearen Zusammenhang zwischen der zu rekonstruierenden örtlichen Verteilung der Quellintensitäten im Objekt und den gemessenen Strahlsummen zerstört. Wird diese Störgröße ignoriert, so ergeben sich Objektverzerrungen, die für das Beispiel einer homogenen Scheibe und verschiedene Gammaenergien in Abb. 102 dargestellt sind. Weitere Störeinflüsse stellen Streustrahlung und, für die Positronentomographie PET, zufällige Koinzidenzen dar, welche die Auswirkungen des Absorptionseinflusses bei Objekten wie in Abb. 102 dargestellt, rein visuell abmildern und im nächsten Abschnitt diskutiert werden sollen.

Durch das Vorhandensein der Absorption erhält die in Gl. (2) angegebene Radontransformation eine komplexere Form („attenuated Radon transform")

$$
p_\gamma(l, \theta) = \iint\limits_{-\infty}^{+\infty} \left\{ f(x, y) \exp\left[- \iint\limits_{xy}^{\text{Detektor}} \mu(x', y') \delta(l - x' \cos\theta - y' \sin\theta) \, dx' dy' \right] \right.
$$
$$
\left. \cdot \delta(l - x \cos\theta - y \sin\theta) \right\} dx \, dy \tag{50}
$$

Im Vergleich mit Gl. (2) wird deutlich, daß jeder Objektpunkt auf dem Projektionsstrahl nur bewichtet mit der Gesamtabsorption zwischen dem Emissionsort und dem Detektor in die entsprechende Strahlsumme eingeht. GULLBERG (1979) veranschaulicht Gl. (50) so, daß jeder Nukleus auf der Integrationslinie eine unterschiedliche Detektionswahrscheinlichkeit besitzt (ausgedrückt durch den Exponentialfaktor), welche abhängig ist von den Absorptionseigenschaften zwischen Nukleus und Detektor und damit nicht unabhängig ist von der Position der Quelle auf dem Integrationswege.

Eine Sonderstellung nimmt dagegen die Positronenemissionstomographie ein. Durch das Prinzip der Kollimation durch elektronische Koinzidenz ist das Meßergebnis nicht von der Position der Quelle innerhalb des Absorbers abhängig (vgl. Abschnitt E.II.), und so lassen sich die Integrale in Gl. (50) separieren

$$
p_{\gamma\gamma}(l, \theta) = \exp\left[- \iint\limits_{-\infty}^{+\infty} \mu(x, y) \cdot \delta(l - x \cos\theta - y \sin\theta) \, dx \, dy \right]
$$
$$
\cdot \iint\limits_{-\infty}^{+\infty} f(x, y) \cdot \delta(l - x \cos\theta - y \sin\theta) \, dx \, dy \tag{51}
$$

Der Exponentialterm stellt gerade die auf einer Transmissionsmessung mit einer externen Quelle beruhenden Projektionen dar, während der zweite Term die in Gl. (2) vorausgesetzten Projektionen ohne Absorber bildet.

$$
p_{\gamma\gamma}(l, \theta) = p_T(l, \theta) \cdot p(l, \theta) \tag{51a}
$$

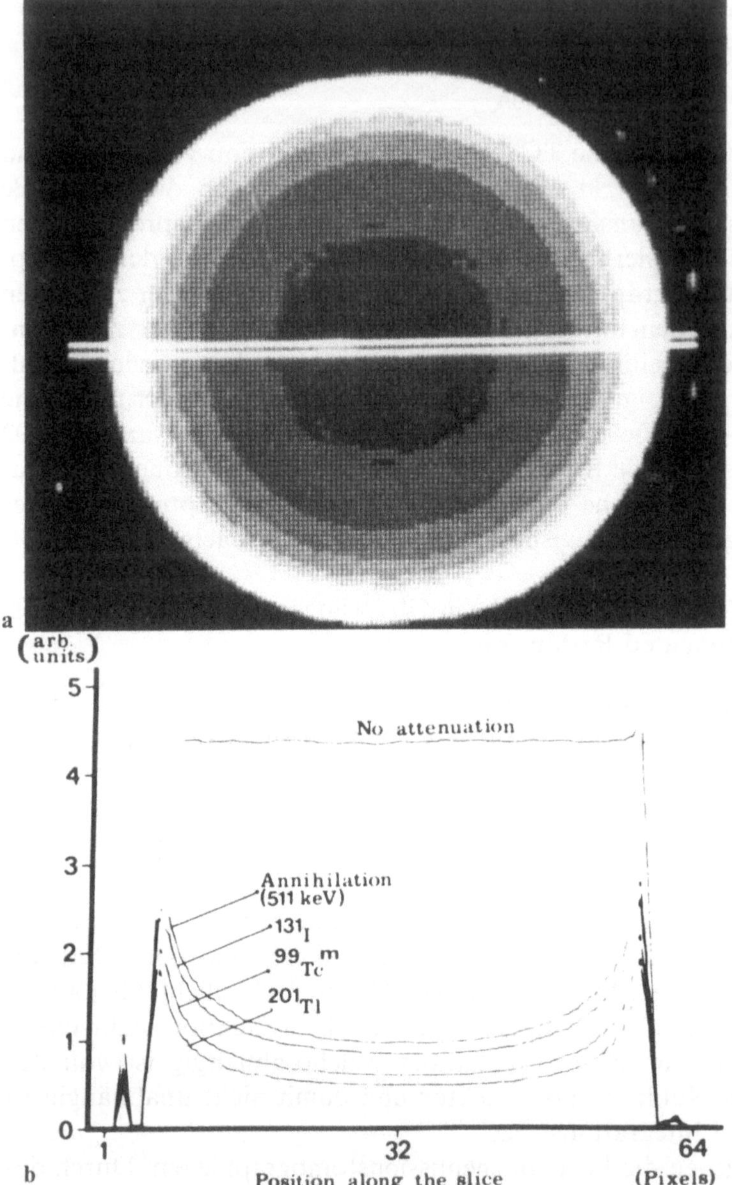

Abb. 102a, b. Einfluß der Absorption auf die Rekonstruktion einer homogenen aktivitätsgefüllten Scheibe (aus LARSSON 1980). **a** zeigt das rekonstruierte Bild für das Nuklid ^{99m}Tc, **b** zeigt Profilschnitte durch das Zentrum der transversalen Schicht für unterschiedliche Radionuklide und ohne Absorption

Somit kann bei der PET-Anwendung der Einfluß der Absorption über eine Transmissionsmessung durch einfache Quotientenbildung der entsprechenden Strahlsummen eliminiert werden. Dieses Verfahren wird detailliert z.B. von HUANG et al. (1979, 1981) untersucht, wobei die Autoren darauf hinweisen, daß die statistische Qualität der korrigierten Projektionen und damit auch das Signal-Rauschverhältnis des Rekonstruktionsergebnisses von der statistischen Qualität der Transmissionsmessung beeinflußt wird, gleichbedeutend mit einer Reduktion der effektiven Impulszahl der Emissionsmessung. Um diesen Effekt unter die Wahrnehmungsschwelle zu drücken, wären bei der Transmissionsmessung um etwa 1 bis 2 Größenordnungen höhere Impulszahlen als bei der Emissionsmessung erforderlich, abhängig u.a. von Gesichtsfeld- und Objektdurchmesser. Auch ALPERT et al. (1982) befassen sich mit dem Problem des Signal-Rauschverhältnisses bei der Absorptionskorrektur. Diese Rauschverstärkung kann dadurch vermieden werden, daß der Absorber durch eine oder mehrere, meist elliptische

Strukturen mit unterschiedlichen Absorptionskoeffizienten modelliert wird, und die daraus analytisch berechneten Projektionen zur Korrektur verwendet werden. Sowohl die Untersuchungen von HUANG et al. (1979) als auch BERGSTRÖM et al. (1980, 1982) zeigen jedoch, daß Abweichungen dieser Modellbildung nach Form, Lage und Werten des Absorptionskoeffizienten von der Realität eine fehlerverstärkende Wirkung haben. Daher schlagen HUANG et al. (1981) vor, das Modell mit Hilfe eines Konturfindungsalgorithmus aus der Rekonstruktion des Transmissionsbildes zu bilden und geben aufgrund umfangreicher Testuntersuchungen eine mögliche Reduktion der Impulszahl der Transmissionsmessung um etwa den Faktor 3 bis 10 gegenüber der direkten meßtechnischen Methode an. Für die Anwendung am Schädel verwenden auch BERGSTRÖM et al. (1980, 1982) einen Konturfindungsalgorithmus, allerdings nur für das wesentlich einfachere Modell einer Außenkontur.

Während bei der PET eine theoretisch exakte Absorptionskorrektur der gemessenen Projektionen möglich ist, ist das Problem bei der SPECT erheblich komplexer. Wegen der in Gl. (50) angegebenen und nicht separierbaren Nichtlinearität und da bei Inversion der Radontransformation die Rekonstruktion des Objekts im Punkt (x, y) nicht nur vom Wert der Linienintegrale durch diesen Punkt, sondern auch von den Werten aller anderen möglichen Linienintegrale abhängt, können die in Abb. 102 dargestellten Bildverzerrungen nicht durch eine einfache nachträgliche Korrektur des Rekonstruktionsergebnisses allgemein gültig rückgängig gemacht werden. Die daher erforderliche Inversion der „attenuated Radon transform" stellt bis heute das wohl schwerwiegendste Einzelproblem in der SPECT-Anwendung dar und ist für eine beliebige örtliche Verteilung variabler Absorptionskoeffizienten noch nicht analytisch gelöst worden. Die einzige praktikable Lösung für eine beliebige Verteilung $\mu(x, y)$ bieten derzeit iterative Verfahren. Ansonsten ist eine Anzahl mehr oder weniger guter approximativer Lösungen, insbesondere für einen homogenen Absorber mit konstantem μ und konvexer Gestalt, entwickelt worden. Ausgezeichnete Übersichten zu diesem Thema finden sich bei BUDINGER et al. (1979a) und MOORE (1982).

Essentiell für alle SPECT-Korrekturverfahren ist die Bestimmung der Außenkontur des Absorbers. Eine gute Übersicht zu diesem Thema geben GULLBERG et al. (1983). Die Autoren diskutieren die Möglichkeiten zur Festlegung einer elliptischen oder allgemein konvexen Außenkontur aus den Projektionen, aus einer zusätzlichen Akquisition in einem Compton-Fenster oder mit zusätzlichen externen Quellen, sowie die Festlegung einer allgemeinen nicht konvexen Kontur aus einer Transmissions-Rekonstruktion. Eine fehlerhafte Festlegung dieser Kontur (z.B. Verschiebung um 2,5 cm) kann Fehler in der Größenordnung von 10% hervorrufen. Diese Aussage ist in etwa konsistent mit der Angabe von WALTERS et al. (1981), daß ein Fehler entweder in der Kontur oder im Wert von μ von 10% auch etwa einen Fehler von 10% im korrigierten Ergebnis bedeutet.

Eine sehr ausführliche Diskussion der Fehlerfortpflanzung bei Fehlern in den Absorberparametern (Verschiebung, Durchmesser, Zahlenwert für homogenes μ, inhomogenes $\mu(x, y)$) findet sich bei HUANG et al. (1979) und ist an ausgewählten Beispielen in Abb. 103–105 dargestellt. Die genannten Autoren kommen zu dem Schluß, daß sich Fehler in den Absorberparametern um den Faktor 2 bis 3 verstärken können, abhängig von Fehlertyp und Objekt.

Die Korrekturverfahren lassen sich gliedern in prerekonstruktive oder postrekonstruktive approximative Veränderungen der Projektionen, die dann als richtig angesehen und entsprechend Gl. (2) weiterverarbeitet werden, in inhärente Verfahren, die für Spezialfälle die Gl. (50) invertieren und in die erwähnten iterativen Methoden.

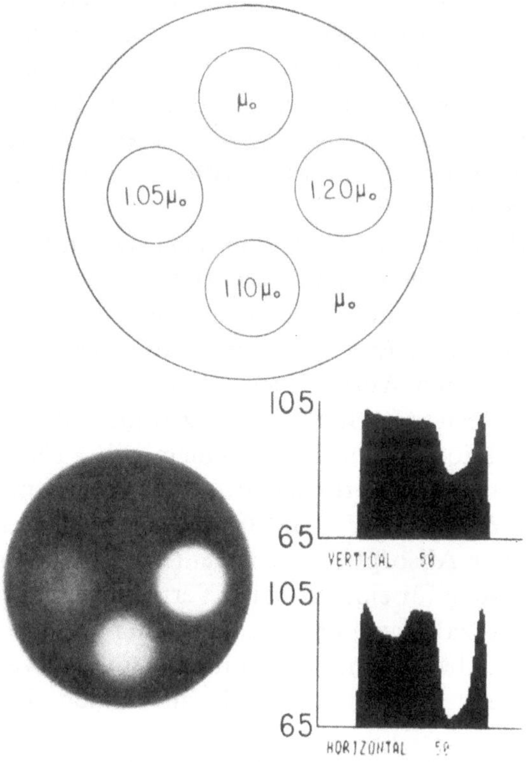

Abb. 103

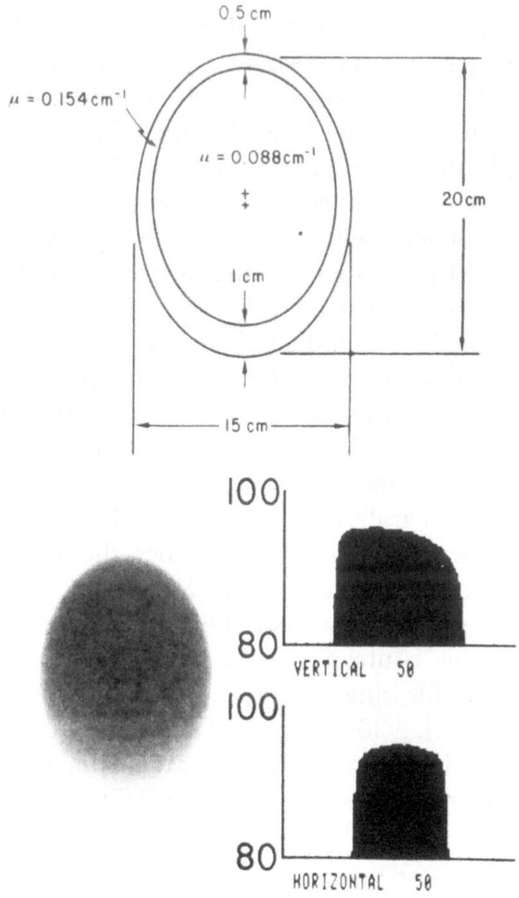

Abb. 104

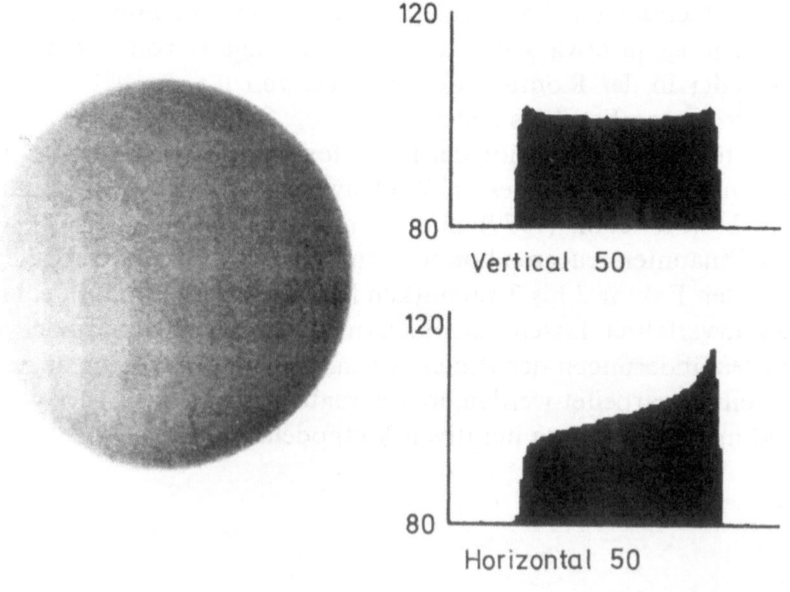

Abb. 105

a) Prerekonstruktive Verfahren

Die einfache Zusammenfassung opponierender Projektionen in Form des arithmetischen bzw. geometrischen Mittels bietet an sich kaum eine Absorptionskorrektur, stellt jedoch in der Regel einen Vorverarbeitungsschritt dar.

Auf der Voraussetzung eines homogenen Absorbers sowie einer ebenfalls homogenen Emissionsquelle von gleicher Ausdehnung basiert die von KAY u. KEYES (1975) angegebene Mittelung des Maximal- und des Minimalwertes des Absorptionsfaktors $(\exp(-\mu t)+\exp(-\mu(L-t)); 0 \leqq t \leqq L$

$$p(l, \theta) \approx \frac{2[p_\gamma(l, \theta)+p_\gamma(-l, \theta+\pi)]}{1+\exp(-\mu L)+2\exp(-0{,}5\,\mu L)} \tag{52}$$

wobei L die Weglänge durch den Absorber ist.

BUDINGER et al. (1979a) schlagen als Korrektur erster Ordnung vor, den Absorptionsfaktor direkt zu mitteln und erhalten

$$p(l, \theta) \approx \frac{\mu L[p_\gamma(l, \theta)+p_\gamma(-l, \theta+\pi)]}{4\exp(-0{,}5\,\mu L)\cdot\sinh(0{,}5\,\mu L)} \tag{53}$$

Diese Beziehung stellt gleichzeitig einen Spezialfall der „hyperbolic sine correction" bei Verwendung des arithmetischen Mittels (Gl. (55)) und der vorstehend genannten Objektkonfiguration dar ($\alpha = 1$, $m = 0{,}5\,L$). Dieses Sinus-Hyperbolicus-Verfahren, welches vielfach in kommerziellen Software-Paketen enthalten ist, basiert wiederum auf einem homogenen Absorber, durch den der Projektionsstrahl eine Weglänge L hat. Die ebenfalls homogene Quelle hat eine mittlere Ausdehnung von αL und eine mittlere Tiefe m innerhalb des Absorbers. Die übliche Form der Korrektur basiert auf der Verwendung des geometrischen Mittels opponierender Projektionen, da sich dann ein von der Tiefe m unabhängiger Korrekturfaktor ergibt

$$p(l, \theta) \approx \frac{[p_\gamma(l, \theta)\cdot p_\gamma(-l, \theta+\pi)]^{0{,}5}}{\sinh(0{,}5\,\mu\alpha L)}\cdot\frac{\mu\alpha L}{2}\cdot\exp(0{,}5\,\mu L) \tag{54}$$

Abb. 103. Fehlerfortpflanzung bei fehlerhaftem Absorptionskoeffizienten. Die Abbildung zeigt die Rekonstruktion einer Scheibe mit homogener Aktivitätsbelegung (Durchmesser 20 cm), aber örtlich variablem Absorptionskoeffizienten. Die Absorptionskorrektur wurde unter der Annahme eines örtlich konstanten $\mu = 0{,}088\ \mathrm{cm}^{-1}$ durchgeführt, der resultierende Fehler der relativen Aktivitätsbestimmung entspricht etwa dem 1,5fachen des relativen Fehlers im Absorptionskoeffizienten (aus HUANG et al. 1979)

Abb. 104. Fehlerfortpflanzung bei fehlerhaften Absorptionskoeffizienten für eine simulierte Schicht durch den Schädel bei homogener Aktivitätsbelegung. Die Korrektur wurde unter der Annahme eines örtlich konstanten Absorptionskoeffizienten durchgeführt, die fehlerhafte Aktivitätsreduktion ist abhängig von der Wandstärke der Schädelkalotte und vom Abstand zur Kalotte (aus HUANG et al. 1979). Insgesamt ist die rekonstruierte Aktivitätsbelegung um 10% gegenüber dem korrekten Wert erniedrigt

Abb. 105. Fehlerfortpflanzung bei fälschlichem Versatz der Absorberkontur. Diese Rekonstruktion einer homogenen Scheibe (Durchmesser 20 cm) wurde absorptionskorrigiert unter Verwendung einer Außenkontur des Absorbers, welche fehlerhaft um 0,5 cm in horizontaler Richtung verschoben war. Der Ordinatenwert 100 entspricht wiederum der korrekten Aktivitätsbelegung (aus HUANG et al. 1979)

Die Weglänge L kann für jeden Projektionsstrahl aus einer geschätzten oder gemessenen Körperkontur berechnet werden, der prozentuale Quellanteil α muß ebenfalls geschätzt oder aus einer Vorrekonstruktion ohne Korrektur bestimmt werden. Das Verfahren, ursprünglich von Sorenson (1974) für den Ganzkörperzähler angegeben, wurde von Budinger u. Gullberg (1974a, b; 1977) für die SPECT-Anwendung diskutiert. Zu erwarten sind relativ gute Ergebnisse bei der Abbildung homogener Quellen von etwa gleicher Intensität (Fehler etwa 10%), bei variablen Quellintensitäten dürften die Ergebnisse schlechter werden (Moore 1982).

Wird anstelle des geometrischen das arithmetische Mittel verwendet, führt die Sinus-Hyperbolicus-Korrektur auf einen tiefenabhängigen Korrekturfaktor

$$p(l, \theta) \approx \frac{[p_\gamma(l, \theta) + p_\gamma(-l, \theta + \pi)] \cdot 0{,}25\,\mu\alpha L \cdot \exp(0{,}5\,\mu L)}{\sinh(0{,}5\,\mu\alpha L) \cdot \cosh(\mu(0{,}5\,L - m))} \tag{55}$$

b) Postrekonstruktive Verfahren

Nach Durchführung der Rekonstruktion mit M Projektionen über 360° ohne Berücksichtigung der Absorption gibt Chang (1978) als ersten Schritt des von ihm vorgeschlagenen iterativen Verfahrens folgende Korrekturmatrix $C(x, y)$ an, die dann punktweise mit der rekonstruierten Verteilung $f(x, y)$ multipliziert wird

$$C(x, y) = \left\{ \frac{1}{M} \sum_{i=1}^{M} \exp(-\mu L(x, y, \theta_i)) \right\}^{-1} \tag{56}$$

Dabei ist $L(x, y, \theta_i)$ der Abstand des Punktes (x, y) von der Grenze des Absorbers entlang des Projektionsstrahles unter dem Winkel θ_i. Dieser Korrekturfaktor entspricht dem Kehrwert der gemittelten Absorption für den Punkt (x, y) und ist exakt für eine einzelne Punktquelle. Dieser Faktor könnte auch für variable Absorptionskoeffizienten $\mu(x, y)$ berechnet werden. Für ausgedehntere Quellen treten jedoch größere Abweichungen auf (Chang 1978, 1979).

Generell steigen sowohl bei den post- als auch bei den prerekonstruktiven Korrekturen die Fehler mit wachsender Abweichung von den zugrunde gelegten Quellenverteilungen, wie auch aus vergleichenden Untersuchungen von Tanaka (1983) und Tanaka et al. (1984) ersichtlich ist. Jaszczak et al. (1981) berichten andererseits über recht gute Ergebnisse bei der Anwendung von Gl. (56).

c) Inhärente Verfahren

Unter der Voraussetzung eines konvexen Absorbers mit konstantem μ aber beliebiger Quellenverteilung ist verschiedenen Autoren die Inversion der „attenuated Radon transform" gelungen. Allen diesen Verfahren gemeinsam ist, daß in einem ersten Schritt die gemessenen Projektionen modifiziert werden. Sei $A(l, \theta)$ der Abstand zwischen der Linie durch das Rotationszentrum (Koordinatenursprung) parallel zum Detektor (der Orientierung der Parallelprojektion) und der Begrenzung des Absorbers ($\mu = $ const.), so werden die modifizierten Projektionen gebildet durch

$$p_\mu(l, \theta) = p_\gamma(l, \theta) \exp(\mu A(l, \theta)) \tag{57}$$

Die Verknüpfung zwischen $p_\mu(l, \theta)$ und $f(x, y)$ wird „modified attenuated Radon transform" genannt. Führt man ein gedrehtes Koordinatensystem ein, wie in Abb. 106 dargestellt, so ergeben sich folgende Transformationsgleichungen

$$x = l \cos \theta - t \sin \theta \qquad l = x \cos \theta + y \sin \theta$$
$$y = l \sin \theta + t \cos \theta \qquad t = -x \sin \theta + y \cos \theta.$$

Dann vereinfacht sich Gl. (50) in Verbindung mit Gl. (57) und $\mu = \text{const.}$

$$p_\mu(l, \theta) = \int\limits_{-\infty}^{+\infty} f(l \cos \theta - t \sin \theta, l \sin \theta + t \cos \theta) \exp(\mu t)\, dt \tag{58}$$

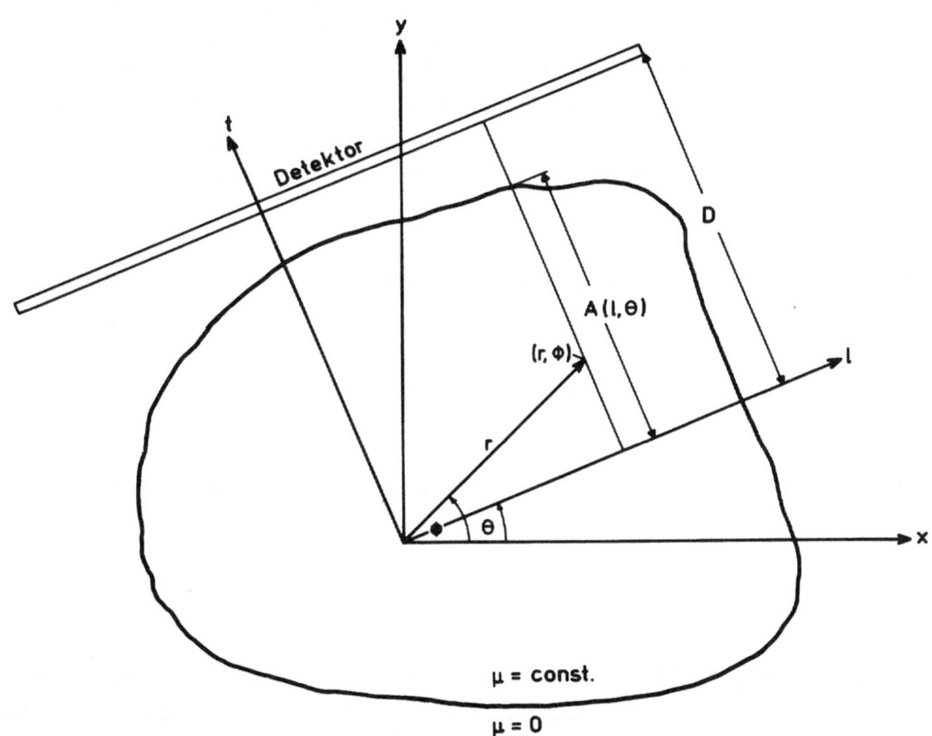

Abb. 106. Geometrie für die Absorptionskorrektur bei der SPECT. Die Projektionen $p(l, \theta)$ werden in einem gegenüber dem ortsfesten Koordinatensystem x, y um den Winkel θ gedrehten System l, t beschrieben. Die Koordinate l ist die laterale Koordinate der Projektion, die Richtung t beschreibt die Integrationsrichtung. Der Abstand $A(l, \theta)$ zwischen l-Achse und der Objektaußenkontur wird zur Berechnung der modifizierten Projektionen verwendet, der Rotationsradius ist D. Gleichzeitig ist aus der Abbildung der Bezug zwischen kartesischen und Polarkoordinaten ersichtlich

Die Vorteile dieser rein mathematisch begründeten Transformation (Gl. (57)) liegen darin, daß der Exponentialfaktor nicht mehr durch ein Integral bestimmt werden muß sowie, daß das obige Integral unabhängig von Detektorposition und Absorberkontur ist (GULLBERG u. BUDINGER 1981).

BELLINI et al. (1979) konnten zeigen, daß zwischen den modifizierten Projektionen und den theoretisch ohne Absorption zu messenden im Frequenzraum folgender Zusammenhang besteht

$$P(k, \theta) = P_\mu\left(\sqrt{k^2 + \frac{\mu^2}{4\pi^2}}, \theta + j \sinh^{-1}\left(\frac{\mu}{2\pi k}\right)\right) \tag{59}$$

Gemäß vorstehender Beziehung lassen sich aus den modifizierten gemessenen Projektionen die idealisierten Projektionen für $\mu=0$ interpolieren. Für die Interpolation im komplexen Winkel geben Bellini et al. (1979) einen Algorithmus an, welcher auf der Zusammenfassung opponierender Projektionen im arithmetischen Mittel beruht (Verwendung in Gl. (57)) und nach Substitution der radialen Frequenzvariablen für jeden Wert von k eine Modifikation der Koeffizienten c_n der Fourierreihenentwicklung über die Winkelvariable mit dem Faktor $\cosh\left(n \sinh^{-1}\left(\dfrac{\mu}{2\pi k}\right)\right)$ beinhaltet. Nach dieser Interpolation erfolgt dann z.B. der normale Algorithmus der Rückprojektion gefilterter Projektionen. Das Verfahren ergibt sehr gute Ergebnisse für $\mu=$const. (Budinger et al. 1979) und ist relativ günstig in der Rauschverstärkung, da die Winkelinterpolation über alle Projektionen eine gewisse Rauschmittelung darstellt. Es sei noch angemerkt, daß Bellini et al. (1979) die Modifikation entsprechend Gl. (57) in leicht veränderter Form gemäß $\exp(\mu(A(l,\theta)-D))$ angeben, wobei D der Abstand Rotationszentrum – Detektor ist. Da der Unterschied nur in dem für alle Projektionen konstanten Faktor $\exp(-\mu D)$ liegt, ergibt sich dadurch kein prinzipieller Unterschied. Der Rechenaufwand wird von den Autoren etwa auf das drei- bis zehnfache einer Rekonstruktion ohne Absorptionsberücksichtigung beziffert.

Zu einer direkten Parallele zur vertrauten Convolution-Methode führt das von Tretiak u. Delaney (1978) entwickelte Verfahren der exponentiell bewichteten Rückprojektion. Nach Faltung der modifizierten Projektionen mit einer geeigneten, absorptionsabhängigen Funktion $g_\mu(l)$

$$p'_\mu(l, \theta) = p_\mu(l, \theta) * g_\mu(l) \tag{60}$$

erfolgt die mit einem exponentiellen Absorptionsterm bewichtete Rückprojektion (vgl. Gl. (6)).

$$f(x, y) = \int\limits_0^{2\pi} p'_\mu(x \cos\theta + y \sin\theta, \theta) \exp(-\mu(-x \sin\theta + y \cos\theta))\, d\theta \tag{61}$$

Diese exponentielle Rückprojektion weist wiederum jedem Punkt (x, y) einen Wert zu, der gleich der Summe der Strahlsummen durch diesen Punkt ist, wobei jede Strahlsumme mit einem Absorptionsfaktor $\exp(-\mu t)$ bewichtet wird. Diese Reihenfolge von Operationen, d.h. Modifikation der Projektionen, Filterung und exponentielle Rückprojektion, ergibt wiederum als Rekonstruktionsergebnis die Faltung des Objekts $f(x, y)$ mit einer shiftinvarianten Punktbildfunktion h_μ, welche sich aus der exponentiellen Rückprojektion der Filterfunktion g_μ ergibt. Für radialsymmetrische Punktbildfunktionen gilt dann in Polarkoordinaten

$$h_\mu(r) = \int\limits_0^{2\pi} g_\mu(r \cos\theta) \exp(-\mu r \sin\theta)\, d\theta \tag{62}$$

Durch iterative Lösung von Gl. (62) (Anpassung im Sinne des kleinsten Fehlerquadrats an eine gewünschte Punktbildfunktion) gibt Gullberg (1979) numerische Werte der Funktion $g_\mu(l)$ für ausgewählte Werte von μ an. Diese numerischen Lösungen führten zu der empirischen Beobachtung, daß deren Darstellung im Frequenzbereich auf Filter führt, die vergleichbar zum bekannten Rampenfilter sind.

$$G_\mu(k) = \begin{cases} |k| & \text{für } \dfrac{\mu}{2\pi} \leq |k| \leq k_{\mathrm{g}} \\[2mm] 0 & \text{sonst} \end{cases} \tag{63}$$

Durch eine analytisch exakte Inversion der „attenuated Radon transform" durch TRETIAK u. METZ (1980) konnte diese Beobachtung verifiziert werden. Basierend auf diesen Arbeiten diskutieren GULLBERG u. BUDINGER (1981) sehr detailliert die Anwendung der bereits in Abschnitt G.IV.1.c.α angegebenen Fensterfunktionen. Den gleichen Ansatz verwenden KIM et al. (1984) für das Shepp-Logan-Filter in Verbindung mit Fehleruntersuchungen für Abweichungen im Wert des Absorptionskoeffizienten und im Verlauf der Objektkontur. Generell gilt für diese Funktionen ohne und mit Absorption

$$
W_\mu(k) = \begin{cases} W\left(\sqrt{k^2 - \dfrac{\mu^2}{4\pi^2}}\right) & \text{für } \dfrac{\mu}{2\pi} \leqq |k| \leqq k_g \\ 0 & \text{sonst} \end{cases} \tag{64}
$$

Interessant erscheint die Beobachtung, daß sowohl nach den Ergebnissen von BELLINI et al. (1979) als auch von TRETIAK u. METZ (1980) sowie GULLBERG u. BUDINGER (1981) die gemessenen Projektionen keine Information im tieffrequenten Bereich $\left(|k| \leqq \dfrac{\mu}{2\pi}\right)$ enthalten.

Speziell für das gaußförmige Fenster werden sehr ausführliche Untersuchungen zur Auflösung und Rauschverstärkung in Abhängigkeit von μ und dem Objektdurchmesser gemacht (GULLBERG u. BUDINGER 1981). Ganz allgemein steigt die Rauschverstärkung mit steigender Auflösung, steigendem μ und steigendem Objektdurchmesser. Die gleichen Autoren weisen darauf hin, daß mit steigendem Zahlenwert für den Absorptionskoeffizienten bei konstant gehaltener Rekonstruktionsauflösung das lineare Abtastintervall verkleinert werden muß, obwohl dieser Effekt in der nuklearmedizinischen Anwendung ($\mu \approx 0{,}10$ bis $0{,}18$ cm^{-1}) noch kaum zu Buche schlägt. Bei hochauflösenden Rekonstruktionen muß das Winkelinkrement ebenfalls verringert werden, da ansonsten aliasing-Fehler durch die numerische Approximation der exponentiellen Rückprojektion auftreten. Die relativ hohe Rauschverstärkung des Verfahrens (die am weitesten vom Detektor entfernten Objektpunkte werden mit einem großen Faktor bewichtet zurückprojiziert), die von GULLBERG (1979) z.B. für eine 30 cm-Scheibe mit etwa einem Faktor 4 höher angegeben wird (für $\mu = 0{,}15$ cm^{-1}) im Vergleich zu $\mu = 0$, führte TANAKA (1983) und TANAKA et al. (1984) zu einer Modifikation der exponentiellen Rückprojektion. Abhängig von einem Rekonstruktionsindex, welcher die Bewichtung innerhalb der Rückprojektion zu verschieben erlaubt und auch den Sonderfall nach Gl. (61) beinhaltet, und von der Wahl eines objektangepaßten Koordinatenursprunges kann das Signal-Rausch-Verhältnis deutlich verbessert werden. Die gleichzeitig erforderliche Modifikation der Filterfunktion wird empirisch nach der „trial and error"-Methode iterativ bestimmt, eine analytische Lösung ist noch nicht bekannt. Die Autoren berichten von guten Ergebnissen für ausgedehnte simulierte Objekte. Beispiele im Vergleich zur exponentiellen Rückprojektion sowie zur prerekonstruktiven (Gl. (54)) und postrekonstruktiven Korrektur (Gl. (56)) sind in Abb. 107 wiedergegeben.

d) Iterative Verfahren

Für variable Absorptionskoeffizienten $\mu(x,y)$ demonstrieren BUDINGER et al. (1977a), BUDINGER u. GULLBERG (1974a, b; 1977), GULLBERG (1979) und BUDINGER et al. (1979a) exakte Rekonstruktionen mit einem iterativen Verfahren. Die Methode bedingt zunächst die Rekonstruktion einer Transmissionsaufnahme, aus der dann für jedes Pixel das Linienintegral der Absorptionskoeffizienten zum Detektor für jeden möglichen Projektionsstrahl berechnet wird. Diese Korrekturfaktoren können dann in die Bewichtungsfaktoren w_{ij} (vgl. Gln. (25), (28)) bei der anschließenden iterativen Rekonstruktion eingebracht werden. GULLBERG (1979) untersucht ausführlich die Konvergenzeigenschaften und die Rauschverstärkung

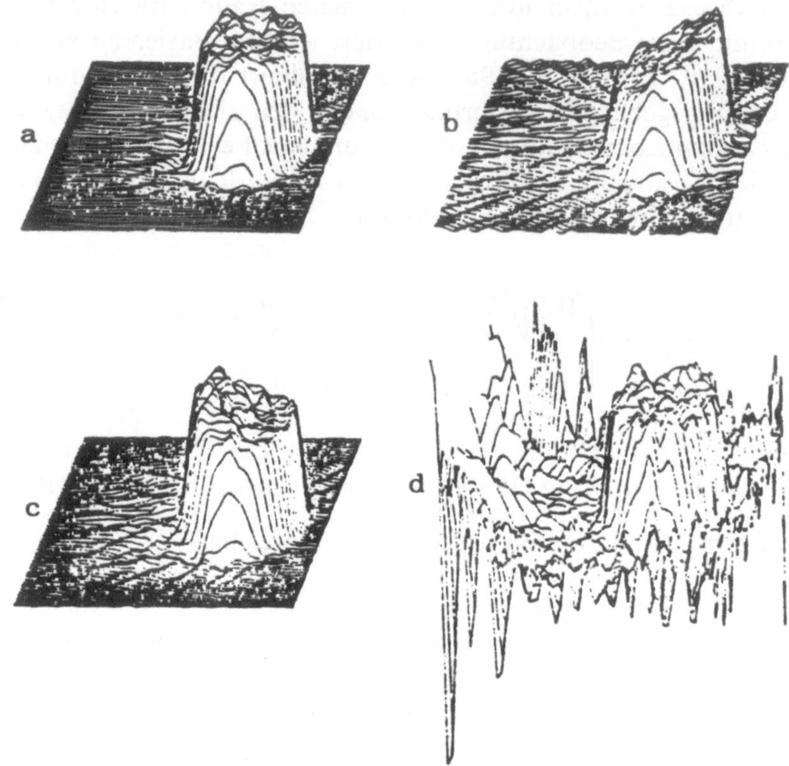

Abb. 107a–d. Vergleich unterschiedlicher Absorptionskorrekturen für die SPECT (aus Tanaka et al. 1984). Die Abbildung zeigt das Rekonstruktionsergebnis für einen Absorber (Durchmesser 30 cm, $\mu = 0{,}15\ \mathrm{cm}^{-1}$) mit einer exzentrisch angeordneten, aktivitätsgefüllten Scheibe (Durchmesser 15 cm) mit einer Gesamtzahl registrierter Photonen von 500000. **a** Tanakas Methode der bewichteten Rückprojektion, **b** Prerekonstruktive Korrektur nach Sorenson (sinus hyperbolicus), **c** Postrekonstruktive Korrektur (nach Chang, 1. Stufe), **d** Inhärente Korrektur mit exponentiell bewichteter Rückprojektion und Fensterfunktion (nach Kim et al. 1984)

des Verfahrens unter Verwendung der Methode der „conjugate gradients" zur Minimierung der Fehlerquadratsumme. Die von ihm durchgeführten Simulationsuntersuchungen lassen eine wesentlich günstigere Beeinflussung des Signal-Rausch-Verhältnisses erwarten als bei der Methode der exponentiellen Rückprojektion. Der Nachteil der Methode ist die sehr viel höhere Rechenzeit.

Ein hybrides Verfahren wird von Chang (1978) vorgeschlagen. Zunächst wird eine Rekonstruktion ohne Absorptionsberücksichtigung mit einem analytischen Verfahren durchgeführt, z.B. durch Rückprojektion gefilterter Projektionen. Nach Anwendung der postrekonstruktiven Korrektur (Gl. (56)) werden Reprojektionen des resultierenden Bildes berechnet und durch Differenzbildung mit den tatsächlich gemessenen Projektionen Fehlerprojektionen gebildet. Diese bilden dann die Basis zur Rekonstruktion eines Fehlerbildes, welches ebenfalls einer Korrektur erster Ordnung gemäß Gl. (56) unterworfen und zum postrekonstruktiv korrigierten Bild addiert wird. Dieser Iterationszyklus, welcher sehr dem iterativen Verfahren zur analytischen Fortsetzung bei eingeschränktem Raumwinkel gleicht (vgl. z.B. auch Chang 1979), konvergiert nach wenigen Iterationen und liefert in der Regel bereits nach einer Iteration bessere Ergebnisse als die Sinus-Hyperbolicus-Korrektur (Chang 1978). Über sehr gute Ergebnisse bei Anwendung des Verfahrens nach einer Modifikation entsprechend der Meßgeometrie des Cleon-Imagers sowie der Einführung eines Dämpfungsfaktors berichten Moore et al. (1982) und Moore (1982).

Eine ähnliche Technik verwenden WALTERS et al. (1981). Ihre Methode vermeidet die Einführung von Interpolationsfehlern, da die Reprojektionen ohne vorhergehende explizite Rekonstruktion eines Zwischenbildes im Verlauf der Iteration berechnet werden.

Eine Methode, die iterativ zur Lösung gelangt durch den Vergleich der einfachen Rückprojektion der modifizierten Projektionen (Gl. (58)) und der Rückprojektion der modifizierten Reprojektionen aus dem vorhergehenden Iterationsschritt schlagen SOUSSALINE et al. (1982) und SOUSSALINE u. LE COQ (1983) vor. Zur Regularisierung beinhaltet das Verfahren eine zusätzliche multiplikative Funktion für die Reprojektionen, die offensichtlich objektabhängig ist. Obwohl generell auch für variables μ geeignet, sind bis jetzt nur Ergebnisse für $\mu = $ const. veröffentlicht worden.

4. Streustrahlung und zufällige Koinzidenzen

Bevor die im vorigen Abschnitt besprochenen Verfahren zur Absorptionskorrektur angewendet werden dürfen, ist zumindest bei quantitativer Zielsetzung die Kontamination der Meßdaten durch Streustrahlung und, bei PET-Systemen, zufällige Koinzidenzen zu eliminieren bzw. zu reduzieren.

Zufällige Koinzidenzen sind zählratenabhängig. Ihre Rate bestimmt sich zu

$$N_{Z1,2} = \tau_{12} \cdot N_1 N_2 \tag{65}$$

mit N_1, N_2 Einzeldetektorrate und τ_{12} Koinzidenzauflösungszeit. Werden diese zufälligen Koinzidenzen nicht aus den Projektionsdaten eliminiert, resultiert eine unter Umständen erhebliche, örtlich variable Überbestimmung des Objekts. Eine sorgfältige Diskussion der zur Zeit bekannten Korrekturverfahren findet sich bei HOFFMAN et al. (1981 b):

1. *Bestimmung der zufälligen Koinzidenzen durch Projektionswerte außerhalb der physikalischen Dimensionen des Objekts.* Werden diese Daten einfach als konstanter Background subtrahiert, können je nach Design des Tomographen Fehler bis zum Faktor 2 auftreten, da die örtliche Verteilung der zufälligen Koinzidenzen nicht unbedingt konstant ist, sondern zur Mitte hin ansteigt. Des weiteren versagt die Methode, wenn die örtliche Verteilung der zufälligen Koinzidenzen nicht radialsymmetrisch ist, z.B. durch stark unsymmetrische Aktivitätsverteilungen im Objekt. Da eventuell vorhandene Empfindlichkeitsunterschiede der Detektorpaare bezüglich des Nachweises zufälliger Koinzidenzen nicht berücksichtigt werden, können Ringartefakte vergleichbar zu einer inadäquaten Inhomogenitätskorrektur erzeugt werden. Das Verfahren wird verwendet bei den Typen PETT III bis PETT VI.
2. *Berechnung der zufälligen Koinzidenzen durch Messung der Einzeldetektorraten gemäß Gl. (65).* Dieses Verfahren, z.B. angewendet von BERGSTRÖM et al. (1980) erfordert eine genaue Kenntnis der Koinzidenzauflösungszeiten der einzelnen Detektorpaare, liefert aber Korrekturfaktoren hoher statistischer Qualität, da die Einzelraten typisch um einen Faktor 100 bis 1000 höher sind als die wahre Koinzidenzrate.
3. *Bestimmung der zufälligen Koinzidenzen durch ein zeitverzögertes Koinzidenzfenster.* Da die zufälligen Koinzidenzen zeitlich gleichverteilt sind, ergibt dieses rein meßtechnische Korrekturverfahren einwandfreie Korrekturfaktoren. Problematisch ist lediglich, daß die so ermittelten Faktoren von statistisch geringerer Güte sind als bei dem vorstehend genannten Verfahren. HOFFMAN et al. (1981 b) zeigen, daß eine Datenglättung problematisch ist und zu ähnlichen Artefakten wie unter 1. beschrieben führen kann.

Während sich zufällige Koinzidenzen noch einfach berücksichtigen lassen, stellt die Kontamination der Meßdaten mit Streustrahlung ein sehr komplexes Problem dar, da deren örtliche Verteilung nicht nur von der Objektverteilung in der betrachteten Schicht abhängig ist, sondern auch von der Aktivitätsverteilung in den benachbarten Objektebenen. Theoretische Untersuchungen, basierend auf der Anwendung der Klein-Nishina Gleichungen und auf Monte Carlo-Simulationen, finden sich z.B. bei PANG u. GENNA (1979), EGBERT u. MAY (1980), BECK (1983) und FLOYD et al. (1984). FLOYD et al. (1984) zeigen, daß für die rotierende Gamma-Kamera (Energieauflösung 12%) bei Verwendung von ^{99m}Tc und einem Energiefenster von $\pm 9\%$ hauptsächlich mit Streustrahlung 1. und 2. Ordnung zu rechnen ist. Es resultiert ein positionsabhängiger Streustrahlungsanteil von etwa 30–40%. Diese Aussage deckt sich auch in etwa mit den Angaben von KING et al. (1981) für eine Positronenkamera, obwohl diese Autoren leider Streustrahlung und zufällige Koinzidenzen zusammenfassen. Für PET-Kameras läßt sich allerdings der Streustrahlungsanteil durch sorgfältiges Design deutlich reduzieren. Diese Zahlenwerte demonstrieren, daß eine Vernachlässigung des Streustrahlungsanteils zu erheblichen Überbestimmungen des Objekts führen muß. Eine exakte Korrektur der Streustrahlung ist zur Zeit noch nicht bekannt, es existieren nur Lösungen für bestimmte Objektkonfigurationen oder mehr oder weniger gute approximative Lösungen. Die einfachste Form der Korrektur ist die Verwendung eines „effektiven" Absorptionskoeffizienten bei der Absorptionskorrektur (z.B. $\mu = 0,12$ bis $0,13$ cm^{-1} für ^{99m}Tc), vgl. beispielsweise LARSSON (1980). Dieses Verfahren ergibt eine eindeutige Unterkompensation des Absorptionseffektes, indem absorbierte Gammaquanten durch gestreute ersetzt werden. Obwohl eventuell in qualitativer Hinsicht akzeptabel ist das Verfahren ungeeignet für quantitative Zwecke. JASZCZAK et al. (1984) berichten, daß die Methode bei einer kalten Kugel von immerhin 6 cm Durchmesser noch eine „Aktivität" von 30% des umgebenden Backgrounds liefert. Die gleichen Autoren setzen sich auch kritisch auseinander mit der von JASZCZAK et al. (1981), MOORE et al. (1982) und MOORE (1982) verwendeten Methode, die Streustrahlung durch Annahme eines mittleren, konstanten Streustrahlungsanteils zu berücksichtigen. Basierend auf Untersuchungen von WHITEHEAD (1977) zur planaren Szintigraphie, wird hier die Voraussetzung einer Streustrahlungsverteilung in Form eines homogenen Backgrounds gemacht. Der Streustrahlungsanteil kann aber durchaus, je nach Objekt, strukturiert sein, vergleiche z.B. TODD-POKROPEK et al. (1984). Diese Aussage wird auch untermauert durch die Feststellung von FLOYD et al. (1984), daß die Linienbildfunktion für Streustrahlung 1. und 2. Ordnung durch Exponentialfunktionen modelliert werden kann, eine Feststellung, die auch schon empirisch von KING et al. (1981) sowie AXELSSON et al. (1984) gemacht wurde. Der Ansatz von BERGSTRÖM et al. (1980), die Streustrahlungs-LSF anhand der Klein-Nishina Gleichungen zu berechnen, durch anschließende Integration die Streustrahlungsverteilung für eine homogene Scheibe zu berechnen und diese Verteilung, normiert über einen aus Strahlsummen außerhalb der physikalischen Objektdimensionen berechneten Skalenfaktor zu subtrahieren, gilt aus den obigen Überlegungen heraus eben nur für diese Objektkonfiguration.

Weitere Ansätze basieren auf Dekonvolution mit einer exponentiellen Streustrahlungs-LSF, z.B. KING et al. (1981) sowie AXELSSON et al. (1984). Basierend auf rechnersimulierten Objektverteilungen berechnen EGBERT u. MAY (1980) mit Hilfe der Klein-Nishina Gleichungen die zugehörigen Streustrahlungsverteilungen und geben ein approximatives, iteratives Verfahren an. ENDO u. IINUMA (1984) entwickeln ein iteratives Korrekturverfahren, basierend auf einer wegen der endlichen Ausdehnung des streuenden Mediums ortsvarianten Streustrahlungs-LSF, für die Meßgeometrie der Positologica. Das Verfahren stützt sich ebenfalls auf die Klein-Nishina Gleichungen.

Auf der Verwendung von Meßdaten der Streustrahlung, die parallel zur Primärstrahlung in einem oder mehreren im Streustrahlungsbereich liegenden Energiefenstern registriert werden, beruhen Verfahren von TODD-POKROPEK et al. (1984) und JASZCZAK et al. (1984). Diese Verfahren dürften zumindest approximativ die aktuellen Streustrahlungsanteile der jeweiligen

Objektverteilung berücksichtigen, und zwar auch die, die von Quellen außerhalb der betrachteten Schicht herrühren. TODD-POKROPEK et al. (1984) rechnen die Streustrahlungsprojektionen durch Dekonvolution von der Streustrahlungs-LSF auf die LSF der Photopeakregistrierung um und führen dann die Streustrahlungskorrektur durch Subtraktion der veränderten Streustrahlungsprojektionen von den im Photopeak inklusive Streustrahlung gemessenen Projektionen durch. JASZCZAK et al. (1984) messen in einem niederenergetischen Fenster ebenfalls zusätzliche Streustrahlungsprojektionen, aus denen anschließend ein Streustrahlungsbild rekonstruiert wird. Die Korrektur erfolgt durch Subtraktion des mit einem Normierungsfaktor bewichteten Streustrahlungsbildes von dem im Primärfenster registrierten Bild. Die Methode wurde auch von BERBERICH et al. (1984a, b) für die planare Szintigraphie untersucht und für die SPECT-Anwendung vorgeschlagen. Folgend einer Übersicht von OPPENHEIM (1984) dürfte unter dem Gesichtspunkt der praktischen Anwendung diesen auf paralleler Streustrahlungserfassung basierenden Verfahren der Vorzug gegeben werden.

5. Quantifizierbarkeit und geometrische Einflüsse

Die Zielsetzung der tomographischen Messung ist neben einer verbesserten Nachweiswahrscheinlichkeit für Läsionen durch Erhöhung des Bildkontrastes die Festlegung von Größe und/oder Volumen der Läsionen und die Quantifizierbarkeit der Aktivitätskonzentration in vivo. Einen fundierten Überblick zu dieser Problematik geben TODD-POKROPEK u. JARRITT (1982). Vorausgesetzt, alle anderen Fehlerquellen wie Digitalisierung, Absorption, Streustrahlung, zufällige Koinzidenzen, statistische Datenqualität und Fehljustierungen des Detektorsystems (z.B. Inhomogenität und Lage des Rotationszentrums) sind berücksichtigt und das System ist linear in der Bestimmung der Aktivitätsmenge, verbleiben noch die geometrischen Einflüsse auf die Quantifizierbarkeit, die auf der begrenzten Auflösung des tomographischen Bildes in allen drei Raumkoordinaten in Relation zur dreidimensionalen Ausdehnung des Objektes (hier der betrachteten Läsion) zurückzuführen sind. Charakterisiert werden diese Einflüsse durch den Begriff des „recovery"-Koeffizienten, welcher definiert ist als Quotient der abgebildeten Aktivitätskonzentration zur tatsächlichen Aktivitätskonzentration. Eine Abweichung dieses RC-Wertes vom Idealwert „eins" bedeutet, daß von der aus dem Bild bestimmten Aktivitätskonzentration nur innerhalb entsprechender Fehlergrenzen auf die wahre Aktivitätskonzentration geschlossen werden kann, oder daß bei bekanntem RC-Wert mit diesem korrigiert werden muß.

Der „recovery"-Koeffizient ist abhängig von den Dimensionen der betrachteten Objektstruktur in allen drei Koordinatenrichtungen in Relation zur dreidimensionalen Auflösung des Meßsystems. Sind die Objektabmessungen in zwei oder einer Koordinatenrichtung hinreichend groß, spricht man von ein- oder zweidimensionalen „recovery"-Koeffizienten. Im eindimensionalen Fall kann der RC-Wert geometrisch veranschaulicht werden durch den Anteil der Fläche der Linienbildfunktion, der vom Objekt überlappt wird. Ist die dreidimensionale Punktbildfunktion des abbildenden Systems separierbar, wie z.B. bei rein gaußförmigen Funktionen, kann der dreidimensionale RC-Wert für einen Würfel durch das Produkt der eindimensionalen RC-Werte (abhängig von der jeweiligen Auflösung) berechnet werden, vergleiche HOFFMAN et al. (1979a).

Für die ECAT-Positronenkamera führen HOFFMAN et al. (1979a) für drei verschiedene Auflösungsmodi detaillierte Untersuchungen (Hotspot-Situation ohne Background) für ein- und zweidimensionale Objekte durch, d.h. für Objekte, deren axiale Dimension (z-Koordinate) so groß ist, daß der Einfluß der meßtechnischen Schichtdicke vernachlässigbar ist, also ohne sogenannte „partial volume"-Effekte. Die Autoren zeigen, daß nach Ausschluß aller anfangs erwähnten Fehlerquellen die meßtechnisch ermittelten RC-Werte gut mit den unter der Voraussetzung gaußförmiger Abbildungsfunktionen ermittelten übereinstimmen.

Am Beispiel des „high resolution"-Modus, der in der LSF geringfügige Penetrationsanteile zeigt (kleiner als 2% der Maximalamplitude), ergeben sich jedoch bereits deutlich zu niedrig liegende meßtechnische RC-Werte (etwa 10%). Die zweidimensionalen RC-Werte für zylindrische Objekte sind in Abb. 108 dargestellt.

In Übereinstimmung mit den Untersuchungen von HOFFMAN et al. (1979a) erweitern KESSLER et al. (1984) die Untersuchungen für den ECAT auf dreidimensionale Objekte unter der Annahme gleicher Auflösung in allen drei Koordinatenrichtungen. Gleichzeitig wird das Konzept von der Abbildung heißer Knoten in kalter Umgebung (hot spot recovery coeffizient HSRC) auch auf kalte Knoten in heißer Umgebung (cold spot recovery coeffizient CSRC) und heiße Knoten in warmer Umgebung (contrast recovery coeffizient CRC) erweitert, wobei die übliche Kontrastdefinition zugrunde gelegt wird ((Läsion − Background) / Background). Für die Relation der verschiedenen RC-Werte gilt

$$HSRC \approx CRC \tag{66a}$$

$$CSRC = 1 - HSRC \tag{66b}$$

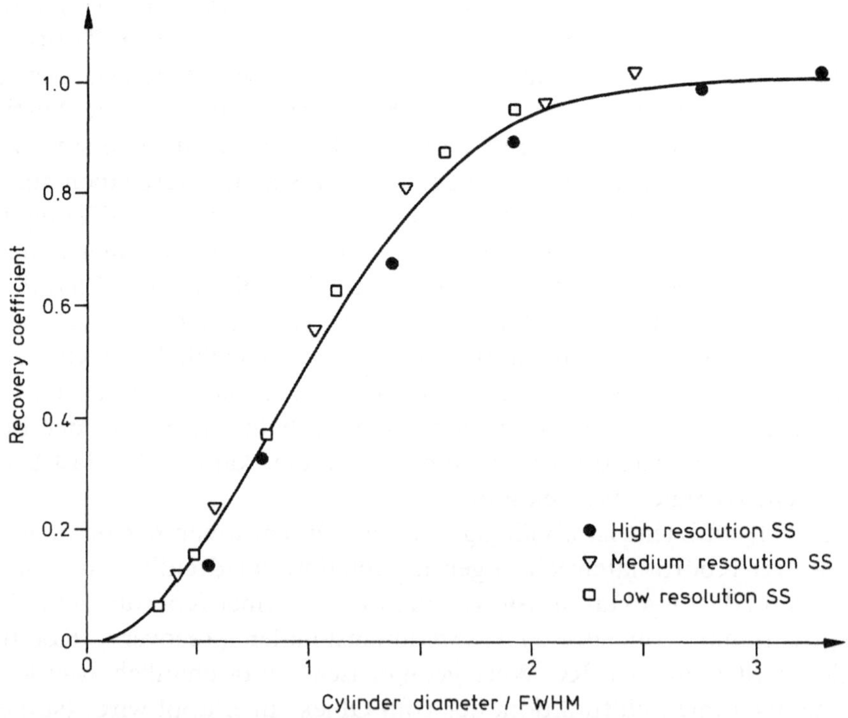

Abb. 108. Einfluß der Auflösung auf die Quantifizierbarkeit. Die Abbildung zeigt die „hot spot recovery"-Koeffizienten für zweidimensionale Objekte (Zylinder) für die verschiedenen Auflösungsmodi des ECAT in Abhängigkeit von Auflösung und Objektdurchmesser. Die durchgezogene Linie entspricht den theoretisch erwarteten Werten für eine gaußförmige LSF gleicher Auflösung. Aufgrund von Septenpenetration (Abweichung von der Gaußförmigkeit) liegen die Meßwerte im hochauflösenden Modus systematisch zu niedrig (aus HOFFMAN et al. 1979a)

Die genannten Autoren weisen ausdrücklich darauf hin, daß eine „recovery"-Korrektur in der üblichen Meßsituation eines nicht vernachlässigbaren Backgrounds nur für den Kontrast vorgenommen werden darf, nicht aber für das Summensignal „heiße Quelle + Background". Es gilt also bei Normierung auf einen Background von „eins"

$$\left(\frac{\text{Läsion}}{\text{Background}}\right)_{\text{Objekt}} = \frac{C_{\text{mess}}}{\text{CRC}} + 1 \tag{67}$$

mit C_{mess} als gemessenem Bildkontrast.

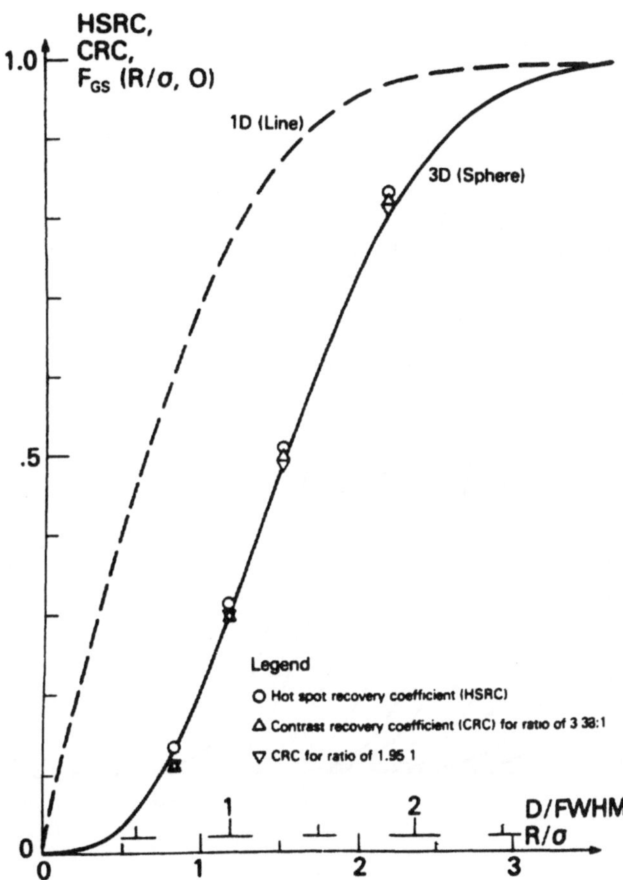

Abb. 109. Einfluß der Auflösung auf die Quantifizierbarkeit. Die Abbildung zeigt „recovery"-Koeffizienten (*„hot spot"* und *Kontrast*) für eindimensionale *(Streifen)* und dreidimensionale *(Kugel)* Objekte in Abhängigkeit vom Verhältnis von Auflösung und Objektdurchmesser (aus KESSLER et al. 1984)

In Abb. 109 sind die Ergebnisse für dreidimensionale (Kugeln) und eindimensionale (Streifen) Objekte dargestellt. Aus diesen Ergebnissen in Verbindung mit Abb. 108 ergibt sich, daß eine „recovery"-Korrektur nicht erforderlich ist (RC = 0,98), wenn mindestens folgende Läsionsabmessungen vorliegen:

1. eindimensionales Objekt: Streifenbreite $\geq 2 \times$ FWHM
2. zweidimensionales Objekt: Zylinderdurchmesser $\geq 2,4 \times$ FWHM
3. dreidimensionales Objekt: Kugeldurchmesser $\geq 2,7 \times$ FWHM

Für Objektdurchmesser in der Größe der Halbwertsbreite liegen die entsprechenden „recovery"-Koeffizienten etwa bei 0,77; 0,5 und 0,3. Die für den Zylinder berechneten Werte korrespondieren recht gut mit den von SHOSA u. KAUFMAN (1981) für die planare Szintigraphie angegebenen Werten, während die Koeffizienten für kugelförmige Läsionen sowohl bei SHOSA u. KAUFMAN (1981) als auch bei WHITEHEAD (1977) zu hoch liegen, da in der planaren Betrachtung die z-Auflösung keinen Einfluß hat. Gestützt auf die von WHITEHEAD (1977) publizierten Daten berichten JASZCZAK et al. (1981) sowie MOORE et al. (1982) über Quantifizierung in der SPECT-Anwendung.

In der Anwendung der „recovery"-Koeffizienten ist ferner zu berücksichtigen, daß alle angegebenen Werte auf dem maximalen bzw. minimalen Pixelinhalt basieren. Aus Gründen des statistischen Rauschens wird in der Anwendung dagegen häufig der Mittelwert einer

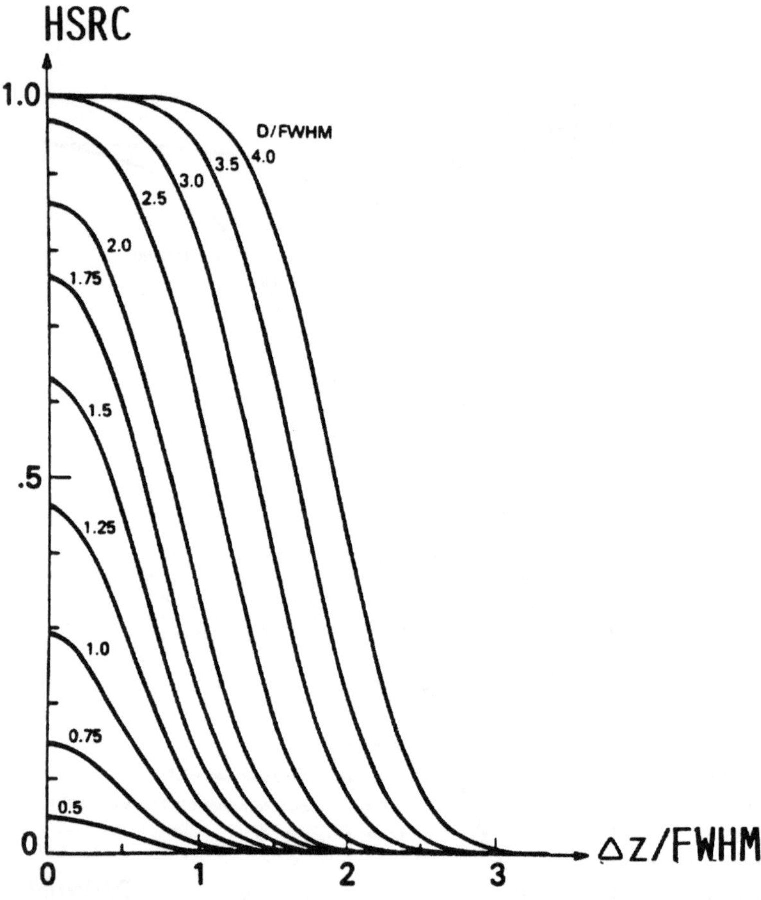

Abb. 110. Einfluß der Objektverschiebung bzw. des Schichtabstandes auf die Quantifizierbarkeit. Die Abbildung zeigt für unterschiedliche Verhältnisse von Kugeldurchmesser zu Auflösung die Reduktion der „recovery"-Koeffizienten in Abhängigkeit von einer Verschiebung Δz des Objekts aus der Schichtebene heraus. Dieser Effekt wiegt besonders schwer bei zu grobem Schichtabstand (aus Kessler et al. 1984)

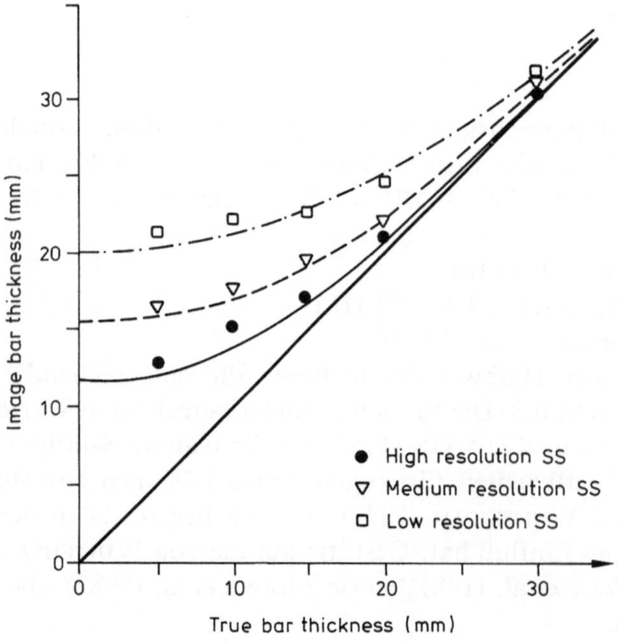

Abb. 111. Einfluß der Auflösung auf die Bestimmung der Objektgröße. Für die drei Auflösungsmodi des ECAT (11,6 mm, 15,5 mm, 19,9 mm FWHM) ist für eindimensionale Objekte die Relation von der aus dem Bild bestimmten zur tatsächlichen Objektgröße dargestellt. Dieser Zusammenhang wird erst linear bei Objektdurchmessern größer als $2 \times$ FWHM. Bei Reduktion der Objektgröße wird die im Bild erscheinende Objektdimension in zunehmendem Maße, unabhängig vom Objekt, lediglich durch die Bildauflösung bestimmt, so daß die Grundlage für eine „recovery"-Korrektur schwindet (aus Hoffman et al. 1979a)

Region benutzt. Hat diese Region einen Durchmesser entsprechend der Halbwertsbreite, schätzen KESSLER et al. (1984) die resultierende Reduktion der „recovery"-Koeffizienten auf 24% ab. Weitere Verfälschungen treten auf, wenn das Abtastintervall in z-Richtung zu grob ist, gleichbedeutend mit einer möglichen Verschiebung des Objekts in z-Richtung relativ zur Bildebene (vgl. Abb. 110).

Voraussetzung der „recovery"-Korrektur ist sowohl eine genaue Kenntnis der Auflösungseigenschaften des Tomographen und des Rekonstruktionsverfahrens wie auch eine Abschätzung der Objektdimensionen aus dem Bild oder aus anatomischem a priori Wissen. Gerade bei kleinen Objektdimensionen wird die anscheinende Größe einer Läsion im Bild mehr von der Auflösungsfunktion als von der tatsächlichen Objektdimension bestimmt (vgl. Abb. 111 für eindimensionale Objekte).

Insgesamt wird von HOFFMAN et al. (1979a) sowie KESSLER et al. (1984) abgeschätzt, daß bei sorgfältiger Anwendung eine „recovery"-Korrektur möglich ist für Objekte, welche größer sind als die Halbwertsbreite. Zu ähnlichen Folgerungen gelangen TODD-POKROPEK u. JARRITT (1982) für den Cleon-Imager. Die Abschätzung von „recovery"-Koeffizienten für anatomische Strukturen und damit die Verbindung zur klinischen Anwendung diskutieren MAZZIOTTA et al. (1981) sowie KESSLER et al. (1984).

Schwieriger wird die Situation, wenn die Auflösung (innerhalb der Schicht und/oder in axialer Richtung) ortsvariant ist. Dieses gilt besonders für Positronen-Ring-Tomographen mit der Erzeugung von Zwischenschichten bei nicht optimalem Design. HOFFMAN et al. (1982) zeigen, daß bereits ein visueller Vergleich von Objekten in echten Schichten und in Zwischenschichten sehr problematisch werden kann, und daß die Voraussetzung einer ortsinvarianten Auflösung für solche Systeme nicht unbedingt gilt. Diese Ortsvarianz der Auflösung bewirkt, wenn sie ausgeprägt ist, schwerwiegende Limitationen in der Fähigkeit zur Quantifizierung; die Autoren berichten von Variationen der „recovery"-Koeffizienten um 30–50%.

Die dargestellten Untersuchungen zur PET-Anwendung zeigen, daß eine Quantifizierung tomographischer Daten große Sorgfalt sowie eine genaue Kenntnis des Tomographen und der mathematischen Zusammenhänge voraussetzt. Leider sind entsprechende umfassende Studien für die rotierende Gammakamera zur Zeit nur ansatzweise bekannt, vermutlich nicht zuletzt deshalb, weil die Probleme der Korrektur von Absorption und Streustrahlung sowie der mit dem Abstand variablen Auflösung für die Routineanwendung noch nicht befriedigend gelöst worden sind.

Literatur

Ahluwalia B, Brownell GL, Hales C, Kazemi H (1981) Regional lung function evaluation with Nitrogen-13. Eur J Nucl Med 6:453–457

Alkhafaji SM (1981) Monte Carlo calculations of a bismuth germanate scintillation detector. Nucl Instr Meth 187:547–551

Allemand R, Gresset C, Vacher J (1980) Potential advantages of a cesium fluoride scintillator for a time-of-flight positron camera. J Nucl Med 21:153–155

Alpert NM, Chesler DA, Correia JA, Ackerman RH, Chang JY, Finklestein S, Davis SM, Brownell GL, Taveras JM (1982) Estimation of the local statistical noise in emission computed tomography. IEEE Trans Med Imag MI-1:142–146

Anger HO, Rosenthal DJ (1959) Scintillation camera and positron camera – technical aspects. In: IAEA (ed) Medical radioisotope scanning. IAEA, Vienna, p 59

Anger HO (1966) Tomographic Gamma-Ray scanner with simultaneous readout of several planes. UCRL-16899 Rep Lawrence Radiation Laboratory

Anger HO (1967) The scintillation camera for radioisotope localization. In: Hoffman G, Scheer KE (Hrsg) Radioisotope in der Lokalisationsdiagnostik (1966). Schattauer, Stuttgart, S 1

Anger HO (1968) Tomographic gamma-ray scanner with simultaneous readout of several planes. In: Gottschalk A, Beck RN (eds) Fundamental problems in scanning. Thomas, Springfield, p 195

Anger HO (1969) Multiplane tomographic Gamma-

Ray scanner. In: IAEA (ed) Medical radioisotope scintigraphy. IAEA, Vienna, p 203

Anger HO (1973) Multiplane tomographic scanner. In: Freedman GS (ed) Tomographic imaging in nuclear medicine. Soc Nucl Med Inc, New York, p 2

Areeda J, Chapman D, Van Train K, Bietendorf J, Friedman J, Berman D, Waxman A, Garcia E (1983) Methods for characterizing and monitoring rotational Gamma camera system performance. In: Esser PD (ed) Emission computed tomography. Soc Nucl Med New York, p 81

Aurich F, Stange R (1982) Streutomographie – Dosimetrie und Aufnahmetechnik mit diagnostischen Röntgenstrahlen. Fortschr Röntgenstr 136:206–210

Axelsson B, Msaki P, Israelsson A (1984) Subtraction of compton-scattered photons in single-photon emission computerized tomography. J Nucl Med 25:490–494

Baron JC, Lebrun-Grandie P, Collard P, Crouzel C, Mestelan G, Bousser MG (1982) Noninvasive measurement of blood flow, oxygen consumption, and glucose utilization in the same brain regions in man by PET: Concise communication. J Nucl Med 23:391–399

Barrett HH (1972) Fresnel zone plate imaging in nuclear medicine. J Nucl Med 13:382–385

Barrett HH, Horrigan FA (1973) Fresnel zone plate imaging of gamma rays: Theory Appl Opt 12:2686–2702

Barrett HH, Meester GD de (1974) Quantum noise in fresnel zone plate imaging. Appl Optics 13:1100–1109

Barrett HH, Swindell W (1977) Analog reconstruction methods for transaxial tomography. Proc of the IEEE 65:89–107

Barrett HH, Wilson DT, Meester GD de (1972) The use of half-tone screens in fresnel-zone plate imaging of incoherent sources. Opt Com 5:398–401

Barrett HH, Stoner WW, Wilson DT, Meester GD de (1974) Coded apertures derived from the fresnel zone plate. Opt Eng 13:539–549

Barrett HH, Gordon SK, Hershel RS (1976) Statistical limitations in transaxial tomography. Comput Biol Med 6:307–323

Bateman JE, Connolly JF, Stephenson R, Flesher AC (1980) The development of the rutherford laboratory MWPC positron camera. Nucl Instr Meth 176:83–88

Bates RHT, Peters TM (1971) Towards improvements in tomography. NZJ Sci 14:883–896

Beck JW (1983) Analysis of a camera based SPECT system. Nucl Instr Meth 213:415–436

Beck JW, Jaszczak RJ, Coleman RE, Starmer CF, Nolte LW (1982) Analysis of SPECT including scatter and attenuation using sophisticated Monte Carlo modeling methods. IEEE Trans Nucl Sci NS-29/1:506–511

Beller GA, Alton WJ, Cochavi S, Hnatowich D, Brownell GL (1979) Assessment of regional myocardial perfusion by positron emission tomography after intracoronary administration of gallium-68 labeled albumin microspheres. J Comput Assist Tomogr 3:447–452

Bellini S, Piacentini M, Cafforio C, Rocca F (1979) Compensation of tissue absorption in emission tomography. IEEE Trans Acoustics, Speech, Signal Process ASSP-27/3:213–218

Berberich R, Schmidt EL, Brill G (1984a) Bildverbesserung durch gewichtete Subtraktion des Comptonanteils. In: Schmidt HAE, Adam WE (Hrsg) Nuklearmedizin 1983. Schattauer, Stuttgart, S 86–90

Berberich R, Brill G, Schmidt EL (1984b) Verbesserung des Auflösungsvermögens der Gammakamera durch gewichtete Subtraktion der Streustrahlung. Nuc Compact 15:246–251

Bergström M, Bohm C, Ericson K, Eriksson L, Litton J (1980) Corrections for attenuation, scattered radiation, and random coincidences in a ring detector positron emission transaxial tomograph. IEEE Trans Nucl Sci NS-27/1:549–554

Bergström M, Litton J, Eriksson E, Blohm C, Blomqvist G (1982) Detamination of object contour from projections for attenuation correction in cranial positron emission tomography. J Comput Assist Tomogr 6:365–372

Bernard AD, Bradstock PA, Milward RC (1978) Transverse-section (tomographic) medical Gamma-Ray imaging using the J&P multipoise tomoscanner. In: Schmidt HAE, Woldring M (Hrsg) Nuklearmedizin 1977. Schattauer, Stuttgart, S 27

Biersack HJ, Fröscher W, Klünenberg H, Reske SN, Rasche A, Reichmann K, Winkler C (1983a) SPECT des Hirns mit J-123-Isoprophyl-Amphetamin bei Epilepsie. NUC Compact 14:62–72

Biersack HJ, Reichmann K, Reske SN, Janson R, Knopp R, Winkler C (1983b) Erste klinische Erfahrungen mit der parametrischen SPECT des Herzbinnenraumes. NUC Compact 14:36–39

Blum AS (1983) Improving SPECT image quality by body contour following. In: Esser PD (ed) Emission computed tomography. Soc Nucl Med, New York, p 163

Boetticher H von, Helmers H, Schreiber P, Schmitz-Feuerhake I (1982) Advances in $\gamma - \gamma$-coincidence scintigraphy with the scintillation camera. Phys Med Biol 27:1495–1506

Bohm C, Eriksson L, Bergström M, Litton J, Sundman R, Singh M (1978) A computer assisted ring-detector positron camera system for reconstruction tomography of the brain. IEEE Trans Nucl Sci NS-25/1:624–637

Bonte FJ, Devous Sr. MD, Stokely EM, Homan RW (1983) Single-photon tomographic determination of regional cerebral blood flow in epilepsy. AJNR 4:544–546

Borrello JA, Clinthorne NH, Rogers WL, Thrall JH, Keyes JW Jr (1981) Oblique-angle tomography: A restructuring algorithm for transaxial tomographic data. J Nucl Med 22:471–483

Bowley AR, Taylor CG, Causer DA, Barber DC, Keyes WI, Undrill PE, Corfield JR, Mallard JR (1973) A radioisotope scanner for rectilinear, arc, transverse section and longitudinal section scanning: (ASS – the Aberdeen Section Scanner). Br J Radiol 46:262–271

Bozzo SR, Robertson JS, Milazzo JP (1968) A data processing method for a multidetector positron scanner. In: Gottschalk A, Beck RN (eds) Fundamental problems in scanning. Thomas, Springfield, p 212

Bracewell RN (1956) Strip integration in radio astronomy. Aust J Phys 9:198–217

Bracewell RN (1978) The fourier transform and its applications. Mc Graw Hill, New York

Bracewell RN (1979) Image reconstruction in radio astronomy. In: Herman GT (ed) Image reconstruction from projections. Springer, Berlin Heidelberg New York, p 81

Bracewell RN, Riddle AC (1967) Inversion of Fan-Beam scans in radio astronomy. The Astrophysical J 150:427–434

Bracewell RN, Wernecke SJ (1975) Image reconstruction over a finite field of view. J Opt Soc Am 65:1342–1346

Britton KE, Shapiro B, Elliott AT (1981) Clinical results of quantitative single photon emission tomography. In: IAEA (ed) Medical radionuclide imaging 1980. vol I. IAEA, Vienna, p 263

Brookeman VA, Maisey MN (1982) Performance characteristics of seven-pinhole tomography. Br J Radiol 55:229–235

Brooks RA, Di Chiro G (1975) Theory of image reconstruction in computed tomography. Radiology 117:561–572

Brooks RA, Di Chiro G (1976) Principles of computer assisted tomography (CAT) in radiographic and radioisotopic imaging. Phys Med Biol 21:689–732

Brooks RA, Weiss GH, Talbert AJ (1978) A new approach to interpolation in CT. J Comput Assist Tomogr 2:577–585

Brooks RA, Sank VJ, Talbert AJ, Di Chiro G (1979a) Sampling requirements and detector motion for positron emission tomography. IEEE Trans Nucl Sci NS-26/2:2760–2763

Brooks RA, Glover GH, Talbert AJ, Eisner RL, Di Bianca FA (1979b) Aliasing: A source of streaks in computed tomograms. J Comput Assist Tomogr 3:511–518

Brooks RA, Sank VJ, Di Chiro G, Friauf WS, Leighton SB (1980) Design of a high resolution positron emission tomograph: The Neuro-PET. J Comput Assist Tomogr 4:5–13

Brooks RA, Sank VJ, Friauf WS, Leighton SB, Cascio HE, Di Chiro G (1981) Design considerations for positron emission tomography. IEEE Trans Biomed Eng BME-28/2:158–176

Brooks RA, Sank VJ, Di Chiro G, Friauf WS, Leighton SB, Cascio HE (1982) The neuro-PET: A new high resolution 7-Slice positron emission tomograph. In: Raynaud C (ed) Nuclear medicine and biology I. Pergamon, Paris, p 550

Brown ML, Keyes JW Jr, Leonard PF, Thrall JH, Kircos LT (1977) Facial bone scanning by emission tomography. J Nucl Med 18:1184–1188

Brownell GL, Burnham CA (1973) MGH positron camera. In: Freedman GS (ed) Tomographic imaging in nuclear medicine. Soc Nucl Med Inc, New York, p 154

Brownell GL, Burnham CA, Wilensky S, Aronow S, Kazemi H, Strieder D (1969) New developments in positron scintigraphy and the application of cyclotron-produced positron emitters. In: IAEA (ed) Medical radioisotope scintigraphy. IAEA, Vienna, p 163

Brownell GL, Burnham CA, Chesler DA, Correia JA, Correll JE, Hoop B Jr, Parker JA, Subramanyam R (1977) Transverse section imaging of radionuclide distributions in heart, lung, and brain. In: Ter-Pogossian MM, et al (eds) Reconstruction tomography in diagnostic radiology and nuclear medicine. Park, Baltimore, p 293

Brownell GL, Correia JA, Zamenhof RG (1978) Positron instrumentation. In: Lawrence JH, Budinger TF (eds) Recent advantages in nuclear medicine, vol 5. Grune & Stratton, New York, pp 1–49

Brownell G, Burnham C, Correia J, Chesler D, Akkerman R, Tavares J (1979) Transverse section imaging with the MGH positron camera. IEEE Trans Nucl Sci NS-26/2:2698–2702

Brownell GL, Kearfott KJ, Kairento AL, Elmaleh DR, Alpert NM, Correia JA, Wechsler L, Ackerman RH (1983) Quantitation of regional cerebral glucose metabolism. J Comput Assist Tomogr 7:919–924

Brunol J, Fonroget J, Roucayrol JC, Beaucoudry N de (1978) A high resolution computed tomography for nuclear medicine using a multipinhole collimator. In: Schmidt HAE, Woldring M (Hrsg) Nuklearmedizin 1977. Schattauer, Stuttgart, S 64

Budinger TF (1977) Instrumentation trends in nuclear medicine. Semin Nucl Med 7:285–297

Budinger TF (1980) Physical attributes of single-photon tomography. J Nucl Med 21:579–592

Budinger TF (1981) Revival of clinical nuclear medicine brain imaging. J Nucl Med 22:1094–1097

Budinger TF (1982a) Single photon emission tomography. In: Raynaud C (ed) Nuclear medicine and biology II. Pergamon, Paris, p 1159

Budinger TF (1982b) Three-dimensional display techniques: Description and critique of methods. In: Raynaud C (ed) Nuclear medicine and biology II. Pergamon, Paris, p 2185

Budinger TF (1983a) Time-of-flight positron emission tomography: Status relative to conventional PET. J Nucl Med 24:73–78

Budinger TF (1983b) Positron emission tomography. In: Moss AA (ed) NMR, interventional radiology, and diagnostic imaging modalities. UCLA, San Francisco, p 149

Budinger TF, Gullberg GT (1974a) Three-dimensional reconstruction in nuclear medicine emission imaging. IEEE Trans Nucl Sci Ns-21: June 2–20

Budinger TF, Gullberg GT (1974b) Three-dimensional reconstruction in nuclear medicine by iterative least-squares and fourier transform techniques. Lawrence Berkeley Lab Rep LBL-2146

Budinger TF, Gullberg GT (1977) Transverse section reconstruction of γ-Ray emitting radionuclides in patients. In: Ter-Pogossian MM, Phelps ME, Brownell GL, Cox JR, Davis DO, Evans RG (eds) Reconstruction tomography in diagnostic radiology and nuclear medicine. University Park Press, Baltimore, pp 315–342

Budinger TF, Macdonald B (1975) Reconstruction of the fresnel-coded gamma camera images by digital computer. J Nucl Med 16:309–313

Budinger TF, Gullberg GT, Nohr ML, McRae J, Anger HO (1973) Quantitative sequential imaging of radionuclide distribution using the whole-body scanner and the gamma camera: Absolute accuracy and aspects of three-dimensional reconstruction. Lawrence Berkeley Lab Rep LBL-2161

Budinger TF, Gullberg GT, Nohr ML, McRae J, Anger HO (1974) Quantitative sequential imaging of radionuclide distribution using the whole-body scanner and the gamma camera: Absolute accuracy and aspects of three-dimensional reconstruction. In: Pabst HW (Hrsg) Nuklearmedizin 1973. Schattauer, Stuttgart, S 2

Budinger TF, Derenzo SE, Gullberg GT, Greenberg WL, Huesman RH (1977a) Emission computer assisted tomography with single-photon and positron annihilation photon emitters. J Comput Assist Tomogr 1:131–145

Budinger TF, Cahoon JL, Derenzo SE, Gullberg GT, Moyer BR, Yano Y (1977b) Three dimensional imaging of the myocardium with radionuclides. Radiology 125:433–439

Budinger TF, Derenzo SE, Greenberg WL, Gullberg GT, Huesman RH (1978) Quantitative potentials of dynamic emission computed tomography. J Nucl Med 19:309–315

Budinger TF, Gullberg GT, Huesman RH (1979a) Emission computed tomography. In: Herman GT (ed) Image reconstruction from projections. Springer, Berlin Heidelberg New York, p 147

Budinger TF, Derenzo SE, Gullberg GT, Huesman RH (1979b) Trends and prospects for circular ring positron cameras. IEEE Trans Nucl Sci NS-26:2742–2745

Budinger TF, Derenzo SE, Huesman RH, Cahoon JL, Yano Y (1980) Dynamic emission transaxial tomography for positron emitters. In: Horst W, Wagner HN Jr, Buchanan J (eds) Frontiers in nuclear medicine. Springer, Berlin Heidelberg New York, p 52

Budinger TF, Derenzo SE, Huesman RH, Cahoon JL (1982) Medical criteria for the design of a dynamic positron tomograph for heart studies. IEEE Trans Nucl Sci NS-29/1:488–492

Büll U, Kirsch CM, Roedler HD (1983a) Die Single-Photon-Emissions-Computertomographie (SPECT). Prinzipien, Ergebnisse, Ausblick. Fortschr Röntgenstr 138:391–402

Büll U, Moser EA, Kirsch CM, Schmiedek P (1983b) Xe-133-DSPECT (Dynamische Single Photon Emission CT). Fortschr Röntgenstr 139:351–358

Burdine JA, Murphy PH, Puey EG de (1979) Radionuclide computed tomography of the body using routine radiopharmaceuticals. II. Clinical applications. J Nucl Med 20:108–114

Burnham CA, Brownell GL (1972) A multi-crystal positron camera. IEEE Trans Nucl Sci NS-19/3:201–205

Burnham C, Bradshaw J, Kaufman D, Chesler D, Brownell GL (1981) One dimensional scintillation camera for positron ECT ring detectors. IEEE Trans Nucl Sci Ns-28/1:109–113

Burnham C, Bradshaw J, Kaufman D, Chesler D, Brownell G (1982) Application of a one-dimensional scintillation camera in a positron tomographic ring detector. IEEE Trans Nucl Nucl Sci NS-29:461–464

Burnham C, Bradshaw J, Kaufman D, Chesler D, Brownell GL (1983) A positron tomograph employing a one dimension BGO scintillation camera. IEEE Trans Nucl Sci NS-30:661–664

Burnham CA, Bradshaw J, Kaufman D, Chesler D, Brownell GL (1984) A stationary positron emission ring tomograph using BGO detector and analog readout. IEEE Trans Nucl Sci NS-31:632–636

Carril JM, Mac Donald AF, Dendy PP, Keyes WI, Undrill PE, Mallard JR (1979) Cranial scintigraphy: Value of adding emission computed tomographic sections to conventional pertechnetate images (512 cases). J Nucl Med 20:1117–1123

Carroll LR (1978) Design and performance characteristics of a production model positron imaging system. IEEE Trans Nucl Sci NS-25/1:606–614

Carroll LR, Kretz P, Orcutt G (1983) The orbiting rod source: Improving performance in PET transmission correction scans. In: Esser PD (ed) Emission computed tomography. Soc Nucl Med, New York, p 235

Cassen B (1969) Image formation by electronic cross-time correlation of signals from angular ranges of unfocused collimating channels. In: IAEA (ed) Medical radioisotope scintigraphy. IAEA, Vienna, p 107

Celsis P, Goldman T, Henriksen L, Lassen NA (1981) A method for calculating regional cerebral blood flow from emission computed tomography of inert gas concentrations. J Comput Assist Tomogr 5:641–645

Chang LT (1978) A method for attenuation correction in radionuclide computed tomography. IEEE Trans Nucl Sci NS-25/1:638–643

Chang LT (1979) Attenuation correction and incomplete projection in single photon emission computed tomography. IEEE Trans Nucl Sci NS-26/2:2780–2789

Chang LT, Mac Donald B, Perez-Mendez V (1976) Axial tomography and three dimensional image reconstruction. IEEE Trans Nucl Sci NS-23/1:568–572

Chang W, Henkin RE (1980) Seven-pinhole multigated tomography and its application to blood-pool imaging: Technical parameters. J Nucl Med 21:682–688

Chang W, Lin SL, Henkin RE (1982) A new collimator for cardiac tomography: The quadrant slant-hole collimator. J Nucl Med 23:830–835

Chen CT, Metz CE (1984) Evaluation and comparison of image reconstruction algorithms for positron emission tomography with time-of-flight information (TOFPET). Proc of the IEEE, Int Symp on Medical Images and Icons, pp 388–393

Chesler DA (1971) Three-dimensional activity distribution from multiple positron scintigraphs. J Nucl Med 12:347–348 (Abs)

Chesler DA (1973) Positron tomography and three-dimensional reconstruction technique. In: Freedman GS (ed) Tomographic imaging in nuclear medicine. Soc Nucl Med Inc, New York, p 176

Chesler DA (1982) Noise power spectrum in time-of-flight tomography. In: IEEE (ed) 1982 workshop on time-of-flight tomography. IEEE Computer Soc, Los Angeles, p 113–116

Chesler DA, Riederer SJ (1975) Ripple suppression during reconstruction in transverse tomography. Phys Med Biol 20:632–636

Chesler DA, Riederer SJ, Pelc NJ (1977) Noise due to photon counting statistics in computed X-Ray tomography. J Comput Assist Tomogr 1:64–77

Cho ZH, Farukhi MR (1977) Bismuth germanate as a potential scintillation detector in positron cameras. J Nucl Med 18:840–844

Cho ZH, Chan JK, Eriksson L, Singh M, Graham S, MacDonald NS, Yano Y (1975) Positron ranges obtained from biomedically important positron-emitting radionuclides. J Nucl Med 16:1174–1176

Cho ZH, Chan JK, Eriksson L (1976) Circular ring transverse axial positron camera for 3-dimensional reconstruction of radionuclides distribution. IEEE Trans Nucl Sci NS-23/1:613–622

Cho ZH, Cohen MB, Singh M, Eriksson L, Chan J, MacDonald N, Spolter L (1977a) Performance and evaluation of the circular ring transverse axial positron camera (CRTAPC). In: IAEA (ed) Medical radionuclide imaging, vol I. IAEA, Vienna, p 269

Cho ZH, Cohen MB, Singh M, Eriksson L, Chan J, MacDonald N, Spolter L (1977b) Performance and evaluation of the circular ring transverse axial positron camera (CRTAPC). IEEE Trans Nucl Sci NS-24/1:532–543

Cho ZH, Nalcioglu O, Farukhi MR (1978) Analysis of a cylindrical hybrid positron camera with bismuth germanate (BGO) scintillation crystals. IEEE Trans Nucl Sci NS-25/2:952–963

Cho ZH, Hong KS, Ra JB, Lee SY (1981) A new sampling scheme for the ring positron camera: Dichotomic ring sampling. IEEE Trans Nucl Sci NS-28/1:94–98

Cho ZH, Yi W, Jung KJ, Lee BU, Min HB, Song HB (1982) Performance of single photon tomographic system – Gammatom-1. IEEE Trans Nucl Sci NS-29:484–487

Cho ZH, Hilal SK, Ra JB, Hong KS, Bigler RE, Yoshizumi T, Wolf AP, Fowler JS (1983a) High-resolution circular ring positron tomograph with dichotomic sampling: dichotom-I. Phys Med Biol 28:1219–1234

Cho ZH, Ra JB, Hilal SK (1983b) True three-dimensional reconstruction (TTR) – Application of algorithm toward full utilization of oblique rays. IEEE Trans Med Imag MI-2:6–18

Cho ZH, Hilal SK, Ra JB, Hong KS, Lee HS (1983c) Experimental results of the dichotomic sampling in circular ring positron emission tomography. IEEE Trans Nucl Sci NS-20/3:1892–1898

Chu G, Tam KC (1977) Three-dimensional imaging in the positron camera using fourier techniques. Phys Med Biol 22:245–265

Chu D, Tam KC, Perez-Mendez V, Lim CB, Lambert D, Kaplan SN (1976) High-efficiency collimator-converters for neutral particle imaging with MWPC. IEEE Trans Nucl Sci NS-23/1:634–639

Chu D, Tam K, Perez-Mendez V, Kaplan SN, Lim C, Hattner R, Kaufman L, Price D, Swan S (1977) High efficiency gamma converters and their application in an MWPC positron camera. In: IAEA (ed) Medical Radionuclide Imaging, vol I. IAEA, Vienna, p 171

Chung V, Chak KC, Zacuto P, Hart HE (1980) Multiple photon coincidence tomography. Semin Nucl Med X:345–354

Coleman RE, Jaszczak RJ, Cobb FR (1982a) Comparison of 180° and 360° data collection in Thallium-201 imaging using single-photon emission computerized tomography (SPECT): Concise communication. J Nucl Med 23:655–660

Coleman RE, Drayer BP, Jaszczak RJ (1982b) Studying regional brain function: A challenge for SPECT. J Nucl Med 23:266–270

Coleman RE, Greer KL, Drayer BP, Albright RE, Petry NA, Jaszczak RJ (1983) Collimation for I-123 imaging with SPECT. In: Esser PD (ed)

Emission computed tomography: Current trends. Soc Nucl Med, New York, p 135

Colsher JG (1980) Fully three-dimensional positron emission tomography. Phys Med Biol 25:103–115

Colsher JG, Muehllehner G (1981) Effects of wobbling motion on image quality in positron tomography. IEEE Trans Nucl Sci NS-28/1:90–93

Condon B, Mills J, Ardley R, Taylor D (1983) A physical comparison of two fixed-angle emission tomographic cardiac imaging systems. Phys Med Biol 28:131–138

Cooke BE, Evans AC, Fanthome EO, Alarie R, Sendyk AM (1984) Performance figures and images from the Therascan 3128 positron emission tomograph. IEEE Trans Nucl Sci NS-31:640–644

Cormack AM (1963) Representation of a function by its line integrals, with some radiological applications. J Appl Physiol 34:2722–2727

Cormack AM (1973) Reconstruction of densities from their projections, with application in radiological physics. Phys Med Biol 18:195–207

Cormack AM (1980) Early two-dimensional reconstruction (CT-scanning) and recent topics stemming from it. Nobel lecture, December 8, 1979. J Comput Assist Tomogr 4:658–664

Cowan RJ, Watson NE (1980) Special characteristics and potential of single photon emission computed tomography in the brain. Semin Nucl Med X:335–344

Crawford CR, Kak AC (1979) Aliasing artifacts in computerized tomography. Appl Opt 18:3704–3711

Del Guerra A, Lim CB, Lum GK, Ortendahl D, Perez-Mendez V (1982a) Medical positron imaging with a dense drift space multi wire proportional chamber. IEEE Trans Med Imag MI-1/1:4–11

Del Guerra A, Bellazzini R, Tonelli G, Venturi R, Nelson WR (1982b) A detailed monte carlo study of multiple scattering contamination in compton tomography at 90°. IEEE Trans Med Imag MI-1:147–152

Derenzo SE (1979) Precision measurement of annihilation point spread distributions for medically important positron emitters. In: Hasiguti RR, Fujiwara K (eds) Proc 5th Int Conf on Positron Annihilation. The Japan Institute of Metals, p 819

Derenzo SE, Zaklad H, Budinger TF (1975) Analytical study of a high-resolution positron ring detector system for transaxial reconstruction tomography. J Nucl Med 16:1166–1173

Derenzo SE, Budinger TF, Cahoon JL, Huesman RH, Jackson HG (1977) High resolution computed tomography of positron emitters. IEEE Trans Nucl Sci NS-24/1:544–558

Derenzo SE, Budinger TF, Cahoon JL, Greenberg WL, Huesman RH, Vuletich T (1979) The donner 280-crystal high resolution positron tomograph. IEEE Trans Nucl Sci NS-26/2:2790–2793

Derenzo SE, Budinger TF, Huesman RH, Cahoon JL, Vuletich T (1981) Imaging properties of a positron tomograph with 280 BGO crystals. IEEE Trans Nucl Sci NS-28/1:81–89

Derenzo SE, Budinger TF, Huesman RH, Cahoon JL (1982) Dynamic positron emission tomography in man using small bismuth germanate crystals. In: Coleman PG, Sharma SC, Diana LM (eds) Positron annihilation. North-Holland, Amsterdam, p 935

Derenzo SE, Budinger TF, Vuletich T (1983) High resolution positron emission tomography using small bismuth germanate crystals and individual photosensors. IEEE Trans Nucl Sci NS-30:665–670

Di Chiro G, Oldfield E, Bairamian D, Patronas NJ, Brooks RA, Mansi L, Smith BH, Kornblith PL, Margolin R (1983) Metabolic imaging of the brain stem and spinal cord: Studies with positron emission tomograph using F-18-2-Deoxyglucose in normal and pathological cases. J Comput Assist Tomogr 7:937–945

Döring V, Hahn R, Sauer J (1983) Meßtechnische Probleme bei der J-123-Szintigraphie. Nuc Compact 14:362–370

Doria D, Singh M (1982) Comparison of reconstruction algorithms for an electronically collimated gamma camera. IEEE Trans Nucl Sci NS-29/1:447–451

Drayer B, Jaszczak R, Friedman A, Albright R, Kung H, Greer K, Lischko M, Petry N, Coleman E (1983) In vivo quantitation of regional cerebral blood flow in glioma and cerebral infarction: Validation of the HIPDm – SPECT method. AJNR 4:572–576

Egbert SD, May RS (1980) An integral-transport method for compton-scatter correction in emission computed tomography. IEEE Trans Nucl Sci NS-27/1:543–548

Eichling JO, Higgins CS, Ter-Pogossian MM (1977) Determination of radionuclide concentrations with positron CT scanning (PETT): Concise communication. J Nucl Med 18:845–847

Ell PJ, Todd-Pokropek A, Williams ES (1978) The future of non-invasive medical imaging. Fortschr Röntgenstr 128:486–490

Ell PJ, Khan O (1981) Emission computerized tomography: clinical applications. Semin Nucl Med XI:50–60

Ell PJ, Williams ES, Deacon JM (1980) Clinical efficacy study of ECAT and TCAT brain scans in 118 patients. In: Höfer R, Bergmann H (Hrsg) Radioaktive Isotope in Klinik und Forschung 14. Egermann, Wien, S 245

Ell PJ, Jarritt J, Cullum I (1982) Present trends of single photon radionuclide tomography. Fortschr Röntgenstr 136:330–336

Endo M, Iinuma TA (1984) Software correction of scatter coincidence in positron CT. Eur J Nucl Med 9:391–396

Ericson K, Bergström M, Eriksson L (1980) Positron emission tomography in the evaluation of subdural hematomes. J Comput Assist Tomogr 4:737–745

Eriksson L, Cho ZH (1976) Efficiency optimization analysis for dynamic function studies with 3-D transaxial positron cameras. Comput Biol Med 6:361–372

Eriksson L, Bohm C, Bergström M, Ericson K, Greitz T, Litton J, Widen L (1980) One year experience with a high resolution ring detector positron camera system: Present status and future plans. IEEE Trans Nucl Sci NS-27/1:435–444

Eriksson L, Bohm C, Kesselberg M, Blomqvist G, Litton J, Widen L, Bergström M, Ericson K, Greitz T (1982) A four ring positron camera system for emission tomograph of the brain. IEEE Trans Nucl Sci NS-29/1:539–543

Feine U, Anger K, Müller-Schauenburg W, Milward RC (1977) Erste klinische Erfahrungen mit einem axialen Emissions-Computer-Tomographen. Fortschr Röntgenstr 127:358–365

Firusian N, Schmidt CG (1979) Ergebnisse der Emissions-Computer-Tomographie der Leber bei 113 bioptisch untersuchten Patienten. Nucl Med XVIII:65–72

Flower MA, Parker RP (1980) Quantitative imaging using the cleon emission tomography system. Radiology 137:535–539

Floyd CE, Jaszczak RJ, Harris CC, Coleman RE (1984) Energy and spatial distribution of multiple order Compton scatter in SPECT: a Monte Carlo investigation. Phys Med Biol 29:1217–1230

Frackowiak RSJ, Lenzi GL, Jones T, Heather JD (1980) Quantitative measurement of RCBF and oxygen metabolism in man using 0–15 and positron emission tomography: Theory, procedure, and normal values. J Comput Assist Tomogr 4:727–736

Freedman GS (1970) Tomography with a gamma camera. J Nucl Med 11:602–604

Freedman GS (1973) Digital gamma camera tomography-theory. In: Freedman GS (ed) Tomographic imaging in nuclear medicine. Soc Nucl Med Inc, New York, p 68

Frieden BR (1975) Image enhancement and restoration. In: Huang TS (ed) Picture processing and digital filtering. Springer, Berlin Heidelberg New York, p 177

Friedland RP, Budinger TF, Ganz E, Yano Y, Mathis CA, Koss B, Ober BA, Huesman RH, Derenzo SE (1983) Regional cerebral metabolic alterations in dementia of the Alzheimer type: Positron emission tomography with (F-18)fluorodeoxyglucose. J Comput Assist Tomogr 7:590–598

Gariod R, Allemand R, Cormoreche E, Laval M, Moszynski M (1982) The „LETI" positron tomograph architecture and time-of-flight improvements. In: IEEE (ed) 1982 workshop on time-of-flight tomography. IEEE Computer Soc, Los Angeles, p 25

Genna S, Pang SC, Smith A (1982) Digital scintigraphy: concepts and designs. IEEE Trans Nucl Sci NS-29:558–562

Gilbert P (1972) Iterative methods for the three-dimensional reconstruction of an object from projections. J Theor Biol 36:105–117

Gindi GR, Arendt J, Barrett HH, Chiu MY, Ervin A, Giles CL, Kujoory A, Miller EL, Simpson RG (1982) Imaging with rotating slit apertures and rotating collimators. Med Phys 9:324–339

Goitein M (1972) Three-dimensional density reconstruction from a series of two-dimensional projections. Nucl Instr Meth 101:509–518

Goldstein RA (1982) Myocardial metabolic imaging: a new diagnostic era – teaching editorial. J Nucl Med 23:641–644

Goodman MM, Elmaleh DR, Kearfott KJ, Ackerman RH, Hoop B, Brownell GL, Alpert NM, Strauss HW (1981) F-18-Labeled 3-Deoxy-3-Fluoro-D-Glucose for the study of regional metabolism in the brain and heart. J Nucl Med 22:138–144

Gordon R (1974) A tutorial on ART. IEEE Trans Nucl Sci NS-21/3:78–93

Gordon R, Herman GT (1974) Three-dimensional reconstruction from projections: a review of algorithms. Int Rev Cytol 38:111–151

Gordon R, Bender R, Herman GT (1970) Algebraic reconstruction techniques (ART) for three-dimensional electron microscopy and X-Ray photography. J Theor Biol 29:471–481

Gore JC, Leeman S (1980) The reconstruction of objects from incomplete projections. Phys Med Biol 25:129–136

Gottschalk S, Salem D (1982) Effect of an elliptical orbit on SPECT resolution and image uniformity. In: Raynaud C (ed) Nuclear medicine and biology I. Pergamon, Paris, p 1026

Gottschalk SC, Salem D, Lim CB, Wake RH (1983) SPECT resolution and uniformity improvements by noncircular orbit. J Nucl Med 24:822–828

Gullberg GT (1979) The attenuated radon transform: theory and application in medicine and biology. Thesis, Univ of California, Berkeley

Gullberg GT, Budinger TF (1981) The use of filtering methods to compensate for constant attenuation in single photon emission computed tomography. IEEE Trans Biomed Eng BME-28/2:142–157

Gullberg GT, Malko JA, Eisner RL (1983) Boundary determination methods for attenuation correction in single photon emission computed tomography. In: Esser PD (ed) Emission computed tomography. Soc Nucl Med, New York, p 33

Harding G (1982) On the sensitivity and application possibilities of a noval compton scatter Imaging System. IEEE Trans Nucl Sci NS-29:1260–1265

Harper PV (1968) The three-dimensional reconstruction of isotope distributions. In: Gottschalk A, Beck TN (eds) Fundamental problems in scanning. Thomas, Springfield, p 191

Harper PV, Beck RN, Charleston DE, Brunsden B, Lathrop KA (1965) The three dimensional mapping and display of radioisotope distributions. J Nucl Med 6:332 (Abs)

Harris FJ (1978) On the use of windows for harmonic analysis with the discrete fourier transform. Proc of the IEEE 66:51

Hart HE, Rudin S (1977) Three-dimensional imaging of multimillimeter sized cold lesions by focusing collimator coincidence scanning (FCCS). IEEE Trans Biomed Eng BME-24:169–177

Hasegawa B, Kirch D, Stern D, Adams M, Sklar J, Johnson T, Steele P (1982) Single-photon emission tomography with a 12-Pinhole collimator. J Nucl Med 23:606–612

Hedde JP, Reischies FM, Felix R, Helmchen H, Kanowski S (1982) Untersuchungen der regionalen Hirndurchblutung mit dem dynamischen Emissions-Computertomographen nach Inhalation von Xenon-133. Nuc Compact 13:309–312

Hedde JP, Reischies FM, Fiegler W, Felix R, Helmchen H, Kanowski S (1984) Tomographische nicht-invasive Messung der regionalen Hirndurchblutung. Fortschr Röntgenstr 140:128–135

Heffernan PB, Robb RA (1983) Image reconstruction from incomplete projection data: Iterative reconstruction-reprojection techniques. IEEE Trans Biomed Eng BME-30/12:838–841

Helmers H, Boetticher H von, Schmitz-Feuerhake I (1982) Depth – discrimination in direct 3D-scanning without image reconstruction using a coincidence technique. Eur J Nucl Med 7:324–326

Henriksen L, Lassen NA, Paulson OB (1980) Dynamic single photon emission tomography of the brain by Xenon-133 inhalation. Preliminary clinical studies. In: Höfer R, Bergman (Hrsg) Radioaktive Isotope in Klinik und Forschung 14. Egermann, Wien, S 463

Herman GT (1979a) The mathematics of wobbling a ring of positron annihilation detectors. IEEE Trans Nucl Sci NS-26/2:2756–2759

Herman GT (1979b) Data collection for cross-sectional image reconstruction by a moving ring of positron annihilation detectors. J Comput Assist Tomogr 3:261–266

Herman GT, Lung HP (1980) Reconstruction from divergent beams: A comparison of algorithms with and without rebinning. Comput Biol Med 10:131–139

Herman GT, Naparstek A (1977) Fast image reconstruction based on a Radon inversion formula appropriate for rapidly collected data. SIAM J Appl Math 33:511–533

Herman GT, Rowland SW (1973) Three methods for reconstructing objects from X-Rays: A comparative study. Comp Graph Image Proc 2:151–178

Herman GT, Lakshminarayanan AV, Naparstek A (1976) Convolution reconstruction techniques for divergent beams. Comput Biol Med 6:259–271

Herman GT, Rowland SW, Yau M (1979) A comparative study of the use of linear and modified cubic spline interpolation for image reconstruction. IEEE Trans Nucl Sci NS-26/2:2879–2893

Herscovitch P, Markham J, Raichle ME (1983) Brain blood flow measured with intravenous H_2O-15. I. theory and error analysis. J Nucl Med 24:782–789

Higa T, Tanada S, Taki W, Fukuyama H, Ishii Y, Fujita T, Yonekawa Y, Odori T, Mukai T, Handa H, Kameyama M, Morita R, Torizuka K (1983) Superimposition of Krypton-81m single photon emission CT and X-Ray CT images for cerebral blood flow evaluation. J Comput Assist Tomogr 7:37–41

Hill TC, Costello P, Gramm HF, Lovett R, McNeil BJ, Treves S (1978) Early clinical experience with a radionuclide emission computed tomographic brain imaging system. Radiology 128:803–806

Hirose Y, Ikeda Y, Higashi Y, Koga K, Hattori H, Kanno I, Miura Y, Miura S, Uemura K (1982) A hybrid emission CT – HEADTOME II. IEEE Trans Nucl Sci NS-29/1:520–523

Hoffman EJ (1982) 180° compared with 360° sampling in SPECT. J Nucl Med 23:745–747

Hoffman EJ, Phelps ME, Mullani NA, Higgins CS, Ter-Pogossian MM (1976) Design and performance characteristics of a whole-body positron transaxial tomograph. J Nucl Med 17:493–502

Hoffman EJ, Phelps ME, Weiss ES, Welch MJ, Coleman RE, Sobel BE, Ter-Pogossian MM (1977) Transaxial tomographic imaging of canine myocardium with C-11-Palmitic acid. J Nucl Med 18:57–61

Hoffman EJ, Huang SC, Phelps ME (1979a) Quantitation in positron emission computed tomography: 1. Effect of object size. J Comput Assist Tomogr 3:299–308

Hoffman EJ, Phelps ME, Wisenberg G, Schelbert HR, Kuhl DE (1979b) Electrocardiographic gating in positron emission computed tomography. J Comput Assist Tomogr 3:733–739

Hoffman EJ, Phelps ME, Ricci AR, Huang SC, Kuhl DE (1979c) Optimization of system design parameters for emission computed tomography. IEEE/EMBS CH 1440-7/79:363–368

Hoffman EJ, Phelps ME, Huang SC, Kuhl DE, Crabtree M, Burke M, Burgiss S, Keyser R, Highfill R, Williams C (1981a) A new tomograph for quantitative positron emission computed tomography of the brain. IEEE Trans Nucl Sci NS-28/1:99–103

Hoffman EJ, Huang SC, Phelps ME, Kuhl DE (1981b) Quantitation in positron emission computed tomography: 4. Effect of accidental coincidences. J Comput Assist Tomogr 5:391–400

Hoffman EJ, Huang SC, Plummer D, Phelps ME (1982) Quantitation in positron emission computer tomography: 6. Effect of nonuniform resolution. J Comput Assist Tomogr 6:987–999

Hoffman EJ, Phelps ME, Huang SC (1983a) Performance Evaluation of a positron tomograph designed for brain imaging. J Nucl Med 24:245–257

Hoffman EJ, Ricci AR, van der Stee L, Phelps ME (1983b) ECAT III – Basic design considerations. IEEE Trans Nucl Sci NS-30:729–733

Holman BL, Idoine JD, Sos TA, Tancrell R, Meester G de (1977) Tomographic scintigraphy of regional myocardial perfusion. J Nucl Med 18:764–769

Holman BL, Hill TC, Wynne J, Lovett RD, Zimmerman RE, Smith EM (1979) Single-photon transaxial emission computed tomography of the heart in normal subjects and in patients with infarction. J Nucl Med 20:736–740

Houle S, Joy MLG (1977) Quantum utilization limits for collimators and coded apertures. IAEA-SM-210/156. In: IAEA (ed) Medical radionuclide imaging, vol 1. IAEA, Vienna, pp 219–229

Hounsfield GN (1972) A method of and apparatus for examination of a body by radiation such as X or gamma radiation. The Patent Office, London, Patent Specification 1283915

Hounsfield GN (1973) Computerized transverse axial scanning (tomography): part I. Description of system. Br J Radiol 46:1016–1022

Huang SC, Hoffman EJ, Phelps ME, Kuhl DE (1979) Quantitation in positron emission computed tomography: 2. Effects of inaccurate attenuation correction. J Comput Assist Tomogr 3:804–814

Huang SC, Hoffman EJ, Phelps ME, Kuhl DE (1980) Quantitation in positron emission computed tomography: 3. Effect of sampling. J Comput Assist Tomogr 4:819–826

Huang SC, Carson RE, Phelps ME, Hoffman EJ, Schelbert HR, Kuhl DE (1981) A boundary method for attenuation correction in positron computed tomography. J Nucl Med 22:627–637

Huang SC, Carson RE, Hoffman EJ, Kuhl DE, Phelps ME (1982a) An investigation of a double-tracer technique for positron computerized tomography. J Nucl Med 23:816–822

Huang SC, Frazee J, Carson RE, Mazziotta J, Phelps ME, Hoffman EJ, MacDonald N, Kuhl DE (1982b) An investigation of a tomographic technique for in vivo measurement of local cerebral blood flow and water partition coefficient. In: Raynaud C (ed) Nuclear medicine and biology II. Pergamon, Paris, p 1965

Huesman RH (1977) The effects of a finite number of projections angles and finite lateral sampling of projections on the propagation of statistical errors in transverse section reconstruction. Phys Med Biol 22:511–521

Huesman RH, Cahoon JL (1980) Data acquisition, reconstruction and display for the donner 280-Crystal positron tomograph. IEEE Trans Nucl Sci NS-27/1:474–478

Huesman RH, Gullberg GT, Greenberg WL, Budinger TF (1977) Donner algorithms for reconstruction tomography. Lawrence Berkeley Laboratory, University of California, PUB 214

Huesman RH, Derenzo SE, Budinger TF (1982) A two position sampling scheme for positron emission tomography. In: Raynaud C (ed) Nuclear medicine and biology I. Pergamon, Paris, p 542

Hundeshagen H (1979) Entwicklung der Gerätetechnik und ihre Reflexion auf die nuklearmedizinische Praxis. In: Schmidt HAE, Ortiz Berrocal J (Hrsg) Nuklearmedizin 1978. Schattauer, Stuttgart, S 2

Inouye T (1979) Image reconstruction with limited angle projection data. IEEE Trans Nucl Sci NS-26/2:2666–2669

Isenberg JF, Simon W (1978) Radionuclide axial tomography by half-backprojection. Phys Med Biol 23:154–158

Jahangir SM, Brill AB, Bizais YJC, Rowe RW (1983) Count-rate variations with orientation of camera detector. J Nucl Med 24:356–359

Jarritt PH, Cullum ID (1983) Quality control of single photon emission tomographic systems. In: Mould RF (ed) Quality control of nuclear medicine instrumentation. The Hospital Physicists, Ass, London, p 81

Jarritt PH, Ell PJ, Myers MJ, Brown NJG, Deacon JM (1979) A new transverse-section brain imager for single-gamma emitters. J Nucl Med 20:319–327

Jarritt PH, Cullum ID, Ell PJ (1981) SPECT I – figures of merit for two multiple detector (single slice) and one area detector (multiple slice) single photon emission tomographic instruments. In: IAEA (ed) Medical radionuclide imaging 1980, vol I. IAEA, Vienna, p 243

Jaszczak RJ (1982) Physical characteristics of SPECT systems, September, 1982. J Comput Assist Tomogr 6:1205–1215

Jaszczak RJ, Coleman RE (1980) Selected processing techniques for scintillation camera based SPECT systems. In: Soc Nucl Med, NY (ed) Single photon emission computed tomography. Soc Nucl Med, New York, p 45

Jaszczak RJ, Murphy PH, Huard D, Burdine JA (1977) Radionuclide emission computed tomography of the head with Tc-99m and a sczintillation camera. J Nucl Med 18:373–380

Jaszczak RJ, Chang LT, Stein NA, Moore FE (1979a) Whole-body single-photon emission computed tomography using dual, largefield-of-view scintillation cameras. Phys Med Biol 24:1123–1143

Jaszczak RJ, Chang LT, Murphy PH (1979b) Single Photon Emission Computed Tomography using Multi-Slice Fan Beam Collimators. IEEE Trans Nucl Sci NS-26/1:610–618

Jaszczak RJ, Coleman RE, Lim CB (1980) Spect:

Single photon emission computed tomography. IEEE Trans Nucl Sci NS-27/3:1137–1153

Jaszczak RJ, Coleman RE, Whitehead FR (1981) Physical factors affecting quantitative measurements using camera-based single photon emission computed tomography (SPECT). IEEE Trans Nucl Sci Ns-28:69–80

Jaszczak RJ, Greer K, Coleman RE (1982a) Lesion detection with SPECT and conventional imaging in the presence of source motion. In: Raynaud C (ed) Nuclear medicine and biology I. Pergamon, Paris, p 461

Jaszczak RJ, Whitehead FR, Lim CB, Coleman RE (1982b) Lesion detection with single-photon emission computed tomography (SPECT) compared with conventional imaging. J Nucl Med 23:97–102

Jaszczak RJ, Greer K, Coleman RE (1983) SPECT system misalignment: Comparison of phantom and patient images. In: Esser PD (ed) Emission computed tomography. Soc Nucl Med, New York, p 57

Jaszczak RJ, Greer KL, Carey CF, Harris CC, Coleman RE (1984) Improved SPECT quantification using compensation for scattered photons. J Nucl Med 25:893–900

Jeavons A (1979) The CERN proportional chamber positron camera. In: Hasiguti RR, Fujiwara K (eds) Proc 5th Int Conf on Positron Annihilation. The Japan Institute of Metals, p 355

Jeavons AP, Charpak G, Stubbs RJ (1975) The high-density multiwire drift chamber. Nucl Instr Meth 124:491–503

Jeavons A, Schorr B, Kull K, Townsend D, Frey P, Donath A (1981) A large-area stationary positron camera using wire chambers. In: IAEA (ed) Medical radionuclide imaging 1980, vol I. IAEA, Vienna, p 49

Johnson TK, Kirch DL, Hasegawa BH, Thompson D, Steele PP (1983) Spatial/temporal/energy dependence of scintillation camera nonlinearities. In: Esser PD (ed) Emission computed tomography: Current trends. Soc Nucl Med, New York, p 71

Jordan K (1980) Grundlagen der Strahlenmeßtechnik. In: Hundeshagen H (ed) Nuklearmedizin. Springer, Berlin Heidelberg New York (Handbuch der medizinischen Radiologie, Bd XV/1A, S 131)

Jordan K (1981) Die Verfahren der Emissions-Computertomographie und ihre Grenzen. In: Pöppl SJ, Pretschner DP (Hrsg) Systeme und Signalverarbeitung in der Nuklearmedizin. Springer, Berlin Heidelberg New York, S 222

Jordan K, Geisler S (1973) Data display in scintigraphy by means of a high-speed electrostatic plotter and special computer averaging techniques. In: IAEA (ed) Medical radioisotope scintigraphy 1972. IAEA, Vienna, p 635

Jordan K, Gettner U (1977) Rechnergesteuerte Über-wachung von 60 Szintillationsmeßsonden in einem Tomographiescanner. In: Schmidt HAE (Hrsg) Nuklearmedizin 1975. Schattauer, Stuttgart, S 300

Jordan K, Gettner U (1981) Einsatz der Flugzeitmessung bei quantitativen dynamischen Untersuchungen mit Positronen-Strahlern. In: Schmidt HAE, Wolf F, Mahlstedt J (Hrsg) Nuklearmedizin 1980. Schattauer, Stuttgart, S 27

Jordan K, Gettner U (1982) Dreidimensionale Ortung von Positronen-Strahlern mit Hilfe der Flugzeitmessung. In: Höfer R, Bergmann H (Hrsg) Radioaktive Isotope in Klinik und Forschung, Bd 15. Egermann, Vienna, S 219

Jordan K, Friel HI, Gettner U, Kaempf E, Geisler S, Harsdorf J von, Nentwig C (1974) A new concept of an experimental tomographic scanner. In: WFNMB (ed) Proceedings of the First World Congress of Nuclear Medicine. WFNMB, Tokyo Kyoto, p 1274

Jordan K, Gettner U, Judas R (1982) A real time functional positron camera using time-of-flight techniques. In: Bleifeld W, Harder D et al. (eds) Proceedings of the World Congress on Medical Physics and Biomedical Engineering 1982. MPBE, Hamburg, p 21.07

Jordan K, Judas R, Gettner U, Knoop BO, Newiger H (1984a) SATOF I: Ein Positronen Ringtomograph der Signalverstärkung (SAT) und Flugzeitmesstechnik (TOF) vereint. In: Höfer R, Bergmann H (Hrsg) Radioaktive Isotope in Klinik und Forschung. 16. Band, Egermann, Wien, S 509

Jordan K, Gettner U, Judas R, Knoop BO (1984b) SATOF I: A new design concept for a whole body positron emission tomograph with small rectangular crystals, high packing fraction, and excellent TOF-resolution. In: Schmidt HAE, Vauramo E (Hrsg) Nuklearmedizin 1984. Schattauer, Stuttgart, S 3

Judas R, Jordan K, Gettner U (1984) Bariumfluorid – Ein schneller anorganischer Szintillator im Vergleich mit CsF und NE 102 A. In: Schmidt HAE, Adam WE (Hrsg) Nuklearmedizin 1983. Schattauer, Stuttgart, S 24

Kairento AL, Brownell GL, Schluederberg J, Elmaleh DR (1983) Regional blood-flow measurement in rabbit soft-tissue tumor with positron imaging using the CO_2-15 steady-state and labeled microspheres. J Nucl Med 24:1135–1142

Kanno I, Uemura K, Miura S, Miura Y (1981) HEADTOME: A hybrid emission tomograph for single photon and positron emission imaging of the brain. J Comput Assist Tomogr 5:216–226

Kaplan SN, Kaufman L, Perez-Mendez V, Valentine K (1973) Multiwire proportional chambers for biomedical applications. Nucl Instr Meth 106:397–406

Kaufman L, Ewins J, Rowan W, Hosier K, Okerlund M, Ortendahl D (1980) Semiconductor gamma-cameras in nuclear medicine. IEEE Trans Nucl Sci NS-27/3:1073–1079

Kay DB, Keyes JW (1975) First order correction for absorption and resolution compensation in radionuclide fourier tomography. J Nucl Med 16:540–541

Kay DB, Keyes JW, Simon W (1974) Radionuclide tomographic image reconstruction using fourier transform techniques. J Nucl Med 15:981–986

Kearfott KJ (1982a) Absorbed dose estimates for positron emission tomography (PET): CO-15, C-110, and COO-15. J Nucl Med 23:1031–1037

Kearfott KJ (1982b) Radiation absorbed dose estimates for positron emission tomography (PET): K-38, Rb-81, Rb-82, and Cs-130. J Nucl Med 23:1128–1132

Kearfott KJ, Junck L, Rottenberg DA (1983) C-11 Dimethyloxazolidinedione (DMO): Biodistribution, radiation absorbed dose, and potential for PET measurement of regional brain pH: Concise communication. J Nucl Med 24:805–811

Kearfott KJ, Carroll LR (1984) Evaluation of the performance characteristics of the PC 4600 positron emission tomograph. J Comput Assist Tomogr 8:502–513

Kessler RM, Ellis JR, Eden M (1984) Analysis of emission tomographic scan data: Limitations imposed by resolution and background. J Comput Assist Tomogr 8:514–522

Keyes WI (1979) Current status of single photon emission computerized tomography. IEEE Trans Nucl Sci NS-26/2:2752–2755

Keyes WI, Chesser R, Undrill PE (1977) Transversection emission tomography. In: Hay G (ed) Medical images. Wiley, Chichester, p 51

Keyes JW Jr (1982) Perspectives on tomography. J Nucl Med 23:633–640

Keyes JW Jr, Orleanda N, Heetderks WJ, Leonard PF, Rogers WL (1977) The humongotron – a scintillation-camera transaxial tomograph. J Nucl Med 18:381–387

Keyes JW Jr, Leonard PF, Svetkoff DJ, Brody SL, Rogers WL, Lucchesi BR (1978a) Myocardial imaging using emission computed tomography. Radiology 127:809–812

Keyes JW Jr, Leonard PF, Brody SL, Svetkoff DJ, Rogers WL, Lucchesi BR (1978b) Myocardial infarct quantification in the dog by single photon emission computed tomography. Circulation 58:227–232

Keyes JW Jr, Rogers WL, Clinthorne NH, Koral KF, Harkness BA (1982) An image quality maintenance program for rotating gamma camera SPECT. In: Höfer R, Bergmann H (Hrsg) Radioaktive Isotope in Klinik und Forschung, Bd 15. Egermann, Wien, S 529

Kim KI, Tewarson RP, Bizais Y, Rowe RW (1984) Inversion for the attenuated radon transform with constant attenuation. IEEE Trans Nucl Sci NS-31/1:538–542

King PH, Hubner K, Gibbs W, Holloway E (1981) Noise identification and removal in positron imaging systems. IEEE Trans Nucl Sci NS-28/1:148–151

Kirch DL, Vogel RA, LeFree MT, Stern DM, Sklar J, Hasegawa BH, Steele PP (1980) An anger camera/computer system for myocardial perfusion tomography using a seven pinhole collimator. IEEE Trans Nucl Sci NS-27/1:412–420

Kirsch CM, Doliwa R, Büll U, Roedler D (1983) Detection of severe coronary heart disease with Tl-201: Comparison of resting single photon emission tomography with invasive arteriography. J Nucl Med 24:761–767

Kloster G, Laufer P, Wutz W, Stöcklin G (1983) Br-75, 77- and I-123-Analogues of D-Glucose as potential tracers for glucose utilization in heart and brain. Eur J Nucl Med 8:237–241

Klug A, Crowther RA (1972) Three-dimensional image reconstruction from the viewpoint of information theory. Nature 238:435–440

Knoll GF, Williams JJ (1977) Application of a ring pseudorandom aperture for transverse section tomography. IEEE Trans Nucl Sci NS-24/1:581–586

Knoop BO (1980) Positronenmessung: Prinzip und Vorteile gegenüber einfacher Gamma-Messung. Der Nuklearmediziner 3:121–129

Knoop BO (1982) Klinische Anwendung digitaler Bildrekonstruktionsverfahren zur Quantifizierung von Profilmessungen im Ganzkörperzähler und zur nichtinvasiven Nierendurchblutungsbestimmung. Diss Universität Bremen

Knoop BO, Jordan K, Schober O (1984a) Überlegungen zur realistischen Definition der räumlichen Auflösung. In: Schütz J (Hrsg) Medizinische Physik 1983. Hüthig, Heidelberg, S 597

Knoop BO, Jordan K, Judas R, Schober O (1984b) Spatial resolution in imaging systems: Equivalent width a realistic measure to replace FWHM. J Nucl Med 25/5:22 (abs)

Kobayashi M, Morimoto K, Yoshida H, Sugimoto S, Kobayashi S, Chiba M, Ishii M, Akiyama S, Ishibashi H (1983) Bismuth silicate as a scintillating material for electromagnetic shower detectors. Nucl Instr Meth 205:133–136

Koral KF, Rogers WL (1979) Application of ART to timecoded emission tomography. Phys Med Biol 24:879–894

Koral KF, Rogers WL, Knoll GF (1975) Digital tomographic imaging with time-modulated pseudorandom coded aperture and anger camera. J Nucl Med 16:402–413

Koral KF, Freitas JE, Rogers L, Keyes JW (1979) Thyroid scintigraphy with time coded aperture. J Nucl Med 20:345–349

Koral KF, Clinthorne NH, Rogers WL, Keyes JW (1982) Feasibility of sharpening limited-angle tomography by including an orthogonal set of projections. Nucl Instr Meth 193:223–227

Kouris K, Garnett ES, Herman GT (1981) Sampling properties of stationary and half-rotation rings in positron emission tomography. J Comput Assist Tomogr 5:744–754

Kouris K, Herman GT, Tuy HK, Nahmias C (1982a) Coincidence time window, ring sampling and attenuation problems in positron emission tomography. Nucl Instr Meth 193:215–222

Kouris K, Spyrou NM, Jackson DF (1982b) Imaging with ionizing radiations. In: Jackson DF, Mayneord WV (eds) Progress in medical and invironmental physics, vol 1. Surrey University Press

Kouris K, Tuy H, Lent A, Herman GT, Lewitt RM (1982c) Reconstruction from sparsely sampled data by ART with interpolated rays. IEEE Trans Med Imag MI-1:161–167

Kuhl DE (1984) Imaging local brain function with emission computed tomography. Radiology 150:625–631

Kuhl DE, Edwards RQ (1962) Body-section radioisotope scanning. J Nucl Med 3:199 (Abs)

Kuhl DE, Edwards RQ (1963) Image separation radioisotope scanning. Radiology 80:653–662

Kuhl DE, Edwards RQ (1964) Cylindrical and section radioisotope scanning of the liver and brain. Radiology 83:926–936

Kuhl DE, Edwards RQ (1968) Reorganizing data from transverse section scans of the brain using digital processing. Radiology 91:975–983

Kuhl DE, Edwards RQ (1969) Digital processing for modifying and rearranging rectilinear and section scan data under direct observation. In: IAEA (ed) Medical Radioisotope Scintigraphy. IAEA, Vienna, p 703

Kuhl DE, Edwards RQ (1970) The Mark III Scanner: A compact device for multiple-view and section scanning of the brain. Radiology 96:563–570

Kuhl DE, Hale J (1965) Transmission scanning for improved orientation of the emission scan. J Nucl Med 6:333 (Abs)

Kuhl DE, Hale J, Eaton WL (1966) Transmission scanning: A useful adjunct to conventional emission scanning for accurately keying isotope deposition to radiographic anatomy. Radiology 87:278–284

Kuhl DE, Edwards RQ, Ricci AR, Reivich M (1973a) Quantitative section scanning. In: IAEA (ed) Medical radioisotope scintigraphy 1972, vol I. IAEA, Vienna, p 347

Kuhl DE, Edwards RQ, Ricci AR, Reivich M (1973b) Quantitative section scanning using orthogonal tangent correction. J Nucl Med 14:196–200

Kuhl DE, Reivich M, Alavi A, Nyary I, Staum MM (1975) Local cerebral blood volume determined by three-dimensional reconstruction of radionuclide scan data. Circ Res 36:610–619

Kuhl DE, Edwards RQ, Ricci AR, Yacob RJ, Mich TJ, Alavi A (1976) The Mark IV system for radionuclide computed tomography of the brain. Radiology 121:405–413

Kuhl DE, Hoffman EJ, Phelps ME, Ricci A, Reivich M (1977) Design and application of Mark IV scanning system for radionuclide computed tomography of the brain. In: IAEA (ed) Medical radionuclide imaging, vol I. IAEA, Vienna, p 309

Kuhl DE, Phelps ME, Engel J Jr (1980) Emission-computed tomography of Fluoride-18-Fluorodeoxyglucose and Nitrogen-13-Ammonia in stroke and epilepsy. In: IAEA (ed) Medical radionuclide imaging 1980, vol II. IAEA, Vienna, p 333

Kuhl DE, Barrio JR, Huang SC, Selin C, Ackerman RF, Lear JL, Wu JL, Lin TH, Phelps ME (1982) Quantifying local cerebral blood flow by N-Isoprophyl-p-(I-123)Iodoamphetamine (IMP) tomography. J Nucl Med 23:196–203

Kwoh YS, Reed IS, Truong TK (1977) Back projection speed improvement for 3-D reconstruction. IEEE Trans Nucl Sci NS-24/5:1999–2005

Lange K, Carson R (1984) EM reconstruction algorithms for emission and transmission tomography. J Comput Assist Tomogr 8:306–316

Larsson SA (1980) Gamma camera emission tomography. Acta Radiol [Suppl] (Stockh) 363

Larsson SA, Israelsson A (1982) Considerations on system design. Implementation and computer processing in SPECT. IEEE Trans Nucl Sci NS-29/4:1331–1342

Lassen NA (1982) Imaging cerebral blood flow by Xe-133 inhalation and dynamic single photon tomography. In: Schmidt HAE, Rösler H (Hrsg) Nuklearmedizin 1981. Schattauer, Stuttgart, S XLV

Lassen NA, Sveinsdottir E, Kanno I, Stokely EM, Rommer P (1978) A fast moving single photon emission tomograph for regional cerebral blood flow studies in man. J Comput Assist Tomogr 2:661–662 (Abs)

Lassen NA, Henriksen L, Paulson O (1981) Regional cerebral blood flow in stroke by Xe-133 inhalation and emission tomography. Stroke 12:284–288

Lassen NA, Henriksen L, Holm S, Barry I, Paulson OB, Vorstrup S, Rapin J, le Poncin-Lafitte M, Moretti JL, Askienazy S, Raynaud C (1983) Cerebral blood-flow tomography: Xenon-133 compared with Isoprophyl-Amphetamine-Iodine-123. J Nucl Med 24:17–21

Lauritzen M, Henriksen L, Lassen NA (1981) Regional cerebral blood flow during rest and skilled hand movements by Xenon-133 inhalation and emission computerized tomography. J Cereb Blood Flow Metab 1:385–389

Lauterbur PC (1973) Measurements of local nuclear magnetic resonance relaxation times. Bull Am Phys Soc Ser II/18:86 (Abs)

Laval M, Allemand R, Campagnolo R, Garderet P, Gariod R, Guinet P, Moszynski M, Tournier E,

Vacher J (1982) Contribution of the time-of-flight information to the positron tomographic imaging. In: Raynaud C (ed) Nuclear medicine and biology III. Pergamon, Paris, p 2315

Laval M, Moszynski M, Allemand R, Cormoreche E, Guinet P, Odru R, Vacher J (1983) Barium fluoride – inorganic scintillator for subnanosecond timing. Nucl Instr Meth 206:169–176

Ledley RS, di Chiro G, Luessenhop AJ, Twigg HL (1974) Computerized transaxial X-ray tomography of the human body. Science 186:207–212

Le Free MT, Vogel RA, Kirch DL, Steele PP (1981) Seven-pinhole tomography – a technical description. J Nucl Med 22:48–54

Leichter I, Karellas A, Craven JD, Greenfield MA (1984) The effect of the momentum transfer on the sensitivity of a photon scattering method for the characterization of tissues. Med Phys 11:31–36

Levy G (1974) Comment on fresnel zone plate imaging in nuclear medicine. J Nucl Med 15:214–215

Lewis SE, Stokely EM, Devous MD, Bonte FJ, Buja LM, Parkey RW, Willerson JT (1981) Quantitation of experimental canine infarct size with multipinhole and rotating-slanthole tomography. J Nucl Med 22:1000–1005

Lewis MH, Bonte FJ, Lewis SE, Stokely EM (1982) Work in progress: A comparison of data collection protocols for single photon emission tomography: 180° versus 360°. Radiology 145:501–504

Lim CB, Chang LT, Jaszczak RJ (1980) Performance analysis of three camera configurations for single photon emission computed tomography. IEEE Trans Nucl Sci NS-27/1:559–568

Lim CB, Cheng A, Boyd DP, Hattner RS (1978) A 3-D iterative reconstruction method for stationary planar positron cameras. IEEE Trans Nucl Sci NS-25/1:196–201

Lim CB, Han KS, Hawman EG, Jaszczak RL (1982) Image noise, resolution and lesion detectability in single photon emission CT. IEEE Trans Nucl Sci NS-29/1:500–505

Llacer J (1979) Theory of imaging with a very limited number of projections. IEEE Trans Nucl Sci NS-26/1:596–602

Llacer J (1982) Tomographic image reconstruction by eigenvector decomposition: Its limitations and areas of applicability. IEEE Trans Med Imag MI-1:34–42

Llacer J, Spieler H, Goulding FS (1982) Theoretical analysis of the use of germanium detectors for time-of-flight emission tomography. In: IEEE (ed) 1982 workshop on time-of-flight tomography. IEEE Computer Soc. Los Angeles, p 75

Lonn AHR, Rowbotham GD, Holman LA (1983) Monitoring rotating gamma camera performance for emission tomography. In: Mould RF (ed) Quality control of nuclear medicine instrumentation. The Hospital Physicists' Ass, London, p 92

Lottes G (1982) Verfahren zur iterativen Rekonstruktion bei der longitudinalen „Single-Photon-Emission-Computed-Tomography (SPECT)" am Beispiel eines Multidetektor-Scanners. Diss Medizinische Hochschule Hannover

Lottes G, Jordan K (1978a) Anwendung von iterativen Korrekturverfahren bei der longitudinalen Tomographie. In: Oeff K, Schmidt HAE (Hrsg) Nuklearmedizin 1976, Bd II. Medico Informationsdienste, Berlin, S 460

Lottes G, Jordan K (1978b) Der Einfluß des statistischen Rauschens auf die Bildrekonstruktion bei der longitudinalen Computer-Emissions-Tomographie. In: Schmidt HAE, Woldring M (Hrsg) Nuklearmedizin 1977. Schattauer, Stuttgart, S 53

Lottes G, Jordan K (1978c) Demonstration von rekonstruierten Schichtbildern der longitudinalen Emissions-Tomographie. In: Schmidt HAE, Woldring M (Hrsg) Nuklearmedizin 1977. Schattauer, Stuttgart, S 69

Lottes G, Jordan K (1979a) Vergleich von verschiedenen Rekonstruktions-Algorithmen bei der longitudinalen Emissions-Tomographie. In: Schmidt HAE, Ortiz-Berrocal J (Hrsg) Nuklearmedizin 1978. Schattauer, Stuttgart, S 57

Lottes G, Jordan K (1979b) Ergebnisse der longitudinalen Emissionstomographie. In: Schmidt HAE, Ortiz-Berrocal J (Hrsg) Nuklearmedizin 1978. Schattauer, Stuttgart, S 81

Lottes G, Jordan K (1980) Möglichkeiten zur Absorptionskorrektur bei der longitudinalen Emissionstomographie. In: Schmidt HAE, Riccabona G (Hrsg) Nuklearmedizin 1979. Schattauer, Stuttgart, S 118

Lottes G, Jordan K (1981) Demonstration von Randfehlereinflüssen bei der longitudinalen Emissionstomographie anhand von klinischen Aufnahmen. In: Schmidt HAE, Wolf F, Mahlstedt J (Hrsg) Nuklearmedizin 1980. Schattauer, Stuttgart, S 23

MacIntyre WJ, Go RT, Houser TS, Sufka B, Napoli C, Cook SA (1982) Evaluation of 180-DEG and 360 DEG reconstruction of the heart by transaxial tomography with thallium-201. In: Esser PD (ed) Digital imaging. Soc of nuclear medicine. Inc, New York, p 197

Marr RB (1974) On the reconstruction of a function on a circular domain from a sampling of its line integrals. J Math Analysis and Applications 45:357–374

Mathieu L, Budinger TF (1974) Pinhole digital tomography. In: WFNMB (ed) Proceedings of the first world congress of nuclear medicine. WFNMB, Tokyo Kyoto, p 1264

Maublant J, Cassagnes J, Le Jeune JJ, Mestas D, Veyre A, Jallut H, Meyniel G (1982) A comparison between conventional scintigraphy and emission tomography with thallium-201 in the detection of myocardial infarction: Concise communication. J Nucl Med 23:204–208

Mazziotta JC, Phelps ME, Plummer D, Kuhl DE (1981) Quantitation in positron emission computed tomography: 5. Physical-Anatomical Effects. J Comput Assist Tomogr 5:734–743

McAffee JG, Mozley JM (1969) Longitudinal tomographic radioisotopic imaging with a scintillation camera: Theoretical considerations of a new method. J Nucl Med 10:654–659

McCready VR, Flower MA, Meller ST (1980) A clinical and physical evaluation of an emission tomographic system. In: Höfer R, Bergmann H (Hrsg) Radioaktive Isotope in Klinik und Forschung 14. Egermann, Wien, S 251

McIntyre JA (1980a) A three-dimensional position-sensitive gamma ray detection system. Nucl Instr Meth 171:19–27

McIntyre JA (1980b) Design features of a positron tomograph with 2.4 mm resolution. IEEE Trans Nucl Sci NS-27/4:1305–1311

McIntyre JA (1980c) Plastic scintillation detectors for high resolution emission computed tomography. J Comp Assist Tomogr 4:351–360

McIntyre JA (1982) Plastic scintillators for time-of-flight tomography. In: IEEE (ed) 1982 workshop on time-of-flight tomography. IEEE Computer Soc, Los Angeles, p 51

McKee BTA (1982) Towards high-resolution positron emission tomography for small volumes. In: Coleman PG, Sharma SC, Diana LM (eds) Positron annihilation. North-Holland, Amsterdam, p 955

Mersereau RM (1973) Recovering multidimensional signals from their projections. Comp Graph Image Proc 1:179–195

Mersereau RM (1976) Direct fourier transform techniques in 3-D image reconstruction. Comput Biol Med 6:247–258

Metz CE, Beck RN (1974) Quantitative effects of stationary linear image processing and noise and resolution of structure in radionuclide images. J Nucl Med 15:164–169

Meyer GJ, Schober O, Gielow P, Hundeshagen H (1982) Functional imaging of the pancreas by positron emission tomography: Routine production of C-11-L-Methionine, quality control, methodology. In: Raynaud C (ed) Nuclear medicine and biology II. Pergamon, Paris, p 1977

Meyer GJ, Schober O, Hundeshagen H (1983) Konstante Infusion von O-15-markiertem Wasser und Inhalation von C-11-markiertem Kohlenmonoxid als methodische Grundlage zur regionalen Bestimmung des Lungenwassers mittels Positronen-Emissionstomographie. Nucl Med XXII:121–127

Mintun MA, Raichle ME, Martin WRW, Herscovitch P (1984) Brain oxygen utilization measured with O-15 radiotracers and positron emission tomography. J Nucl Med 25:177–187

Miraldi F, Chiro G di (1970) Tomographic techniques in radioisotope imaging with a proposal of a new device: The tomoscanner. Radiology 94:513–520

Miraldi F, Chiro G di, Skoff G (1969) Evaluation of current methods of radioisotope tomography and design of a new device: The tomoscanner. J Nucl Med 10:358 (Abs)

Mirell SG, Hecht HS, Hopkins JM, Blahd WH (1981) Biplanar cardiac blood-pool tomography. J Nucl Med 22:913–920

Monahan WG, Beattie JW, Laughlin JS (1970) Operation and use of a scintillation camera system with three-dimensional resolution for positron emitters. J Nucl Med 11:347 (Abs)

Monahan WG, Beattie JW, Powell MD, Laughlin JS (1973) Total organ kinetic imaging monitor. In: IAEA (ed) Medical radioisotope scintigraphy 1972, vol I. IAEA, Vienna, p 285

Moore SC (1982) Attenuation compensation. In: Ell PJ, Holman BL (eds) Computed emission tomography. Oxford University Press, Oxford, p 339

Moore SC, Brunelle JA, Kirsch CM (1982) Quantitative multi-detector emission computerized tomography using iterative attenuation compensation. J Nucl Med 23:706–714

Moore RH, Alpert NM, Strauss HW (1983) A variable angle slant-hole collimator. J Nucl Med 24:61–65

Moszynski M, Gresset C, Vacher J, Odru R (1981) Timing properties of BGO scintillator. Nucl Instr Meth 188:403–409

Moszynski M, Allemand R, Laval M, Odru R, Vacher J (1983) Recent progress in fast timing with CsF scintillators in application to time-of-flight positron tomography in medicine. Nucl Instr Meth 205:239–249

Muehllehner G (1970) Rotating collimator tomography. J Nucl Med 11:347 (Abs)

Muehllehner G (1971) A tomographic scintillation camera. Phys Med Biol 16:87–96

Muehllehner G (1973) Performance parameters for a tomographic scintillation camera. In: Freedman GS (ed) Tomographic imaging in nuclear medicine. Soc Nucl Med Inc, New York, p 76

Muehllehner G (1975) Positron camera with extended counting rate cabability. J Nucl Med 16:653–657

Muehllehner G (1976) Resolution limit of positron cameras. J Nucl Med 17:757

Muehllehner G, Colsher JG (1980) Use of positron sensitive detectors in positron imaging. IEEE Trans Nucl Sci NS-27/1:569–571

Muehllehner G, Colsher J (1981) Single photon imaging. New instrumentation and techniques. In: IAEA (ed) Medical radionuclide imaging 1980, vol I. IAEA, Vienna, p 173

Muehllehner G, Colsher JG (1982) Positron computed tomography: 1. Instrumentation. In: Ell PJ, Holman BL (eds) Computed emission tomography. Oxford Univ Press, Oxford, p 3

Muehllehner G, Hashmi Z (1972) Quantification of the depth effect of tomographic and section imaging devices. Phys Med Biol 17:251–260

Muehllehner G, Wetzel RA (1971) Section imaging by computer calculation. J Nucl Med 12:76–84

Muehllehner G, Buchin MP, Dudek JH (1976) Performance parameters of a positron imaging camera. IEEE Trans Nucl Sci NS-23/1:528–537

Muehllehner G, Atkins F, Harper PV (1977) Positron camera with longitudinal and transverse tomographic capabilities. In: IAEA (ed) Medical radionuclide imaging, vol I. IAEA, Vienna, p 291

Mullani NA, Higgins CS, Hood JT, Currie CM (1978) PETT IV: Design analysis and performance characteristics. IEEE Trans Nucl Sci NS-25/1:180–183

Mullani NA, Ficke DC, Ter-Pogossian MM (1980a) Cesium fluoride: a new detector for positron emission tomography. IEEE Trans Nucl Sci NS-27/1:572–575

Mullani NA, Markham J, Ter-Pogossian MM (1980b) Feasibility of time-of-flight reconstruction in positron emission tomography. J Nucl Med 21:1095–1097

Mullani NA, Gould KL, Gaeta JM (1981) Tomographic imaging of the heart with thallium-201: Seven-pinhole or rotating gamma camera? J Nucl Med 22:925–926

Mullani NA, Wong WH, Hartz RK, Yerian K, Philippe EA, Gould KL (1982) Design of TOFPET: A high resolution time-of-flight positron camera. In: IEEE (ed) 1982 Workshop on time-of-flight tomography. IEEE Computer Soc, Los Angeles, p 31

Mullani NA, Wong WH, Hartz R, Yerian K, Philippe EA, Gaeta JM, Gould KL (1983) Preliminary results with TOFPET. IEEE Trans Nucl Sci NS-30:739–743

Murayama H, Nohara N, Tanaka E, Hayashi T (1982) A quad BGO detector and its timing and positioning discrimination for positron computed tomography. Nucl Inst Meth 192:501–511

Murphy PH, Thompson WL, Moore ML, Burdine JA (1979) Radionuclide computed tomography of the body using routine radiopharmaceuticals. I. System characterization. J Nucl Med 20:102–107

Myers MJ, Buseman Sokole E, Bakker J de (1983) A comparison of rotating slant hole collimator and rotating camera for single photon emission tomography of the heart. Phys Med Biol 28:581–588

Myers WG, Bigler RE, Benua RS, Graham MC, Laughlin JS (1983) PET tomographic imaging of the human heart, pancreas and liver with nitrogen-13 derived from (N-13)-L-Glutamate. Eur J Nucl Med 8:381–384

Nahmias C, Kenyon DB, Garnett ES (1982) Experience with a high efficiency positron emission tomograph. IEEE Trans Nucl Sci NS-29/1:548–550

Nahmias C, Firnau G, Garnett ES (1984) Performance characteristics of the McMaster positron emission tomograph. IEEE Trans Nucl Sci NS-31:637–639

Nalcioglu O, Cho ZH, Lou RY (1979) Limited field of view reconstruction in computerized tomography. IEEE Trans Nucl Sci NS-26/1:546–551

Nassi M, Brody WR, Medoff BP, Macovski A (1982) Iterative reconstruction-reprojection: An algorithm for limited data cardiac-computed tomography. IEEE Trans Biomed Eng BME-29:333–340

Nestor OH, Huang CY (1975) Bismuth germanate: A High-Z gamma-ray and charged particle detector. IEEE Trans Nucl Sci NS-22/1:68–71

Newell RR, Saunders W, Miller ER (1952) Multichannel collimators for gamma-ray scanning with scintillation counters. Nucleonics 10:36

Nichols AB, Cochavi S, Hales CA, Beller GA, Strauss HW (1979) Resolution rates of pulmonary embolism assessed by serial positron imaging with inhaled O-15-labeled carbon dioxide. J Nucl Med 20:281–286

Nickles RJ, Meyer HO (1978) Design of a three-dimensional positron camera for nuclear medicine. Phys Med Biol 23:686–695

Nohara N, Tanaka E, Tomitani T, Yamamoto M, Murayama H, Suda Y, Endo M, Iinuma T, Tateno Y, Shishido F, Ishimatsu K, Ueda K, Takami K (1980) Positologica: A positron ECT device with a continuously rotating detector ring. IEEE Trans Nucl Sci NS-27/3:1128–1132

Ogawa K, Nakajima M, Yuta S (1984) A reconstruction algorithm for truncated projections. IEEE Trans Med Imag MI-3/1:34–40

O'Leary DH, Hill TC, Lee RGL, Clouse ME, Holman BL (1983) The use of I-123-Iodoamphetamine and single-photon emission computed tomography to assess local cerebral blood flow. AJNR 4:547–549

Oppenheim BE (1974) More accurate algorithms for iterative 3-dimensional reconstruction. IEEE Trans Nucl Sci NS-21/3:72–77

Oppenheim BE (1975) Three-dimensional reconstruction from incomplete projections. In: Raynaud C, Todd-Pokropek A (eds) Information processing in scintigraphy. Proceedings of the IVth international Conference, Orsay 1975, p 288–324

Oppenheim BE (1980) Algebraic reconstruction technique (ART) for transaxial emission computed tomography. In: Soc Nucl Med (ed) Single photon emission computed tomography. Proc 10th Symp Soc Nucl Med Computer Council, Soc Nucl Med Inc, NY, p 31–44

Oppenheim BE (1984) Scatter correction for SPECT. J Nucl Med 25:928–929

Ore A, Powell JL (1949) Three-photon annihilation of an electron-positron pair. Phys Rev 75:1696–1699

Osamu I (1983) A new metabolically trapped agent by brain monoamine oxidase: N-methyl labeled (C-14) N-methylphenylethylamine (C-14-MPEA). Eur J Nucl Med 8:385–388

Ott RJ, Bateman JE, Flesher AC, Flower MA, Leach MO, Webb S, Khan O, McCready VR (1983a) Preliminary clinical images from a prototype positron camera. Br J Radiol 56:773–776

Ott RJ, Flower MA, Khan O, Kalirei T, Webb S, Leach MO, McCready VR (1983b) A comparison between 180° and 360° data reconstruction in single photon emission computed tomography of the liver and spleen. Br J Radiol 56:931–937

Pang SC, Genna S (1979) The effect of compton scattered photons on emission computerized transaxial tomography. IEEE Trans Nucl Sci NS-26/2:2772–2774

Patton J, Brill AB, Erickson J, Cook WE, Jonston RE (1969) A new approach to mapping three-dimensional radionuclide destributions. J Nucl Med Med 10:363 (Abs)

Patton JA, Brill AB, King PH (1973) Transverse section brain scanning with a multicrystal cylindrical imaging device. In: Freedman GS (ed) Tomographic imaging in nuclear medicine. Soc Nucl Med Inc, New York, p 28

Patton JA, Price RR, Brill AB, Pehl R (1977) A mosaic intrinsic germanium radioisotope scanning device with longitudinal section scanning capability. In: IAEA (ed) Medical radionuclide imaging, vol I. IAEA, Vienna, p 159

Patton JA, Price RR, Rollo FD, Brill AB, Pehl RH (1978) Clinical and experimental results with a 9 element high purity germanium array. IEEE Trans Nucl Sci NS-25/1:653–656

Patton JA, Price RR, Pickens DR, Brill AB (1980) Techniques for X-Ray fluorescence tomography. IEEE Trans Nucl Sci NS-27:421–424

Pelc NJ, Chesler DA (1979) Utilization of cross-plane rays for three-dimensional reconstruction by filtered back-projection. J Comput Assist Tomogr 3:385–395

Peres A (1979) Tomographic reconstruction from limited angular data. J Comput Assist Tomogr 3:800–803

Perez-Mendez V, Schwartz G, Nelson WR, Bellazini R, Del Guerra A, Massai MM, Spandre G (1983) Further improvements in the design of a positron camera with dense drift space MWPCs. Nucl Instr Meth 217:89–91

Phelps ME (1977a) What is the purpose of emission computed tomography in nuclear medicine? J Nucl Med 18:399–402

Phelps ME (1977b) Emission computed tomography. Semin Nucl Med 7:337–365

Phelps ME (1981) Positron computed tomography studies of cerebral glucose metabolism in man: Theory and application in nuclear medicine. Semin Nucl Med XI:32–49

Phelps ME, Hoffman EJ, Mullani NA, Ter-Pogossian MM (1975a) Application of annihilation coincidence detection to transaxial reconstruction tomography. J Nucl Med 16:210–224

Phelps ME, Hoffman EJ, Huang SC, Ter-Pogossian MM (1975b) Effect of positron range on spatial resolution. J Nucl Med 16:649–652

Phelps ME, Hoffman EJ, Coleman RE, Welch MJ, Raichle ME, Weiss ES, Sobel BE, Ter-Pogossian MM (1976) Tomographic Images of blood pool and perfusion in brain and heart. J Nucl Med 17:603–612

Phelps ME, Hoffman EJ, Kuhl DE (1977) Physiologic tomography (PT). A new approach to in-vivo measure of metabolism and physiological function. In: IAEA (ed) Medical radionuclide imaging, vol I. IAEA, Vienna, p 233

Phelps ME, Hoffman EJ, Huang SC, Kuhl DE (1978) ECAT: A new computerized tomographic imaging system for positron emitting radiopharmaceuticals. J Nucl Med 19:635–647

Phelps ME, Huang SC, Hoffman EJ, Kuhl DE (1979) Validation of tomographic measurement of cerebral blood volume with C-11-labeled carboxyhemoglobin. J Nucl Med 20:328–334

Phelps ME, Hoffman EJ, Huang SC, Kuhl DE (1981) Positron computed tomography. In: IAEA (ed) Medical radionuclide imaging 1980, vol 1. IAEA, Vienna, p 199

Phelps ME, Huang SC, Hoffman EJ, Plummer D, Carson R (1982) An analysis of signal amplification using small detectors in positron emission tomography. J Comput Assist Tomogr 6:551–565

Pickens DR, Price RR, Patton JA, Erickson JJ, Rollo FD, Brill AB (1980) Focal-plane tomography image reconstruction. IEEE Trans Nucl Sci NS-27/1:489–492

Pickens DR, Price RR, Ericson JJ, Patton JA, Partain CL, Rolle FD (1981) Longitudinal and transverse digital image reconstruction with a tomographic scanner. In: IAEA (ed) Medical radionuclide imaging 1980, vol I. IAEA, Vienna, p 325

Politte DG, Snyder DL (1982) A simulation study of design choices in the implementation of time-of-flight reconstruction algorithms. In: IEEE (ed) 1982 workshop on time-of-flight tomography. IEEE Computer Soc, Los Angeles, pp 131–136

Politte DG, Snyder DL (1984) Results of a comparative study of a reconstruction procedure for producing improved estimates of radioactivity distributions in time-of-flight emission tomography. IEEE Trans Nucl Sci NS-31/1:614–619

Price LR (1975) CCA: A high resolution, high sensitivity, three-dimensional imaging system for nuclear medicine. Nucl Instr Meth 131:353–368

Price LR (1978) CCA-II: An improved system for emission computed tomography (ECT). Nucl Instr Meth 152:213–220

Price LR (1979) An improved coded-aperture system for emission computed tomography (ECT). IEEE Trans Nucl Sci NS-26/2:2794–2796

Ra JB, Cho ZH (1981) Generalized true three-dimensional reconstruction algorithm. Proc IEEE 69:668–670

Ra JB, Lim CB, Cho ZH, Hilal SK, Correll J (1982) A true three-dimensional reconstruction algorithm for the spherical positron emission tomograph. Phys Med Biol 27:37–50

Radon J (1917) Über die Bestimmung von Funktionen durch ihre Integralwerte längs gewisser Mannigfaltigkeiten. Ber Verh Sächs Akad Wiss Leipzig, Math Phys Kl 69:262–277

Raichle ME, Martin WRW, Herscovitch P, Mintun MA, Markham J (1983) Brain blood flow measured with intravenous H_2O-15. II. Implementation and validation. J Nucl Med 24:790–798

Ramachandran GN, Lakshminarayanan AV (1971) Three-dimensional reconstruction from radiographs and electron micrographs: Application of convolution instead of fourier transforms. Proc Natl Acad Sci USA 68/9:2236–2240

Rangayyan RM, Gordon R (1982) Streak preventive image reconstruction with ART and adaptive filtering. IEEE Trans Med Imag MI-1/3:173–177

Rankowitz S, Robertson JS, Hihinbotham WA, Rosenblum MJ (1962) Positron scanner for locating brain tumors. IRE Int Con Rec 10/9:49–56

Ratib O, Henze E, Hoffman E, Phelps ME, Schelbert HR (1982) Performance of the rotating slant-hole collimator for the detection of myocardial perfusion abnormalities. J Nucl Med 23:34–41

Renaud L, Joy MLG, Gilday GL (1979) Fourier multiaperture emission tomography (FMET). J Nucl Med 20:986–991

Rhodes CG, Wollmer P, Fazio F, Jones T (1981) Quantitative measurement of extravascular lung density using positron emission and transmission tomography. J Comput Assist Tomogr 5:783–791

Ricci AR, Hoffman EJ, Phelps ME, Huang SC, Plummer D, Carson R (1982) Investigation of a technique for providing a pseudo-continuous detector ring for positron tomography. IEEE Trans Nucl Sci NS-29/1:452–456

Rizi HR, Kline RC, Thrall JH, Besozzi MC, Keyes JW Jr, Rogers WL, Clare J, Pitt B (1981) Thallium-201 myocardial scintigraphy: A critical comparison of seven-pinhole tomography and conventional planar imaging. J Nucl Med 22:493–499

Robertson JS, Marr RB, Rosenblum M, Radeka V, Yamamoto YL (1973) 32-Crystal positron transverse section detector. In: Freedman GS (ed) Tomographic imaging in nuclear medicine. Soc Nucl Med Inc, New York, p 142

Rogers WL, Han KS, Jones LW, Beierwaltes WH (1972) Application of a fresnel zone plate to gamma-ray-imaging. J Nucl Med 13:612–615

Rogers WL, Clinthorne NH, Harkness BA, Koral KF, Keyes JW Jr (1982a) Field-flood requirements for emission computed tomography with an anger camera. J Nucl Med 23:162–168

Rogers WL, Koral KF, Mayans R, Leonard PF, Thrall JH, Brady TJ, Keyes JW Jr (1980) Coded-aperture imaging of the heart. J Nucl Med 21:371–378

Rogers WL, Clinthorne NH, Stamos J, Koral KF, Mayans R, Keyes JW Jr, Williams JJ, Snapp WP, Knoll GF (1982b) SPRINT: A stationary detector single photon ring tomograph for brain imaging. IEEE Trans Med Imag MI-1:63–68

Rollo FD, Patton JA (1980) Teaching editorial: Perspectives on seven pinhole tomography. J Nucl Med 21:888–890

Rosenfeld D, Macovski A (1977) Time modulated apertures for tomography in nuclear medicine. IEEE Trans Nucl Sci NS-24/1:570–576

Rosier DJ de, Klug A (1968) Reconstruction of three-dimensional structures from electron micrographs. Nature 217:130–134

Rowland SW (1979) Computer implementation of image reconstruction formulas. In: Herman GT (ed) Image reconstruction from projections. Springer, Berlin Heidelberg New York, p 9

Rusinek H, Youdin M, Reich T (1978) Reconstruction of isotope distribution in the brain: Error analysis for instrument design. Ann Biomed Eng 6:399–412

Rusinek H, Reich T, Youdin M, Clagnaz M, Kolwicz R (1980) A ultrapure germanium detector array for quantitating three-dimensional distribution of a radionuclide: A study of phantoms. J Nucl Med 21:777–782

Sank VJ, Brooks RA, Friauf WS, Leighton SB, Cascio HE, Di Chiro G (1983) Performance evaluation and calibration of the neuro-PET scanner. IEEE Trans Nucl Sci NS-30:636–639

Schelbert HR, Phelps ME, Hoffman EJ, Huang SC (1980a) Regional myocardial perfusion assessed by nitrogen-13 labeled ammonia and positron emission computerized axial tomography. In: Horst W, Wagner HN Jr, Buchanan J (eds) Frontiers in nuclear medicine. Springer, Berlin Heidelberg New York, p 20

Schelbert HR, Henze E, Phelps ME (1980b) Emission tomography of the heart. Semin Nucl Med X:355–373

Schmidlin P (1972) Iterative separation of sections in tomographic scintigrams. Nuklearmedizin XI:1–16

Schmidlin P (1973) Zerlegung der Aufnahmen der symmetrischen Positronenkamera in einzelne Bildebenen mit Hilfe eines mathematischen Verfahrens. In: Pabst HW (Hrsg) Nuklearmedizin 1971. Schattauer, Stuttgart, S 295

Schmitz-Feuerhake I (1970) Studies on three-dimensional scintigraphy with γ-γ-coincidences. Phys Med Biol 15:649–656

Schober O, Meyer GJ, Bossaller C, Lobenhoffer P, Knoop B, Müller S, Creutzig H, Sturm J, Lichtlen P, Hundeshagen H (1983) Quantitative Messung des regionalen extravaskulären Lungenwassers bei Hunden mit der Positronen-Emissionstomographie. Fortschr Röntgenstr 139:117–126

Schön HR, Schelbert HR, Phelps ME (1983) Positronen-Computertomographie: Eine neue Methode zur quantitativen Bestimmung von Stoffwechsel, Durchblutung und Funktion des Herzens. I. Technische und experimentelle Grundlagen. Nucl Med XXII:171–180

Shepp LA, Logan BF (1974) The fourier reconstruction of a head section. IEEE Trans Nucl Sci NS-21/3:21–43

Shepp LA, Vardi Y (1982) Maximum likelihood reconstruction for emission tomography. IEEE Trans Med Imag MI-1/2:113–122

Shosa D, Kaufman L (1981) Methods for evaluation of diagnostic imaging instrumentation. Phys Med Biol 26:101–112

Singh M (1983) An electronically collimated gamma camera for single photon emission computed tomography. Part I: Theoretical considerations and design criteria. Med Phys 10:421–427

Singh M, Doria D (1981) Computer simulation of image rekonstruction with a new electronically collimated gamma tomography systems. SPIE vol 273. Applicat Optic Instr Med IX:192–200

Singh M, Doria D (1983) An electronically collimated gamma camera for single photon emission computed tomography. Part II. Image reconstruction and preliminary experimental measurements. Med Phys 10:428–435

Smalling RW (1983) The spectrum of Thallium-201 imaging in coronary artery disease. Teaching editorial. J Nucl Med 24:854–858

Smith DB, Cumpstey DE, Evans NTS, Coleman JD, Ettinger KV, Mallard JR (1982) A scanner for single photon emission tomography. In: Raynaud C (ed) Nuclear medicine and biology II. Pergamon, Paris, p 1221

Snyder DL, Cox JR Jr (1977) An overview of reconstructive tomography and limitations imposed by a finite number of projections. In: Ter-Pogossian MM et al (eds) Reconstruction tomography in diagnostic radiology and nuclear medicine. Univ Park Press, Baltimore, p 3

Snyder DL (1982) Some noise comparisons of data-collection arrays for emission tomography-systems having time-of-flight measurements. IEEE Trans Nucl Sci NS-29/1:1029–1033

Snyder DL (1984) Utilizing side information in emission tomography. IEEE Trans Nucl Sci NS-31/1:533–537

Snyder DL, Politte DG (1983) Image reconstruction from list-mode data in an emission tomography system having time-of-flight measurements. IEEE Trans Nucl Sci NS-30/3:1843–1849

Snyder DL, Thomas LJ, Ter-Pogossian MM (1981) A mathematical model for positron-emission tomography systems having time-of-flight measurements. IEEE Trans Nucl Sci NS-28/3:3575–3583

Sorensen JA (1974) Methods for quantitative measurements of radioactivity in vivo by whole body counting. In: Hine GJ, Sorensen JA (eds) Instrumentation in nuclear medicine, vol 2. Academic Press, New York, pp 311–348

Soussaline F, Le Coq G (1983) A regularizing method for quantitative SPECT reconstruction. IEEE Trans Med Imag MI-2/1:24–30

Soussaline F, Todd-Pokropek AE, Comar D, Raynaud C, Kellershohn C (1981a) Potential and limits of quantitative studies in emission tomography. In: IAEA (ed) Medical radionuclide imaging 1980, vol I. IAEA, Vienna, p 231

Soussaline FP, Todd-Pokropek AE, Zurowski S, Huffer E, Raynaud CE, Kellershohn CL (1981b) A rotating conventional gamma camera single-photon tomographic system: Physical characterization. J Comput Assist Tomogr 5:551–556

Soussaline FP, Cao A, Le Coq G, Raynaud C, Kellershohn C (1982) An analytical approach to single photon emission computed tomography with the attenuation effect. Eur J Nucl Med 7:487–493

Stark H, Woods JW, Paul J, Hingorani R (1981) An investigation of computerized tomography by direct fourier inversion and optimum interpolation. IEEE Trans Biomed Eng BME-28/7:496–505

Stoddart HF, Stoddart HA (1979) A new development in single gamma transaxial tomography – union carbide focused collimator scanner. IEEE Trans Nucl Sci NS-26/2:2710–2712

Stokely EM (1982) A contigous-slice design for single-photon emission tomography (SPECT). J Nucl Med 23:355–356

Stokely EM, Sveinsdottir E, Lassen NA, Rommer P (1980) A single photon dynamic computer assisted tomograph (DCAT) for imaging brain function in multiple cross sections. J Comput Assist Tomogr 4:230–240

Strauss L, Bostel F, Clorius JH, Raptou E, Wellman H, Georgi P (1982) Single-photon emission computed tomography (SPECT) for assessment of hepatic lesions. J Nucl Med 23:1059–1065

Syrota A, Comar D, Cerf M, Plummer D, Maziere M, Kellershohn C (1979) C-11 methionine pancreatic scanning with positron emission computed tomography. J Nucl Med 20:778–781

Takami K, Ueda K, Okajima K, Tanaka E, Nohara N, Tomitani T, Yamamoto M, Murayama H, Shishido F, Ishimatsu K, Ohgushi A, Inoue S, Takakusa Y, Hayashi T, Nakase S (1983) Performance study of whole-body, multislice positron computed tomograph – positologica-II. IEEE Trans Nucl Sci NS-30:734–738

Tam KC (1983) Multispectral limited-angle image reconstruction. IEEE Trans Nucl Sci NS-30/1:697–700

Tam KC, Perez-Mendez V (1981) Limits to image reconstruction from restricted angular input. IEEE Trans Nucl Sci NS-28/1:179–183

Tam KC, Perez-Mendez V (1983) Improving gated cardiac scanning using limited-angle reconstruction technique. IEEE Trans Nucl Sci NS-30/1:681–685

Tam KC, Chu G, Perez-Mendez V, Lim CB (1978) Three dimensional reconstruction in planar positron cameras using fourier deconvolution of generalized tomograms. IEEE Trans Nucl Sci NS-25/13:152–159

Tam KC, Perez-Mendez V, Macdonald B (1979) 3-D object reconstruction in emission and transmission tomography with limited angular input. IEEE Trans Nucl Sci NS-26/2:2797–2805

Tam KC, Perez-Mendez V, Macdonald B (1980) Limited angle 3-D reconstruction from continuous and pinhole projections. IEEE Trans Nucl Sci NS-27/1:445–458

Tamaki N, Mukai T, Ishii Y, Yonekura Y, Kambara H, Kawai C, Torizuka K (1981) Clinical evaluation of thallium-201 emission myocardial tomography using a rotating gamma camera: Comparison with seven-pinhole tomography. J Nucl Med 22:849–855

Tamaki N, Mukai T, Ishii Y, Fujita T, Yamamoto K, Minato K, Yonekura Y, Tamaki S, Kambara H, Kawai C, Torizuka K (1982) Comparative study of thallium emission myocardial tomography with 180° and 360° data collection. J Nucl Med 23:661–666

Tanaka E (1982) Line-writing data acquisition and signal-to-noise ratio in time-of-flight positron emission tomography. In: IEEE (ed) 1982 workshop on time-of-flight tomography. IEEE Computer Soc, Los Angeles, pp 101–108

Tanaka E (1983) Quantitative image reconstruction with weighted backprojection for single photon emission computed tomography. J Comput Assist Tomogr 7:692–700

Tanaka E, Iinuma TA (1974) Image formation in coded aperture imaging and its application to a rotating slit aperture. In: WFNBM (ed) Proceedings of the First World Congress of Nuclear Medicine. WFNMB, Tokyo Kyoto, p 9

Tanaka E, Iinuma TA (1976) Image processing for coded aperture imaging and an attempt at rotating slit imaging. In: Raynaud C, Todd-Pokropek A (eds) Information processing in scintigraphy. CEN, Saclay, p 43

Tanaka E, Nohara N, Yamamoto M, Tomitani T, Murayama H, Ishimatsu K, Takami K (1979) Positologica – The search for suitable detector arrangements for a positron ECT with continuous rotation. IEEE Trans Nucl Sci NS-26/2:2728–2731

Tanaka M, Hirose Y, Koga K, Hattori H (1981) Engineering aspects of a hybrid emission computed tomograph. IEEE Trans Nucl Sci NS-28/1:137–141

Tanaka E, Nohara N, Tomitani T, Endo M (1982) Analytical study of the performance of a multiplier positron computed tomography scanner. J Comput Assist Tomogr 6:350–364

Tanaka E, Toyama H, Murayama H (1984) Convolutional image reconstruction for quantitative single photon emission computed tomography. Phys Med Biol 29:1489–1500

Ter-Pogossian MM (1977) Basic principles of computed axial tomography. Semin Nucl Med VII:109–127

Ter-Pogossian MM (1981) Special characteristics and potential for dynamic function studies with PET. Semin Nucl Med XI:13–23

Ter-Pogossian MM, Phelps ME, Hoffman EJ, Mullani NA (1975) A positron-emission transaxial tomograph for nuclear imaging (PETT). Radiology 114:89–98

Ter-Pogossian MM, Phelps ME, Hoffman EJ, Coleman RE (1977) The performance of PETT III. In: Ter-Pogossian MM et al. (eds) Reconstruction tomography in diagnostic radiology and nuclear medicine. Park, Baltimore, p 359

Ter-Pogossian MM, Mullani NA, Wood J, Higgins CS, Currie CM (1978a) A multislice positron emission computed tomograph (PETT IV) yielding transverse and longitudinal images. Radiology 128:477–484

Ter-Pogossian MM, Mullani NA, Hood JT, Higgins CS, Ficke DC (1978b) Design considerations for a positron emission transverse tomograph (PETT V) for imaging of the brain. J Comput Assist Tomogr 2:539–544

Ter-Pogossian NM, Mullani NA, Ficke DC, Markham J, Snyder DL (1981) Photon time-of-flight-assisted positron emission tomography. J Comput Assist Tomogr 5:227–239

Ter-Pogossian MM, Ficke DC, Yamamoto M, Hood Sr JT (1982a) Super PETT I: A positron emission tomograph utilizing photon time-of-flight information. IEEE Trans Med Imag MI-1/3:179–187

Ter-Pogossian MM, Ficke DC, Hood Sr JT, Yamamoto M, Mullani NA (1982b) PETT VI: A positron emission tomograph utilizing cesium fluoride scintillation detectors. J Comput Assist Tomogr 6:125–133

Ter-Pogossian MM, Bergmann SR, Sobel BE (1982c) Influence of cardiac and respiratory motion on tomographic reconstructions of the heart: Implications for quantitative nuclear cardiology. J Comput Assist Tomogr 6:1148–1155

Thompson CJ, Yamamoto YL, Meyer E (1979) Positome II: A high efficiency positron imaging device for dynamic brain studies. IEEE Trans Nucl Sci NS-26/1:583–589

Todd-Pokropek A (1980) Image processing in nuclear medicine. IEEE Trans Nucl Sci NS-27/3:1080–1094

Todd-Pokropek A (1982) Single photon emission computerized tomography (SPECT): Quality control and assurance. In: Höfer R, Bergmann H (Hrsg) Radioaktive Isotope in Klinik und Forschung, 15. Bd. Egermann, Wien, S 539

Todd-Pokropek A (1983a) Non-circular orbits for the reduction of uniformity artefacts in SPECT. Phys Med Biol 28:309–313

Todd-Pokropek A (1983b) The Mathematics and physics of emission computerized tomography (ECT). In: Esser PD (ed) Emission computed tomography: Current Trends. Soc Nucl Med, New York, p 3

Todd-Pokropek AE, Jarritt PH (1982) The noise characteristics of SPECT systems. In: Ell PJ, Holman BL (eds) Computed emission tomography. Oxford Univers Press, Oxford, p 361

Todd-Pokropek A, Soussaline F (1982) Quality control of SPECT systems: Removal of artefacts. In: Raynaud C (ed) Nuclear medicine and biology I. Pergamin, Paris, p 1018

Todd-Pokropek A, Clarke G, Marsh R, Gillardi MC, Fazio F (1984) SPECT quantitation: The need for scatter and attenuation correction. In: Höfer R, Bergmann H (eds) Radioaktive Isotope in Klinik und Forschung, Bd 16/2. Egermann, Wien, pp 613–625

Tomitani T (1981) Image reconstruction and noise evaluation in photon time-of-flight assisted positron emission tomography. IEEE Trans Nucl Sci NS-28/6:4582–4589

Tomitani T (1982) Simulation study of reconstruction with practical writing functions and noise evaluation in time-of-flight assisted positron computed tomography. In: IEEE (ed) 1982 workshop on time-of-flight tomography. IEEE Computer Soc, Los Angeles, p 117

Townsend DW, Zanella P (1980) Computational aspects of positron imaging using multiwire proportional chambers in nuclear medicine. Nucl Instr Meth 176:397–401

Townsend D, Piney C, Jeavons A (1978) Object reconstruction from focused positron tomograms. Phys Med Biol 23:235–244

Townsend D, Schorr B, Jeavons A (1980) Three-dimensional image reconstruction for a positron camera with limited angular acceptance. IEEE Trans Nucl Sci NS-27/1:463–470

Tretiak OJ, Delaney P (1978) The exponential convolution algorithm for emission computed axial tomography. In: Proc 5th Intern Conf on Information Processing in Med Imaging, Oak Ridge Rep ORNL/BCJIC-2, pp 266–268

Tretiak OJ, Metz CE (1980) The exponential radon transform. SIAM J Appl Math 39:341–354

Truong TK, Reed IS, Jonckheere EA, Kwoh YS (1983) A modified reconstruction filter for diverging X-ray beams. IEEE Trans Biomed Eng BME-30/7:423–426

Tsui E, Budinger TF (1978) Transverse section imaging of mean clearence time. Phys Med Biol 23:644–653

Tsui BMW, Jaszczak RJ (1984) Interactions of collimator, sampling and filtering on SPECT spatial resolution. IEEE Trans Nucl Sci NS-31/1:527–532

Turner DA, Ramachandran PC, Ali AA, Fordham EW, Ferry TA (1976a) Brain scanning with the anger multiplane tomographic scanner as a primary examination. Radiology 121:125–129

Turner DA, Fordham EW, Paganow JV, Ali AA, Ramos MV, Ramachandran PC (1976b) Brain scanning with the anger multiplane tomographic scanner as a second examination. Radiology 121:115–124

Uemura K, Kanno I, Miura Y, Miura S, Tominaga S (1982) Tomographic study of regional cerebral blood flow in ischemic cerebrovascular disease by Kr-81m intraarterial infusion and HEADTOME. J Comput Assist Tomogr 6:677–682

Van Sciver, Hofstadter R (1952) Gamma and alpha produced scintillations in cesium fluoride. Phys Rev 87:522

Vogel RA, Kirch DL, Le Free MT, Steele PP (1978) A new method of multiplanar emission tomography using a seven pinhole collimator and an anger scintillation camera. J Nucl Med 19:648–654

Vogel RA, Kirch DL, Le Free MT, Rainwater JO, Jensen DP, Steele PP (1979) Thallium-201 myocardial perfusion scintigraphy: Results of standard and multi-pinhole tomographic techniques. Am J Cardiol 43:787–793

Vogel RA, Le Free MT, Kirch DL (1980) Rapid and inexpensive cardiac tomography using a widefield anger camera. In: Horst W, Wagner Jr HN, Buchanan J (eds) Frontiers in nuclear medicine. Springer, Berlin Heidelberg New York, p 79

Vyska K, Höck A, Freundlieb C, Becker V, Schmidt A, Feinendegen LE, Kloster G, Stöcklin G (1981) Stoffwechseluntersuchung am Herzen mit J-123-Fettsäuren und C-11-Methylglukose. Nucl Med XX:148–155

Vyska K, Freundlieb C, Höck A, Becker V, Schmidt A, Feinendegen LE, Kloster G, Stöcklin G, Heiss WD (1982) Analysis of local perfusion rate (LPR) and local glucose transport rate (LGTR) in brain and heart in man by means of C-11-Methyl-D-glucose (CMG) and dynamic positron emission tomography (DPET). In: Höfer R, Bergmann H (Hrsg) Radioaktive Isotope in Klinik und Forschung. Egermann, Wien, S 129

Wagner HN Jr (1978) Images of the future. J Nucl Med 19:599–605

Wagner HN Jr (1983) Notes and impressions from meetings. Two positron emission tomography meetings. J Comput Assist Tomogr 7:1128–1131

Walters TE, Simon W, Chesler DA, Correia JA (1981) Attenuation correction in gamma emission computed tomography. J Comput Assist Tomogr 5:89–94

Webb S, Flower MA, Ott RJ, Leach MO, Grey LJ (1982) A physical evaluation of three pinhole tomography. In: Raynaud (ed) Nuclear medicine and biology I. Pergamon, Paris, p 469

Webb S, Flower MA, Ott RJ, Leach MO (1983) A comparison of attenuation correction methods for quantitative single photon emission computed tomography. Phys Med Biol 28:1045–1056

Weiss GH, Talbert AJ, Brooks RA (1982) The use of phantom views to reduce CT-streaks, due to insufficient angular sampling. Phys Med Biol 27:1151–1162

Whitehead FR (1977) Quantitative analysis of minimum detectable lesion-to-background uptake ratios for nuclear medicine imaging systems. In: IAEA (ed) Medical radionuclide imaging, vol 1. Vienna, pp 409–434

Williams CW, Crabtree MC, Burgiss SG (1979) Design and performance characteristics of a positron emission computed axial tomograph: ECAT II. IEEE Trans Nucl Sci NS-26/1:619–627

Williams CW, Crabtree MC, Burke MR, Keyser RM, Burgiss SG, Hoffman EJ, Phelps ME (1981) Design of the neuro-ECAT: A high resolution, high efficiency positron tomograph for imaging the adult head or infant torso. IEEE Trans Nucl Sci NS-28/2:1736–1740

Williams DL, Ritchie JL, Harp GD, Caldwell JH, Hamilton GW (1980) In-vivo simulation of Thallium-201 myocardial scintigraphy by seven-pinhole emission tomography. J Nucl Med 21:821–828

Williams DL, Ritchie JL, Harp GD, Caldwell JH, Hamilton GW (1980) In vivo simulation of Thallium-201 myocardial scintigraphy by seven-pinhole emission tomography. J Nucl Med 21:821–828

Williams JJ, Knoll GF (1979) Initial performance of SPRINT: A single photon system for emission tomography. IEEE Trans Nucl Sci NS-26/2:2732–2735

Williams JJ, Snapp WP, Knoll GF (1979) Introducing SPRINT: A single photon ring system for emission tomography. IEEE Trans Nucl Sci NS-26/1:628–633

Wilson BC, Parker RP (1975) Digital processing of images from a zone-plate camera. Phys Med Biol 20:757–770

Wolf AP (1981) Special characteristics and potential for radiopharmaceuticals for positron emission tomography. Semin Nucl Med XI:2–12

Wong WH, Mullani NA, Philippe EA, Hartz R, Gould KL (1983) Image improvement and design optimization of the time-of-flight PET. J Nucl Med 24:52–60

Wood SL, Macovski A, Morf M (1979) Reconstruction with limited data using estimation theory. In: Raviv et al. (eds) Computer aided tomography and ultrasonics in medicine. North-Holland, Amsterdam, p 219

Yamamoto M, Kawaguchi F (1982) Quad-detector arrangement and sampling characteristics in rotary positron tomography: Positologica II. IEEE Trans Med Imag MI-1/2:136–142

Yamamoto M, Ficke DC, Ter-Pogossian NM (1982a) Experimental assessment of the gain-achieved by the utilization of time-of-flight information in a positron emission tomograph (Super PETT I). IEEE Trans Med Imag MI-1/3:187–192

Yamamoto M, Ficke DC, Ter-Pogossian MM (1982b) Performance study of PETT VI, a positron computed tomograph with 288 cesium fluoride detectors. IEEE Trans Nucl Sci NS-29/1:529–533

Yamamoto YL, Thompson CJ, Meyer E, Robertson JS, Feindel W (1977) Dynamic positron emission tomography for study of cerebral hemodynamics in a cross section of the head using positron-emitting GA-69-EDTA and KR-77. J Comput Assist Tomogr 1:43–56

Yamashita Y, Uchida H, Yamashita T, Hayashi T (1984) Recent developments in detectors for high spatial resolution positron CT. IEEE Trans Nucl Sci NS-31:424–428

Yano Y, Chu P, Budinger TF, Grant PM, Ogart AE, Barnes JW, O'Brain HA Jr, Hoop B Jr (1977) Rubidium-82 generators for imaging studies. J Nucl Med 18:46–50

Yen CK, Budinger TF (1981) Evaluation of blood-brain barrier permeability changes in rhesus monkeys and man using Rb-82 and positron emission tomography. J Comput Assist Tomogr 5:792–799

3. Klinische Anwendung der Positronen-Emissionstomographie

Von

O. Schober und G.-J. Meyer

Mit 69 Abbildungen und 9 Tabellen

A. Einleitung

I. Vorteile der Positronen-Emissionstomographie

In der nuklearmedizinischen Diagnostik werden seit über 40 Jahren Radionuklide mit großem Erfolg eingesetzt. Sie finden entweder direkte Anwendung in einfachen anorganischen Formen oder dienen zur Markierung körpereigener Substanzen und geeigneter Pharmaka. Um optimal und routinemäßig in der Diagnostik eingesetzt werden zu können, müssen die Radionuklide bestimmte Voraussetzungen bezüglich ihrer physikalischen Eigenschaften aufweisen. Dazu gehören im wesentlichen eine gute Verfügbarkeit und eine gute Meßmethodik. Darüber hinaus müssen die Strahlungsart und die damit verbundene spezifische Dosisleistung des Nuklid, dem Anwendungszweck möglichst gut angepaßt sein. Nuklide mit Halbwertzeiten unter 12 Stunden sind im allgemeinen nur dann für die Routinediagnostik ausreichend verfügbar, wenn sie über Generatorsysteme mit entsprechend langer Halbwertzeit hergestellt werden können. Um mit dem in der nuklearmedizinischen Diagnostik am weitesten verbreiteten Meßsystem, der Angerkamera, detektiert werden zu können, muß die emittierte Gammastrahlung im Bereich von 80–300 keV liegen. Weil es keine Radionuklide der wichtigsten physiologisch-organischen Elemente Kohlenstoff (C), Stickstoff (N) und Sauerstoff (O) gibt, die diese Voraussetzungen erfüllen, war es bis vor kurzem nicht möglich, entsprechend markierte Radiopharmaka zur Diagnostik einzusetzen.

Die einzigen für diagnostische Zwecke einsetzbaren Isotope dieser drei Elemente, ^{11}C, ^{13}N und ^{15}O, sind Positronenstrahler mit Halbwertzeiten von 2 min (^{15}O), 10 min (^{13}N) und 20 min (^{11}C). Hinzu kommt noch das Nuklid ^{18}F mit 109 min Halbwertzeit, das zwar weitgehend unphysiologisch ist, andererseits aber sehr stabile, kovalente Bindungen mit Kohlenstoff bildet und damit in viele organische Moleküle eingebaut werden kann. Die kurzen Halbwertzeiten machen eine Produktion dieser Radionuklide in unmittelbarer Nähe des Applikationsortes notwendig. Die Herstellung erfordert einen Beschleuniger, möglichst ein Zyklotron. Andererseits erlauben die Eigenschaften dieser Nuklide erstmalig, durch die gezielte Markierung körpereigener Stoffe eine breite Palette physiologischer und metabolischer Vorgänge im Körper ortsabhängig, quantitativ und weitgehend nicht-invasiv zu bestimmen. Das breite Spektrum der chemischen Verbindungen, die heute mit diesen kurzlebigen Nukliden markierbar sind, reicht von Aminosäuren über Zucker und Fettsäuren bis zu Hormonen und pharmakologisch wirksamen Substanzen. Eine Übersicht über den Stand der Radiochemie, die sich mit der Herstellung dieser Radiopharmaka befaßt, findet sich an anderer Stelle in diesem Handbuch.

Die speziellen physikalischen Eigenschaften der Positronenstrahler ermöglichen eine erheblich verbesserte räumliche Auflösung bei der Messung gegenüber der herkömmlichen Detektion mit der Anger-Kamera. Dies bedeutet, daß Verteilungsmuster einer Substanz im Körper genauer und deutlicher dargestellt werden können. Ferner gestattet diese Meßtechnik aufgrund exakt bestimmbarer Absorptionsparameter erstmalig die ortsabhängige, streng quantitative Aktivitätsbestimmung im Körper. Eine detaillierte Beschreibung der Vorteile der Positronen-Emissionstomographie sowie Einzelheiten der Meßtechnik finden sich ebenfalls an anderer Stelle in diesem Handbuch.

Unter Berücksichtigung zeitlicher Veränderungen der Aktivitätskonzentrationen, und bei geschickter Tracerauswahl auch unter physiologischen Gleichgewichtsbedingungen, können damit Stoffwechselvorgänge im Körper exakt quantitativ erfaßt und beschrieben werden. Die Berechnung von Stoffwechselraten setzt allerdings die Kenntnis einer Reihe physiologischer Zusammenhänge voraus, die dann in einem mathematisch beschreibbaren Modell zusammengefaßt werden müssen. Einen Überblick über die Methoden und Ansätze zur Entwicklung solcher physiologisch-kinetischer Modellvorstellungen wird im Abschnitt B dieses Kapitels gegeben. Gelingt es, eine solche Modellvorstellung, etwa zur Durchblutungsmessung oder zum Glukosestoffwechsel zu validieren, so ergibt sich damit die Möglichkeit einer quantitativen Bestimmung von Durchblutungs- und Funktionszuständen in einzelnen Organen mit hoher räumlicher Auflösung. Dies eröffnet die Perspektive zu völlig neuen diagnostischen Aussagen, die mit anderen Methoden, auch den invasiven und den Patienten belastenden Untersuchungsverfahren, gar nicht oder nur teilweise zu gewinnen sind.

II. Indikationen

Die Entwicklung klinischer Verfahren läßt sich in vier verschiedene Stufen oder Phasen einteilen.

1. Im Rahmen der Grundlagenforschung müssen fundamentale Prinzipien der Meßtechnik wie die Genauigkeit, Reproduzierbarkeit und Zuverlässigkeit einer Methode analysiert werden.
2. Aufgabe der klinischen Forschung ist es, physiologische und pathologische Parameter zu trennen.
3. Klinische Studien dienen dazu, den Wert eines Verfahrens im Hinblick auf klinische Fragestellungen in Begriffen wie Sensitivität und Spezifität zu definieren und zu beschreiben.
4. Die letzte und höchste Anforderung an (neue) diagnostische Verfahren beinhaltet Fragen nach Beeinflussungen der Morbidität oder Mortalität, oder auch der ökonomischen Randbedingungen.

Die Indikation zu einer Untersuchung ergibt sich zum einen aus dem unmittelbaren Vorteil für den einzelnen Patienten, zum anderen aber durchaus aus dem Gewinn von Erkenntnissen, die anderen Patienten zugute kommen können.

Die erwünschte Grundinformation, die die Indikation zu einer Untersuchung ist, kann auf die Frage reduziert werden: Wie verhält sich der Stoffwechsel in dem interessierenden Gewebe? Die Frage verlangt also primär nach physiologischen oder biochemischen Informationen. Morphologisch orientierte Verfahren, wie das konventionelle Röntgen, Ultraschall, die Computertomographie oder die Kernspintomographie, geben im allgemeinen Aussagen über Strukturveränderungen in Folge von Stoffwechselstörungen. Prinzipien der Tracerkinetik gestatten es uns dagegen unmittelbar, physiologische, biochemische, pharmakokinetische und hämodynamische Prozesse regional zu messen und zu beschreiben.

Mit der Positronen-Emissionstomographie ist es also möglich, nicht-invasiv biochemische Vorgänge in Organen und Organsystemen quantitativ mit einem in der klinischen Routine ausreichenden regionalen Auflösungsvermögen darzustellen.

Zum gegenwärtigen Zeitpunkt existieren nach Arbeiten an mehr als 50 PET-Zentren in der Welt grundsätzliche klinische Studien, die epidemiologisch und klinisch besonders wichtige Fragestellungen betreffen, wie die der zerebrovaskulären Erkrankung, heredo-degenerativer Erkrankungen, der Epilepsie, der Demenz und der koronaren Herzerkrankung, sowie Lungenerkrankungen und Tumorkrankheiten. Dabei werden klinische Anwendungsbeispiele zur Messung der folgenden physiologischen Funktionsparameter beschrieben: Blutvolumen, Blutfluß, Integrität von Membranen (Blut-Hirn-Schranke), Sauerstoff-Extraktionsrate, Sauerstoffmetabolismus, Glukosemetabolismus, Proteinsynthese, Dichte und Verfügbarkeit von Rezeptoren sowie Gewebe-pH-Wert.

Eine detaillierte Aufstellung der bisherigen Untersuchungsgebiete liefert der Abschnitt D dieses Kapitels.

Die Aussagekraft und der Wert der PET lassen sich bei diesen Untersuchungen nicht nur in Maßen, wie Sensitivität und Spezifität, sondern auch in Hinblick auf den Vergleich und die Kalibrierung anderer Untersuchungsmethoden und ihre mögliche Substitution benennen. Zur Unterstreichung der wachsenden Akzeptanz der Methodik sei schließlich erwähnt, daß sich die Anzahl der jährlichen Original-Publikationen über klinische Anwendungen der Positronen-Emissionstomographie in den vergangenen Jahren von ca. 80 im Jahr 1980 auf über 600 im Jahr 1985 erhöht hat.

III. Forschung

Die klinisch orientierte Forschung konzentriert sich zur Zeit auf drei Schwerpunkte:

Mit den organisch-physiologischen Radioisotopen, wie ^{11}C, ^{13}N, ^{15}O und ^{18}F, können nahezu alle *Pharmaka* markiert werden. Insgesamt sind derzeit mehr als 500 verschiedene Synthesen bekannt. Schon vor der klinischen Kontrolle wird die Wirksamkeit im Sinne einer nicht-invasiven Qualitätskontrolle regional und quantitativ beurteilbar sein. Als Beispiel seien die antibiotische Therapie, etwa bei der Osteomyelitis, und die zytostatische Therapie bei Tumorerkrankungen genannt.

Konventionelle, ubiquitär zur Verfügung stehende Verfahren, die primär insbesondere morphologische Informationen liefern, können gegen funktionelle PET-Studien *kalibriert* werden. Als Beispiel sei die Beurteilung des Lungenödems angeführt. Mit der PET kann das extravaskuläre Lungenwasser (Ödem) regional quantifiziert werden. Von klinischem Interesse ist, bei welcher pathologischen Zunahme des Lungenwassers konventionelles Röntgen und CT positive Befunde anzeigen, aber auch eine Korrelation zu den biochemisch relevanten Relaxationszeiten T1 und T2 sowie der Protonendichte, die mit der Kernspintomographie gewonnen werden können.

Rezeptoren haben in der Diagnostik der Neurologie und Neuropharmakologie, aber auch bei verschiedenen Tumorerkrankungen, in den letzten Jahren wegen der prognostischen Relevanz erheblich an Bedeutung gewonnen. So ist es möglich, Dopaminrezeptoren (Hirndiagnostik der heredo-degenerativen Erkrankungen) und cholinerge/katecholaminerge Synapsen (Herzdiagnostik) regional und quantitativ zu bestimmen.

IV. Substitution

Inwieweit andere Verfahren, wie die Sonographie, das konventionelle Röntgen, die Computertomographie oder auch die Kernspintomographie, von der Positronen-Emissionstomographie substituiert werden können, läßt sich noch nicht beurteilen. Allerdings konnte bei der Einführung der anderen o.g. Verfahren diese Fragestellung auch nicht im voraus beantwortet werden. Die der PET-Methode inhärenten Eigenschaften, die nicht-invasiv die quantitative und regionale Beurteilung natürlicher Stoffwechselvorgänge ermöglichen, läßt aber einen deutlichen Fortschritt in der Diagnostik für den Arzt und damit den Patienten erwarten.

V. Klinik: Interdisziplinäre Zusammenarbeit

Eine entscheidende Voraussetzung für den Nutzen der Positronen-Emissionstomographie, die dem Patienten zugute kommen soll, sind definierte klinische Fragestellungen. Die interdisziplinäre Zusammenarbeit zwischen den Nuklearmedizinern und den Radiologen, Internisten (Kardiologie, Pulmonologie, Gastroenterologie und Onkologie), Neurologen und Chirurgen (Neuro-, Unfall-, Abdominal-, Herz-Thorax- und Transplantations-Chirurgie) muß zu diesen Fragestellungen führen.

In Bezug auf die klinische Routine-Diagnostik steht die Wertigkeit der Positronen-Emissionstomographie für einzelne Fragestellungen noch nicht fest. Sehr große Patientenkollektive mit entsprechend zahlreichen Untersuchungen, die Rückschlüsse auf Meßzahlen wie Mortalität, Morbidität und Ökonomie zulassen, liegen noch nicht vor. Aus diesem Grunde reicht es u.E. nicht aus, sich mit der PET auf eine einzelne klinische Fragestellung zu beschränken. Aus der Klinik, in die das Verfahren PET eingebettet werden soll, müssen deshalb verschiedene Fragestellungen an den Nuklearmediziner herangetragen werden. Grundvoraussetzungen sind nicht nur logistische (z.B. Verbindungswege) Grundstrukturen, sondern auch eine in der klinischen Routine erprobte Zusammenarbeit.

B. Methodische Grundlagen und tracerkinetische Modellvorstellungen zur Bestimmung physiologischer Parameter

Die physiologische Funktion eines Organismus oder eines Teilorgans ist mit der Summe der darin ablaufenden biochemischen Prozesse eindeutig verknüpft. Der Begriff der Funktionsdiagnostik muß sich daher auf eine Überprüfung dieser biochemischen Prozesse beziehen. Meist geschieht dies über eine relative, besser jedoch über eine quantitative Analyse der Konzentrationen von Reaktionspartnern und Stoffwechselprodukten sowie eine Bestimmung ihrer Bildungs- und Verschwinderaten.

Die quantitative Beschreibung des physiologischen Zustands eines Organs oder einer seiner Funktionen erfordert somit die Entwicklung eines mathematischen Modells. Dazu ist es in erster Näherung hilfreich, das Organ als ein Kompartment mit wohl definierten Grenzen zu betrachten. Der physiologische Prozeß wird dann in einer Reihe von biochemischen Reaktionen zerlegt. Schließlich wird angenommen, daß der physiologische Funktionsprozeß mit Hilfe der Zeit- und Konzentrationsabhängigkeit der biochemischen Reaktionspartner beschrieben werden kann. Einen zusammenfassenden Überblick geben Lambrecht u. Rescigno (1983).

Die mathematische Beschreibung der reaktionskinetischen Zusammenhänge kann von zwei Ansätzen ausgehen. Der mathematisch-analytische Ansatz beginnt mit der Bestimmung der Einzelparameter einer gemessenen Zeit-Aktivitätskurve.

Die Zerlegung der Systemgewichtsfunktion („response function") wird auch als das „Inverse Problem der Kompartmentanalyse" bezeichnet (JAQUES 1972). Sie erfolgt üblicherweise durch iterative Verfahren der nichtlinearen Regression. Dabei wird die gemessene Funktion durch eine Modellfunktion approximiert und die Anpassung mit einem Gütekriterium bewertet, etwa der kleinsten quadratischen Abweichung.

Die Aufspaltung der „response function" in einzelne exponentielle Anteile ist eine notwendige, nicht aber eine hinreichende Bedingung zur Beschreibung der zugrundeliegenden physiologischen Funktionsprozesse. Da ein aus drei Differentialgleichungen zusammengesetztes System auf 21 verschiedenen Verknüpfungsstrukturen beruhen kann (BROWN 1980), müssen die physiologischen und biochemischen Randbedingungen festgelegt werden. Dies gelingt durch Zuordnung der Exponentialanteile zu physiologisch abgegrenzten homogenen Strukturen mit einheitlichem Tracerverhalten (BERGNER 1964). Eine eingehende mathematische Behandlung anhand eines Beispiels der Nierenfunktionsdiagnostik wurde von KNOOP (1982) vorgelegt.

Der synthetische Ansatz beginnt mit der Erstellung eines Kompartmentmodells. In einem Kompartment ist die Tracerverteilung homogen und einheitlich. Für Reaktionen erster Ordnung ist dann die Transportrate aus dem Kompartment heraus der Tracerkonzentration proportional. Die Proportionalitätskonstante wird als Transferkonstante ("rate constant") $k(t^{-1})$ bezeichnet. Die inverse Summe aller Transferkonstanten dieses Kompartments ist die "turnover" Zeit T, wobei $T/\ln 2$ der Halbwertzeit des Tracers im Kompartment entspricht, wenn zwischenzeitlich keine Zuführung des Tracers erfolgt.

Obwohl für viele physiologische Vorgänge eine lineare Differentialanalyse streng genommen nicht gültig ist, kann das Tracerverhalten mit einer Kinetik erster Ordnung annähernd beschrieben werden, wenn die Tracerkonzentration sehr klein ist (RESCIGNO u. SEGRE 1966). Für ein System von Kompartmenten ergibt sich damit ein Satz linearer Differentialgleichungen.

Wird der Tracer impulsförmig (bolusmäßig) zugeführt, so ist die Lösung der "response function" eine Summe von Exponentialfunktionen. Ist die „input function" kein Impuls, dann ergibt sich die Zeit-Aktivitätskurve aus der Convolution der „input function" mit der Impuls-„response function" des Systems.

Bei der Reduktion physiologischer Prozesse auf biochemische Reaktionen und deren Reaktionskinetik müssen drei Phänomene beachtet werden:

1. Transportphänomene. Sie umfassen Fluß, Diffusion und katalysierten, „carrier facilitated", Transport und müssen im Kompartmentmodell als Zuführung und Transport regulierende Faktoren berücksichtigt werden.

2. Anreicherungsphänomene. Zu ihnen gehören Prozesse wie das „metabolic trapping" oder die Rezeptorbindung, die eine Akkumulation im Kompartment bewirken.

3. Metabolische Phänomene. Sie resultieren in einer verzögerten oder beschleunigten Passage des Tracers durch das Kompartment.

Im folgenden soll versucht werden, die mathematischen Ansätze zur quantitativen Beschreibung dieser Phänomene für verschiedene Funktionsuntersuchungen mittels der Positronen-Emissionstomographie zu erläutern.

I. Blutvolumen

Zur quantitativen Bestimmung des regionalen Blutvolumens bietet sich vornehmlich die Methode der Isotopenverdünnungstechnik im Gleichgewichtszustand an (Meier u. Zierler 1954). Nach Applikation eines streng intravasal verbleibenden Tracers und dessen gleichmäßiger Verteilung im gesamten Blut kann das regionale Blutvolumen durch eine emissionstomographische Messung des Verteilungsraumes ermittelt werden. Variationsmöglichkeiten in der Methodik ergeben sich vor allem bei der Auswahl des Tracers. Die verschiedenen kurzlebigen Tracer sind in Tabelle 1 zusammengestellt.

Tabelle 1. Intravasalraum-Markierungsarten

Tracer	Anbindung	Literatur
$^{11}C-CO$	Erythrozyten	Phelps et al. (1976, 1979 a/b), Clark u. Buckingham (1975), Glass et al. (1968)
$^{15}O-CO$	Erythrozyten	Eichling et al. (1975), Hnatowitch et al. (1979), Clark u. Buckingham (1975), Meyer u. Hundeshagen (1982)
^{11}C-Albumin	Plasmaprotein	Turton et al. (1984)
^{68}Ga-DTPA	Plasmaprotein	Hnatowitch et al. (1979), Welch et al. (1977)

Die Begrenzung des Verteilungsraumes auf das Intravasalvolumen gelingt durch feste Anbindung eines Tracers an Blutbestandteile oder durch Injektion von komplexen Tracern, die eine vernachlässigbare Membranpermeabilität haben.

Erythrozyten werden durch Beladung mit ^{11}CO oder $C^{15}O$ unter Bildung von Karboxyhämoglobin markiert. Die Markierung kann entweder *in vivo* durch Inhalation (Jones et al. 1976a; Subramanyam et al. 1978) oder *in vitro* durch Gasbeladung autologer Erythrozyten (Clark u. Buckingham 1975; Subramanyam et al. 1977; Meyer u. Hundeshagen 1982) erfolgen. Die Bindung von CO an das Hämoglobin ist sehr stabil und zeigt eine zerfallskorrigierte biologische Halbwertzeit von ca. 180 min (Weinreich et al. 1975).

Nach bolusförmiger wie auch bei kontinuierlicher Applikation dauert es ca. 10 min bis ein Gleichgewichtszustand erreicht ist. Bei der Verwendung von $C^{15}O$ mit nur 2.03 min Halbwertzeit ergeben sich damit Probleme im Hinblick auf die Erreichung eines Gleichgewichtszustandes. Bei Bolusapplikation muß daher $^{15}O-CO$ relativ hoch dosiert werden, um im Gleichgewicht noch genügend Aktivität messen zu können. In jedem Fall muß der Konzentrationsgradient auf Grund des Zerfalls von ^{15}O entlang des Verteilungsweges berücksichtigt werden. Der Effekt kann jedoch bei der Auswertung unter Berücksichtigung von Transitzeiten korrigiert werden (Meyer et al. 1985a). Neben diesen Nachteilen bei der Verwendung von $^{15}O-CO$ bietet es andererseits den Vorteil der schnellst möglichen Wiederholbarkeit der Messung bzw. die Einbindung der Messung als Korrekturfaktor in andere Funktionsmessungen, wie z.B. bei der Bestimmung der Sauerstoffextraktionsrate (Lammertsma u. Jones 1983; Pantano et al. 1985).

Bei Verwendung von ^{11}CO mit 20.3 min Halbwertzeit sind die Gradienteneffekte vernachlässigbar. Andererseits ist die Messung erst nach ein paar Stunden wiederholbar und führt in direkter Verbindung mit anderen Funktionsmessungen zu einem erhöhten Untergrund.

Bei der Blutvolumenmessung mit CO-beladenen Erythrozyten müssen die im Kapillarparenchym auftretenden Hämatokritschwankungen ebenfalls berücksichtigt werden. Diese können zu einer Unterschätzung des Intravasalvolumens führen. Nach OLDENDORF et al. (1965) und LARSEN u. LASSEN (1964) ist der Hämatokrit im Gehirn um ca. 20% erniedrigt, während er in der Lunge um ca. 15% vermindert ist. Regionale Hämatokritschwankungen können durch den Vergleich von Volumenmessungen mit CO-beladenen Erythrozyten und markierten Plasmabestandteilen quantitativ erfaßt werden (LAMMERTSMA et al. 1984).

Andererseits muß bei der Messung des Blutvolumens der physiologische Hintergrund der Fragestellung berücksichtigt werden. Wenn es bei der Messung um die potentielle Sauerstoffversorgung geht und nicht die intravasale Raumforderung im Vordergrund steht, kann die hämatokritabhängige Messung der physiologisch sinnvollere Wert sein. Im Vergleich dazu kann für Funktionsmessungen, die eine Intravasalvolumen-Korrektur erfordern, der Plasmabereich sinnvoller sein. Andererseits ergeben sich bei der Markierung von Plasmabestandteilen wie $^{11}CH_3$-Albumin (TURTON et al. 1984; LAMMERTSMA et al. 1984) oder anderen Verbindungen wie ^{68}Ga-markiertem Transferrin Fehlerquellen durch transkapillären Proteinfluß oder Membranleckagen, die dann in Parenchymbereichen zu einem virtuell vergrößertem Intravasalvolumen führen können.

II. Extravasalräume

Viele kleine Moleküle, wie Ionen, Wasser, Gase und Alkohole, können den Intravasalraum leicht verlassen und diffusiv den interstitiellen und den intrazellulären Raum erreichen. In parenchymartigen Gewebestrukturen mit hoher spezifischer Durchblutung sind die Diffusionsstrecken klein, so daß ein schneller und weitgehender Austausch zwischen Intra- und Extravasalraum stattfindet. Der allgemeine Ansatz zur Messung von Extravasalräumen geht von der Indikatorverdünnungsmethode aus (STEWART 1897; HENRIQUES 1913; HAMILTON et al. 1928); für eine Übersicht siehe LASSEN u. PERL 1979. Zunächst wird das gesamte erreichbare Volumen mit einem frei diffusiblen Tracer bestimmt. Dann wird das intravasale Volumen mit einem nicht-diffusiblen Tracer bestimmt und schließlich der extravasale Raum durch Differenzbildung der beiden Volumina ermittelt.

1. Dynamische Indikatorverdünnungsanalysen

Bei der Passage eines radioaktiven Bolus durch ein Volumen V registriert ein darauf gerichteter Detektor eine typische Dilutionskurve, wie sie beispielhaft in Abb. 1 gezeigt ist.

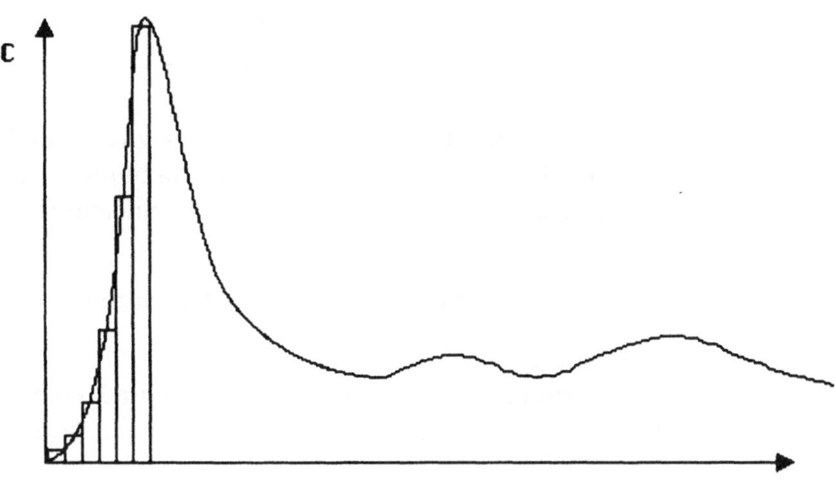

Abb. 1. Dilutionskurve

Die Gesamtaktivität Q des Tracers ergibt sich aus dem Produkt von Fluß F und Konzentration C, d.h. die auf die Volumeneinheit bezogene Aktivität.

$$Q = F \cdot \int C(t)\, dt \tag{1}$$

Somit kann der Fluß aus dem Verhältnis der Gesamtaktivität (Dosis) zur Kurvenfläche berechnet werden (Stewart 1897; Henriques 1913; Hamilton et al. 1928).

$$\text{Fluß} = \frac{\text{Dosis}}{\text{Fläche}} \tag{1a}$$

Betrachtet man das Volumen als ein Kompartment mit einem Ein- und Ausgang (s. Abb. 2) so kann auf das System die „black-box"-Kompartmentanalyse (vgl. Lassen u. Perl 1979) angewandt werden.

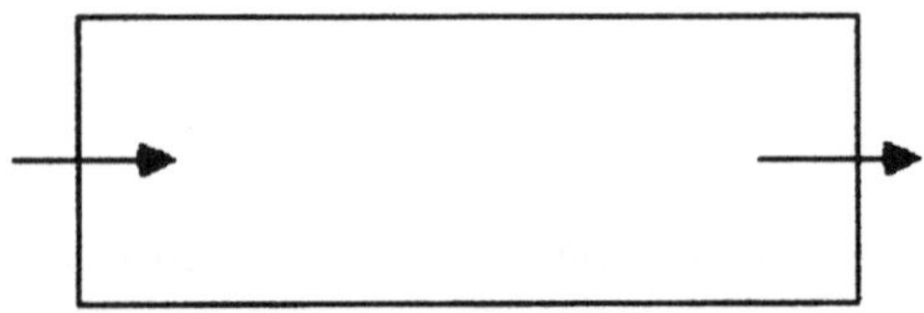

Abb. 2. Schema der „black-box"-Kompartmentanalyse

Dabei ist das Volumen V aus dem Produkt von Fluß F und mittlerer Transitzeit $\bar{t}$ entsprechend Gleichung (2) errechenbar.

$$V = F \cdot \bar{t} \tag{2}$$

Bei Betrachtung der mittleren Transitzeit als dem Integral einer Frequenzfunktion (Meier u. Zierler 1954; Zierler 1961, 1962b, 1963) wird die mittlere Transitzeit aus der Dilutionskurve eindeutig berechenbar und das Volumen durch die Gleichung (3) beschreibbar.

$$V = \frac{Q}{\int C(t) \cdot dt} \cdot \bar{t} \tag{3}$$

Unter der Voraussetzung, daß die gesamte Dosis zu einem beliebigen Zeitpunkt vom Detektor erfaßt wird, gilt ferner, daß die Höhe im Maximum der Dilutionskurve der Dosis proportional ist und damit die Gleichung (3) in der vereinfachten verbalen Form von

$$\text{Volumen} = \frac{\text{Height}}{\text{Area}} \cdot \text{Transittime} \tag{3a}$$

geschrieben werden kann.

Werden zwei Messungen mit je einem diffusiblen und einem intravasal verbleibenden Tracer durchgeführt, so ergeben sich zwei Dilutionskurven, aus denen das gesamte Verteilungsvolumen des diffusiblen Tracers und das intravasale Volumen berechnet werden können. Die Differenz dieser Volumina ist das per Diffusion erreichbare extravaskuläre Volumen.

Um zu einem relativen Wert zu gelangen, der geringeren Meßfehlern unterliegt, führten CHINARD et al. (1962) als relatives Maß das Verhältnis des Volumen des extravaskulären Wassers V_{ew} zum Plasmavolumen V_p ein. Dieser Wert läßt sich nach Normierung der beiden Dosiswerte direkt aus den mittleren Transitzeiten der Tracer nach Gleichung (4) berechnen:

$$\frac{V_{ew}}{V_p} = \frac{\bar{t}_w - \bar{t}_p}{\bar{t}_p}$$
(4)

wobei $\bar{t}_w$ die mittlere Transitzeit der Aktivität durch das Gesamtvolumen und $\bar{t}_p$ die mittlere Transitzeit durch den Intravasalraum bedeuten.

In den folgenden Jahren wurde die Methode zur Bestimmung des extravaskulären Lungenwassers von GORESKY et al. (1969), GIUNTINI (1971), COOPER et al. (1972), JONES et al. (1972), FAZIO et al. (1976a, b), FAZIO u. GIUNTINI (1979), BINSWANGER et al. (1978) und HELMEKE et al. (1982) aufgenommen und weiterentwickelt. Theoretisch zusammenfassend wurde die Methode von ZIERLER (1962a, 1965), CHINARD (1975), von GIUNTINI u. FAZIO (1979) sowie von BASSINGTHWAIGHTE (1985) beschrieben.

Obwohl die Methode unter Zuhilfenahme von Kameratechniken prinzipiell eine regionale Quantifizierung des extravasalen Verteilungsraumes erlaubt, ist ihre Genauigkeit nur begrenzt. Limitierend wirkt sich erstens die relativ geringe Zählstatistik in kleinen Regionen aus. Zweitens wird eine Abhängigkeit des gemessenen Extravasalvolumens vom Herz-Zeit-Volumen gefunden. Drittens ergeben sich bei niedrigen Flußraten aufgrund von geringer Herzleistung Schwierigkeiten bei der Korrektur von Rezirkulationseffekten, und schließlich ist im „single pass" nicht der gesamte Extravasalraum erfaßbar, sondern in Abhängigkeit von der Extraktionsrate und dem Verteilungskoeffizienten nur ca. 60%–80% desselben.

GIUNTINI u. FAZIO (1979) konnten zeigen, daß die Rezirkulation und die Unterbewertung des extravaskulären Lungenwassers mit der Indikator-Verdünnungsmethode eng miteinander verknüpft sind. Durch Messung der „input-" und der „response-function" gelang ihnen eine weitgehende Angleichung der gemessenen und der *post-mortem* bestimmten Lungenwasserwerte in Hunden. Das Verfahren erfordert jedoch ein arterielles „sampling" und ist damit invasiv.

2. Indikatorverdünnungsanalysen im Gleichgewichtszustand: „Steady-State-Methodik"

Die Grundlagen des Steady-State-Modells beruhen auf Ansätzen, die auch von KETY u. SCHMIDT 1945, 1948 für die Entwicklung der Flußmessung nach dem Fick'schen Diffusionsgesetz benutzt wurden. Der von KETY u. SCHMIDT benutzte differentielle Ansatz wurde von vielen späteren Anwendern für den Gleichgewichtszustand vereinfacht. Weitere Anwender, wie BASSINGTHWAIGHTE (1974, 1977), BASSINGTHWAIGHTE u. HOLLOWAY (1976), ORR (1979), LASSEN u. HENRIKSEN (1983), haben die Theorie und das Modell verfeinert und ihren speziellen Fragestellungen angepaßt. Der vereinfachte Ansatz ist im folgenden wiedergegeben. Eine Einführung in den differentiellen Ansatz wird im folgenden Abschnitt 3 im Rahmen der Grundlagen der Flußmessung gegeben.

Unter der Bedingung der konstanten Infusion oder Inhalation eines kurzlebigen Tracers wird ein Gleichgewichtszustand erreicht, der mit der Gleichung (5) beschrieben werden kann.

$$C_{in} \cdot F_{in} = C_{out} \cdot F_{out} + Q \cdot \lambda$$
(5)

Im Gleichgewicht ist das Produkt aus Fluß und Eintrittskonzentration gleich dem Produkt aus Fluß und der Austrittskonzentration plus dem Produkt aus Aktivitätsmenge im Volumen und der Zerfallskonstanten des Isotops. Durch Substitution der Austrittskonzentration C_{out} durch das Verhältnis von Tracermenge zu Volumen und Auflösung nach der Tracermenge oder dem Fluß ergeben sich die Gleichung (6) und für gleiche Einfluß- und Ausflußgeschwindigkeit ($F_{in} = F_{out}$) die Gleichung (6a).

$$Q = \frac{F_{in} \cdot C_{in}}{\dfrac{F_{out}}{V} + \lambda} \tag{6}$$

$$F = \frac{\lambda \cdot Q \cdot V}{C_{in} \cdot V - Q} \tag{6a}$$

Diese Gleichungen stellen die theoretische Grundlage für die meisten Ansätze zur regionalen Blutflußmessung sowie davon abgeleiteter Parameter dar, wie der regionalen Sauerstoffextraktion (Subramanyam et al. 1978; Huang et al. 1979; Lammertsma et al. 1981; Selikson u. Eichling 1982; Lassen u. Henrikson 1983).

Zur Berechnung eines Verteilungsvolumens im Steady State mit kurzlebigen Tracern kann durch Gleichsetzung der Ein- und Ausflußgeschwindigkeit in Gleichung (6) die Gleichung (7) erhalten werden.

$$Q = \frac{V \cdot C_{in}}{1 + V/F \cdot \lambda} \tag{7}$$

Wird in Gleichung (6) der Quotient V/F als die mittlere Transitzeit $\bar{t}$ betrachtet, so kann Gleichung (7) zu Gleichung (7a) umgeformt werden.

$$Q = \frac{V \cdot C_{in}}{1 + \bar{t} \cdot \lambda} \tag{7a}$$

Auflösung nach dem Volumen V ergibt die Gleichung (8)

$$V = \frac{Q}{C_{in}} (1 + \bar{t} \cdot \lambda), \tag{8}$$

die die direkte Proportionalität von Tracermenge und Volumen angibt, mit einem Korrekturglied für den Zerfall der Tracermenge während der Passage durch das Volumen V.

Bei der Messung extravaskulärer Wassermengen werden das Intravasalvolumen und das durch Diffusion erreichbare Volumen in getrennten Messungen ermittelt. Durch Normierung der beiden Volumina auf die gleiche Intravasalaktivität Q ergibt die Differenz der beiden Volumenmessungen das extravasale Wasservolumen V_{ew} nach Gleichung (9).

$$V_{ew} = \frac{Q_w \cdot (1 + \bar{t}_w \cdot \lambda_w) - Q_b \cdot (1 + \bar{t}_b \cdot \lambda_b)}{C_{in}} \tag{9}$$

Bei der Verwendung von ^{11}C-markierten Intravasalraum-Tracern ist λ_b hinreichend klein, um als Korrekturfaktor für den Zerfall während der intravasalen Passage durch ein Gewebevolumen vernachlässigt werden zu können. Damit ergibt sich für die Berechnung des extravasalen Wasserraumes die vereinfachte Formel (9a):

$$V_{ew} = \frac{Q_w - Q_b}{C_{in}} + \frac{Q_w}{C_{in}} \cdot \bar{t}_w \cdot \lambda_w \tag{9a}$$

Tabelle 2. Mittlere Transitzeiten (sek) für intravasale und diffusible Passage durch Lungen und Gehirn

	Lungen				Gehirn			
Literatur	HELMEKE et al. (1982)		FAZIO u. GIUN-TINI (1979)		BINSWANGER et al. (1978)		SZABO u. RITZL (1983)	
Zustand	normal	pathol.	normal	pathol.	normal	pathol	normal	pathol.
Intravasal	7 ± 4	12 ± 5	10 ± 2	25 ± 10	9 ± 3	20 ± 9	11 ± 4	19 ± 7
Diffusibel	12 ± 4	25 ± 10	13 ± 2	30 ± 15	12 ± 4	33 ± 13	–	–

Die notwendige Korrektur für einen kurzlebigen, z.B. mit ^{15}O markierten, frei diffusiblen Tracer, kann anhand vermessener Transitzeiten exakt, bzw. für einen physiologischen Bereich anhand von Normwerten durchgeführt werden. Typische Transitzeiten für Lungen und Gehirn sind in Tabelle 2 wiedergegeben.

Die Fehlerempfindlichkeit dieser Methode, auch im Hinblick auf pathologisch veränderte Extraktionsraten und Verteilungskoeffizienten, wurde von MEYER et al. (1985 a) beschrieben.

Ein vereinfachter Ansatz zu Bestimmung extravasaler Wasserräume, der allerdings auf eine relative Messung des Lungenwassers beschränkt ist, geht von der Annahme aus, daß extravasale Dichteerhöhungen in der Lunge mit extravasalem Wasser korrelieren. Damit kann auf die Bestimmung des Wasserverteilungsvolumens verzichtet werden. Die Dichte wird aus der für beide Methoden notwendigen Transmissionsaufnahme ermittelt. Die extravasale Dichte-Bestimmung wurde von RHODES et al. (1980, 1981) und WOLLMER et al. (1983, 1984) entwickelt und liefert in einem weiten klinischen Bereich vergleichbare Ergebnisse wie die direkte Bestimmung des extravasalen Wasserverteilungsraumes. SCHUSTER et al. (1986) haben die Methode ebenfalls aufgegriffen und deren Fehlerempfindlichkeit speziell im Hinblick auf Dichteschwankungen bezüglich der Atmungstiefe untersucht (SCHUSTER u. MARKLIN 1986). Unter Normalbedingungen wurde dabei eine zufriedenstellende Korrelation mit Dichtebestimmungen durch die Transmissionscomputertomographie gefunden und eine nur geringe Fehlerempfindlichkeit bezüglich der Atmungstiefe. Unter äußerst pathologischen Verhältnissen, wie z.B. unter künstlicher Beatmung, bei einem stumpfen Thoraxtrauma, eingedrücktem Brustkorb oder posttraumatischen nekrotischen Veränderungen, muß jedoch mit ungünstigeren Korrelationen gerechnet werden.

III. Blutfluß

Kurzzeitige Ausfälle in der Energieversorgung sowohl des Herzens wie des Gehirns können zu irreversiblen Organschäden führen. Hauptursache für solche Ausfälle sind kardio- und zerebrovaskuläre Erkrankungen, deren Ausmaß häufig schwer zu diagnostizieren ist. Da angiographisch erkennbare Gefäßverengungen eines bestimmten Grades aufgrund unterschiedlicher Kollateralausbildungen nicht notwendigerweise zu einer korrelierenden Unterversorgung des entsprechenden Versorgungsgebietes führen, ist eine regional quantifizierbare Messung des Blutflusses das Hauptziel der Diagnostik, die zu einer optimalen Therapie dieser Gefäßerkrankungen führt.

Die Ansätze zur Messung des Blutflusses nach der Indikator-Verdünnungsmethode gehen, wie schon bei der Volumenmessung erwähnt, auf STUART, HENRIQUES und HAMILTON zurück. Die erste brauchbare Methode wurde von KETY u. SCHMIDT (1948) durch direkte Messung der arterio-venösen Differenz von Lachgaskonzentrationen im Laufe der Inhalation von N_2O

entwickelt. Die Grundlage dieser Messung bestand in der Anwendung des Fick'schen Prinzips (Fick 1855), das die diffusive Extraktion im Gleichgewichtszustand beschreibt:

$$F \cdot C_{in} - F \cdot C_{out} = J_{ex} \tag{10}$$

Darin sind F der Fluß, C_{in} und C_{out} die Ein- und Ausflußkonzentrationen und J_{ex} die durch nicht konvektiven Fluß, d.h. durch Diffusion entzogene Tracermenge pro Zeiteinheit.

Da im Gleichgewicht der zeitvariable Flux $J = F \cdot C = Q/t$ durch die entsprechende Tracermengen Q ersetzt werden darf, gilt dann für das Gehirn:

$$Q_a = Q_v - Q_c \tag{11}$$

wobei Q die Tracermenge in den Kompartmenten $a =$ arteriell, $v =$ venös und $c =$ Hirn bedeutet.

Wie schon unter Abschnitt II gezeigt, kann bei zeitvariabler Tracerkonzentration C in einem Zeitraum von $t_0 - t_1$ und konstantem Fluß F die gesamte Tracermenge Q für jedes Kompartment ausgedrückt werden als:

$$Q = F \cdot \int_0^1 C \cdot dt \tag{1}$$

Für den speziellen Fall des Hirnkompartments gilt dann:

$$Q_c = F \cdot \int_0^1 (C_a - C_v) \cdot dt \tag{12}$$

Auflösung nach F ergibt:

$$F = \frac{Q_c}{\int_0^1 (C_a - C_v) \cdot dt} \tag{13}$$

Nach hinreichend langer Äquilibrierungszeit wird für einen frei diffusiblen Tracer der Quotient aus Q_c und dem Hirnvolumen, also die Hirnkonzentration, gleich der venösen Konzentration C_v. Die tatsächliche Abweichung dieser Konzentrationen voneinander wird durch den als Konstante angenommenen Verteilungskoeffizienten σ ausgeglichen. Durch zeitabhängige Messung zerebroarterieller und venöser N_2O-Konzentrationen konnten Kety u. Schmidt (1948) den spezifischen Fluß f (Fluß pro Gramm Gewebe) nach Gleichung (14) berechnen:

$$f = \frac{C_v \cdot \sigma}{\int_0^1 (C_a - C_v) \cdot dt} \tag{14}$$

Wie im folgenden gezeigt wird, ist die Kety-Schmidt-Methodik prinzipiell einer „steady state"-Transitzeit-Bestimmung äquivalent.

Eine weitere Kompartmentisierung der Methode über die „black box"-Analyse hinaus zeichnet sich in der gegenwärtigen Diskussion um die Weiterentwicklung und Verbesserung der Blutflußmessung zwar ab (Budinger u. Gjedde 1986), kann im Rahmen dieser Darstellung aber noch nicht ausführlich diskutiert werden, da bisher nur theoretische Grundlagen, aber noch keine Anwendungsmodelle publiziert wurden; entsprechendes gilt für Anwendungsmodelle für Organe mit mehrfachen Einflußfunktionen (PERL et al. 1969).

Eine Unterteilung in Blutflußmessungen am Gehirn und am Herzen erscheint hier nicht sinnvoll, da die Methodik für beide Anwendungsgebiete sehr ähnlich ist. Da die Methodenentwicklung aus meßtechnischen Limitationen heraus vorwiegend auf dem Gebiet der Blutflußmessung im Gehirn stattgefunden hat, stehen in den folgenden Abschnitten entsprechende Arbeiten im Vordergrund.

Zur besseren Übersichtlichkeit sollen die Modellvorstellungen zur Blutflußmessung jedoch in dynamische und steady state-Methoden aufgeteilt und beschrieben werden. Darüber hinausgehende Übersichtsarbeiten sind von BETZ (1972), LASSEN u. PERL (1979), und BASSINGTHWAIGHTE (1976, 1985) erschienen.

1. Dynamische Meßverfahren zur Blutflußbestimmung mittels Bolusinjektion und Transitzeit-Messungen

Bei Flußbestimmungen durch Messung der Passage eines Bolus durch ein zu untersuchendes Volumen können verschiedene Ansätze unterschieden werden. Die zwei als klassisch bezeichenbaren Ansätze gehen von ZIERLERS Überlegungen zur Messung der mittleren Transitzeit $\bar{t}$ aus (MEIER u. ZIERLER 1954; ZIERLER 1961, 1963).

Für einen propfenartigen Fluß durch ein black box-System gilt die Gleichung:

$$\text{Volumen} = \text{Fluß} \cdot \text{Transitzeit} \tag{15}$$

Wird jedoch in einem realistischen Experiment eine Anzahl von Partikeln in ein System mit einem Ein- und Ausgang (black box) injiziert, so werden die individuellen Transitzeiten der Partikel entsprechend einer Häufigkeitsverteilung verteilt sein. Die mittlere Transitzeit ist dann entsprechend Abb. 3 die Fläche unter der Residualkurve geteilt durch die Partikelzahl.

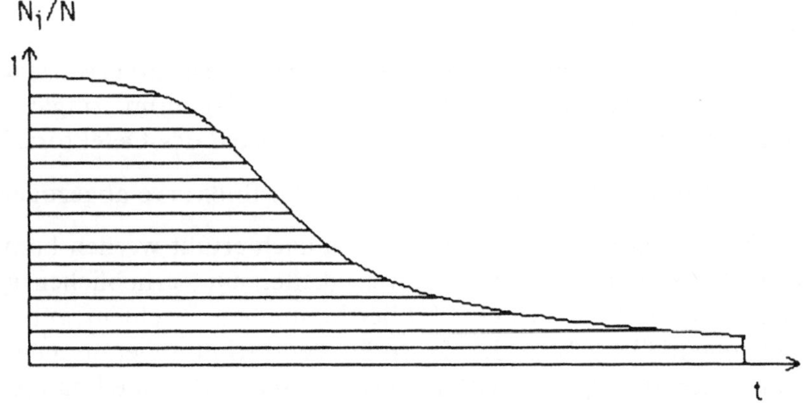

Abb. 3. Zeitlicher Verlauf des Verlassens fraktioneller Anteile N_i einer Partikelanzahl N eines black-box-Systems

Dies zeigt, daß die Transitzeit der Mittelwert einer Häufigkeitsverteilung ist, deren Form nach Gleichung (16) beschrieben werden kann.

$$\bar{t} = \int h \cdot dt \tag{16}$$

wobei h die Häufigkeitsverteilung beschreibt.

Betrachtet man h als den Anteil der Partikel, der ein Volumen pro Zeiteinheit verläßt ($Q(t)/q$), kann die Transitzeit auch in Form von Gleichung (17) geschrieben werden:

$$\bar{t} = \int t \cdot \frac{Q(t)}{q}\, dt = \int t \cdot \frac{F \cdot C(t)}{q}\, dt \tag{17}$$

wobei mit q die Tracereinheitsmenge gemeint ist.

Aufgrund der Äquivalenz der Gleichung (17) mit Gleichung (3) ist damit auch der in Abschnitt II etwas schnelle Sprung in die Transitzeit exakt erklärt.

Mit $\bar{t} \cdot F = V$ und Gleichung (1) ergibt sich die grundlegende Gleichung für die Anwendung der Transitzeitmessungen:

$$\bar{t} = \frac{V \cdot \int C(t)\, dt}{Q} = \frac{V}{F} \tag{18}$$

oder verbal ausgedrückt:

$$\text{Mittlere Transitzeit} = \text{Verteilungsvolumen/Fluß} \tag{18a}$$

Der auf das Verteilungsvolumen bezogene Fluß, also z.B. der Fluß in ml/min · 100 g Gewebe, ist damit der in diesem Gewebe gemessenen Transitzeit umgekehrt proportional.

Zur Messung der auf das Verteilungsvolumen bezogenen Transitzeit können verschiedene Auswertungen von Tracerdilutionskurven herangezogen werden. Meist ergeben sie sich aus der „Area over Height"-Methode nach der Umstellung der Gleichung:

$$\frac{\bar{t}}{V} = \frac{\int C(t) \cdot dt}{Q} = \frac{\text{Fläche}}{\text{Höhe}} \tag{19}$$

Als absolut wichtige und limitierende Voraussetzungen für die Anwendung der „black box"-Analyse müssen jedoch folgende Faktoren beachtet werden:

Erstens: Die Bolusweite muß wesentlich enger sein als die kleinste zu erwartende Transitzeit, damit zu irgendeinem Zeitpunkt die gesamte Dosis, die das Organ im „single pass" erreichen kann, in dem zu untersuchenden Volumen, d.h. im Gesichtsfeld des Detektors, liegt.

Zweitens: Rezirkulationsanteile müssen von der Bolus-Ausflußkurve abgezogen werden.

Während die erste Bedingung im allgemeinen recht einfach erfüllt werden kann, ist die Korrektur von Rezirkulationsanteilen oft mit Schwierigkeiten und erheblichen systematischen Fehlern verbunden. Obwohl für einfache Flußbestimmungen in einem gut durchmischten System ein monoexponentieller Abfall der Tracerkonzentration angenommen werden kann, verhalten sich reale Systeme aufgrund vieler physiologischer Randbedingungen nicht ideal und haben verlängerte Auswaschzeiten. Weiterführende mathematische Behandlungen dieser Limitationen finden sich bei Roberts et al. (1973) und Perl et al. (1985).

Der Rezirkulationsanteil wird dadurch systematisch überschätzt. Nach Lassen u. Perl (1979) liegt der Fehler, der durch semilogarithmische Extrapolation des ersten Abfalls entsteht, bei gut 10%, was zu einer entsprechend erhöhten Transitzeit bzw. einer Unterschätzung des tatsächlichen Flusses führt.

Erste Messungen dieser Art zur Bestimmung des Blutflusses im Gehirn mit Positronenstrahlern, unter Berücksichtigung des später noch zu diskutierenden Verteilungskoeffizienten von Wasser zwischen Plasma und Hirngewebe, wurden von Ter-Pogossian u. Powers (1958) und Ter-Pogossian et al. (1969) durchgeführt.

Wird nicht das perfundierte Gewebe selbst beobachtet, sondern die Ein- und Ausflußstelle je einzeln betrachtet, so kann der Fluß in dem dazwischenliegenden Volumen auch aus der Differenz der Schwerpunkte der Durchflußkurven in diesen Meßpunkten ermittelt werden. Diese Art der Flußbestimmung, wie sie in Abb. 4 dargestellt ist, wird als Einfluß-Ausfluß-Differenzmethode bezeichnet. Die mittlere Transitzeit $\bar{t}$ durch das dazwischenliegende Organ ergibt sich aus $\bar{t}_{out} - \bar{t}_{in}$.

Dynamische Meßmethoden zur Blutflußbestimmung über die Transitzeit sind nach LASSEN u. PERL (1979) auch solche, die das allmähliche Erreichen des Gleichgewichtszustands durch konstante Tracerapplikation oder das Abfallen aus einem Gleichgewichtszustand nach konstanter Tracerapplikation verfolgen.

Zu den Ersteren gehört schließlich auch die Methode von KETY u. SCHMIDT (1945, 1948), deren Schema in Hinblick auf die Transitzeit-Bestimmung in Abb. 5 wiedergegeben ist.

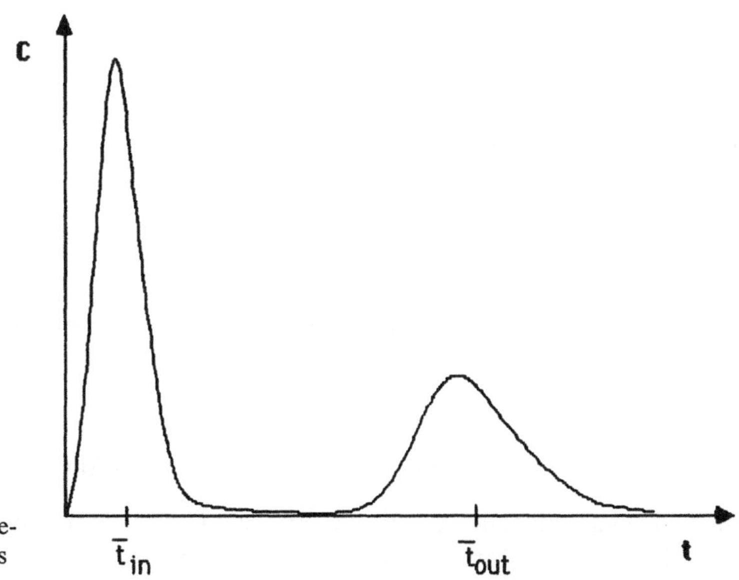

Abb. 4. Ein-, Ausfluß-Differenzmethode zur Bestimmung des Flusses

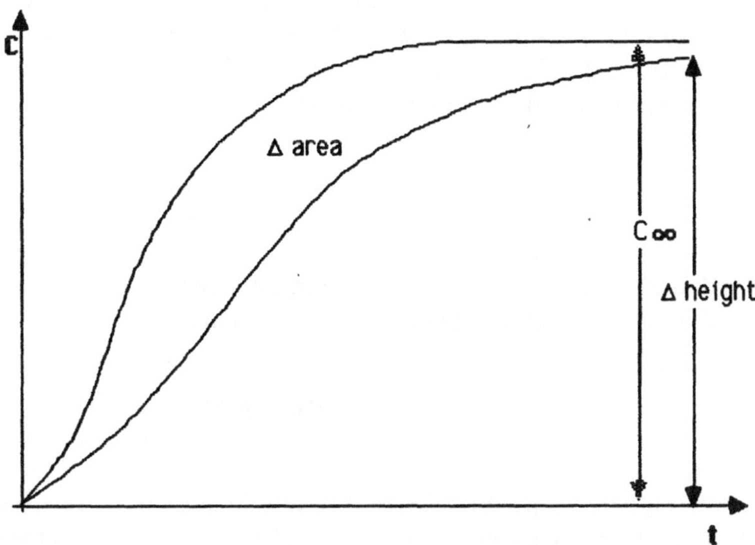

Abb. 5. Kety-Schmidt-Methodik zur Flußbestimmung

Die Desaturierungstechnik haben Ingvar u. Lassen (1962) mit der Krypton-Clearance zu einer klinisch nutzbaren Methode ausgearbeitet, deren Prinzip in Abb. 6 wiedergegeben ist.

Erste Messungen dieser Art zur Bestimmung des Blutflusses im Gehirn mit Positronenstrahlern wurden von Ter-Pogossian et al. (1969) durchgeführt.

Sowohl bei der Kety-Schmidt-Methode als auch bei der Lassen-Technik besteht die Hauptschwierigkeit in der Extrapolation der Endwerte der aufgezeichneten Meßkurven, die durch unvollständige Äquilibrierung bzw. Rezirkulationseffekte maskiert werden, sowie in der genauen Bestimmung des Verteilungskoeffizienten ∂, der, sofern er von 1 abweicht, über $V_d = \partial \cdot V_{\text{gemessen}}$ als Korrekturfaktor berücksichtigt werden muß (s. Abschnitt III.2).

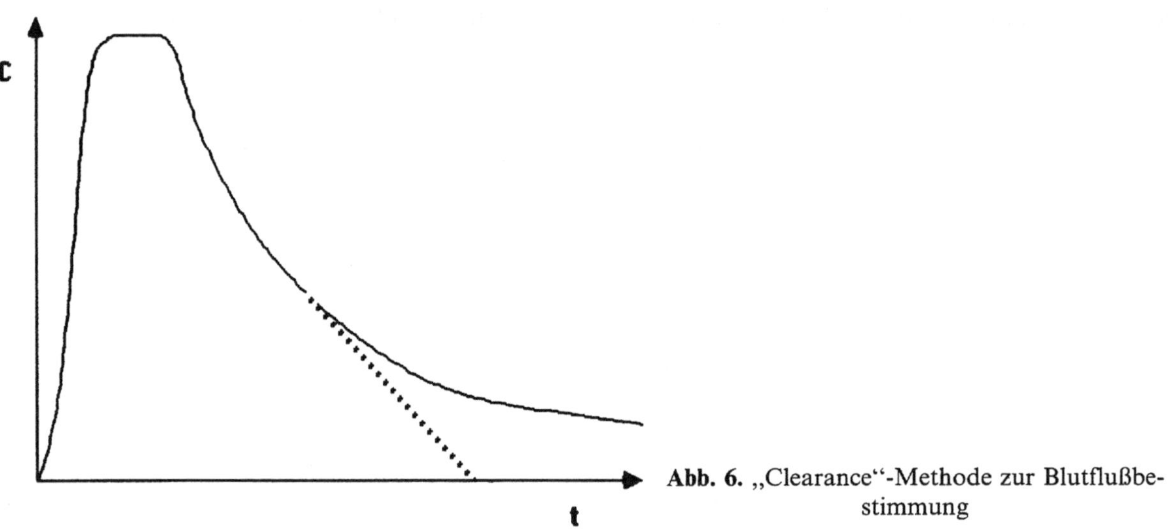

Abb. 6. „Clearance"-Methode zur Blutflußbestimmung

2. Flußmessung im „Steady State" mit kurzlebigen Tracern

Ein Gleichgewichtszustand ist durch eine zeitlich gleichbleibende Tracerkonzentration in den betrachteten Verteilungsräumen gekennzeichnet, wie dies z.B. für die Bestimmung des Blutvolumens beschrieben wurde. Verluste an Tracerkonzentration können einmal durch Abwandern des Tracers in ein anderes Verteilungsvolumen auftreten oder durch Zerfall des Tracers. Um diese Verluste auszugleichen, kann eine konstante Zuführung des Tracers erfolgen. Für den sich daraus entwickelnden Gleichgewichtszustand nach ausreichend langer konstanter Inhalation oder Infusion eines kurzlebigen Tracers gilt die Gleichung (5), deren Auflösung nach dem Fluß zur Gleichung (6a) führt:

$$F = \frac{Q \cdot V \cdot \lambda}{C_{\text{in}} \cdot V - Q} \tag{6a}$$

Wird der Fluß auf eine Volumeneinheit bezogen, so kann der zerebrale Blutfluß als CBF in ml/Volumeneinheit·Minute als F/V geschrieben werden als:

$$\text{CBF} = F/V = \frac{\lambda}{C_{\text{in}}/C_{\text{Hirn}} - 1} \tag{6b}$$

Unter Verwendung von ^{15}O-markiertem Wasser als diffusiblem Flußtracer wurde dieser relativ einfache Ansatz von T. Jones et al. (1976a) für erste quantitative Messungen des regionalen

CBF eingesetzt und validiert (FRACKOWIAK et al. 1980b), sowie auf seine Fehlerempfindlichkeit hin analysiert (LAMMERTSMA et al. 1981). Andere Arbeitsgruppen haben die Methode ebenfalls aufgegriffen und methodisch beschrieben (BARON et al. 1979; ACKERMANN et al. 1980; BIGLER et al. 1981, 1982; S.C. JONES et al. 1985).

Die Grenzen des Modells beruhen im wesentlichen auf der Nicht-Linearität der Operationsgleichung (6b), die bei großen Flüssen zu einer vergrößerten Fehlersensitivität führt. Dies wird leicht ersichtlich wenn man bedenkt, daß bei hohem Fluß die Konzentrationsdifferenz zwischen der arteriellen und der venösen Seite klein wird und damit ein Meßfehler ΔC_{Hirn} zu einem überproportionalen Fehler im berechneten Fluß führt. Abbildung 7 zeigt jedoch, daß selbst bei hohen Flüssen von ca. 100 ml/min · 100 g die relative arterio-venöse Differenz für einen frei diffusiblen Tracer, auch wenn er mit ^{15}O ($\lambda = 0.35$) markiert ist, größer als 20% bleibt.

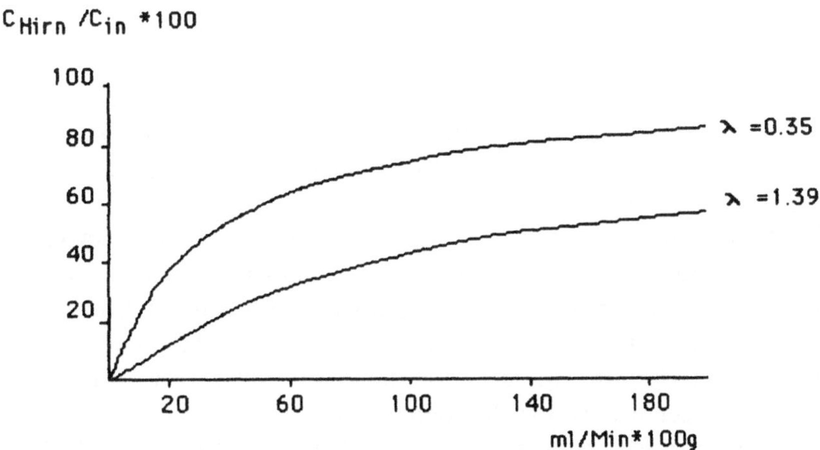

Abb. 7. Relative arteriovenöse Differenz entsprechend Gleichung 6b in Abhängigkeit des Flusses für zwei Tracer mit Halbwertzeiten von 2 min ($\lambda = 0.35$) und 0.5 min ($\lambda = 1.39$)

Weitere Fehleranalysen für die Methode wurden von HUANG et al. (1979), LAMMERTSMA et al. (1982) und JONES et al. (1982) durchgeführt. HUANG et al. (1979) differenzierten die Gleichung (6a) und trugen die Standardabweichung des prozentualen Fehlers gegen die Halbwertzeit des Tracers auf. Dabei zeigte sich, daß die Funktion ein Minimum bei $T_{1/2} = 0.5$ min aufweist. JONES et al. (1982) diskutieren neben der Fehlerempfindlichkeit der Methode an sich auch die resultierende Genauigkeit im Hinblick auf unterschiedliche Meßgeräte-Parameter und die applizierte Strahlendosis, während LAMMERTSMA et al. (1982) die vorherigen theoretischen Arbeiten anhand von Meßwerten statistisch überprüfen.

Eine weitere Limitation der Methode liegt in der Annahme, daß sowohl der Verteilungskoeffizient von Wasser zwischen Plasma und Hirngewebe als auch der Extraktionskoeffizient vernachlässigbar wenig von 1 abweichen und daß dies auch in pathologisch veränderten Bereichen zutrifft. Die mit dieser Annahme verbundene Fehlersensitivität wurde ebenfalls von LAMMERTSMA et al. (1981) analysiert.

Grundlage für eine Berücksichtigung der Extraktionsfraktion und des Verteilungskoeffizienten ist das lineare Kapillarmodell entsprechend den Vorstellungen von RENKIN (1959) und CRONE (1963).

Danach kann die Extraktionsfraktion E durch den Ausdruck:

$$E = e^{-P \cdot S/F} \tag{20}$$

beschrieben werden. Darin stellen $P \cdot S$ das Produkt aus Permeabilität und Oberfläche und F den Fluß dar. Der Verteilungskoeffizient für einen diffusiblen Tracer ergibt sich aus der Vorstellung, daß im Gleichgewicht der Gesamtverteilungsraum V_d aus der Summe von Blutvolumen V_b und einem virtuellen Gewebeverteilungsraum V_x besteht, der sich aus dem Verteilungskoeffizienten ∂ und dem Gewebevolumen V_t zusammensetzt.

$$V_d = \partial \cdot V_t + V_b \tag{21}$$

Eine Übersicht zu verschiedenen Ansätzen zur Berechnung von E und ∂ findet sich bei Crone u. Lassen (1970).

Der als klassisch geltende Ansatz zur Berücksichtigung beider Faktoren im Steady-State-Modell lautet demnach:

$$Q = \frac{C_{\text{in}} \cdot F \cdot E}{\dfrac{F}{V_d} + \lambda} + \frac{C_{\text{in}} \cdot F \cdot (1 - E)}{\dfrac{F}{V_b} + \lambda} \tag{22}$$

Darin ist für das Verteilungsvolumen V_d die Menge der Eintrittsaktivität um den Faktor der Extraktionsfraktion E vermindert worden und der nicht extrahierbare Anteil als vaskulärer Bestandteil addiert worden.

Grundsätzlich kann dazu angemerkt werden, daß die Extraktion im Gleichgewichtszustand wesentlich vollständiger ist als nach der Passage eines Bolus. Der Verteilungskoeffizient bleibt für Wasser und auch für alle anderen Substanzen auch im Gleichgewicht deutlich unter 1.0. Neuere Arbeiten (Herscovitch u. Raichle 1985; Jones et al. 1985) bestätigen dieses Verhalten von Wasser. In einigen Arbeiten wird daher ^{15}O-Butanol als ein besser geeigneter diffusibler Tracer favorisiert, für den ein Verteilungskoeffizient von >0.98 in der Literatur beschrieben wird (Raichle et al. 1976; 1983b; Gjedde et al. 1980; Takagi et al. 1984).

Abgesehen von der oben angeführten Kritik an der Methode, bietet die Steady-State-Flußmessung im Gehirn mit ^{15}O-Wasser aber auch einige Vorteile, die auch in neueren Übersichtsarbeiten anerkannt worden sind (Frackowiak u. Lammertsma 1985; Carson 1986).

Die Vorteile der Methode liegen einmal in der problemlosen kontinuierlichen Traceradministration durch Infusion von ^{15}O-markiertem Wasser oder durch Inhalation von ^{15}O-markiertem Kohlendioxid, zum anderen in der relativ einfachen Meßanordnung, die eine gute Reproduzierbarkeit gewährleistet und die schwierige Erfassung von Zeitaktivitätskurven in kleinen Arealen umgeht.

Diese Vorteile wirken sich besonders bei der Verwendung etwas älterer und damit langsamerer Tomographen aus. Die verbleibenden Unsicherheiten in der absoluten Quantifizierung der Flußdaten können darüberhinaus in vielen klinischen Fragestellungen, bei denen relative Messungen der Flußänderung im Vordergrund stehen, vernachlässigt werden.

Eine weitere Variante der Flußbestimmung mittels kontinuierlicher Traceradministration stellt die Gradienten-Infusion dar, bei der entweder exponentiell oder linear ansteigend der Flußtracer injiziert wird (Selikson u. Eichling 1982; Duncan et al. 1983). Dies erlaubt die Erstellung bzw. die Erhöhung der arterio-venösen Differenz, entsprechend den Anforderungen die aus Randbedingungen wie der Meßzeit und der Halbwertzeit des Tracers entstehen. Theoretisch ist die Methode der konstanten Infusion sowie den Bolus-Injektionsmethoden überlegen, da sie eine statistisch genauere Berechnung der regionalen Verteilungskoeffizienten gestattet. Als Nachteile müssen jedoch gegenüber den Bolustechniken eine höhere Strahlenbelastung sowie die aufwendige Injektionstechnik erwähnt werden.

3. Flußmessungen mit dynamischen Auswaschverfahren („Washout-Analytik")

Grundsätzlich sind in der Aufzeichnung des zeitlichen Verlaufes einer Tracerakkumulation oder Tracerpassage zusätzliche Informationen enthalten, die bei der Beobachtung des Gleichgewichtszustandes nicht erhalten werden können (ROBERTSON 1962). Um diese Zusatzinformationen zu nutzen, betrachten HUANG et al. (1982) in ihrem allgemeinen Ansatz zur Beschreibung des Flusses in einem Einkompartmentmodell entsprechend Gleichung (6a) die Zeitvariablen Q und C_{in} als die Summen ihrer zeitlichen Infinitesimalwerte und schreiben:

$$F = \frac{\lambda \cdot \int Q \cdot dt}{\int C_{\mathrm{in}} \cdot dt - V^{-1} \cdot \int Q \cdot dt} \tag{23}$$

Formal sind die Gleichung (23) und die Gleichung (6a) völlig identisch, sie gelten jedoch unter verschiedenen Randbedingungen. Die Beschreibung des Verteilungsvolumens nach der Gleichung $V = Q/C$ bringt bei kurzlebigen Tracern entsprechend den Ausführungen in Abschnitt B.II. einen Korrekturterm für den Zerfall des Tracers während der Passage durch das Verteilungsvolumen. Für eine Substitution des Volumenterms in Gleichung (23) werden daher von HUANG et al. (1982) die zerfallskorrigierten Formen von Q und C_{in} als $Q^*(t) = Q(t) \cdot e^{-\lambda \cdot t}$ und $C^*(t) = C_{\mathrm{in}}(t) \cdot e^{-\lambda \cdot t}$ eingeführt. Mit der nun gültigen Substitution von $V = \int Q^* \cdot dt / \int C^* \cdot dt$ ergibt sich eine Gleichung der Form:

$$F = \frac{\lambda \int Q \cdot dt \int Q^* \cdot dt}{\int C_{\mathrm{in}} \cdot dt \int Q^* \cdot dt - \int Q \cdot dt \int C_{\mathrm{in}}^* \cdot dt} \tag{24}$$

Bei einer mathematischen Betrachtung zeigt sich, daß diese Gleichung nur für die Integration von 0 bis ∞ gültig ist, d.h. wenn an beiden Integrationsgrenzen $Q(t)$ und $Q^*(t)$ gleich 0 werden. Im Falle eines Abbruchs der Integration zum Zeitpunkt (T) muß $Q(T)$ durch Integration von Gleichung (5a)

$$\frac{dQ}{dt} = F \cdot C_{\mathrm{in}}(t) - F \cdot C_{\mathrm{out}}(t) - \lambda \cdot Q(t) \tag{5a}$$

ermittelt werden.

Die Lösungen für F und V ergeben sich nach HUANG et al. (1982) zu

$$F = \frac{\int Q^* dt [\lambda \int Q dt + Q(T)] - Q^*(T) \int Q dt}{\int C_{\mathrm{in}} dt \int Q^* dt - \int Q dt \int C_{\mathrm{in}}^* dt} \tag{25}$$

$$V = \frac{\int Q^* dt [\lambda \int Q dt + Q(T)] - Q^*(T) \int Q dt}{\int C_{\mathrm{in}}^* dt [\lambda \int Q dt + Q(T)] - Q^*(T) \int C_{\mathrm{in}}^* dt} \tag{25a}$$

wobei nach relativ kurzer Zeit $Q(T)$ vernachlässigbar ist, wohingegen $Q^*(T)$ infolge der Zerfallskorrektur als Rezirkulationsanteil erhalten bleibt. Weil darüberhinaus $Q^*(T)$ nicht punktuell, sondern infolge der PET-Randbedingungen nur über einen Zeitraum ermittelt werden kann, muß die Messung in einem späten Teil des Beobachtungsraumes erfolgen, in dem der zeitliche Verlauf von $Q^*(T)$ nahezu linear ist.

Einen anderen Ansatz verfolgen HOWARD et al. (1983) und HERSCOVITCH et al. (1983), die formal die autoradiographische Methode KETYS zur Messung des CBF (LANDAU et al. 1955) auf die PET übertragen. Dabei gehen sie zunächst von einem nicht zerfallenden Tracer aus, für den nach dem Fickschen Prinzip der Massenerhaltung in einem Einkompartmentmodell der Ansatz nach Gleichung (12) gilt:

$$\frac{dQ}{dt} = F \cdot C_{in}(t) - F \cdot C_{out}(t) \tag{12a}$$

Mit $C_{out} = C/\partial$, $Q = C/V$ und $F/V = f$ wird

$$\frac{dC}{dt} = f\,[C_{in}(t) - 1/\partial \cdot C(t)] \tag{12b}$$

und

$$C(t) = f \int (C_{in}(t) - 1/\partial \cdot C(t)) \cdot dt \tag{12c}$$

Die Gleichung (12c) entspricht zunächst dem klassischen Ansatz von Fick, dessen Lösung von Kety jedoch über Faltung der „input-" und „responsefunction" gesucht wird. Dieser Ansatz wird formal verständlich, da sich $C(t)$ als das Integral zweier Funktionsanteile darstellt, die sich um einen Zeitversatz, nämlich dem zwischen „input" und „response" unterscheiden.

Betrachtet man nun den „input" C_{in} als eine Deltafunktion mit den Eigenschaften $\Delta_{in}(0) = \infty$ und $\int \Delta_{in} = 1$, dann ergibt sich als Lösung für das Restintegral, $(C_r(t) = \int f/\partial \cdot C(t) dt)$, das die „system-response"-Funktion darstellt: $C_r(t) = C_0 e^{-(f/\partial)t}$.

Die Lösung für $C(t)$ für eine beliebige „inputfunction" kann dann als die Faltung (Convolution, dargestellt durch $\otimes$) der „inputfunction" mit der „system-response"-Funktion dargestellt werden:

$$C(t) = f\, C_{in}(t) \otimes e^{-(f/\partial)t} \tag{26}$$

Auf PET-Verhältnisse übertragen, unter denen $C(t)$ nicht punktuell, sondern immer nur in endlichen Zeitintervallen von wenigstens einigen Sekunden erfaßt werden kann, bedeutet dies, daß $C(t)$ durch ein Integral $\int C(t) dt$ in den Grenzen von T_1 bis T_2 ersetzt werden muß. Damit kann der Ansatz entsprechend Gleichung (26) formuliert werden als:

$$\int C(t)\,dt = f \int (C_{in}(t) \otimes e^{-(f/\partial)t}) \cdot dt \tag{26a}$$

Die Lösung dieser Funktion erfolgt am besten numerisch, wobei der Fluß aus Vergleichstabellen für entsprechende gemessene Integralwerte abgelesen wird. Theoretisch ist dabei eine weitgehende Linearität von gemessener Aktivitätskonzentration im Gewebe und dem Fluß gegeben (Herscovitch et al. 1983b). Praktisch führt der Ansatz aufgrund der limitierten Diffusibilität von Wasser bei hohen Flußraten zu einer Unterschätzung des Flusses, weil von einem homogenen und konstanten Verteilungskoeffizienten ausgegangen wird. Da der Verteilungskoeffizient beide Voraussetzungen nicht erfüllt, müssen Korrekturen am Modell angebracht werden. Diese können entweder durch das Einbringen von Wichtungsfunktionen (Alpert et al. 1984) oder durch Einbeziehung gemessener Extraktionswerte (Transitzeitmessung mittels arteriellem Bolus) (Raichle et al. 1983b) erreicht werden. Dies wiederum erfordert schnelle mehrfache arterielle Probennahmen und ist damit als eine relativ invasive und sicher als aufwendige Methodik zu betrachten. Ein Ansatz, der die arterielle Konzentration aus der Anstiegsrate im Gewebe abzuleiten versucht, wurde von Koeppe et al. (1985) beschrieben.

Vorläufige Ergebnisse von Raichle et al. (1983a) zeigen, daß mit ^{11}C-Butanol bzw. auch mit ^{15}O-Butanol bessere Korrelationen zu hohen Flußwerten erhalten werden können, was von den Autoren auf eine bessere Diffusibilität von Butanol im Vergleich zu Wasser zurückgeführt wird. Nach Raichle et al. (1983b) ist es weiterhin entscheidend, daß die Meßzeit bei der Washout-Analyse relativ kurz, d.h. kleiner als 60 s gehalten wird, da sonst bisher nicht erklärbare Umverteilungsprozesse das Flußbild derart verfälschen können, daß es zu Unterbewertungen der tatsächlichen Flußverhältnisse kommt. Zur Überwindung dieser Probleme schlagen LAMBRECHT u. RESCIGNO (1984) eine kontinuierlich ansteigende Infusionsrate vor, die zu einer kontrollierbaren Input-Funktion führt.

Die oben erwähnten Umverteilungsprozesse überlagern wahrscheinlich auch die Verteilungsbilder in Steady-State-Messungen, konnten bisher aber noch nicht quantifiziert werden und fallen daher zunächst in die allgemeine Fehlerdiskussion der Methodik. Wahrscheinlich reicht das zugrundeliegende Einkompartmentmodell nicht aus; auch dann nicht, wenn es um den nichtextrahierten Anteil (LAMMERTSMA et al. 1982) entsprechend dem Modell von RENKIN (1959) und CRONE (1963) erweitert wird. Zur Zeit wird die Notwendigkeit einer Erweiterung des Einkompartmentmodells für die Wasserverteilung diskutiert (BUDINGER u. GJEDDE 1986). Dabei erscheint die Einführung eines Kompartments notwendig, in das das Wasser langsamer hineindiffundiert. Physiologisch könnte ein solches Kompartment mit dem Vorhandensein von proteingebundenem Wasser in hydrophilen Strukturanteilen der Eiweiß- und Membranmoleküle erklärt werden.

Diese Limitationen beider Methoden sind jedoch nur im Hinblick auf Absolutmessungen des Blutflusses von Bedeutung. Relativmessungen, wie sie für klinische Anwendungen häufig ausreichen, können sicher mit Steady State oder auch nicht absolut korrigierten Washout-Messungen durchgeführt werden, weil auch bei diesen Methoden das direkte Verteilungsbild immer einen relativen Eindruck der Flußverhältnisse wiedergibt.

4. Statische Messungen zur Blutflußbestimmung

Statische Messungen des Blutflusses gelingen nur mit Tracern, die während der Meßzeit keine Umverteilung erfahren. Dies bedeutet, daß sie bei der ersten Passage des Kapillarbetts weitgehend abgefangen oder extrahiert werden müssen, und daß sie im Anschluß an diesen Schritt keine oder nur eine sehr langsame Umverteilung erfahren dürfen. Weil Mikrosphären oder Makroaggregate diese Voraussetzungen in nahezu idealer Weise erfüllen, gelten Fluß-messungen mit diesen Partikel-Tracern als goldener Standard, an deren Ergebnissen sich alle anderen Methoden orientieren müssen.

Die Methode hat andererseits eine Reihe von Nachteilen, die eine klinische Anwendung nahezu ausschließen. Die erste Schwierigkeit liegt in der Notwendigkeit der arteriellen Applikation des Tracers, die, wenn sie nicht zentral erfolgt, entsprechend dem Versorgungsgebiet der gewählten Hirnarterie, auch zu einer nur teilweisen Darstellung der Hirnperfusion, führt. Ferner muß zur Absolutkalibrierung der Gesamtfluß über eine dynamische Transitzeitmessung mit einem Intravasalmarker bestimmt werden. Darüberhinaus führt die arterielle Applikation von Teilchen in 5–20 µm Bereich zu einer Mikroembolisierung im Hirn, über deren Folgen nur begrenzte Erfahrungen vorliegen und die daher ein schwer abzuschätzendes Risiko darstellen. Die Methode ist daher nur im Labormaßstab als Vergleichs- und Standardisierungsverfahren für andere Meßmethoden geeignet und bisher nur an Versuchstieren (LAVENDER et al. 1979; STEINLING et al. 1985) durchgeführt worden.

Andere Tracer mit ähnlichen Eigenschaften aber nicht partikulärer Struktur sind in den letzten Jahren systematisch gesucht und gefunden worden. Eine der dabei entwickelten Strategien beruht auf dem pH-shift zwischen Blutplasma und den Hirnzellen. Dabei wurden Substanzen gesucht, die nach Passage der Blut-Hirn-Schranke aufgrund des pH-shifts im Hirn protoniert, dadurch ionisiert werden, und dann aufgrund ihres nun ionischen Charakters an der Rückdiffusion über die Bluthirnschranke gehindert sind (KUNG u. BLAU 1980).

Andere Strategien gehen von neurologisch wirksamen Substanzen aus, die an Rezeptoren oder anderen spezifischen Stellen gebunden werden. Zu den Tracern, die im „first pass" nahezu vollständig extrahiert werden und dann nur eine langsame Umverteilung erfahren, gehören das N-Isopropyl-p-Jod-Amphetamin, das besonders mit ^{123}J markiert in der klinischen Praxis Eingang gefunden hat (Winchell et al. 1980; Holman et al. 1983, 1984a, b; Creutzig et al. 1986), das ^{123}J-HIPDM: ein Trimethyl-Hydroxy-Metyl-Jodbenzyl-Propandiaminderivat (Kung u. Blau 1984; Holman et al. 1984a; Kung et al. 1983) und das Hexamethyl-Propylenamin-Oxim, das ein mit ^{99m}Tc-markierbares Molekül darstellt (Ell et al. 1985; Nowotnik et al. 1985).

Die Genauigkeit dieser Meßmethodik ist aber wiederum durch die Unsicherheit der räumlichen Homogenität der Extraktionskoeffizienten insbesondere in pathologisch verändertem Gewebe limitiert. Diese Substanzen wurden jedoch im wesentlichen zur Messung mit Hilfe der Single Photon Emissionstomographie (SPECT) entwickelt, bei der aufgrund anderer, schwerwiegender und inhärenter Quantifizierungsprobleme diesen Fehlerquellen eine untergeordnete Bedeutung zukommt.

Für Messungen mit der PET wurden vor allem ^{18}F-Fluoromethan (Wagner et al. 1984; Celesia et al. 1983, 1984), ^{18}F-Fluoroantipyrine (Sako et al. 1984) und ^{11}C-Butanol (Raichle et al. 1983b) vorgeschlagen, die alle wesentlich vollständiger als Wasser extrahiert werden, und daher geringere Fehlerempfindlichkeiten gegenüber räumlichen Schwankungen des Verteilungskoeffizienten aufweisen. Andererseits werden alle diese Substanzen auch relativ schnell wieder ausgewaschen und benötigen somit schnelle meßtechnische Systeme. Der Nachteil gegenüber ^{15}O-markiertem Wasser liegt weiterhin in den längeren Halbwertszeiten dieser Tracer, die keine schnelle bzw. nur eine limitierte Wiederholung der Messungen erlauben. Darüberhinaus werden Blutflußmessungen häufig in Verbindung mit anderen metabolischen Funktionsmessungen durchgeführt, die mit längerlebigen Tracern dann nicht in direkter zeitlicher Sequenz erhalten werden können. Eine Möglichkeit diese Probleme zu überwinden, scheint sich jedoch mit der Entwicklung von ^{15}O-markiertem Butanol anzubahnen (Kabalka et al. 1984; Berridge et al. 1986; Takahashi et al. 1986).

IV. Sauerstoffmetabolismus

Für die Bestimmung von Volumina und Flüssen braucht nur das Verteilungsverhalten von Substanzen beschrieben zu werden. Dagegen muß für funktionelle Untersuchungen der metabolischen Umsatzraten zusätzlich das metabolische Schicksal des Tracermoleküls bzw. sogar des Traceratoms quantitativ beschreibbar sein.

Für die regionale Sauerstoffextraktion und den regionalen Sauerstoffverbrauch bieten sich dafür sowohl tracerkinetische Berechnungen im Gleichgewichtszustand mit kurzlebigen Nukliden wie auch dynamische Modellrechnungen an. Erste Ansätze zur dynamischen Bestimmung der regionalen Sauerstoffextraktion mit ^{15}O wurden bereits von Ter-Pogossian et al. (1970) beschrieben, in dessen Arbeitsgruppe die Methode auch weiterentwickelt wurde (s.u.). Die Entwicklung der Steady-State-Methodik erfolgte durch Jones et al. (1976a) und Subramanyam et al. (1978). Über Weiterentwicklungen und Validierungen wurde von Frackowiak et al. (1980a, b), Jones et al. (1982) und Bigler et al. (1981, 1982) berichtet. Für beide Ansätze wird das folgende 2-Kompartmentmodell angenommen.

In der dynamischen wie in der Gleichgewichtstechnik wird von zwei Messungen ausgegangen. Zunächst wird die Verteilung von Sauerstoff in Form von ^{15}O$-$O$_2$ nach Inhalation bestimmt. Dabei wird O$_2$ an Hämoglobin gebunden und dann arteriell ins Kapillarparenchym transportiert. Dort wird der Sauerstoff entweder in das energieverbrauchende Gewebe extrahiert, um dort als Elektronen-Akzeptor zu Wasser metabolisiert zu werden, oder er wird im Kapillarbett verbleiben und als nichtextrahierter Sauerstoff-Hämoglobinkomplex in den venösen Kreislauf zu gelangen. Das metabolisch gebildete Wasser diffundiert teilweise in den Blutkreislauf zurück, wird dort rezirkulieren und sich den Flußverhältnissen entsprechend verteilen. Die Verteilung des Wassers ist natürlich analog der, die sich auch bei Infusion von ^{15}O-Wasser oder nach Inhalation von ^{15}O$-$CO$_2$ einstellt. Bei der zweiten Messung wird daher eben diese Verteilung bestimmt und damit eine Möglichkeit zur Trennung des Metaboliten vom Substrat geschaffen. Zunächst soll der im wesentlichen von der Arbeitsgruppe am Hammersmith Hospital entwickelte Ansatz zur Messung der Sauerstoffextraktion aus Gleichgewichtsmessungen erläutert werden.

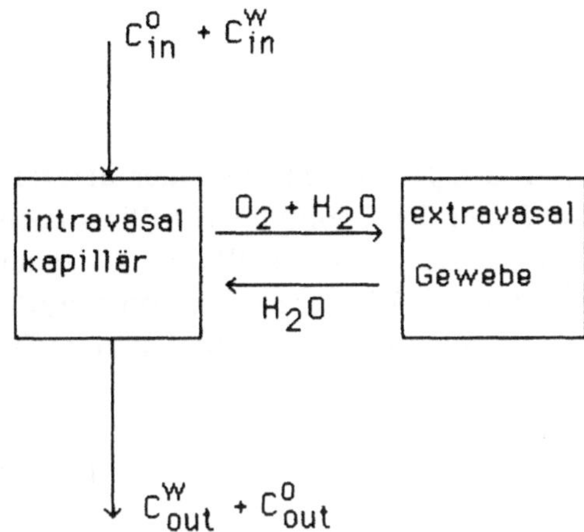

Abb. 8. 2-Kompartmentmodell für Verteilung und Metabolismus von Sauerstoff

1. Gleichgewichts-Methodik

In einem zu untersuchenden Gewebevolumen wird bei Inhalation von ^{15}O-Sauerstoff im Gleichgewicht der Einfluß J_{in} von Aktivität durch die Summe von Sauerstoffzufuhr und Zufuhr von rezirkulierendem Wasser bestimmt.

$$J_{in} = F \cdot C^0_{in} \cdot E^0 + F \cdot C^{Wr}_{in} \tag{27}$$

Dabei sind C^0_{in} die arterielle Sauerstoffkonzentration, E^0 die Sauerstoffextraktion, und C^{Wr}_{in} der rezirkulierende arterielle Wasseranteil.

Der Ausfluß an Aktivität J_{out} wird durch den Abfluß in Form von metabolischem Wasser und den Aktivitätszerfall der das Gewebe passierenden Tracermenge Q^0 während der Passage bestimmt.

$$J_{out} = F \cdot C^W_{out} + Q^0 \cdot \lambda \tag{28}$$

Wird davon ausgegangen, daß der gesamte Sauerstoff zu Wasser metabolisiert wird, so kann die Wasserkonzentration im Gewebe C^W durch die beobachtete Tracermenge Q^0/V ersetzt werden. Damit wird

$$J_{out} = Q^0 (F/V + \lambda) \tag{29}$$

Im Gleichgewicht gilt $J_{in} = J_{out}$ und damit:

$$Q^0 = \frac{F \cdot C^W_{out} + Q^0 \cdot \lambda}{(F/V + \lambda)} \tag{30}$$

Bei der Gleichgewichtsverteilung von ^{15}O-Wasser durch direkte Infusion oder Inhalation von ^{15}O$-$CO$_2$ ergibt sich die beobachtbare Tracermenge Q^W zu:

$$Q^W = \frac{F \cdot C^W_{in}}{F/V + \lambda} \tag{6}$$

Die Division der beiden beobachtbaren Tracermengen Q^0 und Q^W führt zu:

$$Q^0/Q^W = \frac{C_{in}^0 \cdot E^0 + C_{in}^{Wr}}{C_{in}^W} \tag{31}$$

Die Auflösung nach E^0 liefert folgenden Ausdruck für die Sauerstoffextraktion:

$$E^0 = \frac{(Q^0/Q^W) \cdot C_{in}^W - C_{in}^{Wr}}{C_{in}^0} \tag{32}$$

C_{in}^0 und C_{in}^{Wr} können aus einer arteriellen Blutprobe während der Sauerstoffinhalation und nachfolgender Trennung von Plasma- und Erythrozytenaktivität bestimmt werden. Der Verteilungskoeffizient von Wasser zwischen Plasma und Erythrozyten wird aus einer Blutprobe während der Wasserapplikation ermittelt, die dann auch C_{in}^w liefert.

Der regionale, zerebrale Sauerstoffverbrauch $CMRO_2$ (cerebral metabolic rate of oxygen) ergibt sich dann als:

$$CMRO_2 = F \cdot E^0 \cdot [O_2] \cdot Q^0 \tag{33}$$

Dieser klinisch verwertbare Ansatz enthält jedoch eine Reihe von Annahmen, wie die Vernachlässigung von arteriellen und venösen Aktivitätsanteilen, die einer exakten Quantifizierung nicht genügen. Sowohl rOER (regional oxygen extraction rate) wie auch $CMRO_2$ werden systematisch überschätzt, und zwar um ca. 14% in grauem und um 8% in weißem Hirngewebe (Raichle 1985; Huang u. Phelps 1986).

Eine weitgehende Analyse der Fehlerempfindlichkeit bezüglich verschiedener Faktoren wurde von Lammertsma et al. (1981a, 1981b, 1983) und Lammertsma u. Jones (1983) vorgenommen. Von den verschiedenen Vereinfachungen erwies sich die Vernachlässigung der nicht extrahierten Sauerstoffmenge im venösen Verteilungsraum am schwerwiegendsten. Lammertsma u. Jones (1983) entwickelten dafür eine Korrekturmöglichkeit über die Messung des regionalen Blutvolumens gemäß Gleichung (34):

$$rOER = (E^0 - X)/(1 - X) \tag{34}$$

wobei

$$X = (rCBF/100 + \lambda)/(rCBF/rCBV + \lambda) \tag{34a}$$

ist. Dazu muß also eine weitere Aktivitätsmessung nach Applikation von ^{15}O- bzw. ^{11}C-markiertem Kohlenmonoxid durchgeführt werden.

2. Dynamische Meßmethodik

Ausgehend von den Messungen mit Kopfsonden durch Ter-Pogossian et al. (1969, 1970), wurde die dynamische Meßmethode auf der Grundlage von Ketys „washout"-Analytik von der Arbeitsgruppe in St. Louis von Mintun et al. (1984), Herscovitch u. Raichle (1985) und Raichle (1985) weiterentwickelt.

Im Falle einer bolusförmigen Sauerstoffapplikation können für das Einfluß- und Ausflußverhalten im Gewebekompartment die Gleichungen (27–29) in folgender Form geschrieben werden.

Für den Einfluß in das Gewebekompartment gilt:

$$J_{\text{in}} = F \cdot E^0 \cdot C_{\text{in}}^0(t) + F \cdot C_{\text{in}}^w(t) \tag{27a}$$

wobei der zweite Summand den bereits rezirkulierenden Wasseranteil beschreibt. Für den Ausfluß aus dem Gewebe gilt:

$$J_{\text{out}} = F \cdot C^w(t)/\partial \tag{28a}$$

Dabei wird wiederum vorausgesetzt, daß aller extrahierter Sauerstoff zu Wasser metabolisiert wird.

Die beobachtbare Tracermenge $Q(t)$ im Gewebekompartment ist nun gleich der Differenz der integrierten Ein- und Ausflüsse:

$$Q(t) = \int J_{\text{in}}\,dt - \int J_{\text{out}}\,dt \tag{35}$$

Unter Benutzung der Konvolutionsmethode ergibt sich die folgende Lösung:

$$Q(t) = F \cdot E^0 \cdot C_{\text{in}}^0(t) \otimes e^{-kt} + F \cdot C_{\text{in}}^w(t) \otimes e^{-kt} \tag{36}$$

Die im Gewebekompartment beobachtbare Tracermenge muß noch um den im venösen Kapillarbett befindlichen Aktivitätsanteil des Sauerstoffs korrigiert werden. Das venöse Kapillarvolumen kann annäherungsweise durch einen fraktionellen Anteil des Gesamtblutvolumens, CBV, ausgedrückt werden. Dieser Anteil liegt nach MINTUN et al. (1984) bei 0.83. Das Gesamtblutvolumen muß darüberhinaus um den verringerten Hämatokrit, R, im Kapillarsystem korrigiert werden, so daß das zur Signalgebung beitragende Blutvolumen, $V_{b(\text{korr})}$, geschrieben werden kann als:

$$V_{b(\text{korr})} = 0.83 \cdot \text{CBV} \cdot R \tag{37}$$

Der darin verbliebene nicht extrahierte Sauerstoffanteil ergibt sich damit zu:

$$Q^{0(\text{korr})} = C_{\text{in}}^0 \cdot [\text{CBV} \cdot R - E^0 \cdot (0.83 \cdot \text{CBV} \cdot R)] \tag{38}$$

Da für PET-Untersuchungen die Aktivität über eine Zeitspanne gemessen werden muß, gilt für die PET – beobachtbare Aktivitätsmenge:

$$Q_{\text{PET}} = \int Q_{\text{gesamt}}(t)\,dt \tag{39}$$

$$Q_{\text{PET}} = F \cdot E^0 \cdot \int C_{\text{in}}^0(t) \otimes e^{-kt}\,dt + F \cdot \int C_{\text{in}}^w(t) \otimes e^{-kt}\,dt$$
$$+ [\text{CBV} \cdot R - E^0 \cdot (0.83 \cdot CBV \cdot R)] \cdot \int C_{\text{in}}^0 \cdot dt \tag{40}$$

Die Sauerstoffextraktionsrate ergibt sich durch Auflösung nach E^0 zu:

$$E^0 = \frac{Q_{\text{PET}} - F \cdot \int C_{\text{in}}^w(t) \otimes e^{-kt}\,dt - R \cdot \text{CBV} \cdot \int C_{\text{in}}^0 \cdot dt}{F \cdot \int C_{\text{in}}^0(t) \otimes e^{-kt}\,dt - (0.83 \cdot \text{CBV} \cdot R) \cdot \int C_{\text{in}}^0 \cdot dt} \tag{41}$$

Wie bei der Steady-State-Methode wird schließlich der Sauerstoffverbrauch entsprechend Gleichung (33) berechnet.

$$\text{CMRO}_2 = E^0 \cdot F \cdot [\text{O}_2]_{\text{art}} \tag{33a}$$

V. Glukosestoffwechsel

Der Energieverbrauch des Gehirns liegt höher als der aller anderen Organe, zumindest im Ruhezustand. Unter Normalbedingungen verbraucht das menschliche Gehirn mit ca. 2% der Gesamtkörpermasse über 20% des Sauerstoffumsatzes, bei Kindern sogar bis zu 50%. Die Sauerstoffverbrauchsrate eines durchschnittlichen Gehirns von 1400 g liegt bei 2,2 mMol/min, entsprechend 156 µMol/min · 100 g. Die CO_2-Produktionsrate liegt ebenfalls bei 156 µMol/min · 100 g, was auf eine ausschließliche Verwendung des Sauerstoffverbrauchs zur Verbrennung von Kohlehydraten hinweist (Sokoloff 1986).

Während andere Organe ihren Stoffwechsel unterschiedlichen Angebotssituationen anpassen können, ist die Energieversorgung des Gehirns ausschließlich von der Zufuhr von Glukose abhängig. Gesamt-hemisphärische Messungen von zerebralem Blutfluß, Sauerstoffverbrauch und Glukoseverbrauch mittels der Ketyschen Methodik zeigten in Tierexperimenten und Untersuchungen an hypoglykämischen Patienten, daß der Glukoseverbrauch und die Gehirnaktivität streng gekoppelt sind (Kety 1950, 1957). Der mittlere Glukoseverbrauch liegt bei 31 µMol/100 g · min. Entsprechend der Umsetzungsgleichung: $C_6H_{12}O_6 + 6O_2 = 6H_2O + 6CO_2$ ergibt sich damit ein Atmungskoeffizient für das Gehirn von 0,84. Der tatsächliche Glukoseverbrauch liegt demnach um ca. 5 µMol über dem Sauerstoffäquivalent, was auf zusätzliche Glukoseverbrauchsprozesse, wie z.B. für die Synthese von Glykoproteinen, hinweist. Bezogen auf die Verbrennung von Glukose entspricht die tatsächliche Sauerstoffverbrauchsrate einem Energieäquivalent von 20 Watt bzw. 0,25 Kcal/min. Untersuchungen von Sloviter u. Kamimoto (1970) zeigten, daß abgesehen von wenigen pathologischen Ausnahmezuständen nur Mannose ein Glukosedefizit substituieren kann (Sokoloff 1986).

Die strenge Korrelation von Hirnfunktion und Glukoseverbrauch führte zur Suche nach Möglichkeiten, um diesen Parameter regional mit einer Auflösung von bis zu wenigen mm quantifizieren zu können. Die von Sokoloff et al. (1977) entwickelte autoradiographische Methode beruht auf der Kombination der Ketyschen Methode zur Flußbestimmung mit den biochemischen Eigenschaften des Glukosederivats 2′-Desoxyglukose (DG).

Grundsätzlich ist die Methode nicht auf das Gehirn beschränkt, sondern kann auch auf andere Organe, wie z.B. das Herz angewandt werden (Phelps et al. 1978). Da die Methodik bei der Anwendung am Herzen jedoch von der im Gehirn nicht abweicht und die Methodenentwicklung sich weitgehend auf den zerebralen Glukoseverbrauch bezieht, soll im weiteren Verlauf der methodischen Beschreibung auf Betrachtungen, die sich speziell auf Herzanwendungen beziehen, verzichtet werden. Zusammenfassende Arbeiten über die Anwendung der Methode am Herzen wurden von Schelbert (1985), Geltman et al. (1985) sowie von Schelbert u. Schwaiger (1986) publiziert.

1. 2′-Desoxyglukose

Der Transport von 2′-Desoxyglukose über die Blut-Hirn-Schranke wird von demselben enzymatischen Transportsystem katalysiert, das auch den Glukosetransport selbst steuert (Bachelard 1971; Oldendorf 1971). Im Hirngewebe wird 2′-Desoxyglukose ebenso wie Glukose von Hexokinase zu 2′-Desoxyglukose-6-Phosphat phosphorylisiert. Der Transport von 2′-Desoxyglukose-6-Phosphat über die Blut-Hirn-Schranke in das Plasma ist vernachlässigbar. Der weitere Abbau von 2′-Desoxyglukose-6-Phosphat über den Angriff von Dehydrogenase zum Fruktose-6-Phosphat-Derivat ist jedoch gehemmt. Die Phosphatase-Aktivität, die zu einer Rückreaktion führen könnte, ist im Gehirn nur sehr gering (Sokoloff et al. 1977; Sokoloff 1986). Umlagerungen zu 2′-Desoxyglukose-1-Phosphat mit Folgereaktionen zu Glykoproteinen etc. sind ebenfalls vernachlässigbar (Nelson et al. 1984). Folglich wird

2′-Desoxyglukose-6-Phosphat effektiv im Hirngewebe festgehalten. Dieser als „metabolic trapping" bezeichnete Mechanismus ist in Abb. 9 schematisch wiedergegeben.

Für diesen physiologischen Zusammenhang läßt sich das folgende vereinfachte 3-Kompartmentmodell aufstellen (Abb. 10).

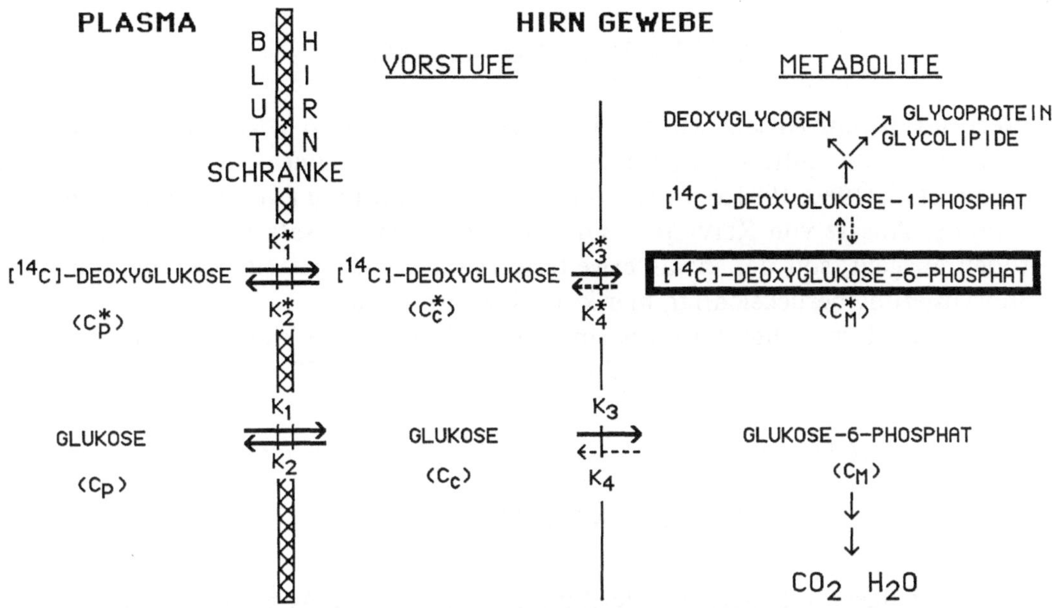

Abb. 9. Reaktionsschema für den Metabolismus von Glukose und Desoxyglukose

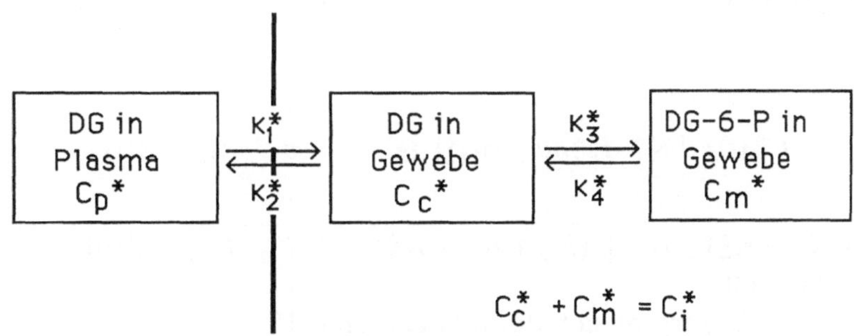

Abb. 10. Kompartmentmodell zur Beschreibung des Stoffwechselverhaltens von Desoxyglukose

Darin kann C_p über einen Zeitraum T_0 bis T_1 gemessen werden. C_i^* kann integral über einen Zeitraum T_0 bis T_1 bestimmt werden. K_4^* soll zunächst vernachlässigbar sein. Die Reaktionskonstanten $K_1^* - K_3^*$ können in unabhängigen Experimenten ermittelt werden (SOKOLOFF et al. 1977; REIVICH et al. 1985; GJEDDE u. DIEMER 1985).

Auf der Grundlage der Michaelis-Menten-Beziehung für enzymkatalysierte Reaktionen läßt sich dann für das vereinfacht dargestellte 3-Kompartment-Modell die folgende Beziehung (Gl. 42) für die Reaktionsrate von Desoxyglukose-6-Phosphat (R_i) herleiten (SOKOLOFF et al. 1977; SOKOLOFF 1986):

$$R_i = \frac{C_i^* - K_1 \cdot e^{-(K_2^* + K_3^*) \cdot T} \cdot \int C_p^* \cdot e^{(K_2^* + K_3^*) \cdot t} dt}{\frac{\lambda \cdot V_m^* \cdot K_m}{\Phi \cdot V_m \cdot K_m^*} \int (C_p^*/C_p) \cdot dt - e^{-(K_2^* + K_3^*) \cdot T} \cdot \int (C_p^*/C_p) \cdot e^{(K_2^* + K_3^*) \cdot t} \cdot dt} \tag{42}$$

Darin sind λ das Verhältnis des Verteilungsraumes von Deoxyglukose zu Glukose und Φ die Glukose-Umsetzungsrate; V_m^* und K_m^* sind die Michaelis-Menten-Konstanten für Deoxyglukose und V_m und K_m die entsprechenden Konstanten für Glukose. Der ganze erste Term aus diesen Konstanten im Nenner der Gleichung wird zur sogenannten „lumped constant" zusammengefaßt.

2. ^{18}F-2-Fluor-2′-Desoxyglukose

Entsprechend diesem Ansatz wurden Lösungen für die in vivo Messung der zerebralen Glukoseverbrauchsrate mittels ^{18}F-2′-Desoxyglukose von Reivich et al. (1979), Reivich (1985), Huang et al. (1980, 1981 a), Phelps et al. (1979 b) und Phelps (1981) entwickelt.

Während der Ansatz von Reivich wie der Sokoloffsche Ansatz vom klassischen Ketyschen Modell ausgeht, soll der etwas erweiterte Ansatz von Huang und Phelps, der die Dephosphorylisierung berücksichtigt, hier kurz skizziert werden:

Das in Abb. 10 dargestellte 3-Kompartmentmodell liefert die kinetischen Reaktionsgleichungen für die Bildungsraten von C_c und C_m entsprechend den Gleichungen 43 a, b:

$$dC_c^*(t)/dt = K_1^* \cdot C_p^*(t) - (K_2^* + K_3^*) \cdot C_c^*(t) + K_4^* \cdot C_m^*(t) \tag{43a}$$

$$dC_m^*(t)/dt = K_3^* \cdot C_c^*(t) - K_4^* \cdot C_m^*(t) \tag{43b}$$

Die Lösung dieser linearen Differentialgleichungen liefert für die Abhängigkeit der intrazellulären Kompartimentkonzentrationen von der Plasmakonzentration die Ausdrücke:

$$C_c^*(t) = [K_1^*/(\alpha_2 - \alpha_1)] \cdot [(K_4^* - \alpha_1) \cdot e^{-\alpha_1 \cdot t} + (\alpha_2 - K_4^*) \cdot e^{-\alpha_2 \cdot t}] \otimes C_p^*(t) \tag{44a}$$

und

$$C_m^*(t) = [K_1^* \cdot K_3^*/(\alpha_2 - \alpha_1)] \cdot (e^{-\alpha_1 \cdot t} - e^{-\alpha_2 \cdot t}) \otimes C_p^*(t) \tag{44b}$$

wobei $\alpha_{2,1} = (K_2^* + K_3^* + K_4^*) \pm 1/2 \cdot \sqrt{(K_2^* + K_3^* + K_4^*)^2 - 4 \cdot K_2^* \cdot K_4^*}$ bedeuten, und $\otimes$ den Convolutionsoperator darstellt.

Mit $C_i^*(t) = C_c^*(t) + C_m^*(t)$ ergibt sich dann Gleichung (45):

$$C_i^*(t) = \frac{K_1^*}{\alpha_2 - \alpha_1} \cdot [(K_3^* + K_4^* - \alpha_1) \cdot e^{-\alpha_1 \cdot t} + (\alpha_2 - K_3^* - K_4^*) \cdot e^{-\alpha_2 \cdot t} \otimes C_p^*(t) \tag{45}$$

Für den inaktiven Fall gilt im Gleichgewicht für die Phosphorylisierungsrate, d.h. für die Bildungsrate von Glukose-6-Phosphat:

$$dC_m/dt = \text{LCMRGl} = K_3 \cdot C_c - K_4 \cdot C_m \tag{46}$$

Durch Definition des durch Metabolismus verschwindenden Anteils von Glukose-6-Phosphat als $\Phi = 1 - K_4 C_m/K_3 \cdot C_c$ kann Gleichung (46) vereinfacht werden zu:

$$\text{LCMRGl} = \Phi \cdot K_3 \cdot C_c \tag{46a}$$

Da im Gleichgewicht weiterhin gilt:

$$K_1 \cdot C_p + K_4 \cdot C_m = K_2 \cdot C_c + K_3 \cdot C_c \tag{47}$$

ergibt sich daraus

$$C_c = K_1 \cdot C_p / K_2 + \Phi \cdot K_3 \tag{48}$$

und weiterhin:

$$\text{LCMRGl} = K_1 \cdot K_3 \cdot \Phi \cdot C_p / K_2 + \Phi \cdot K_3 \tag{49}$$

Da Glukose und FDG im Phosphorylisierungsschritt gemeinsam auf das Enzym Hexokinase angewiesen sind, kann aus der allgemeinen Michaelis-Menten-Beziehung für eine durch Tracer unbeeinflußte Kinetik:

$$V = dC_m / dt = K_3 \cdot C_c = \frac{V_m / K_m \cdot C_c}{1 + C_c / K_m} \tag{50}$$

die spezielle Beziehung für K_3 und K_3^* abgeleitet werden:

$$K_3 = \frac{V_m / K_m}{1 + C_c / K_m + C_c^* / K_m^*} \tag{51a}$$

$$K_3^* = \frac{V_m^* / K_m^*}{1 + C_c / K_m} + C_c^* / K_m^* \tag{51b}$$

mit $V_m = K_3 \cdot [\text{Hexokinase}]$ und $V_m^* = K_3^* \cdot [\text{Hexokinase}]$

sowie $K_m = (K_2 + K_3)/K_1$ und $K_m^* = (K_2^* + K_3^*)/K_1^*$

Durch Erweiterung der rechten Seite von Gleichung (51a) mit $K_1^* \cdot K_3^* / (K_1^* + K_3^*)$ und der Zusammenfassung von K_3^* / K_3 zu f sowie von $[K_1^* / (K_2^* + K_3^*)]/K_1^* / [(K_2^* + K_3^* \cdot \Phi)]$ zu X ergeben sich:

$$f = V_m^* \cdot K_m / V_m \cdot K_m^* \tag{52a}$$

und

$$X \cdot f / \Phi = \frac{X \cdot V_m^* \cdot K_m}{\Phi \cdot V_m \cdot K_m^*} = \text{LC} \tag{52b}$$

Dieser Ausdruck entspricht formal der „lumped constant" in der Sokoloffschen Gleichung und führt zu der Gleichung:

$$\text{LCMRGl} = \frac{C_p}{\text{LC}} \cdot \left(\frac{K_1^* \cdot K_3^*}{K_2^* + K_3^*} \right) \tag{53}$$

Durch Erweiterung von Gleichung (53) mit $C_m^*(t)$ und Substitution von $C_m^*(t)$ durch $C_i^*(t) - C_c^*(t)$ und schließliches Einsetzen der Gleichungen (45) und (44a) für $C_i^*(t)$ bzw. $C_c^*(t)$

läßt sich die Glukoseverbrauchsrate LCMRGl in folgender Form ausdrücken:

$$\text{LCMRGl} = \frac{C_p\left\{C_i^*(T) - \dfrac{K_1^*}{\alpha_2 - \alpha_1} \cdot [(K_4^* - \alpha_1)\cdot e^{-\alpha_1 \cdot t} + (\alpha_2 - K_4^*)\cdot e^{-\alpha_2 \cdot t}] \otimes C_p^*(t)\right\}}{\text{LC}\left(\dfrac{K_2^* + K_3^*}{\alpha_2 - \alpha_1}\right)(e^{-\alpha_1 \cdot t} - e^{-\alpha_2 \cdot t}) \otimes C_p^*(t)} \tag{54}$$

Aus dieser Gleichung kann die Glukoseverbrauchsrate über die Meßgrößen C_p, C_p^* und C_i^* bestimmt werden, wobei für die Reaktionskonstanten $K_1^* - K_4^*$ Mittelwerte aus normalem Gewebe eingesetzt werden können, die durch iterative Anpassung an eine Hilfsfunktion wie z.B. Gleichung (45) (Huang et al. 1980) ermittelt werden können.

Entsprechend der Entwicklung dieses Modells zur Messung von LCMRGl könnte diese auch nach der in ihrer Form wesentlich einfacheren Gleichung (53) berechnet werden. Dies setzt aber die Kenntnis der regionalen Verteilung der K^*-Werte voraus, die wiederum nur über gemessene C_i^*-Werte ermittelt werden können.

Diskussionen über die Gültigkeit der Modellvorstellung sowohl von Sokoloff wie auch des daraus weiterentwickelten Ansatzes von Phelps und Huang konzentrierten sich auf die Fragestellung, inwieweit die Konstante LC auch in pathologisch verändertem Gewebe als Konstante angesehen werden darf. Dabei zeigte sich in einer Reihe von Arbeiten, daß der physiologischen Modellvorstellung entsprechend LC solange konstant bleibt, wie der Phosphorylisierungsschritt geschwindigkeitsbestimmend ist (Phelps et al. 1983; Crane et al. 1981; Pardridge 1983; Gjedde 1982; Wienhard et al. 1983; Pettigrew et al. 1983). Dies trifft nur in Fällen extremer Hypoglykämie nicht zu, in denen der Transport von Glukose über die Blut-Hirn-Schranke zum geschwindigkeitsbestimmenden Schritt wird (Kato et al. 1985).

Weitere Verbesserungen an der Modellvorstellung, die darauf abzielen, den vaskulären Anteil von FDG zu berücksichtigen, wirken sich im wesentlichen auf kinetische Messungen in der frühen Phase nach der Applikation aus und haben damit Einfluß auf die Berechnung der Transportkonstanten. Dies gilt besonders in stark vaskularisierten Hirnarealen, wie auch in ebenso vaskularisierten Tumoren (Hawkins et al. 1986). Kinetische Messungen während der Extraktionsphase bis zum Erreichen des Gleichgewichtszustands dienen vorwiegend zur Erstellung von parametrischen Bildern der K-Wert-Verteilung, der sogenannten K-Maps. Arbeiten hierzu wurden von Carson (1986), Heiss et al. (1984), Hawkins et al. (1983a) und Wienhard et al. (1985) vorgelegt.

3. $[^{18}\text{F}]$-3-Fluor-3′-Desoxyglukose und 3-O-^{11}C-Methyl-D-Glukose

Die Glukosederivate $[^{18}\text{F}]$-3-Fluor-3′-Desoxyglukose (3-FDG) und 3-O-^{11}C-Methyl-glukose (CMG) verhalten sich biochemisch sehr ähnlich und sollen daher hier gemeinsam behandelt werden. Vom Blut kommend werden beide Zuckerarten an der Blut-Hirn-Schranke von demselben Transportenzym erfaßt, das auch Glukose und 2′-Desoxyglukose transportiert (Betz u. Gilboe 1974; Pardridge u. Oldendorf 1975). Im Gegensatz zu Glukose und 2′-Desoxyglukose werden diese beiden Derivate aber nicht (CMG) (Pardridge 1983), oder nur in sehr geringem Maße (3-FDG) (Halama et al. 1983) phosphorylisiert, bieten sich also nicht als Substrate für die Hexokinase an. Dagegen sind beide Zuckerderivate einem freien Rücktransport über die Blut-Hirn-Schranke unterworfen.

Entsprechend einer Modellvorstellung von Vyska et al. (1984, 1985) können aus der zeitabhängigen Messung der Plasmakonzentration $C_p(t)$, der Gewebekonzentration $C_2(t)$ und der Gleichgewichtskonzentration die lokale Glukosetransportrate im Hirn (LCTRGl) sowie der Blutfluß ermittelt werden. Dazu geht VYSKA von einem einfachen 2-Kompartmentmodell aus. Unter der Voraussetzung, daß für den Einfluß Φ_i^* gilt:

$$\Phi_i^* = m \cdot K_1^* \cdot f \cdot C_p^* \tag{55}$$

und der Ausfluß durch Φ_e^* mit

$$\Phi_e^* = K_2^* \cdot C_2^* \tag{56}$$

beschrieben werden kann, ergibt sich:

$$dC_2^*/dt = m \cdot K_1^* \cdot f \cdot C_p^* - K_2^* \cdot C_2^* \tag{57}$$

Dabei sind C_p^* und C_2^* die Plasma- und Gewebekonzentrationen des Zuckerderivates, K_1^* und K_2^* die Reaktionskonstante, f ist der Plasmafluß in ml/min·g, und m ist eine Proportionalitätskonstante mit der Dimension min^{-1}.

Nach VYSKA et al. (1984, 1985) kann gezeigt werden, daß $K_1^* = K_2^*$ ist. Aus der Messung des Anstiegs der Glukosederivat-Konzentration im Hirngewebe sowie den Gleichgewichtskonzentrationen im Gewebe und im Blut erlaubt das Modell danach eine Berechnung des unidirektionalen Glukosetransports und des Flusses. Dabei ergibt sich der Fluß direkt aus dem Verhältnis von Gewebe- zu Blutkonzentration, während die lokale Transportrate für die Glukosederivate eine dazu proportionale Größe darstellt.

Zu einer durchaus unterschiedlichen Interpretation der 3-FDG und CMG Daten kommen GJEDDE et al. (1985) und BROOKS et al. (1986). Nach ihrer Auffassung beschränkt sich der Wert der 3-FDG Daten auf die Möglichkeit, im Vergleich mit den 2-FDG Daten eine Trennung von Fluß- und Transportphänomenen vornehmen zu können. Auf diese Weise können die Schwankungen der „lumped constant" und deren Bandbreite in pathologischen Zuständen überprüft werden.

Die noch anhaltende Diskussion um die Interpretation der mit diesen Glukosederivaten erhaltbaren Daten schließt eine detailliertere Behandlung im Rahmen dieses Handbuches aus.

4. ^{11}C-Glukose

^{11}C-markierte Glukose wurde bereits lange vor der Entwicklung des SOKOLOFFschen Desoxyglukose-Modells hergestellt (LIFTON u. WELCH 1971). Die auch heute noch aktuelle Methode beruht auf der Assimilation von ^{11}CO$_2$ durch Algen oder schnellwachsende Blattpflanzen und führt zu einer statistisch verteilten Markierung in allen 6 Kohlenstoffpositionen des Zuckers. Anfängliche Probleme bei der Reinigung der Glukose von anderen Assimilationsprodukten sowie der Sterilisation des Endproduktes konnten mittlerweile gelöst werden (DENCE et al. 1982; EHRIN et al. 1983).

Bei der Verwendung von ^{11}C-Glukose als Tracer für die Untersuchung des Glukosestoffwechsels muß beachtet werden, daß die Verstoffwechselung über den Hexokinase-Schritt hinausgeht und zu einer Reihe markierter Metabolite führt, von denen ^{11}CO$_2$ am wichtigsten ist. Um die Einflüsse aus diesem Stoffwechselverhalten möglichst klein zu halten, gehen RAICHLE et al. (1975) davon aus, daß innerhalb sehr kurzer Zeitintervalle nach der Injektion von ^{11}C-Glukose die Bildung von Metaboliten vernachlässigt werden kann.

Für den Versuch, den Glukosestoffwechsel modellhaft quantitativ zu beschreiben, muß ein erweitertes Kompartmentmodell erstellt werden, da die Metabolite eine von Glukose unterschiedliche Verteilung erfahren (Abb. 11).

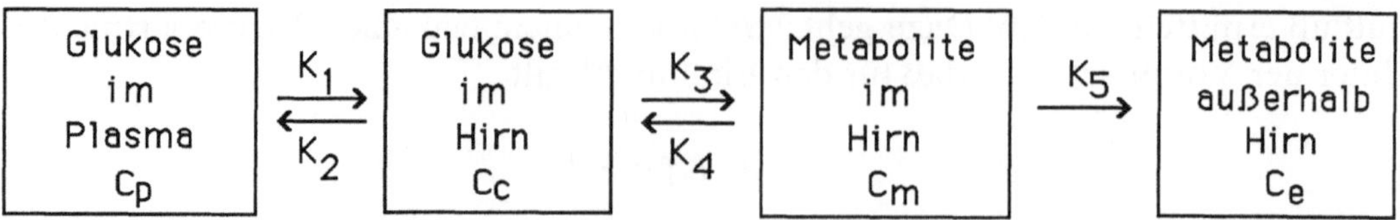

Abb. 11. Kompartmentmodell für die Beschreibung des Stoffwechselverhaltens von Glukose

Eine Betrachtung von Blomqvist et al. (1985) benutzt dazu konstante Parameter aus Kalibriermessungen zur Beschreibung des Metabolitenverlusts. Dabei wird aus Messungen der arteriovenösen Differenz des $^{11}CO_2$ eine globale Egress-Funktion für das Hirn berechnet. Zur Vereinfachung des Modells muß dann aber die durch K_4 gekennzeichnete Dephosphorylierung vernachlässigt werden. Nach Blomqvist et al. (1985) und Gjedde (1982) ergibt sich die Glukoseverbrauchsrate LCMR zu:

$$\text{LCMR} = \frac{\{C_s^*(t) - C_p^*(t) + C_e^*(t) - [K_2/(K_2+K_3)] \cdot C_c^*(t)\} \cdot C_p}{\int C_p^*(t)\,dt} \tag{58}$$

Darin sind die mit * versehenen Konzentrationen die der aktiven Produkte und C_p die Gesamtkonzentration von Glukose im Plasma. C_s^* stellt die meßbare Gesamtaktivität im Gehirn entsprechend $C_s^* = C_p^* + C_c^* + C_m^*$ dar. Der kumulative Verlust an Tracer $C_e^*(t)$ wird über eine Hilfsfunktion aus dem zeitlichen Verlauf der arteriovenösen Differenz von $^{11}CO_2$ ($\Delta C_e^*(t)$) approximiert:

$$C_e^*(t) = f \cdot \int \Delta C_e^*(t) \cdot dt \tag{59}$$

Der Vorteil der Glukose-Methode im Vergleich zur Desoxyglukose-Methode beruht auf dem Fortfall der „lumped constant" im physiologisch kinetischen Modell. Der Nachteil beruht andererseits auf der notwendigen Vereinfachung des Zuckerabbaus unter Vernachlässigung einiger Nebenprodukte und der Gleichbehandlung aller markierten Positionen im Glukosemolekül, sowie der Neueinführung des kumulativen Verlustes von Tracer in das kinetische Modell.

VI. Fettsäurestoffwechsel

Anders als das Gehirn kann das Herz seinen Energiehaushalt über verschiedene Stoffwechselprozesse ausgleichen. Der größte Anteil des Energieverbrauchs wird jedoch durch die Verbrennung von Fettsäuren gedeckt. Dieser Anteil beträgt unter Normalbedingungen ca. 80%. Der Rest des Energiebedarfs wird durch Glykolyse und die Verstoffwechslung von Aminosäuren zur Verfügung gestellt, deren Anteile unter Normalbedingungen ca. 15% bzw. 5% ausmachen. Die Verteilung der Anteile an der Energieversorgung sind jedoch von Faktoren wie der Sauerstoffverfügbarkeit, der Konzentration freier und gebundener Fettsäuren im Plasma sowie dem Belastungszustand des Herzens abhängig. Unter Belastung oder Sauerstoffmangel kann auch die Glykolyse zum dominierenden Energielieferanten werden. Für eine Übersicht vgl. Taegtmeyer (1986).

Ein Schema des Fettsäurestoffwechsels ist in Abb. 12 wiedergegeben. Die freie Fettsäure, die im Plasma weitgehend als Albuminkomplex vorliegt, passiert die Kapillarmembran wahrscheinlich über einen trägerkatalysierten Transportprozeß (Rose et al. 1977; Rose u. Goresky 1977; Bieber u. Fiol 1985; Abumrad et al. 1984). Im Sarkoplasma der Herzzelle wird die

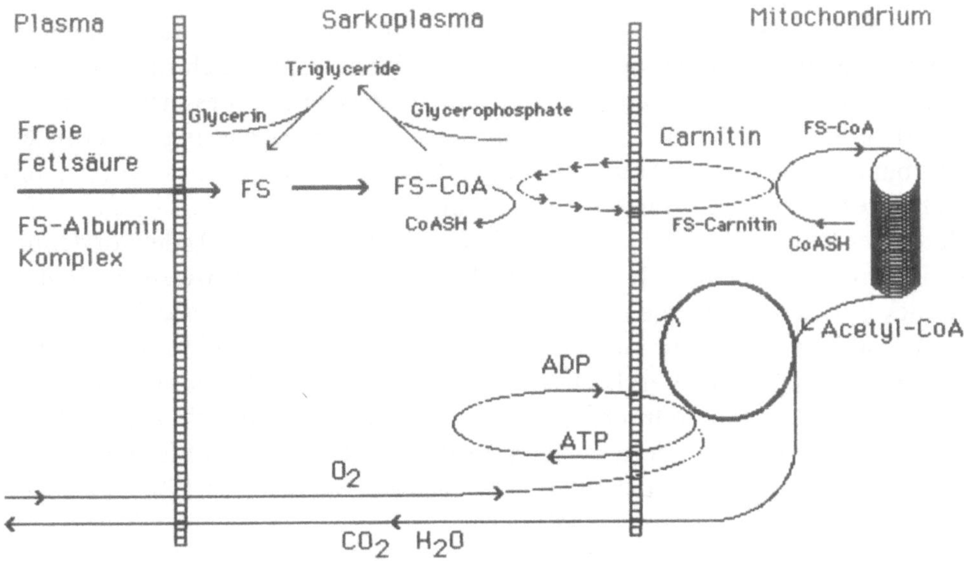

Abb. 12. Schematische Darstellung des Fettsäureabbaus

freie Fettsäure durch CoA aktiviert und kann je nach Energiebedarfslage der Zelle entweder im Triglyzerid-Speicher zwischengelagert werden oder weiter in den Carnitinkomplex überführt werden, der das Fettsäuremolekül auf dem Weg des sogenannten „Carnitin-Shuttle" in das Mitochondrium einschleust. Dort wird die CoA aktivierte Fettsäure der β-Oxidation unterworfen, bei der sie schrittweise in Azetyl-CoA Einheiten, und diese weiter im Zitronensäure-Zyklus zu CO_2 und Wasser abgebaut wird.

Obwohl der Mechanismus der β-Oxydation weitgehend geklärt ist (LEHNINGER 1970; BREMER 1983; BING 1965), sind die kinetischen Zusammenhänge bisher nicht quantitativ beschreibbar. Die größte Schwierigkeit besteht dabei in der Relativierung des kinetischen Verhaltens der Einzelprozesse sowie in der Beurteilung des geschwindigkeitsbestimmenden Schritts des Modellschemas. Da der Gesamtprozeß relativ schnell abläuft, überlagern sich die Einflußkinetik, die eigentlichen Stoffwechselprozesse und die Elimination der Stoffwechselprodukte sehr stark.

Wesentliche Erkenntnisse über das kinetische Verhalten des Fettsäurestoffwechsels wurden durch ausführliche Untersuchungen an jodierten Fettsäurederivaten erhalten (FEINENDEGEN et al. 1981; OKADA et al. 1983; RESKE et al. 1985; VISSER et al. 1985a, b). Die Problematik wird jedoch dadurch verdeutlicht, daß trotz sehr ähnlichem gesamtkinetischen Verhaltens von [123]J-Heptadekansäure und ^{11}C-Palmitinsäure, bei der Jodfettsäure nicht die β-Oxidation der geschwindigkeitsbestimmende Schritt ist, sondern die Elimination des Metaboliten [123]J⁻ aus dem Herzmuskel, während für ^{11}C-Palmitinsäure die β-Oxidation als der geschwindigkeitsbestimmende Schritt angesehen wird und nicht die Elimination von [11]CO_2.

Die mit der Positronen-Emissionstomographie im Herzmuskel beobachtbare Tracerkinetik nach ^{11}C-Palmitinsäure Applikation verläuft dreiphasig (WEISS et al. 1976; GOLDSTEIN et al. 1980; LERCH et al. 1982). Nach einer schnellen Aufnahme im Gewebe erfolgt zunächst eine schnelle Eliminationsphase, an die sich eine weitere langsamere Auswaschphase anschließt. Die beiden Auswaschphasen lassen sich zwei unterschiedlichen Umsetzungsarten zuordnen. Während die schnelle Eliminierung als β-Oxidation freier Fettsäure interpretiert werden kann, wird die zweite langsamere Phase der Umsetzung von Fettsäure aus dem Triglyzerid-Pool zugeordnet (GELTMAN et al. 1985; SCHELBERT 1985; SCHELBERT u. SCHWAIGER 1986).

Versuche, die Stoffwechselprozesse durch Verwendung von Fettsäurederivaten voneinander zu trennen, die ein metabolisches "Trapping" erfahren, sind noch nicht über erste Versuchs-Studien hinausgekommen, lassen jedoch für die Zukunft verbesserte Quantifizierungsansätze erwarten. So kann z.B. der Angriff von CoA durch Verwendung β-methylierter Fettsäuren unterbunden und so die Einflußkinetik des Fettsäurederivates von nachfolgenden Stoffwechselprozessen getrennt werden (Livni et al. 1982). Kürzere Fettsäuren wie Essigsäure lassen andererseits keine wesentliche Vereinfachung der kinetischen Modellvorstellung erwarten, da sie einer großen Vielfalt sich überlagernder metabolischer Prozesse zugänglich sind.

Im Hinblick auf diese Probleme erscheint es sinnvoll, den Fettsäurestoffwechsel im Herzen nicht isoliert, sondern im Zusammenhang mit Glykolyse und Aminosäurestoffwechsel zu betrachten. Entsprechend sind Vergleichsuntersuchungen mit Palmitinsäure und Fluorodesoxyglukose bzw. auch Glutamat durchgeführt worden, die bisher jedoch noch nicht zu quantifizierbaren Aussagen führen, sondern nur qualitative Beurteilungen des Ischämiegrades erlauben (Knapp et al. 1982; Taegtmeyer 1986; Schelbert u. Schwaiger 1986).

VII. Aminosäurestoffwechsel

Physiologische Kompartmentmodelle für den Aminosäurestoffwechsel im Gehirn wurden in den letzten Jahren von Smith et al. (1980), Bustany u. Comar (1985), Bustany et al. (1981, 1982, 1983a, b, 1986), Phelps et al. (1984, 1985b) und Barrio (1986) vorgestellt. Hauptziel dieser Arbeiten ist die Entwicklung quantitativer Methoden zur Beschreibung der Proteinsynthese in verschiedenen Organen, die einen wichtigen Funktionsfaktor für die Beurteilung physiologischer und pathologischer Zustände darstellen kann.

Im Vergleich zur Verstoffwechselung von Fettsäuren sind die physiologisch-chemischen Voraussetzungen für die quantitative Beschreibung des Aminosäurestoffwechsels etwas günstiger. Zunächst sind die Transporteigenschaften der Aminosäuren über die Blut-Hirn-Schranke recht genau untersucht worden (Oldendorf 1971, 1973a, b; Oldendorf u. Szabo 1976). Der Prozeß ist trägerkatalysiert, weitgehend unidirektional und relativ schnell. Für eine Reihe von Aminosäuren ist die Inkorporation in Protein der dominierende Reaktionweg. Die Proteine erfahren nur eine sehr langsame Umverteilung, so daß sich für die tracerkinetische Betrachtung eine der Deoxyglukose sehr ähnliche Situation ergibt. Nebenreaktionen, die weitgehend zum Abbau des Moleküls führen, sind relativ gut bekannt und müssen im Modell berücksichtigt werden, sofern sie nicht in erster Näherung als vernachlässigbar eingestuft werden können.

Von den bisher beschriebenen Aminosäuren Alanin (Ropchan u. Barrio 1984), Leucin (Barrio et al. 1983b), Phenylalanin (Barrio et al. 1983a) und Methionin (Bustany et al. 1981) soll hier am Beispiel des Methionins die mit der Aufstellung eines Kompartmentmodells verbundene Problematik aufgezeigt werden. In Abb. 13 sind die wesentlichen biochemischen Prozesse des Methioninstoffwechsels zusammengefaßt.

Nach dem Transport des Methionins vom Plasma in den Intrazellulärraum ergeben sich zwei konkurrierende Reaktionsmöglichkeiten. Zum ersten kann die Aminosäure durch Aminoacyl-tRNA-Synthesase für die Inkorporation in Protein aktiviert werden. Zum zweiten kann Methionin in einen metabolischen Abbau geraten. Dieser wird ebenfalls durch eine ATP verbrauchende Aktivierung des Methionins zum S-Adenosyl-Methionin eingeleitet. Der Abbau beginnt mit dem Angriff von Methyltransferase, wobei als erstes Abbauprodukt S-Adenosyl-Homocystein entsteht. Als Methylakzeptoren treten Adrenalin, Nikotinamid, Cholin, Kreatin, Vitamin B 12 und viele andere auf (Bender 1975; Anhalt et al. 1981). Der weitere stufenweise Abbau verläuft über Cystathionin, Homoserin und α-Ketobutyrsäure zum Propionyl-CoA und CO_2. Letzteres wird in dem vorwiegend aus dem Kohlehydrat-

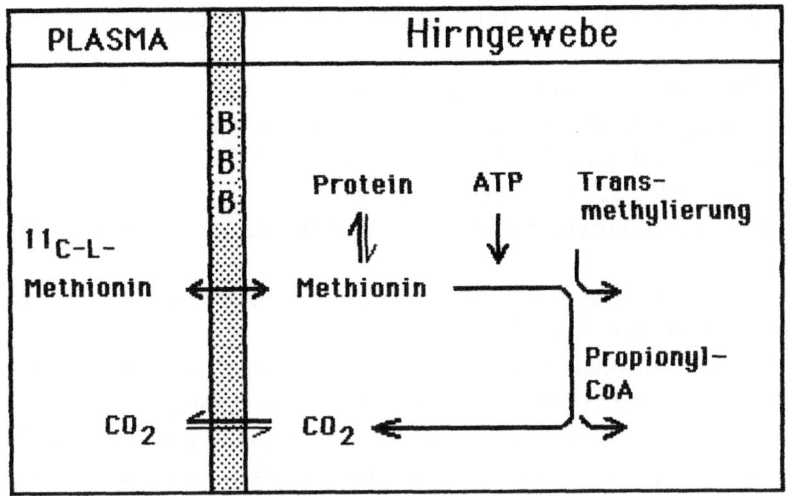

Abb. 13. Schematische Darstellung des Methioninstoffwechsels

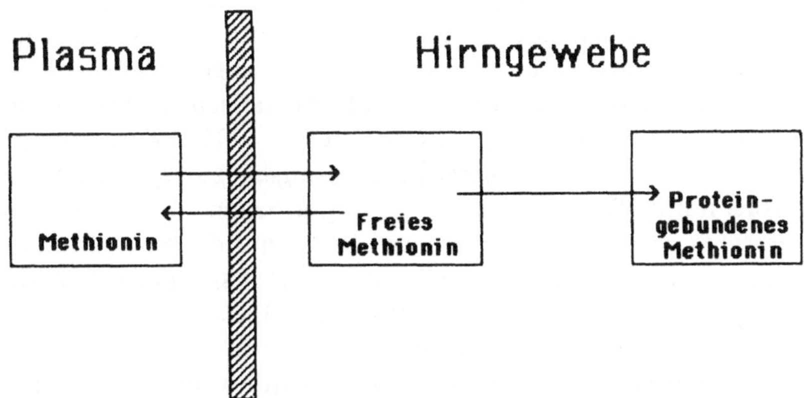

Abb. 14. Vereinfachtes Kompartmentmodell zur Berechnung der Methionin-Inkorporation in Hirnprotein

und Fettsäure-Abbau resultierenden Karbonat-Pool verdünnt, ins Plasma zurückgeführt und über die Lunge abgeatmet.

Für die oben angeführten Aminosäuren, die in der Carboxyl-Gruppe mit ^{11}C markiert sind, erfolgt die Tracerelimination aus Abbaureaktionen über $^{11}CO_2$. Für in der S-Methyl Gruppe markiertes Methionin ist die Transmethylierungsreaktion ein kritischer Reaktionsschritt. Die Verzweigung der darauffolgenden Reaktionen ist unübersichtlich und quantitativ nicht beschreibbar. Eine Weiterentwicklung des Kompartmentmodells über den Transmethylierungsschritt hinaus ist damit unmöglich. Entsprechend dieser Limitation ist das in Abb. 14 wiedergegebene Kompartmentmodell von BUSTANY et al. (1983) derart vereinfacht, daß der Transmethylierungsschritt vernachlässigt wird. Dies geschieht unter der Voraussetzung, daß der Transmethylierungsprozeß nicht mehr als 4% des Gesamtumsatzes von Methionin ausmacht (BUSTANY u. COMAR 1985).

Zusätzlich muß bei dem Modell vorausgesetzt werden, daß die einzige Tracerquelle für das Hirngewebe aus Methionin im Plasma besteht. Da aber in anderen Organen wie der Leber sehr hohe Transmethylierungsraten zu erwarten sind (HOLLOWAY 1981), wird das Plasma-Kompartment bald mit anderen markierten Metaboliten kontaminiert, so daß diese Voraussetzung nur unzureichend erfüllt ist. So haben LUNDQVIST et al. (1985) nach Applikation von S-[^{11}C]-Methyl-Methionin auch andere ^{11}C-markierte Aminosäuren im Plasma nachgewiesen.

Da die Extraktion von Aminosäuren im Gehirn mit nur ca. 1% zwar sehr gering ist, jedoch relativ schnell erfolgt, und die Transmethylierungsprodukte erst nach längerer Zeit (ca. 30 min) im Plasma auftreten (LUNDQVIST et al. 1985), kann die Störung der Kinetik durch Metabolite erst in der Spätphase auftreten. Dort und im „quasi"-Gleichgewichtszustand nach 30 min wird die Transmethylierung nicht ohne Einfluß auf die verfolgbare Tracerkinetik sein.

Die Markierung der Aminosäuren in der Carboxylgruppe vermeidet die Komplikationen durch solche Nebenreaktionen. Ein Kompartmentmodell für diese Tracer muß jedoch das $^{11}CO_2$ aus den Abbaureaktionen berücksichtigen. Ein entsprechendes Modell wurde von SMITH et al. (1980), PHELPS et al. (1984, 1985b) und BARRIO (1986) vorgestellt (Abb. 15).

Limitierende Voraussetzungen für dieses Modell sind die folgenden Annahmen:

1. Das Kompartment der freien Aminosäure im Gehirn wird nur durch das Plasma Kompartment und nur durch eine markierte Aminosäure gespeist.
2. Die synthetisierten markierten Proteine sind während der Meßperiode stabil und ortsfest.
3. Die metabolische Abbausequenz zum markierten CO_2 ist unidirektional.

Eine vorläufige Validierung des Modells für L-Leucin wurde von PHELPS et al. (1984) berichtet. Dabei wurde eine zweiphasige Kinetik der Aminosäure-Abnahme im Gehirn beobachtet, deren schneller Anteil dem metabolischen Abbau zugeschrieben wurde. Dazu muß einschränkend angemerkt werden, daß im Gegensatz zu statischen Messungen an Tumorpatienten zur Identifikation von Tumoren (BERGSTRÖM et al. 1986; ERICSON et al. 1985; MEYER et al. 1985b; SCHOBER et al. 1986b), kinetische Messungen zur quantitativen Analyse der Proteinsynthese bisher nur im Rahmen von Forschungsarbeiten durchgeführt wurden (PHELPS et al. 1984). Andererseits verläuft die Weiterentwicklung auf diesem Anwendungssektor der Positronen-Emissionstomographie sehr schnell. Einige Arbeitsgruppen unter der Leitung von F. BUDINGER (Berkley), H. HUNDESHAGEN (Hannover), B. LANGSTRÖM (Upsalla), H. WAGNER (Baltimore) betreiben intensive Grundlagenarbeiten an Tiermodellen und an in vitro Proben zur Klärung weiterer kinetischer Parameter der Proteinsynthese im Hirn. Dabei werden neben der Bestimmung der Transportkinetik und deren Blockierbarkeit durch Sättigung des „Carrier Enzyms" auch die Stereospezifität des Transportsystems untersucht. Als Beispiel ist in Abb. 16a–c das kinetische Verhalten von L-Leucin und D-, L-Methionin im Rattenkortex wiedergegeben (LAUENSTEIN et al. 1987).

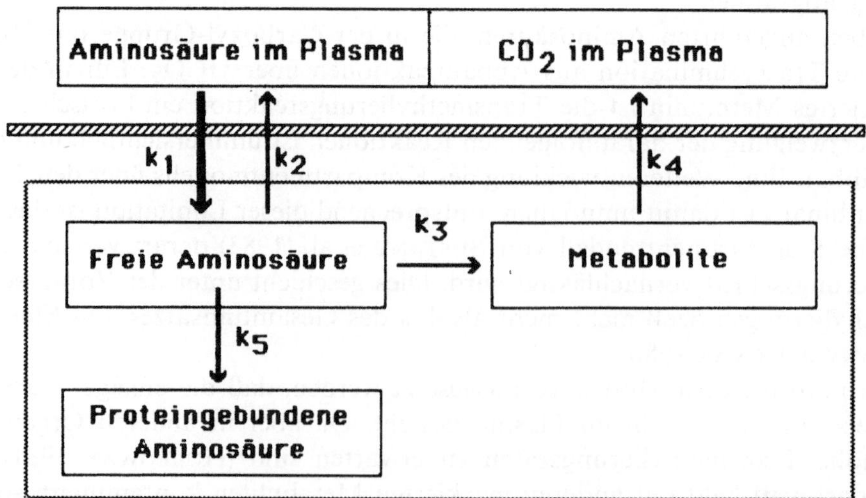

Abb. 15. Kompartmentmodell zur quantitativen Beschreibung der Proteinsyntheserate im Gehirn

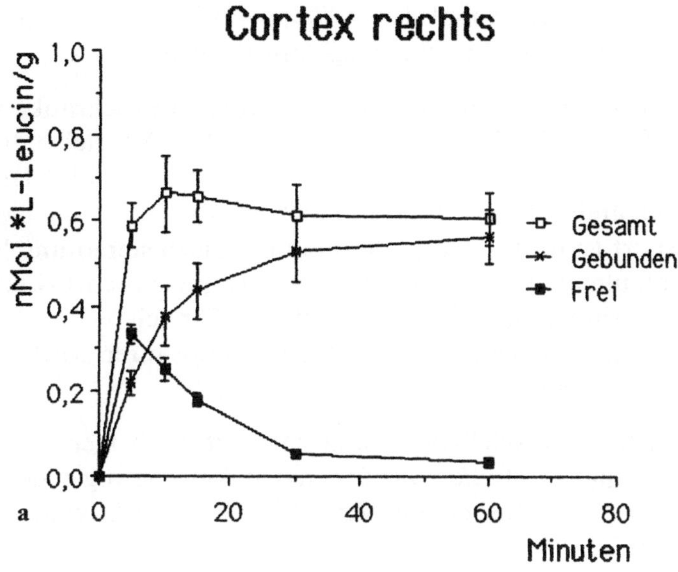

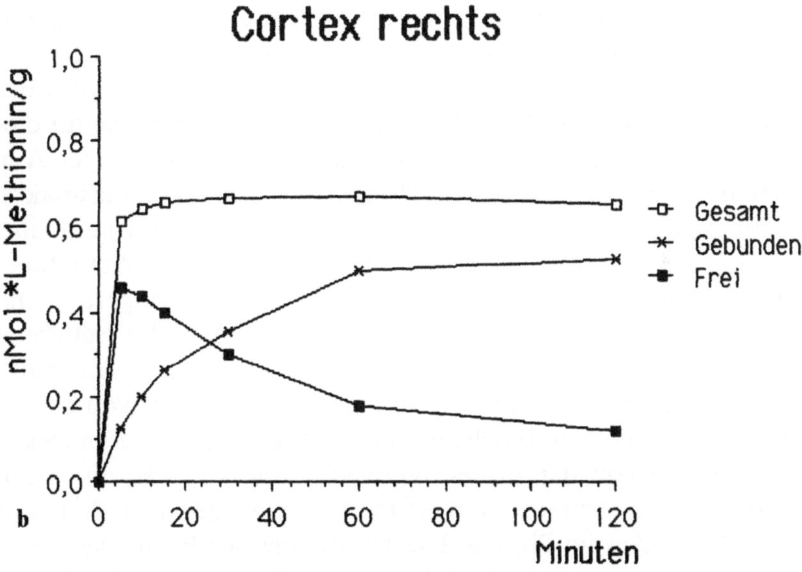

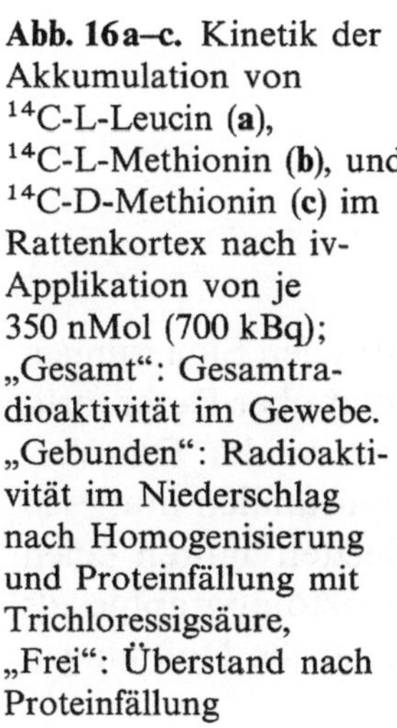

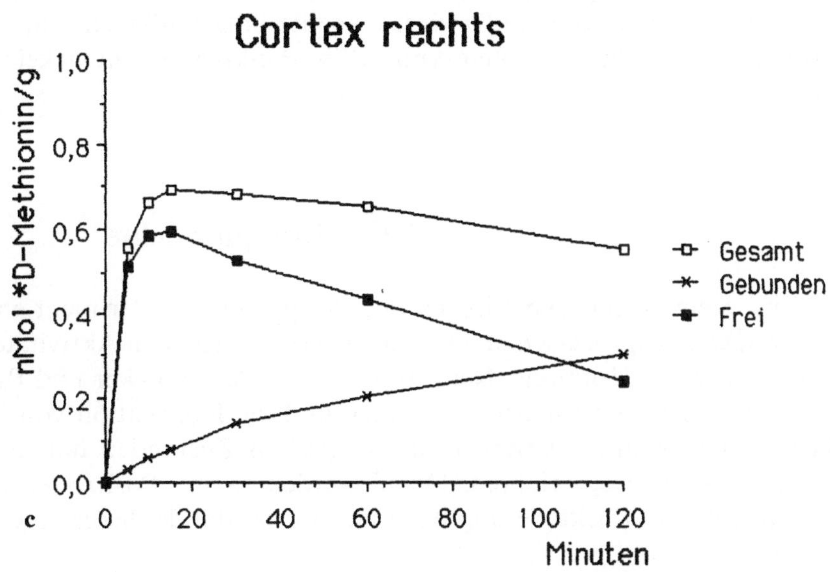

Abb. 16a–c. Kinetik der Akkumulation von ^{14}C-L-Leucin (**a**), ^{14}C-L-Methionin (**b**), und ^{14}C-D-Methionin (**c**) im Rattenkortex nach iv-Applikation von je 350 nMol (700 kBq); „Gesamt": Gesamtradioaktivität im Gewebe. „Gebunden": Radioaktivität im Niederschlag nach Homogenisierung und Proteinfällung mit Trichloressigsäure, „Frei": Überstand nach Proteinfällung

Aus diesen Ergebnissen und den Arbeiten der anderen Arbeitsgruppen können z.Z. folgende Schlüsse gezogen und zusammengefaßt werden.

1. Der Transport der Aminosäure über die Blut-Hirn-Schranke ist der geschwindigkeitsbestimmende Schritt, die Proteinsynthese verläuft im Vergleich dazu langsam.
2. Der Transport von markierten Aminosäuren über die Blut-Hirn-Schranke ist durch größere Mengen anderer Aminosäuren blockierbar.
3. Der Transport ist für D- und L-Methionin nahezu stereo-unselektiv.
4. Die Gesamtaufnahme und Verteilung der Aminosäuren L-Leucin, L-Phenylalanin, sowie D-, und L-Methionin im Hirngewebe ist sehr ähnlich.
5. Von den in diesen Arbeiten untersuchten Aminosäuren wird L-Leucin am vollständigsten in Proteine eingebaut.

Da die kinetische Modellvorstellung zur Zeit noch nicht weit genug entwickelt ist, um quantitative Aussagen zu treffen, werden in den Anwendungen der Messung von Aminosäure-Aufnahme in Tumoren bisher nur Verhältnisse von Aktivitäten in Tumor zu non-Tumor Regionen angegeben.

Da besonders in der Entwicklungsphase der Messung von Aminosäure-Aufnahmen Untersuchungen am Pankreas im Vordergrund standen, soll hier kurz auf die Möglichkeiten neuer Quantifizierungsansätze in diesem Bereich hingewiesen werden.

Pankreas und Leber weisen erheblich höhere Extraktionsraten für Aminosäuren auf als alle anderen Organe. Aufgrund der Regelfunktion der Leber für die Aminosäurekonzentration im Plasma kann bereits aus der Plasmakonzentration einiger Aminosäuren eine Leberfunktionsanalytik entwickelt werden (Holloway 1981). Die Plasmakonzentration von Methionin liegt im Normbereich zwischen 20 und 40 µMol/l und kann in pathologischen Fällen auf über 1000 µMol/l ansteigen. Kinetische Daten über die Aufnahme und die Umsetzung könnten hier auch unter den Problemaspekten der Überlagerung mehrerer Vorgänge zu einer verbesserten Aussage über die Regelfunktion führen. Als weiteres Beispiel kann die Überprüfung von Enttoxifizierungsprozessen gelten. Hier bietet sich mit S-[^{11}C]-Methyl-Methionin ein hervorragendes Substrat zur Messung der Aktivität von S-Methyl-Transferase an.

Das Spektrum der biochemischen Reaktionen im Pankreas ist deutlich schmaler und wird eindeutig von der Proteinsynthese dominiert. Der in anderen Organen beobachtbare Abbauanteil der Aminosäuren ist hier nur von geringer Bedeutung wie auch das Auftreten anderer Vorstufen im Plasma. Die Dominanz der Proteinsynthese führt zu einer, wenn auch nur scheinbar geringeren, Selektivität, so daß die Zeitaktivitätskurve im Gewebe von Nebenreaktionen weniger beeinflußt wird. Es sollte daher möglich sein, ein relativ einfaches Kompartmentmodell für die Proteinsynthese im Pankreas zu entwickeln.

VIII. Rezeptordichte

Eine Reihe von enzymatischen und der größte Teil der nicht-enzymatischen Steuerungen von Stoffwechselprozessen und besonders von neuronalen Aktivitäten erfolgt über Rezeptorliganden, wie z.B. Hormone, Neurotransmitter, Beta-Blocker und Psychopharmaka. Das Verständnis dieser Steuerungsmechanismen und die Korrelation von Defektzuständen in diesen Steuereinheiten mit definierten pathologischen Zuständen hat in den letzten Jahren einen großen Aufschwung erfahren. Dabei werden in die Positronen-Emissionstomographie als Instrument zur Objektivierung der Funktionszustände dieser Regelkreise große Hoffnungen gesetzt.

Die Wirkungsweise der Rezeptoren kann vereinfacht folgendermaßen dargestellt werden: Rezeptormoleküle stellen Relaissysteme dar, die durch Kopplung mit spezifischen Substanzen aktiviert oder desaktiviert werden. Die Aktivierung führt zu einer Aktion, die je nach Regeltyp inhibierend oder stimulierend auf eine weitere biochemische Reaktion oder neuronale Schaltvorgänge wirkt. Liganden, die durch spezifische Kopplung mit dem Rezeptor eine solche Aktion auslösen, werden Agonisten genannt. Liganden, die zwar spezifisch mit dem Rezeptor koppeln, aber keine Aktion auslösen, ihn desaktivieren, werden Antagonisten genannt. Aufgrund der sehr geringen Konzentration von Rezeptoren werden nur sehr geringe Konzentrationen von Liganden benötigt, um ein Aktionspotential auszulösen oder abzublocken. Die Rezeptorkonzentration liegt in den meisten Fällen in der Größenordnung von einigen pico-Mol pro Gramm Gewebe. Es wird angenommen, daß nicht die Ligandenkonzentration das Potentialniveau reguliert, sondern daß die Anzahl der aktivierbaren Rezeptoren variiert und so das Potentialniveau kontrolliert wird. Die Lokalisation der Rezeptoren mit spezifischen Eigenschaften ist häufig auf ein bestimmtes Organ oder gar nur Teile davon begrenzt. Ziel der Untersuchungen mit Positronen-markierten Liganden und der PET ist demnach eine quantitative Beschreibung der aktiven Rezeptordichte in örtlich begrenzten Arealen.

Da die Rezeptorliganden ihre Wirkung schon bei sehr niedrigen Konzentrationen entfalten, ergeben sich sehr hohe Anforderungen an die spezifische Aktivität der Tracer. Hohe Konzentrationen der markierten Liganden würden nur zu einer unspezifischen Belegung des umgebenden Gewebes mit überschüssigem Tracer führen, den Kontrast erniedrigen und eine quantitative Auswertung erschweren oder gar unmöglich machen.

Da die Rezeptorliganden im Normalfall keinem schnellen Stoffwechsel unterliegen und die Bindung an den Rezeptor sehr stabil ist, kann das kinetische Verhalten mit einem relativ einfachen Modell beschrieben werden, wie es in Abb. 17 gezeigt ist (WAGNER et al. 1985; SYROTA et al. 1984; HUANG u. PHELPS 1986).

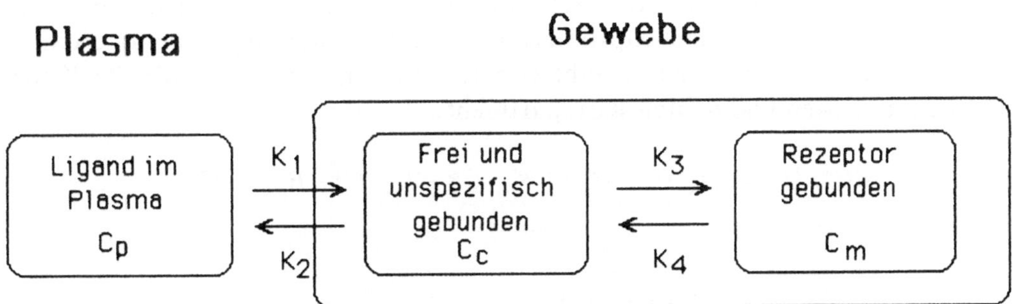

Abb. 17. Kompartmentmodell zur Beschreibung der Rezeptordichte

Voraussetzung für die Gültigkeit dieses vereinfachten Ansatzes ist die Annahme, daß weder der Transport (Diffusion) des Liganden in der Zelle zum Rezeptor, noch die Kopplung und Redissoziation des Liganden an unspezifischen Bindungsstellen geschwindigkeitsbestimmende Schritte darstellen (HUANG u. PHELPS 1986).

Unter Vernachlässigung der Dissoziationskonstanten des Rezeptor-Liganden Komplexes K_4 ergibt sich dann ein Modell, das dem der 2′-Fluoro-Desoxyglukose unter Vernachlässigung der Dephosphorylierung bzw. dem Glukosemodell von BLOMQVIST et al. (1985), unter Vernachlässigung des weiteren Metabolismus, sehr ähnlich ist.

Mit

$$dC_c^*/dt = K_1 C_p^*(t) - (K_2 + K_3) \cdot C_c^*(t) \tag{60}$$

und

$$dC_m^*/dt = K_3 C_c^*(t) \tag{61}$$

ergibt sich die Nettobindungsrate K an den Rezeptoren zu:

$$K = \frac{C_i^* - K_2 \cdot C_c^*/(K_2 + K_3)}{\int C_p^*(t) \cdot dt} \tag{62}$$

dabei sind $C_i^* = C_c^* + C_m^*$ und $K = K_1 \cdot K_2/(K_1 + K_3)$ (Wagner et al. 1985).

Mit $C_c = C_p \cdot K_1/(K_2 + K_3)$ ergibt sich für das Verhältnis von C_i^* zu C_c^*:

$$\frac{C_i^*}{C_c^*} = K_3 \cdot \frac{\int C_p^*(t) \cdot dt}{C_p(t)} + \frac{K_2}{K_2 + K_3} \tag{63}$$

Über die Berechnung des meßtechnisch direkt zugänglichen Verhältnisses von C_i/C_c, das dem Verhältnis der Aktivitätskonzentrationen in rezeptorreichen zu rezeptorarmen Regionen entspricht, und das über einen weiten Bereich zeitlich linear verläuft, kann dann aus der Steigung die Bindungsrate K_3 des Liganden zum Rezeptor berechnet werden.

In der bisherigen Literatur für in vivo Messungen der Bindungseigenschaften von Liganden an Rezeptoren ist die Definition der quantitativ zu erfassenden bzw. zu beschreibenden Größen uneinheitlich und reicht von klassischen in vitro Ansätzen bis zur rechneroptimierten Kompartmentanalyse (Schafer 1983; Mintum et al. 1984a; Young et al. 1986).

Verfeinerte Modellvorstellungen wie die von Mintum et al. (1984a) berücksichtigen die Dissoziation der Liganden-Rezeptor Komplexe und den Anteil des Plasmas im Gesamtsignal aus dem Gewebe. In ihrem differentiellen Ansatz werden unter der Annahme eines rein diffusiven Transports über die Blut-Hirn-Schranke die Gleichgewichtskonstanten K_1 und K_2 durch das Permeabilitäts-Oberflächenprodukt PS ersetzt. Unter der Annahme einer Sättigungsgrenze infolge der begrenzten Anzahl von Rezeptoren ergibt sich für die Konzentrationsänderung im zweiten und dritten Kompartment:

$$dC_c^*/dt = PS/V_c \cdot (C_b - C_c) + K_4 \cdot C_m^* - K_3 \cdot C_c^* \cdot (B_{max} - C_m^*) \tag{64}$$

und

$$dC_m^*/dt = K_3 \cdot C_c^*(B_{max} - C_m^*) - K_4 \cdot C_m^* \tag{65}$$

Mintum et al. (1984a) kommen dabei zu dem Schluß, daß unter realen Bedingungen, bei denen die Ligandenkonzentration aufgrund der ebenfalls sehr niedrigen Rezeptorkonzentrationen nicht vernachlässigbar sind, die Gesamtanzahl der aktiven Rezeptoren nicht unabhängig von der Bindungsaffinität bestimmt werden kann. Sie führen daher als neuen bestimmbaren Term das Bindungspotential BP ein, das als das Verhältnis der maximalen spezifischen Bindungskonzentration B_{max} und der Bindungsaffinität $K_d = K_3/K_4$ definiert wird.

$$BP = B_{max}/K_d \tag{66}$$

Erfahrungen an Patienten liegen mit dieser Auswertemethode jedoch bisher nicht vor.

IX. pH-Messungen im Gehirn

Regionale Gewebe-pH-Werte gestatten die Beurteilung einer Reihe von Funktionszuständen, die in vielen Fällen nicht oder nur schwer mit einzelnen physiologisch-chemischen Prozessen beschrieben bzw. korreliert werden können. So sind pH-Veränderungen in Tumorgewebe bekannte Indikatoren für Thermoempfindlichkeit, Strahlenresistenz und Proliferationsgeschwindigkeit (GERSON et al. 1982).

Zur Berechnung des pH-Wertes mittels der Positronen Emissionstomographie kann von folgendem Ansatz ausgegangen werden:

In einem definierten chemischen Kompartment, in dem die Reaktion

$$AH \rightleftarrows A^- + H^+ \tag{67}$$

zu einem Gleichgewichtszustand gekommen ist, kann der pH Wert im Kompartment über die Anfangskonzentration von AH und deren spezifische Dissoziationskonstante K_d berechnet werden. Nach dem Massenwirkungsgesetz und der Hasselbach-Henderson-Gleichung gilt:

$$[AH] = K_d \cdot [A^-] \cdot [H^+] \tag{68}$$

und

$$pH = pK_d + \log[A^-]/[AH] \tag{68a}$$

Mit diesem Ansatz wurde schon von RAICHLE et al. (1979) vorgeschlagen, den intrazellulären pH-Wert des Gehirns entsprechend der Reaktionsgleichung:

$$^{11}CO_2 + H_2O \rightleftarrows H^{11}CO_3^- + H^+ \tag{69}$$

zu bestimmen.

Das Modell geht dabei von folgender Kompartmentvorstellung aus: $^{11}CO_2$ ist ein diffusibles Gas, dessen intra- und extrazelluläre Konzentration im „Steady State" gleich groß ist. Intra- und extrazellulär dissoziiert $^{11}CO_2$ zu Karbonat und Wasserstoffionen. Karbonationen können die Blut-Hirn-Schranke jedoch nicht passieren. Durch Bestimmung des intravasalen $^{11}CO_2$ Gehaltes und der regionalen zellulären $H^{11}CO_3^-$ Konzentration kann damit der intrazelluläre pH-Wert entsprechend Gleichung (68a) bestimmt werden.

Der Ansatz birgt allerdings einige Probleme in sich, da $^{11}CO_2$ nicht inert ist und nicht ausschließlich in der gewünschten Weise reagiert, sondern sowohl in metabolische Reaktionswege eingeschleust werden kann, als auch teilweise über die Lunge abgeatmet wird. Der aus ebensolchen Gründen von LOCKWOOD u. FINN (1982) formulierten Kritik an diesem Ansatz begegneten BUXTON et al. (1984) und BROOKS et al. (1984a) mit einem erweiterten „Steady State" Modell, das die Metabolisierungsrate (Fixierung) von $^{11}CO_2$ berücksichtigt.

Eine elegante Variante dieses Ansatzes zur regionalen pH-Wert Bestimmung im Gehirn mittels PET wurde von KEARFOTT et al. (1983a) und ROTTENBERG et al. (1983, 1985) auf der Grundlage einer Arbeit von WADDELL u. BUTLER (1959) durch Verwendung von ^{11}C-markiertem Dimethyloxazolidendion (DMO) entwickelt. Dieses Molekül ist metabolisch neutral, passiert in protonierter Form die Blut-Hirn-Schranke rein diffusiv und hat die Eigenschaft entsprechend Gleichung (67) zu dissoziieren:

$$HDMO \rightleftarrows DMO^- + H^+ \tag{70}$$

Die anionische Form kann die Blut-Hirn-Schranke nicht passieren. In einem 2-Kompartment-modell aus Plasma und Hirngewebe kann dann der Gewebe-pH (pH_c) als Funktion des Plasma-pH (pH_p) sowie der Plasma- (C_p) und der Hirngewebekonzentration (C_c) von DMO^- entsprechend Gleichung (71) ausgedrückt werden:

$$pH_c = pH_p + \log C_c - \log C_p \qquad (71)$$

Dabei wird angenommen, daß die Konzentration HDMO in Plasma und Hirngewebe gleich groß ist. Entsprechend kann die gemessene Gesamtkonzentration im Hirngewebe, die sich aus HDMO und DMO^- zusammensetzt, um den protonierten Anteil korrigiert werden, der unter Berücksichtigung des Wasseranteils des Plasmas und des Hämatokrit aus den arteriellem Blutwerten erhalten werden kann. Die Benutzung arterieller Blutwerte erwies sich als erforderlich, da die Gleichgewichtseinstellung zwischen Blut und Hirngewebe nur sehr langsam erfolgt. Die Methode wurde mit ^{14}C-markiertem DMO validiert (Junck et al. 1981). Die Fehlerempfindlichkeit der Methodik wird von Rottenberg et al. (1985) für pH-Werte $>6{,}5$ mit ± 0.1 pH angegeben. Für kleinere pH-Werte ist die Genauigkeit aufgrund des zunehmenden Einflusses des Blutvolumens und der schlechteren Statistik geringer. Eine Übersicht über die allgemeine Problematik der Messung intrazellulärer pH-Werte geben Roos u. Boron (1981).

X. Messungen von Blut-Hirn-Schrankenstörung

Die Blut-Hirn-Schranke wird von einer dichten Endothelzellenschicht ohne die sonst üblichen Zwischenräume an den Zellverbindungslinien gebildet. Übersichten und eine Einführung in die Funktionsweise dieser komplizierten Membran geben Rapoport (1976), Bradbury (1979, 1985), Pardridge (1983) sowie Goldstein u. Betz (1986). Die Blut-Hirn-Schranke ist unter normalen physiologischen Bedingungen für ionische Verbindungen und die meisten Makromoleküle undurchlässig und nur für hoch lipophile Substanzen diffusiv passierbar. Für einige wasserlösliche Substanzen existieren spezielle Transportmechanismen. Die Störung der Blut-Hirn-Schranke ist ein sensitiver Indikator für pathologische Veränderungen im Gehirn und kann mit verschiedenen Methoden, wie CT und Szintigraphie beobachtet werden. Eine quantitative Beurteilung der Störung gelingt jedoch nur mit der Positronen-Emissionstomographie. Dabei wird versucht, das Ausmaß der Störung durch Berechnung der Änderung des Permeabilitäts-Oberflächen Produktes für eine sonst nicht passierende Substanz auszudrücken. Als Substanzen zur Messung der Permeabilitätsstörung wurden ^{68}Ga-EDTA (Kessler et al. 1983, 1984; Hawkins et al. 1984; Blasberg et al. 1984; Bergström et al. 1983), ^{82}Rb (Yen u. Budinger 1981; Yen et al. 1982; Lammertsma et al. 1984b; Brooks et al. 1984b) und ^{13}NH$_3$ (Lockwood et al. 1984) vorgeschlagen.

Physiologisch-kinetische Modellvorstellungen zur Quantifizierung wurden für ^{68}Ga-EDTA von Kessler et al. (1983) und für ^{82}Rb von Lammertsma et al. (1984b) entwickelt. Beiden liegt zunächst ein 2-Kompartmentmodell im Gleichgewichtszustand entsprechend Abb. 18 zugrunde, das aus Intravasalraum und dem Gehirngewebe besteht.

Bei der konstanten Infusion des kurzlebigen ^{82}Rb ($T_{1/2} = 75$ s) ergibt sich für die Aktivität im Intravasalbereich analog zu Gleichung (5), jedoch unter Einbeziehung der Extraktionsfraktion E:

$$F \cdot C_{in(r)} \cdot (1 - E) = F \cdot C_{out(r)} + Q_{b(r)} \cdot \lambda_{(r)} \qquad (72)$$

wobei E die Extraktionsfraktion, F den Fluß, $C_{in(r)}$ und $C_{out(r)}$ die arterielle und venöse Blutkonzentration des ^{82}Rb, $Q_{b(r)}$ die Aktivitätsmenge des ^{82}Rb im fraktionellen Blutvolumen

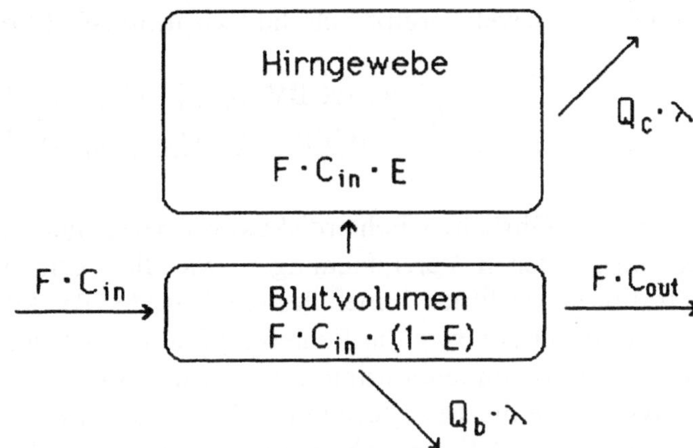

Abb. 18. Zweikompartmentmodell zur Bestimmung der Permeabilitätsstörung der Blut-Hirn-Schranke durch Messung im „Steady State"

und $\lambda_{(r)}$ die Zerfallskonstante des Tracers ^{82}Rb darstellen. Durch Gleichsetzung des fraktionellen Blutvolumens mit dem venösen Anteil (dieser entspricht über 90% des parenchymalen Blutvolumens) kann die venöse Konzentration $C_{\text{out}(r)}$ durch das Verhältnis von Tracermenge $Q_{b(r)}$ zu Volumen V_b (s. Gleichung (6a)) ersetzt werden. Damit ergibt sich:

$$F \cdot C_{\text{in}(r)} \cdot (1 - E) = F \cdot Q_{b(r)}/V_b + Q_{b(r)} \cdot \lambda_{(r)} \tag{73}$$

Wegen der kurzen Halbwertzeit des ^{82}Rb wird eine Rückdiffusion des Tracers im 2. Kompartment, dem Gehirngewebe, zunächst vernachlässigt. Für die Gehirnkonzentration gilt dann analog zur Gleichung (5):

$$F \cdot C_{\text{in}(r)} \cdot E = Q_{c(r)} \cdot \lambda_{(r)}, \tag{73a}$$

mit $Q_{c(r)}$ als der Aktivitätsmenge im Gehirngewebe.

Die Gesamtaktivitätsmenge im Gesichtsfeld eines Tomographen setzt sich dann aus der Blutaktivität und der Gehirngewebeaktivität zusammen und kann folgendermaßen beschrieben werden:

$$Q_{\text{ges}(r)} = Q_{c(r)} + Q_{b(r)} = \frac{C_{\text{in}(r)} \cdot F \cdot E}{\lambda_{(r)}} + \frac{C_{\text{in}(r)} \cdot F \cdot (1 - E)}{F/V_b + \lambda_{(r)}} \tag{74}$$

Die Berechnung des Flusses mittels konstanter Infusion von $H_2^{15}O$ kann nach Gleichung (6a, 7) erfolgen.

$$Q_{(w)} = \frac{V \cdot C_{\text{in}(w)}}{1 + V/F \cdot \lambda_{(w)}} \tag{7}$$

Division von Gleichung (74) durch Gleichung (7) ergibt die Gleichung (75).

$$E = \frac{\lambda_{(r)}}{F/V_{b(r)}} \cdot \left(\frac{Q_{\text{ges}(r)} \cdot C_{\text{in}(w)} \cdot (F/V_b + \lambda_{(r)})}{Q_{(w)} \cdot C_{\text{in}(r)} \cdot (F/V + \lambda_{(w)})} - 1 \right) \tag{75}$$

Die Messung des regionalen Blutvolumens V_b kann durch separate Messung mit ^{11}CO erfolgen. Durch Einsetzen der Werte für F und V_b als rCBF in ml/min · 100 g Gewebe und rCBV in ml/100 g Gewebe ergibt sich die Extraktionsfraktion zu:

$$E = \frac{\lambda_{(r)} \cdot rCBV}{rCBF} \cdot \left(\frac{Q_{ges(r)} \cdot C_{in(w)} \cdot (rCBF/rCBV + \lambda_{(r)})}{Q_w \cdot C_{in(r)} \cdot (rCBF/100 + \lambda_{(w)})} - 1 \right) \tag{76}$$

In einer ausführlichen Fehlerdiskussion berechnen Lammertsma et al. (1984b) die Einflüsse der verschiedenen Vereinfachungen, wie die Vernachlässigung der arteriellen Komponente im fraktionellen Blutvolumen des Gehirns, der Rückdiffusion von ^{82}Rb und der Inhomogenität des Gewebes sowie die Fehlerempfindlichkeit gegenüber Unsicherheiten in der Blutfluß- und der Blutvolumenbestimmung und den Einfluß der Zählstatistik. Auf die Details dieser Analyse sowie die Erweiterung des Modells um ein arterielles Kompartment, kann im Rahmen dieser Darstellung nicht eingegangen werden. Zusammenfassend kommen Lammertsma et al. (1984b) zu dem Ergebnis, daß der Gesamtfehler auch in dem vereinfachten hier erörterten Modell auf 5–10% beschränkt werden kann, wenn die Blut-Hirn-Schrankenstörung in relativ großen Arealen, speziell beim Vergleich zweier Hemisphären, angegeben werden soll. In Fällen mit Arealen hoher Permeabilität kann die Extraktion mit einer Genauigkeit von ca. 10% auch in kleineren Regionen quantifiziert werden.

C. Meßtechnische Limitationen

Die pharmakokinetischen Modellvorstellungen sind trotz Rücksichtnahme auf die grundsätzlichen Limitationen der meßtechnischen Methodik weitgehend idealisiert. Daher führt die Anwendung realer Daten auf die Berechnungsformeln zu zusätzlichen Fehlern, deren Größe nur über die Kenntnis meßtechnischer Korrekturparameter abgeschätzt und damit reduziert werden kann. Eine Beseitigung dieser Fehlerquellen ist praktisch nicht möglich. Ihre Verringerung ist das Ziel aller Verbesserungen in der Auslegung und Konstruktion neuer Positronen-Emissionstomographen und der Optimierung von Anwendungsprotokollen. Details der Konstruktionsmerkmale von Positronentomographen, die entsprechende meßtechnische Limitationen beeinflussen, werden an anderer Stelle in diesem Handbuch erörtert.

Neben einer Zusammenstellung dieser Limitationen soll hier auf deren praktische Auswirkungen hingewiesen werden, wie sie sich besonders bei der Methoden-Standardisierung mittels Normalbefunden sowie bei der Beurteilung klinischer Befunde bemerkbar machen.

I. Auflösungsvermögen

Das Auflösungsvermögen eines Positronen-Emissionstomographen wird zunächst von den Dimensionen des Szintillationskristalls bestimmt. Hinzu kommen Faktoren wie die Ortungsgenauigkeit des angesprochenen Szintillationskristalls und die Eigenschaften des Rekonstruktionsalgorithmus.

Das Auflösungsvermögen von Positronen-Emissionstomographen ist derzeit auf 5–8 mm in der Schichtebene und auf ca. 6–12 mm in der Schichtdicke begrenzt. Dies führt zu einer Reihe meßtechnischer Limitationen, die sich bei der quantitativen Auswertung rekonstruierter Schichtaufnahmen durch Über- oder Unterschätzung von Aktivitätskonzentrationen bemerkbar machen.

Eine der Fehlerquellen ist der sogenannte Teilvolumeneffekt. Er tritt auf, wenn Volumenelemente beurteilt werden müssen, die inhomogene Gewebestrukturen enthalten, aber als homogenes Gewebe in Berechnungsformeln einhergehen. Beispiele dafür sind Schwierigkeiten bei der Beurteilung von Randzonen des Herzens, sehr kleine Funktionsdefekte (heiß oder kalt) in allen Organen sowie Unterschiede zwischen grauer und weißer Hirnsubstanz an deren Grenzflächen. Der Effekt kann folgendermaßen veranschaulicht werden: Beträgt die abgebildete Voxelgröße $10 \times 10 \times 15$ mm^3 = 1,5 cm^3 und hat ein heißer Knoten eine Ausdehnung von 1 cm^3 mit einer Aktivitätskonzentration von 1500 cps/cm^3, so wird die errechnete Aktivitätskonzentration nur 1000 cps/cm^3 betragen.

Sogenannte „Spill-over"-Effekte beruhen auf den Eigenschaften der Abbildungsfunktionen. Sie entstehen durch heiße Areale, die aufgrund der begrenzten Auflösung an den Grenzflächen in benachbarte Gebiete hineinstrahlen und damit zu scheinbar vergrößerten Verteilungsvolumina führen.

Schließlich ist die Auflösung im Gesichtsfeld nicht homogen, sondern ortsvariant, mit besserer Auflösung im Zentrum des Gesichtsfeldes und sich zum Rand hin verschlechternden Abbildungseigenschaften. Diese Variation der Auflösung beruht auf der Ortsvarianz verschiedener Konstruktionsparameter des Tomographen. Sie führt zu einer Inhomogenität der Abbildungsgröße und damit zu einer Art sekundärem Teilvolumeneffekt. Aktivitäten kleiner Ausdehnung werden damit in den Randgebieten des Gesichtsfeldes eher unterschätzt.

II. Empfindlichkeit

Unter Empfindlichkeit wird die Anzahl der gemessenen echten Koinzidenzen pro Zeiteinheit je Aktivitätseinheit im Gesichtsfeld verstanden. Da die Empfindlichkeit von der geometrischen Verteilung der Aktivität im Gesichtsfeld nicht völlig unabhängig ist, wird die Empfindlichkeit nahezu immer auf eine homogene, zentriert zylindrische Verteilung von 20 cm Durchmesser bezogen. Die Empfindlichkeit moderner Geräte für eine direkte Koinzidenzschicht von ca. 6 mm Schichtdicke liegt bei 4000–5000 cps/µCi/cm^3.

Die Empfindlichkeit wird im wesentlichen von drei Faktoren bestimmt:

Erstens dem Kristallmaterial der Szintillationsdetektoren. Die relativ hohe Energie der Positronenvernichtungsstrahlung von 511 keV erfordert ein möglichst dichtes Material mit darüberhinaus guten Szintillationseigenschaften. Das heute am weitesten verbreitete und dichteste Material ist Bismut-Germanat ($Bi_2Ge_2O_7$), das im nicht-chemischen Sprachgebrauch als BGO abgekürzt wird.

Zweitens der Packungsdichte des Kristallmaterials. Um pro Zeiteinheit möglichst viele der in alle Raumwinkel emittierten Gamma-Quanten zu erfassen, ist es notwendig die Kristalle auf einem geschlossenen Ring möglichst eng anzuordnen. Durch die Wahl rechteckiger Kristalle werden dabei heute Packungsdichten von über 90% erreicht. Der Ringdurchmesser ist für die Empfindlichkeit von zweitrangiger Bedeutung. Zwar haben kleine Ringe formal größere Empfindlichkeiten als große Ringe, der Empfindlichkeitsgewinn beruht aber zu einem großen Teil auf erhöhter Streustrahlungsempfindlichkeit. Die Ringdicke in achsialer (Z) Richtung geht dagegen direkt in die Gesamtempfindlichkeit ein. Da die Gesamtdicke in Z-Richtung in unterschiedlich viele Schichten aufgeteilt sein kann, ist die Angabe der Empfindlichkeit pro Schicht solange irreführend, wie nicht die Schichtdicke berücksichtigt wird. Beim Vergleich von Empfindlichkeiten unterschiedlicher Tomographen sollte daher eine Empfindlichkeit pro cm Schichtdicke als Maßzahl dienen.

Drittens wird die Empfindlichkeit von den Blei-Septen zur Abschirmung von Strahlung aus Regionen außerhalb des Gesichtsfeldes sowie zur Kollimierung in Z-Richtung beeinflußt. Geeignete Wahl von Material und geometrischer Anordnung können das Signal zu Rausch-

Verhältnis entscheidend verbessern, führen aber auch zu einer Reduktion der Empfindlichkeit. Bei entsprechender Optimierung beruht die Empfindlichkeitsreduktion im wesentlichen auf einer Reduktion unerwünschter Streustrahlungsanteile.

Aus der begrenzten Empfindlichkeit ergeben sich meßtechnische Limitationen speziell für die Untersuchung von relativ langsamen Stoffwechselprozessen. So sind beispielsweise Untersuchungen mit ^{11}C-markierten Verbindungen über Zeiträume von mehr als 60 Minuten fast nicht mehr zu verfolgen. Darüberhinaus können Untersuchungssequenzen nach bolusförmiger Applikation von besonders kurzlebigen Radiopharmaka wie ^{15}O-Wasser oder -Butanol nur schwer bis in den Gleichgewichtszustand hinein verfolgt werden. Der sich dagegen anbietenden Lösung der Applikation höherer Anfangsaktivitäten stehen neben Strahlenschutz-Gründen manchmal auch eine begrenzte Zählratenverarbeitungskapazität des Gerätes in der Anfangsphase der Meßzeit entgegen.

III. Signal- zu Rauschverhältnis, und Zählratenverarbeitungs-Kapazität

Unechte Koinzidenzereignisse verschlechtern das Signal- zu Rauschverhältnis. Die Hauptquellen solcher unechter Koinzidenzereignisse stellen die Streustrahlung (Scatter) und zufällige Koinzidenzen dar.

Die Verringerung gestreuter Anteile gelingt durch drei voneinander unabhängige Maßnahmen. Zunächst kann viel Streustrahlung durch Verlängerung der Septen und der Randabschirmung schon an dem Erreichen der Detektoren gehindert werden. Sodann kann durch Hochsetzen der Schwellenenergie am Diskriminator ein weiterer Teil der Streustrahlung erkannt und unterdrückt werden. Beide Faktoren wirken sich aber auch auf die Empfindlichkeit aus und müssen daher optimiert werden. Schließlich kann durch Berechnung der resultierenden Streustrahlung aus einem bekannten Verteilungsvolumen mit bekannten Streueigenschaften eine nachträgliche Korrektur der Meßdaten bezüglich der Streuanteile erfolgen.

Die Anzahl zufälliger Koinzidenzen ist von der Detektorgröße und dem zeitlichen Auflösungsvermögen des Tomographen sowie von der Aktivitätsmenge im Gesichtsfeld abhängig. Da die Detektorgröße schon aus Gründen des geometrischen Auflösungsvermögens so klein wie möglich gemacht wird, bleibt die zeitliche Auflösung als limitierendes Kriterium für die Anzahl zufälliger Koinzidenzen. Da die zufälligen Koinzidenzen sowohl aus der Einzelrate der Impulse jedes Detektors errechnet werden können als auch in einem zeitversetzten Fenster gemessen werden können, ergeben sich, bis auf den Grenzbereich sehr hoher Aktivitäten, recht brauchbare Korrekturmöglichkeiten für die zufälligen Koinzidenzen. In diesem Grenzbereich jedoch, der durch hohe Totzeitverluste und schließliche Sättigung der Detektoren gekennzeichnet ist, werden die meßtechnischen Limitationen für bestimmte Anwendungsprotokolle gravierend.

Die Empfindlichkeit des Meßsystems bezüglich der Totzeitverluste, d.h. die Zählratenverarbeitungskapazität beruht nicht nur auf dem zeitlichen Auflösungsvermögen des Koinzidenzfensters, sondern darüberhinaus auf der Anzahl voneinander unabhängiger Detektoren je Koinzidenzkanal. Neuere Positronen-Emissionstomographen enthalten häufig Blockdetektoren, in denen die Ortszuordnung nach dem Angerkamera-Prinzip erfolgt. Dabei werden Einschränkungen hinsichtlich der Zählratenverarbeitungskapazität zugunsten der Empfindlichkeit und der Auflösung bewußt in Kauf genommen.

Bei bolusförmigen Applikationen können jedoch in den ersten Sekunden sehr hohe Aktivitäten im Gesichtfeld auftreten, die dann auf Grund der oben angeführten meßtechnischen Limitationen nicht mit genügender Genauigkeit quantitativ erfaßt werden können.

Während die Zählratenkapazität jedoch nur in wenigen Anwendungsprotokollen und speziell schnellen dynamischen Studien limitierend wirkt, beeinflussen hohe Streustrahlungsanteile grundsätzlich die quantitative Auswertung aller Untersuchungen.

IV. Absorptionskorrektur

Im Gegensatz zur Messung einzelner Photonen ist bei der Messung koinzidenter Gammaquanten gleicher Energie die Kenntnis des Absorptionsverhaltens in Richtung des Meßstrahls hinreichend, um eine Absorptionskorrektur durchzuführen. Insbesondere ist demnach die gemessene Koinzidenzzählrate unabhängig von der Verteilung der Aktivität im untersuchten Streumedium. Die Absolutberechnung der Aktivität setzt demnach nur die Kenntnis des Gesamtabsorptionsverhaltens des untersuchten Mediums voraus. Zur Bestimmung dieses Absorptionsverhaltens gibt es prinzipiell zwei Methoden.

Die erste Möglichkeit besteht in der Messung des Absorptionsverhaltens mittels einer Transmissionsaufnahme. Meßtechnische Limitationen ergeben sich aus der Tatsache, daß eine Transmissionsaufnahme wie auch jede Emissionsaufnahme grundsätzlich Rauschanteile enthält, die bei der Korrekturrechnung das korrigierte Emissionsbild zusätzlich verrauschen. Um diesen Störeffekt geringer als 10% zu halten, muß die Transmissionsaufnahme eine ca. 10fach bessere statistische Güte aufweisen als das zu korrigierende Emissionsbild. Dies bedeutet, daß Transmissionsmessungen relativ lange dauern und daß sie die Anwendungprotokolle komplizieren.

Die zweite Möglichkeit besteht in der rein rechnerischen Absorptionskorrektur. Dabei wird die äußere Form des Streumediums aus den Emissionsdaten gewonnen und eine meist homogene Verteilung des Absorptionskoeffizienten angenommen. Unter Berücksichtigung einer gleichmäßig dicken Kalottenschicht führt diese Vereinfachung im Schädelbereich zu nur relativ geringen Fehlern. Prinzipiell können auch komplexe, ineinander verschachtelte und unregelmäßige Absorptionsgeometrien, wie sie beispielsweise im Thorax vorliegen, berechnet werden; Modellannahmen über solche Absorptionsgeometrien führen in der Praxis jedoch zu erheblichen Fehlern.

Zur Vermeidung solcher Fehler bietet sich eine Kombination beider Korrekturverfahren an. Dabei wird zunächst eine kurze Transmissionsaufnahme angefertigt. Diese enthält zwar relativ hohe Rauschanteile, sie erlaubt aber trotzdem die Aufstellung eines individuellen Absorptionsmodells, in dem dann die anatomischen Bereiche mit gleichen Absorptionskoeffizienten zusammengefaßt werden. Das sich daraus ergebende Korrekturmodell hat eine der Wirklichkeit recht genau entsprechende Geometrie und ist abgesehen von Randunschärfen rauschfrei.

V. Patientenpositionierung und Bewegungskoordination

Die Bedeutung der Reproduzierbarkeit der Patientenpositionierung und der Fixierung des Patienten im Tomographen für eine quantitative Interpretation von PET-Daten wird häufig unterschätzt. Vor allem bei Anwendungsprotokollen, die eine Verrechnung mehrerer Aufnahmen erfordern, wie z.B. die regionale Sauerstoff-Verbrauchsrate oder Blutvolumenkorrigierte Funktionsdarstellungen, müssen die Schichtebenen der Einzelaufnahmen sehr genau übereinstimmen. Dies erfordert eine genaue Ausrichtungsmöglichkeit und Positionierungskontrolle in allen drei Raumebenen sowie eine Fixierungseinrichtung, die auch bei der Absorptionskorrektur Berücksichtigung findet. Unzureichende Vorkehrungen in dieser Hinsicht führen sowohl zu einer Verschlechterung der Auflösung als auch zu größerer Ungenauigkeit in der Quantifizierung der Daten.

Während diese Anforderungen für Aufnahmen am Kopf relativ einfach erfüllt werden können, ergeben sich in Thorax und Abdomen zusätzliche Probleme. Für Aufnahmen mit hoher Auflösung in diesen Körperregionen müssen die aus Herzbewegung und Atemtätigkeit resultierenden Bewegungsartefakte durch entsprechende Triggereinrichtungen minimalisiert werden. Dies wiederum erfordert erheblich verlängerte Aufnahmezeiten, die mit den Anforderungen einiger Anwendungprotokolle, wie der schnellen dynamischen Flußmessung mittels Bolusapplikation, nicht vereinbar sind. Darüberhinaus muß auf den erheblichen apparativen und datenverarbeitungsmäßigen Aufwand bei dennoch begrenzter Genauigkeit der Einrichtungen zur Bewegungskorrektur hingewiesen werden.

VI. Konstitution und Rekonstitution des Patienten

Schließlich muß auf Limitationen hingewiesen werden, die sich aus der Nicht-Uniformität der Untersuchungsobjekte ergeben. Für viele Funktionsuntersuchungen sind nicht nur dietätische und sensorische Einflüsse auf die Normalwerte unbekannt, sondern häufig ist sogar die Schwankungsbreite der Normalwerte in einem Kontrollkollektiv nur unzureichend dokumentiert. Hinzu kommen konstitutionelle Unterschiede der Patienten, die zu unterschiedlichen Basiswerten der zu untersuchenden Funktionsparameter führen.

So wird beispielsweise in den meisten veröffentlichten Anwendungsprotokollen zur Bestimmung der regionalen Glukose-Verbrauchsrate darauf hingewiesen, daß die Patienten standardisierten sensorische Einflüsse unterworfen werden müssen. Dazu werden eine leichte Abdunkelung des Untersuchungsraumes und eine Geräuschdämpfung bzw. auch eine gezielte Geräusch- oder Musikbeschallung (evtl. über Kopfhöhrer) empfohlen. Dies kann zu erheblichen, aber nicht quantifizierbaren emotionalen Belastungen der Patienten führen, deren Verminderung evtl. durch vorangehendes Durchüben der Untersuchungssituation erreicht werden kann. Für eine Anzahl von Patienten mag andererseits auch das Durchüben der Untersuchungssituation zu erhöhtem Streß führen. Wiederholungsuntersuchungen nach Stimulation können unter Berücksichtigung dieser Einflüsse somit nur relative Aussagen über die Reizgröße geben.

Über diätetische Einflüsse liegen bisher nur wenige systematische Untersuchungen vor. So ist allgemein bekannt, daß bei Herzstoffwechseluntersuchungen Aufnahme und Kinetik der Fettsäureverbrennung wie auch die Glukoseaufnahme vom Zeitpunkt und der Zusammensetzung der letzten Mahlzeit beeinflußt sein können. Ebensolche Beeinflussungen scheint es auch bei der Untersuchung der Aminosäure-Aufnahme sowohl im Gehirn wie auch in anderen Organen zu geben.

D. Physiologische und klinische Anwendungen

I. Hirn

1. Physiologie

Allgemeine Physiologie. Die quantitative Charakterisierung regionaler zerebraler Funktionen und Strukturen wird ermöglicht durch die Implementierung von Tracerkinetiken mit den entsprechenden Modellen. Voraussetzung ist ein Verständnis der Biochemie der Tracer, die auf regionale, physiologische und pathologische Veränderungen im Zentralnervensystem schließen läßt. Die Prozesse können folgende Stoffwechselvorgänge und Randbedingungen beinhalten:

a) Blut-Hirn-Schranke
b) Blutfluß
c) Blutvolumen

d) Sauerstoffmetabolismus und Sauerstoff-Extraktionsrate
e) Glukosemetabolismus
f) Protein-Synthese
g) Neurorezeptoren und Pharmaka
h) Gewebe-pH
i) Funktionelle Aktivierungen
k) Altersabhängigkeit

Fehler und Variationen mit der PET bestimmter metabolischer Parameter können auf methodische Probleme der PET und der Anatomie, wie die Abhängigkeit von Größe und Form einer Struktur, auf solche der Datenanalyse, d.h. den Weg von der Messung des Signals bis zur Interpretation über eine Modellvorstellung, wie Signal-zu-Rausch-Verhältnis, Absorptionskorrekturen und Teilvolumeneffekte, bis hin zu nicht definierbaren der subjektiven Auffassung und Interpretation inhärenten Analysen zurückzuführen sein. Dabei spielen insbesondere die Test-Bedingungen eine erhebliche Rolle (Tabelle 3).

Radiologische, neuropsychologische und elektrophysiologische Verfahren haben bisher die diagnostischen Möglichkeiten bestimmt. Verstehen und Dokumentation des physiologischen Verhaltens sind aber zumindest komplementäre Voraussetzungen der Diagnose neurologischer Krankheitsbilder.

Tabelle 3. Fehler und Variationen bei der Positronen-Emissionstomographie.
(Nach MAZZIOTTA u. PHELPS 1984)

PET-Methode	Anatomie und Datenanalyse	Untersuchung
1. Räumliche Auflösung	1. Bewegungsartefakt	1. Biologische Varianz
2. Zeitliche Auflösung	2. Anatomische Positionierung	2. Definition, Beobachtung des Zustandes
3. Tracerkinetik vs. zeitliche Sequenz der funkt. Aktivität	3. Anatomische Struktur und Identifizierung	3. Nicht gewünschte Aktivität Angst, Streß, ablenkende Stimuli, Gewöhnung, Motivation
4. Validität des Tracer-Modells	4. Verknüpfung versch. Aktivitäten (z.B. additiv, unabhängig)	
5. Anzahl der tomogr. Schichten	5. Mehrdeutigkeit (z.B. PET vs. EEG)	
6. Kalibrierung		

a) Blut-Hirn-Schranke

Die Blut-Hirn-Schranke (BBB: blood brain barrier) dient als funktionelle Schranke (interface) zwischen dem Hirngewebe und dem Blutsystem. Vier verschiedene Mechanismen sind für einen Transport über die Blut-Hirn-Schranke hinaus zu diskutieren: passive Diffusion, „carrier facilitated transport", aktiver Transport und Pinozytose (LAJTHA u. FORD 1968). Theoretische Modellvorstellungen gehen in erster Linie auf Überlegungen von RENKIN (1959) und CRONE (1963) zurück. Verschiedene Modelle wurden mit den Positronenstrahlern $^{13}NH_3$, ^{68}Ga-EDTA und ^{82}Rb untersucht. Die charakterisierenden Parameter sind analog zur Transmissions-Computertomographie mit Kontrastmitteln oder der statischen Hirnszintigraphie die Extraktionsrate und das Permeabilitätsoberflächenprodukt (BERGSTRÖM et al. 1983; BROOKS et al. 1984b; ERICSON et al. 1985; LAMBRECHT u. RESSIGNO 1983; LAMMERTSMA et al. 1984; LOCKWOOD et al. 1980, 1984; YANO et al. 1981; YEN et al. 1982).

Mit ^{68}Ga-EDTA stellen sich im Normalfall nur die perfundierten Gebiete dar, insbesondere die mimische Muskulatur und die Galea aponeurotica, Dach und Basis des Schädels und die Blutleiter der harten Hirnhaut (Sinus sagittalis, transversus und sigmoideus, Sinus occipitalis und petrosus, Sinus cavernosus) (HEISS et al. 1985b).

b) Blutfluß

Eine der Basis-Funktionen ist die regionale Perfusion; Tracer, die mehr oder weniger direkt ein Maß für die Perfusion sind, lassen sich einteilen in solche, die frei diffusibel die Blut-Hirn-Schranke passieren, und solche, die wie Mikrosphären „getrappt" werden.

Die direkte Meßmethode zur Bestimmung der absoluten Durchblutung F (ml/min), die eine bolusförmige Injektion des intravasalen Tracers direkt in das zuführende Gefäß und die Bestimmung der venösen Konzentration in Abhängigkeit von der Zeit erfordert, setzt eine vollständige arterielle Durchmischung, die Erfassung des gesamten venösen Ausflusses und eine während des Untersuchungszeitraumes konstante Durchblutung voraus (Stewart 1897; Hamilton et al. 1928; Kety u. Schmidt 1945). Mit der Positronen-Emissionstomographie wird dagegen in der Regel die spezifische Durchblutung (ml/100 g/min) der untersuchten Strombahn angegeben (Knoop 1982).

Als frei diffusible Tracer wurden bisher in der Klinik in erster Linie Gammastrahler, wie ^{133}Xe, ^{127}Xe, ^{77}Kr, aber auch das kurzlebige Zyklotronprodukt ^{81m}Kr ($T_{1/2} = 13$ sec) verwendet (Fazio et al. 1980; Lassen 1985; Roland et al. 1981; Yamamoto et al. 1977). Die Beurteilung tiefer gelegener Hirnstrukturen ist mit dem relativ weichen Gammastrahler ^{133}Xe ($E_\gamma = 81$ keV) nicht möglich. Von den Positronenstrahlern haben ^{18}F-Fluoromethan, ^{11}C-Butanol, ^{11}C-Iodoantipyrin, ^{11}C-Methyl-Glukose, ^{11}C-Methan und ^{11}C-Azetylen eine gewisse Bedeutung erlangt (Büll et al. 1984b Celesia et al. 1983, 1984; Ginsberg et al. 1981; Heiss et al. 1981; Holden et al. 1981a, b; Koeppe et al. 1985; Madsen et al. 1981).

Der klassische Positronenstrahler, der zur Bestimmung des regionalen zerebralen Blutflusses (CBF) verwendet wird, ist das ^{15}O in Form des frei diffusiblen Wassers. Seit der ersten Anwendung von ^{15}O in der Medizin (Ter-Pogossian et al. 1958) wurden systematische Studien in den Zentren an der Washington University in St. Louis, USA (Ter-Pogossian et al. 1969; Ter-Pogossian 1981) und im Hammersmith Hospital, London (Frackowiak et al. 1980a, b, 1985) durchgeführt (Abb. 19, Tabelle 4). Das Meßprinzip besteht entweder in einer Gleichgewichtsstudie mit Tracerinhalation kontinuierlich applizierten C^{15}O$_2$ (Ficksches Prinzip, Erhaltung der Masse, Verwendung diffusibler Tracer) (Kety u. Schmidt 1948; Alpert et al. 1977; Parker et al. 1978; Orr 1979; Frackowiak et al. 1980a, b; Jones

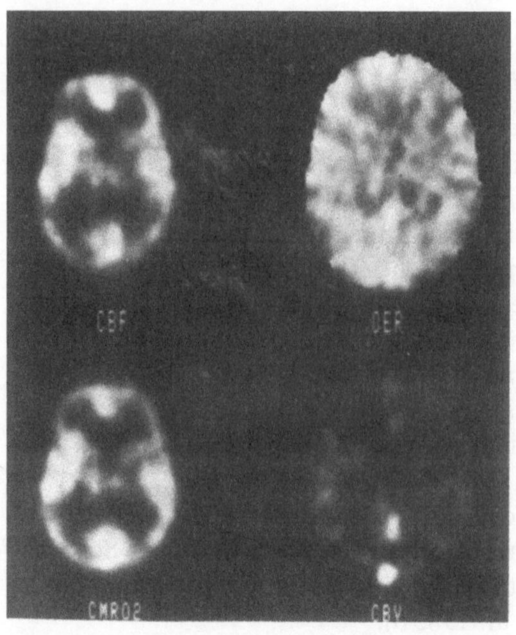

Abb. 19. Zerebraler Blutfluß (*CBF*), Sauerstoff-Extraktion (*OER*), Sauerstoff-Verbrauch (*CMRO₂*) und Blutvolumen (*CBV*) in einer Schnittebene einer normalen Kontrollperson (Grauskala den Meßwerten entsprechend; weiß: hohe Werte). Die Studie wurde mit der O₂-Gleichgewichtsmethode bei Inhalation durchgeführt (MRC Cyclotron Unit, Hammersmith Hospital, London). (Aus Mazziotta u. Phelps 1986)

Tabelle 4. Zerebraler Blutfluß, Sauerstoffmetabolismus und Sauerstoffextraktionsfraktion. Alle Werte wurden mit dem ECAT-II-Tomographen bestimmt. Die Größe der Regions of Interest (ROI) variiert erheblich. Angegeben sind Mittelwerte und Standardabweichungen, die Daten enthalten keine Korrektur für das Blutvolumen. (Nach Mazziotta u. Phelps 1986)

	n	14	7	14	27	13	7
	Alter (J)	26–74	Mittel 43	49–74	*	32–54	Mittel 27
	Methode	$^{15}O-CI$	$^{15}O-CI$	$^{15}O-CI$	$^{15}O-CI$	$^{18}F-CH_3$	$H_2{}^{15}O$
	Zitat	a: 1980	b: 1981	c: 1982	d: 1981	e: 1983	f: 1983
Kortex: Insular, Temporal	LCBF	65 ± 7	61 ± 10	–	65 ± 17	55 ± 8	39 ± 7
	LOER	49 ± 2			47 ± 9		
	LCMRO$_2$	263 ± 26	109 ± 33	–	256 ± 50		
Kortex: Frontal	LCBF			45	52 ± 6		
	LOER			50			
	LCMRO$_2$			185			
Kortex: Visuell	LCBF	63 ± 17		46	60 ± 8		
	LOER			52			
	LCMRO$_2$	242 ± 60		204			
Thalamus	LOER				55 ± 10		
	LCMRO$_2$	149 ± 26					
Weiße Substanz Zentrum	LCBF	21 ± 2	20 ± 7		21 ± 3	26 ± 5	19 ± 3
	LOER	48 ± 4			47 ± 9		
	LCMRO$_2$	80 ± 10	71 ± 14		82 ± 15		
Global Zentrum	LCBF	48**		39 ± 6	43 ± 4		31 ± 5
	LOER	49**		0.56 ± 0.06			
	LCMRO$_2$	188**	167 ± 27				

Abkürzungen: LCBF: Zerebraler Blutfluß (ml/min/100 g); LCMRO$_2$: Sauerstoff-Metabolismus (µmol/min/100 g); LOER: Sauerstoff-Extraktionsrate (%). CI: Kontinuierliche Inhalation von $C^{15}O_2$ und $^{15}O_2$, ansonsten bolusförmige Injektion. Variationen der Normalwerte können teilweise auf die Anhängigkeiten vom p_{aCO_2} zurückgeführt werden.
*: n=16: <50 Jahre, n=11: >50 Jahre.
**: Angenommenes Verhältnis zwischen Grauer und Weißer Substanz: 60:40
a: Frackowiak et al. (1980b), b: Baron et al. (1981a), c: Lenzi et al. (1982), d: Lenzi et al. (1981a), e: Celesia et al. (1983), f: Huang et al. (1983).

et al. 1976b; Lenzi et al. 1981a, b; Leenders et al. 1984a; Meyer u. Yamamoto 1984) oder in einer Bestimmung des regionalen zerebralen Blutflusses (LCBF) nach einer Bolusinjektion (Huang et al. 1981b). Biochemische Grundlage ist die Umwandlung des CO_2 durch die in der Lunge vorhandene Carboanhydrase zu H_2O (West u. Dollery 1960). Die Randbedingungen und meßtechnischen Limitationen, wie Rezirkulationseffekte und Reproduzierbarkeit, werden in Abschnitt B.III im Einzelnen beschrieben.

Die Extraktion des Kationes $^{13}NH_3/^{13}NH_4^+$ ist wegen der Abhängigkeit von Blutfluß und Permeabilitätsoberflächenprodukt nicht zu einer quantitativen Beurteilung des zerebralen Blutflusses geeignet, so werden bei Normalpersonen etwa 40% des Tracers im „first pass" extrahiert (Lockwood et al. 1984; Phelps et al. 1977, 1981a).

Mit der Einführung der Gamma-Strahler N-Isopropyl-^{123}I-p-Iodoamphetamin (IMP) und ^{99m}Tc-Hexamethylpropylen-Aminoxim (HM-PAO) liegen für die klinische Routine Radiopharmaka vor, die bei entsprechender Fragestellung, d.h. Problemen aus dem zerebrovaskulären Formenkreis, ein Maß für die Perfusion geben. Wegen grundsätzlicher, der SPECT inhärenter Randbedingungen ist allerdings eine absolute Quantifizierung nur bei exakter Kenntnis der regionalen Absorptionskoeffizienten möglich (Budinger 1980, 1985; Chaplin et al. 1985; Creutzig et al. 1986; Hill et al. 1982; Jordan 1987; Kuhl et al. 1982a; Kuhl 1984; Sharp et al. 1986).

c) Blutvolumen

Die Messung des zerebralen Blutvolumens (CBV) beruht auf der Bildung von Karboxyhämiglobin nach einer Bolusinhalation von ^{11}CO oder einer kontinuierlichen Inhalation von $C^{15}O$, wobei die Tracerkonzentrationen unter 1 ppm liegen und pharmakologische Nebenwirkungen nicht zu erwarten sind (Phelps et al. 1979a, b). Ein Korrekturfaktor (0.85) berücksichtigt, daß der mittlere zerebrale Hämatokrit niedriger ist als der in peripheren Gefäßen (Larsen u. Lassen 1964).

Neben der grundsätzlichen physiologischen Bedeutung ist die absolute Bestimmung des zerebralen Blutvolumens notwendig als Korrekturterm bei der Bestimmung der lokalen Sauerstoff-Extraktionsrate (OER), insbesondere bei niedrigem zerebralem Fluß und großem arteriellen Anteil (Frackowiak u. Lammertsma 1985; Lammertsma et al. 1983b). Die Berücksichtigung des mittleren zerebralen Blutvolumens führt bei Kontrollpersonen (4.3 ± 0.4 ml/100 g) zu einer Korrektur der Sauerstoff-Extraktionsrate (OER) der grauen Substanz um 14%, für die der weißen Substanz um 8% (Frackowiak et al. 1980a), nach anderen Studien um 20–30% (Mazziotta u. Phelps 1986). Bei Hirntumoren ist dieser Korrekturterm von noch größerer Bedeutung (Lammertsma et al. 1983a; Lammertsma u. Jones 1983). Der Anteil des CBV teilt sich bei Normalbefunden auf in: 70% Venen und Venolen, 10% Arterien, 20% Kapillaren (Phelps et al. 1979b). Der mittlere zerebrale Hämatokrit muß nach Lammertsma et al. (1984a) mit 0.69 und nicht mit 0.85 angenommen werden. Die mittleren Normwerte in der Literatur für Kontrollpersonen sind in Tabelle 4 zusammengestellt (Nach Mazziotta u. Phelps 1986).

d) Sauerstoffmetabolismus ($CMRO_2$) und Sauerstoff-Extraktionsrate (OER)

30–40% des arteriell zugeführten zerebralen Sauerstoffes werden vom normalen Hirngewebe extrahiert. Physiologische und pathophysiologisch veränderte metabolische Zustände können dazu führen, daß der Gewebebedarf an Sauerstoff erhöht wird. Diesem kann durch veränderte hämodynamische Bedingungen Rechnung getragen werden (CBF), in Zuständen ohne diese kompensatorische Regulationsmöglichkeit aber auch durch eine erhöhte Extraktionsrate. Eine Erhöhung des pCO_2, des Gewebe-pH oder der Temperatur begleiten das Absinken der Sauerstoffkonzentration im Gewebe. Allgemein ist der regionale Sauerstoffverbrauch $CMRO_2$ abhängig von dem Fluß (CBF), der Extraktionsrate (OER) und der arteriellen Sauerstoffkonzentration $[O_2]_A$:

$$LCMRO_2 = LCBF \times LOER \times [O_2]_A.$$

Die Bestimmung des zerebralen Blutflusses und der Sauerstoffextraktionsrate allein gibt daher nur ungenügende Auskunft über Angebot und Bedarf des Hirngewebes an Sauerstoff. Über einen weiten Bereich besteht zwischen dem zerebralen Blutfluß und dem Sauerstoffmetabolismus eine hohe lineare Korrelation (Abb. 20) (Baron et al. 1983a, 1985a).

Dieser Ansatz wurde von Jones et al. (1976) entwickelt und von Ter-Pogossian u. Powers (1958), Dyson et al. (1959, 1960), Dollery et al. (1960) und Dollery u. West (1960) in grundsätzlichen Vorarbeiten ermöglicht. Die Variabilität der Parameter ist regional unterschiedlich und liegt in der Größenordnung von $\pm 5\%$ bis $\pm 20\%$ (FRACKOWIAK et al. 1980 b; LENZI et al. 1981 a, b).

Für den Kliniker sind diese Parameter besonders interessant, wenn es um Zustände wie Ischämie und Perfusionsreserve geht. Bei Kontrollpersonen wird die Sauerstoff Extraktionsrate mit 0.37 für die graue Substanz und 0.41 für die weiße Substanz angegeben (HUANG et al. 1983; LEBRUN-GRANDIÉ et al. 1983). Bei Normalpersonen besteht zwischen Perfusion und Metabolismus eine enge Korrelation, die sich dem Bedarf anpaßt (Abb. 20) (BARON et al. 1982, 1983 a, 1985 a; RAICHLE et al. 1976).

e) Glukosemetabolismus

Das normale Gehirn entnimmt mehr als 95% der Energie über den Glukosemetabolismus, der somit häufig synonym mit der Bestimmung zerebraler Funktionen gleichgesetzt wird. Andererseits sind Methoden zur Bestimmung des Glukosestoffwechsels relativ unspezifisch im Hinblick auf komplexe Aufgaben, wie funktionelle Aktivierungen, Wachheitszustände,

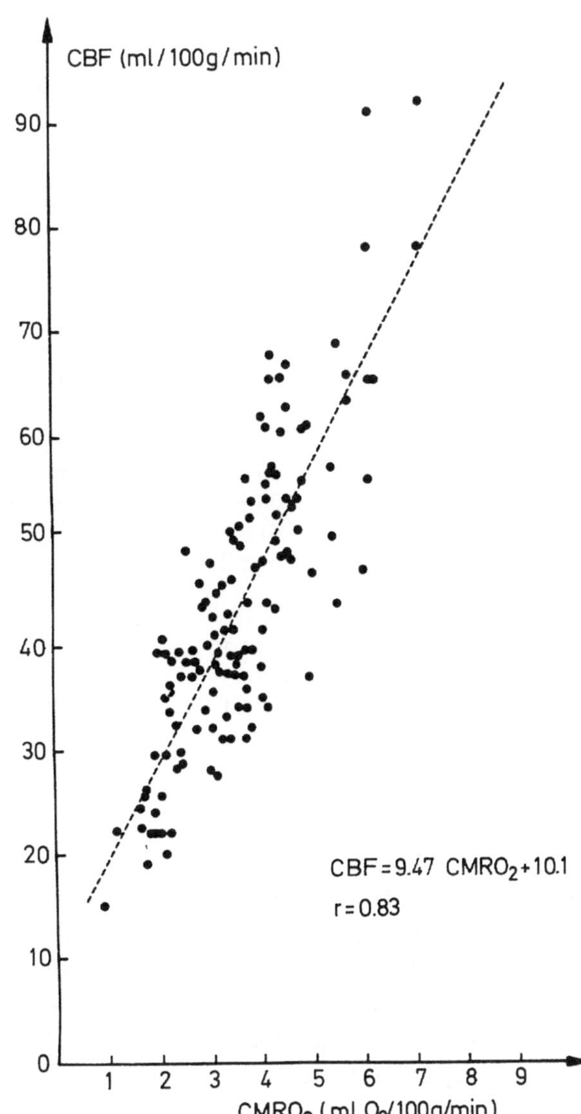

Abb. 20. Weitgehend lineare Abhängigkeit des lokalen zerebralen Blutflusses (*LCBF*) vom Sauerstoff-Verbrauch (*CMRO$_2$*) in 131 Hirnregionen bei 19 Kontrollpersonen über einen physiologisch weiten Bereich. (Aus BARON 1983)

aber auch Krankheitszustände, wie etwa heredo-degenerative Erkrankungen, Epilepsien und Psychosen.

Zwei Ansätze haben sich in der quantitativen Bestimmung des zerebralen Glukosestoffwechsels (CMRGlc) durchgesetzt, nachdem ursprünglich die Kety-Schmidt-Methode mit der Bestimmung des zerebralen Blutflusses und der arterio-venösen Glukose-Differenz verwendet wurde (Kety u. Schmidt 1948; Kety 1960).

Bei dem *Deoxyglukosemodell* werden als Tracer das Glukose-Analogon ^{18}F-2-Fluoro-2-Deoxy-D-Glukose (FDG) oder die 2-Deoxy-D-(1-^{11}C)-Glukose (^{11}C-DG) benutzt (Bessel et al. 1972; Brownell et al. 1980; Alavi et al. 1981a; Ido et al. 1978; Reivich et al. 1979; Sacks et al. 1983). Über die ersten Ergebnisse am Menschen wurde von Reivich et al. (1979) und Phelps et al. (1979b) berichtet (Tabelle 5). Die Modellvorstellung beruht auf folgenden Axiomen:

1. Kompetitive Wechselwirkung des Substrates mit der Glukose, 2. Der „precursor pool" des FDG im zerebralen Gewebe hat eine relativ schnelle Turnover-Rate, 3. das Endprodukt der FDG, (FDG-6-PO$_4$), wird nicht weiter metabolisiert und hat nur eine geringe Dephosphorilisierungsrate (Gallagher et al. 1978; Phelps et al. 1979b), und 4. die Plasmaaktivität kann der FDG zugeordnet werden.

Tabelle 5. Lokale metabolische Raten des Glukosestoffwechsels (LCMRGl) bei gesunden Kontrollpersonen. Mittelwerte (µmol/100 g/min) und Standardabweichung

	Reivich et al. (1979)	Mazziotta et al. (1981)	Schwartz et al. (1983)	Heiss et al. (1984)
Frontaler Kortex	46±1	43±10	32±7	40±6
Parietaler Kortex	38±6	43±10	30±6	36±4
Okzipitaler Kortex		37±9	24±5	32±6
Primär visuell	57±8	47±11	31±6	43±7
Temporaler Kortex	45	44±11	24±6	33±6
Insularer Kortex			33±6	39±7
Gyrus cinguli		43±12	34±7	42±6
Nucleus lentiformis	36±2	44±8	33±4	42±10
Nucleus caudatus	38±3	38±8	30±6	40±8
Thalamus	41±10	36±7	28±7	37±9
Hippocampus	34±2		25±7	28±5
Pons				19±6
Mesenzephalon				23±6
Frontale weiße Substanz	20±10			18±5
Okzipitale weiße Substanz	24±3			17±6
Centrum semiovale	21±1	29±7	15±4	16±3

Diese Ansätze wurden vom Sokoloff-Modell übernommen, das mit der traumatischen ^{14}C-Methode entwickelt wurde (Sokoloff et al. 1977; Sokoloff 1981).

Das *Glukosemodell* wurde von Raichle et al. (1975, 1978) vorgeschlagen, und von Heiss et al. (1981, 1983a), Vyska et al. (1985) und Blomquist et al. (1985) in klinischen Studien angewandt. Den theoretischen Vorteilen des kinetischen Modelles und der kürzeren Halbwertszeit des ^{11}C gegenüber der des ^{18}F bei der FDG-Methode stehen Nachteile in der Meßbarkeit, z.B. der Berücksichtigung der Metabolite und der Rückdiffusion, entgegen.

Normalwerte können sowohl für mehr anatomisch orientierte Verteilungen, aber auch entsprechend physiologischen Funktionen angegeben werden (Abb. 21). In Tabelle 5 sind Glukose-Stoffwechselstudien bei gesunden Versuchspersonen zusammengefaßt. Bei diesen „Normalwerten" müssen insbesondere neben physiologischen Schwankungen aufgrund funktioneller Aktivierungen (abgedunkelter Raum etc.) die meßtechnischen Limitationen mit den regionalen und tracerabhängigen Variabilitäten und Reproduzierbarkeiten, so etwa der „lumped constant" berücksichtigt werden. So wird die „lumped constant" für $[^{18}F]$FDG mit 0.52 ± 0.03 und für $[^{11}C]$DG mit 0.56 ± 0.04 angegeben (METTER et al. 1983a, MAZZIOTTA u. PHELPS 1986). BARON et al. (1982) bestimmten die Extraktionsfraktionen der Glukose bei kombinierter Messung der zerebralen Perfusion zu 17% für die graue Substanz und 24% für die weiße Substanz, bei einem Mittelwert von $19 \pm 3\%$.

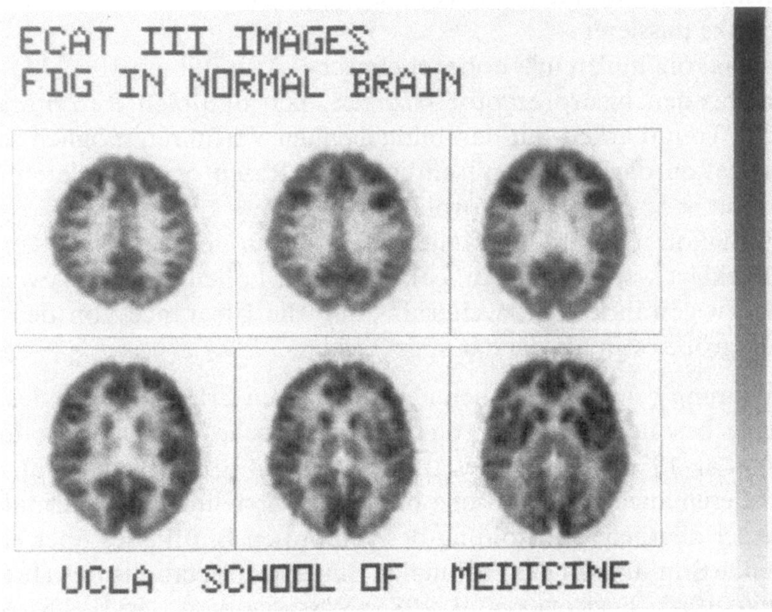

Abb. 21. ^{18}F-FDG-Funktionsbilder, die mit dem ECAT-III-Tomographen gewonnen wurden. 8 transaxiale Schnitte in gleichen 5 mm Abständen parallel zur Kanthomeathal-Linie (*CML*). Das Auflösungsvermögen beträgt in der transversalen Richtung etwa 5 mm, in der axialen Richtung etwa 9 mm. Es läßt sich besonders an der Darstellung der Basalganglien abschätzen. Die Grauwerte geben die metabolischen Raten für Glukose (*CMRGl*) in µmol/100 g/min an. (Aus MAZZIOTTA u. PHELPS 1986)

f) Proteinsynthese

Der Aminosäuremetabolismus ist weniger für verschiedene kurzzeitige funktionale Zustände, sondern für die Synthese der Proteine und Neurotransmitter von Bedeutung. Die Möglichkeiten zur quantitativen Beurteilung der Proteinsynthese (PS) werden mit ihren Randbedingungen bestimmt durch die Stoffwechselwege und die Annahme und Validisierung eines kinetischen Modells. Nach grundsätzlichen autoradiographischen Studien von SMITH et al. (1980), haben insbesondere PHELPS et al. (1982, 1984) und BUSTANY et al. (1981, 1982, 1983a, b) quantitative „Normalwerte", so für ^{11}C-L-Methionin mit 0.18 ± 0.06 nmol/min/g und für ^{11}C-L-Leucin mit 0.61 ± 0.18 nmol/min/g, angegeben. Die grundsätzlichen Kriterien, die diese quantitativen Daten beleuchten, werden in Abschnitt B.VII diskutiert.

g) Neurorezeptoren und Pharmaka

Die Positronen-Emissionstomographie ermöglicht die bildliche Darstellung und die Quantifizierung von Neurotransmittern und ihren Rezeptoren im Gehirn. Charakteristisch für diese Rezeptoren sind (Mintun et al. 1984):

I. Die Rezeptorplätze sind bzgl. der Zahl begrenzt (B_{max}), haben eine hohe Affinität zum Liganden K_D^{-1} und werden schon bei relativ kleinen Liganden-Mengen gesättigt ($B_{max}K_D^{-1}$).
II. Die Bindungen sind sehr spezifisch.
III. Die gebundenen Liganden haben spezifische pharmakologische Eigenschaften.

Voraussetzungen sind folgende Randbedingungen (Young et al. 1986):

1. Das Radiopharmakon muß nach intravenöser Applikation bei hoher Extraktionsrate die Blut-Hirn-Schranke passieren.
2. Das Radiopharmakon muß eine hohe chemische Affinität ($>10^{-9}$ M) und Spezifität zu dem entsprechenden Neurorezeptor besitzen; bei multiplen Rezeptorsystemen sollte eine anatomische Trennbarkeit mit den bildgebenden Verfahren möglich sein.
3. Das Radiopharmakon darf nur unwesentlich vom Rezeptor dissoziieren (Dissoziationskonstante) und nur $<5\%$ der Rezeptorplätze besetzen.
4. Das Radiopharmakon oder seine Metabolite müssen in niedriger Konzentration im Plasma schnell geklärt werden (Clearance), um einen hohen Kontrast zwischen Rezeptor und Umgebung zu gewährleisten; weiterhin muß die Clearance von den unspezifischen Rezeptorplätzen größer sein als die der spezifischen.

Wegen der Bedeutung bei verschiedenen neurologischen Erkrankungen des dopaminergen Stoffwechsels wurde besonders intensiv das präsynaptische ^{18}F-6-Fluorodopa untersucht (Abb. 22) (Firnau et al. 1975; Garnett et al. 1983, 1984a, b; Leenders et al. 1984b). Neben Normalwerten existieren auch systematische bildliche Darstellungen. Pharmakologisch führt das L-DOPA zu einer deutlichen Erhöhung des zerebralen Blutflusses über eine Vasodilatation, ohne begleitende Stimulation des regionalen Sauerstoffmetabolismus (Inoue et al. 1985; Larson u. Di Chiro 1985; Leenders et al. 1985; Wagner et al. 1983). Die postsynaptische Rezeptorverteilung wurde mit ^{11}C-3-N-Methyl-Spiperon und ^{18}F-Spiperon untersucht (Leenders et al. 1984b; Mintun et al. 1984; Wagner et al. 1984; Wong et al. 1984a, b). Weitere Liganden für Dopaminrezeptoren sind: ^{11}C-Pimozid (Baron et al. 1983c, 1985b), ^{18}F-Spiroperidol (Welch et al. 1984), $^{76/77}$Br-Spiroperidol (Larson u. DiChiro 1985; Mazière et al. 1984), ^{11}C-Racloprid (Farde et al. 1985) und ^{11}C-3-Acetylcyclofoxy (Larson u. DiChiro 1985).

Untersucht wurden weitere Liganden, wie ^{18}F-Haloperidol (Tewson et al. 1980; Zanzonico et al. 1983), ^{11}C-Diphenylhydantoin (Baron et al. 1983b), ^{11}C-Chlorpromazin, Imipramin (Soussaline et al. 1979; Syrota et al. 1981b), ^{11}C-Propanolol (Berger et al. 1982), der Serotonin-Antagonist ^{11}C-Ketanserin (Berridge et al. 1983), Butyrophenonderivate (Stöcklin 1985), ^{11}C-Flunitrazepam als Benzodiazepinrezeptor und ^{11}C-RO 15.1788 als Benzodiazepinantagonist (Mazière et al. 1984).

Das durch Naloxan spezifisch inhibierbare Opiat ^{11}C-Carfentanil (Endorphinrezeptor) wurde eingehend von Frost et al. (1985) untersucht (Abb. 23) wie auch das ^{11}C-Diprenorphin (Jones et al. 1985) sowie ^{11}C-Quinuclidinyl-Benzylat-Methiodid und ^{123}I-IQNB für muskarinerge Azetylcholin-Rezeptoren (Drayer et al. 1982; Eckelmann et al. 1984). Diese teilweise auch systemisch (u.a. kardial und pulmonal) wirksamen Antagonisten bzw. Rezeptoren sind intensiv in Einzelbeispielen dokumentiert, klinische Studien, die die pharmakologischen und neurologischen Erwartungen belegen könnten, stehen jedoch noch nicht zur Verfügung.

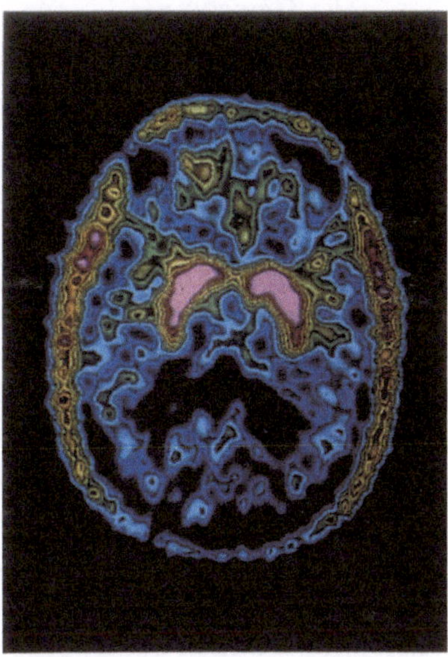

Abb. 22. Selektive Darstellung der präsynaptischen Dopaminverteilung in den Basalganglien nach Applikation (i.v.) von 40 mCi 6-^{18}F-Fluoro-L-Dopa durch Dopamin und seine Metabolite bei einer Kontrollperson. Die postsynaptische Rezeptorwechselwirkung läßt sich mit ^{11}C-Methylspiperon dokumentieren. (Aus GAR-NETT et al. 1983)

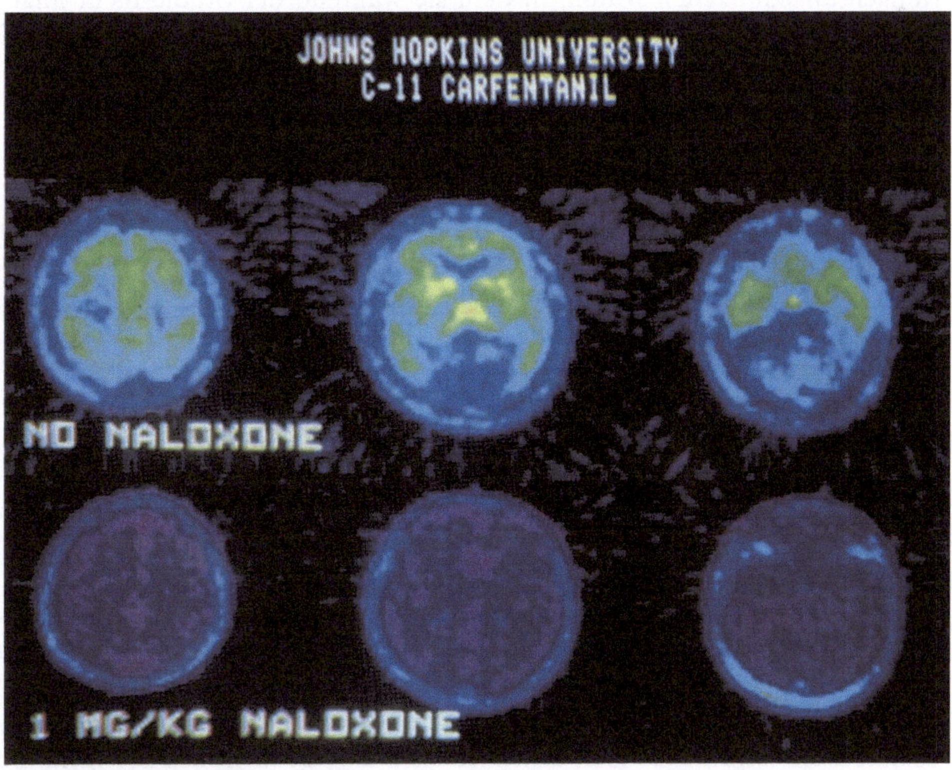

Abb. 23. Darstellung von Opiat-Rezeptoren im menschlichen Gehirn, 30–60 min nach i.v.-Applikation von 25 mCi ^{11}C-Carfentanil (80 ng/kg). Die Transversalschnitte liegen 7.2, 4.0 und 0.8 cm oberhalb der Kantho-meatal-Linie. Die mittlere Reihe zeigt, daß > 90% der spezifischen Rezeptoren in Thalamus und Basalgan-glien durch den Antagonisten (+) Naloxon blockiert werden. (Aus FROST et al. 1984a, b)

h) Gewebe-pH

Der zelluläre Metabolismus, so etwa die Glykolyse (Phosphofruktokinase, Hexokinase), ist vom intrazellulären pH abhängig, für den als Normwert 7.0–7.1 angegeben wird (Syrota et al. 1983a, 1985a, b). Darüberhinaus moduliert der pH die elektrische Leitfähigkeit axonaler Membrane (Berridge et al. 1982; Rottenberg et al. 1983, 1985). Das nicht metabolisierte ^{11}C-DMO (5,5-Dimethyloxazolidin-2,4-Dion) wird als Indikator bei der PET verwendet, mit dem Hintergrund, daß bei verschiedenen Erkrankungen (Ischämie, Tumore, Anfallsleiden) der pH und infolgedessen auch verschiedene metabolische Funktionen verändert sind (Raichle 1983; Siesjö et al. 1981). Wegen meßtechnischer Limitationen des metabolisierten CO_2 ist dieses Pharmakon zur pH-Bestimmung nicht sicher geeignet (Brooks et al. 1984a; Buxten et al. 1984; Raichle et al. 1979).

i) Funktionelle Aktivierungen

Roy u. Sherrington (1890) und Alexander (1912) postulierten bereits vor nahezu 100 Jahren die enge Beziehung zwischen Änderungen funktionaler Aktivität des Gehirnes und denen des Blutflusses und Metabolismus. Vor einer Beurteilung des pathologischen Zustandes gilt es demnach, zunächst die Auswirkungen sensorischer Stimulationen und der Deprivation zu untersuchen. Studien über den Glukosemetabolismus und den Blutfluß zu dieser Problematik wurden vornehmlich in den Zentren in Los Angeles (Mazziotta et al. 1981, 1984, 1985b; Mazziotta u. Phelps 1984, 1986). St. Louis (Reivich et al. 1985) und Köln (Heiss et al. 1985a, b) durchgeführt.

Bei der Basisuntersuchung liegen die Kontrollpersonen nach eingehender Aufklärung in einem ruhigen abgedunkelten Raum, in dem sie während der Studie nicht angesprochen werden. Die Ohren sind lautdicht verschlossen, die Augen sind geschlossen und 15–30 Minuten nach Legen der Zugänge wird der Tracer appliziert. In der Regel wird bei diesem Zustand eine Seitendifferenz des Metabolismus (links > rechts) beobachtet (Mazziotta u. Phelps 1986).

Die Ergebnisse lassen sich wie folgt strukturieren und zusammenfassen:

1. Stärke und Symmetrie (anterior-posterior, links-rechts) des Glukosemetabolismus in Abhängigkeit von den *Basis-Testbedingungen* (Mazziotta et al. 1982a, b).
2. Quantitative Korrelation des regionalen zerebralen Glukosemetabolismus mit verschieden komplexen Stadien *visueller Aktivierung* (Abb. 26) (Greenberg et al. 1981; Mazziotta et al. 1983a, b; Phelps et al. 1981b; Reivich et al. 1981) wie auch Sakkaden (Fox et al. 1985b).
3. Hemisphären-Lateralisation mit Einfluß auf den Stimulus-Inhalt. *Visuelles System* (Mazziotta et al. 1983a), *auditives System* (Abb. 25) (Mazziotta et al. 1982b).
4. Effekt der Lateralisation nach verschiedenen, rationalen teilweise komplexen Aufgaben. *Auditives und visuelles System* (Abb. 24) (Phelps et al. 1981b, 1982; Mazziotta et al. 1982a, b).
5. Subkortikale Antwort (Nucleus caudatus, Thalamus) auf sensorische Stimuli. *Auditives System* (Mazziotta et al. Neurology, in press), sensorische Stimuli (Zerebellum) (Fox et al. 1985c)
6. Korrelation zwischen der *Physiologie,* der *Klinik* und der PET mit den durch sie dokumentierten *somatosensorischen und motorischen Bahnen*, u.a. Gedächtnisleistungen, motorische Leistungen (Greenberg et al. 1981; Phelps et al. 1981a, b; Reivich et al. 1979, 1981, 1983; Reivich u. Gur 1985; Buchsbaum et al. 1983).
7. Korrelation zu *kognitiven und emotionalen* Effekten (Gur et al. 1983; Mazziotta et al. 1985b; Mazziotta u. Phelps 1986; Reivich et al. 1983).

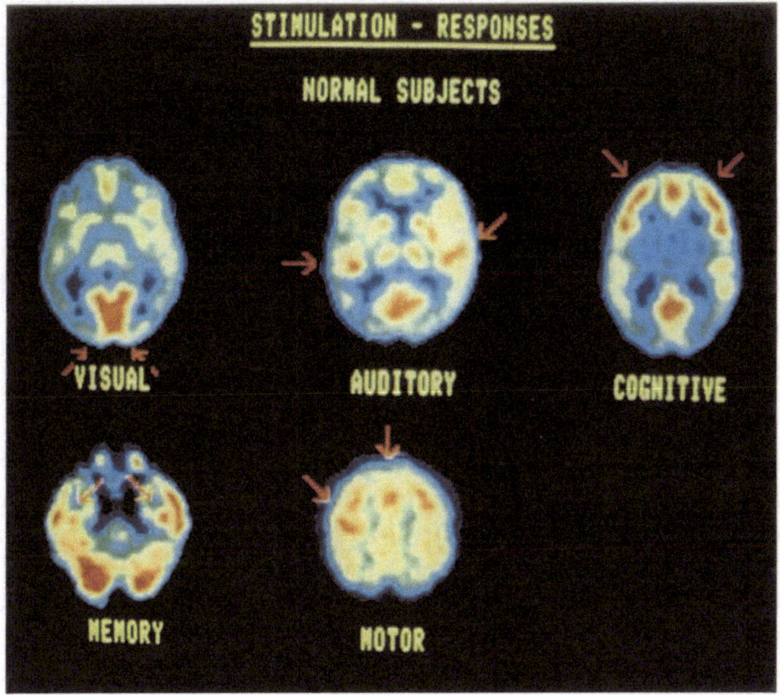

Abb. 24. Topographische und quantitative Darstellung der Hirnregionen während differenzierter sensorischer, sensomotorischer, motorischer und kognitiver Reizungen und Aufgaben. (UCLA, School of Medicine, USA)

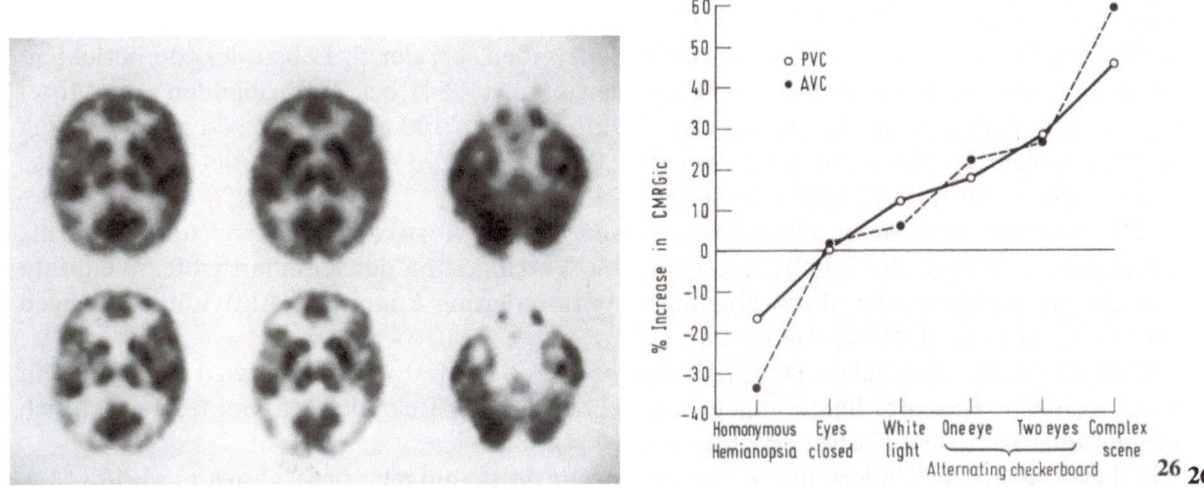

Abb. 25. Während des Hörens einer Erzählung werden bei einer Versuchsperson (*untere Rẹihe*) gegenüber einer Kontrollperson ohne auditive Reizung (*obere Reihe*) der auditive Kortex in der hinteren Henleschen Querwindung des Temporallappens und nach Aufforderung des Erinnerns der Hippokampus aktiviert. (Aus MAZZIOTTA et al. 1983)

Abb. 26. Relative Änderung des Glukosestoffwechsels im visuellen Kortex in Anhängigkeit von der Reizung. *PVC:* primärer visueller Kortex, *AVC:* visueller Assoziationskortex. (Aus PHELPS et al. 1981 b)

Ohne Hinweise auf ein lokalisierbares Schlafzentrum beobachten Heiss et al. (1985a) bei schlafenden Versuchspersonen einen global verminderten Glukosemetabolismus im Bereich der Großhirnrinde und der basalen Strukturen gegenüber dem Wachzustand. In Traumzuständen weisen in erster Linie der visuelle Kortex und Anteile des Temporal- und Frontallappens einen erhöhten Glukosemetabolismus auf.

Entsprechende Untersuchungen wurden auch für die Bestimmung des zerebralen Blutflusses (CBF) durchgeführt, wobei teilweise die bekannte Kopplung des CBF an neuronale Funktionen und den Metabolismus beobachtet wird. (Fox et al. 1984; Fox u. Raichle 1985; Kearfott et al. 1983b; Lauter et al. 1983; Lebrun-Grandié et al. 1983; Raichle et al. 1976; Roland et al. 1981, 1982).

k) Altersabhängigkeit

Während mit der Transmissions-Computertomographie deutlich unterschiedliche morphologische Strukturen im Sinne von Dilatationen und Atrophien der Ventriculi und Sulci mit zunehmendem Alter bei gesunden Kontrollpersonen beobachtet werden, ist der globale und regionale *Glukosemetabolismus* weitgehend unabhängig vom Alter, wie De Leon et al. (1984) an etwa 40 Personen zeigen konnten (Highes u. Grado 1981; Zatz et al. 1982). Metter et al. (1984) berichten von diskreten regionalen Umverteilungen. Statistisch nicht signifikant, aber konstant wird über einen „hypofrontalen" Zustand berichtet, im Mittel: $\Delta = -26\%$ (Kuhl et al. 1982c), der aber von anderen Beobachtern nicht gefunden wird (De Leon u. George 1983; De Leon et al. 1983a, b; Duara et al. 1983, 1984; Ferris et al. 1983; Hawkins et al. 1983a; Rapoport et al. 1983).

Für den *Sauerstoffmetabolismus* geben Davis et al. (1983) bei vier älteren Personen niedrigere Werte als bei Jüngeren an, während bei 8 Kontrollpersonen keine Unterschiede gefunden werden. Zu ähnlichen Ergebnissen kommen in einer systematischen Studie an 32 Kontrollpersonen Lammertsma et al. (1981) und Frackowiak et al. (1985), die von einem Einschnitt im Stoffwechsel der grauen Substanz, nicht der weißen, bei der 5. Lebensdekade berichten, sowie Pantano et al. (1984) bei 27 Probanden et al. (1984) bei 27 Probanden (im Mittel $\Delta = -17\%$). Während die $CMRO_2$ (ab 180 µmol O_2/min/100 g) und der *zerebrale Blutfluß* im Alter erniedrigt sind, werden die *Sauerstoffextraktionsrate (OER)* und der arteriovenöse Sauerstoffgradient normal oder erhöht beobachtet.

Die Autoren diskutieren einen progressiven Verlust kortikaler Neurone und/oder eine verminderte Aktivität der erhaltenen sowie eine Verringerung der Kapillardichte. Weiterhin muß die Möglichkeit eine altersabhängigen Verminderung kognitiver Aktivitäten erwogen werden (Cutler et al. 1984; Riege et al. 1985).

Für den postsynaptischen *Dopaminrezeptor* ^{11}C-3-N-Methylspiperon wird eine mit dem Alter geringere Rezeptordichte angegeben, wobei dieser Effekt bei Männern offensichtlich ausgeprägter ist als bei Frauen (Wong et al. 1984a, b).

Über Studien an Kindern liegen nur vereinzelte Mitteilungen vor (Cremer et al. 1982).

2. Zerebro-vaskuläre Erkrankungen

Fragestellung. Vaskuläre Erkrankungen des Nervensystems stellen die häufigsten Probleme innerhalb der neurologischen Erkrankungen dar. Der traditionelle diagnostische Weg führt über Computertomographie, Kernspintomographie und Angiographie, ist also morphologisch orientiert, während ein pathophysiologisches Verstehen Daten quantifizierbarer, regionaler und metabolischer Funktionen erfordert.

Nicht ein einzelnes Ereignis, sondern eine Reihe pathophysiologischer Vorgänge in Folge einer Ischämie sind verantwortlich für die Frage, ob die Funktionsstörung reversibel bleibt, oder ob irreversible morphologische Zerstörungen folgen, wobei Dauer, Lage, Ausdehnung und Schweregrad der Durchblutungsstörung von entscheidender Bedeutung sind (MAZZIOTTA u. PHELPS 1986).

Unabhängig von dem pathophysiologischen Verständnis, der Prognose und der konservativen Therapie haben diese Untersuchungen nach den Schlußfolgerungen einer EC/IC Bypass Study keine Bedeutung für das chirurgische Vorgehen. Die extra-intrakranielle Anastomose ist danach nicht effektiv in der Prävention zerebraler Ischämien bei Patienten mit arteriosklerotischen Veränderungen, die die Versorgungsgebiete der Aa. carotis et cerebri media betreffen. In einer internationalen randomisierten Studie wurden 1377 Patienten über einen mittleren Zeitraum von 56 Monaten beobachtet. Operativ versorgte Patienten mit schweren Stenosen der A. cerebri media und solche mit persistierenden ischämischen Symptomen hatten sogar eine signifikant schlechtere Prognose als eine Kontrollgruppe (EC/IC Bypass Study Group 1985).

Kritisch ist dieser wichtigen Studie gegenüber anzumerken, daß keine metabolischen Parameter bei der Beurteilung und Diskriminierung herangezogen wurden. So zeigen Ergebnisse einer Untersuchung der Perfusion und des Sauerstoffwechsels an 12 Patienten mit Insult, daß eine nach diesen funktionellen Kriterien gestellte Indikation zur oder Ablehnung der Bypass-Operation noch nicht abschließend beurteilt werden sollte (SAMSON et al. 1985). Vielmehr wird die Notwendigkeit der Bestimmung regionaler, quantitativer und metabolischer Größen deutlich, die nur mit Hilfe der Positronen-Emissionstomographie möglich erscheint (MEHDORN et al. 1985; HEISS 1986). Dabei müssen jedoch wegen der instabilen pathophysiologischen Situation, die bei akutem Insult besteht, insbesondere Randbegrenzungen von Seiten der physiologischen Modelle und der Meßtechnik berücksichtigt werden (MIES et al. 1983).

a) Pathophysiologie

Eine unzureichende Blut- und Sauerstoffzufuhr impliziert Veränderungen des Metabolismus, beim Hirn in erster Linie der Glykolyse und der weiteren primären (ATP, PCr) und sekundären Energiereserven. Erst dieses führt zu elektrophysiologischen Änderungen der Nervenzelle nach homöostatischen Störungen (Kalium, Natrium, Kalzium) an der Zellmembran. Daraufhin werden weitere pathogene Mechanismen induziert, wie die Freisetzung und Produktion von Fettsäuren, Leukotrienen, Prostaglandinen und Endoperoxidasen. Mit der Laktat-Produktion und der pH-Veränderung ist schließlich auch eine Störung der Blut-Hirn-Schranke verbunden (HEISS 1985).

b) Blutfluß, Blutvolumen und Sauerstoffmetabolismus

Im folgenden soll versucht werden, den zeitlichen Ablauf einer verschiedengradigen Perfusionsstörung mit den entsprechenden metabolischen Veränderungen aufzuzeigen (Tabelle 6). Das Primärereignis ist ein Abfall des zerebralen Perfusionsdruckes (CPP), der zunächst im Sinne einer Autoregulation kompensatorisch durch eine Vasodilation der präkapillaren Gefäße ausgeglichen wird (LCBV erhöht), wobei der Sauerstoffmetabolismus ($LCMRO_2$, LOER) normal bleibt (Abb. 27) (POWERS u. RAICHLE 1985). Neurologische Symptome treten dann relativ diskret, teilweise in Form von transitorischen ischämischen Attacken (TIA) auf. Reichen die hämodynamischen Reserven, etwa infolge zu geringer Gefäßreagibilität im Anfangsstadium eines Infarktes, nicht aus, oder sind die Grenzen der Autoregulation erreicht, so wird ein fast normaler Sauerstoffverbrauch ($LCMRO_2$) trotz verminderten zerebralen Blutflusses (CBF) in einem Übergangsstadium durch eine gesteigerte Extraktion (LOER) bei vermehrtem Blutvolumen (LCBV) gewährleistet (WISE et al. 1983a, b). Diese Anpassung an den Bedarf etwa innerhalb von 3 Tagen nach dem Primärereignis wird mit

Tabelle 6. Mögliche pathophysiologische Abfolge metabolischer Parameter im menschlichen Gehirn bei Erniedrigung des zerebralen Perfusionsdruckes, von geringer Hypoperfusion bis zum Infarkt. (Nach Frackowiak u. Wise 1983; Mazziotta u. Phelps 1986)

	LCMRO$_2$	LCBV/LCBF	LOER	LCBF
Erniedrigte hämodyn. Reserve	Normal	Gesteigert	Normal	Normal
Erniedrigter Sauerstoff Extraktionsreserve	Normal	Gesteigert	Gesteigert	Erniedrigt
Ischämie	Erniedrigt	Gesteigert	Gesteigert	Erniedrigt
Früher Infarkt	Erniedrigt	Variabel	Erniedrigt	Variabel
Später Infarkt	Erniedrigt	Variabel	Normal	Erniedrigt

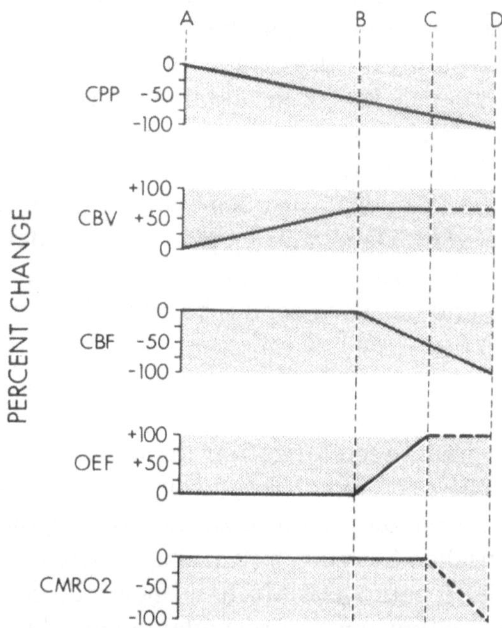

Abb. 27. Kompensatorische Regulationen nach regionaler zerebraler Minderperfusion. Auf eine Abnahme des zerebralen Perfusionsdruckes (*CPP*) erfolgt im Sinne einer Autoregulation eine Dilatation der präkapillären Widerstandsgefäße. Der zerebrale Blutfluß (*CBF*) und der Sauerstoff-Metabolismus (*CMRO$_2$*) bleiben so noch erhalten. Nach maximaler kompensatorischer Dilatation führt ein weiterer Abfall des regionalen Perfusionsdruckes zu einer Erniedrigung des Blutflusses. Zur Aufrechterhaltung des Sauerstoffmetabolismus erhöht sich die Sauerstoff-Extraktionsrate (*OEF*). Erst wenn dieser kompensatorische Mechanismus nicht mehr ausreicht, beginnt das klinische Bild des Infarktes. (Nach Powers u. Raichle 1985)

dem Begriff „misery" oder „critical perfusion" beschrieben (Abb. 28, Tabelle 6) (Baron et al. 1981 b, c; Frackowiak et al. 1984; Gibbs et al. 1983 a, b, 1984; Powers et al. 1983, 1984, 1985 a, b; Powers u. Raichle 1985).

Frühe Stadien eines Infarktes zeichnen sich durch einen erniedrigten Sauerstoff-Metabolismus aus, während Blutvolumen (BV) und Sauerstoff-Extraktionsrate (CMRO$_2$) in dieser Übergangsphase nicht einheitlich verändert sind (Lenzi et al. 1981 a, b; 1982). Bei einer weitergehenden Ischämie (LCBF erniedrigt) sind die funktionellen Reserven erschöpft, der Sauerstoffbedarf (LCMRO$_2$) wird trotz teilweise erhöhter Extraktionsrate (LOER; LCBF/LCBV >5.5; Norm: LCBF/LCBV$=10$) nicht mehr ausreichend gedeckt. Dieses geschieht in deutlicher Abhängigkeit von der Dauer und dem Schweregrad der Minderperfusion und

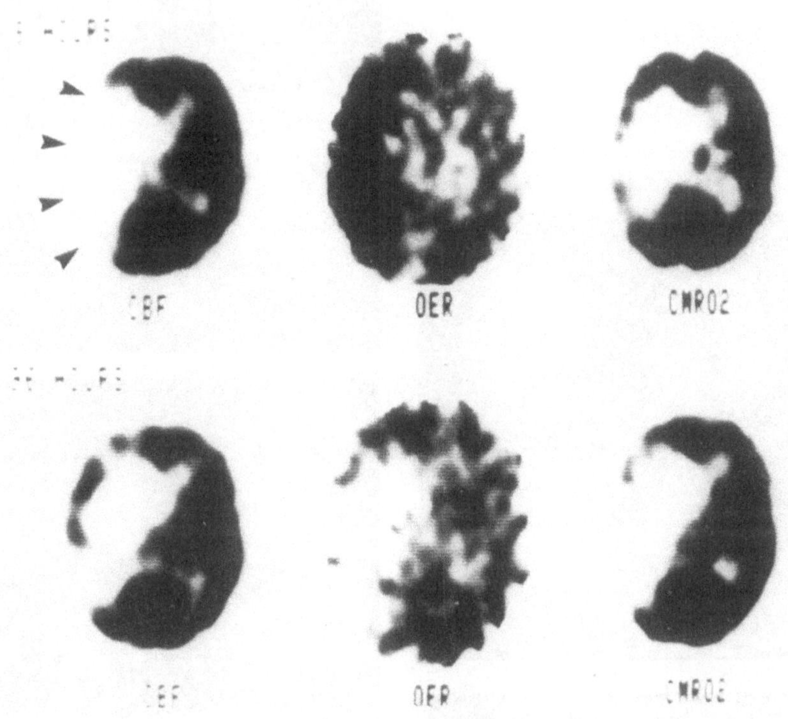

Abb. 28. Kritische Perfusion (*oben*) und „Luxus-Perfusion" (*unten*). Das klinische Beispiel zeigt den Übergang von erhöhter Sauerstoff-Extraktion (*LOER*) zu einer erniedrigten LOER mit erniedrigtem Sauerstoff-Metabolismus (*LCMRO₂*) (8 Stunden und 96 Stunden nach Beginn der neurologischen Symptomatik aufgrund einer Ischämie, ohne Änderung des klinischen Zustandes). (Aus Frackowiak u. Wise 1983)

ist mit neurologischen und klinischen Symptomen verbunden (Frackowiak u. Wise 1983; Wise et al. 1983).

Besonders eine gelegentlich erhöhte zerebrale Perfusion zu diesem Zeitpunkt oder später bei bereits eingetretenem Zelltod, der Lassen (1966) das Attribut „*Luxus-Perfusion*" gegeben hat, wird auf eine gestörte vaskuläre Autoregulation, kapilläre Hyperplasie oder auch eine Postinfarkt-Hyperperfusion zurückgeführt. Diese relative Luxusperfusion kann mit hohen, niedrigen oder normalen Werten des CBF korreliert sein. Der Zelluntergang ist mit einer zerebralen Minderperfusion gekoppelt, wobei die Schwelle in der Größenordnung von 20 ml/min/100 g liegt (Ackerman et al. 1983a, b; Wise et al. 1983).

Im weiteren Verlauf, etwa 24 Stunden nach dem Primärereignis, sinkt der Sauerstoffmetabolismus weiter ab, während die Extraktionsrate schließlich fast „normale" oder nur leicht erniedrigte Werte erreicht. Die Perfusion ist gelegentlich höher als es der Stoffwechsel erfordert. Das Gewebe ist irreversibel zerstört, eine Nekrose ist eingetreten, die mit morphologischen Verfahren, wie der CT, nachgewiesen werden kann, soweit nicht das Stadium des „Fogging" vorliegt.

Es hat sich gezeigt, daß der zerebrale Blutfluß allein kein geeignetes Maß für die Prognose eines Hirnareals und des Patienten bei zerebraler Ischämie bietet, dagegen sind Parameter des Sauerstoffmetabolismus (CMRO₂, OER) verläßlichere Prädiktoren des pathologischen und klinischen Befundes (Abb. 29). Sind beide Werte unter einer kritischen Schwelle (LCMRO₂ <58 μmol O₂/min/100 g oder <40% im Vergleich zur kontralateralen Seite, LOER), so ist dieses synonym mit dem Zelltod (Ackerman et al. 1981b, c; Baron et al.

F10494.IMF
MAX PLANCK INSTITUT KOELN
FLOW   (ML/100G/MIN)
12
18
25
32
38
45
52
59
65
72
79

MTHO1.IMM
MAX PLANCK INSTITUT KOELN
METABOLISM (UMOL GLU/100G/MIN)
7
10
13
16
19
22
25
28
31
34
37

F12514.IMF
MAX PLANCK INSTITUT KOELN
FLOW   (ML/100G/MIN)
12
18
25
32
38
45
52
59
65
72
79

MTHO6 IMM
MAX PLANCK INSTITUT KOELN
METABOLISM (UMOL GLU/100G/MIN)
7
10
13
16
19
22
25
28
31
34
37

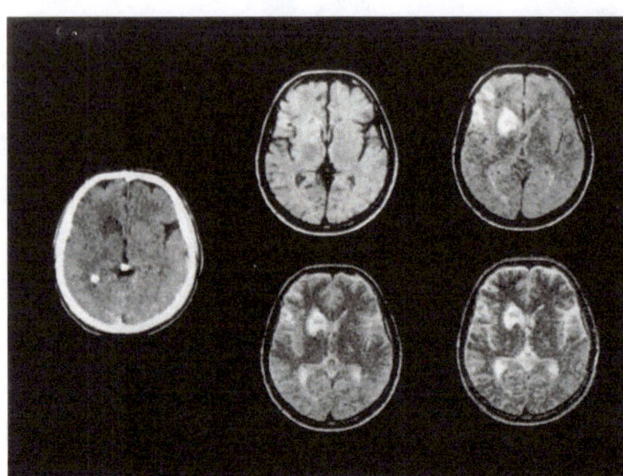

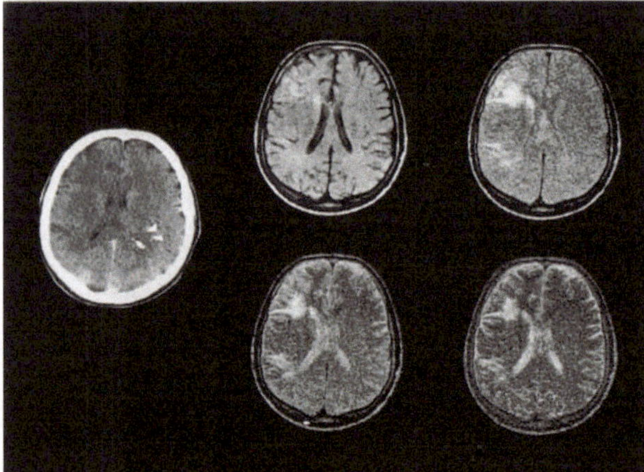

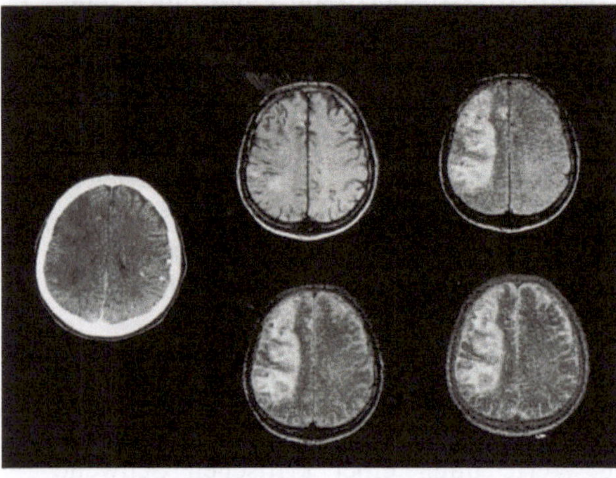

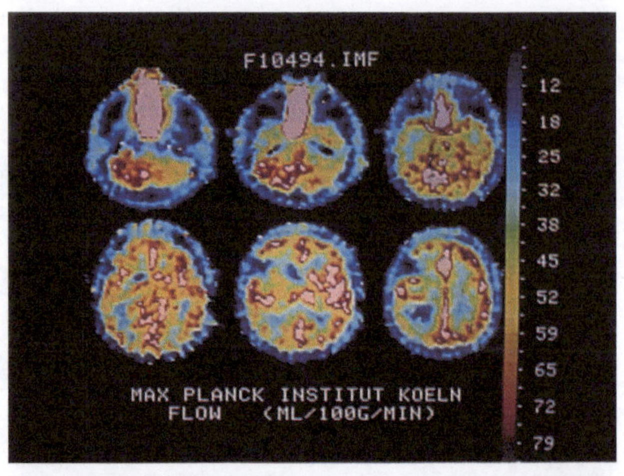

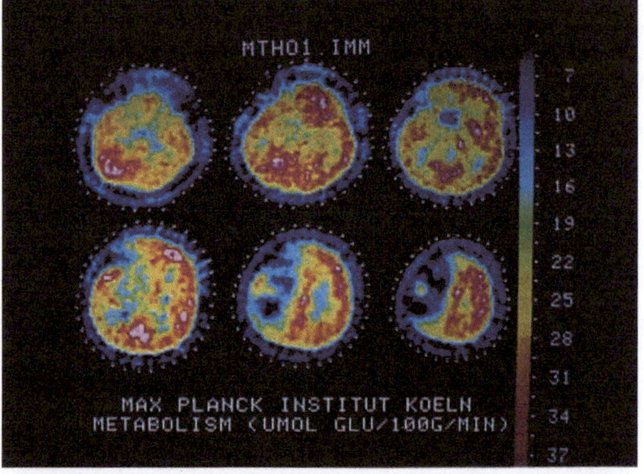

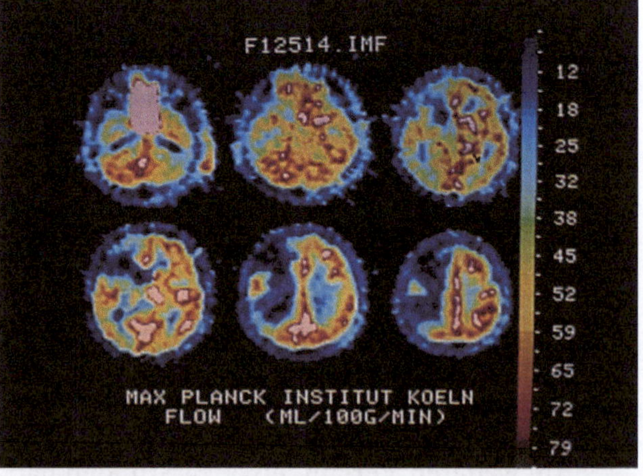

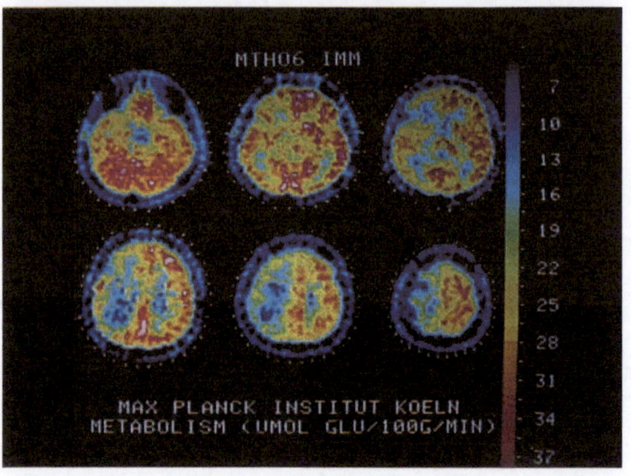

Abb. 29 a–g

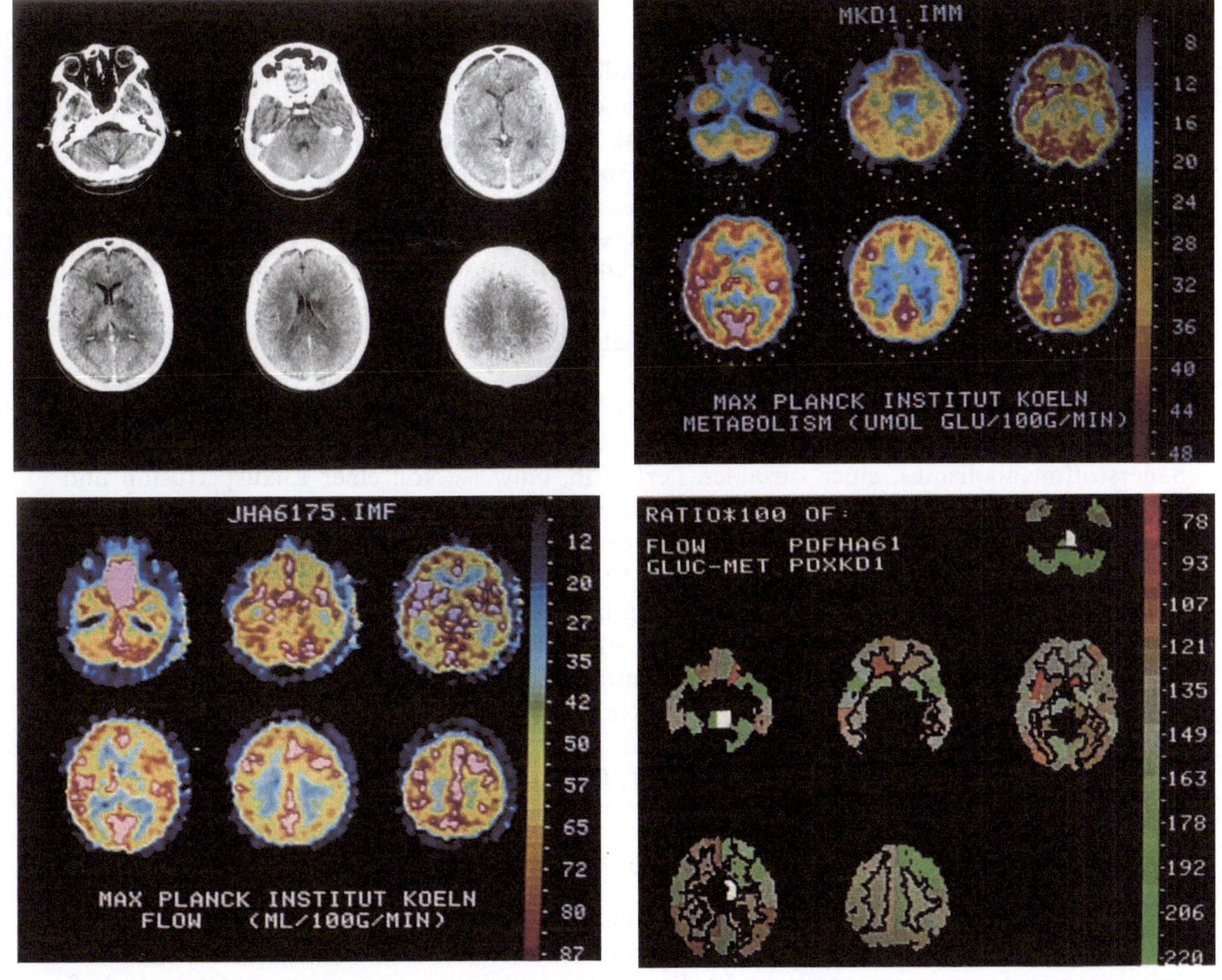

Abb. 30. CT-(a), ^{18}F−CH$_3$- und ^{18}FDG-PET-Bilder einer 49jährigen Patientin mit Infarkt in der Capsula interna links. **b** Verminderte Durchblutung im Infarkt, in benachbarten Basalganglien und durch Inaktivierung im kontralateralen Kleinhirn; im darüberliegenden Frontallappen Hyperperfusion durch kompensatorische Steigerung der Kollateraldurchblutung. **c** Verminderung der Stoffwechselraten im Infarkt, in Basalganglien und Thalamus, in weiten Teilen der homolateralen Hirnrinde – auch im hyperperfundierten Frontallappen – und im kontralateralen Kleinhirn. **d** Bild der Relation von Durchblutung zu Stoffwechsel in einzelnen Regionen: Entkoppelung mit maximaler Durchblutungsminderung im Infarkt und relativer Hyperperfusion im linken Frontallappen und im Kleinhirn. (Aus HEISS et al. 1985b)

Abb. 29a–g. Unterschiedliche Darstellung eines Infarktes im Gebiet der A. cerebri media rechts bei einem 56jährigen Patienten in CT, MRI, ^{18}F−CH$_3$ und ^{18}FDG-PET. **a–c** CT und MRI 45, 55 und 65 mm über CML: Im CT stellt sich das infarzierte Areal dar; in MRI-Multi-Echo-Technik mit einer Repetitionszeit von 650 ms und Echozeiten von 50, 100, 150 und 200 ms stellten sich in den T$_1$-gewichteten Bildern (kurze Echozeiten) anatomische Details mit hohem Auflösungsvermögen, in den T$_2$-gewichteten Bildern pathologische Veränderungen mit maximalem Kontrast dar: zusätzlich zum infarzierten Gewebe bildet sich das perifokale Ödem in den T$_2$-gewichteten Aufnahmen ab. **d** ^{18}F−CH$_3$-Bilder 3 Tage nach Insult zeigen Ausdehnung der primären Durchblutungsstörung und inaktivierungsbedingte Perfusionsminderung im kontralateralen Kleinhirn. **e** In den FDG-Bildern nach Insult reicht die Stoffwechselstörung weit über das Gebiet der verminderten Durchblutung hinaus; die Verteilung ist ähnlich den T$_2$-gewichteten MR-Bildern, zusätzlich zeigen aber Basalganglien, Thalamus und kontralaterales Kleinhirn durch Inaktivierung verminderte Stoffwechselraten. **f** ^{18}F−CH$_3$-Bilder 17 Tage nach Insult zeigen Reperfusion in einigen Infarktbereichen. **g** In den ^{18}FDG-Bildern zeichnet sich die Ausdehnung des Defektes ab. (Aus HEISS et al. 1985b)

1979, 1981a–c; 1985a; FRACKOWIAK u. WISE 1983; LENZI et al. 1978a, b, 1979; SHISHIDO et al. 1984; WISE et al. 1983).

Metabolische Beurteilungen revaskulierender chirurgischer Maßnahmen anhand klinischer Kriterien bestätigen diese Ergebnisse und führen zu entsprechenden therapeutischen (EC-IC-bypass)-Indikationen (ACKERMAN et al. 1983; BARON et al. 1981c; FRACKOWIAK u. WISE 1983; GRUBB et al. 1979; WISE et al. 1983b; YAMAMOTO et al. 1977).

Dieser zeitliche Verlauf der fokalen zerebrovaskulären Erkrankung hat noch Variationen bzgl. kortikaler und subkortikaler Areale, z.B. was die tieferen Bereiche der Basal-Ganglien betrifft. So beträgt im Basalganglienbereich die OER etwa 0.45, verglichen mit 0.67 im kortikalen Bereich. Die Autoren interpretieren diese lokalen Unterschiede mit den verschiedenen Versorgungstypen, entsprechend der Möglichkeit kollateraler Versorgung (WISE et al. 1983a, b).

Die ersten wissenschaftlichen und klinischen PET-Studien wurden in der Regel erst mehr als 3 Tage nach dem Insult durchgeführt und haben dementsprechend von einem geringeren Sauerstoffmetabolismus, einer variablen Perfusion, teilweise von einer Luxusperfusion und einer erniedrigten Sauerstoffextraktionsrate berichtet. Die Korrelation zur morphologisch orientierten CT war dem Zeitpunkt entsprechend meistens relativ gut (ACKERMAN et al. 1981a, 1984; BARON et al. 1978, 1979, 1981a, b; LENZI et al. 1978a, b, 1981a, b; 1982).

Zur Problematik der transitorisch ischämischen Attacken (TIA) liegen nur relativ wenige metabolische Studien vor. Entsprechend der Vielzahl der möglichen pathophysiologischen Mechanismen werden nach der meist intermittierenden neurologischen Symptomatik unauffällige Befunde (CBF, OER), aber auch kombinierte und entkoppelte funktionelle Veränderungen (CBF, $CMRO_2$) mit erhöhter und erniedrigter OER beschrieben (BARON et al. 1978; CELESIA et al. 1983; DONNAN et al. 1983; ROUGEMONT et al. 1982).

c) Blutfluß, Sauerstoffmetabolismus und Glukosemetabolismus

Über die gleichzeitige Bestimmung des zerebralen Blutflusses und des Glukosemetabolismus liegen nur Studien zu einem relativ späten Zeitpunkt nach dem Primärereignis des Infarktes vor. Gemeinsam ist diesen Beobachtungen, daß nie eine gesteigerte Glukose-Aufnahme in ischämischen Bereichen gefunden wurde. Allerdings war der Glukosmetabolismus, ähnlich dem Sauerstoffmetabolismus, teilweise relativ weniger erniedrigt als die entsprechende Perfusion. Die Ausdehnung des Befundes war im Funktionsbild der PET immer ausgedehnter als die entsprechenden morphologischen Veränderungen in der CT oder dem MRI (Abb. 30, 31) (CELESIA et al. 1983; HEISS et al. 1985b; KUHL et al. 1980b; PHELPS et al. 1981a).

Die gleichzeitige Bestimmung der zerebralen Perfusion (LCBF), des Glukose (LCMRGlc)- und Sauerstoffmetabolismus ($LCMRO_2$) hat gezeigt, daß die Glukose-Aufnahme in infarzierten Bereichen in der Regel weniger erniedrigt ist als die $LCMRO_2$, allerdings liegen noch keine differenzierten Studien über die zeitliche Abhängigkeit des Geschehens auch für den CBF und die $CMRO_2$ vor (FRACKOWIAK u. WISE 1983; GIBBS et al. 1983a, b; WISE et al. 1983).

In Hypothesen für diese Entkopplung der metabolischen Parameter werden diskutiert: 1. irreversible Störung des oxidativen mitochondrialen Metabolismus der Karbonsäuren bei Erhalt des Embden-Meyerhof-Zyklus, 2. anaerobe Glykolyse der Makrophagen im Infarkt-Bereich und 3. Invalidität des Glukose-Modells (FDG, lumped constant) (BARON et al. 1985a; GIBBS et al. 1983a, b; MAZZIOTTA u. PHELPS 1986; SIESJÖ 1978). Die Schwelle von der Ischämie zum irreversiblen Infarkt wird bei einem zerebralen Blutfluß (CBF) von 15 ml/100 g/min und einem Sauerstoffmetabolismus ($CMRO_2$) von 1.3 ml/100 g/min angegeben (POWERS et al. 1985a, b).

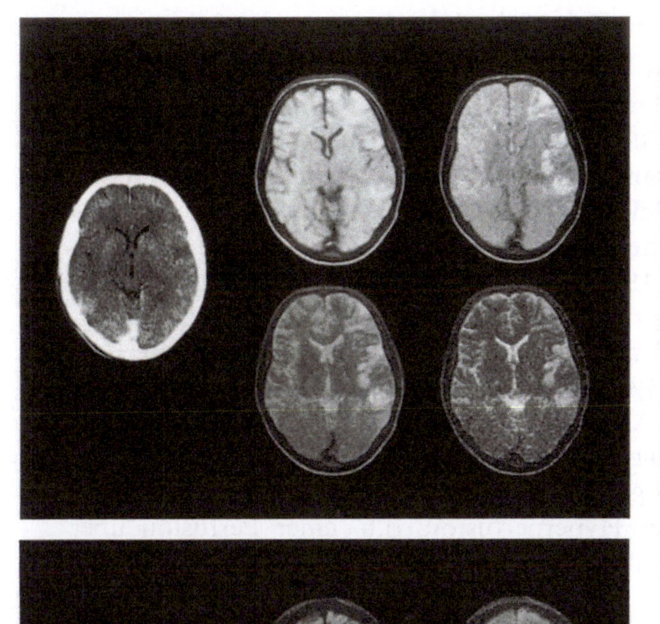

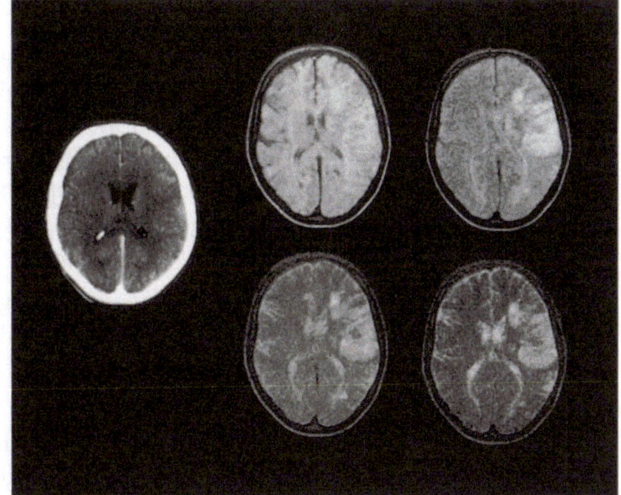

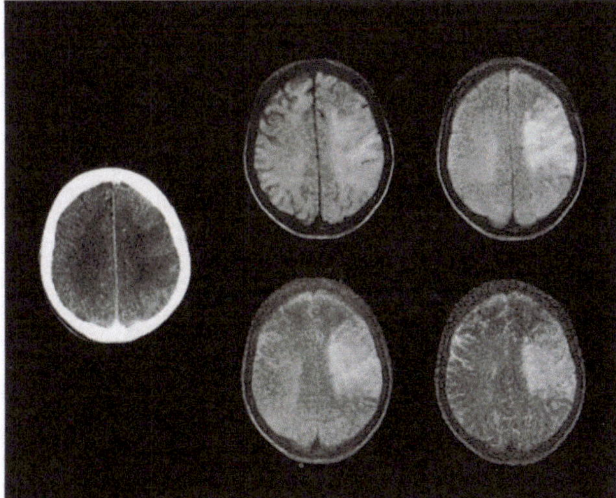

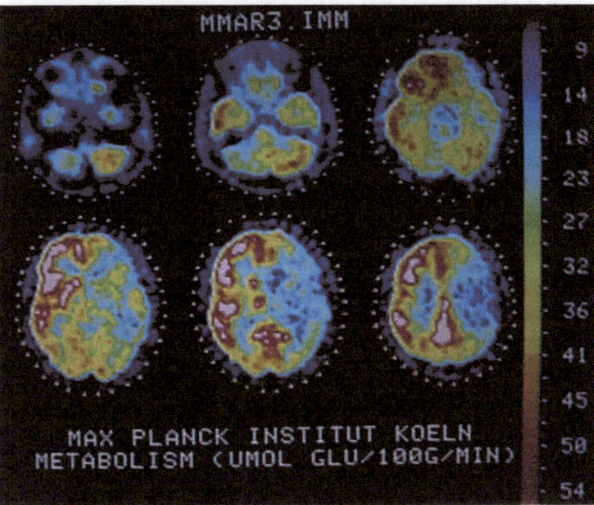

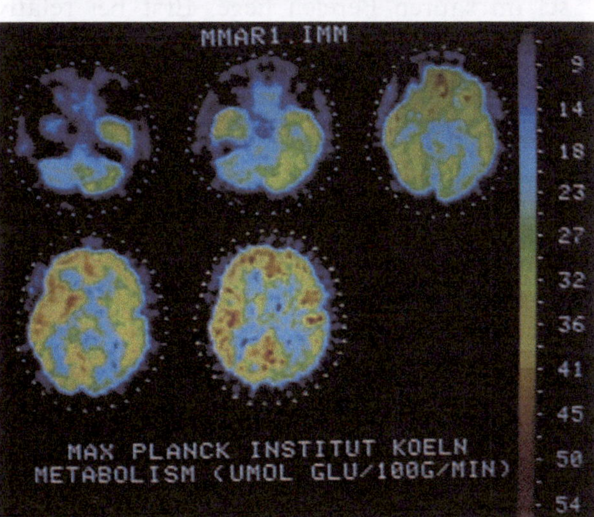

Abb. 31 a–e. CT- (**a**) und MRI-(Multi-Echo-Technik) (**b**) und FDG-PET-Bilder (**c**) einer 26jährigen Patientin mit Infarkt nach Verschluß der A. cerebri media links. Am 2. Tag nach Insult ist die Ausdehnung des Infarktes im CT noch nicht erkennbar, im T_2-gewichteten MRI deutlich abgrenzbar. Im frühen Stadium (**d**) ist der Stoffwechsel im gesamten Gehirn stark beeinträchtigt, im infarzierten Bereich finden sich Areale mit gesteigerter Glukoseaufnahme als Hinweis auf anaerobe Glykolyse. **e** 31 Tage nach dem Insult findet sich ein ausgedehnter Defekt mit vermindertem Stoffwechsel und Inaktivierung morphologisch intakter Hirnstrukturen (Thalamus, kontralaterales Kleinhirn). Der Stoffwechsel in den anderen Hirnregionen hat sich mit Besserung der Bewußtseinslage normalisiert. (Aus HEISS et al. 1985 b)

d) Blut-Hirn-Schranke, Gewebe-pH

Neben den Wechselwirkungen von Blutfluß, Sauerstoff- und Glukosemetabolismus sowie dem Blutvolumen ist auch der zerebrale Gewebe-pH mit der Blut-Hirn-Schranke in infarzierten Bereichen verändert (Kogure et al. 1980; Siesjö 1978).

Infarkte mit verminderten Stoffwechselparametern (CBF, $CMRO_2$ und CMRGlc) zeigen nach Syrota et al. (1985a, b) eine lokale Gewebsalkalose, wobei das Maß der Alkalose (pH) invers mit der Sauerstoffextraktion korrelieren soll (LOER) (Mabe et al. 1983; Rottenberg et al. 1983, 1985; Syrota et al. 1983a, 1985b). Ob eine geringere Produktion saurer Stoffwechselprodukte oder eine Vergrößerung des Extrazellulärraumes (^{76}Br) dafür verantwortlich sind, kann derzeit nicht abschließend beurteilt werden, zumal der vergrößerte Bromidraum gerade beim Infarkt und „sick cell syndrome" zumindest nicht die anatomischen Kompartimente wiedergibt und intrazelluläre Anreicherungen angenommen werden müssen (Schober et al. 1982). Dagegen berichten Heiss et al. (1985b), daß der pH in typischen Infarkten mit verminderter Durchblutung und gestörtem Sauerstoff- und Glukosestoffwechsel im sauren Bereich liege. Erst bei relativer Hyperperfusion, d.h. einer Perfusion über den Bedarf des Gewebes an Stoffwechselsubstraten hinaus, entwickle sich eine lokale Gewebsalkalose (Yamamoto et al. 1985).

Mit dem Positronenstrahler ^{68}Ga-EDTA wurden Störungen der Blut-Hirn-Schranke (BBB) untersucht. Zwischen 6 und 60 Tage nach dem Infarktereignis wurden mit der PET bei 6 von 14 Patienten sensitiver Störungen der Blut-Hirn-Schranke nachgewiesen als mit der CT mit Kontrastmitteln. Neben Unterschieden in der Größe und den chemischen Eigenschaften der Pharmaka mögen kinetische Gründe im Sinne einer langsamen Diffusion für diese Ergebnisse verantwortlich sein (Ericson et al. 1981, 1985). Regionen mit Störungen der Blut-Hirn-Schranke konnten mit dem Kation ^{82}Rb dargestellt werden, während das perifokale Ödem keine Kontrastanhebung bot (Brooks et al. 1984b).

e) Desaktivierung entfernter Hirnstrukturen

Mit der Positronen-Emissionstomographie wurde beobachtet, daß morphologisch unauffällige entfernte Hirnstrukturen abnorme Perfusions- oder metabolische Verhältnisse aufweisen können (Metter et al. 1983a). Diese Regionen betreffen subkortikale Strukturen ipsilateraler kortikaler Läsionen, kortikale Strukturen ipsilateraler subkortikaler Läsionen, diffuse und fokale Veränderungen der kontralateralen zerebralen Hemisphäre und Veränderungen des kontralateralen Zerebellums.

Beschrieben wurde der Begriff *Diaschisis* von von Monakow bereits 1914. „Die *Diaschisis* stellt eine meist plötzlich eintretende, auf bestimmte weit verzweigte zentrale Funktionskreise sich beziehende „Betriebseinstellung" dar, die ihren Ursprung aus der örtlichen Läsion nimmt, ihre Angriffspunkte aber nicht (wie der apoplektische Insult) im ganzen Kortex (Stabkranz, etc.), sondern nur an solchen Stellen hat, wo aus der Gegend der Läsionsstelle fließende Fasern in primär nicht lädierte graue Substanz des ganzen Zentralnervensystems auslaufen. Bei der Diaschisis handelt es sich im wesentlichen um Herabsetzung oder Aufhebung, Refraktärwerden der Anspruchsfähigkeit, resp. der zentralen Elemente (Neuronengruppen) für Reize üblicher Stärke, und zwar innerhalb eines bestimmten, physiologisch wohl definierten Erregungskreises. Dieser Kreis fällt indessen mit den gewöhnlichen, von der Peripherie und vom Zentrum aus sich ausdehnenden physiologischen Innervationswegen nicht zusammen".

Gemeinsame Verringerungen des LCBF und der $LCMRO_2$ entfernter Hirnstrukturen, bei denen die *kontralaterale Hemisphäre* aufgrund supratentorieller Infarkte betroffen ist, werden Desaktivierungen transhemisphärischer kallöser Fasersysteme zugeschrieben. Bei ausgedehnteren Desaktivierungen korrelieren die metabolischen Größen und Parameter zur Klinik (CELESIA et al. 1983; FRACKOWIAK u. WISE 1983; HEISS et al. 1983b; LENZI et al. 1981b, 1982).

Kortikal-subkortikale (Nucleus caudatus, Thalamus) Wechselwirkungen im Sinne gegenseitiger Desaktivierungen werden kompressions-induzierten Ischämien, Wallerschen Degenerationen, Verschlüssen selektiver tiefer Arterien und funktionellen Desaktivierungen, etwa kortiko-ponto-zerebellaren Bahnen, zugeschrieben (CELESIA et al. 1983; HEISS et al. 1983b; KUHL et al. 1980b; METTER et al. 1981).

Die sog. gekreuzte *zerebellare Diaschisis* entspricht einer Verringerung der Perfusion und der metabolischen Parameter im Zerebellum aufgrund eines supratentoriellen Infarktes auf der kontralateralen Seite. Der Fluß (LCBF) ist um 19–27%, der Sauerstoffmetabolismus um 16–25%, der Glukosemetabolismus um etwa 22% reduziert (BARON et al. 1980, 1981d, 1982, 1983, 1985a; CELESIA et al. 1983; HEISS et al. 1983b; KANAYA et al. 1983; MARTIN u. RAICHLE 1983a, b).

Der nach einem Infarkt zeitliche Verlauf der zerebellaren Diaschisis, die auch mit dem Flow-Marker ^{123}I-Amphetamin nachgewiesen werden kann (CREUTZIG et al. 1986), ist noch nicht ausreichend geklärt. Frontale Infarkte scheinen eine größere Ausprägung dieses Phänomens zu begünstigen als parieto-okzipitale Insulte (MARTIN u. RAICHLE 1983b), wobei die Ergebnisse von KUSHNER et al. (1984) auch bei parietalen Infarkten eine deutliche Reduktion des Glukose-Metabolismus des kontralateralen Zerebellums beschreiben. Das gleiche Phänomen wird auch bei supratentoriellen Tumoren gesehen (Abschnitt D.I.6).

f) Verschiedene (zerebrovaskuläre) neurologische Erkrankungen

Intrazerebrale Blutungen, wie subarachnoidale Blutungen nach Vasospasmen (POWERS et al. 1985a, RAICHLE 1980), intraparenchymale Blutungen (ACKERMAN et al. 1983b; KELLY et al. 1982), subdurale Hämatome (^{68}Ga-EDTA: ERICSON et al. 1980) und ventrikuläre Blutungen (HERSCOVITCH et al. 1983a) wurden untersucht, wobei offensichtlich zwischen der Perfusionseinschränkung und der Prognose eine positive Korrelation besteht (ACKERMAN et al. 1983b, 1985). Insbesondere gingen die Perfusionsstörungen über das Ausmaß der Blutungen und der morphologischen Veränderungen hinaus.

BEWERMEYER et al. (1985) berichten über einen Patienten mit beidseitigem Thalamus-Infarkt, vergleichend mit PET, CT und MRI. Bei Patienten mit benigner intrakranieller Hypertension sind Sauerstoffmetabolismus und -Extraktion, Blutfluß und -Volumen gegenüber einem Kontrollkollektiv und auch im Vergleich zum Zustand nach Dekompression durch einen lumboperitonealen Shunt nicht verändert (BROOKS et al. 1985). BOSLEY et al. (1985) und CELESIA et al. (1982b) analysieren okzipitale ischämische Läsionen und ihre Wirkungen auf die optischen Bahnen. VOLPE et al. (1983, 1985), HERSCOVITCH et al. (1983a) und PERLMAN et al. (1985) untersuchten Frühgeborene mit perinataler Asphyxie und Kleinkinder mit intrakraniellen Blutungen.

15 Patienten mit Multipler Sklerose zeigten eine signifikante Erniedrigung des Blutflusses und des Sauerstoff-Metabolismus sowohl im Bereich der weißen als auch in den peripheren kortikalen Bereichen der grauen Substanz (BROOKS et al. 1984c). Über eine Patientin mit systemischem Lupus Erythematodus (SLE) berichten HIRAIWA et al. (1983).

3. Heredo-degenerative Erkrankungen

Fragestellung. Der Begriff degenerativ sei hier für eine Gruppe von Erkrankungen angewandt, die in der Regel symmetrisch und progressiv strukturelle Elemente des Nervensystems betrifft. Wegen der familiären Häufung wird häufig von heredo-degenerativen Erkrankungen gesprochen, auch wenn etwa für das Creutzfeld-Jakob-Syndrom eine virale Ursache angenommen werden kann. Unabhängig von den metabolischen Untersuchungen durch die Positronen-Emissionstomographie werden die auf Degenerationen von Neuronen in komplexen Funktionskreisen verursachten, klinisch manifesten Krankheitsbilder ohne größere Schwierigkeiten durch spezifische Symptome diagnostiziert.

Mit der PET wurden bisher Syndrome untersucht, bei denen eine progressive Demenz klinisch im Vordergrund steht (Senile Demenz, Multi-Infarkt-Demenz; M. Alzheimer), solche, bei denen eine Demenz mit extrapyramidalen Syndromen kombiniert ist (Chorea Huntington; M. Wilson) und Krankheiten mit spastisch-atrophischer Muskellähmung (Amyotrophe Lateralsklerose, ALS). Weiterhin liegen Studien zu Syndromen vor, bei denen die Bewegungs-Anomalien deutlich dominieren (M. Parkinson, Paralysis agitans).

a) Morbus Parkinson

Für den M. Parkinson ist ein Zellverlust der Zona compacta der substantia nigra mit einer erniedrigten striatalen Dopamin-Konzentration charakteristisch (Garnett et al. 1984a; Hornykiewicz 1980, 1982).

Zum Glukosemetabolismus beim M. Parkinson liegen nur wenige Studien vor. Während unter L-Dopa-Medikation keine Änderung des Glukosemetabolismus (LCMRGlc) im Vergleich zu einer entsprechenden Altersgruppe gesehen wurden, war die Glukoseaufnahme nach Absetzen der Medikation global, ohne Hinweise auf lokale Änderungen, um 20% verringert (Kuhl et al. 1983b, 1984a, b; Lenzi et al. 1979; Rougemont et al. 1984).

Leenders et al. (1983, 1985) und Wolfson et al. (1985) untersuchten 18 Patienten mit M. Parkinson und verglichen die Ergebnisse mit einem Kontrollkollektiv (n = 6). Nach klinisch wirksamer L-Dopa-Therapie beobachteten sie eine diffuse Erhöhung des kortikalen Blutflusses (CBF) um 13% ohne entsprechende Steigerung der Sauerstoff-Utilisation. Sie interpretieren diese Beobachtung als vereinbar mit einer Vasodilatation der zerebralen Gefäße. Allerdings beobachteten sie keine Korrelation der metabolischen Parameter zur Klinik, trotz deutlicher Verbesserung unter der Therapie. Im Bereich der Basal-Ganglien zeigte sich unter einer L-Dopa-Medikation bei vornehmlich einseitiger Erkrankung eine Verbesserung des CBF um 20% bei unverändertem Sauerstoffmetabolismus (LCMRO$_2$), im Zerebellum dagegen eine Erniedrigung des LCBF bei konstanter CMRO$_2$. Perlmutter u. Raichle (1984, 1985) bestätigen diese Beobachtungen, beschreiben jedoch keine globalen Unterschiede vor und nach Therapie, bzw. im Vergleich zu einer Kontrollgruppe.

Bustany et al. (1983b, 1985) konnten diese Ergebnisse für die Aminosäure-Aufnahme (^{11}C-L-Methionin) bestätigen und fanden bei Patienten mit M. Parkinson keine signifikante Änderung gegenüber einer Kontrollgruppe.

Der Gruppe um Firnau u. Garnett ist es zuerst gelungen, die Dopamin-Rezeptoren mit dem entsprechenden präsynaptischen Analogon [^{18}F]-6-fluoro-L-dopa ‚in vivo' darzustellen (Firnau et al. 1975, 1981; Garnett et al. 1983). Gerade bei einem Hemi-Parkinson zeigte es sich, daß die ^{18}F-Aufnahme im Bereich des kontralateralen Striatum erniedrigt war, vornehmlich im Putamen. Die Darstellung der ^{18}F-Verteilung des Striatum auf der betroffenen Seite war inhomogen. Autoradiographische Untersuchungen entsprechen diesen Ergebnissen (Hornykiewicz et al. 1980). Diese Beobachtung wird mit einem intrazerebralen Kompensationsmechanismus erklärt, der die Manifestation des Dopaminmangels bis zu einem relativ späten klinischen Stadium hinausschiebt. In einem subklinischen Zustand der Zerstörung der Substantia nigra konnten bereits Defekte des dopaminergen Systems nachgewiesen werden (Calne et al. 1985). Die Berichte von Frost et al. (1984b) aus der Gruppe am NIH in Baltimore unterstützen diese Ergebnisse. Das Putamen ist offensichtlich stärker in Bewegungsstörungen involviert, während die Nuclei caudati mehr die kognitiven Prozesse beeinflussen (Nahmias et al. 1985).

Beim Rhesus-Affen konnte gezeigt werden, daß etwa 50% des ^{18}F-Dopa nach Reserpin-Applikation aus dem Striatum verdrängt werden können (FIRNAU et al. 1981). Dieses mag ein Beispiel für eine biologische Qualitätskontrolle sein.

b) Morbus Wilson

Beim M. Wilson handelt es sich um eine seltene Form einer hepatolentikulären Degeneration, die auf eine massiv erhöhte Kupferspeicherung (Coeruloplasmin) in vielen Organen, besonders in der Leber, aber auch in den basalen Ganglien zurückzuführen ist. Die neurologische Symptomatik manifestiert sich in der Regel erst nach den hepatischen und hämatologischen Symptomen.

Neben einer Verminderung des Glukosemetabolismus im Bereich des Nucleus lentiformis, weniger deutlich im Bereich des Nucleus caudatus, wurden mit einer Tendenz entsprechend der Klinik auch globale Verminderungen der Glukose-Stoffwechsels (LCMRGlc) kortikal und subkortikal beschrieben (HAWKINS et al. 1983b).

c) Amyotrophe Lateralsklerose (ALS)

Bei fünf Patienten mit Amyotropher Lateralsklerose fand die Gruppe am NIH, Bethesda, einen erniedrigten Glukosestoffwechsel in sensomotorischen Arealen und relativ ausgedehnte Bereiche kortikaler Suppression (MANSI et al. 1983).

d) Chorea Huntington

Das Gehirn des Patienten mit Chorea Huntington ist mit Betonung des Frontallappens insgesamt atrophiert. Charakteristisch ist eine schwere bilaterale Atrophie the Nucleus caudatus, weniger ausgeprägt die des Putamens oder des Globus pallidus.

KUHL et al. (1981, 1982b, 1984b) untersuchten 13 Patienten mit Chorea Huntington und 15 Angehörige von Chorea-Familien (dominant-autosomale Vererbung). Schon vor morphologischen Veränderungen im CT war bei leichteren Fällen der Glukosemetabolismus vornehmlich im Caudatus vermindert, während schwere Veränderungen, die auch kortikale Regionen betrafen, im CT nachgewiesen werden konnten. Die Klinik korrelierte eher mit den morphologischen Parametern als denen des Metabolismus, wobei aber meßtechnische Limitationen berücksichtigt werden müssen (Abb. 32).

Gerade bei den familiär belasteten Risikopatienten erwiesen sich die funktionellen Studien der Positronen-Emissionstomographie, besonders im Caudatus-Bereich, bei noch unauffälliger Klinik als sehr sensitiv (GARNETT et al. 1984b). Diese auch in Hinblick auf die Prognose wichtigen Ergebnisse konnten von MAZZIOTTA et al. (1985a) bestätigt werden.

e) Demenz

Die Demenz bildet beim alten Menschen das häufigste Krankheitsbild aus dem psychiatrischen Formenkreis. Schon aus epidemiologischen Gründen hat sie deshalb eine erhebliche Bedeutung in der westlichen Welt. In den Vereinigten Staaten von Amerika leiden etwa 1,3 Millionen Patienten an schwerer Demenz, wobei mindestens 50–60% vom Alzheimer Typ sind. Eine Differentialdiagnose der Demenz bietet aus Ansätzen der verschiedenen Ätiologie therapeutisch sehr unterschiedliche Möglichkeiten, dabei muß aber insbesondere eine noch nicht einheitlich beurteilte normalen Altersabhängigkeit der Stoffwechselparameter berücksichtigt werden (ALAVI u. DELEON 1985).

Klinisch orientierte und morphologische bildgebende Verfahren, wie die Transmissions-Computertomographie (CT) und die Kernspintomographie (MRI), haben bisher in der Beurteilung und der Korrelation zur Klinik besonders in frühen Stadien wenig diagnostisch rele-

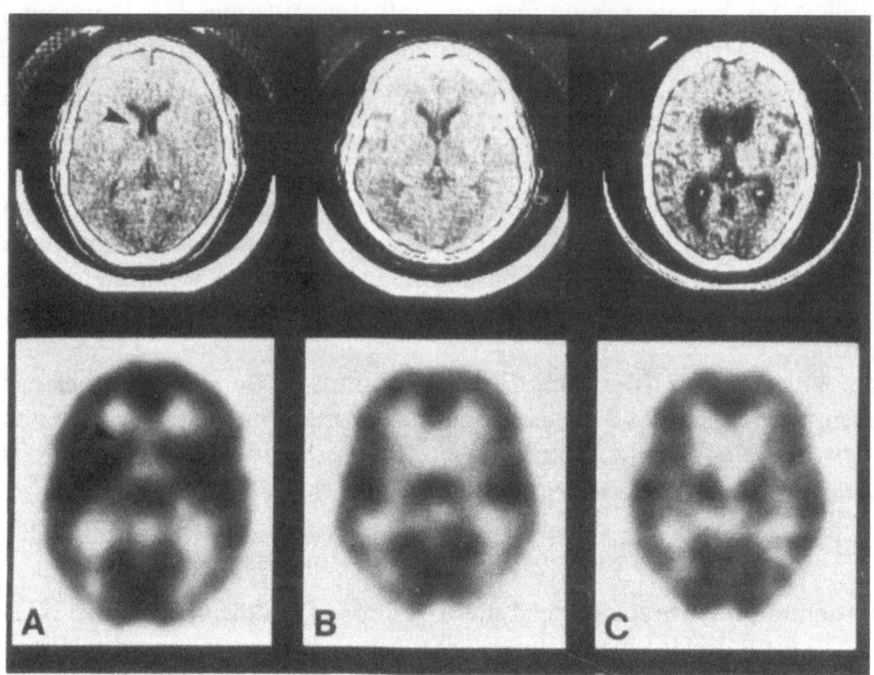

Abb. 32A–C. Morphologisch dokumentierte Atrophie und Darstellung des Glukose-Stoffwechsels bei der Chorea Huntington. **A** Normale Kontrollperson, insbesondere unauffällige Nucleus caudatus und Putamen (*Pfeil*). **B** Patient mit Frühsymptomen. Während im Bereich der Basalganglien noch keine strukturellen Veränderungen zu beobachten sind, ist die Glukose-Aufnahme bilateral im Bereich des Caudatus und des Putamen bereits erniedrigt. **C** In einem späteren Stadium der Chorea Huntington kommen strukturelle Veränderungen zu den funktionellen Störungen hinzu. (Aus Kuhl et al. 1981, 1982b)

vante Informationen beitragen können. Erst bei ausgeprägten klinischen Zuständen von Demenz werden regional unterschiedliche Veränderungen der Rinde im Sinne einer Atrophie, vor allem des Temporallappens, und Erweiterungen der Sulci und signifikanter der Ventrikel beobachtet (De Leon et al. 1983c, 1984; Gado et al. 1982; Zatz et al. 1982).

Wenn bei dieser Fragestellung die PET angewandt wird, so stellt insbesondere aus methodischen Gründen der Teilvolumeneffekt ein Problem dar. So gilt es zu differenzieren, ob eine Minderanreicherung auf eine Hirnatrophie und den Ersatz des Volumens durch zerebrospinale Flüssigkeit zurückzuführen ist oder die funktionale Aktivität vermindert ist (De Leon et al. 1983a, b; De Leon u. George 1983; Herscovitch et al. 1984a). Aus morphometrischen Untersuchungen weiß man, daß bei der senilen Demenz vom Alzheimer-Typ (SDAT) in einem späten Stadium die Zahl der Neurone um über 40% verringert ist, vornehmlich frontal und temporal (Terry et al. 1981).

Pathophysiologische Studien haben gezeigt, daß etwa 50% der chronischen und irreversiblen Demenzen solche vom Alzheimer-Typ (SDAT) sind und 20% auf ein zerebrovaskuläres Multi-Infarkt-Geschehen (MID) zurückgeführt werden können, während bei etwa 12% der Patienten beide Ursachen gefunden werden konnten (Jellinger 1976; Tomlinson u. Kitchner 1972; Tomlinson 1980). Die übrigen Ursachen einer Demenz spielen eine relativ geringere Bedeutung. Untersuchungen liegen vor über Patienten mit Chorea Huntington (Kuhl et al. 1981, 1982b), M. Wilson (Hawkins et al. 1983b), M. Parkinson (Kuhl et al. 1983b, 1984a) und M. Creutzfeld-Jakob (Friedland et al. 1983, 1984). Diese vom klinischen Standpunkt aus gesehen eher vorläufigen Mitteilungen berichten in der Regel von einer verringerten Glukoseaufnahme vornehmlich im Bereich der basalen Ganglien, wobei hier die Effekte beim M. Parkinson am wenigsten ausgeprägt sind mit einer entsprechenden extrapyramidalen Symptomatik, oder in globaleren Bereichen.

Voraussetzung der Schlußfolgerungen aus der PET über den Metabolismus ist die Validität des Modells. Dabei ist eine immer wiederkehrende Frage die nach den kinetischen Konstanten und der experimentell bestimmten „lumped constant". Die kinetischen Konstanten können durch dynamische Messungen spezifisch für das pathologische Gewebe bestimmt werden (WIENARD et al. 1985). Für den Korrekturfaktor „lumped constant", der die Differenz zwischen der gemessenen ^{18}FDG-Konzentration und der arteriovenösen Glukose-Konzentration berücksichtigt und der bei Patienten mit Demenz unverändert sein soll, können „normale Werte" angenommen werden (FRIEDLAND et al. 1983). Messungen mit den Positronen-Tomographen der neueren Generation mit einem Auflösungsvermögen < 10 mm (FWHM) werden diese Beobachtungen in Zukunft bestätigen müssen.

α) *Morbus Alzheimer (SDAT)*. In zahlreichen Studien ist bei Patienten mit M. Alzheimer eine Verringerung der metabolischen Aktivität im parieto-okzipitalen Kortex, aber auch im Bereich der Basalganglien beschrieben worden mit Bevorzugung des motorischen und sensorischen Kortex (Abb. 33). Die kognitiven Fähigkeiten korrelieren invers mit der verringerten Glukoseaufnahme ($\Delta = -17–37\%$) (ALAVI et al. 1980, 1981 b; BENSON et al. 1981, 1983; DE LEON u. GEORGE 1983; DE LEON et al. 1983 a–c; FARKAS et al. 1982, 1984; FERRIS et al. 1983; FOSTER et al. 1983, 1984). So wurde bei insgesamt 55 Patienten mit SDAT eine Verminderung des Glukosemetabolismus um 27%, vornehmlich temporo-parietal, sowie im auditiven Zentrum gefunden (FRIEDLAND et al. 1985; GRIMES et al. 1985).

Insbesondere von den Arbeitsgruppe am NIH, Bethesda, und an der UCLA, Los Angeles, wurden Untersuchungen des regionalen Stoffwechsel im Vergleich zu differenzierten neurologischen Befunden in Abhängigkeit von familiär gehäuften subklinischen und klinischen Schweregraden durchgeführt. Bei jungen Patienten mit Down-Syndrom wurde dagegen sogar eine im Vergleich zu einer entsprechenden Altersgruppe erhöhte Glukoseaufnahme im Gehirn beschrieben, bei erwachsenen Patienten dagegen ein erniedrigter Glukosemetabolismus (CHASE et al. 1985; CUTLER et al. 1984, 1985a, b; KUHL et al. 1983a).

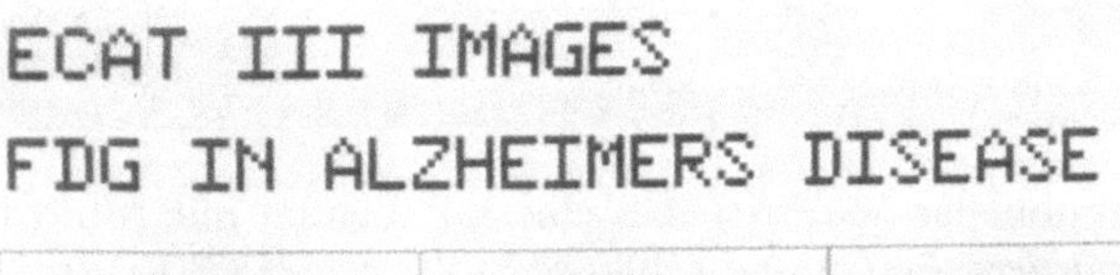

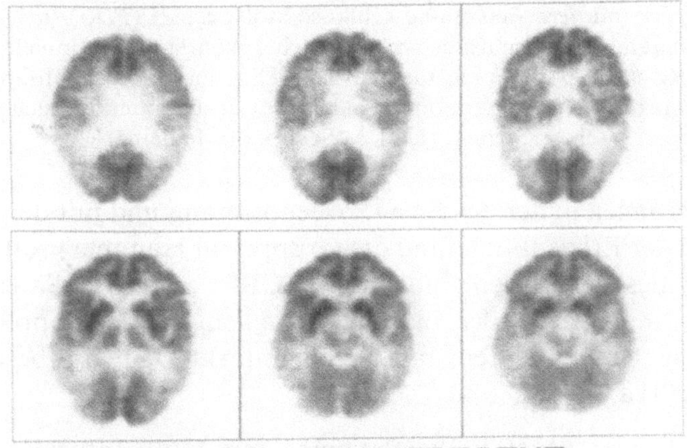

Abb. 33. FDG-PET-Studie bei einem Patienten mit M. Alzheimer mit typischen Veränderungen der Glukose-Aufnahme. Besonders deutlich ist der verminderte Metabolismus in den kortikalen Bereichen infero-frontal und postero-parietal. Weitgehend unverändert zeigen sich der primär auditive und visuelle Kortex sowie subkortikale Bereiche (UCLA, School of Medicine)

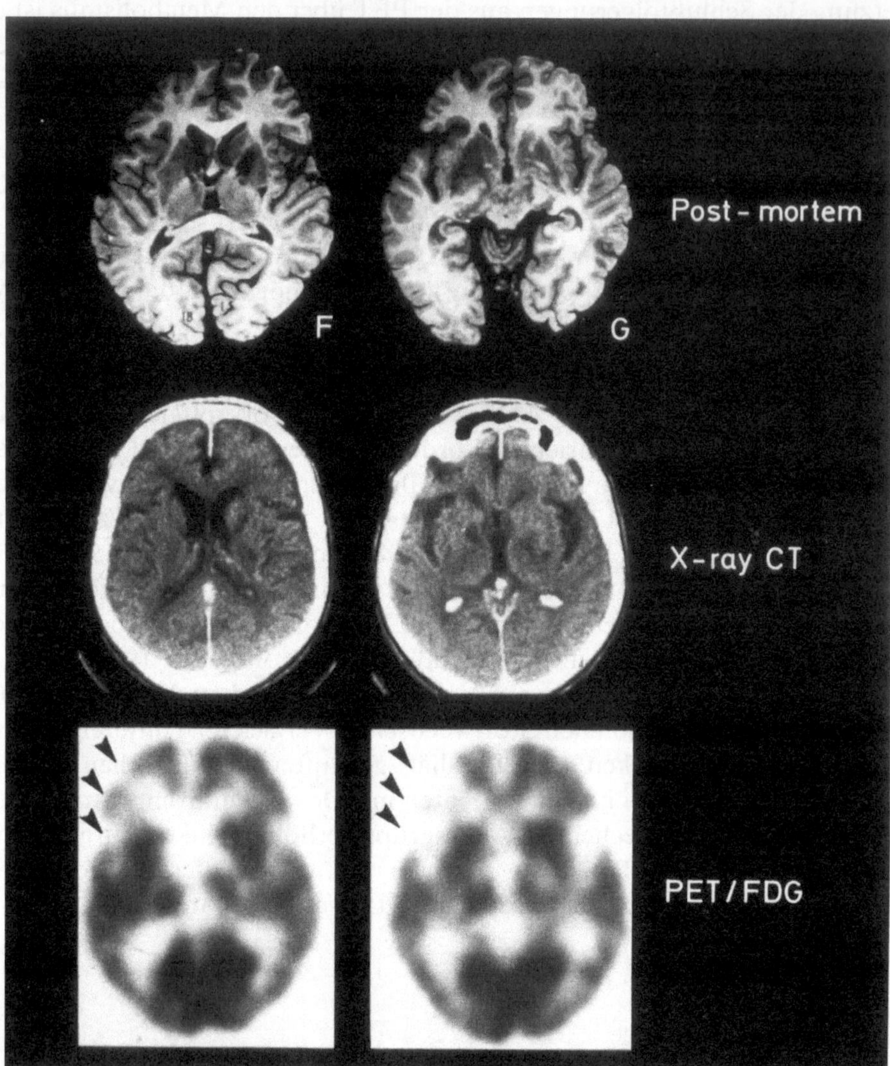

Abb. 34. Struktureller und funktioneller Vergleich bei einem Patienten mit Multi-Infarkt-Demenz (*MID*). Pathologie (*obere Reihe*), CT (*mittlere Reihe*) und Glukose-Stoffwechsel (*FDG*) (*untere Reihe*). 7 Tage nach den Studien starb der Patient aus nicht-neurologischer Ursache. Während funktionelle Störungen im Frontallappen nur mit der PET nachzuweisen waren und auf eine Diaschisis zurückzuführen sein mögen, fanden multiple Infarkte tieferer Hirnstrukturen (Striatum, Thalamus, Capsula interna) auch im CT ihr morphologisches Korrelat (UCLA, School of Medicine)

Quantitative Änderungen in der gleichen Größenordnung und mit der gleichen Abhängigkeit vom Schweregrad der Erkrankung fand die Gruppe am Hammersmith Hospital, London, bei der Bestimmung des zerebralen Blutflusses (CBF) und des Sauerstoffmetabolismus (CMRO$_2$), besonders im Bereich der basalen Ganglien. Diese Kopplung von CBF und CMRO$_2$ wurde auch bei Patienten mit Multi-Infarkt-Demenz beschrieben (Abb. 35) (Frackowiak et al. 1981 a, b).

β) Multi-Infarkt-Demenz (MID). Bei Patienten mit Multi-Infarkt-Demenz fanden sich Erniedrigungen der Glukose-Aufnahme und des mit dem Blutfluß korrelierten Sauerstoffmetabolismus wie bei den Patienten mit M. Alzheimer (SDAT). Dabei waren die Veränderungen im parietalen Kortex (29–37%) deutlicher als im frontotemporalen und frontoparietalen Kortex und den Basalganglien (20–25%), insgesamt aber fokaler und asymmetrischer als bei der SDAT (Abb. 34) (Benson et al. 1983; Frackowiak et al. 1981 a, b). Da sowohl

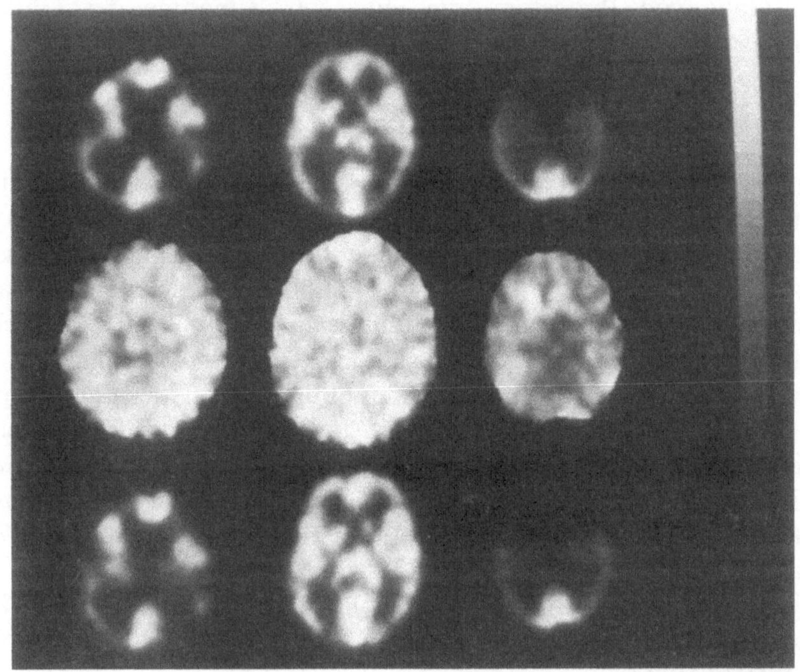

Abb. 35. Sauerstoff-Studien (^{15}O) bei Patienten mit Multi-Infarkt-Demenz im Vergleich zu einer normalen Kontrollperson (mittlere Säule). *Obere Reihe:* Zerebraler Blutfluß (*LCBF*), *mittlere Reihe:* Sauerstoff-Extraktion (*LOEF*), *untere Reihe:* Sauerstoff-Metabolismus ($LCMRO_2$). *Linke Säule:* Patient mit Multi-Infarkt-Demenz und gemeinsamer inhomogener, regional unterschiedlicher Erniedrigung des Flusses und Sauerstoff-Metabolismus, *rechte Säule:* Patient mit schwerer degenerativer Demenz und generalisierter Erniedrigung des Sauerstoff-Metabolismus und des Flusses, insbesondere in den frontalen Regionen. (Aus FRACKOWIAK et al. 1981b)

bei der Multi-Infarkt-Demenz (MID) als auch bei beim M. Alzheimer keine Erhöhung der Sauerstoff-Extraktionsrate gefunden wurde, schließen die Autoren darauf, daß Ischämien primär nicht zur Pathogenese beitragen. Dieses steht in gewissem Widerspruch zu der klinischen Beobachtung, daß bei Patienten mit MID gehäuft arterielle Hypertension, Infarkte und ein diskontinuierlicher klinischer Verlauf vorliegen (ROSEN et al. 1980).

KUHL et al. (1983a) verglichen systematisch PET und CT und fanden im Mittel im Bereich der grauen Substanz mit der FDG-PET eher als mit der CT Läsionen, wobei im Bereich der weißen Substanz die Computertomographie aus methodischen Gründen überlegen war. Klinisch und pathophysiologisch interessant dürfte sein, daß lokale im CT dokumentierte Läsionen funktionelle Desaktivierungen entfernter Hirnstrukturen im Sinne einer Diaschisis verursachen sollen. Andererseits sind die metabolischen Änderungen bei der Multi-Infarkt-Demenz teilweise ausgedehnter als die entsprechenden morphologischen, durch das CT dokumentierten (METTER et al. 1983a, 1985).

Zur Korrelation der Ergebnisse der PET mit klinischen Aufgaben beim M. Alzheimer liegt eine Reihe von Ergebnissen vor, die die motorische Apraxie (FOSTER et al. 1983), Aphasie und Apraxie (FRACKOWIAK et al. 1981; METTER et al. 1981, 1983b) und Gedächtnisleistungen betreffen (FOSTER et al. 1983).

Entsprechende Beobachtungen wurden bei seniler Demenz für die Methionin-Aufnahme mitgeteilt. Patienten mit Demenz zeigten vornehmlich frontal eine Verringerung der Aufnahme um bis zu 67% (BUSTANY et al. 1983a, b).

γ) Pharmakologie. HEISS et al. (1985b) berichteten über eine deutliche Verbesserung der Vigilanz bei Patienten mit Demenz vom Alzheimer-Typ oder nach einem Multi-Infarkt-

Geschehen nach Gabe von Piracetam, die mit einer Zunahme der Glukoseaufnahme (CMRGl) in den Basalganglien korrelierte.

4. Epilepsien und andere anfallsartige Erkrankungen

Fragestellung. Die Epilepsie und anfallsartige Erkrankungen werden charakterisiert durch meist paroxysmale Störungen der Gehirnfunktion im Sinne einer verstärkten neuralen Tätigkeit, die elektrophysiologisch mit der EEG dokumentiert werden kann. Anfallsweise auftretende Bewußtlosigkeit und abnorme motorische Phänomene begleiten eine abnorme synchrone Entladung von Ganglienzellen. Im anfallsfreien Intervall sind die elektrophysiologischen Befunde nicht einheitlich, insbesondere gibt es keine von der klinischen Fragestellung her befriedigende Korrelation zu morphologischen bildgebenden Verfahren wie der Computertomographie, der Kernspinotomographie, der Angiographie und früher der Pneumenzephalographie. Bei genuinen oder idiopathischen Formen ist der CT-Befund häufig unauffällig, trotz im EEG oder auch der ^{123}I-Amphetamin-Szintigraphie mit SPECT positiver fokaler Herde (Biersack et al. 1986; Gastaut 1970, 1976; Gastaut u. Michel 1978; Hofmann 1986; Ishida et al. 1983; Loiseau et al. 1983; Markland 1977; Merlis 1970).

Die Epilepsie kommt in der Bundesrepublik Deutschland etwa gleich häufig vor wie der Diabetes mellitus und die Tuberkulose, derzeit leiden etwa 300000 Menschen an dieser Erkrankung (Hofmann 1986).

In neuerer Zeit stehen Untersuchungen der metabolischen Störungen im Vordergrund. Bis zum diagnostischen Einsatz der Positronenstrahler war man auf Flußuntersuchungen vornehmlich mit Gamma-Strahlern, wie ^{133}Xe, ^{123}IMP, ^{99m}Tc-HM-PAO, und den damit verbundenen inhärenten Problemen angewiesen. Die Ergebnisse waren aber teilweise nicht konsistent, so wurden Hypo- und Hyperperfusionen im Bereich fokaler Herde beobachtet (Ingvar 1973, 1975; Ingvar u. Franzen 1971; Ingvar u. Lassen 1965; Lavy et al. 1976; Sakai et al. 1978; Schwartzkroin u. Wyler 1980).

Da der pathophysiologische Zustand bei der Epilepsie deutlich mit funktionellen Störungen gekoppelt ist, bietet die Positronen-Emissionstomographie hervorragende Möglichkeiten, regionale Änderungen des zerebralen Blutflusses und Stoffwechsels im Anfall und im anfallsfreien Intervall zu untersuchen.

Meßtechnische Probleme stellen die Aquisitionszeiten unter Berücksichtigung der Anfallssequenzen dar, die ein abgestimmtes Meßprotokoll erfordern (Gur et al. 1985; Mazziotta u. Phelps 1986). Die Arbeitsgruppen an der UCLA, Los Angeles, und am Hammersmith Hospital, London, haben sich deshalb auch aus diesen Gründen mit ^{15}O-markierten Radiopharmaka (Fluß und Sauerstoff-Metabolismus) beschäftigt (Engel 1984; Engel et al. 1982a–d, 1983). Gerade die Technik der Bolus-Injektion ^{15}O-markierter Verbindungen scheint den Gleichgewichtsstudien (^{18}FDG, $C^{15}O_2$, $H_2^{15}O$) bei dieser klinischen Fragestellung überlegen zu sein.

Die Ziele sind zum einen die funktionelle Darstellung der Hirnstrukturen im Anfall und im anfallsfreien Intervall, auch in Hinblick auf die therapeutischen Möglichkeiten, andererseits eine Verbesserung der Lokalisations-Genauigkeit mit der Abklärung invasiver therapeutischer Möglichkeiten, wie stereotaktischer oder chirurgischer Eingriffe zur Entfernung der epileptogenen Herde (Abb. 37) (Bohm et al. 1983; Engel et al. 1984; Fox et al. 1985; Kuhl et al. 1980a; Mazziotta u. Engel 1984).

Die Klassifizierung der Epilepsieformen kann nach der Ätiologie, dem Erscheinungsbild oder nach EEG-Kriterien vorgenommen werden. Da die Einteilung der Erscheinungsformen und ihrer teilweise komplizierten Semantik des klinischen Bildes (Generalisierte Anfälle: Grand mal, Absencen; partielle Anfälle mit elementarer und komplexer Symptomatik) nicht immer befriedigend erscheint, sei die Strukturierung und Besprechung mehr nach metabolischen Kriterien aufgeführt (Gastaut 1970; Hofmann 1986; Merlis 1970).

a) Anfallsfreies Intervall

Mehr als 200 Patienten-Studien liegen inzwischen über den Glukosemetabolismus im anfallsfreien Intervall vor (Abb. 36, 37) (ENGEL et al. 1984; THEODORE et al. 1983, 1984; MAZZIOTTA u. PHELPS 1986). Gemeinsam ist diesen Untersuchungen, daß mehr als 70% der Patienten einen oder mehrere fokale Herde mit einer Glukose-Minderanreicherung zeigten, wobei Größe, Zahl, Lage und Form variieren, aber eine deutliche Bevorzugung des Temporallappens zu beobachten ist. Korrelationen zu elektrophysiologischen Untersuchungen wurden nicht gesehen, wohl aber zu therapeutischen Erfolgen (THEODORE et al. 1983).

Sowohl mit der PET als auch mit der EEG fanden sich, wie erwartet, wenig falsch positive intraoperativ kontrollierte Ergebnisse (ENGEL et al. 1982a). Allerdings ist neben der geringen Korrelation der Befunde zum CT besonders interessant, daß die morphologisch-anatomischen Läsionen in der Regel geringer sind, als die entsprechenden Ausdehnungen der verminderten Stoffwechselaktivität im anfallsfreien Intervall (Abb. 37). Eine Interpretation dieser Befunde mag das Phänomen einer funktionellen und anatomischen Desaktivierung entfernter Hirnstrukturen bieten. Andererseits sind gerade diese Bereiche häufig im Anfall besonders stoffwechselaktiv (KUHL et al. 1980a; ENGEL et al. 1982a, 1983).

BERNARDI et al. (1983) bestätigten diese Ergebnisse quantitativ für den zerebralen Blutfluß (CBF), den Sauerstoff-Metabolismus ($CMRO_2$) und die Sauerstoff-Extraktionsrate (OER) mit ^{15}O-markierten Pharmaka und wiesen besonders auf gleichzeitige Veränderungen im Kleinhirn hin. Bei Epileptikern mit Psychosen wird eine medikamentös teilweise reversible Erniedrigung der Stoffwechselparameter beobachtet, besonders frontal, temporal und im Bereich der basalen Ganglien (GALLHOFER et al. 1985).

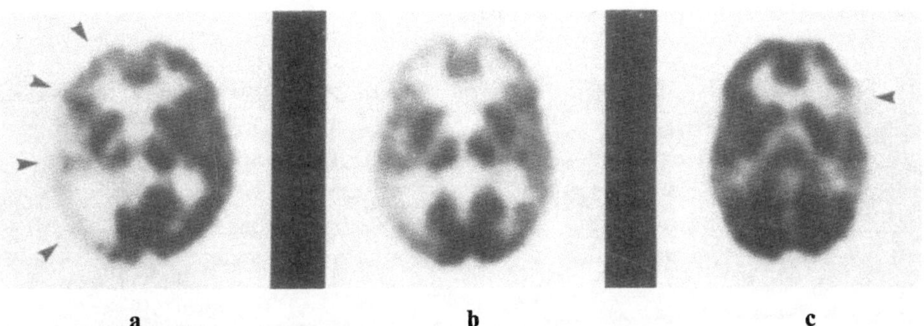

a   b   c

Abb. 36a–c. Studien des Glukose-Stoffwechsels (FDG-PET) bei Kindern mit einem Lennox-Gastaut-Syndrom im anfallsfreien Intervall. **a** 8jähriger Junge mit einem in der linken Hemisphäre diffus verminderten Glukosestoffwechsel bei unauffälligem CT, klinisch waren rechts-betonte klonische Krämpfe dominant, die von einer nachfolgenden rechtsseitigen Hemiparese begleitet wurden; **b** 6jähriges Kind mit bilateral vermindertem Glukose-Metabolismus bei diffuser kortikaler Atrophie in der CT; **c** 5jähriges Kind mit rechts-frontalem Hypometabolismus, wobei im CT lateral des Nucleus caudatus eine kleine kalzifizierte Läsion vorlag. (Aus CHUGANI et al. 1984a)

b) Anfall

Trotz der oben erwähnten meßtechnischen Limitationen wurden auch Studien über Patienten veröffentlicht, die epileptogene Herde während des Anfalles quantitativ beschreiben. Im anfallsfreien Intervall hypometabolische Läsionen, teilweise auch in der anatomischen Umgebung der Läsion, zeigten einen deutlich gesteigerten Glukose-Stoffwechsel im Bereich der Läsion und teilweise seiner Umgebung (Abb. 38). Allerdings sind diese Resultate weniger einheitlich als diejenigen, die im anfallsfreien Intervall gewonnen wurden (THEODORE et al. 1983; ENGEL et al. 1983). Ein noch ungelöstes Problem stellen insbesondere elektro-physiologisch auffällige Daten im Sinne verstärkter neuronaler Aktivität in Bereichen dar, die im

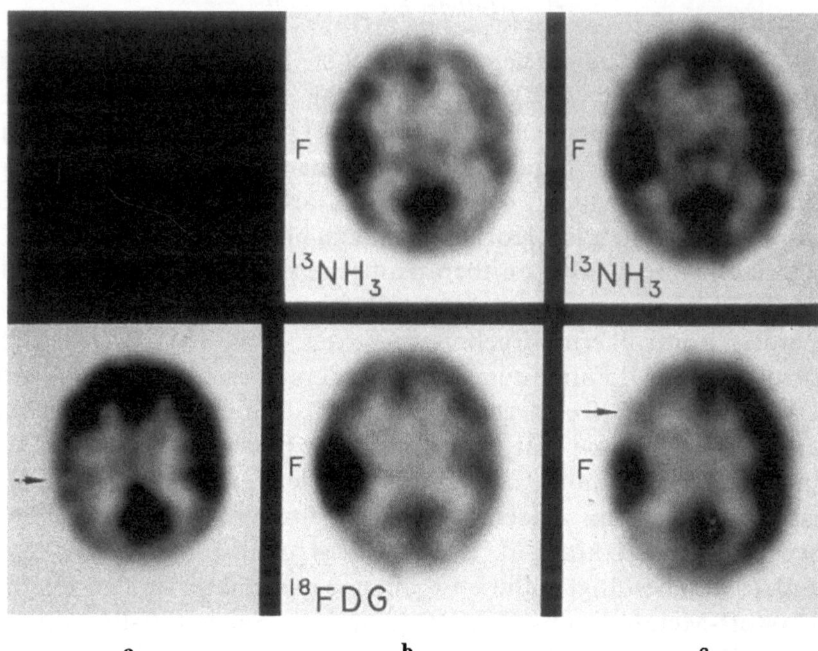

Abb. 37 a–c. Durchblutung (^{13}NH$_3$) und Glukose-Metabolismus (^{18}FDG) bei Patienten während des epileptogenen Anfalls und im anfallsfreien Intervall. Während der Fokus im anfallsfreien Intervall durch eine Läsion mit verminderter Stoffwechselaktivität charakterisiert wird (**a**) findet sich während des Anfalls (**b**) ein verstärkter Glukose-Metabolismus bei verstärkter Durchblutung. Später bilden sich hypometabole Regionen (Desaktivierungen entfernter Hirnstrukturen?) in der Umgebung des epileptogenen Fokus (**c**). (Aus Kuhl et al. 1980a)

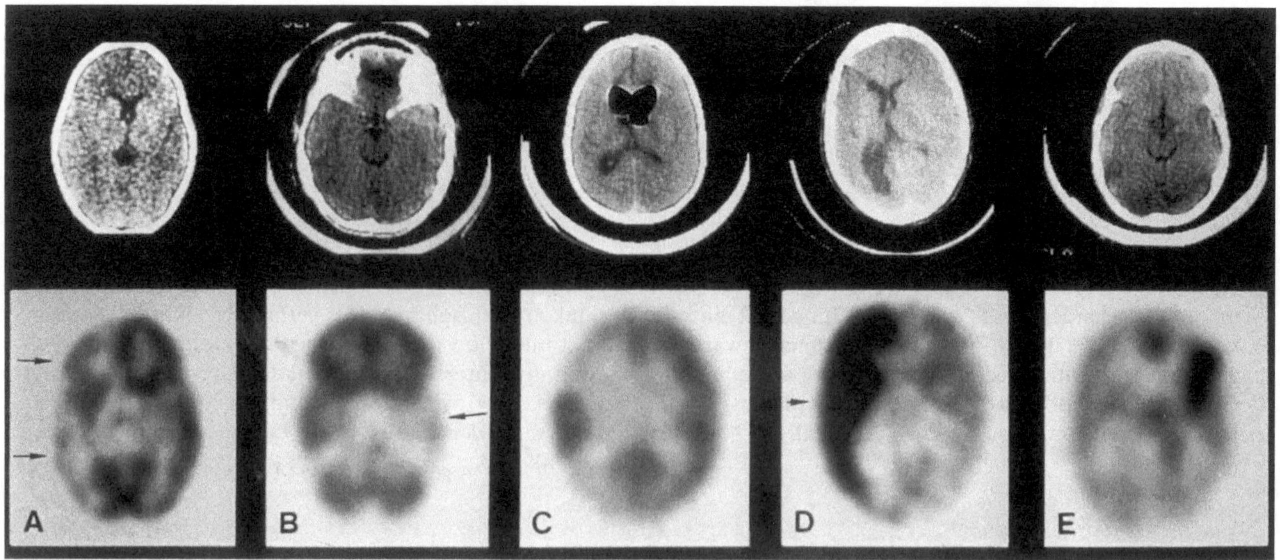

Abb. 38 A–E. Befunde in CT und ^{18}FDG-PET bei Patienten mit Epilepsie. **A** Bei einem Patienten mit nichtfokalen Anfällen fand sich im anfallsfreien Intervall eine große hypometabole Region (*Pfeile*) bei unauffälligem CT. **B** Ein Patient mit fokalen Anfällen zeigte im anfallsfreien Intervall temporal Hypometabolismus (*Pfeil*) bei normalem CT; diese fokale Stoffwechselverminderung ist typisch für epileptogene Herde (Herd im EEG bestätigt). **C** Bei einem Patienten mit motorischen Anfällen rechts zeigte das CT keine strukturellen Änderungen (Luft im Ventrikel nach Pneumenzephalographie), im PET fand sich während des Anfalls (klinisch und im EEG dokumentiert) eine starke Stoffwechselsteigerung in der linken Präzentralregion. Im anfallsfreien Intervall zeigte diese Region verminderten Stoffwechsel. **D** Bei einem Patienten mit nicht lokalisierten Anfällen fand sich im CT eine linksseitige Hemiatrophie des Gehirns. Im PET war während des

PET-Scan hypometabolisch erscheinen (GUR et al. 1985). Entsprechende Ergebnisse liegen für die zerebrale Perfusion (LCBF) und den Sauerstoff-Metabolismus ($LCMRO_2$) vor (DEPRESSEUX et al. 1984).

Wenige Patienten mit nicht fokalen Anfällen, sowie solche vor, während und nach Elektrokrampf-Therapie wegen schwerer endogener Depression, wurden insbesondere an der UCLA, Los Angeles, untersucht (Abb. 39). Die Glukoseaufnahme ist in der iktalen Phase diffus gesteigert, während sie in der postiktalen Phase insgesamt erniedrigt ist (ENGEL et al. 1982d, 1984, 1985; ENGEL 1984; GUR et al. 1982). Eine Hyperventilation allein ruft zwar Änderungen im EEG, dagegen nicht solche des regionalen Glukose-Metabolismus hervor (THEODORE et al. 1985).

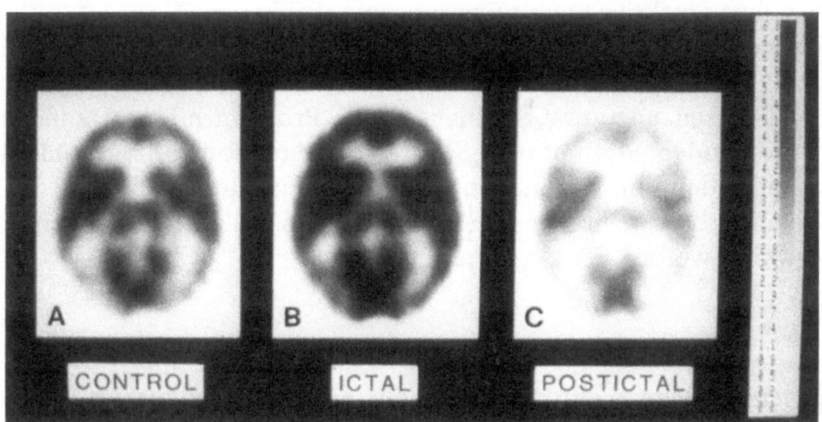

Abb. 39 A–C. [18]FDG-PET-Bilder bei einem Patienten vor, während und nach Elektrokrampftherapie wegen endogener Depression. Im Vergleich zum Kontrollbefund vor der Elektrokrampftherapie ist während des Krampfes der Glukose-Metabolismus diffus gesteigert, in der postiktalen Phase (postiktale Abflachung im EEG) besonders kortikal diffus vermindert (*Graukeil:* Angaben in mg/min/100 g) (ENGEL et al. 1983). (Nach HEISS et al. 1985b)

c) Tumorepilepsie

Obwohl epileptische Anfälle bei Hirntumoren, je nach Tumorart und Lokalisation, mit Bevorzugung der frontalen und temporalen Großhirnrinde, in 10–50% der Fälle vorkommen und die Tumorepilepsien unter den Spätepilepsien 10–20% ausmachen, liegen hier keine systematischen klinischen Studien vor (HOFMANN 1986; NEUNDÖRFER 1986).

d) Pharmaka

Die zerebrale Aufnahme von ^{11}C-markiertem Phenylhydantoin wurde bei Epileptikern (n = 10) und Kontrollpersonen untersucht. Allerdings gab es keine Unterschiede, wobei 60 min p.i. noch kein Gleichgewichtszustand der Kinetik erreicht war. Die Markierung mit längerlebigen Positronen-Strahlern, wie ^{18}F, erscheint notwendig und sinnvoll (BARON et al. 1983b–c).

Anfalls (*Pfeil*) der Stoffwechsel in der ganzen linken Hemisphäre gesteigert (im anfallsfreien Intervall vermindert). E Bei normalem CT zeigte die PET während eines fokal beginnenden und dann generalisierten Anfalls mehrere hypermetabole Herde (rechts frontal, Gyrus cinguli, Insel, rechter Thalamus, basaler temporookzipitaler Kortex) entsprechend der Ausbreitung der Krampfaktivität (UCLA, School of Medicine, nach HEISS et al. 1985b)

Von der Gruppe am NIH in Bethesda, USA, liegen Studien zur ^{18}F-FDG-Aufnahme an neun Patienten mit Schizophrenie vor und nach neuroleptischer Therapie vor. Während im Bereich des gesamten Kortex, besonders temporal und im Bereich der basalen Ganglien, der Glukose-Metabolismus gesteigert wurde, blieb der anterior-posteriore Gradient unbeeinflußt (De Lisi et al. 1985).

5. Psychosen

Fragestellung. Psychiatrische Erkrankungen repräsentieren Syndrome, die häufig in ihrer Ätiologie bisher unbekannt sind. Ihre Diagnostik basiert auf Beschreibungen nicht spezifischer Symptome ohne objektive Quantifizierungsmöglichkeiten (Kaplan et al. 1980). Unabhängig von regionalen, physiologischen Variationen bei der Bestimmung verschiedener Parameter des Hirnmetabolismus kommt bei den Fragestellungen aus dem psychiatrischen Formenkreis noch die Abgrenzung zur „Normalität" als Problem hinzu. Dennoch können mit der nicht traumatisierenden Methode der Positronen-Emissionstomographie gerade wegen der relativ geringen Bedeutung der morphologisch orientierten Techniken in Hinblick auf Ätiologie und lokalisierbare regionale Veränderungen in Zukunft erhebliche diagnostische Möglichkeiten erwartet werden (Volkow et al. 1985).

a) Schizophrenie

Die Schizophrenie ist ein nicht sehr gut definiertes Krankheitsbild, das mit der PET zuerst von Farkas et al. (1980, 1984) untersucht wurde. Buchsbaum et al. (1981, 1982, 1983, 1984) fanden bei unbehandelten Patienten Hinweise auf eine erniedrigte (60% der Norm) Glukoseaufnahme vornehmlich frontal (frontal vs. parietal) und im Bereich der basalen Ganglien, die sich unter einer geeigneten Therapie teilweise normalisierte (Wolfkin et al. 1985). Während Brodie et al. (1983, 1984) diese Ergebnisse für den Glukosemetabolismus und Bustany et al. (1983) für die Methioninaufnahme weitgehend bestätigen, machen Widen et al. (1983) darauf aufmerksam, daß bei akut erkrankten Patienten ohne neuroleptische Therapie der Stoffwechsel des frontalen Kortex weitgehend normal ist. Die oben beschriebenen Veränderungen entwickelten sich erst im chronischen Zustand unter entsprechender Therapie.

Bei zwölf Patienten mit Schizophrenie und akutem Krankheitsbild fand sich dagegen, insbesondere frontal, keine Änderung des zerebralen Blutflusses (LCBF) und des Sauerstoff-Metabolismus (LCMRO$_2$) (Sheppard et al. 1983).

b) Affektive Störungen, Zyklothymien

Entsprechende regionale Veränderungen werden bei affektiven Erkrankungen beobachtet, wobei der Glukosestoffwechsel deutlich von der Phase der Erkrankung abhängig ist (Abb. 40). Studien an kleinen Patientengruppen liegen für unipolare und bipolare Depressionen sowie manische Phasen vor (Baxter et al. 1985; Buchsbaum et al. 1984; Phelps et al. 1985a). Klinisch spontan oder nach therapeutischer Intervention unauffällige Patienten zeigen ein normales zerebrales Stoffwechselverhalten.

Neben kontrollierten Tests lassen sich insbesondere mit der Darstellung und Kinetik spezifischer Liganden, wie ^{11}C-Chlorpromazin (Comar et al. 1979) oder ^{11}C-Racloprid (Sedvall et al. 1986), Erkenntnisse zu Pathogenese und geeigneter Therapie erwarten.

Bei 10 Patienten mit Attacken panischer Angst konnten Reiman et al. (1984) im Vergleich zu 6 Kontrollpersonen zeigen, daß signifikante Hinweise auf eine Minderperfusion (LCBF) im Bereich des linken parahippokampalen Gyrus vorliegen. REIVICH et al. (1983) fanden bei einer kontrollierten Studie an 18 Patienten, daß bis zu einem definierten Maß an Angst (nach SPIELBERGER) der Glukosemetabolismus in frontalen kortikalen Strukturen ansteigt, um dann jedoch abzufallen.

RUMSEY et al. (1985) berichten über 10 erwachsene Patienten mit Autismus-Anamnese in der Kindheit. Es zeigte sich ein regional deutlich gesteigerter Glukose-Metabolismus, Minderanreicherungen von ^{18}FDG wurden bei keinem der Patienten beobachtet.

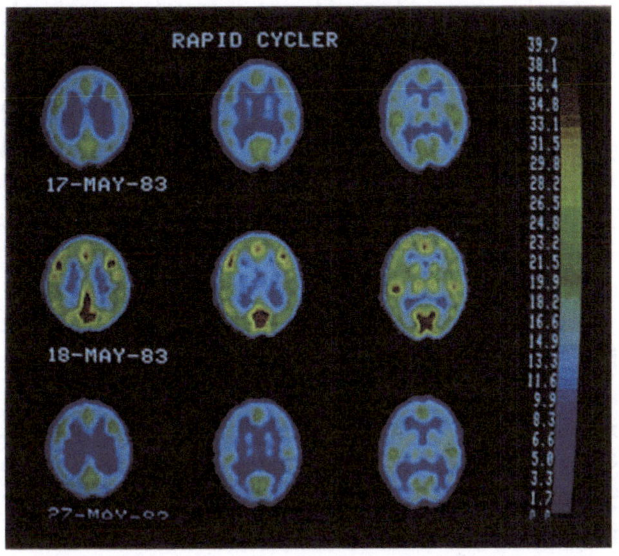

a

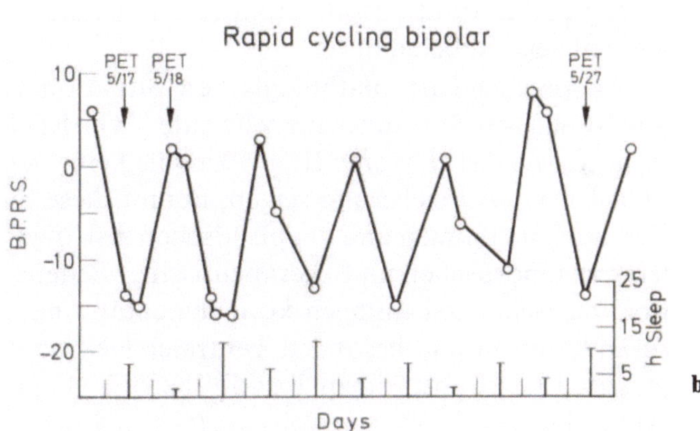

b

Abb. 40. a Affektive Störungen, Zyklothymien. Darstellung verschiedener in kurzen Zeitabständen (24–48 h) wechselnder manisch-depressiver Phasen bei einem Patienten. **b** Während in den manischen Zuständen der Glukose-Stoffwechsel relativ erhöht ist und entsprechenden Werten einer normalen Kontrollgruppe entspricht, wurde in depressiven Phasen eine globale und diffuse supratentorielle Verminderung beobachtet. Die Skalierung gibt die absoluten Werte in µmol/min/100 g an. (Aus BAXTER et al. 1985)

6. Tumoren

Fragestellung. Die Anreicherungsmechanismen von Radiopharmaka in neoplastischen Zellen können wie folgt strukturiert werden:

1. Von besonderer Bedeutung ist die Anreicherung über Stoffwechselwege, etwa wie bei der anaeroben Glykolyse, die schon WARBURG (1926) als spezifisch bei der Transformation in malignes Gewebe diskutiert hat.
2. Weiterhin existieren weniger spezifische Mechanismen, wie die Perfusion, deren Kenntnis allerdings bei speziellen Berechnungen, wie der regionalen Messung des Sauerstoffmetabolismus, eine „conditio sine qua non" ist.
3. Die metabolische Ankopplung des Tumorgewebes an das normale hirneigene Gewebe erfolgt über die Blut-Hirn-Schranke.

4. Bindungen an Rezeptoren werden gemessen und diskutiert, wie bei Untersuchungen mit spezifischen Tumormarkern, z.B. ^{18}F-5-Fluorouridin oder ^{11}C-BCNU.

a) Blut-Hirn-Schranke

Die ersten PET-Studien zur Diagnostik intrakranieller Tumoren hatten eine Beurteilung und Beschreibung der Blut-Hirn-Schranke (BBB) mit ^{68}Ga ($T_{1/2} = 68$ min) markiertem EDTA zum Inhalt (Phelps et al. 1978; Yamamoto et al. 1977). Dieser mit einer hohen Proteinbindung (Transferrin) intravasal verbleibende Tracer reichert sich in Hirntumoren entsprechend der Störung der Blut-Hirn-Schranke und der Vaskularisation an (Lambrecht 1983; Moerlein u. Welch 1981).

Im allgemeinen wird analog zu den Untersuchungen der Transmissions-Computertomographie mit Kontrastmittel die räumliche Ausdehnung der Schrankenstörung mit ^{68}Ga-EDTA oder einem ähnlichen Komplex beschrieben, wobei das peritumoröse Ödem mit der CT oder der MRI deutlicher dargestellt wird (Ericson et al. 1981, 1985; Lilja et al. 1985). Hawkins et al. (1984) machen in einer kinetischen Studie darauf aufmerksam, daß der Intravasalraum nicht vernachlässigt werden darf.

Weniger Anwendung hat bisher das Rubidium-82 ($T_{1/2} = 75$ Sek) gefunden, das wegen der relativ kurzen Halbwertszeit in erster Linie für „first pass"-Studien geeignet ist (Thomas et al. 1984; Yen et al. 1982). Das kann zu Problemen führen, da die Aufnahme des Tracers bei dieser Fragestellung flußlimitiert ist, wobei die Extraktion E nach einem Modell von Renkin (1959) und Crone (1963) über den folgenden Ausdruck abgeschätzt werden kann: $E = \exp[-P \times S/F]$, wobei $P \times S$: Permeabilitätsoberflächenprodukt und F: Fluß sind. Dennoch muß eine verminderte Perfusion nicht notwendigerweise aufgrund einer höheren Extraktionsrate zu einer vermehrten Aufnahme führen, da die Aufnahme einem Produkt aus Vaskularisierung und Extraktionsrate proportional ist und dieses, besonders in pathologischen Zuständen, teilweise unbekannt ist.

Entsprechend der pathologischen Situation zeigen die gut perfundierten Meningeome ohne Blut-Hirn-Schranke eine sehr gute ^{68}Ga-EDTA-Anreicherung. Während relativ benigne Tumore, wie Astrozytome II, großenteils keine gegenüber dem normalen Gewebe gesteigerte ^{68}Ga-EDTA-Anreicherung zeigen, nimmt diese mit zunehmendem Malignitätsgrad, wie höhergradigen Gliomen und anaplastischen Astrozytomen (III–IV), in der Regel zu. Von besonderer diagnostischer und therapeutischer Bedeutung ist, daß CT, MRI, ^{68}Ga-EDTA und Stoffwechseluntersuchungen komplementär sind, was z.B. auch die Beurteilung regressiver Veränderungen und besonders zentraler Nekrosen etwa nach einer Therapie differentialdiagnostisch gegenüber einem Rezidiv betrifft (La France et al. 1986; Schober et al. 1985a) (Abb. 41).

Untersucht wurden bisher auf Störungen der Blut-Hirn-Schranke hin Meningeome, Astrozytome, Oligoastrozytome, Gliome, Glioblastome und Metastasen, wobei die Metastasen, den unterschiedlichen Primärtumoren entsprechend, das relativ uneinheitlichste Bild bieten (Ericson et al. 1981, 1985; Ilsen et al. 1984; Herholz et al. 1985; Lilja et al. 1985; Yen et al. 1982).

Der Tumor-pH, mit ^{11}C-DMO bestimmt und definiert, ist von der normalen grauen oder weißen Substanz nicht verschieden (Rottenberg et al. 1985).

Jarden et al. (1985) untersuchten in einer kinetischen Studie den Transport von ^{82}Rb vom Blut in normales Hirngewebe und in Tumorgewebe. Dabei wurde insbesondere der Effekt der Dexamethason-Therapie und perkutanen Radiatio analysiert. Sie schließen aus ihren Beobachtungen, daß Kortikosteroide die Permeabilität gerade der Tumorkapillaren für kleine hydrophile Moleküle, auch für Zytostatika, erniedrigen, und bei Bestrahlungen eine so induzierte Steigerung der Permeabilität verhindern.

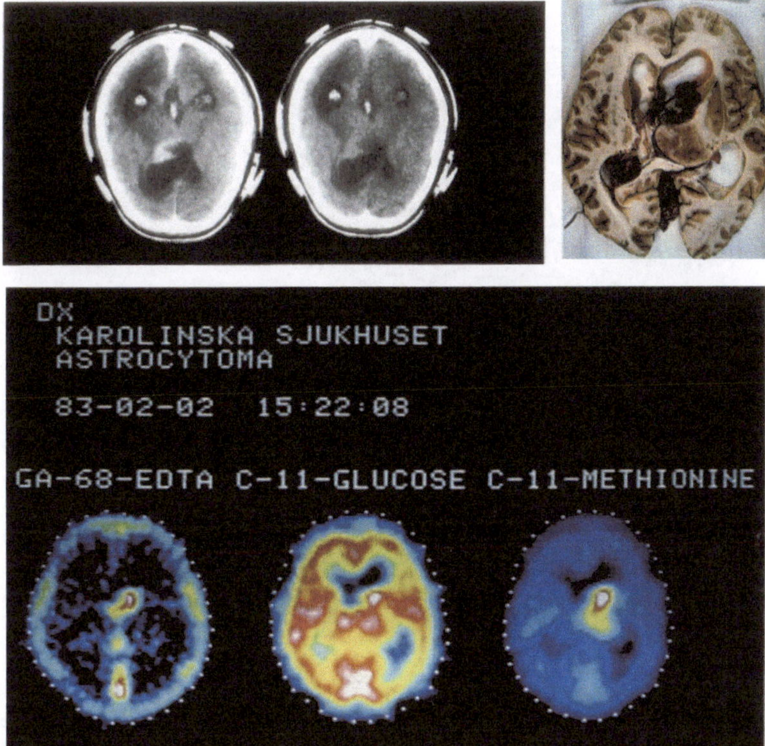

Abb. 41. Bei einem Patienten mit einem Astrozytom II zeigt die PET-Studie mit ^{68}Ga-EDTA nur relativ geringe Störungen der Blut-Hirn-Schranke an. Der Glukosestoffwechsel, berechnet über die ^{11}C-Methyl-Glukose-Aufnahme, ist gegenüber dem normalen Hirngewebe im Tumorbereich vermindert. Im ^{11}C-L-Methionin-PET ist die Aufnahme der Aminosäure, angegeben als Maß für die Proteinsynthese, ausgedehnter als mit ^{68}Ga-EDTA erhöht. (Aus BERGSTRÖM et al. 1983)

b) Blutfluß, Blutvolumen, Sauerstoffmetabolismus

Veränderungen des regionalen oder lokalen zerebralen Blutflusses (LCBF) und des regionalen Blutvolumens (LCBV), verglichen mit dem regionalen Sauerstoff (LCMRO$_2$)- oder Glukosemetabolismus (LCMRGc) in Tumorgewebe und im benachbarten Hirngewebe, sind insbesondere von den Gruppen am Hammersmith Hospital, London, am National Institute of Health, Bethesda, USA, und am Massachusetts General Hospital, Boston, USA, mitgeteilt worden (ACKERMAN et al. 1981b; BROOKS et al. 1986; DI CHIRO et al. 1982; LAMMERTSMA et al. 1981a, 1983).

Bei Patienten mit Gliomen wurde keine Korrelation zwischen dem lokalen zerebralen Blutfluß (LCBF) und dem lokalen Sauerstoffmetabolismus gefunden (ACKERMAN 1981b). Die Gruppe am Hammersmith Hospital fand regionale Unterschiede bzgl. des Glukose- und Sauerstoffmetabolismus und konnte anaerobe und aerobe Glykolyse innerhalb eines Tumors (Astrozytom IV) zeigen sowie ein gegenüber normalem Hirngewebe zusätzliches Glukosestoffwechselkompartment definieren. Sie führen dieses auf einen ineffektiven Phosphorilierungs-Dephosphorilierungs-Zyklus oder eine unspezifische Traceraufnahme zurück (Abb. 42) (BROOKS et al. 1986). Insgesamt weisen die Untersuchungen bei malignen Hirntumoren (Gliom, n=7) häufig bei einer Verminderung der Sauerstoffextraktion (OER: 0.21 ± 0.07 Tumorgewebe vs. 0.47 ± 0.05 kontralateraler Kortex) und des Sauerstoffmetabolismus bei weitgehend erhaltener Perfusion auf eine anaerobe Glykolyse hin, während im

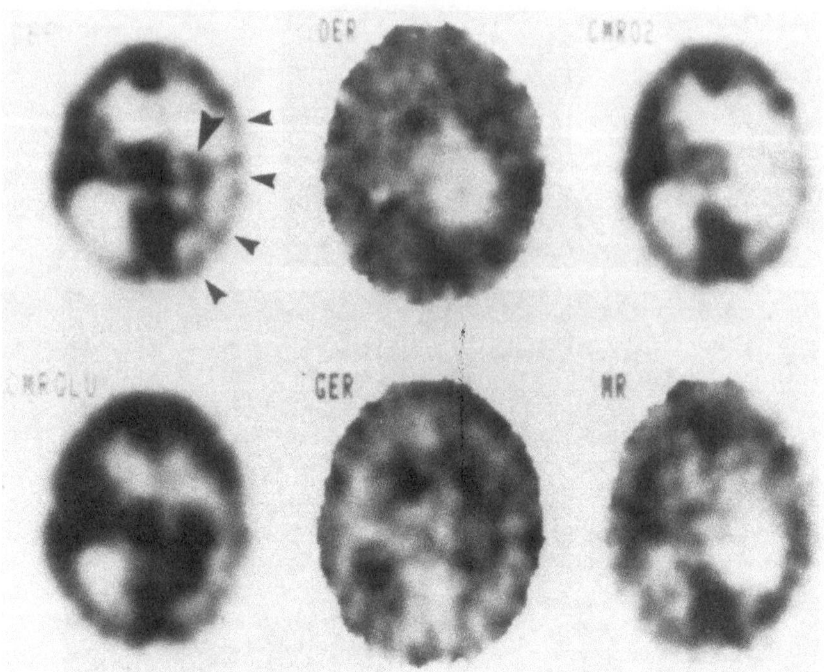

Abb. 42. Metabolische Parameter eines Patienten mit Astrozytom IV. Während der zerebrale Blutfluß (*CBF*) eine inhomogene, heterogene Verteilung zeigt (Gebiet des Tumors: *großer Pfeil*), ist der Fluß über der entsprechenden kortikalen Region diffus erniedrigt (*kleine Pfeile*). Sauerstoffextraktionsrate (*OER*) und Sauerstoffmetabolismus (*CMRO₂*) sind bei weitgehend normaler Perfusion im Tumorgebiet vermindert. Im angrenzenden Kortex sind im Sinne eines „mismatch" die OER normal, die $CMRO_2$ dagegen erniedrigt. Im Glukose-PET werden ein erhöhter Stoffwechsel (*CMRGLU*) und eine erhöhte Glukose-Extraktion (*GER*) im Tumorgebiet deutlich. Das niedrige Utilisationsverhältnis (*MR*: O_2/Glukose) weist auf eine Verschiebung vom oxidativen zum anaeroben Metabolismus. (Aus Rhodes et al. 1983)

peritumorösen Gewebe LCBF und $LCMRO_2$ erniedrigt sind. Bei einem Meningeom scheint der CBF bei normalem Sauerstoffmetabolismus erhöht zu sein (Ito et al. 1982; Lammertsma et al. 1981; Rhodes et al. 1981, 1983).

c) Glukosemetabolismus

Größere Studien an insgesamt mehr als 100 Patienten liegen über den Glukosemetabolismus hirneigener Tumoren vor, insbesondere von den Gruppen am NIH, Bethesda (Di Chiro et al. 1982, 1983, 1984, 1985; Patronas et al. 1982), am Hammersmith Hospital, London (Rhodes et al. 1983) und am Karolinska, Stockholm (Ericson et al. 1985; Kato et al. 1985). Die metabolischen Raten korrelieren mit dem Malignitätsgrad der Tumoren und damit auch der Prognose der Patienten, wenn die Gebiete höchster Traceranreicherung berücksichtigt und Nekrosen und Zysten ausgespart werden. Letztere sind insbesondere differentialdiagnostisch gegenüber Rezidiven durch morphologische Verfahren wie der CT häufig nicht exakt abzugrenzen (Patronas et al. 1985; La France et al. 1986). Während in Tumoren niedrigen Malignitätsgrades der Glukosestoffwechsel mit 23 ± 9 µmol/min/100 g dem der weißen Hirnsubstanz relativ nahe kommt und teilweise gegenüber der normalen benachbarten Substanz erniedrigt ist, findet man die maximale Glukoseaufnahme bei Grad IV Astrozytomen und Glioblastomen mit 46 ± 21 µmol/min/100 g deutlich, insgesamt etwa um einen Faktor 2, erhöht (Di Chiro et al. 1983). Ähnliche Beobachtungen wurden für nicht-gliomatöse zerebrale Tumore beschrieben (Hatazawa et al. 1981).

Diese Ergebnisse entsprechen Schlußfolgerungen aus in-vitro-Studien (WEBER 1977), in denen für schnell wachsende Tumorzellen eine verstärkte Hexokinase-Aktivität gefunden wurde. Die Quantifizierbarkeit der Meßergebnisse für pathologische Gewebe hängt allerdings von der Validität des physiologischen Modells ab. Insbesondere müssen Einflüsse durch Störungen der Blut-Hirn-Schranke, Veränderungen der „lumped constant" und der einzelnen Transportkonstanten berücksichtigt werden (HAWKINS et al. 1983a; PHELPS 1981; RHODES et al. 1983). Insofern sind Verfahren zu einer direkten Bestimmung der kinetischen Konstanten und der Abschätzung der lokalen Glukose-Extraktionsrate, wie sie für Probleme bei zerebrovaskulären Erkrankungen entwickelt wurden, von besonderer Bedeutung (GJEDDE u. DIEMER 1985; HAWKINS et al. 1981; WIENHARD et al. 1985). In einem Homogenisat von „low grade"- und „high grade"-Gliomen führten GRAHAM et al. (1985) kinetische Studien mit ^{18}F-FDG durch. Sie fanden in „high grade"-Gliomen eine verstärkte Hexokinase-Aktivität, die über reversible subzelluläre Kompartimente gesteuert wird.

Wie bei Patienten mit fokaler zerebraler Ischämie werden auch bei mehr als 50% der Patienten mit Hirntumoren funktionelle Desaktivierungen entfernter Hirnstrukturen nach Unterbrechung verbindender Nervenbahnen (kortiko-thalamo-ponto-olivo-zerebellares System) beobachtet (DI CHIRO et al. 1981; PATRONAS et al. 1984). Inwieweit diese häufig mit EEG-Veränderungen korrelierenden Phänomene, z.B. die zerebellare Diaschisis und die ipsilaterale thalamische Depression, Gesamtklinik und Rehabilitationsmaßnahmen beeinflussen, wird seit den Erstbeschreibungen durch VON MONAKOW (1914) und für Hirntumoren durch RIESE (1947) diskutiert (BARON et al. 1981d; HEISS 1983b; KUHL et al. 1980b; PATRONAS et al. 1984).

Eine partielle Reversibilität der Einschränkung des kontralateralen Flusses und Sauerstoffmetabolismus nach Dekompression durch Kraniotomie und Biopsie wird bei 14 Patienten mit verschiedenen Hirntumoren beschrieben (BEANEY et al. 1985; BEANEY u. LAMMERTSMA 1985).

d) Aminosäuremetabolismus

Im zentralen Nervensystem sind freie Aminosäuren Vorläufer (precursor) und katabolische Produkte der Proteine, aber auch Vorläufer bioaktiver Amine. Ziel der Studien mit markierten Aminosäuren ist eine regionale Quantifizierbarkeit der Proteinsynthese, die nur eine geringe Abhängigkeit vom funktionalen Zustand des Gehirns hat, oder zumindest ein Maß für das zu finden, was einen wesentlichen Teil der Proteinsynthese ausmacht.

^{11}C-markierte Aminosäuren, DL-Valin und DL-Tryptophan, wurden zuerst von SMITH et al. (1980) und HÜBNER et al. (1982) zum metabolischen „mapping" von Hirntumoren verwandt.

Aus in-vitro-Studien (ROGERS et al. 1978; SHIBASIKI et al. 1979) und diätetischen Untersuchungen (GADISSEUX et al. 1984) ist bekannt, daß Methionin bei Gliomen und sekundären Hirntumoren die höchsten Tumor/Nicht-Tumor-Gewebeverhältnisse aufweist. Darüberhinaus wurde für Methionin eine hohe Extraktionsrate im Gehirn gefunden, die nur von Phenylalanin, Leucin und Tyrosin übertroffen wird (ROBERTS 1968; OLDENDORF et al. 1981). Verglichen mit anderen Aminosäuren ist die Menge freien L-Methionins im Hirngewebe relativ gering.

In einer Fallstudie zeigten BERGSTRÖM et al. (1983) qualitative und quantitative Unterschiede in der CT-Darstellung, verglichen mit der PET, wobei ^{68}Ga-EDTA, ^{11}C-Glukose und die nicht razemische Form von ^{11}C-L-Methionin als Radiopharmaka verwendet wurden (Abb. 41).

SCHOBER et al. (1985a, b, 1986a) nahmen theoretische Überlegungen von BUSTANY et al. (1983) und PHELPS et al. (1984) auf, und untersuchten in einer kontrollierten prospektiven Studie bei 36 Patienten mit Hirntumoren und sechs Patienten mit Hirninfarkt die relative

Aufnahme von ^{11}C-Methyl-L-Methionin (Abb. 43–45). Die ^{11}C-Aufnahme (T/NT: Tumor/ kontralateral Non-Tumor) korrelierte mit dem Malignitätsgrad primärer hirneigener supratentorieller Tumoren und war bei einem Glioblastom IV (T/NT = 3.2) am höchsten (Abb. 46). Bei den Infarkten wurde eine erniedrigte Aufnahme gefunden. Die konventionelle Hirnszintigraphie (^{99m}Tc-DTPA) zeigte bei zwei Patienten mit Tumor und den 6 Patienten mit Infarkt eine Störung der Blut-Hirn-Schranke ohne bzw. mit geringerer Methionin-Aufnahme als im kontralateralen normalen Hirngewebe, während die Patienten mit Astrozytom II bei negativem ^{99m}Tc-DTPA-Scan, teilweise ohne direkte Darstellung im CT, einen positiven Befund bei der PET boten.

Ohne klinische und zusätzliche Informationen morphologisch orientierter Verfahren läßt sich aber mit der Methionin-PET-Szintigraphie keine Artdiagnose betreiben, wie auch die ähnlichen Kontraste primärer und sekundärer Tumoren zeigen (Abb. 46).

Die Hannoversche Arbeitsgruppe konnte zeigen, daß sich PET, MRI und CT in ihren Aussagen bezüglich Nachweis und Ausdehnung von Tumorgewebe und Ödem ergänzen (Abb. 45). Diese Beobachtungen wurden unabhängig von den Gruppen am Karolinska, Stockholm (Ericson et al. 1985; Lilja et al. 1985) und in Orsay-Paris (Bustany et al. 1983a, 1986) an insgesamt mehr als 40 Patienten mit supratentoriellen Tumoren bestätigt. Auch Ericson et al. (1985) wiesen darauf hin, daß die Methionin-Aufnahme unabhängig von einer Kontrast-Anhebung im CT oder einer positiven Anreicherung von ^{68}Ga-EDTA im Sinne einer Störung der Blut-Hirn-Schranke war. Weiterhin war die relative Methionin-Aufnahme in Hirntumoren deutlicher als die der Glukose, wie auch die Hannoversche Arbeitsgruppe bestätigen konnte (Abb. 47). Eine Sonderrolle spielen wegen ihrer histologischen Struktur die Meningeome, die besonders kontrastreich dargestellt werden. Dieses ist bei fehlender Blut-Hirn-Schranke und Hyperperfusion erklärbar.

Der Wert der semiquantitativen ^{11}C-Methionin-PET wird insbesondere in der präoperativen Vorbereitung und in der Verlaufskontrolle bei der Therapie, z.B. der Differentialdiagnose

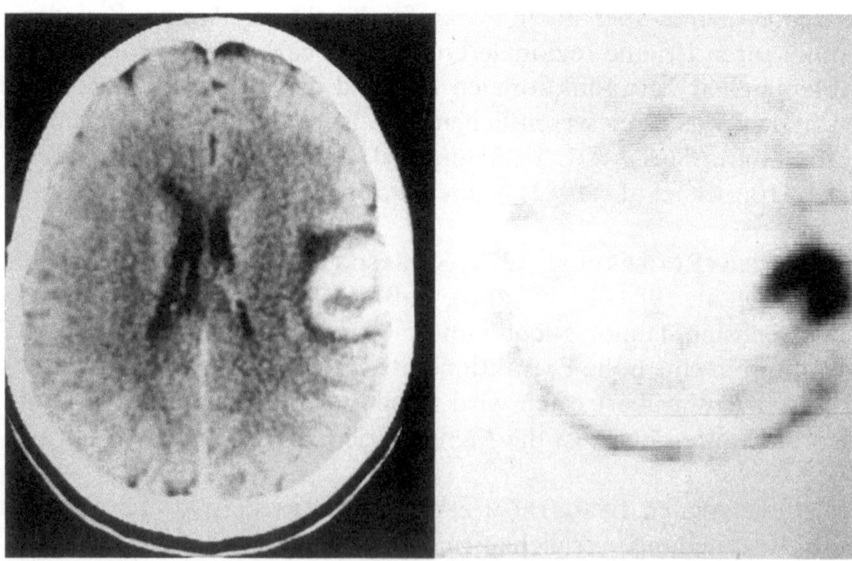

Abb. 43. Vergleichender Befund mit der Computertomographie (*CT*) nach Kontrastmittel-Applikation und der Positronen-Emissionstomographie (*PET*) mit ^{11}C-L-Methionin. In den frontalen Abschnitten des Tumors war die Methionin-Aufnahme als Maß für den Transport der Aminosäure mit einem T/NT-Wert (Tumor/ Non-Tumor) von 2.1 deutlich erhöht, nicht jedoch in den umliegenden Ödemzonen und der zentralen Nekrosezone. Histologisch ergab sich postoperativ der Befund eines Glioblastom IV

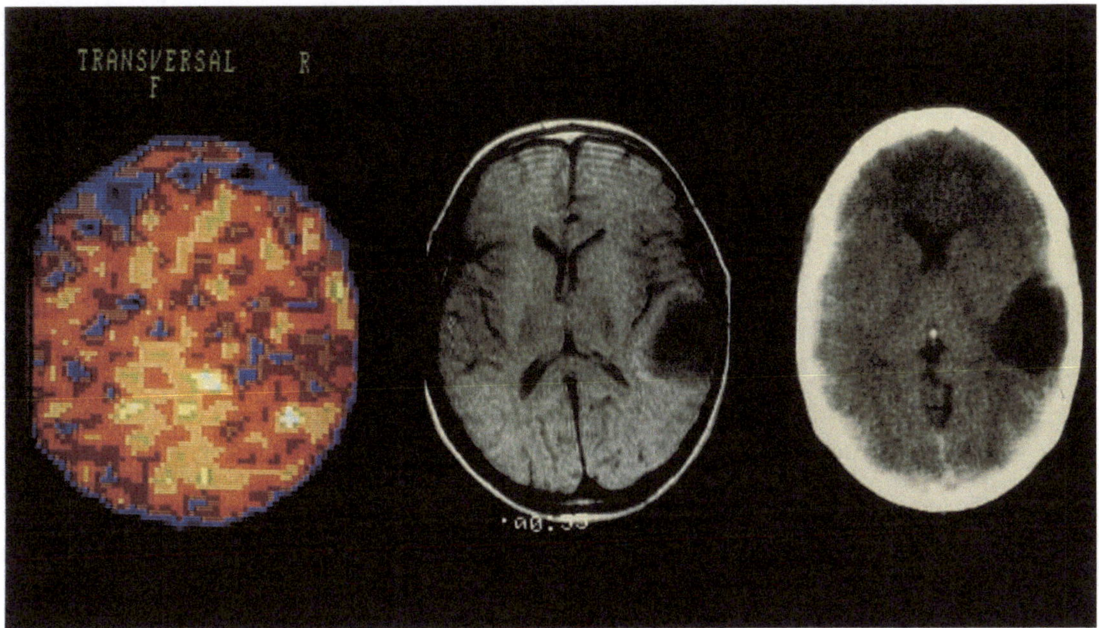

Abb. 44. Die morphologischen Abbildungsverfahren CT (*rechts*) und MRI (*Mitte*) führen zu der Differentialdiagnose Arachnoidalzyste vs. hirneigener Tumor vs. Erweichungsherd. Im ^{11}C-L-Methionin PET (*links*)
ist die Methionin-Aufnahme leicht vermindert, aber homogen verteilt. Mit einem T/NT-Wert (Tumor/Non-
Tumor) von 0.9 spricht der PET-Befund eher für einen niedriggradigen malignen Tumor als für eine Zyste.
Der histologische Befund ergab ein solides, abgekapseltes Astrozytom II

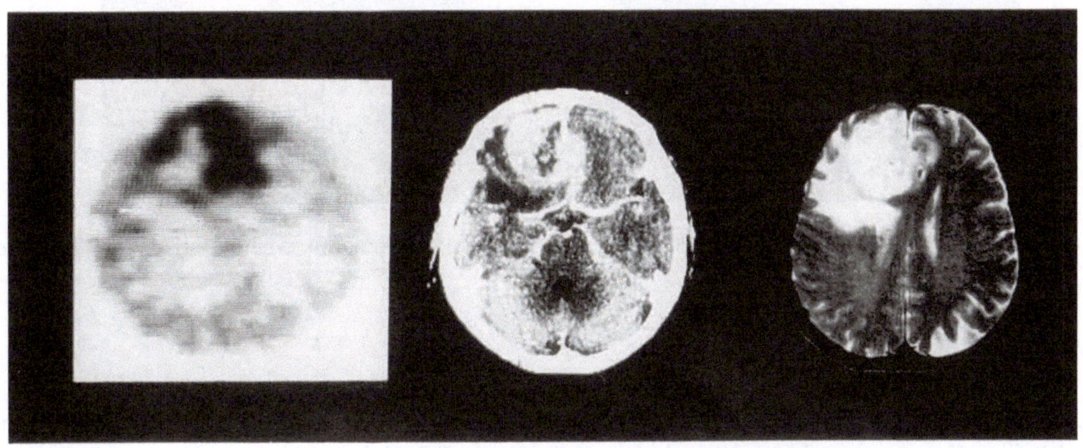

Abb. 45. Ein Patient mit einem Astrozytom IV, temporo-parieto-okzipital rechts, mit Infiltration der Mittelli-
nie und intensiver Kontrastanhebung nach Applikation von Kontrastmittel (*CT*). Das MRI-Bild zeigt im
T_2-gewichteten Spinechomode (TR/TE = 1600/204 msek) eine hohe Signalintensität in der Tumorregion. Im
Gegensatz zum CT-Befund erscheint auch die linke Seite infiltriert. Dieses wird auch im Methionin-PET-Scan
deutlich und semiquantitativ dokumentiert. (Aus SCHOBER et al. 1985a)

Strahlennekrose vs. Rezidiv gesehen. Ähnliche Ergebnisse werden von der ^{18}F-FDG-PET
von der Gruppe am NIH, Bethesda, mitgeteilt (LA FRANCE et al. 1986). Neuere Arbeiten
von DIKSIC et al. (1984) und TYLER et al. (1986) berichten vom Wert der regionalen, quantitativen ^{11}C-Harnstoff und ^{11}C-BCNU-Diagnostik mit der PET.

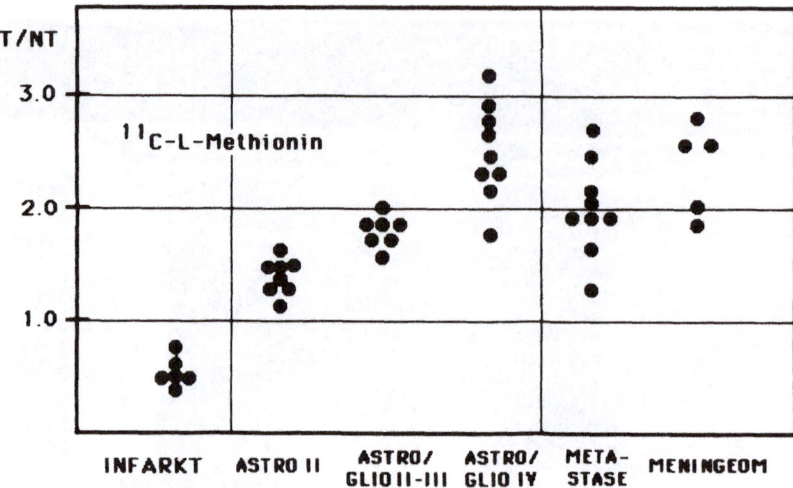

Abb. 46. T/NT-Werte (Tumor/Non-Tumor) der ^{11}C-L-Methionin-Positronen-Emissionstomographie bei verschiedenen Hirntumoren und Infarkten

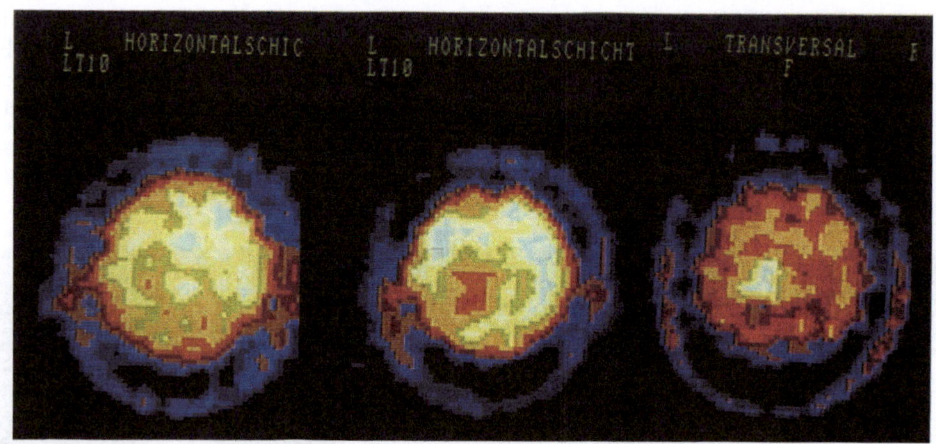

Abb. 47. $H_2{}^{15}O$, ^{18}F-FDG, ^{11}C-L-Methionin-PET bei einem Patienten mit einem Astrozytom III, hochparietal

Das komplexe Schicksal intravenös injizierten ^{11}C-Methyl-L-Methionins, besonders wenn die S-Methyl-Gruppe markiert ist, wird in Abschnitt B.VII beschrieben. Wir schließen aus den Analysen, daß vorerst eine Angabe des Proteinmetabolismus in absoluten Größen und Angaben kinetischer Konstanten nicht sinnvoll erscheint (Bustany et al. 1981; Meyer et al. 1985; Phelps et al. 1984).

II. Herz

1. Physiologie

a) Einleitung

Die Betrachtungsweise der physiologischen Grundlagen in der Kardiologie hat sich in den letzten 30–40 Jahren von der Basis des klinischen Bildes und der Pathologie zu einer quantitativen und rationellen Diagnostik und Therapie entwickelt. Ausgangspunkt dieses Wandels sind diagnostische Methoden, sowie eine Strukturierung der Herzfunktion in ihre *hämodynamischen Leistungen als Pumpe* und die dazu notwendigen *metabolischen Muskelfunktionen* mit dem Koronarkreislauf, dem Stoffwechsel und dem Kontraktionsverhalten.

Während die Drucke im Rahmen einer invasiven Herzkatheter-Untersuchung bestimmt werden, können derzeit die globalen Volumina mit Indikatorverdünnungsmethoden, regionale Werte mit der Angiokardiographie, der Computertomographie (CT), dem Ultraschall (US), der Kernspintomographie (MRI) und der Funktionsszintigraphie bestimmt werden.

Von den charakterisierenden physiologischen Parametern der regionalen Muskelfunktion wird die Durchblutung mit der Koronarangiographie, markierten Tracern und Kaliumanalogen untersucht. Zu Stoffwechseluntersuchungen stehen von den Gammastrahlern in der Klinik nur ^{123}I-markierte Fettsäuren zur Verfügung. Das regionale Kontraktionsverhalten kann mit der Angiokardiographie und der Computertomographie sowie der Sonographie beurteilt werden. Indirekte Hinweise gibt hierzu das EKG (LICHTLEN et al. 1979, 1985; SCHICHA 1986; SCHICHA u. EMRICH 1983).

Der Beitrag der Nuklearmedizin begann bereits 1927 mit Arbeiten von BLUMGART u. WEISS mit Radium C, während PRINZMETAL et al. (1948) erste Untersuchungen mit ^{24}Na durchführten, die die Bezeichnung Radiokardiographie verdienten. Die Entwicklung führte über Studien von FUCKS u. KNIPPING (1955), ANGER (1958) und HARPER et al. (1965) zu STRAUSS et al. (1971), die die Problematik der zeitlich sich verändernden Geometrie mit der Anwendung EKG-getriggerter Aufnahmen angingen. Bei der Beurteilung des Herzmuskels führt der Weg von SAPIRSTEIN et al. (1956) mit der Verwendung von ^{42}K über KAWANA et al. (1970) mit der Einführung des ^{201}Tl zur klinischen Anwendung durch LEBOWITZ et al. (1975) (SCHICHA u. EMRICH 1983).

Mit der Positronen-Emissionstomographie wurde eine nicht invasive, regionale und quantitative Bestimmung biologischer Tracer in Abhängigkeit von der Zeit möglich, nachdem bis dahin nur „in-vitro"-Studien und invasive „in-situ"-Tierexperimente zu vergleichbaren Aussagen geführt haben. Die intrakoronare Injektion von ^{133}Xe oder $^{81m/85}$Kr bietet mit den inhärenten Problemen der Gamma-Strahler begrenzte Möglichkeiten der Bestimmung des absoluten regionalen Blutflusses (CANNON et al. 1972; KLEIN et al. 1965; LICHTLEN et al. 1985).

Technische Randbedingungen in Verbindung mit der Positronen-Emissionstomographie, insbesondere Probleme des Auflösungsvermögens, des respiratorischen und kardialen Gating, werden in Abschnitt C beschrieben und diskutiert.

b) Fluß und Perfusion

Primär ist für die Aufrechterhaltung der Pumpfunktion ein intakter Koronarkreislauf notwendig. Der myokardiale Blutfluß beträgt beim Gesunden etwa 80–100 ml/min/100 g und sichert einen Sauerstoffmetabolismus von etwa 25–30 ml O_2/min. Wegen des niedrigen venösen Sauerstoffpartialdruckes wird ein vermehrter Sauerstoffverbrauch fast ausschließlich über einen weiten Bereich durch eine Erhöhung des Koronarflusses gewährleistet. Insofern korrelieren und entsprechen Messungen der Blutflusses denjenigen des Sauerstoff-Angebotes.

Eine nicht-invasive Quantifizierung der regionalen myokardialen Perfusion unter Ruhe- und Belastungsbedingungen ist von besonderer klinischer Bedeutung bei der Charakterisierung der koronaren Herzerkrankung und zur objektiven Beurteilung pharmakologischer und interventioneller Therapien. PET-Studien mit kurzlebigen Radiopharmaka (^{15}O, ^{13}N) sind insofern zu aufeinanderfolgenden Messungen, etwa der quantitativen Bestimmung der regionalen Koronarreserve, besonders geeignet (s. Abschn. B.III.).

α) *Mikrosphären.* Zur Verfügung stehen mit ^{68}Ga (Beller et al. 1979; Wisenberg et al. 1981), ^{62}Cu oder ^{11}C (Selwyn et al. 1984; Wilson et al. 1983, 1984) markierte Albumin-Mikrosphären, die als nahezu optimale Tracer zur Bestimmung der Perfusion über einen weiten physiologischen Bereich (0–450 ml/min/100 g) weitgehend im „first pass" im arteriolaren oder kapillaren Gefäßbett extrahiert (Trapping) werden. Weniger als 3% der Mikrosphären (9 µm $\varnothing$) passieren das myokardiale Endstromgebiet über arterio-venöse Shunts oder kapilläre Passagen.

Wegen der invasiven Applikation in den linken Ventrikel oder linken Vorhof haben diese Radiopharmaka aber in der Klinik nur eine begrenzte Bedeutung (Hnatowich et al. 1975, 1976). Eine der entscheidenden Randbedingungen ist, daß der Einstrom flußäquivalent markiert sein muß („mixing", Aggregation der Mikrosphären). Berücksichtigt werden müssen weiterhin mögliche biologische Nebenwirkungen. Ansonsten erfordert die Quantifizierung eine Kenntnis des Blutflusses (Flow) in einem Referenzorgan mit arterieller Blutentnahme. Gerade bei Tierexperimenten gilt diese Methode als der „Goldene Standard" (Beller et al. 1979, 1982; Fan et al. 1979; Geltman et al. 1985; Jugdutt et al. 1979).

β) *Sapirstein.* Der zweite Ansatz zur Bestimmung des Blutflusses geht davon aus, daß intravenös applizierte Tracer, wie Kationen, von allen Zellen des Organismus in der gleichen Weise unabhängig vom Fluß und verschiedenen metabolischen Parametern aufgenommen und freigelassen werden (Sapirstein 1956, 1958). Der regionale Fluß wird dann aus dem Anteil des Herzzeitvolumens errechnet. Zu diesen Tracern gehören Thallium, Cäsium, aber auch die Positronen-Strahler $^{81/82}$Rb, ^{38}K, ^{13}NH$_3$/^{13}NH$_4^+$, ^{38}K oder ^{52m}Mn (Abb. 48–50) (Atcher et al. 1980; Atkins et al. 1979; Beller et al. 1982; Budinger et al. 1975; Budinger 1979; Grant et al. 1975; Myers 1973).

^{13}NH$_3$/^{13}NH$_4^+$ wurde von Walsh et al. (1976, 1977) und Schelbert et al. (1979) schon wegen der relativ kurzen physikalischen Halbwertzeit ($T_{1/2} = 10$ min) als Tracer zur Darstel-

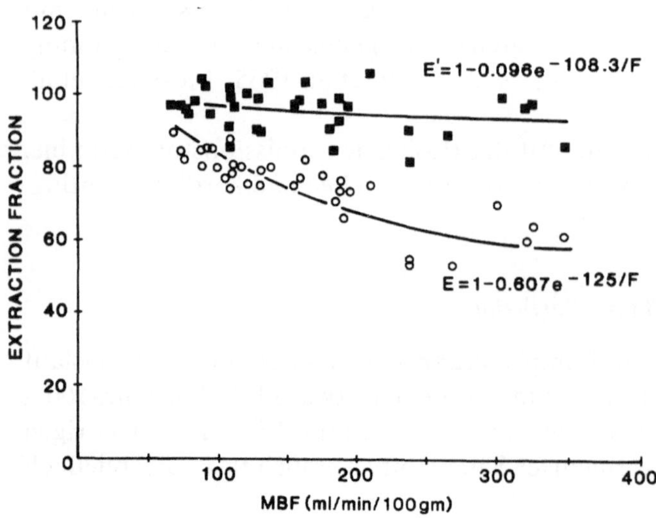

Abb. 48. Relative initiale kapilläre Extraktionsfraktion (E', ■) und Retentionsfraktion (E, o) von Ammoniak (^{13}NH$_4^+$) im Myokard, verglichen mit der regionalen myokardialen Perfusion. (Aus Schelbert et al. 1981)

lung der regionalen myokardialen Perfusion vorgeschlagen. Bei physiologischem pH liegt das $^{13}NH_3$ zu 95% in der Form des Ammoniak, $^{13}NH_4^+$, vor. Wegen der schnellen Konversion innerhalb von 20 µsek ist das Kation bei Transitzeiten in der Größenordnung von 2–3 Sekunden als transkapillärer Tracer geeignet (BUDINGER et al. 1975; HARPER et al. 1972, 1973; LOVE u. BURCH 1959; POE 1972; SCHELBERT et al. 1981; SCHELBERT u. SCHWAIGER 1986; WALSH et al. 1977; WEICH et al. 1977).

Die Gewebe-Clearance ($T_{1/2}$) wird mit 80–400 min angegeben. 2–3 min nach der Applikation stellt bei Vernachlässigung der Rezirkulation die $^{13}NH_3/^{13}NH_4^+$ Anreicherung ein Maß für die regionale Verteilung des myokardialen Blutflusses dar. Die anfängliche kapilläre Extraktion erreicht fast 100%, wegen der Rückdiffusion muß die relative Retention aber mit etwa 80% angenommen werden, und liegt damit in der gleichen Größenordnung wie Kalium (K^+) mit etwa 70% (POE 1972). Als entscheidender Trapping-Mechanismus wird die Glutamat-Glutamin-Reaktion angenommen (KRIVOKAPICH et al. 1983). BERGMAN et al. (1980) diskutieren die Abhängigkeit der Aufnahme des $^{13}NH_3/^{13}NH_4^+$ von hämodynamischen und metabolischen Randbedingungen, wie dem pH. Es ist bisher nicht ausreichend untersucht, ob der beobachtete geringe Einfluß auch für chronische myokardiale Ischämien oder Kardiomyopathien gilt.

Nach der ersten Anwendung durch HARPER et al. (1972) berichteten WALSH et al. (1976) von Untersuchungen bei Patienten mit kardialer Ischämie. Bei den diffusiblen Tracern ist die Extraktion eine Funktion des Flusses; der klinischen Anwendung sind aber erst bei teilweise unphysiologisch hohen Flüssen Grenzen gesetzt, wobei sich die Netto-Extraktion aus dem Produkt der Retentionsfraktion und dem Fluß errechnet (Abb. 51) (SCHELBERT et al. 1979, 1981; SHAH et al. 1985). In diesem Sinne sind einige Grundvoraussetzungen zum Modell von SAPIRSTEIN nicht streng erfüllt.

Klinische Studien liegen vor über Dipyridamol-induzierte Untersuchungen der Koronarreserve, wobei die $^{13}NH_3/^{13}NH_4^+$-Aufnahme mit der Thermo-Farbstoff-Methode verglichen wurde (BROWN et al. 1981; SCHELBERT et al. 1982a, b).

γ) $^{81/82}Rb$, ^{82}Sr-^{82}Rb. Im „first pass" werden mehr als 50% des applizierten Rubidiums extrahiert. Wegen der relativ günstigen physikalischen Halbwertzeit des ^{82}Sr ($T_{1/2}=23$ d) kann das ^{82}Rb ($T_{1/2}=78$ sec) auch an Kliniken ohne eigenes Zyklotron benutzt werden. Schon aus diesen logistischen Gründen hat das Rubidium in der PET eine Bedeutung erhalten (Abb. 49) (BELLER et al. 1982; KNOEBEL et al. 1978; LOVE u. BURCH 1959).

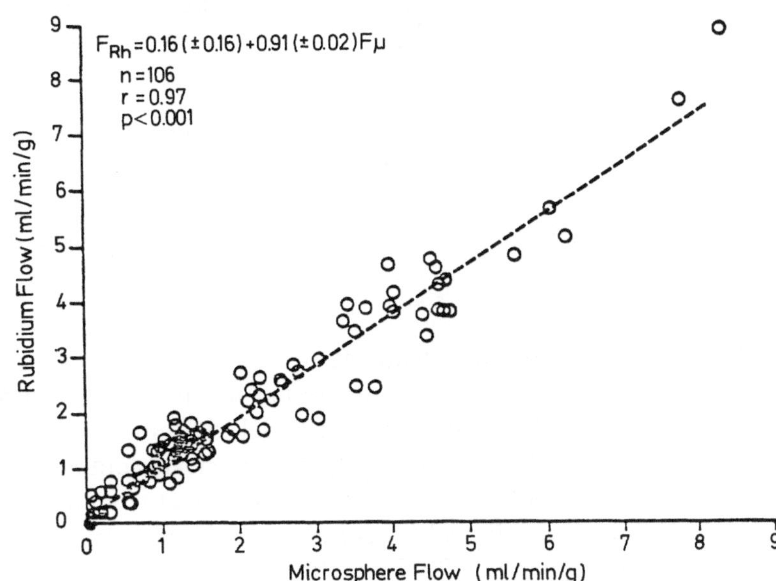

Abb. 49. Bestimmung der regionalen myokardialen Perfusion mit Mikroaggregaten verglichen mit einem First-pass-Extraktionsverfahren (^{82}Rb) über einen weiten Perfusionsbereich beim Hund. *Fµ*: Sample Volumen, *gestrichelte Linie:* Regressionsgrade. (Aus GOLDSTEIN et al. 1983)

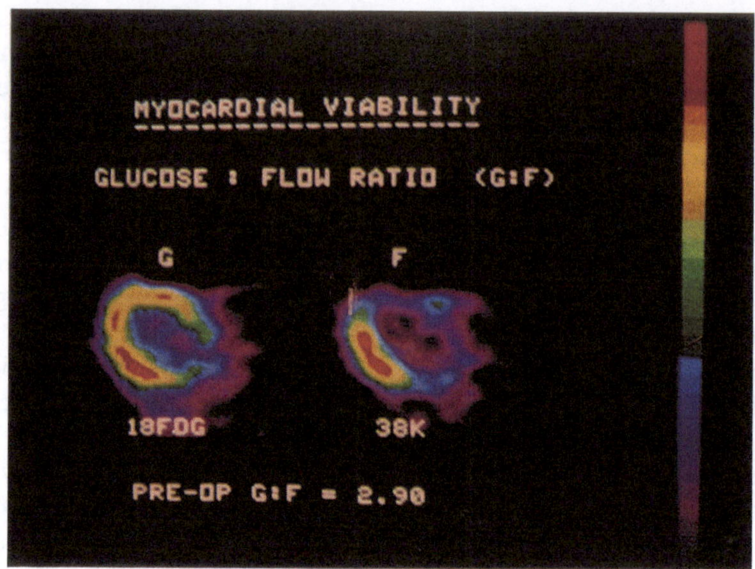

Abb. 50. ^{38}K und ^{18}F-FDG bei myokardialer Ischämie (Rigo, 1986).

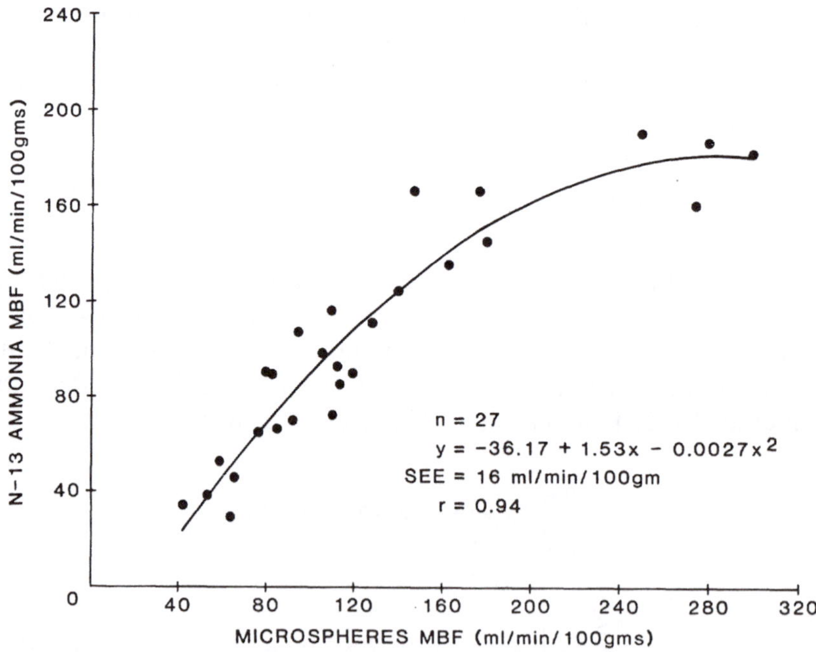

Abb. 51. Bestimmung der regionalen myokardialen Perfusion mit Mikroaggregaten verglichen mit einem First-pass-Extraktionsverfahren (^{14}NH$_4^+$) beim Hund. (Aus Sha et al. 1985)

Bei der Applikation im „steady state" wird das Rubidium zunächst bis zu einer Gleichgewichtseinstellung über etwa 180 Sekunden infundiert, daraufhin wird eine Gleichgewichtsaufnahme, „steady state", über etwa 120 Sek dokumentiert und 30 Sekunden nach Absetzen der Injektion ein 2-Minuten-Bild aufgenommen, das ein Maß für die myokardiale Perfusion ist. Die gemessene Netto-Extraktion ergibt sich aus dem Produkt von Extraktionsrate und Fluß pro Volumen, die Extraktionsfraktion wird aus den arteriellen und myokardialen Rubidium-Konzentrationen der PET errechnet (Budinger et al. 1975; Selwyn et al. 1982).

Messungen im Tierexperiment zur relativ schwachen Korrelation zwischen dem „Goldenen Standard" der Mikrosphären-Methode und der Rubidium-Aufnahme liegen vor (FUKUYAMA et al. 1978; SELWYN et al. 1982). Weiterhin wird eine Interferenz mit der reduzierten Aktivität der membranösen $Na^+ - K^+$-ATPase in ischämischen Arealen, und folglich auch bei Digitalis-Therapie diskutiert (HOUGEN u. SMITH 1978; KU et al. 1974).

Die Bolus-Technik basiert auf der Indikatorverdünnung und erfordert eine Injektion in das Gefäß oder Messung der Input-Funktion des zuführenden Gefäßes sowie die Bestimmung des zeitlichen Verlaufes der venösen Konzentration. Unter Voraussetzung der vollständigen arteriellen Durchmischung, der Erfassung des gesamten venösen Abflusses, einer während der Meßdauer konstanten Durchblutung und einem vernachlässigbaren bzw. korrigierbaren Rezirkulationsfluß ergibt sich die absolute Durchblutung (ml/min) des zwischen Zu- und Abfluß liegenden Gebietes nach STEWART und HAMILTON. Die Kenntnis der arteriellen Konzentration kann durch die venöse ersetzt werden, wenn die Extraktionsfraktion bekannt ist. Gerade das stellt aber ein Fundamentalproblem dar, da die Extraktionsfraktion nicht konstant ist, sondern nicht-linear bei höheren Flüssen und kürzeren Transitzeiten des Tracers in den Kapillaren abnimmt (YANO et al. 1981; GOLDSTEIN 1983; KNOOP 1982; MULLANI 1983; MULLANI u. GOULD 1983; MULLANI et al. 1983; SCHELBERT u. SCHWAIGER 1986).

δ) *Kety-Schmidt.* Der dritte allgemeine Ansatz zur Flußbestimmung wurde von KETY und SCHMIDT unter Berücksichtigung des Fickschen Prinzips der Erhaltung der Massen im Jahre 1945 vorgeschlagen. Die erste Voraussetzung dieser Methode ist, daß die Aufnahme des Tracers flußabhängig und nicht diffusions-limitiert ist (EICHLING et al. 1974; RAICHLE et al. 1978; ROSE et al. 1977). Weiterhin dürfen keine signifikanten Shunts existieren (Quellen, Senken) (FAN et al. 1979). Letztlich muß die Löslichkeit des Tracers ortsunabhängig sein, was nur für kleine Bereiche des Myokards gelten kann (HERSCOVITCH u. RAICHLE 1983; RAICHLE 1983). Ursprünglich wurden diffusible Tracer, wie N_2O (ECKENHOFF et al. 1948; KETY 1960), ^{133}Xe (CANNON et al. 1972), ^{85}Kr (HERD et al. 1962) und ^{14}C-Antipyrin (MALSKY et al. 1977) vorgeschlagen. Von den Positronen-Strahlern wurden in erster Linie ^{11}C-Butanol und $H_2^{15}O$ verwendet (BERGMAN et al. 1982b–c, 1984; HACK et al. 1980).

Die Verwendung von Wasser, $H_2^{15}O$, wurde ursprünglich für die Bestimmung der zerebralen Perfusion von der Gruppe am Hammersmith Hospital, London, vorgeschlagen (FRACKOWIAK et al. 1980a, b; LENZI et al. 1978; PARKER et al. 1978; CHEVIGNE et al. 1983). Sie hat die Vorteile einer fast 100%igen Extraktion im Myokard, $97 \pm 3\%$ über einen weiten Bereich der Perfusion von 13–314 ml/min/100 g Gewebe, und der Unabhängigkeit der Aufnahme des Tracers von metabolischen Funktionen. Andererseits stellen die hohen Aktivitäten im Intravasalraum ein meßtechnisches Problem dar, das eine Darstellung des Blutpools mit ^{11}CO markierten Erythrozyten grundsätzlich erfordert: cross contamination, Totzeitverluste (Abschnitt C.) (ALLAN et al. 1981; BERGMAN et al. 1984). Kalibrierungen dieser Technik mit der Mikrosphären-Methode liegen vor (BERGMAN et al. 1984).

Um die den Äquilibrium-Methoden inhärenten Probleme teilweise zu überwinden, schlugen HACK et al. (1980) eine exponentielle Applikation und HUANG et al. (1982) eine Bolus-Applikation vor (Abschnitt B.III.). Systematische Unterschätzungen des Flusses gegenüber der Mikrosphären-Methode wurden auf Teilvolumeneffekte zurückgeführt (HUANG et al. 1982).

c) Fettsäuren-Stoffwechsel

Das Myokard utilisiert verschiedene Substrate zur Energiegewinnung, darunter freie Fettsäuren, Glukose, Laktat, Pyruvat, Ketone und Aminosäuren. Die Aufnahme dieser Substrate ist allerdings abhängig von vielen Variablen und Parametern, darunter Perfusion und Zusammensetzung der Substrate und Metabolite sowie vom Sauerstoffmetabolismus und der Möglichkeit des Organismus, auf einen alternativen Stoffwechselweg auszuweichen.

Unter normalen Stoffwechselbedingungen stellen die über Proteine (in erster Linie Albumine) transportierten freien Fettsäuren und Triglyzeride mit einem Anteil von 60–80% das primäre Substrat zur Energieversorgung des Myokards dar. Dabei beträgt die Extraktionsfraktion im Mittel etwa 28%, mit deutlicher Bevorzugung der längerkettigen Fettsäuren: Ölsäure 46%, Palmitinsäure 32%, Stearinsäure 10% (Ballard et al. 1960; Bing et al. 1949; Cannon et al. 1969; Evans et al. 1965; Neely et al. 1972; Rothlin u. Bing 1961; Spector u. Steinberg 1965; Stöcklin u. Kloster 1982).

Die nuklearmedizinische Diagnostik führte von Untersuchungen $^{131/123}$I-markierter Öl- und Heptadekan-Säuren (Beierwaltes et al. 1975; Poe et al. 1976, 1977; Robinson u. Lee 1975), über die Markierung verschiedener Fettsäuren mit den Positronenstrahlern ^{34m}Cl und ^{77}Br zu solchen, die mit ^{11}C markiert sind (Knust et al. 1979; Machulla et al. 1978; Wolf 1981). Die relativ kurze physikalische Halbwertszeit des ^{11}C mag in Zukunft die Anwendung ^{18}F-markierter Verbindungen, trotz der teilweisen Abkehr vom Konzept physiologischer Fettsäuren, begünstigen.

Der metabolische Weg der Fettsäuren von der Protein-Bindung im Plasma durch das Sarkolemm in die Myokardzelle ist bisher nicht ausreichend beschrieben. Der weitere Stoffwechselweg kann über eine β-Oxidation einer gebildeten Palmityl-CoA-Verbindung (Enzym: Thiokinase), die Energie verbraucht, in den Mitochondrien mit Bildung von CO_2 führen. Möglich ist jedoch ebenfalls eine Veresterung zu Triglizeriden, und damit ein Stoffwechselweg, der zu einer Speicherungsform führt. Eine genauere biochemische Beschreibung der Stoffwechselwege wird in Abschnitt B.VI. gegeben.

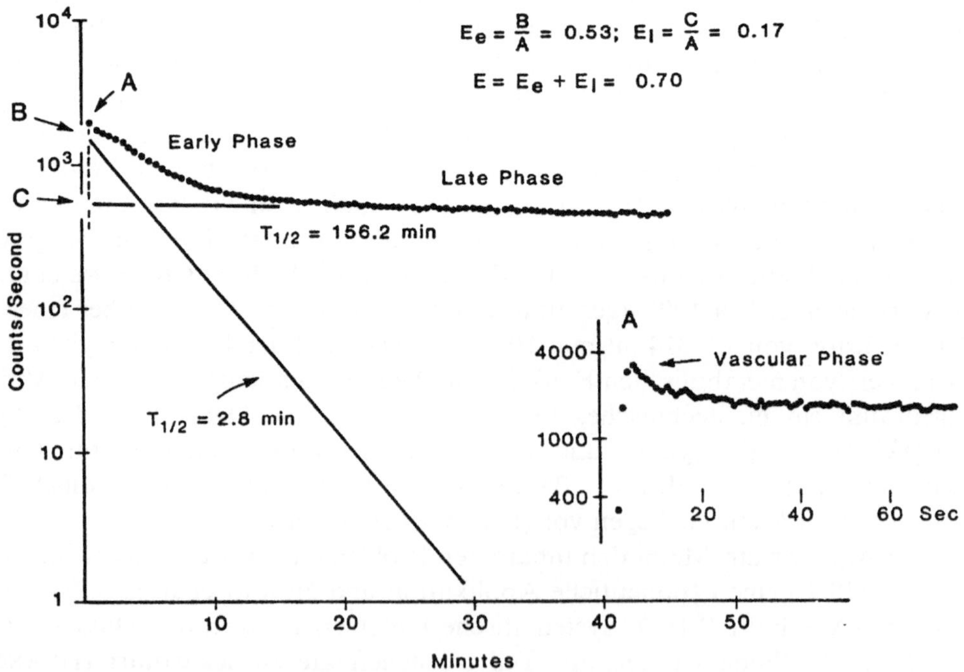

Abb. 52. Myokardiale ^{11}C-Aktivität nach intrakoronarer Injektion von [1-^{11}C]-Palmitat. Zweiphasige Clearance mit einer frühen, schnellen Komponente ($T_{1/2} = 2.8$ min) und einer langsameren, späten Komponente ($T_{1/2} = 156$ min). Bis auf die Anfangsphase (1 s/Meßpunkt) entspricht jeder Punkt einer Meßzeit von 30 s. Das gemessene Maximum A ist proportional zur applizierten Aktivität. Die Parameter B, C, E_1 und E_e werden mit dem „Peeling"-Verfahren bestimmt, das vorwiegend zur graphischen Analyse von Exponentialsummen bestimmt wird. Neben verschiedenen Nachteilen ist der Methode anzumerken, daß sich durch sukzessive Bestimmung der Teilkomponenten alle Fehler fortpflanzen, so daß die zuletzt bestimmte schnellste Komponente, die im Anwendungsfall häufig die wichtigste Information darstellt, mit der größten Fehlerbreite behaftet ist. (Aus Schön et al. 1982a)

α) [^{11}C]-Palmitin-Säure. Die Stoffwechseluntersuchungen der [^{11}C]-Palmitin-Säure sind vornehmlich in den Zentren der UCLA, Los Angeles, und an der Washington University, St. Louis, im Tierexperiment und am Menschen durchgeführt worden (Abb. 54). Diese Studien haben gezeigt, daß die Kinetik der [^{11}C]-Palmitin-Säure, entsprechend den verschiedenen metabolischen Verteilungsräumen, in drei Phasen eingeteilt werden kann (Abb. 52, 53) (GELTMAN et al. 1985; SCHELBERT u. SCHWAIGER 1986).

In der initialen Phase, innerhalb von 20 Sekunden nach der bolusförmigen Applikation, wird der Tracer aus dem vaskulären Verteilungsraum ausgewaschen, zusätzlich werden rückdiffundierte nicht-metabolisierte Tracer beobachtet. Die Clearance-Halbwertzeit beträgt etwa 1.5–7 Sekunden. Hiernach wird von einigen Autoren ein Kurvenbuckel („hump") ohne weitere physiologische Interpretation beschrieben.

Die zweite Phase, auch Frühphase genannt, wird durch eine monoexponentielle Abnahme der kardialen Aktivität mit einer Halbwertzeit von 1–15 min charakterisiert. Diese Phase gibt wahrscheinlich den Anteil der Oxidation wieder, hauptsächlich der β-Oxidation, über eine lineare Beziehung zum Sauerstoffverbrauch, über die Steigung (slope) und die $^{11}CO_2$-Produktion. Auch die Clearance dieser Metabolite ist in dieser Phase berücksichtigt. Eine

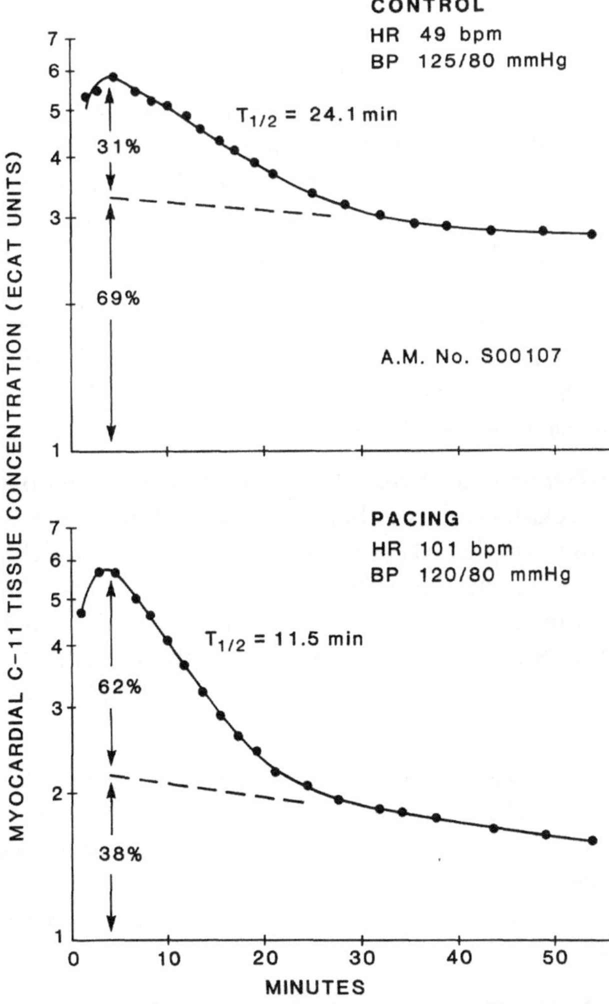

Abb. 53. Veränderungen der [1-^{11}C]-Palmitat-Kinetik im menschlichen Myokard bei einem Arbeitsversuch mit atrialem Pacing. Bei verdoppelter Herzfrequenz und unverändertem Blutdruck (*RR*) weist die Analyse der Zeitaktivitätskurve auf einen um den Faktor 2 vergrößerten Anteil des gegenüber der Studie unter Ruhebedingungen schnelleren (T$_{1/2}$) Oxidationspools. (Aus SCHELBERT u. SCHWAIGER 1986)

Tabelle 7. Änderungen hämodynamischer und funktioneller Parameter der [1-^{11}C]-Palmitat-Kinetik bei Kontrollpersonen und Patienten mit koronarer Herzerkrankung (KHK) unter Ruhebedingungen und nach atrialem Pacing. Bei unveränderten Konzentrationen der Substrate im Plasma, bis auf erhöhte Werte der Fettsäuren bei den Patienten mit KHK, unterscheiden sich beide Gruppen signifikant bzgl. der kinetischen Parameter der schnellen Oxidationsphase des Palmitat. (Aus Schelbert et al. 1983a, b).

	Ruhe	Pacing	Δ (%)
Kontrolle (n = 7)			
Herzfrequenz (1/min)	59 ± 8	104 ± 10	$+78$
Double Produkt (RR × HR)	7200 ± 1130	12800 ± 1000	$+77$
Frühe Phase (%)	36 ± 10	55 ± 12	$+61$
Frühe Phase ($T_{1/2}$: min)	25 ± 9	15 ± 8	-40
Patienten mit KHK (n = 5)			
Herzfrequenz (1/min)	64 ± 12	110 ± 17	$+72$
Double Produkt (RR × HR)	$7050 + 990$	13459 ± 1300	$+91$
Frühe Phase (%)	54 ± 14	48 ± 18	-11
Frühe Phase ($T_{1/2}$: min)	26 ± 5	35 ± 41	$+35$

mathematische Rück-Extrapolation dieser zweiten Phase erlaubt eine Abschätzung der Extraktionsfraktion und der relativen Anteile der Kompartimente über einen weiten Bereich verschiedener Blutflüsse. Die auf diese Weise ermittelte Extraktionsfraktion ist auch relativ unempfindlich gegenüber Änderungen des Sauerstoffmetabolismus. Allerdings verringert sich die Extraktionsfraktion bei deutlicher Erhöhung des Flusses, etwa im Rahmen eines Dipyridamol-Testes.

Die dritte Phase, auch Spätphase, mag ein Maß für den Umsatz des relativ stabilen Pools darstellen, d.h. der neutralen Lipide und veresterten Palmitin-Säuren (Geltman et al. 1985; Goldstein et al. 1980; Hoffman et al. 1977; Lerch et al. 1982; Schön et al. 1982a, b; Schelbert u. Schwaiger 1986; Weiss et al. 1976).

β) β-Methyl-[1-^{11}C]-Heptadekan-Säure. Untersuchungen mit halogenierten und mit ^{11}C-markierten Hepta/Penta-Dekan-Säuren haben eine relativ homogene Anreicherung und Akkumulation des Tracers im normalen Myokard und eine Minderanreicherung mit verlängerter Kinetik in ischämischem bzw. infarziertem Gewebe gezeigt. Nur 5% des Tracers werden zu CO_2 oxidiert, während mehr als 30% metabolisch unverändert rückdiffundieren. 20 min nach der Injektion befinden sich etwa 20% in den Phospholipiden, der entscheidende Anteil in der Größenordnung von 55% dagegen in der Form von Triglyzeriden (Höck et al. 1983; Livini et al. 1982; Morgan et al. 1983).

γ) [1-^{11}C]-Palmitin-Säure und Normalwerte. Semiquantitative Werte und PET-Darstellungen sind in Tabellen und Abbildungen zusammengestellt (Tabelle 7–9 und Abb. 52–54). Dabei muß berücksichtigt werden, daß sich die Meßdaten teilweise nicht anhand der oben skizzierten Modellvorstellungen evaluieren lassen und insbesondere die entsprechenden exponentiellen Fits nicht dem Kompartment-Modell anpassen lassen (Most et al. 1969; Schelbert u. Schwaiger 1986).

δ) [1-^{11}C]-Palmitin-Säure und Arbeitsversuch. Beim Pacing ändern sich bei konstanten Plasmaparametern der Verteilungsraum und die Gewebeclearance (Henze et al. 1982b; Schelbert et al. 1983a, b). Der Anteil der über die β-Oxidation verstoffwechselten Fettsäure vergrößert sich und paßt sich damit dem Energiebedarf an (Abb. 53).

Tabelle 8. Myokardiale [1-^{11}C]-Palmitat-Kinetik. Unter Kontrollbedingungen liegt die O_2-Extraktionsfraktion für die freien Fettsäuren bei $56\pm35\%$, nach Glukose-Insulin-Infusion sinkt sie auf $9\pm33\%$; anders für Laktat und Glukose: für diese Substrate steigt die O_2-Extraktionsfraktion unter diesen Bedingungen von 41% auf 94% (Tierexperiment am Hund, SCHELBERT u. SCHWAIGER 1986).
Die Parameter der [1-^{11}C]-Palmitat-Kinetik wurden mit der PET und teilweise mit, teilweise ohne Kurven-Peeling gewonnen. 50 g orale Glukose hatten keinen Einfluß auf die hämodynamischen Parameter

Kontrollpersonen ($n=5$)	Nüchtern	Postglukose	p
Herzfrequenz (1/min)	64 ± 4	69 ± 6	n.s.
Systol. Blutdruck (mmHg)	121 ± 11	119 ± 17	n.s.
Glukose-Plasma$_\text{venös}$ (mmol/l)	5.1 ± 0.3	8.7 ± 2.7	<0.01
Freie Fettsäuren-Plasma$_\text{venös}$ (mmol/l)	0.53 ± 0.45	0.15 ± 0.09	<0.05
[1-^{11}C]-Palmitat: schnelle Phase			
Relative Größe (%)	47 ± 13	27 ± 9	<0.05
$T_{1/2}$ (min)	19 ± 7	28 ± 6	<0.01

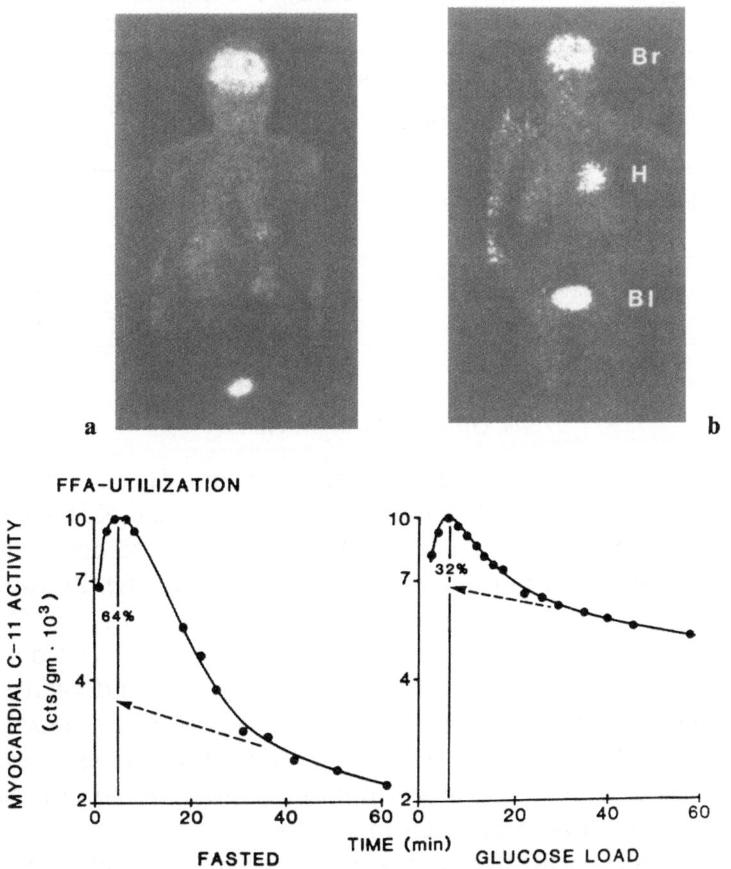

Abb. 54a, b. Darstellung der kardialen Glukose-Verwertung und der Utilisation freier Fettsäuren am Beispiel des [1-^{11}C]-Palmitat beim nüchternen Menschen (**a**). Etwa 2/3 des [1-^{11}C]-Palmitat werden in einem schnellen Stoffwechselverteilungsraum metabolisiert, etwa 50% davon, 1/3 des Gesamtangebotes, nur noch nach zusätzlichem Angebot von 50 g Glukose. Dieser Wechsel vom Fettsäuremetabolismus zu einem Glukosemetabolismus zeigt sich auch in der Studie mit ^{18}F-FDG (**b**, Br: Gehirn, H: Herz, Bl: Blase). (Aus SCHELBERT u. SCHWAIGER 1986)

ε) *[1-^{11}C]-Palmitin-Säure und andere Substrate.* Untersuchungen von Henze et al. (1982 a–c) konnten auch mit der PET am Menschen zeigen, daß die myokardiale Extraktionsfraktion und die Clearanceraten der Palmitinsäure, die primär vom Herzen als Energiesubstrat bevorzugt wird, sehr stark vom arteriellen Substratangebot abhängen. Im Vergleich zum Stoffwechsel nach mehr als 14stündiger Nahrungskarenz ist die Palmitat-Utilisation nach 50 g Glukoseapplikation bei unveränderten hämodynamischen Parametern deutlich vermindert, die Glukoseutilisation (^{18}FDG) entsprechend erhöht (Abb. 53) (Phelps et al. 1978). Normales, funktionstüchtiges Myokard hat danach die Fähigkeit, verschiedene Substrate zur Energiegewinnung zu verwenden. Diese Ergebnisse wurden vorher bereits im Tierexperiment am Hund beobachtet. Bei der Interpretation der kinetischen Parameter der Modellvorstellungen sind demnach die biochemischen Randbedingungen (Pyruvat, Laktat, Glukose etc.) zu berücksichtigen (Schelbert et al. 1983a, b).

Tabelle 9. Die Netto-Aufnahme eines Substrates ergibt sich aus dem Produkt von Fluß, Extraktionsfraktion und arterieller Konzentration. Fluß und Extraktion sind aber nicht grundsätzlich unabhängige Parameter. Mit ‚E‘ ist der in der Myokardzelle metabolisch getrappte, effektive Anteil des [1-^{11}C]-Palmitat bezeichnet. Mit dem Maß FD geben Henze et al. (1982a–b) das Verhältnis der Größe der „Kompartimente" der sehr frühen und der späten Phase an (fractional distribution). $T_{1/2}$ bedeutet die entsprechende Halbwertzeit, 0 zeigt keinen Effekt an, ▲ eine positive und ▼ eine negative, inverse Korrelation. Die Bestimmung der Substrate erfolgte in arteriellen Konzentrationen. (Aus Schelbert u. Schwaiger 1986)

	Frühe Phase				Späte Phase	
	‚E‘	FD	Größe	$T_{1/2}$	Größe	$T_{1/2}$
Myokardialer Blutfluß	▼	0	0	0	0	0
Sauerstoffmetabolismus, MYO$_2$	▲	▲	▲	▼	▼	?
Glukose, Laktat	▼	▼	▼	▲	▲	?
Freie Fettsäuren	▲	▲	▲	▼	▼	?
Ischämie	▼	▼	▼	▲	▲	?

d) Glukose-Stoffwechsel

Obwohl die Fettsäuren unter aeroben Bedingungen das Hauptsubstrat zur Erhaltung des Energiestoffwechsels im Myokard darstellen, stehen mit den Kohlehydraten (Glukose, Laktat etc.) wichtige Energiereserven, auch unter ischämischen Bedingungen, zur Verfügung.

Ohne die zentrale Regulation durch das Insulin ist der transmembranöse Glukosetransport durch eine weitgehend energieunabhängige „carrier-facilitated"-Diffusion limitiert (Neely et al. 1972). Mit Insulin, das den transmembranösen Transport der Fettsäuren inhibiert, wird die Phosphorilierung durch eine Hexokinase geschwindigkeitsbestimmend. Für den Pyruvat-Metabolismus gilt entsprechendes (Park et al. 1968; Geltman et al. 1985).

Wegen der zentralen Bedeutung auch des Glukosemetabolismus wurden verschiedene Glukosen, Glukoseanaloga und Intermediärprodukte hergestellt und untersucht.

Die „natürliche" [^{11}C]-Glukose hat sich in der PET des Herzens wegen des komplexen Modells und der verschiedenen Stoffwechselprodukte nicht durchsetzen können. So diffundieren markierte Milchsäure und Pyruvat vom Gewebe zurück in den Blutverteilungsraum und werden in Aminosäuren eingebaut (Goldstein et al. 1980). Entsprechende Untersuchungen liegen über die [3-^{11}C]-Methyl-D-Glukose vor (Schelbert u. Schwaiger 1986; Weiss et al. 1976).

Wie bei den Hirnstudien erscheint den meisten Arbeitsgruppen derzeit die [18]F-2FDG (^{18}F-2-Fluoro-2-Deoxy-Glukose) als das Radiopharmakon der Wahl (GALLAGHER et al. 1977; PHELPS et al. 1978; RATIB et al. 1982). Die FDG wird über das Sarkolemm transportiert und phosphoriliert. Das Produkt, [18]F-2FDG-6-Phosphat, wird fast vollständig intrazellulär „getrappt" und nicht weiter verstoffwechselt, da das Sarkolemm für phosphorilierte Hexosen nicht permeabel ist. Das FDG-6-Phosphat kann weder als Glykogen gespeichert noch für die Glykolyse oder den Pentose-Shunt herangezogen werden. Innerhalb der Myokardzelle ist die Aktivität über mehr als 120 min relativ konstant (Abb. 55a–c).

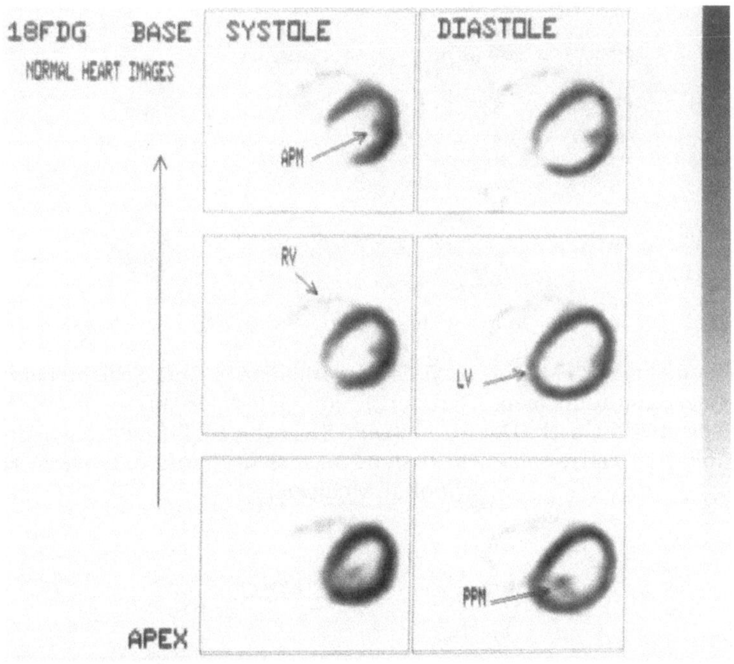

Abb. 55a. EKG-getriggerte PET-Schichtbilder der kardialen Glukose-Aufnahme (10 mCi, 370 MBq ^{18}F-FDG), bei einer normalen Kontrollperson. In den drei Schichten in Systole (8 Zyklen) und Diastole (8 Zyklen) sind der linke und rechte Ventrikel (*LV, RV*) sowie die anterioren und posterioren Papillarmuskel (*APM, PPM*) gekennzeichnet (UCLA, School of Medicine)

Das kinetische Modell wurde von SOKOLOFF übernommen und von PHELPS et al. (1978) und HUANG et al. (1980) der myokardialen Situation angepaßt. In dem Kompartmentmodell werden drei Verteilungsräume, der des Plasma, der der FDG und der Glukose im Gewebe und der der phosphorilierten FDG angenommen. Einzelheiten werden in Abschnitt B.V. beschrieben. In Tierexperimenten und Studien am Menschen wird über eine relativ große Streuung der quantitativen Ergebnisse berichtet. Dieses ist zum einen darauf zurückzuführen, daß neben der Glukose auch Fettsäuren und Milchsäure als Substrat der Energieversorgung zur Verfügung stehen. Andererseits kann in den Myokardzellen auch Glukose über vorhandene Glykogenspeicher oxidativ entstehen. Letztlich gilt es, die Modellvorstellungen als solche, insbesondere den von physiologischen Randbedingungen abhängigen Wert der „lumped constant" abzuschätzen (GELTMAN et al. 1985; HENZE et al. 1981; KRIVOKAPICH et al. 1983; MARSHALL et al. 1981, 1983a–b; SCHWAIGER et al. 1983).

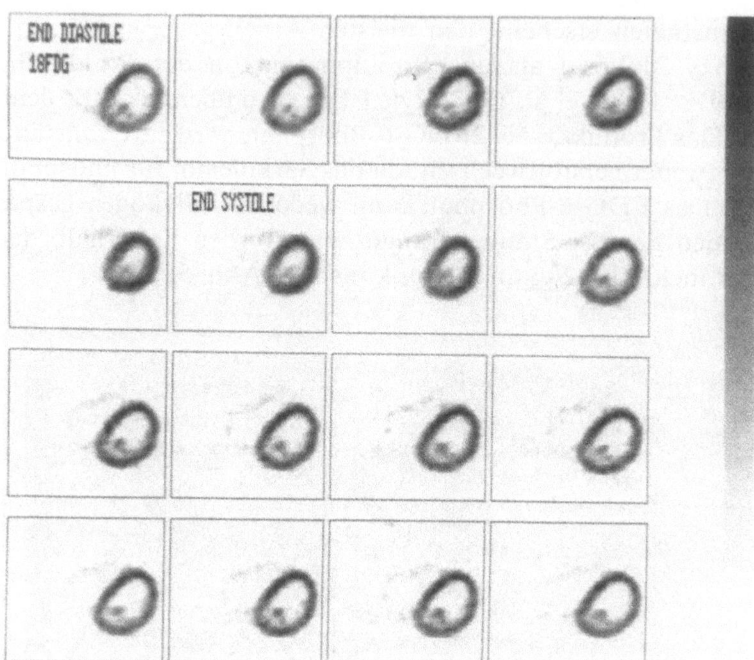

Abb. 55b. Die Glukoseaufnahme (^{18}F-FDG) nach Gleichverteilung in einer Schichtebene durch den mittleren linken Ventrikel bei einer Kontrollperson. Die Herzaktion (RR-Intervall) ist in 16 Abschnitte eingeteilt, jeder mit einer Dauer von etwa 50 msek. Die fortlaufende Serie von PET-Funktionsbildern erfaßt die Phasen vom enddiastolischen bis zum endsystolischen Zustand in diesem „repräsentativen" Herzzyklus (UCLA, School of Medicine)

e) Zwischenprodukte des Kohlenhydrat-Stoffwechsels

Natürliche Zwischenprodukte des Kohlenhydrat-Stoffwechsels, wie insbesondere [^{11}C]-Pyruvat, das Endprodukt der anaeroben Glykolyse als Metabolit bei ischämischen Randbedingungen, [^{11}C]-Laktat oder [^{11}C]-Azetat stellen Tracer dar, die in der Beurteilung des myokardialen Metabolismus von besonderem Wert sind (COHEN 1978; COHEN et al. 1980; GOLDSTEIN et al. 1980; PIKE et al. 1982; SELWYN et al. 1981).

So berichteten KEUL et al. (1965a, b), daß die arterielle Pyruvat-Plasma-Konzentration bei Gesunden von 0.074 µmol/ml unter Ruhe auf 0.174 µmol/ml unter Belastung steigt und die Extraktionsfraktionen unter den entsprechenden Bedingungen von 43% auf 1% sinken, wobei die Änderungen des Laktatstoffwechsels gleichsinnig sind (SCHELBERT u. SCHWAIGER 1986).

Wegen der hohen Extraktionsraten des Azetat von etwa 63% ergibt sich für das „metabolic imaging" ein optimales Verhältnis Myokard/Blut (5:1). Die Clearance des Tracers aus ischämischen Bereichen ist gegenüber normalem Gewebe deutlich verlangsamt ($T_{1/2}=4.1\pm$ 0.2 min vs. 10 ± 0.4 min). Bei einem Arbeitsversuch ist in normalem Myokardgewebe die mit einer mono-exponentiellen Anpassung beschreibbare Clearance beschleunigt, nicht dagegen in elektrokardiographisch definiertem pathologischen Gewebe (PIKE et al. 1982). Das Clearance-Verhalten des Azetat ist dagegen von der Belastung relativ unabhängig (SELWYN et al. 1981).

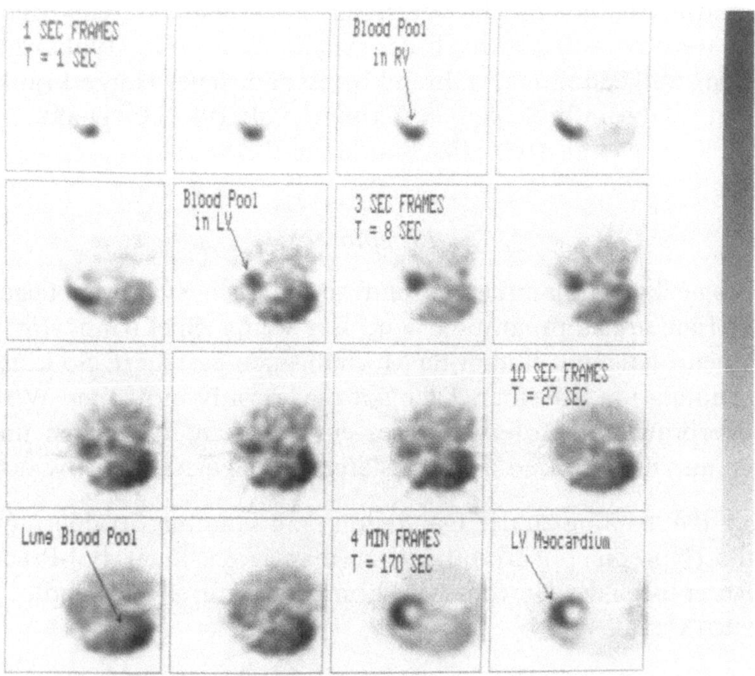

Abb. 55c. Erste Passage durch das zentrale Kreislaufsystem (rechter Ventrikel: *RV*, Lungen und linker Ventrikel: *LV*) und relative Gleichverteilung nach bolusartiger Applikation von ^{13}NH$_3$ (370 MBq) bei einer normalen Kontrollperson. Während die ersten Tomogramme mit einer Aquisitionszeit von jeweils 3 s aufgenommen wurden, ist die Integrationszeit für die weiteren Bilder mit 5 Sek/Frame bzw. 60 Sek/Frame länger (UCLA, School of Medicine)

f) Aminosäuren-Stoffwechsel

Aminosäuren spielen im myokardialen Metabolismus eine zentrale Rolle, besonders im Rahmen der zur Kontraktilität notwendigen Proteinsynthese der Myozyten sowie bei kongestiver und hypertropher Kardiomyopathie (BUDINGER 1979). Sie sind darüberhinaus wichtig im Stoffwechsel der Kohlenhydrate mit den entsprechenden Zwischenprodukten (CAHILL 1978; GELBARD et al. 1980, 1981; GOODWIN 1978; HENZE et al. 1982a; LATHROP et al. 1973; NEELY et al. 1972; SCHELBERT 1985).

Zu den Aminosäuren, deren Metabolismus sehr speziesabhängig ist, gehören ^{13}N-Glutamat, ^{13}N-Glutamin, ^{13}N-Alanin, ^{13}N-Leucin, ^{13}N-Valin, ^{11}C-Aspartat, ^{11}C-Oxalazetat, ^{11}C-Methionin, ^{11}C-Phenylalanin und ^{18}F-p-Fluoro-Phenylalanin. Weiterhin hängt das berechnete Stoffwechselverhalten ab von der einzelnen Aminosäure und der Position der Markierung.

Im Mittel zeigen die ^{13}N-markierten Aminosäuren eine höhere Extraktionsfraktion als die ^{11}C-markierten. Besonders im Tierexperiment am Hund wurden detaillierte Untersuchungen, teilweise mit intrakoronarer Tracerapplikation, durchgeführt. Beim Hund werden beim initialen kapillären Transit etwa 40–60% extrahiert, unter Berücksichtigung der Rückdiffusion in chemisch geänderter oder unveränderter Form bleiben etwa 7–23% der Aminosäure in metabolisierter Form in der Myokardzelle zurück. Die Kinetik wird durch eine schnelle ($T_{1/2}$ = 20–70 Sek) und eine langsame ($T_{1/2}$ = 14–170 min) Phase charakterisiert, während sich bei den ^{11}C-markierten Aminosäuren noch eine zusätzliche Intermediärphase ($T_{1/2}$ = 100–140 Sek) bei einer triexponentiellen Kurvenanpassung definieren läßt (^{13}N: alpha-Position vs. ^{11}C: Position 4). Die verschiedenen Ansätze der Kompartmentanalysen müssen bisher noch teilweise als spekulativ angesehen werden.

Die ^{13}N-Glutamat-Aufnahme im Herzen ist derzeit wohl am systematischsten untersucht. 2–6% der Aktivität werden 5–10 min nach der Applikation vom Myokard mit einer relativ homogenen Verteilung aufgenommen, während bei ischämischer Herzerkrankung die Kinetik und Aufnahme relativ unbeeinflußt bleiben (Cohen et al. 1982; Gelbard et al. 1980, 1981; Henze et al. 1982a; Knapp et al. 1982; Washburn et al. 1982).

g) Rezeptoren

Zur Pharmakologie katecholaminerger und cholinerger Synapsen liegen erste Studien mit der Positronen-Emissionstomographie vor. Ein weites Spektrum von Funktionen des Herzens wird über neuronale und humorale Mechanismen gesteuert. So kommt es z.B. beim Herzen durch β_1-Stimulation zu einer Tachykardie, positiv-inotroper Wirkung und einer Zunahme des O_2-Verbrauchs. Insofern muß es ein Ziel sein, Agonisten und Antagonisten von Herzrezeptoren darzustellen und zu analysieren (Schelbert u. Schwaiger 1986).

α) *β-Sympatholytika.* Analog zu der Darstellung mit Gamma-Strahlern ($^{123/131}$I-MIBG), gelang es, Adrenalin (Norepinephrin) mit ^{11}C zu markieren. Die [^{11}C]-Practolol-Aufnahme der β-adrenergen Rezeptoren des Herzens wird kompetetiv durch Propanolol gehemmt (Fowler et al. 1975; Syrota et al. 1983b).

β) *Parasympathomimetika.* Cholinerge Rezeptoren vom Muscarin-Typ wurden in erster Linie am Affen und in wenigen Studien am Menschen untersucht. Die Arbeitsgruppe in Orsay, Frankreich, untersuchte [^{11}C]-MQNB mit der PET, wobei eine zur Klinik korrelierende Blockade des Parasympathomimetikums durch Atropin möglich war. Bei guter bildlicher Darstellung des Septums und der Seitenwand wurden keine Unterschiede bei gesunden Kontrollpersonen und Patienten mit Kardiomyopathie oder koronarer Herzerkrankung gefunden. Das ist insofern nicht anders zu erwarten, als die höchste Rezeptordichte im Bereich der beiden, relativ dünnen, Vorhöfe beobachtet wurde (Mazière et al. 1981; Syrota et al. 1982b, 1983b, 1984).

Der Beitrag der PET bei der Analyse verschiedener Rezeptoren über die Reaktion markierter Pharmaka läßt Erkenntnisse in bezug auf experimentelle und klinische Pharmakologie erwarten. Voraussetzung sind jedoch Verständnis und quantitative Modelle der Rezeptoren, die ein meßtechnisches Auflösungsvermögen von < 10 mm verlangen. Weiterhin gilt es, den Metabolismus der Substanzen und zell- bzw. gewebsspezifischer Reaktionsketten zu verstehen, an deren Ende erst eine gewebsspezifische Wirkung steht.

2. Koronare Herzerkrankungen

Fragestellung. Die Positronen-Emissionstomographie ermöglicht neben Informationen über das physiologische Verhalten Einsichten in pathophysiologische Erkenntnisse verschiedener kardiovaskulärer Erkrankungen. Für den Kliniker sind insbesondere Probleme des *Koronarkreislaufes* von Interesse, so Koronarstenosen, Ischämien und Infarkte. Weiterhin stellen die *Kardiomyopathien* eine nicht einheitliche Gruppe einer Herzerkrankung dar, die bislang vorwiegend funktionell und nicht ätiologisch klassifiziert wird. Des weiteren bieten Probleme aus dem Kreis der speziellen Pathophysiologie, der *Herzklappenfehler* und der *Myokardhypertrophie* gerade in der Frühdiagnostik myokardialer Dekompensation und der Entscheidung des therapeutischen Vorgehens Möglichkeiten, insbesondere wenn metabolische Veränderungen vor funktionellen Störungen auftreten. Letztlich geht es bei allen Herzerkrankungen um Entscheidungen zur oder Beurteilungen der Therapie sowie prognostischer Möglichkeiten.

a) Koronarkreislauf

Koronarstenosen werden häufig unter Ruhebedingungen nicht beobachtet. Diagnostische Methoden, auch das EKG, machen in der Regel die Beurteilung der koronaren Funktions- oder Flußreserve notwendig, die bei Stenosen durch einen dem Bedarf nicht angepaßten Fluß charakterisiert wird. Notwendig sind dann ergometrische Belastungstests oder pharmakologisch induzierte Erweiterungen der Koronargefäße (Dipyridamol-Test). Nachdem in der klinischen Routine die parametrische ^{201}Thallium-Szintigraphie bei dieser Fragestellung Eingang gefunden hat (BÜLL et al. 1984a; KIRSCH et al. 1983; SCHICHA 1986; SCHICHA u. EMRICH 1983) gibt es erste Ansätze zur Beantwortung dieser Fragestellungen mit der Positronen-Emissionstomographie.

In Tierexperimenten konnten Stenosen von weniger als 50% in Hinblick auf Änderungen des Flusses mit $^{13}NH_3/^{13}NH_4^+$ von GOULD et al. (1979) nachgewiesen werden. Aus meßtechnischen Gründen ist der Dipyridamol-Test bei diesen Fragestellungen den sonst überlegenen ergometrischen Belastungen vorzuziehen. Weiterhin liegen bestätigende Studien auch am Menschen mit $H_2^{15}O$ und ^{82}Rb vor (HARPER et al. 1972; KNABB et al. 1984, 1985; SCHELBERT et al. 1982a, b; SCHELBERT u. SCHWAIGER 1986; WALSH et al. 1976). SCHELBERT et al. (1982b), geben eine Sensitivität von 97% an, die in der gleichen Größenordnung wie die der ^{201}Tl-Szintigraphie liege. Vorteile der PET in der regionalen Identifizierung der Versorgungsgebiete dürften auch nach Einführung der SPECT bei Positronenkameras der neuesten Generation (FWHM < 10 mm) weiterhin bestehen. Grundsätzlich bleibt festzustellen, daß der Dipyridamol-Test eine relativ große intra- und interindividuelle Varianz besitzt und das Kation $^{13}NH_3/^{13}NH_4^+$ wegen der in Abschnitt D.II.1 dargestellten Randbedingungen keine echt quantitativen Daten ergibt (Abb. 56).

b) Ischämie. Änderungen des Flusses

Systematische Untersuchungen der Aufnahme des Kations ^{82}Rb zeigten im Vergleich zu Mikrosphärenstudien und klinischen Parametern (Angina pectoris, EKG), daß sich bei Ischämien der erniedrigte Rubidium-„uptake" erst verzögert nach Beseitigung der Ischämie normalisiert (SELWYN et al. 1982, 1984). Gerade in Hinblick auf die häufig klinisch stummen, nicht ergometrisch induzierten Ischämien, die teilweise im EKG ihr Korrelat haben und bei 75% der Patienten mit stabiler Angina durch mentalen Streß ausgelöst werden können, ist die PET mit ^{82}Rb, die bei mehr als 95% der Patienten positiv und pharmakologisch reversibel ist sowie eine hohe Sensitivität besitzt, von großem Wert (DEANFIELD et al. 1983a–c, 1984a–b).

In Regionen distal von Stenosen, die 50–70% des Durchmessers ausmachen, konnten mit $H_2^{15}O$ unter Ruhebedingungen unauffällige Fluß-Werte gemessen werden, die jedoch nach Dipyridamol eine geringere Steigerung des Flusses als vergleichbare normale Bereiche zeigten (KNABB et al. 1985).

c) Ischämie. Änderungen des Metabolismus

Bei Ischämien ist die β-Oxidation der Fettsäuren reduziert und gehemmt, während der glykolytische Flux in die Myozyten im Sinne einer Verschiebung des Substratstoffwechsels steigt und die Glukose teilweise, geregelt über die Laktat-Konzentration und den lokalen pH, anaerob metabolisiert wird und das wesentliche Substrat für die ATP-Produktion darstellt. Der Krebs-Zyklus und Sauerstoff-Verfügbarkeit sind in diesem Stadium vermindert (OPIE 1976, 1979).

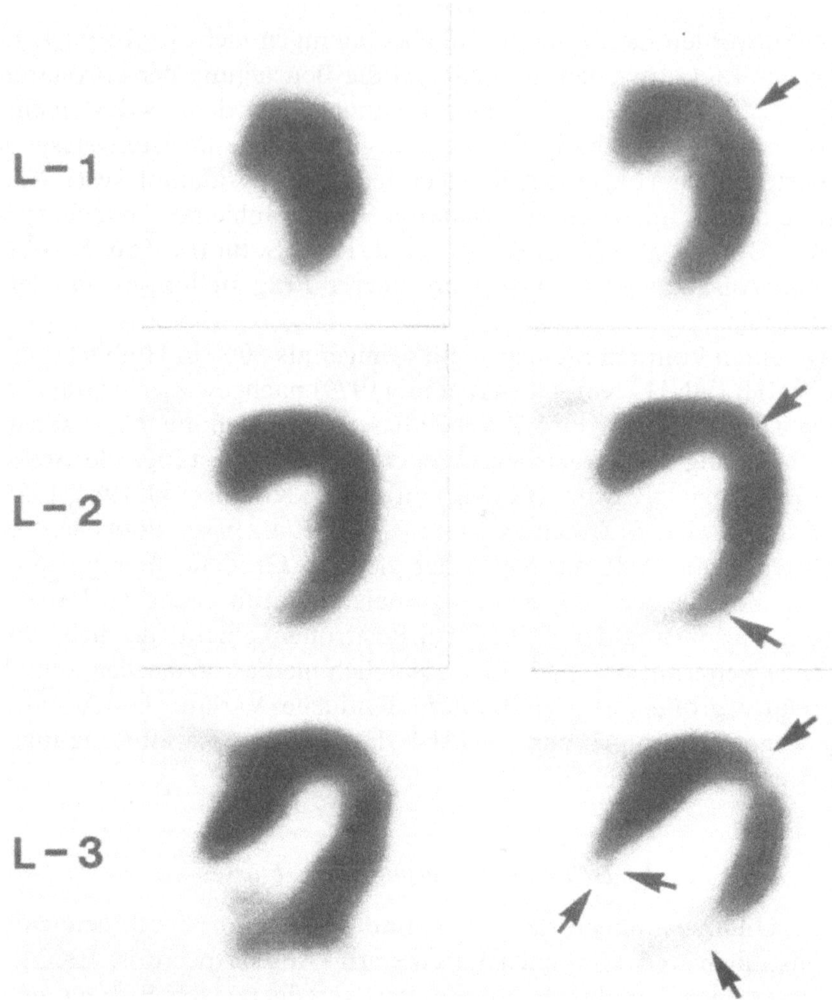

Abb. 56. Dokumentation einer koronaren Herzerkrankung mit der PET und $^{13}NH_3$ als Flußmarker in drei verschiedenen Schichten. Eine Minderperfusion (*Pfeile*) bei Stenosen des R. interventricularis anterior (RIVA: 70%), des R. circumflex sinister (RCX: 95%) und des R. posterolateralis (RPLS: 90%) zeigt sich erst bei einer durch Dipyridamol induzierten Hyperämie (rechts) in den entsprechenden Segmenten. (Aus Schelbert et al. 1982a)

d) Fettsäuren

Die Folge der verminderten β-Oxidation der Fettsäuren bei Sauerstoffmangel führt zur Fragestellung der 1-^{11}C-Palmitinsäure-Aufnahme, -Clearance und -Verstoffwechselung bei Ischämien. Die initiale Aufnahme der Fettsäuren ist offensichtlich weitgehend flußlimitiert, dennoch muß der Fluß wegen der vorhandenen funktionalen Abhängigkeit der Extraktion bei den mangels validen Modells noch immer qualitativen oder semiquantitativen Aussagen mitbestimmt werden (Fox et al. 1985c; Lerch et al. 1981; Schelbert et al. 1983a, b).

Experimentell induzierte Ischämien und Hypoxien werden in minderdurchbluteten Regionen durch eine verlangsamte 1-^{11}C-Palmitinsäure-Clearance charakterisiert (Abb. 57). Bei Ischämien diffundiert offensichtlich ein größerer Teil der Fettsäuren (40% vs. 10% bei Normalen) bei der ersten kapillären Tracerpassage nicht-metabolisiert aus den Myozyten in das Plasma zurück. Dieses wird mit der entsprechenden Verringerung des Sauerstoffmetabolismus (MVO$_2$) verständlich, der sich in Form einer erniedrigten ^{11}CO$_2$-Konzentration meßtechnisch nachvollziehen läßt. Normale Bereiche zeigen dagegen beim Pacing eine verstärkte Anreicherung, die dem schnellen Umsatz der β-Oxidation zugeordnet werden kann. Diese metabolischen Studien korrelieren gut zu klinischen Ergebnissen, die mit komplementären Verfahren, so etwa der Echokardiographie oder der Radionuklid-Ventrikulographie, bestätigt wurden. Die Arbeitsgruppe in St. Louis, USA, gibt mit der PET der Fettsäuren für die Diagnostik der koronaren Herzkrankheit eine Sensitivität von 97% an, die höher als die der planaren ^{201}Thallium-Szintigraphie mit nur 61% liege, und in Bezug auf das infarzierte Volumen sehr gut zur integralen CPK korreliere (Abb. 58) (GELTMAN et al. 1979, 1982; GROYER et al. 1984; LERCH et al. 1982; SCHELBERT et al. 1983a, b; SCHÖN et al. 1982a, b).

Vereinbar sind diese Befunde mit einem verringerten Anteil der Fettsäuren als Energiesubstrat, da die Aktivierung z.B. der Palmitinsäure selbst zu Palmitin-CoA Energie erfordert. In diesem Sinne wird der Anteil der Glykolyse an der Energieversorgung größer, während die Fettsäuren, etwa in in Form der Triglyzeride, „getrappt" werden.

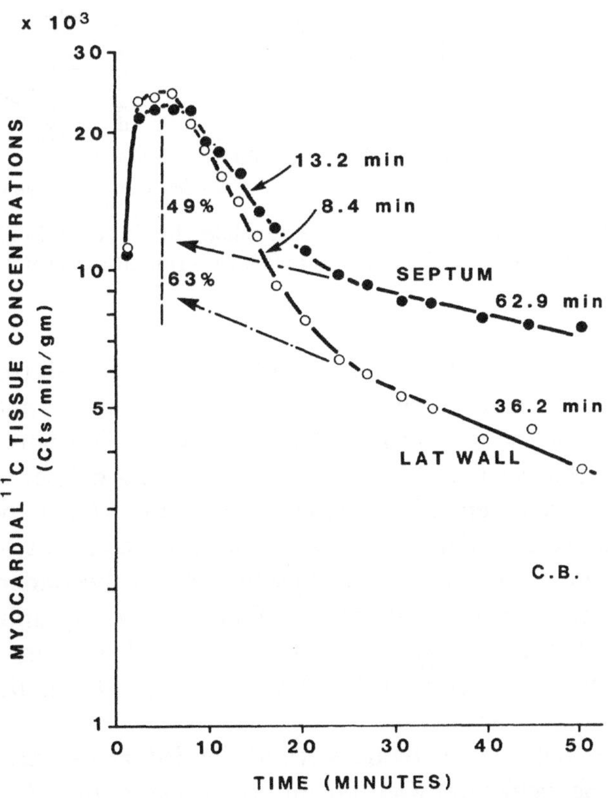

Abb. 57. Geringere Aufnahme und verlangsamte Clearance des [1-^{11}C]-Palmitat bei einem Patienten mit koronarer Herzerkrankung. Eine Ischämie des Septums, im Vergleich zur unauffälligen Seitenwand, wurde durch Pacing erreicht. (Aus SCHELBERT u. SCHWAIGER 1986)

e) Transitorische Ischämien

Bei transitorischen Ischämien, die LERCH et al. (1981) und SCHWAIGER et al. (1985a, b) im Tierexperiment untersuchten, zeigte es sich, daß der Blutfluß nach Reperfusion eines ischämischen Bereiches reversibel ist und sich deutlich schneller erholte als der Palmitat-Metabolismus, der wie die regionale myokardiale Funktion eine zeitliche Verzögerung gegenüber dem Fluß zeigte.

f) Infarkte

Infarkte werden durch eine flußabhängige deutlich erniedrigte Aufnahme der ^{11}C-Palmitin-Säure charakterisiert, wie Sobel et al. (1977) an 12 Patienten im Vergleich zu einem Kontroll-Kollektiv (n = 10) zeigen konnten. Im Tierexperiment konnte eine gute Korrelation zwischen der mit der PET gemessenen Infarktgröße, der integral bestimmten CPK und den morphologischen Bestimmungen gefunden werden (Abb. 58). Entsprechende Untersuchungen am Menschen liegen von der Arbeitsgruppe in St. Louis, USA, vor. Die tomographisch bestimmte Infarktgröße korreliert gut (r = 0.92) mit der CPK-Methode (Billadello et al. 1983; Sobel et al. 1977; Weiss et al. 1977).

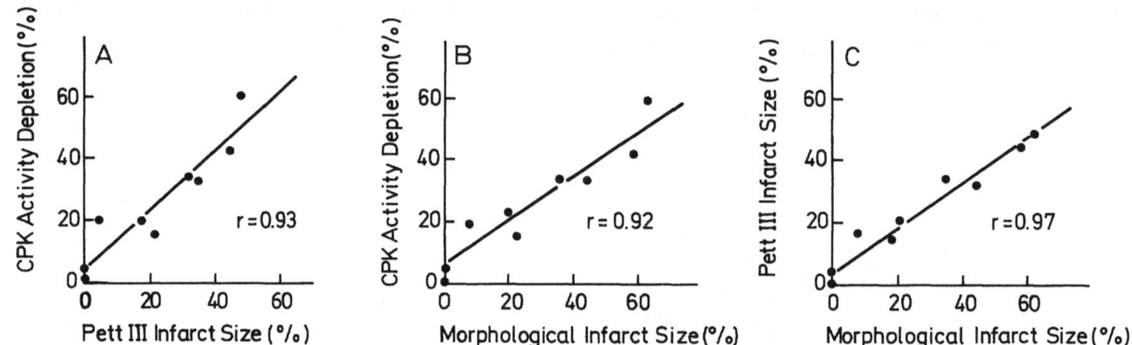

Abb. 58. Korrelationen der morphologischen, der funktionellen (PET: [1-^{11}C]-Palmitat) und der nach der CPK-Freisetzung abgeschätzten Infarktgrößen in einem Tierexperiment am Hund. (Aus Weiss et al. 1976)

Bei diesen Untersuchungen stellt sich insbesondere die Frage, ob transmurale oder nicht-transmurale Infarkte vorliegen. Meßtechnisch ist auch hier unbedingt die Darstellung des Intravasalraumes erforderlich (^{11}CO-Inhalation, Carboxyhämiglobin) (Abb. 59). Transmurale Infarkte sind im Mittel bei der PET um den Faktor 2.5 größer als nicht-transmurale. Die QRS-Gruppe ist bei kleineren, nicht transmuralen Infarkten teilweise wenig oder gar nicht verändert. Diese unspezifischen Änderungen, die zu falsch negativen Diagnosen führen, werden durch die PET sensitiver und genauer beschrieben. Insbesondere können noch vitale Bereiche nekrotischer Areale sensitiver als bei der Thallium-Szintigraphie abgegrenzt werden („match" vs. „mismatch", s. myokardialer Glukose-Metabolismus im Verhältnis zum Blutfluß) (Geltman et al. 1982; Lee et al. 1981; Parodi et al. 1984a, b; Reimer et al. 1977; Schwaiger et al. 1984).

Ein weiteres Problem stellt der zeitliche Verlauf des Infarktes dar, das insbesondere die Analyse der regionalen Bereiche zum Ziel hat, um die noch vitalen Bereiche von den bereits irreversiblen nekrotischen Arealen zu unterscheiden. Schwaiger et al. (1984), Sobel et al. (1984) und Sobel (1985) korrelierten Parameter des Flusses (^{13}NH$_3$) und des Metabolismus (^{18}FDG, ^{11}C-Palmitat) mit klinischen und echokardiographischen Daten. Sie konnten zeigen, daß gerade in Hinblick auf invasive therapeutische Ansätze, wie die *intrakoronare Thrombolyse* oder die *chirurgische Revaskularisierung*, die PET wertvolle, regional unterschiedliche, Hinweise geben kann (Abb. 60). Klinisch ist dabei insbesondere von Bedeutung, daß funktionelle Störungen des Myokards den metabolischen mit zeitlicher Verzögerung folgen (Bergman et al. 1982a, b; Braunwald u. Kloner 1982; Schober et al. 1985c). Bergman et al. (1982a) und Schwaiger et al. (1985a, b) untersuchten dieses semiquantitativ in Tierexperimenten anhand der Streptokinase-Thrombolyse nach Okklusion der LAD mit der 1-^{11}C-Palmitin-Säure und mit ^{13}NH$_3$ in Abhängigkeit einzelner Parameter der Stoffwechselmodelle, wie der Aufnahme und der Clearance einzelner Kompartimente. Die Zusammenhänge zwi-

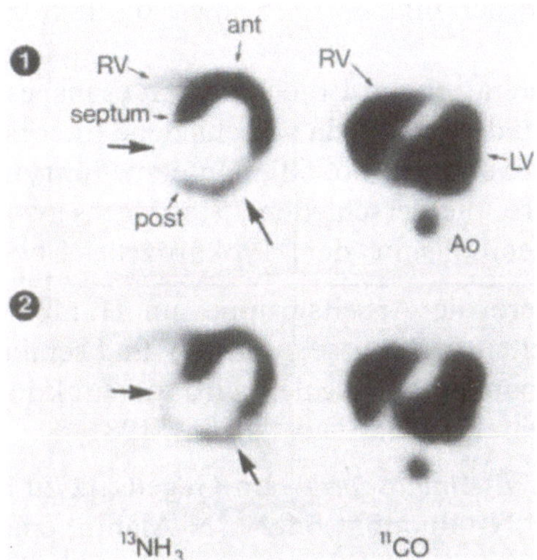

Abb. 59. Anatomische und funktionelle Darstellung des regionalen myokardialen Blutflusses mit $^{13}NH_3$ und des Blutverteilungsraumes, nach Inhalation von ^{11}CO und Bildung von Carboxyhämiglobin, bei einem Patienten mit einem alten Myokardinfarkt und vergrößertem Myokard. In zwei Schichtebenen ist der verminderte Blutfluß in Projektion auf die posterolaterale Wand und das posteriore Septum zu erkennen. *Ao:* Aorta, *RV, LV:* rechter und linker Ventrikel. (Aus SCHELBERT u. SCHWAIGER 1986)

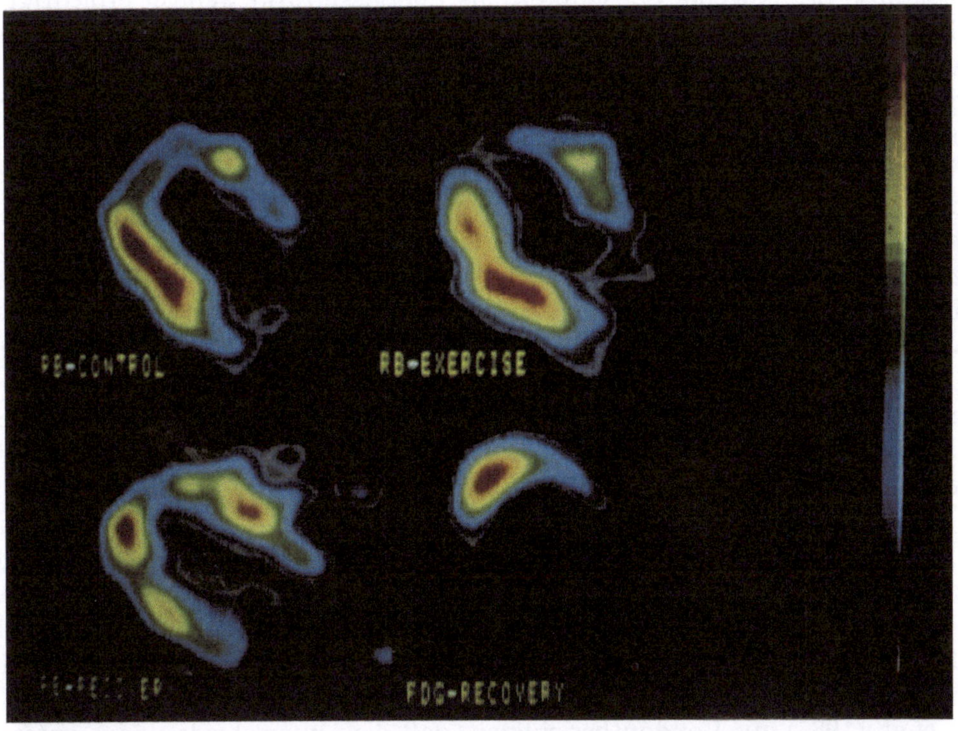

Abb. 60. Patient mit koronarer Herzerkrankung. Die myokardiale Minderperfusion der Vorderwand wurde mit ^{82}Rb unter Ruhe- und Belastungsbedingungen dokumentiert. Die unter Belastungsbedingungen gemessene Glukoseaufnahme weist auf eine teilweise anaerobe Glykolyse. Unter Ruhebedingungen (rechts unten) ist die Glukoseaufnahme im Bereich der Vorderwand deutlich gegenüber dem normalen Gewebe gesteigert. Für diesen Effekt („mismatch") werden ein Persistieren des anaeroben Metabolismus oder eine Wiederauffüllung der Glykogenspeicher diskutiert (P. CAMICI, Hammersmith Hospital, H.R. SCHELBERT, UCLA, School of Medicine)

schen Dauer der Ischämie und der Infarktgröße sowie die Erfolge der Reperfusion wurden analysiert.

Vor einer klinischen Interpretation der Ergebnisse gilt es insbesondere, den metabolischen Zustand des Patienten genau zu definieren, da verschiedene Energiesubstrate eine signifikante gegenseitige Beeinflussung aufweisen (Abb. 60). Untersuchungen über Fettsäuren, wie die ^{11}C-β-Methyl-Heptadekansäure, die verschiedene Stoffwechselwege haben, versprechen zusätzliche Einsichten in dem Metabolismus der Myokardzelle (Livni et al. 1982).

α) ^{11}C-Acetat. Insbesondere die Arbeitsgruppe am Hammersmith Hospital, London, konnte die an Fettsäuren erzielten Ergebnisse qualitativ und semiquantitativ bestätigen. Eine verlangsamte Clearance in ischämischen Arealen wird auf funktionelle Störungen im Krebs-Zyklus zurückgeführt (Raets et al. 1984; Selwyn et al. 1981).

β) ^{11}C- und ^{13}N-markierte L-Aminosäuren. Im Gegensatz zu den Fettsäuren zeigen verschiedene Aminosäuren, wie ^{13}N-Glutamat oder ^{13}N-Alanin, einen im Vergleich zum myokardialen Blutfluß teilweise geringen relativen Anstieg der jeweiligen Extraktionsfraktionen unter induzierten ischämischen Bedingungen (Henze et al. 1982a; Knapp et al. 1982). Allerdings liegen, siehe Abschnitt D.II.1., systematische Studien nur in Tierexperimenten vor.

γ) ^{18}FDG. Glukose. Im Tierversuch wurde von Opie et al. (1973) und Schelbert et al. (1982c) beschrieben, daß induzierte, regionale Ischämien von einer, teils auch gegenüber normalem Gewebe, erhöhten arterio-venösen Glukosedifferenz und einer erniedrigten oder negativen Differenz für Laktat begleitet werden. Dieses sind Hinweise für eine Laktat-Produktion bei anaerober Glykolyse. Im Vergleich zu dem myokardialen Blutfluß und zu den Fettsäuren ist also das Angebot der Glukose als Energiesubstrat weniger erniedrigt. Dieser „mismatch" ist nach Untersuchungen von Marshall et al. (1981, 1983b) typisch für Ischämien, während infarzierte Bereiche durch eine Minderung der Perfusion und der Glukoseaufnahme charakterisiert werden („match") (Abb. 61). Die Bereiche mit „mismatch" wurden in erster Linie bei Postinfarkt-Angina und schwerer koronarer Herzerkrankung beobachtet und mit elektrokardiographischen Veränderungen und Motilitätsstörungen dokumentiert und definiert, trotz teilweise klinisch stummer Angina.

Wie schon erwähnt, ist es klinisch von besonderem Interesse, ob es sich bei Gewebe mit dissoziiertem Verhalten von Fluß und Glukosemetabolismus um reversibel ischämische Bereiche handelt, oder sich nekrotisches Gewebe entwickelt. Tillisch et al. (1985) von der Gruppe an der UCLA, Los Angeles, untersuchten diese Fragestellung prospektiv an 17 Patienten vor einer aorto-koronaren Bypass-Operation mit ^{13}NH$_3$ und ^{18}FDG.

Bei der Klassifizierung und Definition mit der PET entspricht auch beim Menschen „mismatch" vitalem Gewebe und „match", d.h. gleichsinnige Reduktion von Fluß und FDG-Aufnahme, infarziertem Gewebe. Es ergab sich bei ischämischen Segmenten und gleichzeitiger Verbesserung der Motilität ein positiver Voraussagewert von 85% (35/41 Segmenten) im Vergleich zu 92% bei nekrotischen Segmenten (24/26). Entsprechende Beobachtungen und Korrelationen wurden für Veränderungen im EKG (Voraussagewert 42%) untersucht, wobei sich die PET als das sensitivere Verfahren zeigte. In der klinischen Routine ist zu berücksichtigen, daß der positive Voraussagewert eine Wahrscheinlichkeit angibt, daß beim so definierten Untersuchungsergebnis die so definierte Erkrankung vorliegt.

Camici et al. (1983) aus London berichteten, daß die Unterschiede und Kontraste zwischen normalen und ischämischen Regionen nach ergometrischer Belastung besonders deutlich zu dokumentieren sind. Sie führen das, durch Tierstudien unterstützt, auf die poststenotischen ^{18}F-Glykogenspeicher zurück. Andererseits mag die Erholung des Sauerstoffmetabolismus, insbesondere die β-Oxidation, im Sinne einer mitochondrialen Dysfunktion verzögert sein. Ein weiterer beeinflussender Parameter ist das Pyruvat, als Endprodukt der Glykolyse, das für den Aminosäure-Metabolismus und den Krebs-Zyklus von Bedeutung ist.

Ansätze zur direkten positiven Szintigraphie in frisch infarzierten oder nekrotischen Myo-kard-Bereichen existieren mit ^{68}Ga-DTPA und ^{68}Ga-DTPA-Antimyosin-Antikörpern sowie Na^{18}F. Eine klinische Bedeutung kommt diesen Studien allerdings noch nicht zu (COCHAVI et al. 1979; KHAW et al. 1979).

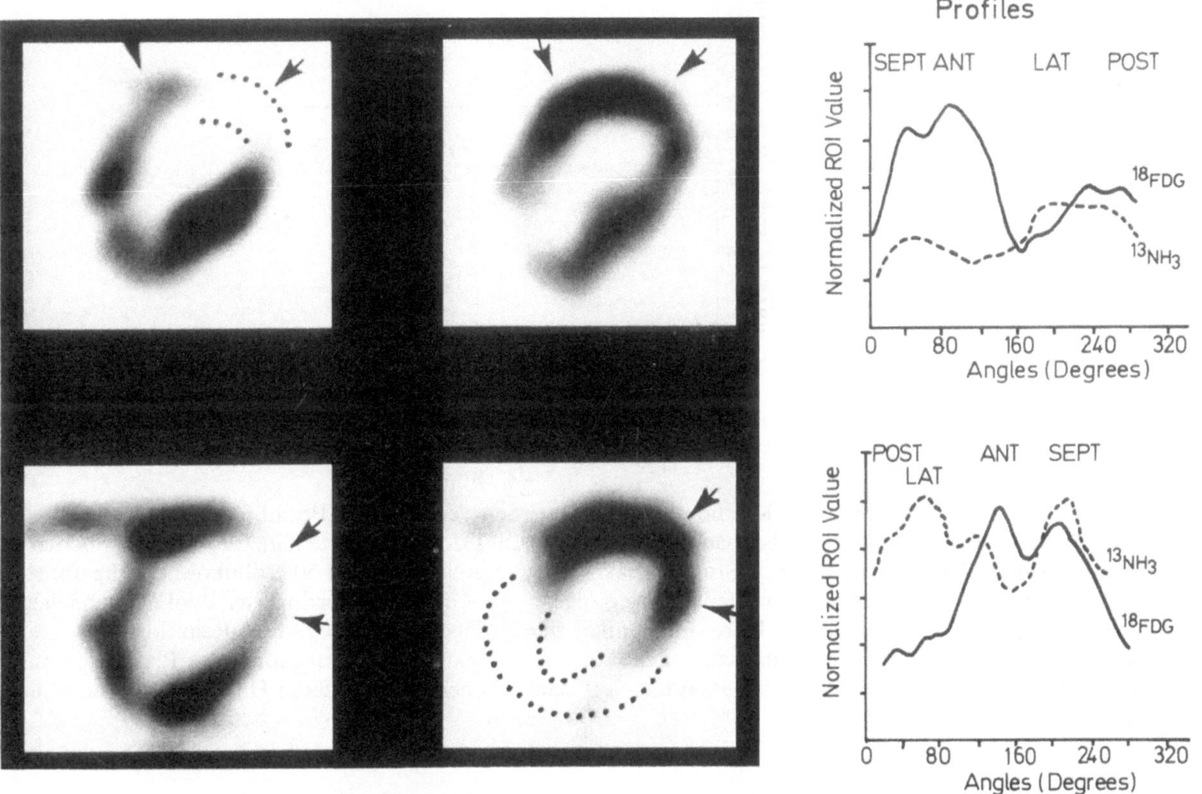

Abb. 61. Myokardiale Perfusion (^{13}NH$_3$) (links) und Glukoseaufnahme (^{18}F-FDG) (rechts) mit der PET bei zwei Patienten mit myokardialer Ischämie. *Oben:* Akinesie der Vorderwand mit deutlicher Minderung der Perfusion bei leicht verstärkter Glukoseaufnahme. *Unten:* Patient mit einer globalen Ejektionsfraktion unter 20% und deutlicher Perfusionseinschränkung der Vorderwand und Teilen der Seitenwand, aber deut-licher, gesteigerter Glukoseaufnahme in diesen Segmenten. Die nicht gleichsinnige Änderung von Perfusion und Glukoseaufnahme („mismatch") weist auf vitales Gewebe hin (UCLA, School of Medicine)

3. Kardiomyopathie

a) Primäre Kardiomyopathie

Die primären oder idiopathischen Kardiomyopathien sind keine einheitliche Gruppe von Erkrankungen. Sie werden nach ihrer Pumpfunktion und der Morphologie eingeteilt in re-striktive und hypertrophe, kongestive und dilatative Formen. Die oben skizzierten Regelvor-gänge verschiedener Energiesubstrate funktionieren nicht, offensichtlich liegen primär Stö-rungen des Metabolismus vor (SHABETAI 1983).

GELTMAN et al. (1983) untersuchten Patienten mit dilatativer Kardiomyopathie und fan-den eine inhomogene Anreicherung der ^{11}C-Palmitin-Säure, wobei der regionale „uptake" nicht zum Fluß korrelierte (Abb. 62, 63).

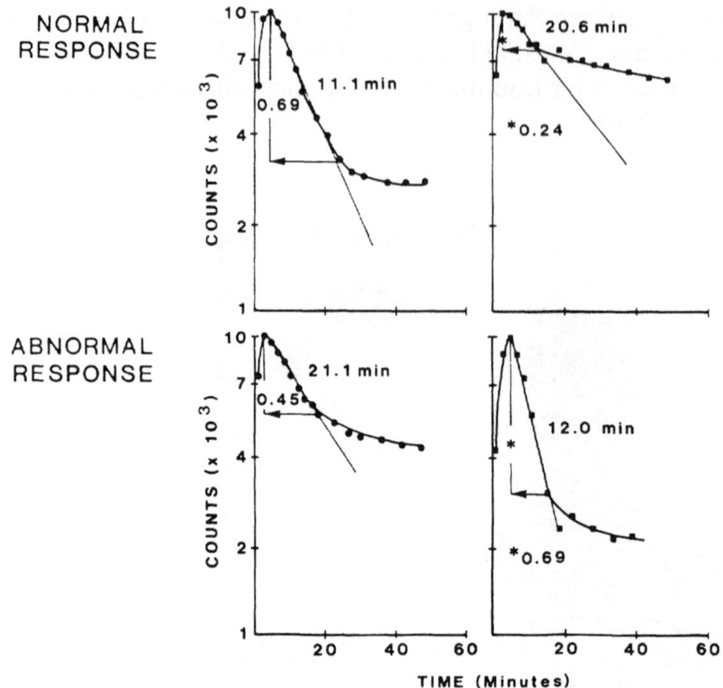

Abb. 62. Bei Patienten mit dilatativen Kardiomyopathien werden verschiedene Beeinflussungen des [1-^{11}C]-Palmitat-Stoffwechsels durch Glukose beobachtet. Die mit der PET dokumentierte Kinetik wurde im nüchternen Zustand (über-Nacht-Fasten) bzw. 2 Stunden nach oraler Applikation von 50 g Glukose durchgeführt. Bei einer normalen Wechselwirkung wird bei einer verlangsamten Kinetik ein verringerter Pool der schnellen β-Oxidation beobachtet. Patienten mit Kardiomyopathie zeigen dagegen eine paradoxe Reaktion. Bei einer Erniedrigung der Freien-Fettsäuren- und einer Erhöhung der Glukose-Konzentrationen im Plasma nimmt der Anteil der schnellen Phase des [1-^{11}C]-Palmitat-Stoffwechsels bei einer kürzeren Halbwertszeit zu. (Aus Henze et al. 1982a, b)

b) Sekundäre Kardiomyopathie

·Sekundäre Kardiomyopathien sind häufig Folgen von Erkrankungen des Koronarkreislaufes, Hypertonie, Vitien oder kongenitalen Herzerkrankungen. Vorläufige Studien an Patienten mit kongestiver Herzinsuffizienz zeigen, daß die metabolischen Parameter nicht einheitlich verändert sind. So werden bei etwa 50% der Patienten die Fettsäuren und alternativ bei entsprechendem Angebot die Glukose „normal" verstoffwechselt. Daneben gibt es aber auch Patienten mit erniedrigter Fettsäureaufnahme im Nüchternzustand, wobei nach Glukoseangebot der Fettsäuremetabolismus „paradox" zunahm. Die klinischen, hämodynamischen Parameter waren bei diesem relativ inhomogenen Patientengut nicht signifikant verschieden. Die pathophysiologischen Interpretationen setzen eine Validität der Modelle voraus, die bisher nicht geprüft wurde (Henze et al. 1982a, b). Erste Ergebnisse zur alkoholtoxischen Kardiomyopathie wurden von Bergman et al. (1982c) mitgeteilt.

Am Beispiel der Muskeldystrophie vom Typ Duchenne konnten Henze et al. (1982c) bei 15 Patienten zeigen, daß biochemische Veränderungen des Herzmuskels vor funktionellen Veränderungen auftreten. Die klinisch manifest erkrankten männlichen Kinder und Jugendlichen weisen eine hohe Prävalenz von Myokarderkrankungen auf zellulärer Ebene auf (Abb. 64) (Perloff et al. 1966, 1984). Bei 14/15 Patienten wurden regionale Minderungen der Perfusion (^{13}NH$_3$) und bei 11/12 Patienten eine verstärkte Glukoseaufnahme (^{18}FDG) in verschiedenen Segmenten beobachtet. Die konventionellen Verfahren, wie EKG, sowie Thallium- und Herzbinnenraum-Szintigraphie erwiesen sich als nicht spezifisch, so waren entsprechende EKG-Veränderungen auch bei den klinisch nicht manifesten erkrankten Müttern zu beobachten.

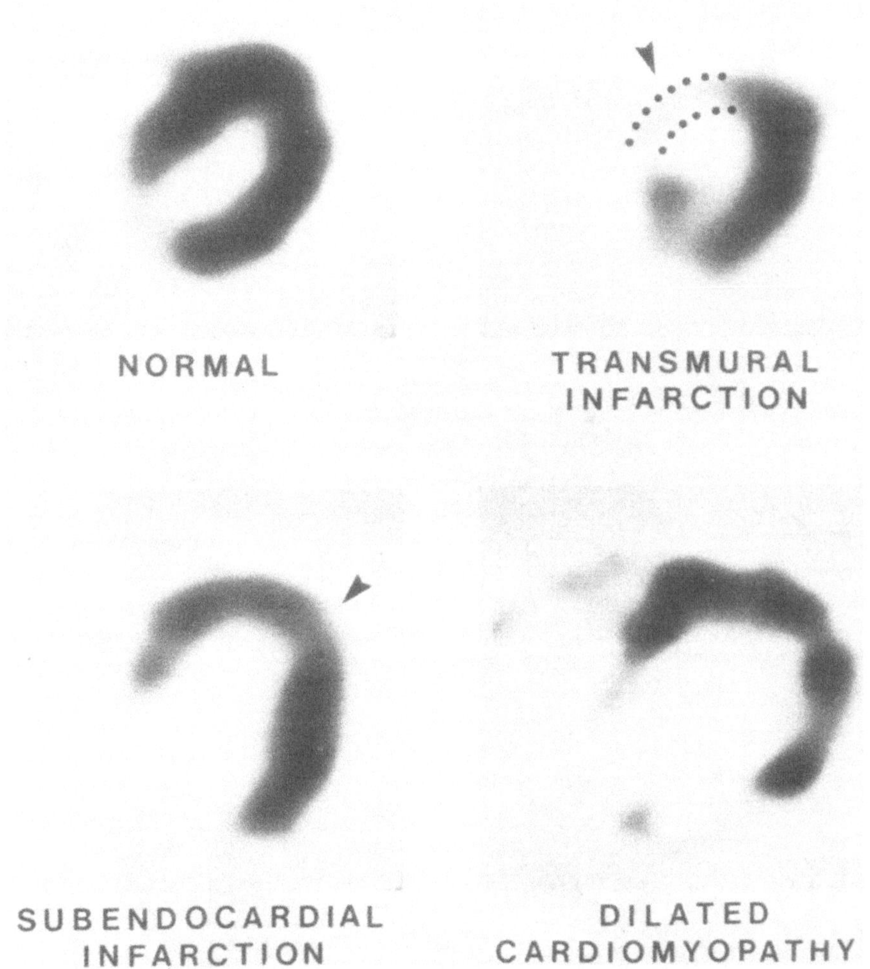

Abb. 63. Der [1-^{11}C]-Palmitat-Stoffwechsel bei dilatativer Kardiomyopathie zeigt im Myokard deutliche regionale Inhomogenitäten. Im Vergleich dazu sind Studien bei Patienten mit subendokardialem und transmuralem Infarkt dargestellt. (Aus GELTMAN et al. 1983)

III. Lunge

1. Physiologie

Die primäre physiologische Aufgabe der Lunge besteht in der Arterialisierung des venösen Blutes. Die Pathophysiologie der dazu notwendigen regionalen Lungenfunktionen, wie Perfusion und Ventilation, sowie entsprechender Verteilungsräume, wie Alveolärvolumina und Verschlußvolumen (trapped air), Blutvolumen, Blutfluß und deren Bestimmung mit Gamma-Strahlern werden seit 30 Jahren diskutiert und beschrieben (BALL et al. 1962; KNIPPING et al. 1955; RAMOS u. RÖSLER 1978). Klinisch steht dabei die Diagnose der Lungenembolie mit Gamma-Strahlern wie einem Tracer zur Ventilationsbestimmung und ^{99m}Tc-markierten Mikrosphären zur Dokumentation der regionalen Perfusion im Vordergrund.

Quantitative dreidimensionale Studien, die mit der Technik der Positronen-Emissionstomographie möglich sind, haben klinisch noch keinen Sinn, wenn nur Aktivitäten pro Einheit

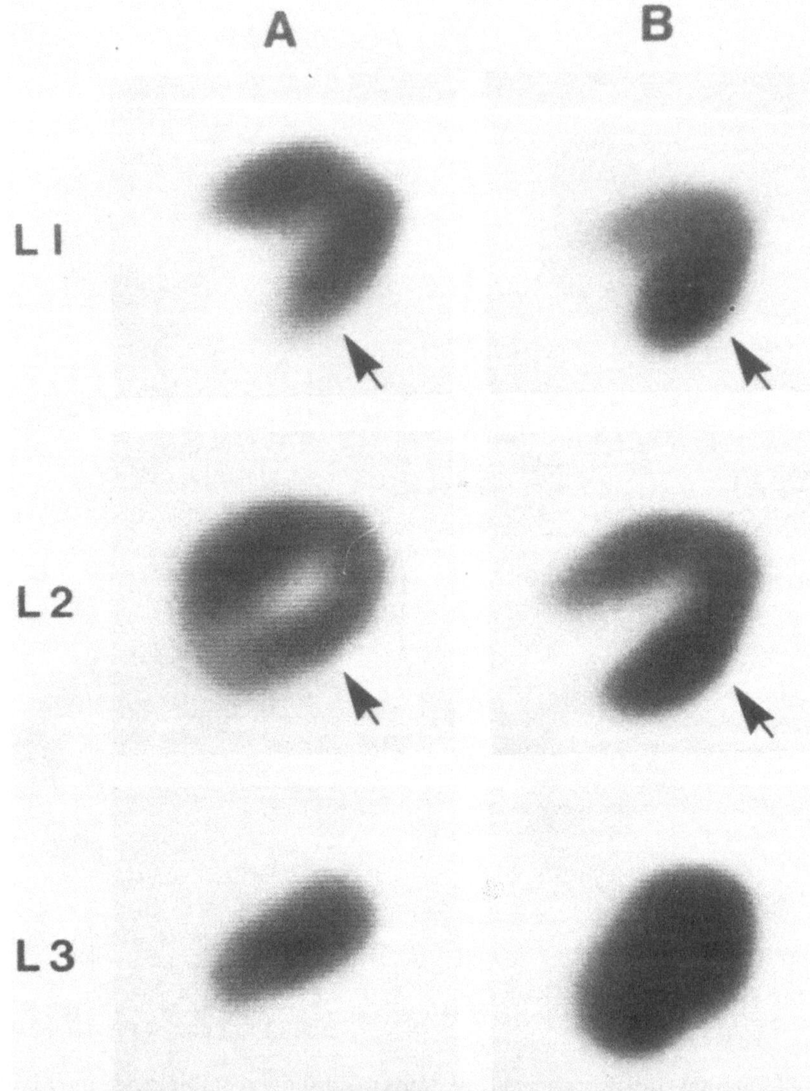

Abb. 64A, B. Myokardiale Perfusion (**A** $^{13}NH_3$) und Glukoseaufnahme (**B** ^{18}F-FDG) bei einem Patienten mit Duchenne Muskelatrophie in drei verschiedenen Schnittebenen. Bei diesem 14jährigen Jungen wurde eine normale globale und regionale linksventrikuläre Funktion bei unauffälliger ^{201}Thallium-Szintigraphie gefunden. In der PET zeigt sich dagegen eine Minderperfusion der posterolateralen Wand (*Pfeil*) bei verstärkter Glukoseaufnahme („mismatch"). (Aus Perloff et al. 1984)

Thoraxvolumen angegeben werden. Erst spezifische morphologische Strukturen oder Funktionen, etwa pro Verteilungsvolumen, Alveolärraum oder extravaskuläres Lungenwasser, Oberfläche oder spezifische Zelldichte, ermöglichen die sinnvolle Angabe physiologisch relevanter Parameter. Es ist daher notwendig, verschiedene Kompartimente örtlich, und wenn möglich auch in ihrem kinetischen Verhalten, zu unterscheiden.

Positronenstrahler, wie $^{15}O_2$, $CO^{15}O$ und $C^{15}O$, werden bereits seit 1960 vor allem von der Gruppe am Hammersmith Hospital, London, eingesetzt (Dollery et al. 1960; Dyson et al. 1960; West u. Dollery 1960). Ansätze zur quantitativen Bestimmung des extravaskulären Lungenwassers mit der „first-pass"-Methode werden seit 1976 beschrieben (Binswanger et al. 1978; Fazio et al. 1976). Rhodes et al. (1981) und Schober et al. (1983) begannen mit Untersuchungen im „steady state", um die den „first-pass"-Studien inhärenten Probleme teilweise zu lösen. Die Ventilationsszintigraphie mit dem Zyklotronprodukt ^{81}Rb/^{81m}Kr wird in der klinischen Routine seit etwa 10 Jahren durchgeführt (Amis et al. 1975; Amis u. Jones 1980; MacCarther et al. 1980; Ahluwalia et al. 1981a, b; Fazio u. Jones 1975; Müller et al. 1983).

Daneben haben verschiedene metabolische Funktionen der Lunge, wie die Inaktivierung zirkulierender vasoaktiver Verbindungen und das retikuloendotheliale System (RES), eine noch weitgehend in Einzelproblemen dargestellte, zunehmend größer werdende Bedeutung (Junod 1972; Gallagher et al. 1977; Skort et al. 1979; Berger et al. 1982; Pang et al. 1982; Pascal et al. 1982; Pistolesi et al. 1985; Said 1982; Syrota et al. 1981b).

2. Ventilation und Perfusion

Die Messung der regionalen Ventilation wird in der Klinik in erster Linie mit ^{133}Xe und ^{81m}Kr durchgeführt. Andere im Blut gut und schlecht lösliche radioaktive Gase sind von untergeordneter Bedeutung (^{15}O$_2$, C^{15}O, C^{15}O$_2$, ^{11}CO$_2$, ^{13}N$_2$, ^{19}Ne, ^{77}Kr, ^{85}Kr, ^{85m}Kr, ^{123}Xe, ^{127}Xe, ^{133}Xe, ^{135}Xe). Von den Positronenstrahlern sind in einzelnen Literaturangaben die Nuklide ^{13}N und ^{19}Ne zur Beurteilung der Ventilation verwandt worden (Rosenzweig et al. 1969; Ramos u. Rösler 1978; Hughes 1979; Susskind et al. 1981; Williams 1981; Modell u. Graham 1982; Megnan et al. 1984).

Valind et al. (1983) untersuchten nach Inhalation von ^{19}Ne ein Kontrollkollektiv und fanden ein dorsal gegenüber ventral um 25–30% vergrößertes Alveolarvolumen und erklärten dieses mit der regionalen Compliance. Aus kinetischen Studien errechnen sie weiterhin ein Maß für die Ventilation. Die Perfusion bestimmen sie nach intravenöser Injektion von ^{13}N, wobei die Applikation ^{11}C-markierter Mikrosphären sicherlich optimaler wäre.

3. Pathophysiologie: Lungenödem

Das Lungenödem wird nach physiologischen Kriterien eingeteilt in ein solches hydrostatischer Genese (kardiogen, high pressure) oder ein solches mit Permeabilitätsstörungen (nichtkardiogen, low pressure) sowie anatomisch klassifiziert in ein interstitielles und/oder alveoläres Ödem (Crandall et al. 1983; Staub 1974, 1978; Stender 1961; Stender u. Schermuly 1969; West 1977). Starlings (1896) Hypothese zur Beschreibung der Ödementstehung in der Lunge über die transvaskulären treibenden Kräfte zur Erhaltung der Flüssigkeitsgleichgewichte ist, wenn auch in modifizierter Form, immer noch Basis jeder rationalen Diskussion und Therapie.

$dQ/dt = K[(P_{mv} - P_{pmv}) - S(\pi_{mv} - \pi_{pmv})]$

dQ/dt = netto transvaskuläre Filtrationsrate
K   = Transportkonstante der mikrovaskulären Barriere
P   = hydrostatischer Druck
mv   = mikrovaskuläres Lumen
pmv = perimikrovaskuläre interstitielle Flüssigkeit
S   = Reflexionskoeffizient (O > S > 1)
π = Protein osmotischer Druck (kolloid, onkotisch)

In der klinischen Praxis wird der Schweregrad dieser Veränderungen anhand des physikalischen Befundes und des Röntgenbildes abgeschätzt. Dabei sind theoretische Modellvorstellungen von ebenso relativ untergeordneter Bedeutung, wie morphologisch orientierte und indirekte nicht-destruktive Meßverfahren:

Compton-Scatter (Gamsu et al. 1979; Guzzardi u. Mey 1979), Absorption von Gamma-Strahlern (Simon et al. 1979), transvaskulärer Proteinfluß (Creutzig et al. 1984; Sturm et al. 1985; Sugerman et al. 1981, 1982a, b), Blutpool-Markierungen im Gleichgewicht (Ba-

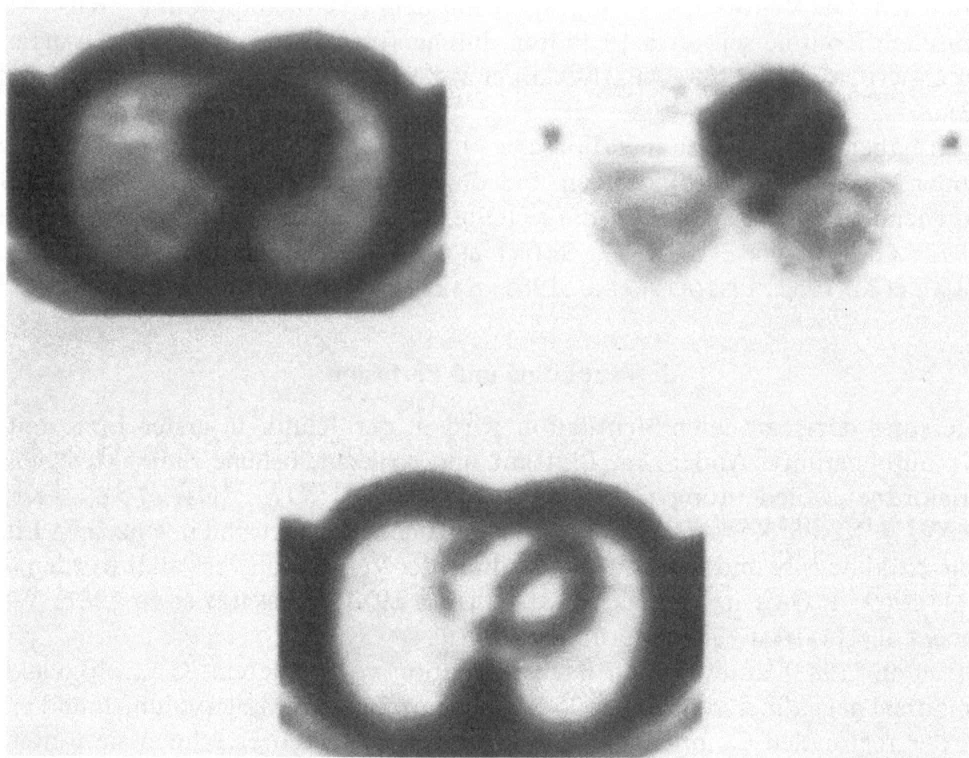

Abb. 65. Transaxiale Schichtaufnahmen der Lungendichte (*oben links*), des regionalen Blutvolumens (rBV, *oben rechts*) und der errechneten regionalen extravaskulären Lungendichte (rELD, *unten*) bei einer Kontrollperson. (Aus Rhodes et al. 1981)

Teman et al. 1983) und Transmissionscomputertomographie (Döhring et al. 1981; Wegener et al. 1978) oder Thallium-201 Auswaschkinetiken (Tamaki et al. 1982). Auch Indikatorverdünnungsmethoden haben, besonders wegen ihrer ausschließlich globalen Aussagen bei methodisch einschränkenden Randbedingungen in der Klinik, nur unter Intensivpflegebedingungen eine Bedeutung (Chinard 1973; Chinard u. Enns 1954; Chinard et al. 1955, 1962; Cooper et al. 1972; Critchley et al. 1981; Fazio et al. 1976; Goresky et al. 1969, 1970; Helmecke et al. 1982; Hughes 1977; Jones et al. 1976; Lewis et al. 1982; Schober et al. 1983).

4. Extravaskuläre Lungendichte (ELD), extravaskuläres Lungenwasser (ELW), thorakales Blutvolumen (BV)

a) Normalpersonen

Rhodes et al. (1981) entwickelten eine Methode zur regionalen, quantitativen Bestimmung des Intravasalraumes mit der Positronen-Emissionstomographie (PET), nach Inhalation von ^{11}CO und der in-vivo-Markierung der Erythrozyten über die Bildung von Carboxyhämiglobin (Phelps et al. 1979), und der extravaskulären Lungendichte mit der Transmissions-Computertomographie (CT) (Abb. 65). Bei Kontrollpersonen beträgt die mittlere Lungendichte 0.29 ± 0.08 g/cm^3 mit einem anterio-posteriorem Gradienten von 0.20–0.38 g/cm^3, während die ELD einen leichten ventrodorsalen Gradienten, von 0.12 g/cm^3 auf 0.16 g/cm^3, aufwies. Dieser Gradient wird auf den Einfluß der Gravidität zurückgeführt. Die Variation der räum-

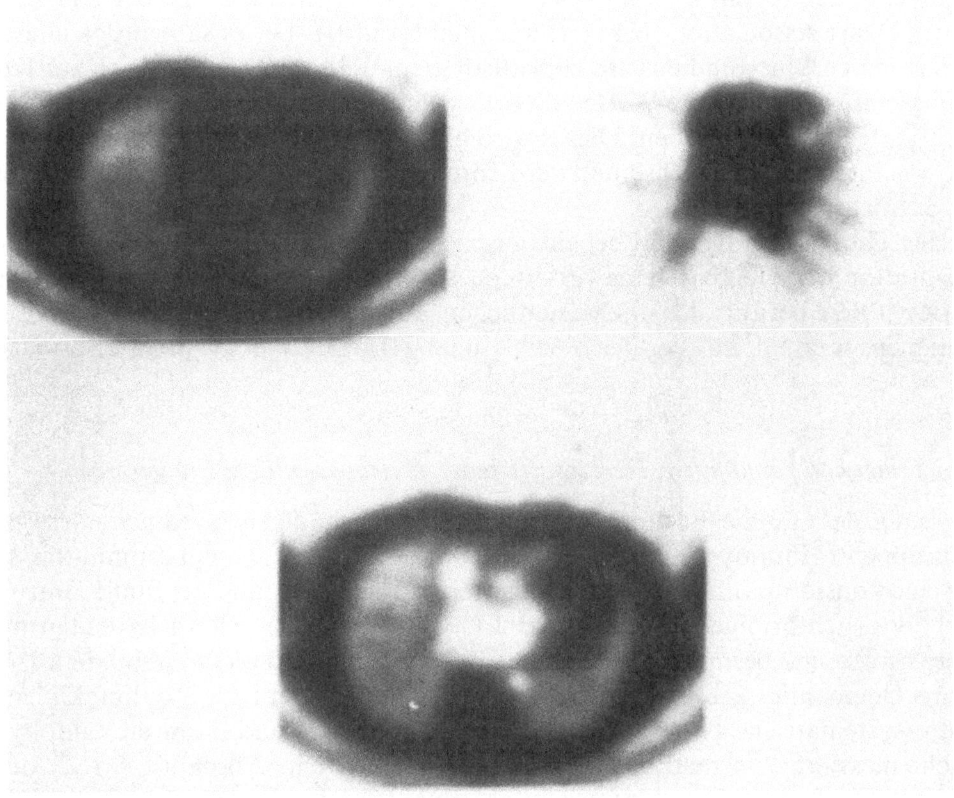

Abb. 66. Transaxiale Schichtaufnahmen der Lungendichte (*oben links*), des regionalen Blutvolumens (rBV, *oben rechts*) und der regionalen extravaskulären Lungendichte (rELD, *unten*) bei einem Patienten mit chronischer pulmonaler Hypertension. Das regionale Blutvolumen ist vermindert, der normale ventro-dorsale Gradient aufgehoben. Die extravaskuläre Lungendichte ist besonders in den posterioren Anteilen erhöht. (Aus WOLLMER et al. 1983)

lichen Blutdichte, bezogen auf das Thoraxvolumen, folgt einer ähnlichen Verteilung mit 0.08 ml/cm³ anterior bis 0.21 ml/cm³ posterior. Verantwortlich für diesen Gradienten sind im wesentlichen der transmurale, hydrostatische Druck des Gefäßsystems (intravaskulär vs. perivaskulär) und die elastischen Eigenschaften der Gefäße (WEST et al. 1964). Die Unterschiede zwischen einer kaudalen und einer kranialen Ebene sind relativ gering bzgl. der ELD, aber deutlich in bezug auf das Blutvolumen ($\triangle = 30\%$).

Die absoluten Werte wurden von der Arbeitsgruppe in Hannover bzgl. des regionalen intrathorakalen Blutvolumens bestätigt. Das regionale Blutvolumen wurde mit 0.21 ± 0.02 g/cm³ und einem deutlichen baso-apikalen Gradienten bestimmt (0.25–0.17). Das extravaskuläre Lungenwasser wurde allerdings im „steady state" mit $H_2^{15}O$ bestimmt. Der Mittelwert wurde mit 0.13 ± 0.02 g/cm³ und einem geringen baso-apikalen Gradienten (0.12–0.14) angegeben (SCHOBER et al. 1985d).

b) Lungenerkrankungen, Herzinsuffizienz: Regionales Blutvolumen

Die Arbeitsgruppe vom Hammersmith Hospital, London, fand bei Patienten mit pulmonaler Hypertension einen Anstieg der ELD um 40%, vorwiegend basal, während das regionale Blutvolumen hier um 25% reduziert war (Abb. 66) (WOLLMER et al. 1983, 1984).

Die gleiche räumliche Verteilung des regionalen Blutvolumens fand die Arbeitsgruppe in Hannover bei Patienten mit kongestiver Herzinsuffizienz, entsprechend der Klassifizierung der New York Heart Association (NYHA) maximal Grad III–IV. Basal wurden eine Erniedrigung des regionalen Blutvolumens um 20% (0.18 g/cm^3), kranial im Vergleich zur Kontrollgruppe (0.16 g/cm^3) unveränderte Werte von 0.17 g/cm^3, und damit eine relativ gleichförmige apico-basale Verteilung beschrieben. Dieses wird auf strukturelle Veränderungen im Lungenparenchym, wie interstitielle Fibrose und verdichtete Gefäßwände zurückgeführt (Bossaller et al. 1985; Schober et al. 1985 d).

Die für das Thorax-Röntgenbild bei chronischer Herzinsuffizienz und Lungenödem typische Kranialisation der Gefäßsysteme (Pistolesi et al. 1978, 1982; Stender 1961; Stender u. Schermuly 1969) beruht also im wesentlichen auf dem Effekt der relativen Zunahme des Blutvolumens kranial im Vergleich zu kaudal (Bateman et al. 1983; Schober et al. 1985 d).

c) Lungenerkrankungen, Herzinsuffizienz: Extravaskuläres Lungenwasser

Zur Messung des für die Bestimmung des ELW notwendigen Gesamtwassers benutzte die Arbeitsgruppe in Hannover nicht die indirekte Methode der Dichtebestimmung, sondern entwickelte eine konstante Infusion ^{15}O-markierten Wassers. Sie fand bei fünf Kontrollpersonen eine relativ gleichförmige Verteilung des ELW (0.11 g/cm^3), bei 14 Patienten mit kongestiver Herzinsuffizienz besonders basal eine Erhöhung auf 0.20 g/cm^3 (Abb. 67). Inwieweit das alveoläre Ödem mit „steady-state"-Methoden und kurzlebigen Radionukliden erfaßt werden kann (systematische Unterschätzung um bis zu 30%), und dann die „unphysiologischere" Dichtemessung von methodischem Vorteil ist, wird in Abschnitt B.II.2. diskutiert (Meyer et al. 1983, 1984, 1985 b; Schober et al. 1983, 1985 d).

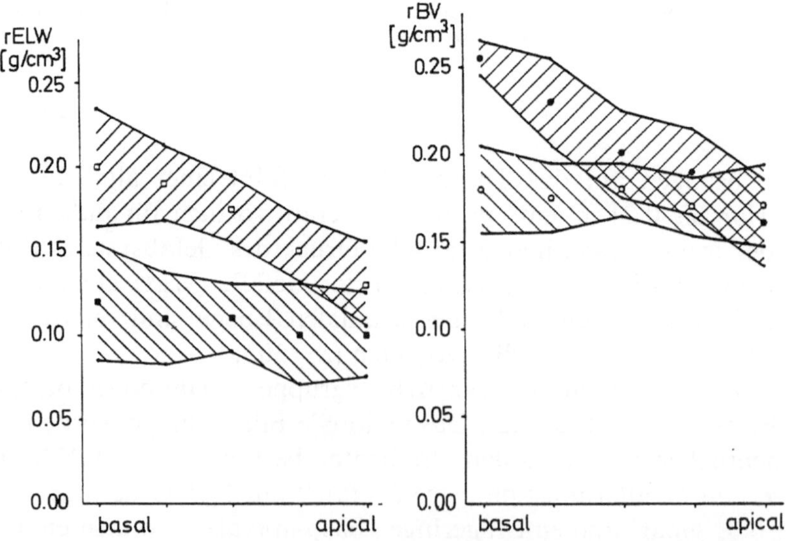

Abb. 67. Bei Kontrollpersonen ist das regionale extravaskuläre Lungenwasser (*rELW*) von basal nach apikal relativ homogen verteilt. Bei Patienten mit chronischer Herzinsuffizienz findet sich ein im Vergleich zu den Kontrollpersonen erhöhtes rELW. Während das apikale rELW bei der Herzinsuffizienz fast unverändert bleibt, steigt es besonders basal auf etwa doppelte Werte an. Mit zunehmender Herzinsuffizienz bleibt das apikale regionale Blutvolumen (*rBV*) weitgehend unverändert, während es basal abnimmt. Aus den Veränderungen läßt sich schließen, daß die im Röntgenbild der Lungen gefundene „Kranialisation der Lungengefäße" nicht auf einer Zunahme des regionalen pulmonalem Blutvolumens in den kranialen Anteilen der Lungen, sondern auf einer Abnahme des rBV in den kaudalen Anteilen beruht. (Aus Schober et al. 1983, 1985 d)

Im Vergleich zu hämodynamischen Parametern (Cardiac-Index, Pulmonalis-Druck, Ejektionsfraktion etc.) zeigte sich die beste Korrelation zwischen regionalem ELW (rELW) und der klinischen Klassifizierung entsprechend der NYHA ($r = 0.69$). Das auf das regionale Blutvolumen bezogene rELW weist mit $r = 0.87$ eine besonders hohe Korrelation zur „Klinik" auf. Dieser Quotient ist bzgl. systematischer Fehler, wie Teilvolumeneffekt und unzureichende Absorptionskorrektur, weniger empfindlich.

Ein Vergleich mit konventionellen Röntgenaufnahmen des Thorax zeigt, daß regionale Erhöhungen des ELW um 30% von einem erfahrenen Untersucher als spezifische Veränderungen erkannt werden (retikuläre Strukturvermehrung, interlobuläre Septumlinien, peribronchiale und perivaskuläre Verdichtungen, unscharfe perihiläre Zonen, subpleurale Verdichtungen) (SCHOBER et al. 1985 d).

WOLLMER et al. (1984) fanden Erhöhungen der ELD und Erniedrigungen des pulmonalen Blutvolumens bei interstitiellen Lungenerkrankungen, wie fibrosierender Alveolitis und Sarkoidose. Diese Veränderungen korrelierten gut mit globalen Lungenfunktionsprüfungen.

5. Pharmakologie

a) Nicht-biogene Amine

PASCAL et al. (1982) untersuchten die Aufnahme und das Auswaschverhalten ^{11}C-markierter lipophiler Amine, Imipramin und Propanolol, bei Patienten mit Sarkoidose, Tuberkulose und chronisch obstruktiver Lungenerkrankung (BERGER et al. 1982). Die flußbestimmte Aufnahme führt zu einem „uptake" von etwa 70% im „first pass". Bei Kontrollpersonen und Patienten beobachtete er die gleiche maximale Tracer-Konzentration in den Lungen. Bei Patienten mit infiltrativen Lungenerkrankungen und vergrößertem Extravasalraum waren jedoch die Aufnahme verringert und der Auswaschvorgang verzögert. Trotz der pharmakologisch faszinierenden Möglichkeiten in der Zukunft zeigt gerade dieses Beispiel bei Halbwertszeiten der Clearance in der Größenordnung von 30–40 h und einer physikalischen Halbwertzeit des Tracers von 20 min die Grenzen auf, die es nur spekulativ erlauben, in diesem Fall auf einen möglichen Endothelschaden als Ursache zu schließen.

b) Aminosäuren, Glukose

^{11}C-L-Methionin wird von primären Lungen- und Mediastinal-Tumoren aufgenommen. KUBOTA et al. (1982, 1983, 1985) diskutieren die Aufnahme über einen verstärkten Aminosäure-Metabolismus und sehen die Möglichkeit der Diskrimination zwischen malignem und benignem, nekrotischem und vitalem Gewebe. SUZUKI u. IDO (1982) sehen ähnliche differentialdiagnostische Möglichkeiten für ^{11}C-Glukose und ^{11}C-Fruktose.

c) Erythromycin

^{11}C-markiertes Erythromycin wurde zum quantitativen, regionalen Nachweis der Verteilung des Antibiotikums bei Lobär-Pneumonien verwandt (WOLLMER et al. 1982). In-vivo Studien dieser Art versprechen einen neuen, grundsätzlichen Ansatz zur Beurteilung von Pharmaka.

d) Bleomycin

^{55}Co-Bleomycin wurde bei Patienten mit Bronchial-Karzinom und Hirnmetastasen untersucht (BEEKHUIS u. NIEWEG 1984; NIEWEG et al. 1981, 1982). Die physikalische Halbwertzeit von 18 Stunden läßt bei geeigneter Detektortechnik sowohl diagnostische Hilfen als auch eine Beurteilung der Therapie erwarten.

IV. Tumoren und entzündliche Veränderungen

Das pathophysiologische Verständnis führt zu Merkmalen der Neoplasien, die Störungen der Homöostasie betreffen, aber auch die Problematik der *Vaskularisierung*, des *nutritiven Blutflusses* und des damit verbundene *Metabolismus*. Ziel der Untersuchungen mit der Positronen-Emissionstomographie ist es, diese funktionelle Verflechtung, d.h. die stoffwechselbedingten Wechselwirkungen zwischen Organismus und Tumor, darzustellen und zu analysieren.

1. Pankreas

Das Pankreas utilisiert freie Aminosäuren zur Synthese von Verdauungsenzymen. Da die Bauchspeicheldrüse das Organ mit der höchsten Proteinsyntheserate des Organismus in den exokrinen Azinuszellen ist, erfolgte der Ansatz zur regionalen Funktionsdarstellung über Aminosäuren oder ihre Analoga. Das Radiopharmakon, das bisher am häufigsten angewandt wurde, ist das ^{75}Se-L-Methionin, das aber aufgrund seiner Gamma-Energie (Hauptenergie: 0.27 MeV) und seiner physikalischen Halbwertszeit ($T_{1/2} = 120$ d) bei dem heutigen Entwicklungsstand der Radiopharmazie und Nuklearmedizin, aber auch gegenüber den übrigen bildgebenden Verfahren, wie Sonographie, Computertomographie (CT) und Kernspintomographie (MRI), als sehr ungeeignet einzustufen ist (Blau 1961; Blau u. Manske 1961; Hundeshagen 1978; Kirchner et al. 1980; Smith et al. 1982; Stark et al. 1984).

Aminosäuren. Mit der Positronen-Emissionstomographie wurde es möglich, natürliche Aminosäuren, wie DL-Tryptophan, DL-Valin, oder L-Methionin mit ^{11}C zu markieren.

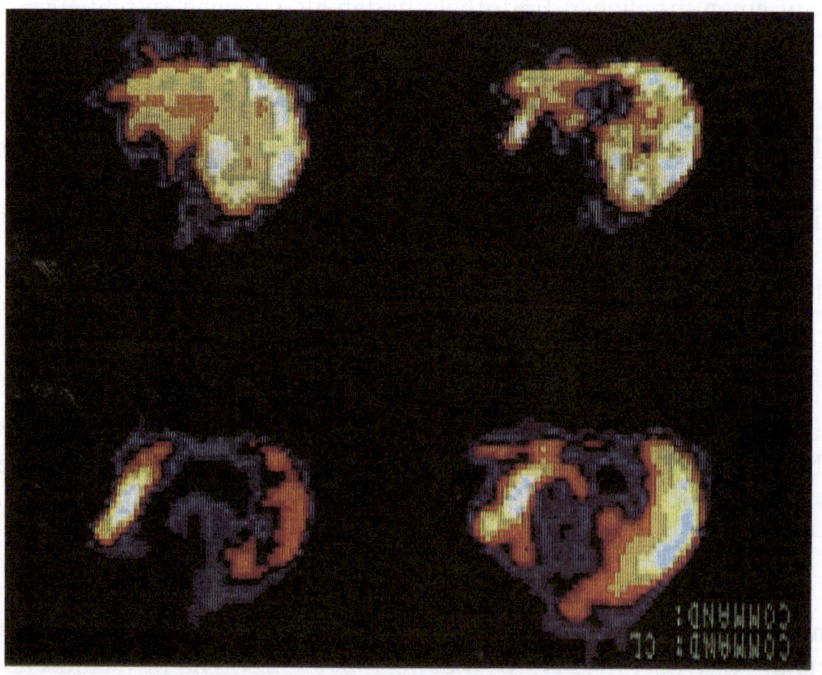

Abb. 68. Tomographische Schichtaufnahmen mit ^{11}C-L-Methionin bei einer Kontrollperson. Entsprechend der Proteinsynthese ist die Leber ebenfalls dargestellt

Wegen des ungeklärten und komplizierten Modelles des Aminosäure-Metabolismus ist es bisher nicht möglich, quantitative Angaben zu erhalten, vielmehr liegen Berichte über qualitative Aufnahmewerte vor.

Nach intravenöser Applikation ist die initiale Clearance relativ schnell, so verbleiben 15 min p.i. weniger als 20% der Aktivität im Plasmaraum, während die Demethylierung beim Menschen offensichtlich innerhalb der 1. Stunde p.i. keine große Rolle spielt und die ^{11}C-Konzentration relativ konstant bleibt (HÜBNER et al. 1979; KIRCHNER et al. 1980)

^{11}C-DL-Valin: HÜBNER et al. (1979), WASHBURN et al. (1976, 1978, 1979)
^{11}C-DL-Tryptophan: HÜBNER et al. (1979)
^{11}C-L, DL-Methionin: MEYER et al. (1982), SYROTA et al. (1979, 1981a, 1982a)
^{13}N-L-Glutamat: LAUGHLIN et al. (1980), MYERS et al. (1983)

Diskutiert wird, ob die Aufnahme des ^{11}C-L, D-Tryptophans wegen des höchsten Target/Nicht-Target-Verhältnisses, d.h. der relativ geringsten Untergrundaktivität, am optimalsten zur Pankreasdarstellung geeignet ist (BUSCH et al. 1959). Tatsächlich wird sogar eine verstärkte Aufnahme des nicht racemischen Tryptophans in einzelnen Pankreastumoren von der Gruppe in Oak Ridge, Tennesse, berichtet (BUONOCORE u. HÜBNER 1979; HÜBNER et al. 1979). Diese Ergebnisse konnten von den Gruppen in Chicago (COOPER u. HARPER et al. 1980; KIRCHNER et al. 1980), Orsay, Frankreich (1982) und Hannover (MEYER et al. 1982; SCHOBER et al. 1986b) nicht bestätigt werden.

^{11}C-L-Methionin. Die größten Erfahrungen aus klinischen Studien an mehr als 150 Patienten liegen aus Orsay, Frankreich und Hannover über die ^{11}C-L-Methionin-Aufnahme vor (Abb. 68) (MEYER et al. 1982; SYROTA et al. 1982a).

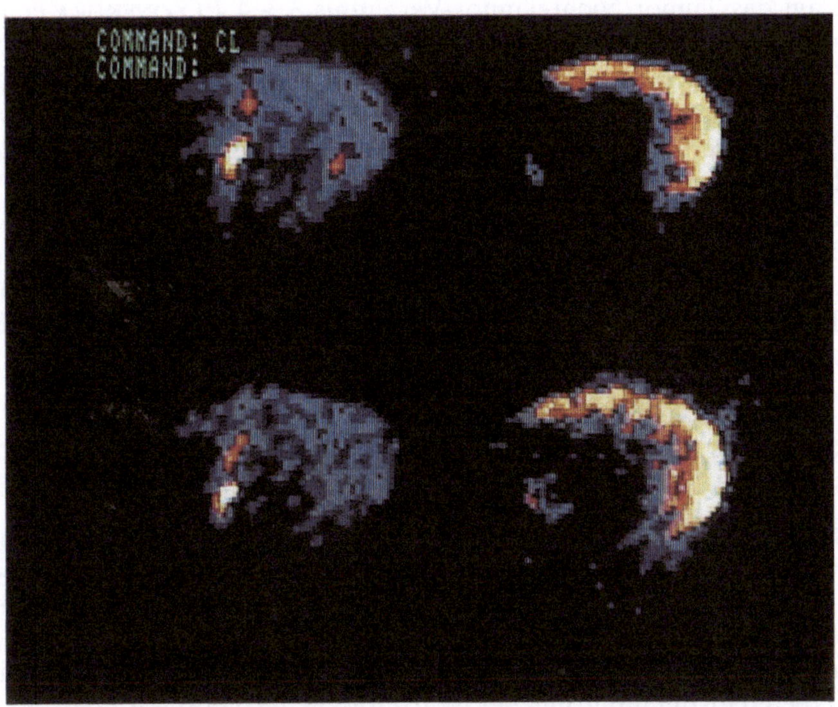

Abb. 69. Tomographische Schichtaufnahmen mit ^{11}C-L-Methionin bei einem Patienten mit chronischer Pankreatitis. Die Anreicherung der Aminosäure im Pankreas ist deutlich erniedrigt

So war bei einem Patientenkollektiv mit akuter und chronischer Pankreatitis sowie Pankreaskarzinom gegenüber einer Kontrollgruppe die ^{11}C-Methionin-Aufnahme stets vermindert gegenüber normalem Gewebe (Abb. 69). Bei Normalpersonen wurden 0.011 ± 0.003 %/ml Lebergewebe und 0.015 ± 0.005%/ml Pankreasgewebe der applizierten Aktivität gefunden. Das führt zu einer relativen Pankreas/Leber-Konzentration von 1.4 ± 0.4, bei einer allerdings großen Spannweite von 0.9–2.9. Bei akuter Pankreatitis war dieses Verhältnis bei einer kleinen Patientengruppe nicht wesentlich verringert, bei chronischer Pankreatitis (0–1.5) und Pankreaskarzinom (0–0.9) allerdings unspezifisch deutlich verringert bzw. keine Aktivität nachweisbar (Syrota et al. 1982a).

Gerade von der Gruppe in Orsay werden eine größere Sensitivität (85%) und Spezifität (98%) der Methionin-PET als bei der CT und der Sonographie angegeben. Dieses wird darauf zurückgeführt, daß funktionelle Änderungen vor morphologischen Veränderungen zu erwarten sind. Allerdings sind, wie die Arbeitsgruppe aus Hannover zeigte, neben einer bisher fehlenden Modellvorstellung, die Selektion des Patientenkollektivs, die Vergleichbarkeit der Meßgeräte mit den entsprechenden räumlichen Auflösungsvermögen und eine endgültige klinische Diagnose zu berücksichtigen. Tatsächlich werden von dieser Gruppe keine signifikanten Unterschiede zwischen normalen und transformierten Zellen beobachtet (Holley 1972; Meyer et al. 1982).

2. Leber

Zu PET-Untersuchungen der Leber liegen nur vereinzelte Berichte und intensive Fallstudien vor. So berichten Hayashi et al. (1985) über eine positive Darstellung des häufigsten malignen primären Lebertumors, des Hepatoms, mit ^{13}NH$_3$/^{13}NH$_4^+$ bei 5 Patienten. Sie diskutieren primär die vaskuläre Versorgung und Perfusion bei guter Tracer-Extraktion.

Bei Patienten mit Lebermetastasen eines Kolon-Karzinoms wird über eine positive Darstellung mit ^{18}F-FDG der Lebermetastasen gegenüber normalen Lebergewebe berichtet, 50 min p.i. beträgt das Tumor/Nicht-Tumor-Verhältnis 3.3–4.7 (Yonekura et al. 1982). Bei einem hypervaskularisierten, entdifferenzierten Hepatom war das Tumorgewebe, nicht aber der zentrale nekrotische Bereich, mit ^{18}F-FDG positiv dargestellt (Paul et al. 1985). Dieses kann auf die Schlüsselenzyme des Glukosemetabolismus (Hexokinase, Phosphofruktokinase, Pyruvatkinase) zurückgeführt werden, zumal in Hepatomata die Hexokinaseaktivität um das zwei- bis dreifache gegenüber dem Normalgewebe vergrößert ist (Weber 1977). Absolute quantitative Angaben können jedoch nicht gemacht werden, da das Sokoloff-Modell nicht angewandt werden kann. Im Gehirn werden mehr als 95% der FDG in Form der FDG-6-P gespeichert, in der Leber dagegen nur weniger als 40%. Die genauen Konzentrationen der Enzyme Hexokinase und Glukose-6-Phosphatase in den verschiedenen Tumoren sind unbekannt (Welch 1982; Lawrence u. Jullien 1982; Fukuda et al. 1982).

3. Mamma-Karzinom

Bei neun Patienten mit Mamma-Karzinom wurden Blutvolumen (BV), Blutfluß (BF), Sauerstoff-Extraktion (OER) und Sauerstoffmetabolismus (MRO$_2$) untersucht. Die regionale Perfusion war in nicht-nekrotischem Gewebe deutlich, etwa um einen Faktor 4, höher als in dem normalen umgebenden Gewebe und auf der kontralateralen Seite, während der Sauerstoffmetabolismus (MRO$_2$) leicht erhöht war und die relative Extraktion erniedrigt beobachtet wurde. In Übereinstimmung mit der Warburgschen Hypothese fand die Gruppe am Hammersmith Hospital einen im Vergleich zum Sauerstoffverbrauch deutlicher erhöhten Glukosestoffwechsel (Beaney 1984; Beaney u. Lammertsma 1985; Beaney et al. 1984).

4. Non-Hodgkin Lymphom

Auch bei einem Patienten mit Non-Hodgkin Lymphom wurden in einem inguinalen Lymphknoten eine deutlich erhöhte Perfusion, eine erniedrigte Sauerstoffextraktion und ein relativ hoher Sauerstoffmetabolismus beschrieben (BEANEY u. LAMMERTSMA 1985).

5. Knochentumoren

REIMAN et al. (1982b) untersuchten die Aufnahme von ^{13}N-L-Glutamat bei Patienten mit *Ewingsarkom,* vor und nach Chemotherapie. Dieselbe Arbeitsgruppe berichtet über ^{13}N-L-Glutamat-Aufnahme bei einem Patienten mit *embryonalen Rhabdomyosarkom* (SORDILLO et al. 1982), und einem Patienten mit *Weichteil-Sarkom* (SORDILLO et al. 1983) und einem *osteogenen Sarkom* (GELBHARD et al. 1979; REIMAN et al. 1981). Hier werden eine erhöhte Perfusion, eine erniedrigte Sauerstoffextraktion und ein leicht erhöhter Sauerstoffmetabolismus außerhalb der nekrotischen Bereiche dokumentiert. Unter einer Chemotherapie werden veränderte Stoffwechselparameter beobachtet (BEANEY u. LAMMERTSMA 1985; GRONEMEYER et al. 1980; KNAPP et al. 1984; KNAPP u. VYSKA 1984).

6. Metastasen verschiedener Tumoren

Bei Patienten mit Metastasen unterschiedlicher Primärtumoren beobachteten HÜBNER et al. (1977, 1981) eine Anreicherung alizyklischer Aminosäuren, der ^{11}C-ACPC und ^{11}C-ACBC.

Verschiedenes. Mit ^{124}I gelang die tomographische Darstellung dieser Schilddrüse (FREY et al. 1985). Der Ammoniakstoffwechsel, insbesondere bei Lebererkrankungen, wurde von LOCKWOOD et al. (1979) untersucht. Diagnose und Lokalisation zerebrospinaler Fisteln wurde mit ^{68}Ga-EDTA erfolgreich durchgeführt (BERGSTRAND et al. 1982). Der periphere Blutfluß bei Diabetikern wurde von SPINKS et al. (1984, 1985) beschrieben.

Literatur

Abumrad NA, Park PH, Park CR (1984) Permeation of long-chain fatty acids into adipocytes: Specificity and evidence for involvement of a membrane protein. J Biol Chem 259:8945–8953

Ackerman RH, Correia JA, Alpert NM, Baron JD, Gouliamos A, Grotta A, Brownell GL, Taveras JM (1981a) Positron imaging in ischemic stroke disease using compounds labeled with oxygen 15. Arch Neurol 38:537–543

Ackerman RH, Davis SM, Correia JA, Alpert NM, Buonanno F, Finkelstein S, Brownell GL, Taveras JM (1981b) Positron Imaging of CBF and metabolism in patients with cerebral neoplasms. J Cereb Blood Flow Metab 1:575–576

Ackerman RH, Alpert NM, Correia JA, Finkelstein S, Buonanno F, Davis SM, Chang JY, Brownell GL, Taveras JM (1981c) Importance of monitoring metabolic function in assessing the severity of a stroke insult (CBF: an epiphenomenon?). J Cereb Blood Flow Metab 1:502–503

Ackerman RH, Alpert NM, Davis SM, Celly RE, Correia JA, Brownell GL, Taveras JM (1983a) Positron emission tomography of stroke patients. In: Heiss WD, Phelps ME (eds) Positron emission tomography of the brain. Springer, Berlin Heidelberg New York Tokyo, pp 113–119

Ackerman RH, Kelley RF, Davis SM, Alpert NM, Correia JA, Brownell GL (1983b) Positron imaging of CBF and metabolism in nontraumatic intracerebral hemorrhage. In: Mizukami M et al. (eds) Hypertensive intracerebral hemorrhage. Raven, New York, pp 165–176

Ackerman RH, Alpert NM, Correia JA, Finkelstein S, Davis SM, Kelley RE, Donnan GA, D'Alton JG, Taveras JM (1984) Positron imaging in ischemic stroke disease. Ann Neurol 15:S126–S130

Ackerman RH, Correia JA, Alpert NM, Haley EC, Buxton RB, Elmaleh DR, Taveras JM (1985) PET studies of stroke. In: Reivich M, Alavi A (eds) Positron emission tomography. Liss, New York, pp 249–262

Ahluwalia B, Brownell GL, Hales C, Kazemi H (1981a) An index of pulmonary edema measured with emission computed tomography. J Comput Assist Tomogr 5:690–694

Ahluwalia B, Brownell GL, Hales C, Kazemi H (1981b) Regional lung function evaluation with Nitrogen-13. Eur J Nucl Med 6:453–457

Alavi A, Leon MJ de (1985) Studies of the brain in aging and dementia with positron emission tomography and X-ray computed tomography. In: Reivich M, Alavi A (eds) Positron emission tomography. Liss, New York, pp 273–290

Alavi A, Ferris S, Wolf A, Reivich M, Farkas T, Dann R, Christman D, Fowler J (1980) Determination of cerebral metabolism in senile dementia using F-18-deoxyglucose and positron emission tomography. J Nucl Med 21:P21

Alavi A, Reivich M, Greenberg J, Hand P, Rosenquist A, Rintelman W, Christman D, Fowler J, Goldman A, MacGregor R, Wolf A (1981a) Mapping of functional activity in brain with 18-F-Fluoro-Desoxyglucose. Semin Nucl Med 11:24–31

Alavi A, Ferris S, Wolf A et al. (1981b) Determination of regional cerebral metabolism in dementia using F-18 deoxyglucose and positron emission tomography. In: Meyer JS, Lechner H, Reivich M, Ott ED, Aranibar A (eds) Cerebral vascular disease. Excerpta Medica, Amsterdam, pp 109–112

Alexander FG (1912) Untersuchungen über den Blutgaswechsel des Gehirnes. Biochem Z 44:127

Allan RM, Selwyn AP, Pike VW, Eakins MN, Maseri A (1980) In vivo experimental and clinical studies of normal ischemic myocardium using 11-C-Acetate. Circulation [Suppl III] 72:74

Allan RM, Jones T, Rhodes CG, Heather JD, Maseri A, Facc MD, Selwyn AP (1981) Qantitation of myocardial perfusion in man using oxygen-15 and positron tomography. Am J Cardiol 47:481

Alpert NM, Ackerman R, Correia JA et al. (1977) Measurement of rCBF and rCMRO$_2$ by continuous inhalation of ^{15}O-labeled CO$_2$ and O$_2$. Acta Neurol Scand [Suppl 2] 56:186–187

Alpert NM, Ericsson L, Chang JY, Bergstrom M, Litton JE, Correia JA, Bohm C, Ackerman RH, Taveras JM (1984) Strategy for the measurement of regional cerebral blood flow using short-lived tracers and emission tomography. J Cereb Blood Flow Metab 4:28–34

Amis TC, Jones T (1980) Krypton-81m as a flow tracer in the lung: theory and quantitation. Eur Physiopath Resp 16:245–259

Amis TC, Ciofetta G, Clark JC, Hughes JMB, Jones HA, Pratt TA (1975) Use of Krypton 81m and 85m for the measurement of ventilation and perfusion distribution within the lungs. Br J Radiol 15:52–58

Anger HO (1958) Scintillation camera. Rev Sci Instrum 29:27

Anhalt E, Tegtmeier F, Holloway YJ (1981) Biochemische Aspekte des Methioninstoffwechsels. HEK-Forum 11:21–24

Atcher RW, Friedman AM, Huizenge JR, Rayudo GYS, Silverstein EA, Turner DA (1980) Manganese-52m, a new short lived, generator produced radionuclide. A potential tracer for positron tomography. J Nucl Med 21:565–569

Atkins HL, Som P, Fairchild RG, Hui J, Schachner E, Goldman A, Kla T (1979) Myocardial positron tomography with manganese-52m. Radiology 133:769–774

Bachelard HS (1971) Specific and kinetic properties of monosaccharide uptake into guinea pig cerebral cortex in vitro. J Neurochem 18:213–233

Ball WC Jr, Stewart PB, Newskham LGS, Bates DY (1962) Regional pulmonary function studied with xenon-133. J Clin Invest 41:519–531

Ballard F, Danforth W, Nagele S, Bing R (1960) Myocardial metabolism of fatty acids. J Clin Invest 39:717–723

Baron JC (1983) The interrelationsships of cerebral blood flow and cerebral metabolism and its study with positron emission tomography in man. In: Reba RC, Goodenough DJ, Davidson HF (eds) Diagnostic imaging in medicine. Nijhoff, Boston, pp 407–435

Baron JC, Comar D, Bousser MG, Soussaline F, Crouzel C, Plummer D, Kellershon C, Castaigne P (1978) Etude tomographique, chez l'homme, du débit sanguin et de la consommation d'oxygène du cerveau par inhalation continué dòxygène 15. Rev Neurol (Paris) 134:545–556

Baron JC, Comar D, Bousser MG et al. (1979) Patterns of CBF and oxygen extraction fraction (EO$_2$) in hemispheric infarcts: A tomographic study with ^{15}O continuous inhalation technique. Acta Neurol Scand [Suppl 72] 60:324–325

Baron JC, Bousser MG, Comar D, Castaigne P (1980) "Crossed cerebellar diaschisis" in human supratentorial brain infarction. Trans Am Neurol Assoc 105:459–461

Baron JC, Steinling M, Tanaka T, Cavalheiro E, Soussaline F, Collard P (1981a) Quantitative measurement of CBF, oxygen extraction fraction (OEF) and CMRO$_2$ with O-15 continous inhalation techniques and positron emission tomography (PET): Experimental evidence and normal values in man. J Cereb Blood Flow Metab 1:S5–S6

Baron JC, Bousser MG, Comar D, Soussaline F, Castaigne P (1981b) Noninvasive tomographic study of cerebral blood flow and oxygen metabolism in vivo. Potentials, limitations and clinical applications in cerebral ischemic disorders. Eur Neurol 20:273–284

Baron JC, Bousser MG, Rey A, Guillard A, Comar D, Castaigne P (1981c) Reversal of focal misery-perfusion syndrome by extra-intracranial arterial bypass in hemodynamic cerebral ischemia. Stroke 12:454–459

Baron JC, Bousser MG, Comar D et al. (1981d) Crossed cerebellar diaschisis: a remote functional depression secondary to supratentorial infarction in man. J Cereb Blood Flow Metab 1:500–501

Baron JC, Lebrun-Grandie Ph, Collard Ph, Crouzel C, Mestelan G, Bousser MG (1982) Noninvasive measurement of blood flow, oxygen consumption, and glucose utilisation in the same brain regions in man by positron emissions tomography. J Nucl Med 21:391–399

Baron JC, Rougemont D, Bousser MG, Lebrun-Grandie P, Iba-Zizen MT, Chivas JC (1983a) Local CBF, oxygen extraction fraction (OEF), and $CMRO_2$: Prognostic value in supratentorial infarction in humans. J Cereb Blood Flow Metab 3:S1–S2

Baron JC, Roeda D, Munari C, Crouzel C, Chodkiewicz JP, Comar D (1983b) Brain regional pharmacokinetics of ^{11}C-labeled diphenylhydantoin: Positron emission tomography in humans. Neurology (NY) 33:580–585

Baron JC, Comar D, Crouzel C, Roeda D, Mestelan G, Zarifian E, Munari C, Stoffels C, Bancaud J, Chodkiewicz JP, Loo H, Agid Y (1983c) Brain regional pharmacokinetics of C-11-labeled diphenylhydantoin and pimozide in man. In: Heiss WD, Phelps ME (eds) Positron emission tomography of the brain. Springer, Berlin Heidelberg New York Tokyo, pp 212–224

Baron JC, Rougemont D, Soussaline F, Bustany P, Crouzel C, Bousser MG, Comar D (1984) Local interrelationships of cerebral oxygen consumption and glucose utilization in normal subjects and in ischemic stroke patients: A positron tomography study. J Cereb Blood Flow Metab 4:140–149

Baron JC, Rougemont D, Samson Y, Pantano P, Collard P, Collard P, Citavy M, Bustany P, Crouzel C, Bousser MG, Comar D (1985a) The local interrelationships of cerebral oxygen consumption and glucose utilization in normals and in ischemic stroke patients. In: Greitz T, Ingvar DH, Widén L (eds) Raven, New York, pp 377–386

Baron JC, Comar D, Zarifian E, Agid Y, Crouzel C, Loo H, Deniker P, Kellershon C (1985b) Dopaminergic receptor sites in human brain: Positron emission tomography. Neurology 35:16–24

Barrio JR (1986) Biochemical principles in radiopharmaceutical design and utilization. In: Phelps ME, Mazziotta JC, Schelbert HR (eds) Positron emission tomography and autoradiography. Raven, New York, pp 451–492

Barrio JR, Keen R, Chugani H, Ackerman R, Chugani DC, Phelps ME (1983a) L-(1-C-11)phenylalanine for the determination of cerebral protein synthesis rates in man with positron emission tomography. J Nucl Med 24:70

Barrio JR, Keen RE, Ropchan JR, MacDonald NS, Baumgartner FJ, Padgett HC, Phelps ME (1983b) L-(1-C-11)Leucine: Routine synthesis by enzymatic resolution. J Nucl Med 24:515–521

Bassingthwaighte JB (1974) The measurement of blood flows and volumes by indicator dilution. In: Ray CD (ed) Medical engineering in research, diagnosis and treatment. Year Book Medical Pub, Chicago, pp 246–260

Bassingthwaighte JB (1977) Physiology and theory of tracer washout techniques for the estimation of myocardial blood flow: flow estimation from tracer washout. Prog Cardiovasc Dis 20:165–189

Bassingthwaighte JB (1985) Overview of the process of delivery: flow, transmembrane transport, reaction, and retention. Circulation [Suppl] 72:IV39–IV46

Bassingthwaighte JB, Holloway GA (1976) Estimation of blood flow with radioactive tracers. Semin Nucl Med 6:141–161

Bateman TM, Gray RJ, Czer LS, Levy RL, Stewart ME, DeRobertis MA, Brown DE, Matloff JM, Swan HJ, Berman DS (1983) Regional distribution of pulmonary blood volume: an index of pulmonary capillary wedge pressure determined from blood pool scintigraphy. Am J Cardiol 51:1404–1408

Baxter LR, Phelps ME, Mazziotta JC, Schwartz JM, Gerner RH, Selin CE, Sumida RM (1985) Cerebral metabolic rate for glucose in mood disorders studied with PET and (F-18)-fluorodeoxyglucose (FDG). Arch Gen Psychiatry 42:441–447

Beaney RP (1984) Positron emission tomography in the study of human tumors. Semin Nucl Med 14:324–341

Beaney RP, Lammertsma AA (1985) Use of PET in oncology. In: Reivich M, Alavi A (eds) Positron emission tomography. Liss, New York, pp 425–450

Beaney RP, Lammertsma AA, Jones T, McKenzie CG, Halnan KE (1984) Positron emission tomography for in-vivo measurement of regional blood flow, oxygen utilisation, and blood volume in patients with breast carcinoma. Lancet 1:131–134

Beaney RP, Brooks DJ, Leenders KL, Thomas DG, Jones T (1985) Blood flow and oxygen utilisation in the contralateral cerebral cortex of patients with untreated intracranial tumours as studied by positron emission tomography, with observations on the effect of decompressive surgery. J Neurol Neurosurg Psychiatry 48:310–319

Beekhuis H, Nieweg OE (1984) Radiation absorbed doses from Co-57- and Co-55-Bleomycin. J Nucl Med 25:478–485

Beierwalters WJ, Ice RD, Shar JM, Shaw MJ, Ryo UY (1975) Myocardial uptake of labeled oleic acid and linoleic acids. J Nucl Med 16:842–845

Beller GA, Alton WJ, Cochavi S, Hnatowich D,

Brownell G (1979) Assessment of regional myocardial perfusion by positron emission tomography after intracoronary administration of gallium-68 labeled albumin micorspheres. J Comput Assist Tomogr 3:447–452

Beller GA, Cochavi S, Smith T, Brownell GL (1982) Positron emission tomographic imaging of the myocardium with ^{81}Rb. J Comput Assist Tomogr 6:341–349

Bender DA (1975) Amino Acid Metabolism. Wiley, London

Benet LZ (1972) General treatment of linear capillary models with elimination from any compartment as used in pharmacokinetics. J Pharm Sci 61:536–541

Benson DF, Kuhl DE, Phelps ME et al. (1981) Positron emission computed tomography in the diagnosis of dementia. Trans Am Neurol Assoc 106:1–4

Benson DF, Kuhl DE, Hawkins RA, Phelps ME, Cummings JL, Tsai SY (1983) The fluorodeoxyglucose ^{18}F scan in Alzheimer's disease and multi-infarct dementia. Arch Neurol 40:711–714

Berger G, Mazière M, Prenant C, Sastre J, Syrota A, Comar D (1982) Synthesis of C-11-propanolol. J Radioanal Chem 74:301–306

Bergman SR, Hack S, Tewson T, Welch MJ, Sobel RE (1980) The dependance of accumulation of ^{13}NH$_3$ by myocardium on metabolic factors and its implications for the quantitative assessment of perfusion. Circulation 61:34–43

Bergman SR, Lerch RA, Fox KAA, Ludbrook PA, Welch MJ, Ter-Pogossian MM, Sobel BE (1982a) Temporal dependance of beneficial effects of coronary thrombolysis characterized by positron tomography. Am J Med 73:573–581

Bergman SR, Fox KAA, Rand AL, McElvany KD, Ter-Pogossian MM, Sobel BE (1982b) Non-invasive measurement of regional myocardial perfusion by positron tomography. Circulation [Suppl II] 66:148

Bergman SR, Nomura H, Rand AL, Sobel BE, Lange LG (1982c) Extern detectable changes in fatty acid utilization by perfused hearts from rabbits exposed to alcohol. Circulation [Suppl II] 66:109

Bergman SR, Fox KAA, Rand AL, McElvany KD, Welch MJ, Markham J, Sobel BE (1984) Quantification of regional blood flow in vivo with H$_2$^{15}O. Circulation 70:724–733

Bergner P (1964) Tracer dynamics and the determination of pool-sizes and turnover factors in metabolic systems. J Theor Biol 6:137–158

Bergstrand G, Bergström M, Eriksson L, Edner G, Widen L (1982) Positron emission tomography with ^{68}Ga-EDTA in the diagnosis and localization of CSF fistulas. J Comput Assist Tomogr 6:320–324

Bergström M, Collins VP, Ehrin E, Ericson K, Eriksson L, Greitz T, Halldin C, Holst H v, Langström B, Lilja A, Lundquist H, Nagren K (1983) Discrepancies in brain tumor extent as shown by computed tomography and positron emission tomography using ^{68}Ga-EDTA, ^{11}C-Glucose, and ^{11}C-Methionine. J Comput Assist Tomogr 7:1062–1066

Bergström M, Mosskin M, Ericson K, Lilja A, Blomqvist G, Collins VP, Eriksson L, Ehrin E, Holst H von, Johnström P, Lundqvist H, Langström B (1986) Accumulation kinetics of C-11-D-Glucose, [Methyl-C-11]-L-Methionine, and Ga-68-EDTA in brain tumors measured with positron emission tomography. J Comput Assist Tomogr (in press)

Bernardi S, Trimble MR, Frackowiak RSJ et al. (1983) An interictal study of partial epilepsy using positron emission tomography and the oxygen-15 inhalation technique. J Neurol Neurosurg Psychatry 46:473–477

Berridge M, Comar D, Roeda D, Syrota A (1982) Synthesis and in vivo characteristics of (2-^{11}C)-5,5-dimethyloxazolidine-2,4-dione (DMO). Int J Appl Radiat Isot 33:647–651

Berridge M, Comar D, Crouzel C, Baron JC (1983) C-11-labeled ketanserin: A selective serotonin S$_2$ antagonist. J Lab Comp Radiopharm 20:73–78

Berridge M, Franceschini M, Tweson T, Gould L (1986) Preparation of ^{15}O-Butanol for positron emission tomography. J Nucl Med 27:834–837

Bessel EM, Foster AB, Westwood JH (1972) The use of deoxyfluoro-D-glucopyranose and related compounds in a study of yeast hexokinase specifity. Biochem J 128:199–204

Betz E (1972) Cerebral blood flow: Its measurement and regulation. Physiol Rev 52:595–630

Betz LA, Gilboe DD (1974) Kinetics of cerebral glucose transport in vivo. Inhibition of 3-O-methylglucose. Brain Res 65:368–372

Bewermeyer H, Dreesbach HA, Rackl A, Nevelling M, Heiss WD (1985) Presentation of bilateral thalamic infarction on CT, MRI and PET. Neuroradiology 27:414–419

Bieber LL, Fiol CJ (1985) Fatty acid and ketone metabolism. Circ [Suppl IV] 72:9–12

Biersack HJ, Hartmann A, Friedrich G, Fröscher M, Reichmann K, Reske SN, Knopp R (1984) Zur Ursache der gekreuzten cerebellaren Diaschisis bei cerebrovaskulären Erkrankungen. Nucl Med 23:227–230

Biersack HJ, Reichmann K, Stephan H, Kuhnen U, Neirinckx R, Tyrell D, Penin H, Winkler C (1986) Brain SPECT with ^{99m}Tc-labeled Hexamethylpropyleneamineoxime (HM-PAO): Results in epilepsy. Radioakt Isot Klinik Forsch 17:33–38

Bigler RE, Kostick FA, Gillespie JR (1981) Compartmental analysis of the steady-state distribution of ^{15}O$_2$ and ^{15}O$-$H$_2$O in total body. J Nucl Med 22:959–965

Bigler RE, Gillespie JR, Kostick J (1982) Re: Compartmental analysis of the steady-state distribution of $^{15}O_2$ and $^{15}O-H_2O$ in the total body. J Nucl Med 23:750–751

Billadello JJ, Smith JL, Ludbrook PA, Tiefenbrunn AJ, Jaffe AS, Sobel BE, Geltman EM (1983) The implications of "reciprocal" ST segment depression associated with acute myocardial infarction identified by positron tomography. J Am Coll Cardiol 2:614–624

Bing RJ (1965) Cardiac metabolism. Physiol Rev 45:171–213

Bing RJ, Hammond MM, Handelsmann JC, Powers SR, Spencer FC, Eckenhoff JE, Goodale WT, Hafkenschiel JH, Kety SS (1949) The measurement of coronary blood flow, oxygen consumption, and efficiency of the left ventricle in man. Am Heart J 38:1–24

Binswanger RO, Rösler H, Noelpp U, Matter L, Härtel M (1978) The bedside determination of extravascular lung water. A non-invasive double indicator using ^{123}I-antipyrine, ^{113m}In-transferrin and external counting. Eur J Nucl Med 3:109–114

Blasberg RG, Wright DC, Patlak CS et al. (1984) Determination of regional blood tissue transfer constants and initial plasma volume in brain tumors using Ga-68-EDTA and dynamic positron emission tomography. J Nucl Med 25:P51

Blau M (1961) Biosynthesis of ^{75}Se-Selenomethionine and ^{75}Se-Selenocystine. Biochim Biophys Acta 49:389–390

Blau M, Manske RF (1961) The pancreas specifity of ^{75}Se-Selenomethionine. J Nucl Med 2:102–105

Blomquist G, Bergström K, Bergström M, Ehrin E, Eriksson L, Garmelius B, Lindberg B, Lilja A, Litton JE, Lundmark L, Lundqvist H, Malmborg P, Moström U, Stone-Elander S, Widen L (1985) Models for C-11-glucose. In: Greitz T, Ingvar DH, Wiedén L (eds) The metabolism of the brain studied with positron emission tomography. Raven, New York, pp 185–194

Blumgart HL, Weiss S (1927) Studies on the velocity of blood flow. I. The method utilized. J Clin Invest 4:1–14

Bohm C, Greitz T, Kingsley D, Berggren BM, Olsson L (1983) Adjustable computerized stereotaxic brain atlas for transmission and emission tomography. AJNR 4:731–733

Bosley TM, Rosenquist AC, Kushner M, Burke A, Stein A, Dann R, Cobbs W, Savino PJ, Schatz NJ, Alavi A (1985) Ischemic lesions of the occipital cortex and optic radiations: positron emission tomography. Neurology 35:470–484

Bossaller C, Schober O, Meyer G-J, Hundeshagen, Lichtlen PR (1985) Positronenemissionstomographie des regionalen extravaskulären Lungenwassers und des regionalen Blutvolumens bei chronischer Herzinsuffizienz. Z Kardiol 74:5–14

Bradbury M (1979) The concept of a blood-brain barrier. Wiley, Chichester

Bradbury M (1985) The blood brain barrier: transport across the cerebral endothelium. Circ Res 57:213–222

Braunwald E, Kloner RA (1982) The stunned myocardium: Prolonged, postischemic ventricular dysfunction. Circulation 66:1146–1149

Bremer J (1983) Carnitine – metabolism and function. Physiol Rev 63:1420–1480

Brodie JD, Wolf AP, Volkow N, Christman DR, DeFina P, DeLeon P, Farkas T, Ferris SH, Fowler JS, Gomez-Mont F, Jaeger J, Russel JAG, Stamm R, Yonekura Y (1983) In: Heiss WD, Phelps ME (eds) Positron emission tomography of the brain. Springer, New York, pp 201–206

Brodie JD, Christman DR, Corona JF, Fowler JS, Gomez-Mont F, Jaeger J, Micheels PA, Rotrosen J, Russel JAG, Volkow ND, Wikler A, Wolf AP, Wolkin A (1984) Patterns of metabolic activity in the treatment of schizophrenia. Ann Neurol 15:S166–S169

Brooks DJ, Lammertsma AA, Beaney RP, Leenders KL, Buckingham PD, Marshall J, Jones T (1984a) Measurement of regional cerebral pH in human subjects using continuous inhalation of $^{11}CO_2$ and positron emission tomography. J Cereb Blood Flow Metab 4:458–465

Brooks DJ, Beaney RP, Lammertsma AA, Leenders KL, Horlock PL, Kensett MJ, Marshall J, Thomas DG, Jones T (1984b) Quantitative measurement of blood-brain barrier permeability using ^{82}Rb and positron emission tomography. J Cereb Blood Flow Metab 4:535–545

Brooks DJ, Leenders KL, Head G, Marshall J, Legg NJ, Jones T (1984c) Studies on regional cerebral oxygen utilisation and cognitive function in multiple sclerosis. J Neurol Neurosurg Psychiatry 47:1182–1191

Brooks DJ, Beaney RP, Leenders KL, Marshall J, Thomas DJ, Jones T (1985) Regional cerebral oxygen utilization, blood flow, and blood volume in benign intracranial hypertension studied by positron emission tomography. Neurology 35:1030–1034

Brooks DJ, Beaney RP, Lammertsma AA, Herold S, Turton DR, Luthra SK, Frackowiak RSJ, Thomas DG, Marshall J, Jones T (1986) Glucose transport across the blood-brain-barrier in normal human subjects and patients with cerebral tumours studied using [^{11}C]3-O-methyl-D-glucose and positron emission tomography. J Cereb Blood Flow Metab 6:230–239

Brooks RA (1982) Alternative formula for Glucose utilisation using labeled Deoxyglucose. J Nucl Med 23:538–539

Brown BG, Josephson MA, Peterson RB, Pierce CD, Wong M, Hecht HS, Bolson E, Dodge HT (1981) Intravenous dipyridamole combined with isometric handgrip for near maximal acute increase in coronary flow in patients with coronary artery disease. Am J Cardiol 48:1077–1085

Brown RF (1980) Compartmental system analysis:

state of the art. IEEE Trans Biomed Eng BME-27:1–11

Brownell GL, Ackermann RH, Strauss HW, Elmaleh DR, Cochavi S, Alpert N, Correia JA, Kearfott KJ, Taveras J (1980) Preliminary imaging results with 18-F-2-fluoro-2-deoxy-D-glucose. J Comput Assist Tomogr 4:473–477

Buchsbaum MS, Kessler R, Bunney WE et al. (1981) Simultaneous electroencephalography and cerebral glucography with positron emission tomography (PET) in normals and patients with schizophrenia. J Cereb Blood Flow Metab 1:S457–S458

Buchsbaum MS, Kessler R, Bunney WE et al. (1982) Cerebral glucography with positron tomography: Use in normal subjects and patients with schizophrenia. Arch Gen Psychatry 39:251–259

Buchsbaum MS, Holocomb HH, Johnson J, King AC, Kessler R (1983) Cerebral metabolic consequences of electrical cutaneous stimulation in normal individuals. Hum Neurobiol 2:35–38

Buchsbaum MR, Cappletti J, Ball R, Hazlett E, King AC, Johnson J, Wu J, DeLisi LE (1984) Positron emission tomographic image measurement in schizophrenia and affective disorders. Ann Neurol 15:S157–S165

Budinger TF (1979) Amino acid uptake by the myocardium. In: Willerson JT (ed) Nuclear cardiology. Davis, Philadelphia, pp 59–60

Budinger TF (1980) Physical attributes of single-photon tomography. J Nucl Med 21:579–592

Budinger TF (1981) Revival of clinical nuclear medicine brain imaging. J Nucl Med 22:1094–1097

Budinger TF (1985) Quantitative single-photon-emission tomography for cerebral flow and receptor distribution imaging. In: Reivich M, Alavi A (eds) Positron emission tomography. Liss, New York, pp 227–240

Budinger TF, Gjedde A (1986) Background of the kinetik approach. Teaching session: 33rd annual meeting of the Soc Nucl Med, Washington

Budinger TF, Yano Y, Hoop B (1975) A comparison of $^{82}Rb^+$ and $^{13}NH_3$ for myocardial positron scintigraphy. J Nucl Med 16:429–431

Büll U, Doliwa R, Kirsch CM, Roedler HD, Strauer BE (1984a) Die ^{201}Thallium-Single-Photon-Emissions-Computertomographie (SPECT) in der funktionellen Beurteilung koronarstenotischer Veränderungen. Ergebnisse des Vergleichs von Belastungszintigraphischen mit koronarangiographischen Befunden. Z Kardiol 73:313–320

Büll U, Moser EA, Schmiede P, Leinsinger G, Kreisig T, Kirsch CM, Einhäupl K (1984b) Dynamic SPECT with ^{133}Xe: Regional cerebral blood flow in patients with unilateral cerebrovascular disease. J Nucl Med 25:441–446

Buoncore E, Hübner KR (1979) Positron emission computed tomography of the pancreas: A preliminary study. Radiology 133:195–201

Bush H, Davis JR, Honig GR, Anderson DC, Nair PV, Nyhan WL (1959) The uptake of a variety of amino acids into nuclear proteins of tumors and other tissues. Cancer Res 19:1030–1039

Bustany P, Comar D (1985) Protein synthesis evaluation in brain and other organs in humans by PET. In: Reivich M, Alavi A (eds) Positron emission tomography. Liss, New York, pp 183–201

Bustany P, Sargent T, Saudubray JM, Henry JF, Comar D (1981) Regional human brain uptake and protein incorporation of ^{11}C-L-Methionine studied in vivo with PET. J Cereb Blood Flow Metab 1:517–518

Bustany P, Henry J, Cabanis E, Soussaline F, Grouzel M, Comar D (1982) Incorporation of L-C-11-methionine in brain proteins studied by PET in dementia. In: Raynaud C (ed) Proc 3rd World Congr Nucl Med Biol, Paris. Pergamon, Paris, pp 2276–2279

Bustany P, Henry JF, Sargent T, Zarifian E, Cabanis E, Collard P, Comar D (1983a) Local brain protein metabolism in dementia and schizophrenia: In vivo studies with C-11-L-methionine and positron emission tomography. In: Heiss WD, Phelps ME (eds) Positron emission tomography of the brain. Springer, Berlin Heidelberg New York Tokyo, pp 208–211

Bustany P, Henry JF, deRotrou J et al. (1983b) Local cerebral metabolic rate of ^{11}C-L-methionine in early stages of dementia, schizophrenia and Parkinson's disease. J Cereb Blood Flow Metab 3:S492–S493

Bustany P, Henry JF, DeRotrou J, Signoret P, Cabanis E, Zarifian E, Ziegler M, Derlon JM, Crouzel C, Soussaline F, Comar D (1985) Correlations between clinical state and PET measurement of local protein synthesis in Alzheimer's dementia, Parkinson's disease, schizophrenia and gliomas. In: Greitz T, Ingvar DH, Wiedén L (eds) The metabolism of the human brain studied with positron emission tomography. Raven, New York, pp 247–249

Bustany P, Chatel M, Derlon JM, Darcel F, Sgouropoulos P, Soussaline F, Syrota A (1986) Brain tumor protein synthesis and histological grades: a study by positron emission tomography (PET) with C-11-L-methionine. J Neurooncol 3:397–404

Buxton RB, Wechsler LR, Alpert NM, Ackerman RH, Elmaleh DR, Correia JA (1984) Measurement of brain pH using $^{11}CO_2$ and positron emission tomography. J Cereb Blood Flow Metab 4:8–16

Cahill GF Jr (1978) Protein and amino acid metabolism. Circ Res 38:1109–1114

Calne DB, Langston JW, Martin WR, Stossl AJ, Ruth TJ, Adam MJ, Pate BD, Schulzer M (1985) Positron emission tomography after MPTP: Observations relating to the cause of Parkinson's disease. Nature 317:246–248

Camici P, Kaski JC, Shea MJ, Selwyn AP, Jones T, Maseri A (1983) Increased myocardial glucose utilization in excertional angina. Circulation [Suppl III] 68:324

Cannon PJ, Haft JI, Johnson PM (1969) Visual assessement of regional myocardial perfusion using radioactive xenon and scintillation photography. Circulation 40:277–288

Cannon PJ, Dell RB, Dwyer Jr EM (1972) Measurement of regional myocardial perfusion in man with ^{133}Xenon and a scintillation camera. J Clin Invest 51:964–977

Carson RE (1986) Parameter estimation in positron emission tomography. In: Phelps ME, Mazziota JC, Schelbert H (eds) Positron emission tomography and autoradiography. Raven, New York, pp 347–390

Carson RE, Mazziotta JC, Huang SC (1984) Factors affecting the estimation of the rate constants for the fluorodesoxyglucose model from positron emission tomography data. J Nucl Med 25:P63

Celesia GG, Polcyn RE, Holden JE et al. (1982a) Visual evoked potentials and positron emission tomographic mapping of regional cerebral blood flow and cerebral metabolism: Can the neuronal potential generators be visualized: Electroencephalogr Clin Neurophysiol 54:243–256

Celesia GG, Polcyn RE, Nickles RJ, Holden JE, Gatley SJ (1982b) Residual visual function in cortical blindness evaluated by positron emission tomography. Neurology 32:A95

Celesia GG, Polcyn RE, Holden J et al. (1983) ^{18}F-Fluoromethane positron emission tomography determination of regional cerebral blood flow in cerebral infarction. J Cereb Blood Flow Metab 3:S23–S24

Celesia GG, Polcyn RE, Holden JE, Nickles RJ, Koeppe RA, Gatley SJ (1984) Determination of regional cerebral blood flow in patients with cerebral infarction. Use of fluoromethan with fluorine-18 and positron emission tomography. Arch Neurol 41:262–267

Chaplin SB, Oberle PO, Hoffman TJ, Volkert WA, Holmes RA (1985) Regional brain uptake and retention of Tc-99m-Propylene amine oxime derivates. J Nucl Med 26:P18

Chase TN, Brooks RA, DiChiro G et al. (1985) Focal cortical abnormalities in Alzheimer's disease. In: Greitz T et al. (eds) The Metabolism of the human brain studied with positron emission tomography. Raven, New York, pp 433–440

Chevigne M, Quaglia L, Delfiore G, Peters JM, Rigo P (1983) Radiocardiographic evaluation of left ventricular function after inhalation of ^{15}O–CO_2. Eur J Nucl Med 8:155–158

Chinard FP (1975) Estimation of extravascular lung water by indicator-dilution techniques. Circ Res 37:137–145

Chinard FP, Enns T (1954) Transcapillary pulmonary exchange of water in the dog. Am J Physiol 178:197–202

Chinard FP, Vosburgh GJ, Enns T (1955) Transcapillary exchange of water and of other substances in certain organs of the dog. Am J Physiol 183:221–234

Chinard FP, Enns T, Nolan MF (1962) Pulmonary extravacular water volumes from transit time and slope data. J Appl Physiol 17:179–183

Chugani HT et al. (1984) PET with ^{18}F-2-fluorodeoxyglucose in infantile spasms. Ann Neurol 16:336–377

Chugani HT, Engel J Jr, Mazziotta JC, Phelps ME (1984) ^{18}F-2-fluorodeoxyglucose positron emission tomography in medically refrectory childhood epilepsy. Neurology 34:S107

Clark JC, Buckingham PD (1975) Short-lived radioactive gases for clinical use. Butterworth, London

Cochavi S, Pohost GM, Elmaleh DR, Strauss HW (1979) Transversal-sectional imaging with Na^{18}F in myocardial infarction. J Nucl Med 20:1013–1017

Cohen MB (1978) Synthesis and utilization of ^{13}N compounds for positron scanning. Int J Nucl Med Biol 5:201

Cohen MB, Spolter L, Chang CC, Cooks JS, McDonald NS (1980) Enzymatic synthesis of ^{11}C pyruvic acid and ^{11}C-DL-lactic acid. Int J Appl Radiat Isot 31:45–49

Cohen MB, Spolter L, Chang CC, Behrendt D, Cook J, McDonald NS (1982) The variing tissue distribution of L-glutamic acid labeled at three different sites. Int J Appl Radiat Isot 33:613–617

Comar D, Zarifian E, Verhas M, Soussaline F, Maziere M, Berger G, Loo H, Cuche H, Kellershon C, Deniker P (1979) Brain distribution and kinetics of ^{11}C-chloropromazine in schizophrenics: PET studies. Psychiatry Res 1:23–29

Cooper JD, McCullogh NJ, Lowenstein E (1972) Determination of pulmonary extravascular water using oxygen 15-labeled water. J Appl Physiol 33:842–845

Cooper MD, Harper PV (1980) Radionuclide scintigraphy of the pancreas: Perspectives on its role in the diagnosis of pancreatic neoplasms. In: Mossa AR (ed) Tumors of the pancreas. Williams and Wilkins, Baltimore, Md, pp 245–257

Crandall ED, Staub NC, Goldberg HS, Effros RM (1983) UCLA Conference. Recent developments in pulmonary edema. Ann Intern Med 99:808–822

Crane PO, Pardridge WM, Nyerges AM, Oldendorf WH (1981) The interaction of transport and metabolism on brain glucose utilization: A reevaluation of the lumped constant. J Neurochem 36:1601–1604

Cremer JE (1982) Substrate utilization and brain development. J Cereb Blood Flow Metab 2:394–407

Creutzig H, Sturm JA, Schober O, Nerlich ML, Kant

CJ (1984) Nuklearmedizinische Diagnostik des "Pulmonary Capillary Protein Leakage". Nucl Med 23:253–256

Creutzig H, Schober O, Gielow P, Friedrich R, Bekker H, Dietz H, Hundeshagen H (1986) Cerebral dynamics of N-isopropyl-(I-123)p-iodoamphetamine. J Nucl Med 26:178–183

Critchley M, Prichard H, Grime JS, Patten M, Ansell I (1981) Radionuclide assessment of extravascular lung water in minimal pulmonary oedema. Clin Radiol 32:607–609

Crone C (1963) The permeability of capillaries in various organs as determined by use of the indicator diffusion method. Acta Physiol Scand 58:292–305

Crone C, Lassen NA (1970) Cappilary permeability: The transfer of molecules and ions between capplilary blood and tissue. Academic, New York

Cutler NR, Duara R, Creasy H, Grady CL, Haxby JV, Shapiro MB, Rapoport SI (1984) Brain imaging: Aging and dementia. Ann Intern Med 101:355–369

Cutler NR, Haxby JY, Duara R, Grady CL, Moore AM, Parisi JE, White J, Heston L, Margolin RM, Rapoport SI (1985a) Brain metabolism as measured with positron emission tomography: Serial assessment in a patient with familial Alzheimer's disease. Neurology 35:1556–1561

Cutler NR, Heston LL, Davies P, Haxby JV, Shapiro MB (1985b) NIH Conference. Alzheimer's disease and Down's syndrome: new insights. Ann Intern Med 103:566–578

Davis SM, Ackerman RH, Correia JA, Alpert NM, Chang J, Buonanno F, Kelly RE, Rosner B, Taveras JM (1983) Cerebral blood flow and cerebrovascular CO_2 reactivity in stroke-age normal controls. Neuroradiology 33:391–399

Deanfield JE, Selwyn AP, Chierchia S, Maseri A, Ribeiro P, Krikler S, Morgan M (1983a) Myocardial ischemia during daily life in patients with stable angina: Its relation to symptoms and heart rate changes. Lancet: 2:753–758

Deanfield JE, Shea M, Wilson R, de Landsheere CM, Jones T, Maseri A, Selwyn AP (1983b) ST segment changes as a marker of ischemia in stable angina: A patient study using positron tomography. Circulation [Suppl III] 68:22

Deanfield JE, Shea M, Wilson R, Horlock P, Selwyn AP (1983c) Mental stress and ischemia in patients with coronary disease. Circulation [Suppl III] 68:258

Deanfield JE, Shea M, Ribiero P, Landsheere CM de, Wilson RA, Horlock P, Selwyn AP (1984a) Transient ST-segment depression as a marker of myocardial ischemia during daily life. Am J Cardiol 54:1195–1200

Deanfield JE, Shea M, Kensett M, Horlock P, Wilson RA, deLandsheere CM, Selwyn AP (1984b) Silent myocardial ischemia due to mental stress. Lancet 2:1001–1005

Dence CS, Kilbourn MR, Ter-Pogossian MM, Welch MJ (1982) A remote system for the routine production of uniformly labeled carbon-11-glucose for metabolism studies. J Nucl Med 23:P107

Depresseux JC, Granck G, Sadzot B (1984) Regional cerebral blood flow and oxygen uptake rate in human focal epilepsy. In: Blady-Moulinier M, Ingvar DH, Meldrum BS (eds) Current problems in epilepsy. Libby, London, pp 76–81

Di Chiro G, DeLaPaz RL, Smith BH, Patronas NJ, Kufta CV, Kessler RM, Johnston GS, Manning RG, Wolf AP (1981) ^{18}F-2-fluoro-2-deoxyglucose positron tomography of human cerebral gliomas. J Cereb Blood Flow Metab 1:S11–S12

Di Chiro G, DeLaPaz RL, Brooks RA, Sokoloff L, Kornblith PL, Smith BH, Patronas NJ, Kufta CV, Kessler RM, Johnston GS, Manning RG, Wolf AP (1982) Glucose utilization of cerebral gliomas measured by 18-F-fluorodeoxyglucose and positron emission tomography. Neurology 32:1323–1329

Di Chiro G, Oldfield E, Bairamian D, Patronas NJ, Brooks RA, Mansi L, Smith BH, Kornblith PL, Margolin R (1983) Metabolic imaging of the brain stem and spinal cord: Studies with positron emission tomography using 18-F-2-deoxyglucose in normal and pathological cases. J Comput Assist Tomogr 7:937–945

Di Chiro G, Brooks RA, Patronas NJ, Bairamian D, Kornblith PL, Smith BH, Mansi L, Barker J (1984) Issues in the in vivo measurement of glucose metabolism of human central nervous system tumors. Ann Neurol 15:S138–S146

Di Chiro G, Brooks RA, Bairamian D, Patronas NJ, Kornblith PL, Smith BH, Mansi L (1985) Diagnostic and prognostic value of positron emission tomography using (F-18)-fluorodeoxyglucose in brain tumors. In: Reivich M, Alavi A (eds) Positron emission tomography. Riss, New York, pp 291–309

Diksic M, Sako K, Feindel W, Kato A, Yamamoto YL, Farrokhzad S, Thompson C (1984) Pharmacokinetics of positron-labeled 1,3-bis(2-chloroethyl)nitrosourea in human brain tumors using positron emission tomography. Cancer Res 44:3120–3124

Döhring W, Linke G, Stender HSt (1981) CT densitometry of the lung. In: Donner MW, Heuck FHW (eds) Radiology today. Springer, Berlin Heidelberg New York, pp 99–112

Dollery CT, West JB (1960) Regional uptake of radioactive oxygen, carbon monoxide and carbon dioxide in the lung of patients with mitral stenosis. Circ Res 8:765–771

Dollery CT, Dyson NA, Sinclair JD (1960) Regional variations in uptake of radioactive $C^{15}O$ in the normal lung. J Appl Physiol 15:411–417

Donnan G, D'Alton JG, Chang JY et al. (1983) Alterations in cerebral blood flow (CBF) and metabolism (CMRO$_2$) after transient ischemic attacks. Neurology [Suppl 2] 33:115

Drayer B, Jaszczak R, Coleman E, Storni A, Greer K, Petry N, Lischko M, Flanagan S (1982) Muscarinic cholinergic receptor binding: In vivo depiction using single photon emission computed tomography and radioiodinated quinuclidinyl benzilate. J Comput Assist Tomogr 6:536–543

Duara R, Margolin RA, Robertson-Tchabo EA, London ED, Schwartz M, Renfrew JW, Koziarz BJ, Sundaram M, Grady C, Moore AM et al. (1983) Cerebral glucose utilization as measured with positron emission tomography in 21 resting healthy men between ages of 21 and 83 years. Brain 106:761–775

Duara R, Grady C, Haxby, Ingvar D, Sokoloff L (1984) Human brain glucose utilization and cognitive function in relation to age. Ann Neurol 16:703–713

Duncan CC, Lambrecht RN, Rescigno A, Shiue CY, Bennett GW, Ment LR (1983) The ramp injection of radiotracers for blood flow measurements by emission tomography. Phys Med Biol 28:963–972

Dyson NA, Hugh-Jones P, Newbery GR (1959) Preparation and use of O-15 with particular reference to its value in study of pulmonary malfunction. Proc Second UN Int Conf Peacefule Uses Atomic Energy (UN, Geneva, Sept 1958) Pergamon, New York

Dyson NA, Hugh-Jones P, Newbery GR, Sinclair JD, West JB (1960) Studies of regional lung function using radioactive oxygen. Br Med J 1:231–238

EC/IC Bypass Study Group (1985) Failure of extracranial-intracranial arterial bypass to reduce the risk of ischemic stroke. N Engl J Med 313:1191–1200

Eckelman WC, Gibson RE (1984) Receptor binding of ^{18}F-haloperidol and spiroperidol. J Nucl Med 25:532–533

Eckelman WC, Reba RC, Rzeszotarski WJ, Gibson RE, Hill T, Holman BL, Budinger T, Conklin JJ, Eng R, Grissom MP (1984) External imaging of cerebral muscarinic acetylcholine receptors. Science 223:291–293

Eckenhoff JE, Hafkenschiel JH, Harmel MH, Goodale WT, Lubin M, Bing RJ, Kety SS (1948) Measurement of coronary blood flow by the nitrous oxide method. Am J Physiol 152:356–364

Ehrin E, Stone-Elander S, Nilsson JL, Bergström M, Blomqvist G, Brismar T, Ericsson L, Greitz T, Jansson PE, Litton JE, Malmborg P, Ugglas M, Widen L (1983) C-11-labeled glucose and its utilization in positron emission tomography. J Nucl Med 24:326–331

Eichling JO, Raichle ME, Grubb Jr RL, Ter-Pogossian MM (1974) Evidence of the limitations of water as a freely diffusible tracer in brain of the rhesus monkey. Circ Res 35:358–364

Eichling JO, Raichle ME, Grubb RL, Larson KB,

Ter-Pogossian MM (1975) In vivo determination of cerebral blood volume with radioactive oxygen-15 in the monkey. Circ Res 37:707–714

Ell PJ, Hocknell JML, Jarritt PH, Cullum I, Lui D, Campos-Costa, Nowotnik DP, Picket RD, Canning LR, Neirinckx RD (1985) A ^{99m}Tc-labelled radiotracer for the investigation of cerebral vascular disease. Nucl Med Com 6:437–441

Engel J Jr (1984) The use of PET scanning in epilepsy. Ann Neurol 15:S180–S191

Engel J Jr, Brown WJ, Kuhl DE, Phelps ME, Mazziotta JC, Crandall PH (1982a) Pathological findings underlying focal temporal lobe hypometabolism in partial epilepsy. Ann Neurol 12:518–528

Engel J Jr, Kuhl DE, Phelps ME (1982b) Patterns of human local cerebral glucose metabolism during epileptic seizures. Science 218:64–66

Engel J Jr, Kuhl DE, Phelps ME, Crandall PH (1982c) Comparative localization of epileptic foci in partial epilepsy by PCT and EEG. Ann Neurol 12:529–537

Engel J Jr, Kuhl DE, Phelps ME, Mazziotta JC (1982d) Interictal cerebral glucose metabolism in partial epilepsy and its relation to EEG changes. Ann Neurol 12:510–517

Engel J Jr, Kuhl DE, Phelps ME, Rausch R, Nuwer M (1983) Local cerebral metabolism during partial seizures. Neurology 33:400–413

Engel J Jr, Crandall PH, Rausch R (1984) Surgical treatment of the partial epilepsies. In: Rosenberg RN, Grossman RG (eds) The clinical neurosciences. Churchill-Livingston, New York, pp 1349–1380

Engel J Jr, Lubens P, Kuhl DE, Phelps ME (1985) Local cerebral metabolic rate for glucose during petit mal absences. Ann Neurol 17:121–128

Ericson K, Bergström M, Eriksson L (1980) Positron emission tomography in the evaluation of subdural hematomas. J Comput Assist Tomogr 4:737–745

Ericson K, Bergström M, Eriksson L, Hatam A, Greitz T, Söderström CE, Widèn L (1981) Positron emission tomography with (Ga-68)EDTA compared with transmission computed tomography in the evaluation of brain infarcts. Acta Radiol 22:385–398

Ericson L, Lilja A, Bergström M, Collins VP, Eriksson L, Ehrin E, Holst H von, Lundquist H, Langström B, Mosskin M (1985) Positron emission tomography with (C-11)-methyl-L-methionine, (C-11)-D-glucose, and (Ga-68)-EDTA in supratentorial tumors. J Comput Assist Tomogr 9:683–689

Evans JR, Gunton RW, Baker RG, Beanlands DS, Spears JC (1965) Use of radioiodinated fatty acid for photoscans of the heart. Circ Res 16:1–10

Fan FC, Schuessler GB, Chen RYZ, Chien S (1979) Determination of blood flow and shunting of 9- and 15 µm spheres in regional beds. Am J Physiol 244 (Suppl): H25–H33

Farde L, Ehrin E, Eriksson L, Greitz T, Hall H, Hedström CG, Litton JE, Sedvall G (1985) Substituted benzamines as ligands for visualization of dopamine receptor binding in the human brain by positron emission tomography. Proc Natl Acad Sci USA 82:3863–3867

Farkas T, Reivich M, Alavi A, Greenberg JH, Fowler JS, MacGregor RR, Christman DR, Wolf AP (1980) The application of [^{18}F]-2-deoxy-2-fluoro-D-glucose and positron emission tumography in the study of psychatric conditions. In: Passonneau JV, Hawkins R, Lust WD et al. (eds) Cerebral metabolism and neural function. Williams & Wilkins, Baltimore, pp 403–408

Farkas T, Ferris SH, Wolf AP, deLeon MJ, Christman DR, Reisberg B, Alavi A, Fowler JS, George AE, Reivich M (1982) ^{18}F-2-deoxy-2-fluoro-D-glucose as a tracer in the positron emission tomographic study of senile dementia. Am J Psychiatry 139:3

Farkas T, Wolf AP, Jaeger J, Brodie JD, Christman DR, Fowler JS (1984) Regional brain glucose metabolism in chronic schizophrenia. A positron emission transaxial tomographic study. Arch Gen Psychiatry 41:293–300

Fazio F, Giuntini C (1979) Determination of extravascular lung water by dilution method. II. Technique and results in dog and man. J Nucl Med Allied Sci 23:97–107

Fazio F, Jones T (1975) Assessment of regional ventilation by continuous inhalation of radioactive krypton-81m. Br Med J 3:673–676

Fazio F, Jones T, MacArther CGC, Rhodes CG, Steiner RE, Hughes JMB (1976a) Measurement of regional pulmonary oedema in man using radioactive water (H$_2$^{15}O). Br J Radiol 49:393–397

Fazio F, Jones T, Rhodes CG, Hughes JMB (1976b) Measurements of extravascular lung water in vivo by external counting. J Nucl Biol Med 20:81–83

Fazio F, Fieschi C, Collice M, Nardini M, Banfi F, Possa M, Spinelli F (1980) Tomographic assessment of cerebral perfusion using a single-photon emitter (krypton-81m) and a rotating gamma camera. J Nucl Med 21:1139–1145

Fazio F, Wollmer P, Lavender JP, Barr MM (1982) Clinical ventilation imaging with In-113m aerosol: A comparison with Kr-81m. J Nucl Med 23:305–314

Feinendegen LE, Vyska K, Freundlieb C, Höck A, Machulla H-J, Kloster G, Stöcklin G (1981) Non invasive analysis of metabolic reactions in body tissues: The case of myocardial fatty acids. Eur J Nucl Med 6:191–200

Ferris SH, deLeon MJ, Wolf AP, George AE, Reisberg B, Brodie J, Gentes C, Christman D, Fowler JS (1983) Regional metabolism and cognitive deficits in aging and senile dementia. In: Samuel D, Algeri S, Gershon S, Grimm YE, Toffano G (eds) Aging of the brain, vol 22. Raven, New York, pp 133–142

Fick A (1855) Über Diffusion. Annalen der Physik 94:59–86

Firnau G, Garnett ES, Sourkes TL, Missala K (1975) (18-F)Fluoro-dopa: a unique gamma emitting substrate for dopa decarboxylase. Experientia 31:1254–1255

Firnau G, Chirakal R, Sood S, Garnett ES (1981) Radioflurination with xenon difluoride: L-6[^{18}F]fluorodopa. J Labelled Comp Radiopharm 18:7–8

Foster NL, Chase TN, Fedio P, Patronas NJ, Brooks RA, DiChiro C (1983) Alzheimer's disease: Focal cortical changes shown by positron emission tomography. Neurology 33:961–965

Foster NL, Chase TN, Mansi L, Brooks R, Fedio P, Patronas NJ, DiChiro C (1984) Cortical abnormalities in Alzheimer's disease. Ann Neurol 16:649–654

Fowler JS, Wolf AP, Christman RD, McGregor RR, Ansari AA, Atkins H (1975) Carrier-free ^{11}C labeled catecholamines. In: Subramanian J, Rhodes BA, Cooper JT, Sodd VJ (eds) Radiopharmaceuticals. Soc Nucl Med, New York, pp 196–204

Fowler JS, Arnett CD, Wolf AP, MacGregor RR, Norton EF, Finley AM (1982) ^{11}C-Spiroperidol: synthesis, specific activity determination, and biodistribution in mice. J Nucl Med 23:437–445

Fox KAA, Abendschein DR, Ambos HD, Sobel BE, Bergman SR (1985) Efflux of metabolized and nonmetabolized fatty acids from canine myocardium. Implications for quantifying myocardial metabolism tomographically. Circ Res 57:232–243

Fox PT, Raichle ME (1984) Stimulus rate dependence of regional cerebral blood flow in human striate cortex, demonstrated by positron emission tomography. J Neurophysiol 51:1109–1120

Fox PT, Raichle ME (1985) Stimulus rate determines regional brain blood flow in striate cortex. Ann Neurol 17:303–305

Fox PT, Perlmutter JS, Raichle ME (1985a) A stereotactic method of anatomical localization for positron emission tomography. J Comput Assist Tomogr 9:141–153

Fox PT, Fox JM, Raichle ME, Burde RM (1985b) The role of cerebral cortex in the generation of voluntary saccades: a positron emission tomography study. J Neurophysiol 54:348–369

Fox PT, Raichle ME, Thach WT (1985c) Functional mapping of the human cerebellum with positron emission tomography. Proc Natl Acad Sci USA 82:7462–7466

Frackowiak RSJ, Lammertsma AA (1985) Clinical measurement of cerebral blood flow and oxygen consumption. In: Reivich M, Alavi A (eds) Positron emission tomography. Liss, New York, pp 153–181

Frackowiak RSJ, Wise RJ (1983) Positron tomography in ischemic cerebrovascular disease. Neurol Clin 1:183–200

Frackowiak RSJ, Jones T, Lenzi GL, Heather JD (1980a) Regional cerebral oxygen utilisation and blood flow in normal man using oxygen-15 and positron emission tomography. Acta Neurol Scand 62:336–344

Frackowiak RSJ, Lenzi GL, Jones T, Heather JD (1980b) Quantitative measurement of regional cerebral blood flow and oxygen metabolism in man using ^{15}O and positron emission tomography: theory, procedure, and normal values. J Comput Assist Tomogr 4:727–736

Frackowiak RSJ, Pozzili C, Legg NJ et al. (1981a) A prospective study of regional cerebral blood flow and oxygen utilization in dementia using positron emission tomography and oxygen-15. J Cereb Blood Flow Metab 1:S453–S454

Frackowiak RSJ, Pozzilli C, Legg NJ, DuBoulay GH, Marshall J, Lenzi GL, Jones T (1981b) Regional cerebral oxygen supply and utilization in dementia – A clinical and physiological study with oxygen-15 and positron tomography. Brain 104:753–778

Frackowiak RSL, Wise RJ, Gibbs JM, Jones T (1984) Positron emission tomographic studies in aging and cerebrovascular disease at Hammersmith Hospital. Ann Neurol 15:S112–S118

Frey P, Townsend D, Jeavons A, Donath A (1985) In vivo imaging of the human thyroid with a positron camera using ^{124}I. Eur J Nucl Med 10:472–476

Friedland RP, Budinger TF, Ganz E, Vano V, Mathis CA, Koss B, Ober BA, Huesman RH, Derenzo SE (1983) Regional cerebral metabolic alterations in dementia of the Alzheimer type: Positron emission tomography with [^{18}F]fluorodeoxyglucose. J Comput Assist Tomogr 7:590–598

Friedland RP, Prusiner SB, Jagust WJ, Budinger TF, Davis RL (1984) Bitemporal hypometabolism in Creutzfeld-Jakob disease measured by positron emission tomography with [^{18}F]-2-fluorodeoxyglucose. J Comput Assist Tomogr 8:978–981

Friedland RP, Budinger TF, Koss E, Ober BA (1985) Alzheimer's disease: anterior-posterior and lateral hemispheric alterations in cortical glucose utilization. Neurosci Lett 53:235–240

Frost JJ, Dannals RF, Duelfer T, Burns HD, Ravert HT, Langström B, Balasubramanian V, Wagner HN (1984a) In vivo studies of opiate receptors. Ann Neurol 15:S85–S92

Frost JJ, Uhl GE, Wong DF, Preziosi TJ, Dannals RF, Ravert HT, Wagner HN (1984b) Dopamine receptor alterations in asymmetrical and symmetrical Parkinsonism measured by positron emission tomography. Ann neurol 16:128

Frost JJ, Wagner HN, Dannals RF, Ravert HT, Links JM, Wilson AA, Burns HD, Wong DF, McPherson RW, Rosenbaum AE, Kuhar MJ, Snyder SH (1985) Imaging opiate receptors in the human brain by positron tomography. J Comput Assist Tomogr 9:231–236

Fucks W, Knipping HW (1955) Eine Gamma-Retina zur Bestimmung der raum-zeitlichen Verteilung radioaktiver Substanzen. Naturwiss 42:493

Fukuda H, Matsuzawa Z, Abe Y, Endo S, Ymada K, Kubota K, Hatazawa J, Sato T, Ito M, Takahashi T, Iwata R, Ido T (1982) Experimental study for cancer diagnosis with positron-labeled fluorinated glucose analogs: 18-F-2-fluorodeoxy-D-mannose: A new tracer for cancer detection. Eur J Nucl Med 7:294–297

Fukuyama T, Nakamura M, Nakagaki O, Matsuguchi H, Mitsutake A, Kikuchi Y, Kuroiwa A (1978) Reduced reflow and diminished uptake of ^{82}Rb after temporary coronary occlusion. Am J Physiol [Suppl] 234:H274–H279

Gadisseux P, Ward JD, Young HF, Becker DP (1984) Nutrition and the neurosurgical patient. J Neurosurg 60:219–232

Gado M, Hughes CP, Danziger W, Chi D, Jost G, Berg L (1982) Volumetric measurements of the cerebrospinal fluid spaces in demented subjects and controls. Radiology 144:535–538

Gallagher B, Christman D, Fowler J et al. (1977) Radioisotope scintigraphy for the study of dynamics of amine regulation by the human lung. Chest 71:282–284

Gallagher BM, Fowler JS, Gutterson NI, MacGregor RR, Wan CN, Wolf AP (1978) Metabolic trapping as a principle of radiopharmaceutical design. The factors responsible for the bio-distribution of ^{18}F-2-deoxy-2-fluoro-D-glucose (^{18}FDG). J Nucl Med 19:1154–1161

Gallhofer B, Trimble MR, Frackowiak RSJ, Gibbs J, Jones T (1985) A study of cerebral blood flow and metabolism in epileptic psychosis using positron emission tomography and oxygen. J Neurol Neurosurg Psychiatry 48:201–206

Gamsu G, Kaufman L, Swann S, Brito AC (1979) Absolute lung density in experimental canine pulmonary edema. Invest Radiol 14:261–269

Garnett ES, Firnau G, Nahmias C (1983) Dopamine visualized in the basal ganglia of living man. Nature 305:137–138

Garnett ES, Nahmias C, Firnau G (1984a) Central dopaminergic pathways in hemiparkinsonism examined by positron emission tomography. Can J Neurol Sci 11:174–179

Garnett ES, Firnau G, Nahmias C, Carbotte R, Bartolucci G (1984b) Reduced striatal glucose consumption and prolonged reaction time are early features in Huntingtons's disease. J Neurol Sci 65:231–237

Gastaut H (1970) Clinical and electroencephalographic classification of epileptic seizure. Epilepsia 17:102–113

Gastaut H (1976) Conclusions: Computerized transverse axial tomography in epilepsy. Epilepsia 17:337–338

Gastaut JL, Michel B (1978) The impact of cranial CT on electroencephalography. Electroencephalogr Clin Neurophysiol 34:123–132

Gelbard AS, Benua RS, Laughlin JS, Rosen G, Reiman RE, McDonald JM (1979) Quantitative scanning of osteogenic sarcoma with nitrogen-13-labeled L-glutamate. J Nucl Med 20:782–784

Gelbard AS, Buena RS, Reiman RE, McDonald JM, Vomero JJ, Laughlin JS (1980) Imaging of the human heart after administration of L-(N-13)glutamate. J Nucl Med 21:988–991

Gelbard AS, Cooper AJL, Rieman RE, Buena RS (1981) Synthesis of N-13-labeled monocarboxylic amino acids suitable for patient studies with immobilized glutamate dehydrogenase. J Nucl Med 22:P74

Geltman EM, Klein MS, Biello D, Siegel BA, Ter-Pogossian MM, Sobel BE (1979) Dependance of impaired, regional, ventricular function on underlying, persistent metabolic manifestations of infarction. Circulation [Suppl II] 60:232

Geltman EM, Biello D, Welch MJ, Ter-Pogossian MM, Roberts R, Sobel BE (1982) Characterization of nontransmural myocardial infarction by positron-emission tomography. Circulation 65:747–755

Geltman EM, Smith JL, Beecher D, Ludbrook PA, Ter-Pogossian MM, Sobel BE (1983) Altered regional myocardial metabolism in congestive cardiomyopathy detected by positron tomography. Am J Med 74:773–785

Geltman EM, Bergman SR, Sobel BE (1985) Cardiac positron emission tomography. In: Reivich M, Alavi A (eds) Positron emission tomography. Liss, New York, pp 345–385

Gerson DF, Kiefer H, Eufe W (1982) Intracellular pH mitogen-stimulated lymphocytes. Science 216:1009–1010

Gibbs JM, Wise R, Leenders K et al. (1983a) The relationship of regional cerebral blood flow, blood volume, and oxygen metabolism in patients with carotid occlusion: Evaluation of perfusion reserve. J Cereb Blood Flow Metab 3:S590–S591

Gibbs JM, Rhodes CG, Wise RJ et al. (1983b) The relationship of regional cerebral blood flow, oxygen metabolism and glucose metabolism following acute stroke. In: Heiss WD, Phelps ME (eds) Positron emission tomography of the brain. Springer, Berlin Heidelberg New York Tokyo, pp 234–235

Gibbs JM, Wise RJS, Leenders KL, Jones T (1984) Evaluation of cerebral perfusion reserve in patients with carotid-artery occlusion. Lancet 1:182–186

Ginsberg MD, Lockwood AH, Busto R, Finn RD, Campbell JA, Boothe TE (1981) 11-C-iodoantipurine for the measurement of regional cerebral blood flow by positron emission tomography. Stroke 12:745–750

Giuntini C (1971) Theoretical considerations on the measure of pulmonary blood volume and extravascular lung water in man. Bull Eur Physiopathol Respir 7:1125–1160

Giuntini C, Fazio F (1979) Determination of extravascular lung water by dilution method. J Nucl Med 23:85–93

Gjedde A (1982) Calculation of cerebral glucose phosphorilation from brain uptake of glucose analogues in vivo: A reexamination. Brain Res Rev 4:237–274

Gjedde A, Diemer NH (1985) Relationship between unidirectional and net uptake of glucose and glucose analogs into brain: On the variability of tansfer and lumped constants. In: Greitz T, Ingvar DH, Wiedén L (eds) The metabolism of the human brain studied with positron emission tomography. Raven, New York, pp 207–214

Gjedde A, Hansen AJ, Siemkowicz E (1980) Rapid simultaneous determination of regional blood flow and blood brain glucose transfer in brain of rat. Acta Physiol Scand 108:321–330

Gjedde A, Wienhard K, Heiss WD, Kloster G, Diemer NH, Herholz K, Pawlik G (1985) Comparative regional analysis of 2-fluorodeoxyglucose and methylglucose uptake in brain of four stroke patients. J Cereb Blood Flow Metab 5:163–178

Glass H, Brant A, Clark JC (1968) Measurement of blood volume using red cells labelled with radioactive carbonmonoxyde. J Nucl Med 9:571–575

Goldstein GW, Betz AL (1986) The blood-brain barrier. Sci Am 255/3:70–79

Goldstein RA, Klein MS, Welch MJ, Sobel BE (1980) External assessment of myocardial metabolism with C-11 palmitate in vivo. J Nucl Med 21:342–348

Goldstein RA, Mullani NA, Marani SK, Fisher DJ, Gould L, O'Brien HA (1983) Myocardial perfusion with rubidium-82. II Effects of metabolic and pharmacologic interventions. J Nucl Med 24:907–915

Goodwin JF (1978) Daunorubicin cardiomyopathy. In: Hurst JW (ed) The heart. McGraw Hill, New York, pp 1573–1574

Goresky CA, Cronin RFP, Wangel BA (1969) Indicator dilution measurements of extravascular water in the lungs. J Clinic Invest 48:487–501

Goresky CA, Ziegler WH, Bach GG (1970) Barrier-limited and flow-limited distribution. Circ Res 27:739–764

Gould KL, Schelbert HR, Phelps ME, Hoffman EJ (1979) Noninvasive assessment of coronary stenosis with myocardial perfusion imaging during pharmacologic coronary vasodilatation. V. Detection of 47 percent diameter coronary stenosis with intravenous nitrogen-13 ammonia and emission-computed transaxial tomography in intact dogs. Am J Cardiol 43:200–208

Gould KL, Goldstein RA (1984a) Cardiovascular

imaging metabolic and functional. Physiologist 27:27–39

Gould KL, Mullani N (1984b) Dynamic cardiac imaging. J Nucl Med 25:1380–1386

Graham JF, Cummins CJ, Smith BH, Kornblith PL (1985) Regulation of hexokinase in cultured gliomas. Neurosurgery 17:537–542

Grant PM, Erdal BR, O'Brien HA (1975) A ^{82}Sr–^{82}Rb isotope generator for use in nuclear medicine. J Nucl Med 16:300–304

Greenberg HJ, Reivich M, Alavi A, Hand P, Rosenquist A, Rintelmann W, Stein A, Tusa R, Dann R, Christman D, Fowler J, MacGregor B, Wolf A (1981) Metabolic mapping of functional activity in human subjects with the ^{18}F-Fluorodeoxyglucose technique. Science 212:678–680

Grimes AM, Grady CL, Foster NL, Sunderland T, Patronas NJ (1985) Central auditory function in Alzheimer's disease. Neurology 35:352–358

Gronemeyer SA, Brownell GL, Elmaleh DR, Athanasoulis CA (1980) Transverse section imaging of soft tissue tumors and peripheral vascular disease. Semin Nucl Med 10:392–399

Grover M, Schwaiger M, Sochor H, Guzy PM, Child JS, Krivokapich J, Schelbert HR (1984) C-11-palmatic acid kinetics and positron emission tomography detect pacing-induced ischemia in patients with coronary artery disease. Circulation [Suppl II] 70:340

Grubb RL, Phelps ME, Ter-Pogossian MM (1973) Regional cerebral blood volume in humans. Arch Neurol 28:38–44

Grubb RL, Ratcheson RA, Raichle ME et al. (1979) Regional cerebral blood flow and oxygen utilization in superficial temporal-middle cerebral artery anastomosis patients. J Neurosurg 50:733–741

Gur RC, Sussman NM, Alavi A, Gur RE, Rosen AD, O'Connor M, Goldberg HI, Greenberg JH, Reivich M (1982) Positron emission tomography in two cases of childhood epileptic encephalopathy (Lennox-Gastaut syndrome). Neurology 32:1191–1194

Gur RC, Gur RE, Rosen AD, Warach S, Alavi A, Greenberg J, Reivich M (1983) A cognitive-motor network demonstrated by positron emission tomography. Neuropsycologia 21:601–606

Gur RC, Gur RE, Sussman NM, Selzer ME (1985) Positron emission tomography in epilepsy. In: Reivich M, Alavi A (eds) Positron emission tomography. Liss, New York, pp 263–271

Gurpide E, Mann J, Lieberman S (1963) Analysis of open systems of multiple pools by administration of tracers at a constant rate or as a single dose as illustrated by problems involving steroid hormones. J Clin Endocrinol Metab 23:1155–1176

Guzzardi R, Mey M (1979) Further appraisal and improvements of 90′ compton scattering tomography of the lung. Phys Med Biol 26:261–269

Hack SN, Eichling JO, Bergman SR, Welch MJ, Sobel BE (1980) External quantification of myocardial perfusion by exponential infusion of positron-emitting radionuclides. J Clin Invest 66:918–927

Hales CA, Kanarek DJ, Ahluwalia B, Latty A, Erdmann J, Javaheri S, Kazemi H (1981) Regional edema formation in isolated perfused dog lungs. Circ Res 48:121–127

Hamala JR, Holden JE, Gatley SJ, Bernstein D, O'Hara KT, DeGrado TP (1983) Validation of F-18-3-deoxy-3-fluoro-D-glucose (3-FDG) as an agent for measurement of glucose transport by positron emission tomography. J Nucl Med 24:P52

Hamilton WF, Moore JW, Kinsman JM, Spurling RG (1928) Simultaneous determination of the greater and lesser circulation times, of the mean velocity of blood flow through the heart and lungs, of the cardiac output, and an approximation of the amount of blood activity circulating in the heart and lungs. Am J Physiol 85:377–378

Harper PV, Lathrop KA, Andros G, McArdle R, Goodman A, Beck RN, Covell J (1965) Technetium-99m as a clinical tracer material. Strahlentherapie 60:136

Harper PV, Lathrop KA, Krizek H, Lembares N, Stark V, Hoffer PB (1972) Clinical feasability of myocardial imaging with ^{13}NH$_3$. J Nucl Med 13:278–280

Harper PV, Schwartz J, Beck RN, Lathrop KA, Lembares N, Krizek H, Gloria I, Dinwoodie R, McLaughlin A, Stark VJ, Bekerman C, Hoffer PB, Gottschalk A, Resnekov L, Al-Sedir J, Mayoorga A, Brooks HL (1973) Clinical myocardial imaging with nitrogen-13 ammonia. Radiology 108:613–617

Hatazawa J, Bairamian D, Fishbein DS, Brooks RA, Di Chiro B (1981) Glucose utilization of non-gliomatous cerebral neoplasmsas an index of tumor agressivity. J Nucl Med 27:901

Hawkins RA, Phelps ME, Huang SC, Kuhl DE (1981) Effect of ischemia on quantification of local cerebral glucose metabolism rate in man. J Cereb Blood Flow Metab 1:37–51

Hawkins RA, Mazziotta JC, Phelps ME, Huang SC, Carson RE, Metter RJ, Riege WH (1983a) Cerebral glucose metabolism as a function of age in man: Influence of the rate constants in a fluorodeoxyglucose method. J Cereb Blood Flow Metab 3:250–253

Hawkins RA, Phelps ME, Mazziotta JC, Kuhl DE (1983b) A study of Wilson's disease with F-18-FDG and positron tomography. J Cereb Blood Flow Metab 3:S498–S499

Hawkins RA, Phelps ME, Huang SC, Wapenski JA, Grimm PD, Parker RG, Juillard G, Greenberg P (1984) A kinetic evaluation of blood-barrier permeability in human brain tumors with [^{68}Ga]EDTA and positron computed tomography. J Cereb Blood Flow Metab 4:507–515

Hawkins RA, Phelps ME, Huang SC (1986) Effects of temporal sampling, glucose metabolic rates, and disruption of blood brain barrier on the FDG-model with and without a vascular compartment: Studies in human brain tumors with PET. J Cereb Blood Flow Metab 6:170–183

Hayashi N, Tamaki N, Yonekura Y, Senda M, Saji H, Yamamoto K, Konishi J, Torizuka K (1985) Imaging of the hepatocellular carcinoma using dynamic positron emission tomography with nitrogen-13 ammonia. J Nucl Med 26:254–257

Heiss WD, Kloster G, Vyska K et al. (1981) Regional cerebral distribution of ^{11}C-methyl-D-glucose compared with CT perfusion patterns in stroke. J Cereb Blood Flow Metab 1:S506–S507

Heiss WD (1985) The purpose of functional mapping in focal cerebral ischemia. In: Heiss WD (ed) Functional mapping of the brain in vascular disorders. Springer, Berlin Heidelberg New York Tokyo, pp 1–3

Heiss WD (1986) Ansatzpunkte zur Therapie zerebraler Durchblutungsstörungen. DMW 111:186–190

Heiss WD, Ilsen HW, Wagner R, Pawlik G, Wienhard K (1983a) Remote functional depression of glucose metabolism in stroke and its alterations by activating drugs. In: Heiss WD, Phelps ME (eds) Positron emission tomography of the brain. Springer, Berlin Heidelberg New York Tokyo, pp 162–168

Heiss WD, Pawlik G, Wagner R, Ilsen HW, Herholz K, Wienhard K (1983b) Functional hypometabolism in noninfarcted brain regions in ischemia stroke. J Cereb Blood Flow Metab 3:S582–S583

Heiss WD, Pawlik G, Herholz K, Wagner R, Göldner H, Wienhard K (1984) Regional kinetic constants and cerebral metabolic rate for glucose in normal human volunteers determined by dynamic positron emission tomography of [^{18}F]-2-fluoro-2-deoxy-D-glucose. J Cereb Blood Flow Metab 4:212–223

Heiss WD, Pawlik G, Herholz K, Wagner R, Wienhard K (1985a) Regional cerebral glucose metabolism in man during wakefulness, sleep and dreaming. Brain Res 327:362–366

Heiss WD, Beil C, Herholz K, Pawlik G, Wagner R, Wienhard K (1985b) Atlas der Positronen-Emissions-Tomographie des Gehirns. Springer, Berlin Heidelberg New York Tokyo

Helmeke H-J, Schober O, Lehr L, Junker D, Meyer G-J, Fitschen J, Bossaller C, Hundeshagen H (1982) Measurements of regional lung water with O-15 labeled water and CO-15 labeled Carboxyhemoglobin. Radioact Isot Klinik Forsch 15:635–644

Henriques V (1913) Über die Verteilung des Blutes vom linken Herzen zwischen dem Herzen und dem übrigen Organismus. Biochem Zeitschr 56:230–248

Henze E, Perloff JK, Schelbert HR (1981) Alterations of regional myocardial perfusion and metabolism in Duchenne's muscular dystrophy (DMD) detected by positron computed tomography (PCT). Circulation 64:279

Henze E, Schelbert HR, Barrio JR, Egbert JE, Hansen HW, MacDonald NS, Phelps ME (1982a) Evaluation of myocardial metabolism, with N-13- and C-11-labeled amino acids and positron computed tomography. J Nucl Med 23:671–681

Henze E, Grossman RG, Huang SC, Barrio JR, Phelps ME, Schelbert HR (1982b) Myocardial uptake and clearance of C-11 palmatic acid in man: Effects of substrate availibility and cardiac work. J Nucl Med 23:P12

Henze E, Grossman RG, Najafi A, Barrio JR, Phelps ME, Schelbert HR (1982c) Measurement of C-11 palmitate kinetics after metabolic interventions in normals and patients with cardiomyopathy using positron emission computed tomography. Am J Cardiol 49:1023

Herd JA, Hollenberg M, Thornburn GD, Kopald HH, Barger AC (1962) Myocardial blood flow determination with 85-Krypton in unanesthetized dogs. Am J Physiol 203:122–124

Herholz K, Wienhard K, Pawlik G, Seldon L, Beil C, Heiss W-D (1985) Functional imaging of reversible and irreversible ^{68}Ga-EDTA uptake in brain tumors. Acta Neurol Scand 72:105

Herscovitch P, Raichle ME (1983) Effect of tissue heterogeneity on the measurement of cerebral blood flow with the equilibrium C^{15}O$_2$ inhalation technique. J Cereb Blood Flow Metab 3:407–415

Herscovitch P, Raichle ME (1985) What is the correct value for the brain-blood partition coefficient for water? J Cereb Blood Flow Metab 5:65–69

Herscovitch P, Perlan JM, Volpe JJ et al. (1983a) The assessment of regional cerebral blood flow in the newborn with positron emission tomography. J Cereb Blood Flow Metab 3:S502–S503

Herscovitch P, Markham J, Raichle ME (1983b) Brain blood flow measured with intravenous H$_2$^{15}O. I. Theory and error analysis. J Nucl Med 24:782–789

Herscovitch P, Mintum MA, Raichle ME (1984a) Brain blood-flow measurement with bolus intravenous H$_2$^{15}O. J Nucl Med 25:730–731

Herscovitch P, Gado M, Mintum MA, Raichle ME (1984b) The necessity for correcting for cerebral atrophy in global positron emission tomography measurements. Monogr Neurol Sci 11:93–97

Hill, TC, Holman L, Lovett R, O'Leary DH, Front D, Magistretti P, Zimmerman RE, Moore S, Clouse ME, Wu JL, Lin TH, Baldwin RM (1982) Initial experience with SPECT (Single-Photon Computerized Tomography) of the brain using N-isopropyl I-123-p-iodamphetamine: concise communication. J Nucl Med 23:191–195

Hiraiwa M, Nonaka C, Abe T, Iio M (1983) Positron emission tomography in systemic lupus erythematodus. AJNR 4:541–543

Hnatowich DJ (1975) A method for the preparation and quality control of Ga-68 radiopharmaceuticals. J Nucl Med 16:764–768

Hnatowich DJ (1976) Labeling of human albumin microspheres with Ga-68. J Nucl Med 17:57–60

Hnatowich DJ, Kulprathipanja S, Evans G, Elmaleh D (1979) A comparison of positron-emitting blood pool imaging agents. Int J Appl Radiat Isot 30:335–340

Höck A, Freundlieb C, Vyska K, Lösse B, Erbel R, Feinendegen LE (1983) Myocardial imaging and metabolic studies with [17-^{123}I]-Iodoheptadecanoic acid in patients with iodopathic congestive cardiomyopathy. J Nucl Med 24:22–28

Hoffman EJ, Phelps ME, Weiss ES, Welch MJ, Coleman RE, Sobel BE, Ter-Pogossian MM (1977) Transaxial tomographic imaging of canine myocardium with ^{11}C-palmatic acid. J Nucl Med 18:57–61

Hofmann H (1986) Das Epilepsie-Risiko in der Lebensversicherung. Lebensversicherungsmedizin 38:26–30

Holden JE, Gatley SJ, Hichwa RD, Ip WR, Shaughnessy WJ, Nickles RJ, Polcyn RE (1981a) Regional cerebral blood flow using positron emission tomographic measurements of Fluoromethane kinetics. J Cerebr Blood Flow Metab 1:S463–S464

Holden JE, Gatley SJ, Hichwa RD, Ip WR, Shaughnessy WJ, Nickles RJ, Polcyn RE (1981b) Cerebral blood flow using PET measurements of Fluoromethane kinetics. J Nucl Med 22:1084–1088

Holley RW (1972) A unifying hypothesis concerning the nature of malignant growth. Proc Natl Acad Sci USA 69:2840

Holloway CJ (1981) The biochemistry of hepatic detoxification. In: Brunner G, Schmidt FW (eds) Artificial liver support. Springer, Berlin Heidelberg New York, pp 32–48

Holman BL, Hill TC, Lee RGL, Zimmerman RE, Moore SC, Royal HD (1983) Brain imaging with radiolabeled amines. In: Freeman LM, Weissmann HS (eds) Nuclear medicine annual 1983. Raven, New York

Holman BL, Lee RGL, Hill TC, Lovett RD, Lister-James J (1984a) A comparison of two cerebral perfusion tracers, N-Isopropyl I-123p-Iodoamphetamine and I-123 HIPDM, in the human. J Nucl Med 25:25–30

Holman BL, Wick MM, Kaplan ML, Hill TC, Lee RGL, Wu J-L, Lin TH (1984b) The relationship of the eye uptake of N-Isopropyl-p-123-I-Iodoamphetamine to melanin production. J Nucl Med 25:315–319

Hornykiewicz O (1980) Biochemical abnormalities in some extrastriatal neuronal systems in Parkinson's disease. In: Rinne UK, Klingler M, Stamm G (eds) Parkinson's disease; current progress, problems and management. Elsevier, Amsterdam

Hornykiewicz O (1982) Brain neurotransmitter changes in Parkinson's disease. In: Marsden CD, Fahn S (eds) Movement Disorders. Butterworth Scientific, London

Hougen TJ, Smith TW (1978) Inhibition of myocardial monovalent cation active transport by subtoxic doses of ouabain in the dog. Circ Res 42:856–863

Howard BE, Ginsberg MD, Hassel WR, Lockwood AH, Freed P (1983) On the uniqueness of cerebral blood flow measured by the in vivo autoradiographic strategy and positron emission tomography. J Cereb Blood Flow Metab 3:432–444

Huang SC, Phelps ME (1986) Principles of tracerkinetic modeling in positron emission tomography and autoradiography. In: Phelps ME, Mazziotta JC, Schelbert HR (eds) Positron emission tomography and autoradiography. Raven, New York, pp 287–346

Huang SC, Phelps ME, Hoffman EJ, Kuhl DE (1979) A theoretical study of quantitative flow measurements with constant infusion of short-lived isotopes. Phys Med Biol 6:1151–1161

Huang SC, Phelps ME, Hoffman EJ, Sideris K, Selin CJ, Kuhl DE (1980) Noninvasive determination of local cerebral metabolic rate of glucose in normal human subjects with 18-F-Fluoro-2'-Desoxyglucose and emission computed tomography. Am J Physiol [Suppl] 238:E69–E82

Huang SC, Phelps ME, Hoffman JE, Kuhl DE (1981a) Error sensitivity of the fluoro desoxyglucose method for measurement of local cerebral metabolic rate of glucose. J Cereb Blood Flow Metab 1:391–401

Huang SC, Phelps ME, Carson RE et al. (1981b) Tomographic measurement of local cerebral blood flow in man with O-15-water. J Cereb Blood Flow Metab 1:S31–S32

Huang SC, Carson RE, Phelps ME (1982a) Measurement of local blood flow and distribution volume with short-lived isotopes: A general input technique. J Cereb Blood Flow Metabol 2:99–108

Huang SC, Schwaiger M, Carson RE, Henze E, Hoffman EJ, Phelps ME, Schelbert HR (1982b) An O-15 water clearance method for quantitative regional myocardial blood flow measurement. J Nucl Med 23:P69

Huang SC, Carson RE, Hoffman EJ, Carson J, MacDonald N, Barrio RJ, Phelps ME (1983) Quantitative measurement of local cerebral blood flow in humans by positron computed tomography and O-15-water. J Cereb Blood Flow Metab 3:141–153

Hübner KF, Andrews GA, Washburn L, Wieland BW, Gibbs WD, Hayes RL, Butler TA, Winebrenner JD (1977) Tumor location with 1-aminocyclopentane [^{11}C]carboxylic acid: Preliminary clinical trials with single-photon detection. J Nucl Med 18:1215–1221

Hübner KF, Andrews GA, Buonocore E, Hayes RL, Washburn LC, Collman IR, Gibbs WD (1979)

Carbon-11-labeled amino acids for the rectilinear and positron tomographic imaging of the human pancreas. J Nucl Med 20:507–513

Hübner KF, King P, Gibbs WD, Partain CL, Washburn LC, Hayes RL, Holloway E (1980) Clinical investigations with carbon-11-labeled amino acids using positron emission computerized tomography in patients with neoplastic diseases. Symposium on Medical Radionuclide Imaging IAEA-SM-247/90

Hübner KF, Krauss S, Washburn LC, Gibbs WD, Holloway EC (1981) Tumor detection with 1-aminocyclopentane and 1-aminocyclobutane C-11-carboxylic acid using positron emission computerized tomography. Clin Nucl Med 6:249–252

Hübner KF, Purvis JT, Mahaley SM, Robertson JT, Rogers S, Gibbs WD, King P, Partain CL (1982) Brain tumor imaging by positron emission computed tomography using 11-C-labeled amino acids. J Comput Assit Tomogr 6:544–550

Hughes CP, Gado M (1981) Computed tomography and aging of the brain. Radiology 139:391–396

Hughes JMB (1977) Pulmonary edema. In: West JB (ed) Regional differences in the lung. Academic, New York San Francisco London, pp 381–418

Hughes JMB (1979) Short-life radionuclides and regional lung function. Br J Radiol 52:353–370

Hundeshagen H (1978) Pankreas. In: Hundeshagen H (Red von) Diagnostik, Therapie, Klinische Forschung, Teil 2. Springer, Berlin Heidelberg New York (Handbuch der medizinischen Radiologie, Bd. XV/2, s 853–877)

Ido T, Wan CN, Casella V, Fowler JS, Wolf AP, Reivich M, Kuhl DE (1978) Labeled 2-deoxy-D-glucose analogs. ^{18}F labeled 2-FDG, 2-FDM and ^{14}C-2-FDG. J Label Comp Radiopharm 14:175–183

Ilsen HW, Sato M, Pawlik G, Herholz K, Wienhard K, Heiss WD (1984) 68-Ga-EDTA positron emission tomography in the diagnosis of brain tumors. Neuroradiology 26:393–398

Ingvar DH (1973) Regional cerebral blood flow in focal cortical epilepsy. Stroke 4:359–360

Ingvar DH (1975) rCBF in focal cortical epilepsy. In: Langfitt TW, McHenry LC, Reivich M (eds) Cerebral circulation and metabolism. Springer, Berlin Heidelberg New York, pp 361–363

Ingvar DH, Franzen G (1971) Abnormalities of cerebral blood flow distributions in patients with chronic schizophrenia. Acta Psychatr Scand 50:425–462

Ingvar DH, Lassen NA (1962) Regional blood flow of the cerebral cortex determined by Krypton-85. Acta Physiol Scand 54:325–338

Inoue Y, Wagner HN, Wong DF, Links JM, Frost JJ, Dannals RF, Rosenbaum AE, Takeda K, Di-Chiro G, Kuhar MJ (1985) Atlas of dopamine receptor images (PET) of the human brain. J Comput Assist Tomogr 9:129–140

Ishida S, Yaji K, Fujiwara T et al. (1983) A correlative study of CT with EEG findings in epilepsy. J Comput Assist Tomogr 2:524

Ito M, Lammertsma AA, Wise RJS, Bernardi S, Frackowiak RSJ, Heather JD, McKenzie CG, Thomas DGT, Jones T (1982) Measurement of regional cerebral blood flow and oxygen utilization in patients with cerebral tumors using ^{15}O and positron emission tomography: Analytical techniques and preliminary results. Neuroradiology 23:62–74

Jaques JA (1972) Compartmental analysis in biology and medicine. Elsevier, New York

Jarden JO, Dhawan V, Poltorak A, Posner JB, Rottenberg DA (1985) Positron enmission tomographic measurement of blood-to-brain and blood-to-tumor transport of ^{82}Rb: The effect of dexamethasone and whole-brain radiation theraphy. Ann Neurol 18:636–646

Jellinger K (1976) Neuropathological aspects of dementia resulting from abnormal blood and cerebrospinal fluid dynamics. Acta Neurol Belg 76:83–102

Jones AKP, Luthra SK, Pike VW, Herold S, Brady F (1985) New labelled ligand for in-vivo studies of opoid physiology. Lancet II:665–666

Jones SC, Greenberg JH, Dann R, Robinson G Jr, Kushner M, Alavi A, Reivich M (1985) Cerebral blood flow with the continuous infusion of oxygen-15-labeled water. J Cereb Blood Flow Metab 5:566–575

Jones T, Clark JC, Buckingham PD, Grant BJB, Hughes JMB (1972) The use of oxygen 15 labelled water for the measurement of pulmonary extravascular water. Brit J Radiol 45:630

Jones T, Chesler DA, Ter-Pogossian MM (1976a) The continuous inhalation of oxygen-15 for assessing regional oxygen extraction in the brain of man. Brit J Radiol 49:339–343

Jones T, Jones HA, Rhodes CG, Buckingham PD, Hughes JMB (1976b) Distribution of extravascular fluid volumes in isolated perfused lungs measured with $H_2^{15}O$. J Clinic Invest 57:706–713

Jones T, Frackowiak RSJ, Lammertsma AA, Rhodes CG (1982) Compartmental analysis of the steady-state distribution of 15-O_2 in the body. J Nucl Med 23:750

Jordan K, Knoop BO (1987) Meßtechnik in der Emissions-Computertomographie. In: Hundeshagen H (Hrsg) Emissions-Computertomographie mit kurzlebigen zyklotron-produzierten Radiopharmaka. Springer, Berlin Heidelberg New York Tokyo (Handbuch der medizinischen Radiologie, Bd XV/1B)

Jugdutt BI, Hutchins GM, Bulkley BH, Becker LC (1979) The loss of radioactive microspheres from canine necrotic myocardium. Circ Res 45:746–756

Junck L, Blasberg R, Rottenberg DA (1981) Brain

and tumor pH in experimental leptomeningeal carcinomatosis. Trans Am Neurol Assoc 106:298–301

Junod AF (1972) Uptake, metabolism and efflux of C-14-5-hydroxytryptamine in isolated perfused rat lungs. J Pharmacol Exp Ther 183:341–355

Kabalka GW, McCollum GW, Fabirkiewicz AS, Lambrecht RM, Fowler JS, Sajjad M, Wolf AP (1984) Synthesis on ^{15}O-labelled butanol via organoborane chemistry: Preliminary report. J Labeled Comp Radiopharm 21:1247–1249

Kanaya H, Endo H, Sugiyama T et al. (1983) Crossed cerebral diaschisis in patients with putaminal hemorrhage. J Cereb Blood Flow Metab 3:S27–S28

Kaplan HI, Freedman AM, Sadock BJ (eds) (1980) Comprehensive textbook in psychatry. Williams & Wilkins, Baltimore

Kato A, Menon D, Diksic M, Yamamoto VL (1984a) Influence of the input function on the calculation of local cerebral metabolic rate for glucose in the deoxyglucose method. J Cereb Blood Flow Metab 4:41–46

Kato A et al. (1984b) An improved approach for measurement of regional cerebral rate constants in the deoxyglucose method with positron emission tomography. J Cereb Blood Flow Metab 4:555–563

Kato A, Diksic M, Yamamoto YL, Feindel WC (1985) Quantification of glucose utilization in an experimental brain tumor model by the deoxyglucose method. J Cereb Blood Flow Metab 5:108–114

Kawana M, Krizek H, Porter J, Lathrop D, Charleston D, Harper PV (1970) Use of ^{199}Tl as a potassium analog in scanning. J Nucl Med 11:333

Kearfott KJ, Junck L, Rottenberg DA (1983a) ^{11}C-dimethyloxzolidinedione (DMO): biodistribution, estimates of radiation absorbed dose, and potential for positron emission tomographic (PET) measurements of regional brain tissue pH. J Nucl Med 24:805–811

Kearfott KJ, Rottenberg DA, Volpe BT (1983b) Design of steady-state positron emission tomography protocols for neurobehavioral studies: CO^{15}O and ^{19}Ne. J Comput Assist Tomogr 7:51–58

Kelly RE, Ackerman RH, Alpert NM et al. (1982) Positron emission tomography in nontraumatic intracerebral hemorrhage. Neurology 32:A88

Kessler RM, Goble JC, Barranger JA, Bird JH, Rapoport SI (1983) Quantitative measurement of blood-brain barrier permeability following osmotic opening. J Nucl Med 24:107

Kessler RM, Goble JC, Bird JH, Girton ME, Doppman JL, Rapoport SI, Baranger JA (1984) Measurement of blood-brain barrier permeability with positron emission tomography and [^{68}Ga]EDTA. J Cereb Blood Flow Metab 4:323–328

Kety SS (1950) Circulation and metabolism of the human brain in health and disease. Am J Med 8:205–217

Kety SS (1957) The general metabolism of the brain in vivo. In: Richer D (ed) The metabolism of the nervous system. Pergamon, London

Kety SS (1960) Theory of blood-tissue exchange and its application to measurement of blood flow. Meth Med Research 8:223–227

Kety SS, Schmidt CF (1945) The determination of cerebral blood flow in man by the use of nitrous oxide in low concentrations. Am J Physiol 143:53–66

Kety SS, Schmidt CF (1948) The nitrous oxide method for the quantitative determination of cerebral blood flow in man: theory, procedure and normal values. J Clin Invest 27:476–483

Keul J, Doll E, Steim H, Homburger H, Kern H, Reindell H (1965a) Über den Stoffwechsel des menschlichen Herzens. III Der oxidative Stoffwechsel des menschlichen Herzens unter verschiedenen Arbeitsbedingungen. Pflügers Arch 282:43–53

Keul J, Doll E, Steim H, Homburger K, Kern H, Reindell H (1965b) Über den Stoffwechsel des menschlichen Herzens. I Substratversorgung des gesunden Herzens in Ruhe, während und nach körperlicher Arbeit. Pflugers Arch 282:1–27

Khaw BA, Fallon JT, Katus H, Elmaleh D, Strauss HW, Locke E, Pohost GM, Haber E (1979) Positron imaging of experimental myocardial infarction with ^{68}Ga-DTPA-antimyosin antibody. Circulation [Suppl II] 60:135

Kirchner PT, Ryan J, Zalutsky M, Harper PV (1980) Positron emission tomography for the evaluation of pancreatic disease. Semin Nucl Med 10:374–391

Kirsch CM, Doliwa R, Büll U, Rödler D (1983) Detection of severe coronary heart disease with Tl-201: comparison of resting single photon emission tomography with invasive arteriography. J Nucl Med 24:761–767

Klein MD, Cohen LS, Gorlin R (1965) Krypton-85 myocardial blood flow: Precordial scintillation versus coronary sinus sampling. Am J Physiol 209:705–710

Knabb RM, Fox KAA, Bergman SR (1984) Detection of coronary stenoses by positron emission tomography with H$_2$^{15}O. Circulation 70:11340

Knabb RM, Fox KA, Sobel BE, Bergman SR (1985) Characterization of the functional significance of subcritical coronary stenoses with H$_2$^{15}O and positron-emission tomography. Circulation 71:1271–1278

Knapp WH, Vyska K (eds) (1984) Currents topics in tumor cell physiology and positron-emission tomography. Springer, Berlin Heidelberg New York Tokyo

Knapp WH, Helus F, Ostertag H, Tillmans H, Kübler W (1982) Uptake and turnover of L-(13N)-glutamate in the normal human heart and patients with coronary artery disease. Eur J Nucl Med 7:211–215

Knapp WH, Helus F, Sinn H, Ostertag H, Georgi P, Brandeis WE, Braun A (1984a) N-13-L-glutamate uptake in malignancy: Its relationship to blood flow. J Nucl Med 25:989–997

Knipping HW, Bolt W, Venrath H, Valentin H, Ludes H, Endler P (1955) Eine neue Methode zur Prüfung der Herz- und Lungenfunktion. Die regionale Funktionsanalyse in der Lungen- und Herzklinik mit Hilfe des radioaktiven Edelgases Xenon-133 (Isotopen-Thorakographie). Dtsch Med Wochenschr 80:1146–1147

Knoebel SB, Lowe DK, Lovelace DE, Friedman JJ (1978) Myocardial blood flow as measured by fractional uptake of rubidium-84 and microspheres. J Nucl Med 19:1020–1026

Knoop BO (1982) Klinische Anwendung digitaler Bildrekonstruktionsverfahren zur Quantifizierung von Profilmessungen im Ganzkörperzähler und zur nichtinvasiven Nierendurchblutungsbestimmung, Dissertation, Universität Bremen

Knust EJ, Kupfernagel Ch, Stöcklin G (1979) Longchain F-18 fatty acids for the study of regional metabolism in heart and liver; odd-even effects of metabolism in mice. J Nucl Med 20:1170–1175

Koeppe RA, Holden JE, Polcyn RE, Nickles RJ, Gutchins GD, Weese JL (1985) Quantitation of local cerebral blood flow and partition coefficient without arterial sampling: Theory and validation. J Cereb Blood Flow Metab 5:214–223

Kogure K, Busto R, Schwartzmann RJ, Scheinberg P (1980) The dissociation of cerebral blood flow, metabolism, and function in the early stages of developing cerebral infarction. Ann Neurol 8:278–290

Krivokapich J, Barrio JR, Phelps ME, Watanabe CR, Keen RE, Padgett HC, Douglas A, Shine KI (1983) Kinetic characterization of $^{13}NH_3$ and ^{13}N-glutamine metabolisnm in rabbit heart. Am J Physiol 246:H267–H273 (Heart Circ Physiol 15)

Ku D, Akera T, Pew CL, Brody TM (1974) Cardiac glycosides: Correlations among Na^+, K^+-ATPase, sodium pump and contractility in the guinea pig heart. Naunyn-Schmiedebergs Arch Pharmacol 285:185–200

Kubota K, Ito M, Fukuda H, Abe Y, Ito K, Fujiwara T, Yoshioka S, Hatazawa J, Matsuzawa T, Iwata R, Watanuki S, Ishiwata K, Ido T (1983) Cancer diagnosis with positron computed tomography and Carbon-11-labelled L-Methionine. Lancet II:1192

Kubota K, Yamada K, Fukada H, Endo S, Abe Y, Yamaguchi T, Fujiwara T, Sato, Ito K, Yshioka S, Hatazawa J, Matsuzawa T, Iwata R (1984) Tumor detection with Carbon-11-labelled amino acids. Eur J Nucl Med 9:136–140

Kubota K, Matsuzawa, Ito M, Ito K, Fujiwara, Abe Y, Yoshioka S, Fukuda H, Hatazawa J, Iwata R, Watanuki S, Ido T (1985) Lung tumoor imaging by positron emission tomography using C-11-L-Methionine. J Nucl Med 26:37–42

Kuhl DE (1984) Imaging local brain function with emission computed tomography. Radiology 150:625–631

Kuhl DE, Engel J Jr, Phelps ME, Selin C (1980a) Epileptic patterns of local cerebral metabolism and perfusion in humans determined by emission computed tomography of ^{18}FDG and $^{13}NH_3$. Ann Neurol 8:348–360

Kuhl DE, Phelps ME, Kowell AP, Metter EJ, Selin C, Winter J (1980b) Mapping local metabolism and perfusion in normal and ischemic brain by emission computed tomography of ^{18}FDG and $^{13}NH_3$. Ann Neurol 8:47–60

Kuhl DE, Phelps ME, Markham C et al (1981) Local cerebral glucose metabolism in Huntington's disease determined by emission computed tomography of ^{18}F-fluorodeoxyglucose. J Cereb Blood Flow Metab 1:S459–S460

Kuhl DE, Barrio JR, Huang SC, Selin C, Ackermann RF, Lear JL, Wu JL, Lin TH, Phelps ME (1982a) Quantifying local cerebral blood flow by N-Isopropy-p-(123-I)-Iodoamphetamine (IMP) tomography. J Nucl Med 23:196–203

Kuhl DE, Phelps ME, Markham CH, Metter EJ, Riege WH, Winter J (1982b) Cerebral metabolism and atrophy in Huntington's disease determined by ^{18}FDG and computed tomographic scans. Ann Neurol 12:425–434

Kuhl DE, Metter EJ, Riege WH et al. (1982c) Effect of human aging on patterns of local cerebral glucose utilization determined by the $[^{18}F]$fluorodeoxyglucose method. J Cereb Blood Flow Metab 2:163–171

Kuhl DE, Metter EJ, Riege WH et al (1983a) Local cerebral glucose utilization in elderly patients with depression, multiple infarct dementia and Alzheimer's disease. J Cereb Blood Flow Metab 3:S494–S495

Kuhl DE, Metter EJ, Riege WH, Phelps ME, Winter J (1983b) Local cerebral glucose utilization in Parkinson's disease. J Nucl Med 24:P21

Kuhl DE, Metter EJ, Riege WH, Markham CH (1984a) Pattern of cerebral glucose utilization in Parkinson's disease and Huntington's disease. Ann Neurol 15:S119–S125

Kuhl DE, Metter EJ, Riege WH (1984b) Patterns of cerebral glucose utilization determined in Parkinson's disease by the $[^{18}F]$fluorodeoxyglucose method. Ann Neurol 15:419–424

Kung HF, Blau M (1980) Regional intracellular pH shift: a proposed new mechanism for radiopharmaceutical uptake in brain and other tissues. J Nucl Med 21:147–152

Kung HF, Blau M (1984) A comparison of two cerebral perfusion tracers, N-Isopropyl I-123 p-iodoamphetamine and I-123 HIPDM in the human. J Nucl Med 25:945 (letter to the editor)

Kung HF, Tramposch KM, Blau M (1983) A new brain perfusing imaging agent: (I-123)HIPDM: N,N,N'-Trimethyl-N'-(2-Hydroxy-3-Methyl-5-Iodobenzyl)-1,3-Propanediamine. J Nucl Med 24:66–72

Kushner M, Alavi A, Reivich M, Dann R, Burkke A, Robinson G (1984) Contralateral cerebellar hypometabolism following cerebral insult: A positron emission tomographic study. Ann Neurol 15:425–434

LaFrance ND, Links J, Williams J, Holcomb H, Dannals R, Ravert H, Wilson A, Drew H, Herda S, Wong D, Brem H, Long D, Wagner H (1986) ^{11}C-Methionine and ^{18}F-Deoxylgucose (FDG) in the postoperative management of patients with brain tumors with positron emission tomography. J Nucl Med 27:P890

Lajtha A, Ford DH (1968) Brain barrier systems. Progr Brain Res, vol 29. Elsevier Publishing Comp., Amsterdam London New York

Lambrecht RM (1983) Radionuclide Generators. Radiochim Acta 34:9–24

Lambrecht RM, Rescigno A (1983) Tracer Kinetics and physiological modelling. Springer, Berlin Heidelberg New York Tokyo

Lambrecht RM, Rescigno A (1984) Brain blood flow measurement with bolus intravenous $H_2^{15}O$. J Nucl Med 25:729–730

Lammertsma AA, Itoh M, McKenzi CG, Jones T, Frackowiak RSJ (1981a) Quantitative tomographic measurements of regional cerebral blood flow and oxygen utilization in patients with brain tumors using oxygen-15 and positron emission tomography. J Cereb Blood Flow Metab 1:S567–S568

Lammertsma AA, Jones T, Frackowiak RSJ, Lenzi GL (1981b) A theoretical study of the steady state model for measuring regional cerebral blood flow and oxygen utilisation using oxygen-15. J Comput Assist Tomogr 5:544–550

Lammertsma AA, Frackowiak RSJ, Lenzi GL, Heather JD, Pozilli C, Jones T (1981c) Accuracy of the oxygen-15 steady state technique for measuring rCBF and $rCMRO_2$: Tracer modelling, statistics and spatial sampling. J Cereb Blood Flow Metab [Suppl I] 1:S3–S4

Lammertsma AA, Heather JD, Jones T, Frackowiak RSJ, Lenzi GL (1982) A statistical study of the steady state technique for measuring regional cerebral blood flow and oxygen utilization using ^{15}O. J Comput Assist Tomogr 6:566–573

Lammertsma AA, Jones T (1983a) Correction for the presence of intravascular oxygen-15 in the steady-state technique for measuring regional oxygen extraction ratio in the brain: 1. description of the method. J Cereb Blood Flow Metab 3:416–424

Lammertsma AA, Wise RJS, Heather JD, Gibbs JM, Leenders KL, Frackowiak RSJ, Rhodes CG, Jones T (1983b) Correction for the presence of intravascular oxygen-15 in the steady-state technique for measuring regional oxygen extaction ratio in the brain: 2. Results in normal subjects and brain tumour and stroke patients. J Cereb Blood Flow Metab 3:425–431

Lammertsma AA, Brooks DJ, Beaney RP, Turton DR, Kensett MJ, Heather JD, Marshall J, Jones T (1984a) In vivo measurements of regional cerebral haematocrit using positron emission tomography. J Cereb Blood Flow Metab 4:317–322

Lammertsma AA, Brooks DJ, Frackowiak RSJ, Heather JD, Jones T (1984b) A method to quantitate the fractional extraction of rubidium-82 across the blood-brain barrier using positron emission tomography. J Cereb Blood Flow Metab 4:523–534

Landau WM, Freygang WH, Rowland LP, Kety SS (1955) The local circulation of the living brain. Trans Am Neurol Assoc 80:125–129

Larsen OA, Lassen NA (1964) Cerebral haematocrit in normal man. J Appl Physiol 19:571–574

Larson SM, DiChiro G (1985) Comparative anatomy functional imaging of two neuroceptors and glucose metabolism: A PET study performed in the living baboon. J Comput Assist Tomogr 9:676–681

Lassen NA (1966) The luxury-perfusion syndrome and its possible relation to acute metabolic acidosis localized within the brain. Lancet 2:1113–1115

Lassen NA (1985) Cerebral blood flow tomography with Xenon-133. Semin Nucl Med 15:347–356

Lassen NA, Henriksen O (1983) Tracer studies of peripheral circulation. In: Lambrecht RM, Rescigno A (eds) Tracer kinetics physiological modeling. Springer, Berlin Heidelberg New York Tokyo, pp 235–297

Lassen NA, Perl W (1979) Tracer kinetic methods in medical physiology. Raven, New York

Lassen NA, Henriksen O, Holm S, Barry DI, Paulson OB, Vorstrup S, Poncin-Lafitte Mle, Moretti JL, Askienazy S, Raynaud C (1983) Cerebral blood-flow tomography: Xenon-133 compared with Isopropyl-amphetamine-iodine-123: Concise communication. J Nucl Med 24:17–21

Lathrop KA, Harper PV, Rich BH, Dinwood P, Krizek H, Lembares N, Gloria I (1973) Rapid incorporation of short-lived cyclotron produced radionuclides into radiopharmaceuticals. In: Radiopharmaceuticals and labelled compounds, vol 1. IAEA, Wien, pp 471–483

Lauenstein L, Meyer G-J, Sewing KF, Schober O, Hundeshagen H (1987) Uptake kinetics of ^{14}C L-Leucine and ^{14}C L- and ^{14}C D-methionine in rat brain and incorporation into protein. Neurosurg Rev (in press)

Laughlin JS, Gelbard AS, Benua RS, Reiman RE, Rosen G, Allen J, Helson L, Bigler RE, Hopfan S, Dahl JR, Lee R, Schmall B, Myers WG (1980) Report on compounds labelled with Nitrogen-13 or Carbon-11 used in cancer metabolic studies with quantitative two-dimensional scanning and PET tomography. Medical Radionuclide Imaging 1980. IAEA-SM-247/111. II:497–506

Lauter JL, Formby C, Fox P, Herscovitch P, Raichle ME (1983) Tonotopic organization in human auditory cortex as revealed by regional changes in cerebral blood flow. J Cereb Blood Flow Metab 3:S248–S249

Lavender JP, Khan RAA, Hughes SPF (1979) Blood flow and tracer uptake in normal and abnormal canine bone: Comparisons with Sr-85 Microspheres, Kr-81m, and Tc-99m MDP. J Nucl Med 20:413–418

Lavy S, Melamed E, Portnoy Z et al (1976) Interictal regional blood flow in patients with partial seizures. Neurology (Mineap) 26:418–422

Lawrence DA, Jullien P (1982) Differential uptake of 2-Fluoro-2-deoxyglucose by normal and transformed chicken and mouse fibroblasts as a function of glucose conentration. Eur J Cancer Clin Oncol 18:755–762

Lebowitz E, Greene MW, Fairchild R, Bradley-Moore PR, Atkins HL, Ansari AN, Richards P, Belgrave E (1975) Thallium-201 for medical use. J Nucl Med 16:151

Lebrun-Grandié P, Baron JC, Soussaline F, Loch'h C, Sastre J, Bousser MG (1983) Coupling between regional blood flow and oxygen utilization in the normal human brain. A study with positron tomography and oxygen-15. Arch Neurol 40:230–236

Lett JT, Idaker RE, Reimer KA (1981) Myocardial infarct size and location in relation to the coronary vascular bed at risk in man. Circulation 64:526–534

Leenders K, Wolfson L, Gibbs J, Wise R, Jones T, Legg N (1983) Regional cerebral blood flow and oxygen metabolism in Parkinson's disease and their response to L-dopa. J Cereb Blood Flow Metab 3:S488–S489

Leenders KL, Gibbs JM, Frackowiak RSJ, Lammertsma AA, Jones T (1984a) Positron emission tomography of the brain: New possibilities for the investigation of human cerebral pathophysiology. Prog Neurobiol 23:1–38

Leenders KL, Harold S, Brooks DJ, Palmer AJ, Turton D, Firnau G, Garnett ES, Nahmais C, Veall N (1984b) Pre-synaptic and post-synaptic dopaminergic system in human brain. Lancet 2:110–111

Leenders KL, Wolfson L, Gibbs JM, Wise RSJ, Causon R, Jones T, Legg NJ (1985) The effects of L-Dopa on regional cerebral blood flow and oxygen metabolism in patients with Parkinson's disease. Brain 108:171–191

Lehninger AL (1970) Biochemistry. Worth Publ Inc, New York

Lenzi GL, Jones T, McKenzie CG et al (1978a) Study of regional cerebral metabolism and blood flow relationship in man using the method of continuously inhaling oxygen-15 and oxygen-15 labeled carbon dioxide. J Neurol Neurosurg Psychiatry 41:1–10

Lenzi GL, Jones T, McKenzie CG, et al. (1978b) Non-invasive regional study of chronic cerebrovascular disorders using the oxygen-15 inhalation technique. J Neurol Neurosurg Psychiatry 41:11–17

Lenzi GT, Jones T, Reidl JL, Moss S (1979) Regional impairment of cerebral oxidative metabolism in Parkinson's disease. J Neurol Neurosurg Psychiatry 22:59–62

Lenzi GL, Frackowiak RSJ, Jones T et al (1981a) $CMRO_2$ and CBF by the oxygen-15 inhalation techniques: Results in normal volunteers and cerebrovascular patients. Eur Neurol 20:285–290

Lenzi GL, Frackowiak RSJ, Jones T (1981b) Regional cerebral blood flow (CBF), oxygen utilization ($CMRO_2$) and oxygen extraction ratio (OER) in acute hemispheric stroke. J Cereb Blood Flow Metab 1:S504–S505

Lenzi GL, Frackowiak RSJ, Jones T (1982) Cerebral oxygen metabolism and blood flow in human cerebral ischemic infarction. J Cereb Blood Flow Metab 2:321–335

Leon MJ de, George AE (1983) Computed tomography in aging and senile dementia of the Alzheimer type. In: Mayeux R, Rosèn WG (eds) Advances in neurology, vol 38. The dementias. Raven, New York, pp 103–122

Leon MJ de, George A, Ferris SH, Rosenbloom S, Christman DR, Gentes CI, Reisberg B, Kricheff II, Wolf AP (1983a) Regional correlation of PET and CT in senile dementia of the Alzheimer's type. AJNR 4:553–556

Leon MJ de, Ferris SH, George A, Christman DR, Fowler JS, Gentes C, Reisberg B, Gee B, Emmerich M, Yonekura Y, Brodie J, Kricheff II, Wolf AP (1983b) Positron emission tomographic studies of aging and Alzheimer's disease. AJNR 4:568–571

Leon MJ de, Ferris SH, George A, Reisberg G, Christman DR, Kricheff II, Wolf AP (1983c) Computed tomography and positron emission transaxial tomography evaluation of normal aging and Alzheimer's disease. J Cereb Blood Flow Metab 3:391–394

Leon MJ de, George AE, Ferris SH, Christman DR, Fowler JS, Gentes CI, Brodie J, Reisberg B, Wolf AP (1984a) Positron emission tomography and computed tomography assessments of the aging human brain. J Comput Assist Tomogr 8:88–94

Leon MJ de, George AE, Ferris SH, Rosenbloom S, Christman DR, Gentes CI, Reisberg B, Kricheff II, Wolf AP (1984b) Regional correlation of PET and CT in senile dementia of the Alzheimer type. AJNR 4:553–556

Lerch RA, Ambos HD, Bergmann SR, Ter-Pogossian MM, Sobel BE (1981) Nuclear cardiology-detection and quantitation of myocardial ischemia. Am J Cardiol 47:481

Lerch RA, Bergmann SR, Ambos HD, Welch MJ, Ter-Pogossian MM, Sobel BE (1982) Effect of flow-independent reduction of metabolism on regional myocardial clearence of 11-C-Palmitate. Circulation 65:731–738

Lewis FR, Elings VB, Hill SL, Christensen JM (1982) The measurement of extravascular lung water by thermal-green dye indicator dilution. Ann NY Acad Sci 80:394–410

Lichtlen PR (1979) Koronarangiographie. Straube Perimed, Erlangen

Lichtlen PR, Engel HJ, Hundeshagen H (1985) Assessment of regional myocardial blood flow using invasive techniques, especially the precordial Xenon clearence technique. In: Hundeshagen H (ed) Diagnostik II, Pädiatrische Nuklearmedizin, Teil 3. Springer, Berlin Heidelberg New York Tokyo (Handbuch der medizinischen Radiologie, Bd XV/3, S 65–111)

Lifton JF, Welch MJ (1971) Preparation of glucose labeled with 20 min halflived Carbon-11. Radiat Res 45:35–40

Lilja A, Bergström K, Hartvig P, Spännare B, Halldin C, Lundquist H, Langstrom B (1985) Dynamic study of supratentorial gliomas with L-methyl-11-C-Methionine and positron emission tomography. AJNR 6:505–514

Lisi de, Holcomb HH, Cohen RM, Pickar D, Carpenter W, Morihisa JM, King AC, Kessler R, Buchsbaum MS (1985) Positron emission tomography in schizophrenic patients with and without neuroleptic medication. J Cereb Blood Flow Metab 5:201–206

Livni E, Elmaleh DR, Levy S, Brownell GL, Strauss WH (1982) Beta-methyl[1-^{11}C]heptadecanoic acid: a new myocardial metabolic tracer for positron emission tomography. J Nucl Med 23:169–175

Lockwood AH, Finn RD (1982) ^{11}C-carbon dioxide fixation and equilibration in rat brain: effects on acid base measurements. Neurology (NY) 32:451–454

Lockwood AH, McDonald JM, Reiman RE, Gelbard AS, Laughlin JS, Duffy TE, Plum F (1979) The dynamics of ammonia metabolism in man: Effects of liver disease and hyperammonemia. J Clin Invest 63:449–460

Lockwood AH, Finn RD, Campbell JA (1980) Factors that effect the uptake of N-13 ammonia by the brain: The blood-brain pH gradient. Brain Res 181:259–266

Lockwood AH, Bolomey L, Napoleon F (1984) Blood-brain barrier to ammonia in humans. J Cereb Blood Flow Metab 4:516–522

Loiseau E, Strube E, Broustet D, Bettolechi S, Gomeni C, Morselli PL (1983) Learning impairment of epileptic patients. Epilepsia 24:183–192

Love WD, Burch GE (1959) Influence of the rate of coronary plasma flow on the extraction of ^{86}Rb from coronary blood. Circ Res 7:24–30

Lundqvist H, Stalnacke C-G, Langström B, Jones B (1985) Labeled metabolites in plasma after intravenous administration of [^{11}CH$_3$]-L-Methionine. In: Greitz T, Ingvar DH, Wiedén L (eds) The metabolism of the human brain studied with positron emission tomography. Raven, New York, pp 233–240

Mabe H, Blomquist P, Siesjö BK (1983) Intracellular pH in the brain following transient ischemia. J Cereb Blood Flow Metab 3:109–114

MacCarther CGC, Rhodes CG, Swinburne AJ, Heather JD, Hughes (1980) Measurement of regional lung water using gamma-emitting tracers. Bull Europ Physiopathol Respir 16:321–333

Machulla HJ, Stöcklin G, Kupfernagel CH, Freundlieb CH, Höck A, Vyska K, Feinendegen LE (1978) Comparative evaluation of fatty acids with C-11, Cl-34m, Br-77, I-123, for metabolic studies of the myocardium: concise communication. J Nucl Med 19:298–302

Madsen MT, Hichwa RD, Nickles RJ (1981) An investigation of 11-C-Methane, 13-N-nitrous oxide and 11-C-Acetylene as regional cerebral blood flow agents. Phys Med Biol 26:875–882

Malsky PM, Vokonas PS, Paul SJ, Robbins SL, Hood WB Jr (1977) Autoradiographic measurement of regional blood flow in normal and ischemic myocardium. Am J Physiol [Suppl]:232 H576–H583

Mansi L, Dalakas MC, DiChiro G, Sever JL, Patronas N, Bairamian D, Brooks RA, Jones AE (1983) Evaluation of cerebral glucose metabolism in patients with amyotrophic lateral sclerosis (ALS) by [^{18}F]-fluorodeoxyglucose (FDG) and positron emission tomography (PET). J Nucl Med 24:P21

Markland ON (1977) Slow spike-wave activity in EEG, and associated clinical features: Often called 'Lennox' or 'Lennox-Gastaut' syndrome. Neurology 27:746–757

Marshall RC, Schelbert HR, Phelps ME, Tillisch JH, Henze E, Huang SC (1981) Evaluation of infarcted and ischemic myocardium with ^{18}Fluorodeoxyglucose, ^{13}NH$_3$, and positron computed tomography. Am J Cardiol 47:481

Marshall RC, Huang SC, Nash WW, Phelps ME (1983a) Investigation of the 18-fluorodeoxyglucose tracer kinetic model to accurately measure the myocardial metabolic rate for glucose during ischemia: Preliminary notes. J Nucl Med 24:1060–1064

Marshall RC, Tillisch JH, Phelps ME, Huang SC, Carson R, Henze E, Schelbert HR (1983b) Identification and differentiation of resting myocardial ischemia and infarction in man with positron computed tomography, ^{18}F-labeled fluorodeoxyglucose and ^{13}N-ammonia. Circulation 67:766–778

Martin WR, Raichle ME (1983a) Cerebellar metabolism and blood flow in supratentorial cerebral infarction. J Cereb Blood Flow Metab 3:S584–S585

Martin WR, Raichle ME (1983b) Cerebellar blood flow and metabolism in cerebral hemisphere infarction. Ann Neurol 14:168–176

Mazière B, Comar D, Godot JM, Collard PH, Cepeda C, Naquet R (1981) In vivo characterization of myocardium muscarinic receptors by positron emission tomography. Life Sci 29:2391–2397

Mazière B, Loc'h C, Hantraye P, Guillon R, Duquesnoy N, Soussaline F, Naquet R, Comar D, Mazière M (1984) 76-Br-Bromospiroperidol: A new tool for quantitative In-vivo imaging of neuroleptic receptors. Life Sci 35:1349–1356

Mazziotta JC, Engel J Jr (1984) The use and impact of positron computed tomography scanning in epilepsy. Epilepsia 25:S86–S104

Mazziotta JC, Phelps ME (1984) Human sensory stimulation and deprivation: positron emission tomographic results and strategies. Ann Neurol 15:S50–S60

Mazziotta JC, Phelps ME (1986) Positron emission tomography studies of the brain. In: Phelps ME, Mazziotta JC, Schelbert HR (eds) Raven, New York, pp 493–580

Mazziotta JC, Phelps ME, Miller J, Kuhl DE (1981) Tomographic mapping of human cerebral metabolism: Normal unstimulated state. Neurology (NY) 31:503–515

Mazziotta JC, Phelps ME, Carson RE, Kuhl DE (1982a) Tomographic mapping of human cerebral metabolism: sensory deprivation. Ann Neurol 12:435–444

Mazziotta JC, Phelps ME, Carson RE, Kuhl DE (1982b) Tomographic mapping of human cerebral metabolism: auditory stimulation. Neurology (NY) 32:921–937

Mazziotta JC, Phelps ME, Halgren E (1983a) Local cerebral glucose metabolic responses to audiovisual stimulation and deprivation: Studies in human subjects with positron CT. Hum Neurobiol 2:11–23

Mazziotta JC, Phelps ME, Halgren E et al. (1983b) Hemispheric lateralization and local cerebral metabolic and blood flow response to physiologic stimuli. J Cereb Blood Flow Metab 3:S246–S247

Mazziotta JC, Phelps ME, Carson RE (1984) Tomographic mapping of human cerebral metabolism: Subcortical responses to auditory and visual stimulation. Neurology 34:825–828

Mazziotta JC, Wapenski JA, Phelps ME, Riege W, Baxter LR, Fullerton A, Kuhl De, Selin C, Sumida R (1985a) Cerebral glucose metabolism and blood flow in Huntington's disease: Symptomatic and at-risk subjects. J Cereb Blood Flow Metab (im Druck)

Mazziotta JC, Huang SC, Phelps ME, Carson RE, MacDonald NS, Mahoney K (1985b) A noninvasive positron computed tomography technique using oxygen-15-labeled water for the evaluation of neurobehavioral task batteries. J Cereb Blood Flow Metab 5:70–78

Megnan M, Simonneau G, Oliveira L, Harf A, Cinotti L, Cavellier J-F, Duroux P, Ansquer J-C, Galle P (1984) Computation of ventilation-perfusion ratio with Kr-81m in pulmonary embolism. J Nucl Med 25:149–155

Mehdorn HM, Vyska K, Machulla HJ, Knust EJ (1985) Use of 3-fluoro-deoxyglucose for the assessment of cerebral perfusion and glucose transport. II. Evaluation of patients undergoing EC-IC bypass surgery. Neurol Res 7:68–74

Meier P, Zierler KL (1954) On the theory of the indicator dilution method for measurement of blood flow and volume. J Appl Physiol 12:731–744

Merlis JK (1970) Proposal for an international classification of the epilepsies. Epilepsia 11:114–119

Metter EJ, Riege WH, Hanson WH et al (1981) Correlation of metabolic and language abnormalities in aphasia. Ann Neurol 10:102

Metter EJ, Mazziotta JC, Itobashi H et al (1983a) Pathological comparisons to FDG positron computed tomography in stroke: A case study. Neurology (NY) 33:115

Metter EJ, Riege WH, Hanson WR, Kuhl DE, Phelps ME, Squile LR, Wasterlain CG, Benson DF (1983b) Comparison of metabolic rates, language and memory in subcortical aphasia. Brain Lang 19:33–47

Metter EJ, Riege WH, Kuhl DE, Phelps ME (1984) Cerebral metabolic relationship for selected brain regions in healthy adults. J Cereb Blood Flow Metab 4:1–7

Metter EJ, Mazziotta JC, Itabashi HH, Mankovich NJ, Phelps ME, Kuhl DE (1985) Comparison of glucose metabolism, x-ray CT, and postmortem data in a patient with multiple cerebral infarcts. Neurology 35:1695–1701

Meyer E, Yamamoto YL (1984) The requirement for constant arterial radioactivity in the $C^{15}O_2$ steady-state blood flow model. J Nucl Med 25:455–460

Meyer GJ, Hundeshagen H (1982) An effective method for the preparation of O-15 labeled carboxyhemoglobin. In: Schmidt HAE, Rösler H (Hrsg) Nuklearmedizin. Schattauer, Stuttgart New York, S 340–343

Meyer GJ, Schober O, Gielow P, Hundeshagen H (1982) Functional imaging of the pancreas by positron emission tomography: routine production of C-11-L-methionine, quality control, methodology. In: Raynaud C (ed) Proc Third World Congr Nucl Med Biol. Pergamon, Paris, pp 1977–1980

Meyer GJ, Schober O, Hundeshagen H (1983) Konstante Infusion von O-15-markiertem Wasser und Inhalation von C-11-markiertem Kohlenmonoxid als methodische Grundlage zur regionalen Bestimmung des Lungenwassers mittels Positronen-Emissionstomographie. Nucl Med 22:121–127

Meyer GJ, Schober O, Bossaller C, Hundeshagen H (1984) Quantification of regional extravascular lung water in dogs with positron emission tomography, using constant infusion of O-15-labeled water. Eur J Nucl Med 9:220–228

Meyer GJ, Schober O, Hundeshagen H (1985a) Gradient effects in extravascular water determination using 15-O-labelled water under steady state conditions: Theory and error sensitivity. Eur J Nucl Med 10:77–80

Meyer GJ, Schober O, Hundeshagen H (1985b) Uptake of C-11-L- and D-methionine in brain tumors. Eur J Nucl Med 10:373–376

Mies G, Paschen W, Hossmann KA (1983) Discrepancy between glucose availability and calculated glucose consumption during acute brain ischemia. In: Heiss WD, Phelps ME (eds) Positron emission tomography of the brain. Springer, Berlin Heidelberg New York Tokyo, pp 232–233

Mintun MA, Raichle ME, Kilbourn MR, Wooten GF, Welch MJ (1984a) A quantitative model for the In vivo assessment of drug binding sites with positron emission tomography. Ann Neurol 15:217–227

Mintun MA, Raichle ME, Martin WRW, Herscovitch P (1984b) Brain oxygen utilization measured with O-15 radiotracers and positron emission tomography. J Nucl Med 25:177–187

Modell HI, Graham MM (1982) Limitations of Kr-81m for quantitation of ventilation scans. J Nucl Med 23:301–305

Moerlein SM, Welch MJ (1981) The chemistry of gallium and indium as related to radiopharmaceutical production. Int J Nucl Med Biol 8:277–287

Monakow C von (1914) Die Lokalisation im Großhirn und der Abbau der Funktion durch kortikale Herde. Bergmann, Wiesbaden

Morgan CG, Rellas JS, Corbett JR, Kulkarni P, Devous MD, Parkey RW, Willerson JT, Lewis SE (1983) Quantitative tomographic imaging evaluation of myocardial clearance of I-123 phenyl pentadecanic acid in acute myocardial infarction. J Am Coll Cardiol 1:577

Most AS, Brachfield N, Gorlin R, Wahren J (1969) Free fatty acid metabolism of the human heart at rest. J Clin Invest 48:1177–1188

Müller St, Creutzig H, Hundeshagen H (1983) Vergleich der parametrischen Ventilationsszintigraphie mit Kr-81m und Xe-133. Nuklearmediziner 4(6):479–490

Mullani NA (1983) Myocardial perfusion with rubidium-82. III. Theory relating severity of coronary stenosis to perfusion deficit. J Nucl Med 25:1190–1196

Mullani NA, Gould KL (1983) First pass regional blood flow measurement with external detectors. J Nucl Med 24:577–581

Mullani NA, Goldstein RA, Gould KL, Marani SK, Fisher DJ, O'Brien HAA Jr, Loberg MD (1983) Perfusion imaging with rubidium-82: I. Measurement of extraction and flow with external detectors. J Nucl Med 24:898–906

Myers WG (1973) Radiopotassium-38 for in vivo studies of dynamic processes. J Nucl Med 14:359–360

Myers WG, Bigler RE, Buena RS, Graham MC (1983) PET tomographic imaging of the human heart, pancreas, and liver with nitrogen-13 derived from [^{13}N]-L-glutamate. Eur J Nucl Med 8:381–384

Myers WG, Bigler RE, Graham MC (1984) PET tomography in studies of distributions of 7.6-min potassium 38 in the dog heart. Eur J Nucl Med 9:272–277

Nahmias C, Garnett ES, Firnau G, Lang A (1985) Striatal dopamine distribution in parkinsonian patients during life. J Neurol Sci 69:223–230

Neely JR, Rovetto MJ, Oram JF (1972) Myocardial utilization of carbohydrate and lipids. Prog Cardiovasc Dis 15:289–329

Nelson T, Kaufman EE, Sokoloff L (1984) 2-Deoxyglucose incorporation into rat brain glycogen during measurement of local cerebral glucose utilization by the 2-Deoxyglucose method. J Neurochem 43:949–956

Neundörfer B (1986) Die Bedeutung nicht-invasiver, technischer Untersuchungsverfahren in der Diagnostik der Tumorepilepsie. Lebensversicherungsmedizin 38:22–25

Nieweg OE, Piers DA, Beekhuis H, Paans AMJ, Welleweerd J, Vaalburg W, Woldring MG (1981) Co-55-bleomycin in the detection of lung cancer and brain metastases. J Nucl Med 22:P50

Nieweg OE, Beekhuis H, Paans AMJ, Pier DA, Vaalburg W, Welleweerd J (1982) Detection of lung cancer with 55-Co-bleomycin using a positron camera. A comparison with 57-Co-Bleomycin and 55-Co-bleomycin single photon scintigraphy. Eur J Nucl Med 7:104–107

Nowotnik DP, Canning LR, Cumming SA, Harrison RC, Highley B, Nechvatal G, Pickett RD, Piper JM, Bayne VJ, Forster AM, Weisner PS, Neirinckx RD (1985) Development of a ^{99m}Tc-labelled radiopharmaceutical for cerebral blood flow imaging. Nucl Med Comm 6:499–506

Okada Rd, Elmaleh D, Werre GS, Strauss HW (1983) Myocardial kinetics of ^{123}I-labeled hexadecanoic acid. Eur J Nucl Med 8:211–217

Oldendorf WH (1971) Brain uptake of radiolabeled amino acids, amines, and hexoses after arterial injection. Am J Physiol 221:1629–1638

Oldendorf WH (1973a) Stereospecifity of blood brain barrier permeability to amino acids. Am J Physiol 224:967–969

Oldendorf WH (1973b) Carrier mediated blood brain

barrier transport of short chain monocarboxylic organic acids. Am J Physiol 224:1450–1453

Oldendorf WH (1981) Clearance of radiolabeled substances by brain after artial injection using a diffusible internal standard. In: Marks N, Rodnight R (eds) Research methods in neurochemistry. Plenum, New York, pp 91–112

Oldendorf WH, Szabo J (1976) Amino acid assignment to one of three blood brain barrier amino acid carriers. Am J Physiol 230:94–98

Oldendorf WH, Kitano M, Shimizu S, Oldendorf SZ (1965) Hematocrit of the human cranial blood pool. Circ Res 17:532–539

Opie LH (1976) Effects of regional ischemia on metabolism of glucose and fatty acids. Circ Res 38:152–174

Opie LH (1979) Role of carnitine in fatty acid metabolism of normal and ischemic myocardium. Am Heart J 97:375–388

Opie LH, Owens P, Riemersma RA (1973) Relative rates of oxidation of glucose and free fatty acids by ischemic and non-ischemic myocardium after coronary artery ligation in the dog. Eur J Clin Invest 3:419–435

Orr JS (1979) Continuous administration of short-lived radioisotope tracers and the analogous laplace transform. J Theor Biol 78:101–111

Pang JA, Burtland RJA, Brooks N, Catell M, Geddes DM (1982) Impaired lung uptake of propanolol in human pulmonary emphysema. Am Rev Respir Dis 125:194–198

Pantano P, Baron JC, Lebrun-Grandié, Duquesnoy N, Bousser MG, Comar D (1984) Regional cerebral blood flow and oxygen consumption in human aging. Stroke 15:635–641

Pantano P, Baron JC, Crouzel C, Collard P, Sirou P, Samson Y (1985) The ^{15}O continuous inhalation method: Correction for intravascular signal using ^{15}O $-$ CO. Eur J Nucl Med 10:387–391

Pardridge WM (1983) Brain metabolism: A perspective from the blood brain barrier. Phys Rev 63:1481–1534

Pardridge WM, Oldendorf WH (1975) Kinetics of blood brain barrier transport of hexoses. Biochem Biophys Acta 382:377–382

Park CR, Crofford OB, Kono T (1968) Mediated (non-active) transport of glucose in mammalian cells and its regulation. J Gen Physiol 52:296S–318S

Parker JA, Beller BA, Hoop B, Holman BL, Smith TW (1978) Assessment of regional myocardial blood flow and regional fractional oxygen extraction in dogs, using ^{15}O-water and ^{15}O-hemoglobin. Circ Res 42:511–518

Parodi O, Schelbert HR, Schwaiger M, Hanssen H, Selin C, Hoffman EJ (1984a) Cardiac emission computed tomography: Understimation of regional tracer concentrations due to wall motion abnormalities. J Comput Assist Tomogr 8:1083–1092

Parodi O, Schwaiger M, Krivokapich J, Schelbert HR (1984b) Regional myocardial blood flow and wall motion study in patients with designated acute "subendocardial infarction". J Am Coll Cardiol 3:574

Pascal O, Syrota A, Berger G, Soussaline F, Huchon GJ, Grandory B, Marsac J (1982) In vivo uptake of C-11-labeled amines by human lung. In: Raynaud (ed) Nuclear Medicine and Biology. Proceedings of the Third World Congress of Nuclear Medicine and Biology. Pergamon, Paris, pp 2558–2561

Patronas NJ, Di Chiro G, Brooks RA, DeLaPaz RL, Kornblith PL, Smith LH, Rizzoli HV, Kessler RM, Manning RG, Channing M, Wolf AP, O'Connor CM (1982) (^{18}F)Fluorodeoxyglucose and positron emission tomography in the evaluation of radiation necrosis of the brain. Radiology 144:885–889

Patronas NJ, Di Chiro G, Smith BH, DeLaPaz RL, Brooks RA, Milam HL, Kornblith PL, Bairamian D, Mansi L (1984) Depressed cerebellar glucose metabolism in supratentorial tumors. Brain Research 291:93–101

Patronas NJ, Di Chiro G, Kufta C, Bairamian D, Kornblith DL, Simon R, Larson SM (1985) Prediction of survival in glioma patients by means of positron emission tomography. J Neurosurg 62:816–822

Paul R, Ahonen A, Roeda D, Nordman E (1985) Imaging of hepatoma with ^{18}F-fluorodeoxyglucose. Lancet I:50–51

Perl W, Effros RM, Chinard FP (1969) Indicator equivalence theorem for input rates and regional masses in multi-inlet steady-state systems with partially labeled input. J Theoret Biol 25:297–316

Perl W, Lassen NA, Effros RM (1975) Matrix proof of flow, volume and mean transit time theorems for regional and compartmental systems. Bull Math Biol 37:573–588

Perlman JM, Herscovitch P, Kreusser KL, Raichle ME, Volpe JJ (1985) Positron emission tomography in the newborn: effect of seizure on regional cerebral blood flow in an asphyxiated infant. Neurology 35:244–247

Perlmutter JS, Raichle ME (1984) Pure hemidystonia with basal ganglion abnormalities on positron emission tomography. Ann Neurol 15:228–233

Perlmutter JS, Raichle ME (1985) Regional blood flow in hemiparkinsonism. Neurology 35:1127–1134

Perloff JK, DeLeon AC Jr, Doherty D (1966) The cardiomyopathy of progressive muscular dystrophy. Circulation 69:33–42

Perloff JK, Henze E, Schelbert HR (1984) Alterations in myocardial metabolism, perfusion and wall motion in Duchenne's muscular dystrophy studied by radionuclide imaging. Circulation 69:33–42

Pettigrew KE, Sokoloff L, Patlak CS (1983) A theoretical derivation of the lumped constant for the 2-deoxyglucose method for measuring local glucose metabolism in the brain. J Cereb Blood Flow Metab [Suppl 1] 3:89–90

Phelps ME, Hoffman EJ, Coleman RE, Welch MJ, Raichle ME, Weiss ES, Sobel BE, Ter-Pogossian MM (1976) Tomographic images of blood pool and perfusion in brain and heart. J Nucl Med 17:603–612

Phelps ME, Hoffman EJ, Raybaud C (1977) Factors which affect cerebral uptake and retention of 13-NH_3. Stroke 8:694–702

Phelps ME, Hoffman EJ, Selin CE, Huang SC, Robinson G, MacDonald N, Schelbert HR, Kuhl DE (1978) Investigation of $[^{18}F]$2-fluoro-2-deoxy-D-glucose for the measure of myocardial glucose metabolism. J Nucl Med 19:1311–1319

Phelps ME, Huang SC, Hoffman EJ, Kuhl DE (1979a) Validation of tomographic measurement of cerebral blood volume with C-11-labelled Carboxyhemoglobin. J Nucl Med 20:328–334

Phelps ME, Huang SC, Hoffman EJ, Selin C, Sokoloff L, Kuhl DE (1979b) Tomographic measurement of local cerebral glucose metabolic rate in humans with (F-18)2-Fluoro-2-deoxy-D-glucose: validation of method. Ann Neurol 6:371–388

Phelps ME, Huang SC, Hoffman EJ, Selin C, Kuhl DE (1981a) Cerebral extraction of N-13 ammonia: Its dependence on cerebral blood flow and capillary permeability-surface area product. Stroke 12:607–619

Phelps ME, Mazziotta JC, Kuhl DE et al. (1981b) Tomographic mapping of human cerebral metabolism: visual stimulation and deprivation. Neurology (NY) 31:113–162

Phelps ME (1981c) Positron computed tomography studies of cerebral glucose metabolism in man. Theory and application in nuclear medicine. Semin Nucl Med 11:32–49

Phelps ME, Mazziotta JC, Huang SC (1982) Study of cerebral function with positron computed tomography. J Cereb Blood Flow Metab 2:113–162

Phelps ME, Huang SC, Mazziotta JC, Hawkins RA (1983) Alternate approach for examining stability of the deoxyglucose model lumped constant. J Cereb Blood Flow Metab 3:S13–S14

Phelps ME, Barrio JR, Huang SC, Keen RE, Chugani H, Mazziotta JC (1984) Criteria for the tracer kinetic measurement of cerebral protein synthesis in humans with positron emission tomography. Ann Neurol 15:S192–S202

Phelps ME, Mazziotta JE, Baxter L, Gerner R (1985a) Study design in the investigation of affective disorders: Problems and strategies: Greitz T, Ingvar DH, Widén L (eds) The metabolism of the human brain studied with positron emission tomography. Raven, New York, pp 457–470

Phelps ME, Barrio JR, Huang SC, Keen RE, Chugani H, Mazziotta JC (1985b) Measurement of cerebral protein synthesis in man with positron emission tomography: Model, assumptions, and preliminary results. In: Greitz T, Ingvar DH, Wiedén L (eds) The metabolism of the human brain studied with positron emission tomography. Raven, New York, pp 215–323

Phelps ME, Mazziotta JC, Schelbert HR (eds) (1986) Positron emission tomography and autoradiography. Raven, New York

Pike VW, Eakins MN, Allan TM, Selwyn AP (1982) Preparation of $[1-^{11}C]$acetate-an agent for the study of myocardial metabolism by positron emission tomography. Int J Appl Radiat Isot 33:505–512

Pistolesi M, Giuntini C (1978) Assessment of extravascular lung water. Radiol Clin North Am 16:551–574

Pistolesi M, Miniati M, Ravelli V (1982) Injury versus hydrostatic lung edema: Detection by chest X-ray. Ann NY Acad Sci 80:364–380

Pistolesi M, Miniati M, Ghelarducci L, Mazzuca N, Giuntini C, Taccini E, Renzoni G, Pellegrini N, Gilardi MC, Gerundini P, Fazio F (1985) Lung release of HIPDM: A new index of lung dysfunction for clinical and experimental studies. J Nucl Med 26:P14

Poe ND (1972) Comparative myocardial uptake and clearance characteristics of potassium and cesium. J Nucl Med 13:557–560

Poe ND, Robinson GD Jr, Graham LS, MacDonald NS (1976) Experimental basis for myocardial imaging with ^{123}I-labeled hexadecanoic acid. J Nucl Med 17:1077–1082

Poe ND, Robinson GD Jr, Zielinski FW, Cabeen WR Jr, Smith JW, Gomes AS (1977) Myocardial imaging with 123I-hexadecanoic acid. Radiology 124:419–424

Powers WJ, Raichle ME (1985) Positron emission tomography and its application to the study of cerebrovascular disease in man. Stroke 16:361–367

Powers WJ, Martin WR, Herscovitch P et al (1983) The value of regional cerebral blood volume measurements in the diagnosis of cerebral ischemia. J Cereb Blood Flow Metab 3:S598–S599

Powers WJ, Martin WR, Herscovitch P, Raichle ME, Grubb RL (1984) Extracranial-intracranial bypass surgery: Hemodynamic and metabolic effects. Neurology 34:1168–1174

Powers WJ, Grubb RL Jr, Baker RP, Mintun MA, Raichle ME (1985a) Regional cerebral blood flow and metabolism in reversible ischemia due to vasospasm. Determination by positron emission tomography. J Neurosurg 62:539–546

Powers WJ, Grubb RL Jr, Darriet D, Raichle ME (1985b) Cerebral blood flow and cerebral metabolic rate of oxygen requirements for cerebral function and viability in humans. J Cereb Blood Flow Metab 600–608

Prinzmetal M, Corday E, Bergman HC, Schwartz L, Spritzler RJ (1948) Radiocardiography: a new method for studying the blood flow through the chambers of the heart in human beings. Science 108:340

Raets D, DelFiore G, Quaglia L, Peters JM, Lamotte D, deLandsheere C, Rigo P (1984) Positive visualization of myocardial ischemia using 11C acetate. An experimental study. Eur Heart J 5:328

Raichle ME (1980) Positron emission tomography: A new technology of importance in the study of patients with subarachnoidal hemorrhage. In: Wilkins RH (ed) Cerebral arterial spasm. Williams & Wilkins, Baltimore, 338–350

Raichle ME (1983) The pathophysiology of brain ischemia. Ann Neurol 13:2–10

Raichle ME (1985) Measurement of local brain blood flow and oxygen utilization using ^{15}O-radiopharmaceuticals: A rapid dynamic imaging approach. In: Reivich M, Alavi A (eds) Positron emission tomography. Liss, New York, pp 241–247

Raichle ME, Larson KB, Phelps ME, Grubb RL, Welch MJ, Ter-Pogossian MM (1975) In vivo measurement of brain glucose transport and metabolism employing glucose-^{11}C. Am J Physiol 228:1936–1948

Raichle ME, Eichling JO, Straatman MG, Welch MJ, Larson KB, Ter-Pogossian MM (1976) Blood brain barrier permeability of C-11-labeled alcohols and O-15 labeled water. Am J Physiol 230:543–552

Raichle ME, Welch MJ, Grubb RL Jr, Higgins CS, Ter-Pogossian MM, Larson KB (1978) Measurement of regional substrate utilization rates by emission tomography. Science 199:986–987

Raichle ME, Grubb RL, Higgins CS (1979) Measurement of brain tissue carbon dioxide content in vivo by emission tomography. Brain Res 166:413–417

Raichle ME, Martin WRW, Herscowitch P, Kilbourn M, Welch MJ (1983a) Measurement of cerebral blood flow with ^{11}C-Butanol and PET. J Nucl Med 24:P63

Raichle ME, Martin WRW, Herscovitch P, Mintun MA, Markham J (1983b) Brain blood flow measured with intravenous $H_2^{15}O$. II. Implementation and validation. J Nucl Med 24:790–798

Ramos M, Rösler H (1978) Untersuchungen zu Lungen-Perfusion und -Ventilation mit radioaktiven Edelgasen. In: Hundeshagen H (Hrsg) Diagnostik Therapie, Klinische Forschung, Teil 2. Springer, Berlin Heidelberg New York (Handbuch der medizinischen Radiologie, Bd XV/2, S 265–334)

Rapoport SI (1976) Blood-brain barrier in physiology and medicine. Raven, New York

Rapoport SI, Duara R, Horwitz B, Kessler RM, Sokoloff L, Ingvar DH (1983) Brain aging in 40 healthy mean: rCMRGlc and correlated functional activity in various brain regions in the resting stage. J Cereb Blood Flow Metab 3:484–485

Ratib O, Phelps ME, Huang S-C, Henze E, Selin

CE, Schelbert HR (1982) Positron tomography with Deoxyglucose for estimating local myocardial glucose metabolism. J Nucl Med 23:577–586

Reiman EM, Raichle ME, Butler FK, Herscovitch P, Robins E (1984) A focal brain abnormality in panic disorder, a severe form of anxiety. Nature 310:683–685

Reiman RE, Huvos AG, Buena RS, Rosen G, Gelbard AS, Laughlin JS (1981) Quotient imaging with N-13 L-glutamate in osteogenic sarcoma: Correlation with tumor viability. Cancer 48:1976–1981

Reiman RE, Buena RS, Gelbard AS, Allen JC, Vomero JJ, Laughlin JS (1982a) Imaging of brain tumors after administration of L-(N-13)Glutamate: concise communination. J Nucl Med 23:682–687

Reiman RE, Rosen G, Gelbard AS, Buena RS, Laughlin JS (1982b) Imaging of primary ewing sarcoma with 13-N-L-Glutamate. Radiology 142:495–500

Reimer KA, Lowe JE, Rassmussen MM, Jennings RB (1977) The wavefront phenomenon of ischemic cell death. I. Myocardial infarct size vs duration of coronary occlusion in dogs. Circulation 56:786–794

Reivich M, Kuhl DE, Wolf A, Greenberg J, Phelps ME, Ido T, Casela V, Hoffman E, Alavi A, Sokoloff L (1979) The [18F]fluorodeoxyglucose method for the measurement of local cerebral glucose utilization in man. Circ Res 44:127–137

Reivich M, Cobbs W, Rosenquist A, Stein A, Schatz N, Savino P, Alavi A, Greenberg J (1981) Abnormalities in local cerebral glucose metabolism in patients with visual field defects. J Cereb Blood Flow Metab 1:471–472

Reivich M, Gur R, Alavi A (1983) Positron emission tomographic studies of sensory stimuli, cognitive processes and anxiety. Hum Neurobiol 2:25–33

Reivich M (1985) Cerebral glucose consumption: Methodology and validation. In: Reivich M, Alavi A (eds) Positron emission tomography. Liss, New York, pp 131–151

Reivich M, Gur R (1985a) Cerebral metabolic effects of sensory and cognitive stimuli in normal subjects. In: Reivich M, Alavi A (eds) Positron emission tomography. Liss, New York, pp 329–344

Reivich M, Alavi A, Breenberg J, Wolf A (1985b) Use of ^{18}F-Fluorodeoxyglucose and ^{11}C-Deoxyglucose for the determination of local cerebral glucose consumption in humans. In: Greitz T, Ingvar DH, Wiedén L (eds) The metabolism of the human brain studied with positron emission tomography. Raven, New York, pp 149–157

Renkin EM (1959) Transport of potassium-42 from blood to tissue in isolated mammalian skeletal muscle. Am J Physiol 197:1205–1210

Rescigno A, Segre G (1966) Drug and tracer kinetics. Blaisdell, Woltham/Mass

Reske SN, Sauer W, Machulla HJ, Knust J, Winkler

C (1985) Metabolism of 15-[p-^{123}I-Iodophenyl)]-Pentadecanoic acid in heart muscle and non-cardiac tissues. Eur J Nucl Med 10:228–234

Rhodes CG, Mac Arther CGC, Swinburne AJ, Heather JD (1980) Influence of pulmonary recirculation and the chest wall upon measurements of regional ventilation, perfusion and water volume. Bull Eur Physiopathol Respir 16:383–394

Rhodes CG, Wollmer P, Fazio F, Jones T (1981) Quantitative measurement of regional extravascular lung density using positron emission and emission tomography. J Comput Assist Tomogr 3:783–791

Rhodes CG, Wise RJS, Gibbs JM, Frackowiak RSJ, Hatazawa J, Palmer AJ, Thomas DG, Jones T (1983) In vivo disturbance of the oxidative metabolism of glucose in human cerebral gliomas. Ann Neurol 14:614–626

Riege WH, Metter EJ, Kuhl DE, Phelps ME (1985) Brain glucose metabolism and memory functions: age decrease in factor scores. J Gerontol 40:459–467

Riese W (1947) La diaschisis et les tumeurs cerebrales. L'Encephale 6:183–194

Rikitake T (1979) RI-angiography by the ^{11}CO gas inhalation method comparative study of red blood cell labelling to the in vitro method. Jap J Nucl Med 16:529

Roberts S (1968) Influence of elevated circulating levels of amino acids on cerebral concentration and utilization of amino acids. In: Lajtha A, Ford DH (eds) Brain barrier systems. Elsevier, Amsterdam, pp 235–243

Roberts GW, Larson KB, Spaeth EE (1973) The interpretation of mean transit time measurement for multiphase tissue systems. J Theor Biol 39:447–475

Robertson JS (1962) Mathematical treatment of uptake and release of indicator substances in relation to flow analysis in tissue and organs. In: Hamilton WF, Dow P (eds) Handbook of Physiology, Sec 2, vol 1. Am Physiol Soc, Washington, pp 617–644

Robinson GD, Lee AW (1975) Radioiodinated fatty acids for heart imaging: Iodine monochloride addition compared with iodine replacement labeleing. J Nucl Med 16:17–21

Rogers S, Robertson J (1978) Biochemical subclassification of astrocytoma, grade IV, and its utilization in therapy. Am Assoc Cancer Res 19:98

Roland PE, Meyer E, Yamamoto YL, Thompson CJ (1981) Dynamic positron emission tomography as a tool in neuroscience: Functional brainmapping in normal human volunteers. J Cereb Blood Flow Metab 1:463–464

Roland PE, Meyer E, Shibasaki T et al (1982) Regional cerebral blood flow changes in cortex and basal ganglia during voluntary movements in normal volunteers. J Neurophysiol 48:467–480

Roos A, Boron WF (1981) Intracellular pH. Physiol Rev 61:296–434

Ropchan JR, Barrio JR (1984) Enzymatic synthesis of [1-^{11}C]-Pyruvic acid, L-[1-^{11}C]-Lactic acid and L-[1-^{11}C]-Alanine via DL-[1-^{11}C]-Alanine. J Nucl Med 25:887–892

Rose CP, Goresky CA (1977a) Constraints on the uptake of labeled palmitate by the heart. The barriers at the capillary and sarcolemmal surfaces and the control of intracellular sequestration. Circ Res 41:534–545

Rose CP, Goresky CA, Bach GG (1977a) The capillary and sarcolemmal barriers in the heart. An exploration of labeled water permeability. Circ Res 41:515–533

Rosen WG, Terry RD, Fuld PA, Kathman R, Peck A (1980) Pathological verification of ischaemia score in differentiation of dementias. Ann Neurol 7:486–488

Rosenzweig DY, Hughes JMB, Jones T (1969/70) Uneven ventilation within and between regions of the normal lung measured with nitrogen-13. Respor Physiol 8:86–97

Rothlin ME, Bing RJ (1961) Extraction and release of individual free fatty acids by the heart and fat depots. J Clin Invest 40:1380–1386

Rottenberg DA, Ginoz JZ, Kearfott KJ et al (1983) Determination of regional cerebral acid-base status using ^{11}C-dimethyloxazolidinedione and dynamic positron emission tomography. J Cereb Blood flow Metab 3:150–151

Rottenberg DA, Ginos JZ, Kearfott KJ, Junck L, Dhawan V, Jarden JO (1985) In vivo measurement of brain tumor pH using [^{11}C]DMO and positron emission tomography. Ann Neurol 17:70–79

Rougemont D, Baron JC, Lebrun-Grandié P et al (1982) Débit sanguin cérébral et extraction d'oxygène dans les hémiplégies lacunaires. Path Biol (Paris) 30:295–302

Rougemont D, Baron JC, Collard P, Bustany P, Comar D, Agid Y (1984) Local cerebral glucose utilisation in treated and untreated patients with Parkinson's disease. J Neurol Neurosurg Psychiatry 47:824–830

Roy CS, Sherrington MB (1890) On the regulation of the blood supply of the brain. J Physiol 11:85–108

Rumsey JM, Duara R, Grady C, Rapoport JL, Margolin RA, Rapoport SI, Cutler NR (1985) Brain metabolism in autism. Resting cerebral glucose utilization rates as measured with positron emission tomography. Arch Gen Psychiatry 42:448–455

Sacks W, Sacks S, Fleischer A (1983) A comparison of the cerebral uptake and metabolism of labeled glucose and deoxyglucose in vivo in rats. Neurochem Res 8:661–684

Said SI (1982) Metabolic functions of the pulmonary circulation. Circ Res 50:325–333

Sakai F, Meyer JS, Naritomi H et al (1978) Regional cerebral blood flow and EEG in patients with epilepsy. Arch Neurol 35:648–657

Sako K, Diksic M, Kato A, Yamamoto YL, Feindel W (1984) 18-F Antipyrine for the measurement of cerebral blood flow. J Cereb Blood Flow Metab 4:259–263

Samson Y, Baron JC, Bousser MG, Rey A, Derlon JM, David P, Comoy J (1985) Effects of extra-intracranial arterial bypass on cerebral blood flow and oxygen metabolism in humans. Stroke 16:609–626

Sapirstein LA (1956) Fractionating of the cardiac output in rats with isotopic potassium. Circ Res 4:689

Sapirstein LA (1958) Regional blood flow by fractional distribution of indicators. Am J Physiol 193:161–168

Schafer DE (1983) Measurement of ligand-receptor binding: Theory and practice. In: Lambrecht RM, Rescigno A (eds) Tracer kinetics and physiologic modeling. Springer, Berlin Heidelberg New York Tokyo, pp 445–507

Schelbert HR, Phelps ME, Hoffman EJ, Huang S-C, Selin CE, Kuhl DE (1979) Regional myocardial perfusion assessed with N-13 labeled ammonia and positron emission computerized axial tomography. Am J Cardiol 43:209–219

Schelbert HR, Phelps ME, Huang S-C, MacDonald NS, Hansen H, Selin CE, Kuhl DE (1981) N-13 Ammonia as a indicator of myocardial blood flow. Circulation 63:1259–1272

Schelbert HR, Wisenberg G, Phelps ME, Gould KL, Henze E, Hoffman EJ, Gomes A, Kuhl DE (1982a) Noninvasive assessment of coronary stenoses by myocardial imaging during pharmacologic vasodilation. VI. Detection of coronary artery disease in man with intravenous N-13 ammonia and positron computed tomography. Am J Cardiol 49:1197–1207

Schelbert HR, Henze E, Phelps ME, Kuhl DE (1982b) Assessment of regional myocardial ischemia by positron emission computed tomography. Am Heart J 103:588–597

Schelbert HR, Schön HR, Henze E, Huang SC, Barrio J, Phelps ME (1982c) Effects of substrate availability and acute ischemia on regional myocardial metabolism demonstrated noninvasively with F-18 deoxyglucose, C-11 palmitic acid and positron computed tomography. In: Raynaud C (ed) Nucl Med Biol. Pergamon, Paris, pp 1510–1513

Schelbert HR, Henze E, Schön HR, Keen R, Hansen HW, Selin C, Huang SC, Barrio J, Phelps ME (1983a) C-11 labeled palmitic acid for the noninvasive evaluation of regional myocardial fatty acid metabolism with positron computed tomography. III In vivo demonstration of the effects of substrate availability on myocardial metabolism. Kinetics if C-11 palmatic acid in acutely ischemic myocardium. Am Heart J 105:492–504

Schelbert HR, Henze E, Schön HR, Keen R, Hansen HW, Selin C, Huang SC, Barrio J, Phelps ME (1983b) C-11 labeled palmitic acid for the noninvasive evaluation of regional myocardial fatty acid metabolism with positron computed tomography. IV In vivo demonstration of impaired fatty acid oxidation in acute myocardial ischemia. Am Heart J 106:736–750

Schelbert HR, Henze E, Guzi PM, DonMichael TA, Schwaiger M, Barrio JR (1983c) Noninvasive evaluation of regional myocardial fatty acid metabolism in man with ^{11}C-Palmitic acid and positron CT. J Nucl Med 24:P12

Schelbert HR (1985) Positron emission tomography: Assessment of myocardial blood flow and metabolism. Circ [Suppl IV] 72:122–133

Schelbert HR, Schwaiger M (1986) PET studies of the heart. In: Phelps ME, Mazziotta JC, Schelbert HR (eds) Positron emisssion tomography and autoradiography. Raven, New York, pp 581–661

Schicha H, Emrich D (1983) Nuklearmedizin in der kardiologischen Praxis. GIT, Darmstadt

Schicha H (1986) Nuklearmedizinische Diagnostik in der Kardiologie. Int Welt 2:31–41

Schober O, Lehr L, Hundeshagen H (1982) Bromide space, total body water, and sick cell syndrome. Eur J Nucl Med 7:14–15

Schober O, Meyer G-J, Bossaller C, Lobenhoffer P, Knoop B, Müller St, Creutzig H, Sturm J, Lichtlen P, Hundeshagen H (1983) Quantitative Messung des regionalen extravaskulären Lungenwassers bei Hunden mit der Positronen-Emissionstomographie. Fortschr Röntgenstr 139:117–126

Schober O, Creutzig H, Meyer GJ, Becker H, Schwarzrock R, Dietz H, Hundeshagen H (1985a) 11-C-Methionine-PET, IMP-SPECT, CT und MRI bei Hirntumoren. Fortschr Röntgenstr 143:133–136

Schober O, Meyer GJ, Stolke D, Hundeshagen H (1985b) Brain tumor imaging using C-11-Labeled L-Methionine and D-Methionine. J Nucl Med 26:98–99

Schober O, Schüler S, Gratz K, Warneke H, Lang W, Hetzer R, Creutzig H (1985c) Cardiac function and rejection following transplantation of the heart. J Nucl Med 26:P42

Schober O, Meyer G-J, Bossaller C, Creutzig H, Lichtlen PR, Hundeshagen H (1985d) Quantitative determination of regional extravascular lung water and regional blood volume in congestive heart failure. Eur J Nucl Med 10:17–24

Schober O, Meyer GJ, Creutzig H, Hundeshagen H (1986a) IMP-SPECT and amino acid-PET in brain tumors. In: Biersack HJ, Winkler C (eds) Amphetamines and pH-shift agents for brain imaging. de Gruyter, Berlin New York, pp 157–165

Schober O, Meyer G-J, Gaab MR, Müller JA, Becker H, Schwarzrock R, Hundeshagen H (1986b) 11-C-L-Methionine PET in lesions of the brain. Radioakt Isot Klin Forsch 17:13–20

Schön HR, Schelbert HR, Najafi A, Robinson GR, Huang SC, Barrio J, Phelps ME (1982a) C-11 labeled palmitic acid for the non-invasive evaluation of regional myocardial fatty acid metabolism with positron computed tomography. I: Kinetics of C-11 palmitic acid in normal myocardium. Am Heart J 103:532–547

Schön HR, Schelbert HR, Najafi A, Hansen H, Robinson GR, Huang SC, Barrio J, Phelps ME (1982b) C-11 labeled palmitic acid for the non-invasive evaluation of regional myocardial fatty acid metabolism with positron computed tomography. II: Kinetics of C-11 palmitic acid in acutely ischemic myocardium. Am Heart J 103:548–561

Schuster DP, Marklin GF, Mintun MA, Ter-Pogossian MM (1986) PET measurement of regional lung density: 1. J Comput Assist Tomogr 10:723–729

Schuster DP, Marklin GF (1986) Effect of changes in inflation and blood volume on lung density-a PET study: 2. J Comput Assist Tomogr 10:730–735

Schwaiger M, Huang SC, Krivokapich J, Phelps ME, Schelbert HR (1983) Myocardial glucose utilization measured noninvasively in man by positron tomography. J Am Coll Cardiol 1:688

Schwaiger M, Brunken RC, Grover M, Krivokapich J, Child JS, Tillisch JM, Marshall RC, Schelbert HR (1984) Regional metabolism in patients with acute myocardial infarction determined by positron tomography (PET). Circulation [Suppl II: 70:249

Schwaiger M, Schelbert HR, Ellison D, Hansen H, Yeatman L, Vinten-Johansen J, Selin C, Barrio J, Phelps ME (1985a) Substained regional myocardial abnormalities in cardiac metabolism after transient ischemia in the chronic dog model. J Am Coll Cardiol 6:336–347

Schwaiger M, Schelbert HR, Keen R, Vinten-Johansen J, Hansen H, Selin C, Barrio J, Huang SC, Phelps ME (1985b) Retention and clearance of C-11 palmitic acid and reperfused canine myocardium. J Am Coll Cardiol 6:311–320

Schwartz M, Duara R, Haxby J (1983) Down's syndrome in adults: brain metabolism. Science 221:781–783

Schwartzkroin PA, Wyler AR (1980) Mechanisms underlying epileptiform burst discharge. Ann Neurol 7:95–107

Sedvall G, Farde L, Persson A, Wiesel FA (1986) Imaging of neurotransmitter receptors in the living human brain. Arch Gen psychiatry 43:995–1005

Selikson M, Eichling J (1982) Continuous administration of short-lived isotopes for evaluation dynamic parameters. Phys Med Biol 27:1381–1392

Selwyn AP, Jones T, Turner HJ, Pratt T, Clark J, Lavender P (1978) Continuous assessment of regional myocardial perfusion in dogs using krypton-81m. Circ Res 42:771–780

Selwyn AP, Allan RM, Pike V, Fox K, Maseri A (1981) Positive labeling of ischemic myocardium: a new approach in patients with coronary disease. Amer J Cardiol 47:81

Selwyn AP, Allan RM, L'Abbate A, Horlock P, Camici P, Clark J, O'Brien HA, Grant PM (1982) Relation between regional myocardial uptake of rubidium-82 and perfusion: Absolute reduction of cation uptake in ischemia. Am J Cardiol 50:112–121

Selwyn AP, Shea MT, Foale R, Deanfield JE, Wilson R, Brookes D, de Landsheere C, Brady F, Turton D, Pike V (1984) Myocardial flow in patients with infarction. Circulation 70:11–23

Shabetai R (1983) Cardiomyopathy: How far have we come in years, how far yet to go? J Am Coll Cardiol 5:92–100

Shah A, Schelbert HR, Schwaiger M, Henze E, Hansen H, Selin C, Huang SC (1985) Measurement of regional myocardial blood flow with N-13 ammonia and positron emission tomography in intact dogs. J Am Coll Cardiol 5:92–100

Sharp PF, Smith FW, Gemmell HG, Lyall D, Evans NTS, Gvozdanovic D, Davidson J, Tyrrell DA, Pickett RD, Neirinckx RD (1986) Technetium-99m HM-PAO stereoisomers as potential agents for imaging regional cerebral blood flow: Human volunteer studies. J Nucl Med 27:171–177

Sheppard G, Gruzelier J, Manchanda R, Hirsch SR, Wise R, Jones T, Frackowiak RSJ, Jones T (1983) ^{15}O positron emission tomographic scanning in predominantly never-treated acute schizophrenic patients. Lancet 2:1448–1452

Shibasaki T, Uki J, Kanoh T, Kawafuchi JI (1979) Composition of free amino acids in brain tumors. Acta Neurol Scand 60:301–311

Shishido F, Tatento Y, Takashima T, Tamachi S, Yamaura A, Yamasaki T (1984) Positron CT imaging using a high resolution PCT device (Positologica-I), 11-CO, 13-NH_3, and 18-FDG in clinical evaluation of cerebrovascular diseases. Eur J Nucl Med 9:265–271

Siesjö BK (1978) Brain energy metabolism. Wiley, New York

Siesjö BK (1981) Cell damage in the brain: A speculative synthesis. J Cereb Blood Flow Metab 1:155–185

Simon DS, Murray JF, Staub NS (1979) Measurement of pulmonary edema in intact dogs by transthoracic γ-ray attenuation. J Appl Physiol 47:1228–1233

Skort MD, Dowsett DJ, Heaf PJD, Pavia D, Thomson ML (1979) A comparison between monodisperse Tc-99m-labeled aerosol particles and Kr-81m for the assessment of lung function. J Nucl Med 20:194–200

Sloviter HA, Kamimoto T (1970) The isolated perfused rat brain preparation metabolizes mannose but not maltose. J Neurochem 17:1109–1111

Smith CB, Davidsen L, Deibler G, Patlak C, Pettigrew K, Sokoloff L (1980) A method for the determination of local protein synthesis in brain. Trans Am Soc Neurochem 11:94

Smith W, Reid A, Hutchinson JMS, Mallard JR (1982) Nuclear magnetic resonance imaging of the pancreas. Radiology 142:677–680

Sobel BE (1985) Positron tomography and myocardial metabolism: an overview. Circ [Suppl IV] 72:22–30

Sobel BE, Weiss ES, Welch MJ, Siegel BA, Ter-Pogossian MM (1977) Detection of remote myocardial infarction in patients with positron emission transaxial tomography and intravenous 11-C-Palmitate. Circulation 55:853–857

Sobel BE, Geltman EM, Siefenbrunn AJ, Jaffe AS, Spadaro JJ, Ter-Pogossian MM, Collen D, Ludbrook PA (1984) Improvement of regional myocardial metabolism after coronary thrombolysis induced with tissue-type plasminogen activator or streptokinase. Circulation 69:983–990

Sokoloff L (1981) Localization of functional activity in the central nervous system by measurement of glucose utilization with radioactive deoxyglucose. J Cereb Blood Flow Metab 1:7–36

Sokoloff L (1986) Cerebral circulation, energy metabolism and protein synthesis: General characteristrics and principle measurement. In: Phelps ME, Mazziotta JC, Schelbert HR (eds) Positron emission tomography and autoradiography. Raven, New York, pp 1–71

Sokoloff L, Reivich M, Kennedy C et al (1977) The (C-14)-deoxyglucose method for the measurement of local cerebral glucose utilization: Theory, procedure, and normal values in the conscious and anesthetized albino rat. J Neurochem 28:897–916

Sordillo PP, Reiman RE, Gelbard AS, Buena RS, Magill GB, Laughlin JS (1982) Scanning with L-[^{13}N]glutamate. Assessment of the response to chemotherapy of a patient with embryonal rhabdosarcoma. Am J Clin Oncol (CCT) 5:285–289

Sordillo PP, Reiman RE, Buena RS, Gelhard AS, Magill GB, Rosen G, Laughlin JS (1983) Quantitative scanning of soft-tissue sarcomas with Nitrogen-13-labeled L-glutamate. Cancer Invest 1:387–393

Soussaline F, Todd-Pokropek AE, Plummer D, Comar D, Loch C, Houle S, Kellershohn C (1979) The physical performances of a single slice positron tomographic system and preliminary results in a clinical environment. Eur J Nucl Med 4:237–249

Spector AA, Steinberg D (1965) The utilization of unesterified palmitate by Ehrlich ascites tumor cells. J Biol Chem 240:3747–3753

Spinks IJ, Bateman JE, Flesher AC, Clark JC, Hopkins NF, Jones T (1984) Blood flow in the feet of diabetic patients measured with a MWPC positron camera and inhalation of $C^{15}O_2$. Phys Med Biol 29:873–879

Spinks JT, Lammertsma AA, Jones T, Rhodes CG, Hopkins NF (1985) Influence of intravascular activity on the determination of blood flow and oxygen extraction in normal and ulcerated legs using the ^{15}O steady-state technique and positron emission tomography. J Comput Assist Tomogr 9:342–351

Stark DD, Moss AA, Goldberg HI, Davis PL, Federle MP (1984) Magnetic resonance and CT of the normal and diseased pancreas: A comparative study. Radiology 150:153–162

Starling EH (1896) On the absorption of fluid from the connective tissue spaces. J Physiol (E) 19:312–326

Staub NC (1974) Pulmonary edema. Physiol Rev 54:679–811

Staub NC (ed) (1978) Lung water and solute exchange. Dekker, New York Basel

Steinling M, Baron JC, Maziere B, Lasjaunias P, Loc'h C, Cabanis EA, Guillon B (1985) Tomographic measurement of cerebral blood flow by the Ga-68 labelled microsphere and continuous O−15CO$_2$ inhalation method. Eur J Nucl Med 11:29–32

Stender HSt (1961) Das interstitielle Lungenoedem im Roentgenbild. Forsch Röntgenstr 95:461–471

Stender HSt, Schermuly W (1969) Röntgendiagnostik der Lungengerüsterkrankungen. In: Diethelm L (Hrsg) Encyclopedia of medical radiology. Springer, Berlin Heidelberg New York, pp 226–329

Stewart GN (1897) Researches on the circulation time and on the influences which affect it. IV. The output of the heart. J Physiol (E) 15:159–183

Stöcklin G, Kloster G (1982) Metabolic analogue tracers. In: Ell PJ, Holman BL (eds) Computed emission tomography. Oxford University Press, Oxford, pp 299–338

Strauss HW, Zaret BL, Hurley PJ, Natarajan TK, Pitt B (1971) Ascintigraphic method for measuring left ventricular ejection fraction in man without cardiac catheterization. Am J Cardiol 28:575–584

Sturm JA, Creutzig H, Oestern H-J, Maghsudi M, Wisner DH, Schober O (1985) Die Albuminextravasation als Messverfahren zur klinischen Erfassung einer Permeabilitätsschädigung der Lungenkapillaren. In: Stelzner F (Hrsg) Chirurgisches Forum '85 für experimentelle und klinische Forschung. Springer, Berlin Heidelberg New York, S 69–73

Subramanyam R, Bucelewicz WM, Hoop B, Jones SC (1977) A system for Oxygen-15 labeled blood for medical applications. Int J Appl Radiat Isotopes 28:21–24

Subramanyam R, Alpert NM, Hoop B, Brownell GL, Taveras JM (1978) A model for regional cerebral oxygen distribution during continuous inhalation of $^{15}O_2$, $C^{15}O$, and $C^{15}O_2$. J Nucl Med 9:48–53

Sugerman HJ, Strash AM, Hirsch JI, Glauser FL, Shirazi KK, Sharp DE, Greenfield LJ (1981) Sensitivity of scintigraphy for detection of pulmonary capillary albumin leak in canine oleic acid ARDS. J Trauma 21:520–525

Sugerman HJ, Strash AM, Hirsch JI, Shirazy KL, Tatum JL, Mathers JAL, Greenfield LJ (1982a) Scintigraphy and radiography in oleic acid pulmonary microvascular injury: Effects of positive end-exspiratory pressure (PEEP). J Trauma 22:179–185

Sugerman HJ, Hirsch JI, Tatum JL, Strash AM, Sharp SE, Greenfield LJ (1982b) Comparative scintigraphy in oleic acid pulmonary microvascular injury. Crit Care Med 10:31–33

Susskind H, Atkins HL, Goldman AG, Acevedo JC, Pate HR, Richards P, Brill AP (1981) Sensitivity of Kr-81m and Xe-127 in evaluating nonembolic pulmonary disease. J Nucl Med 22:781–786

Suzuki T, Iio M (1982) The clinical application of ^{11}C-glucose for diagnosis of lung cancer. In: Raynaud C (ed) Proc Third World Congr Nucl Med Biol. Pergamon, Paris, pp 2080–2082

Swinburne AJ, MacArther CGC, Rhodes CG, Heather JD, Hughes JMB (1982) Measurement of lung water in dog lobes using inhaled $C^{15}O_2$ and injected $H_2^{15}O$. J Appl Physiol 52:1535–1544

Syrota A, Comar D, Cerf, Plummer D, Maziere M, Kellershohn C (1979) (11-C)Methionine pancreatic scanning with positron emission computed tomography. J Nucl Med 20:778–781

Syrota A, Dop-Ngassa M, Cerf M, Paraf A (1981a) ^{11}C-L-methionine for evaluation of pancreatic exocrine function. Gut 22:907–915

Syrota A, Pascal O, Crouzel M, Kellershohn C (1981b) Pulmonary extraction of C-11 Chlorpromazine, measured by residue detection in man. J Nucl Med 22:145–148

Syrota A, Duquesnoy N, Paraf A, Kellershohn C (1982a) The role of positron emission tomography in the detection of pancreatic disease. Radiology 143:249–253

Syrota A, Mazière M, Crouzel M, Sastre J, Prenet C (1982b) Visualization of muscarinic acetylcholine receptors in the human heart using ^{11}C-methyl-QNB and positron emission tomography. In: Raynaud C (ed) Nucl Med Biol. Pergamon, Paris, pp 2503–2505

Syrota A, Castaing M, Rougemont D, Berridge M, Baron JC, Bousser MG, Pocidalo JJ (1983a) Tissue acid balance and oxygen metabolism in human cerebral infarction studied with positron emission tomography. Ann Neurol 14:419–428

Syrota A, Dormont D, Betrger J, Mazière M, Prenant C, Sastre J, Davy JM, Aumant MC, Motte J, Gourgon R (1983b) ^{11}C Ligand binding to adrenergic and muscarinergic receptors of the human heart studied in vivo by positron emission tomography. J Nucl Med 24:P20

Syrota A, Paillotin G, Davy JM, Aumont MC (1984) Kinetics of in vivo binding of antagonist to muscarinic cholinergic receptor in the human heart studied by positron emission tomography. Life Sci 35:937–945

Syrota A, Castaing M, Rougemont D et al (1985a) Regional tissue pH and oxygen metabolism in human cerebral infarction studied with positron emission tomography. In: Greitz T, Ingvar DH, Widén L (eds) The metabolism of the human brain studied with positron emission tomography. Raven, New York, pp 285–303

Syrota A, Samson Y, Boullais C, Wajnberg P, Loc'h C (1985b) Tomographic mapping of brain intracellular pH and extracellular water space in stroke patients. J Cereb Blood Flow Metab 5:358–368

Szabo Z, Ritzl F (1983) Mean transittime images, a new method for analyzing brain perfusion studies. Eur J Nucl Med 8:201–205

Taegtmeyer H (1986) Myocardial metabolism. In: Phelps ME, Mazziotta JC, Schelbert HR (eds) Positron emission tomography and autoradiography. Raven, New York, pp 149–195

Takagi S, Ehera K, Kenny PJ, Finn RD, Kothari PJ, Gilson EJ (1984) Butanol for measurement of regional cerebral blood flow. J Cereb Blood Flow Metab 4:275

Takahashi K, Murakami M, Hagami E, Sasaki H, Kondo Y, Mizusawa S, Namishi H, Irda H, Miuras S, Kanno I, Uemura K, Ido T (1986) Radiosynthesis of ^{15}O-labeled Butanol for clinical use. Pro Sixth Int Sympos Radiopharm Chem Boston, June 29–July 3

Tamaki N, Itoh H, Ishii Y, Yonekura K, Yamamoto Y, Torizuky K, Konishi Y, Hikasa Y, Kambara H, Kawai C (1982) Hemodynamic significance of increased lung uptake of thallium 201. Am J Roentgenol 138:223–228

Ter-Pogossian MM, Powers WE (1958) The use of radioactive oxygen-15 in the determination of oxygen content in malignant neoplasms. In: Radioisotopes in scientific research, vol 3. Pergamon, New York, pp 1–11 (Proc First UNESCO Int Conf, Paris 1957)

Ter-Pogossian MM, Eichling JO, Davis DO, Welch MJ, Metzger JM (1969) The determination of regional cerebral blood flow by means of water labeled with radioactive Oxygen-15. Radiology 93:31–40

Ter-Pogossian MM, Eichling JO, Davis DO et al (1970) The measurement in vivo of regional cerebral oxygen utilization by means of oxyhemoglobin labeled with radioactive oxygen-15. J Clin Invest 49:385–391

Ter-Pogossian MM (1981) Special characteristics and potential for dynamic function studies with PET. Semin Nucl Med 11:13–23

Ter-Pogossian MM, Herscovitch P (1985) Radioactive oxygen-15 in the study of cerebral blood flow, blood volume and oxygen metabolism. Semin Nucl Med 15:377–394

Terry RD, Peck A, DeTeresa R, Schecter R, Horoupian DS (1981) Some morphometric aspects of the brain in senile dementia of the Alzheimer type. Ann Neurol 10:184–192

Tewson TJ, Raichle ME, Welch MJ (1980) Preliminary studies with (F-18)-haloperidol: a radioligand for in vivo studies of dopamine receptors. Brain Res 191:291–295

Theodore WH, Newmark ME, Sato S, Brooks R, Patronas N, DeLaPaz R, DiChiro G, Kessler RM, Margolin R, Manning RG, Channing M, Porter RJ (1983) ^{18}F-fluorodeoxyglucose positron emission computed tomography in refrector complex partial seizures. Ann Neurol 13:419–428

Theodore WH, Brooks R, Sato S, Patronas N, Margolin R, DiChiro G, Porter RJ (1984) The role of positron emission tomography in the evaluation of seizure disorders. Ann Neurol 15:S176–S179

Theodore WH, Brooks R, Margolin R, Patronas N, Sato S, Porter SJ, Mansi L, Bairamian D, Di Chiro G (1985) Positron emission tomography in generalized seizures. Neurology 35:684–690

Thomas DG, Beaney RP, Brooks DJ (1984) Positron emission tomography in the study of cerebral tumours. Neurosurg Rev 7:253–258

Thompson HK, Starmer CF, Whalen RE, McIntosh HD (1964) Indicator transit time considered as a gamma variate. Circ Res 14:502–515

Tillisch J, Brunken R, Marshall R, Schwaiger M, Phelps ME, Schelbert HR (1986) Prediction of the reversibility of cardiac wall motion abnormalities using positron tomography, ^{18}fluorodeoxyglucose and ^{13}N-ammonia (submitted for publication)

Tomita M, Gotoh F (1981) Local cerebral blood flow values as estimated with diffusible tracers: Validity of assumptions in normal land ischemic tissue. J Cereb Blood Flow Metabol 1:403–411

Tomlinson BE (1980) The structural and quantitative aspect of the dementias. In: Roberts PJ (ed) Biochemistry of dementia. Wiley, London, pp 15–52

Tomlinson BE, Kitchner D (1972) Granulovascular degeneration of hippocampal pyramidal cells. J Pathol 106:165–185

Turton DR, Brady F, Pike YW, Selwyn AP, Shea MJ, Wilson RA, De Landsheere CM (1984) Preparation of human serum [methyl-^{11}C-]methylalbumin microspheres and human serum [methyl-^{11}C-]methylalbumin for clinical use. Int J Appl Radiat Isot 35:337–344

Tyler JL, Diksik M, Villemure J-G, Evans AC, Yamamoto YL, Feindel W (1986) Metabolic and

hemodynamic studies of gliomas using positron emission tomography (PET). J Nucl Med 27:889

Valind SO, Rhodes CG, Clark J, Burke P, Hughes JMB (1983) Quantitative measurements of regional ventilation using positron computed tomography and a short lived inert gas – neon 19. Nucl Med Commun 4:149

Visser FC, Westera G, vanEenige KJ, vander Wall EE, den Hollander W, Roos PJ (1985a) The myocardial elimination rate of radioiodinated heptadecanoic acid. Eur J Med 10:118–122

Visser FC, van Eenige KJ, van der Wall EE, Westera G, van Engelen CJ, van Lingen A, de Cock CC, den Hollander W, Heidendahl GA, Roos PJ (1985b) The elimination rate of ^{123}I-Heptadecanoic acid after intracoronary and intravenous administration. Eur J Nucl Med 11:114–119

Volkow NA, Brodie JD, Gomez-Mont F (1985) Applications of positron emission tomography to psychatry. In: Reivich M, Alavi A (eds) Positron emission tomography. Liss, New York, pp 311–327

Volpe JJ, Hercovitch P, Perlman JM, Raichle ME (1983) Positron emission tomography in the newborn: Extensive impairment of regional cerebral blood flow with intraventricular hemorrhage and hemorrhagic intracerebral involvement. Pediatrics 72:589–601

Volpe JJ, Herscovitch P, Perlman JM, Kreusser KL, Raichle ME (1985) Positron emission tomography in the asphyxiated term newborn: parasagittal impairment of cerebral blood flow. Ann Neurol 17:287–296

Vyska K, Freundlieb C, Höck A, Becker V, Feinendegen LE, Kloster G, Stöcklin G, Traupe H, Heiss W-D (1981) The assessment of glucose transport across the blood brain barrier in man by use of 2-(11-C)-Methyl-D-glucose. J Cereb Blood Flow Metab 1:S42–S43

Vyska K, Kloster G, Feinendegen LE, Heiss WD, Stöcklin G, Höck A, Freundlieb C, Aulich A, Schuler F, Thal HU, Becker Y, Schmid A (1983) Regional perfusion and glucose uptake determination with ^{11}C-Methyl-glucose and dynamic positron emission tomography. In: Heiss WD, Phelps ME (eds) Positron emission tomography of the brain. Springer, New York, pp 169–180

Vyska K, Profant M, Shuler F, Knust EJ, Machulla HJ, Mehdorn HM, Knapp WH, Spohr G, von Seggern R, Kimmling I, Becker V, Feinendegen LE (1984) In vivo determination of kinetic parameters for glucose influx and efflux by means of 3-O-^{11}C-Methyl-D-Glucose, ^{18}F-3-Deoxy-3-Fluoro-D-Glucose, and dynamic positron emission tomography; theory, method, and normal values. In: Knapp WH, Vyska K (eds) Current topics in tumor cell physiology and positron emission tomography. Springer, Berlin Heidelberg New York Tokyo, pp 37–60

Vyska K, Mehdorn HM, Machulla HJ, Knust EJ

(1985a) Use of 3-Fluoro-Deoxyglucose for the assessment of cerebral perfusion and glucose transport. Neurol Res 7:63–67

Vyska K, Magloire JR, Freundlieb C, Hoeck A, Bekker V, Schmid A, Feinendegen LE, Kloster G, Stöcklin G, Schuier FJ (1985b) In vivo determination of the kinetic parameters of glucose and dynamic positron emission tomography (dPET). Eur J Nucl Med 11:97–106

Waddell WJ, Butler TC (1959) Calculation of intracellular pH from the distribution of 5,5-dimethyl-2,4-oxazolidinedione (DMO): application to skeletal muscle of the dog. J Clin Invest 38:720–729

Wagner HN, Burns HD, Dannals RF et al (1983) Imaging dopamine receptors in the human brain by positron tomography. Science 221:1264–1266

Wagner HN, Burns HD, Dannals RF, Wong DF, Langstrom B, Duelfer T, Frost JJ, Ravert JJ, Links HT, Rosenbloom SB, Lukas SE, Kramer AV, Kuhar MJ (1984) Assessment of dopamine receptor densities in the human brain with carbon-11-labeled N-methylspiperone. Ann Neurol 15:S79–S84

Wagner HN, Burns HD, Dannals RF, Wong DF, Langstrom B, Duelfer T, Frost JJ, Ravert JJ, Links HT, Rosenbloom SB, Lukas SE, Kramer AV, Kuhar MJ (1985) Imaging of dopamine receptors in the human brain by positron tomography. In: Greitz T, Ingvar DH, Wiedén L (eds) The metabolism of the human brain studied with positron emission tomography. Raven, New York, pp 251–267

Wagner R (1984) A fast high yield synthesis of ^{18}F-Fluoromethane from $^{18}F-F_2$. J Labeled Comp Radiopharm 21:1229–1230

Walsh WF, Harper PV, Resnekov L, Fill H (1976) Noninvasive evaluation of regional myocardial perfusion in 112 patients using a mobile scintillation camera and intravenous nitrogen-13 labeled ammonia. Circulation 54:226–275

Walsh WF, Fill HR, Harper PV (1977) Nitrogen-13-labeled ammonia for myocardial imaging. Semin Nucl Med 7:59–66

Warburg OH (1926) Über den Stoffwechsel der Tumoren. Springer, Berlin

Washburn LC, Sun TT, Rafter JJ et al (1976) ^{11}C-labeled amino acids for pancreas visualization. J Nucl Med 17:557–558

Washburn LC, Wieland BW, Sun TT, Hayes RL, Butler TA (1978) [1-^{11}C]DL-Valine, a potential pancreas-imaging agent. J Nucl Med 19:77–83

Washburn LC, Sun TT, Byrd BL, Hayes RL, Butler TA (1979) DL-[carboxyl-^{11}C]tryptophan, a potential agent for pancreatic imaging; production and preclinical investigations. J Nucl Med 20:857–864

Washburn LC, Sun TT, Byrd BL, Callahan AP (1982) Production of L-[1-^{11}C]-valine y HPLC resolution. J Nucl Med 23:29–33

Weber G (1977) Enzymology of cancer cells. II. N Engl J Med 296:541–555

Wegener OH, Koeppe P, Oeser H (1978) Measurement of lung density by computed tomography. J Comput Assist Tomogr 2:263–273

Weich HF, Strauss HW, Pitt B (1977) The extraction of thallium-201 by the myocardium. Circulation 56:188–191

Weinreich R, Ritzl F, Feinendegen LE, Schnippering HG, Stöcklin G (1975) Fixation, retention and exhalation of carrier-free 11-C-labeled Carbonmonoxide by man. Radiat Environm Biophys 12:271–280

Weiss ES, Hoffman EJ, Phelps ME, Welch MJ, Henry PD, Ter-Pogossian MM, Sobel BE (1976) External detection and visualization of myocardial ischemia with 11C-substrates in vitro and in vivo. Circ Res 39:24–32

Weiss ES, Ahmed SA, Welch MJ, Williamson JR, Ter-Pogossian MM, Sobel BE (1977) Quantification of infarction in cross sections of canine myocardium in vivo with positron emission transaxial tomography and ^{11}C-palmitate. Circulation 55:66–73

Welch MJ (1982) New radiopharmaceuticals for studying liver function. J Nucl Med 23:1138–1140

Welch MJ, Thakur ML, Coleman RE, Patel M, Siegel BA, Ter-Pogossian MM (1977) Gallium-68 labeled red cells and platelets, new agents for positron tomography. J Nucl Med 18:558–562

Welch MJ, Raichle ME, Kilbourn MR, Mintun MA (1984) (F-18) Spiroperidol: A radiopharmaceutical for the in vivo study of the dopamine receptor. Ann Neurol 15:S77–S78

West JB, Dollery CT (1960) Distribution of blood flow and ventilation-perfusion ratio in the lung, measured with radioactive CO_2. J Appl Physiol 15:405–410

West JB, Dollery CT, Naimark A (1964) Distribution of blood flow in isolated lung: Relation to vascular and alveolar pressures. J Appl Physiol 19:713–724

West JB (1977) Regional Differences in the Lung. Academic Press, New York

Widén L, Blomquist G, Greitz T, Litton JE, Bergstroem M, Ehrin E, Ericson K, Eriksson L, Ingvar DH, Johansson L, Nilsson L, Stone-Elander S, Sedvall G, Wiesel F, Wiik G (1983) PET studies of glucose metabolism in patients with schizophrenia. AJNR 4:550–552

Wienhard K, Pawlik G, Eriksson L, Wagner R, Ilsen HW, Herholz K, Heiss WD (1983) Kinetic constants for cerebral glucose metabolism in pathological conditions. J Cereb Blood Flow Metab 3:474–475

Wienhard K, Pawlik G, Herholz K, Wagner R, Heiss WD (1985) Estimation of local cerebral glucose utilization by positron emission tomography of ^{18}F-2-fluoro-2-deoxy-D-glucose: A critical appraisal of optimization procedures. J Cereb Blood Flow Metab 5:115–125

Williams LE (1981) On the improvement of analyses of Xenon-133 lung wash-in and wash-out curves. J Nucl Med 22:744–745

Wilson RA, Shea MJ, Landsheere CH de, Turton D, Brady F, Deanfield JE, Maseri A, Selwyn AP (1983) A new method for in vivo quantitation of regional myocardial blood flow using C-11 labeled microspheres and positron tomography. Circulation 68:111–179

Wilson RA, Shea MJ, Landsheere CH de, Turton D, Brady F, Deanfield JE, Selwyn AP (1984) Validation of quantitation of regional myocardial blood flow in vivo using ^{11}C-human albumin microspheres and positron emission tomography. Circulation 70:717–723

Winchell HS, Horst WD, Braun L, Oldendorf WH, Hattner R, Parker H (1980) N-Isopropyl-(123-I)p-iodoamphetamine: single-pass brain uptake and washout; binding to brain synaptosomes; and localization in dog and monkey brain. J Nucl Med 21:947–952

Wise RJS, Rhodes CG, Gibbs JM, Hatazawa J, Palmer T, Frackowiak RSJ, Jones T (1983a) Disturbance of oxidative metabolism of glucose in recent human cerebral infarcts. Ann Neurol 14:627–637

Wise RJ, Bernardi S, Frackowiak RSJ, Legg NJ, Jones T (1983b) Serial observation in the pathophysiology of acute stroke. Brain 106:197–222

Wisenberg G, Schelbert HR, Hoffman EJ, Phelps ME, Robinson GD Jr, Selin CE, Child J, Skorton D, Kuhl DE (1981) In vivo quantitation of regional myocardial blood flow by positron emission computed tomography. Circ 63:1248–1258

Wolf AP (1981) Special characteristics and potential for radiopharmaceuticals for positron emission tomography. Semin Nucl Med 11:2–12

Wolfkin A, Jaeger J, Brodie JD, Wolf A, Fowler AP, Rotrosen J, Gomez-Mont F, Cancro R (1985) Persistence of cerebral metabolic abnormalities in chronic schizophrenia as determined by positron emission tomography. Am J Psychiatry 142:564–571

Wolfson LI, Leenders KL, Brown LL, Jones T (1985) Alterations of regional cerebral blood flow and oxygen metabolism in Parkinson's disease. Neurol 35:1399–1405

Wollmer Per, Rhode CG, Pike VW, Silvester DJ, Pride NB, Sanders A, Palmer AJ, Liss RH (1982) Measurement of pulmonary erythromycin concentration in patients with lobar pneumonia by means of positron tomography. Lancet 18:1361–1364

Wollmer P, Rhodes CG, Allan RM, Maseri A, Fazio F (1983) Regional extravascular lung density and fractional pulmonary blood volume in patients with chronic pulmonary venous hypertension. Clin Physiol 3:241–256

Wollmer P, Rhodes CG, Hughes JMB (1984) Regional extravascular density and fractional blood volume of the lung in interstitial disease. Thorax 39:286–293

Wong DR, Wagner HN, Dannals RF, Links JM, Frost JJ, Ravert HT, Wilson AA, Rosenbaum AA, Gjedde A, Douglass KH et al (1984a) Effects of age on dopamine and serotonin receptors measured by positron tomography in the living human brain. Science 226:1393–1396

Wong DF, Wagner HN, Dannals RF, Frost JJ, Ravert HT, Links JM, Folstein MF, Jensen BA, Kuhar MJ, Toung JT (1984b) Effects of age and sex on dopamin receptors in the living human brain. Ann Neurol 16:128

Yamamoto YL, Thompson CJ, Meyer E, Robertson SJ, Feindel W (1977) Dynamic positron emission tomography for study of cerebral hemodynamics in a cross section of the head using positron-emitting ^{68}Ga-EDTA and ^{77}Kr. J Comp Assist Tomogr 1:43–56

Yamamoto YL, Hakim AM, Diksic M, Pokrupa RP, Meyer E, Tyler J, Evans AC, Worsley K, Thompson CJ, Feindel WH (1985) Focal flow disturbances in acute stroke: Effects on regional metabolism and tissue pH. In: Heiss WD (ed) Functional mapping of the brain in vascular disorders. Springer, Berlin Heidelberg New York Tokyo, pp 85–106

Yano Y, Cahoon JL, Budinger TF (1981) A precision flow-controlled Rb-82 generator for bolus or constant-infusion studies of the heart and brain. J Nucl Med 22:1006–1010

Yen C-K, Budinger TF (1981) Evaluation of blood brain barrier permeability changes in rhesus monkeys and man using Rb-82 and positron emission tomography. J Comput Assist Tomogr 5:792–799

Yen C-K, Yano Y, Budinger TF, Friedland RP, Derenzo SE, Huesman RH, O'Brien HA (1982) Brain tumor evaluation using Rb-82 and positron emission tomography. J Nucl Med 23:532–537

Yonekura Y, Buena RS, Brill AB, Som P, Yeh SDJ, Kemeny NE, Fowler JS, MacGregor RR, Stamm R, Christman DR, Wolf AP (1982) Increased accumulation of 2-Deoxy-2-(^{18}F)fluoro-D-glucose in liver metastases from colon carcinoma. J Nucl Med 23:1133–1137

Young AB, Frey KA, Agranoff BW (1986) Receptor assays: In vivo and in vitro. In: Phelps ME, Mazziotta JC, Schelbert HR (eds) Positron emission tomography and autoradiography. Raven, New York, pp 73–111

Zanzonico PB, Bigler RE, Schmall B (1983) Neuroleptic binding sites: specific labeling in mice with (^{18}F)Haloperidol, a potential tracer for positron emission tomography. J Nucl Med 24:408–416

Zanzonico PB, Bigler RE, Schmall B (1984) F-18 Haloperidol and Spiroperidol. J Nucl Med 25:534–536

Zatz LM, Jernigan TL, Ahumada AJ (1982) Changes

on computed cranial tomography with aging: intracranial fluid volume. AJNR 3:1–11

Zierler KL (1961) Theory of the use of arteriovenous concentration differences for measuring metabolism in steady and non-steady states. J Clin Invest 40:2111–2125

Zierler KL (1962a) Circulation times and the theory of indicator dilution methods for determining blood flow and volume. Handbook of Physiology. Am Physiol Soc (Washington) 1:585–615

Zierler KL (1962b) Theoretical basis of indicator-dilution methods for measuring flow and volume. Circ Res 10:393–407

Zierler KL (1963) Theory of use of indicators to measure blood flow and extracellular volume and calculation of transcapillary movement of tracers. Circ Res 12:464–471

Zierler KL (1965) Equations for measuring blood flow by external monitoring of radioisotopes. Circ Res 16:309–321

Namenverzeichnis – Author Index

Die *kursiv* gesetzten Seitenzahlen beziehen sich auf die Literatur
Page numbers in *italics* refer to the bibliography

Sachverzeichnis

Deutsch – Englisch

Bei gleicher Schreibweise in beiden Sprachen sind die Stichwörter nur einmal aufgeführt

Subject Index

English — German

Where English and German spelling of a word is identical, the German version is omitted

Handbuch der
medizinischen
Radiologie

Encyclopedia of
Medical Radiology

Band 15:

Nuklearmedizin
Nuclear Medicine

Teil 1 A

Radiopharmaka, Gerätetechnik, Strahlenschutz

Radiopharmaceuticals, Instrumentation Technology, Radiation Protection

Von/By R. Berberich, M. Besnard, B. Braun, Y. Cohen,
J. Fitschen, P. Gielow, H. I. Glass, H. Henseler, R. Hindel,
K. Jordan, D. Junker, K. Kasperek, V. Klement, R. A. Krause,
M. Löffler, W. J. Lorenz, R. Maushart, P. Meyer,
P. Oberhausen, R. Wolf

Redigiert von/Edited by **H. Hundeshagen**

1980. 244 Abbildungen in 280 Einzeldarstellungen, 65 Tabellen.
XX, 722 Seiten (146 Seiten in Englisch) Gebunden DM 540,-.
Subskriptionspreis (gilt bei Abnahme des Gesamtwerkes)
Gebunden DM 432,-. ISBN 3-540-08487-8

Für die Bewertung der klinischen Aussagefähigkeit der
Nuklearmedizin bietet dieser Band erstmals eine umfassende
methodische Übersicht über die physikalischen, technischen,
chemischen und strahlenbiologischen Grundlagen und
Voraussetzungen. Das Instrumentarium der Nuklearmedizin
wird in seiner Entwicklung bis zum heutigen Stand abgehandelt. Strahlenmeßtechnik, nuklearmedizinische Gerätetechnik,
die Herstellung von künstlichen Radionukliden mittels Reaktor
und Zyklotron, Datenverarbeitung und Dosisberechnungen für
die Diagnostik und Therapie mit diesen Radionukliden bilden
neben den Problemen des Strahlenschutzes die Hauptschwer-
punkte des Bandes.

Wichtige Kapitel sind weiterhin die Strahlenschutzmeßtechnik,
bauliche Maßnahmen für nuklearmedizinische Untersuchungs-
arbeiten, Normierungsfragen und gesetzliche Bestimmungen.

Springer-Verlag
Berlin Heidelberg
New York London
Paris Tokyo

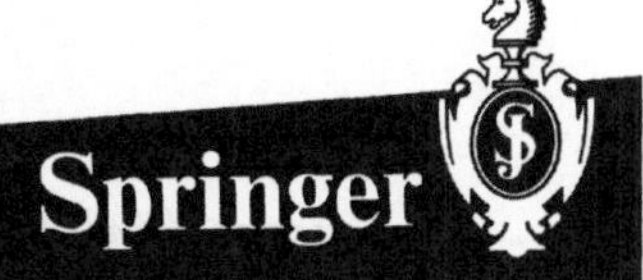

Handbuch der
medizinischen
Radiologie

Encyclopedia of
Medical Radiology

Band 15:

Nuklearmedizin
Nuclear Medicine

Teil 2:

Diagnostik, Therapie, Klinische Forschung

Diagnosis, Therapy, Clinical Research

Von/By K. Anger, D. V. Becker, W. Bessler, A. Bischof-Delaloye,
W. Börner, A. Churchod, B. Delaloye, H. Emde, U. Feine,
W. Finck, M. Friedrich, H. Fritzsche, H. W. Gray, W. R. Greig,
K. Hennig, R. Höfer, G. Hör, H. Hundeshagen, E. Krönert,
P. Mariß, R. Montz, H. W. Pabst, M. Ramos, F. Ritzl, H. Rösler,
K. zum Winkel, F. Wolf, P. Woller, U. Zeidler, E. Zeitler, G. Zita

Redigiert von/Edited by **H. Hundeshagen**

1978. 369 Abbildungen in 1366 Einzeldarstellungen, teilweise in
Farbe, 146 Tabellen. XXVI, 1156 Seiten (51 Seiten in Englisch).
Gebunden DM 780,–
Subskriptionspreis (gilt be Abnahme des Gesamtwerkes):
Gebunden DM 624,–. ISBN 3-540-08388-X

Inhaltsübersicht: Hirn. – Speicheldrüsenfunktions- und Lokalisationsdiagnostik mit Radionukliden. – Schilddrüse. – Thyroid
Gland. – Nuklearmedizinische in vitro-Diagnostik. – Endokrino-
logie. – Lunge. – Hämatologie. – Lymphsystem. – Nephrologie
und Urologie. – Szintigraphische Untersuchungen von Knochen
und Gelenken. – Gastroenterologie. – Die Milz. – Nuklearmedizin in Geburtshilfe und Frauenheilkunde.

Bei diesem Band handelt es sich um den klinischen Teil des
Handbuches für Nuklearmedizin. In ihm sind die wichtigsten
nuklearmedizinischen klinischen Untersuchungsverfahren nach
Organsystemen abgehandelt. Auch die Therapie mit offenen
Radionukliden ist jeweils mitberücksichtigt. Der Band gibt somit
eine Übersicht über die nuklearmedizinische Diagnostik und
Therapie der einzelnen Organe von den Anfängen bis zum jetzi-
gen Stand in der Entwicklung der Methode, den Ergebnissen und
der Bewertung der Ergebnisse für die Klinik wieder.

Springer-Verlag
Berlin Heidelberg
New York London
Paris Tokyo

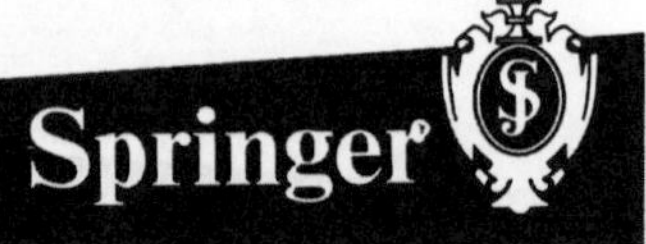